BIRTH EMERGENCIES

for Community Midwives

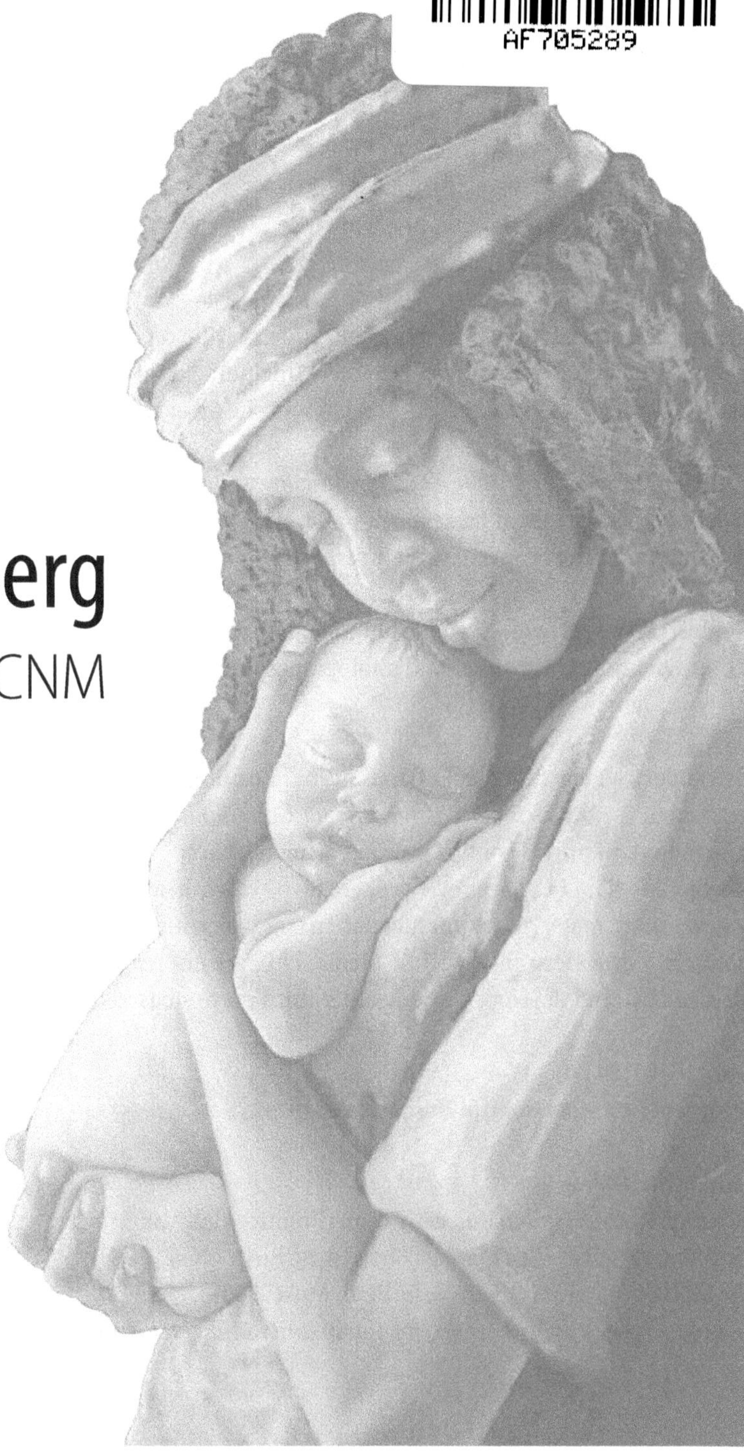

Bonnie U. Gruenberg
MSN, CNM, CRNP, FACNM

SYNCLITIC MEDIA

SYNCLITIC MEDIA, LLC
440 Schoolhouse Road
New Providence, PA 17560
www.syncliticmedia.com
info@syncliticmedia.com
(717) 983-8689

Birth Emergencies for Community Midwives

ISBN: 978-1-941700-47-1
Library of Congress Control Number: 2024921198

Also by the author
Essentials of Prehospital Maternity Care (Prentice Hall, 2005)
Birth Emergency Skills Training (Birth Guru/Birth Muse, 2008)
The Midwife's Journal (Birth Guru/Birth Muse, 2009)
Birth Emergency Skills Training for Community Midwives: Workshop Manual • 2nd Edition (Synclitic Media, LLC, 2025)

To my mother. To all mothers.

Contents

Foreword

It has been my honor to work with community midwives for over four decades. Birth, above all things, is personal. It is an intimate generative act that is the culmination of intimacy. Community midwives honor birth, cherish families, and truly have a holistic view of how childbearing fits within the context of individual people's lives. They get to know their clients, hear their stories, and value them as individuals. Midwives support families in all their reproductive choices, in all their family configurations, and in all their hopes and dreams. They nurture and support each client to have the best birth possible, whatever their given circumstances, through shared decision making and informed choice. When complications arise, they safeguard the lives of the birthing person and the baby, which may include intervening to prevent or treat an emergency, activating emergency medical services, and participating in transfer for medical care.

Pregnancy is a healthy physiologic process, and, like all physiologic processes, it occasionally goes awry. The evidence for physiologic birth shows that the best outcomes and experiences are achieved when these births occur with midwives in a community setting of the client's home, a birth center, or a community health facility. The midwife must be quick to recognize impending complications, know when action is needed, and act promptly when necessary. Optimal midwifery care includes robust coordination among emergency medical services and hospitals that welcome the participation of midwives as part of the health care team.

To promote this vision, we can strive to provide excellent care and to learn to recognize early signs of evolving complications and seek timely medical assistance. We can work with our emergency medical services and health facility staff to build the warm relationships that facilitate smooth transitions of care from one location to another. We can advocate and support postpartum debriefing with our clients and colleagues as an opportunity to improve care and outcomes. We can become involved in our state perinatal quality collaboratives (PQCs) to bring our voices to the table. We can engage with state level workgroups and maternal fetal infant mortality review (MFIMR) panels. And we can be open to the lessons offered through this engagement. When transport does occur, we can be alert for signs of bias or racism that can affect the care and the experiences of birthing families, and we can advocate for our clients as issues arise. When all goes smoothly, we can celebrate an effective transfer of care and share positive feedback to encourage continued client-centered problem-solving.

Birth Emergencies for Community Midwives is a book that supports midwives in every practice setting. While it is written for those who practice community birth, the information provides an important midwifery perspective on potential complications and emergencies that can occur during childbirth in any setting. This information in this book can assist midwives in reducing preventable maternal, fetal, and neonatal complications and deaths. It helps midwives develop the habit of quick systematic review for potential complications as part of every visit. This simple action can promote early diagnosis should some untoward condition develop. Readers are encouraged to soak up every page, every image, every table, and every illustration of the text to build an internal library of information to draw upon when signs or symptoms present or one's intuition guides you to believe that something is wrong. This book will help you trust yourself, trust birth, and trust your network of resources to promote the best possible birth experience.

—Nell Tharpe, MS, CNM, FACNM

Foreword

Although I have now returned to academia, for a few years I had the privilege of working alongside Bonnie Gruenberg in a small community hospital in Ephrata, Pennsylvania. I have seen firsthand that she is highly skilled, and very bright, and that she takes incredible care of her patients.

As a neonatologist, I would naturally prefer that all birth emergencies happen in a hospital. A highly trained team can make a huge difference in the first few minutes of life with a compromised newborn. Nonetheless, many families choose nonhospital settings for deliveries and there are tradeoffs in this decision, not all of which favor delivering in a hospital. With careful patient selection, some communities have demonstrated the same or better outcomes with out-of-hospital deliveries.

Bonnie's excellent book is a valuable resource for community midwives managing out-of-hospital birth emergencies. Her chapters on neonatal resuscitation and prematurity are clear, succinct, and accurate. It is critically important that community midwives be prepared for the hopefully uncommon emergencies that occur in low-risk mothers who elect to deliver in community settings, and Bonnie's work fills an important need. Buy it, read it, reread it, and save lives.

—Joe Livingston, MD, MPH
Neonatologist
Honorary Senior Lecturer, Auckland University
Senior Medical Officer, Waikato Hospital
Hamilton, New Zealand

Author's Note

Midwives appreciate that childbearing is a normal life process and facilitate the physiologic act of birth through holistic, low-intervention support. Natural processes, however, can stall or break down. Any midwife who regularly attends births will eventually encounter complications. Some are very common, including some of the most lethal ones, such as postpartum hemorrhage and hypertensive disorders. Others, such as amniotic fluid embolism, are so rare they might not be encountered by an entire community of midwives in all their years of practice. When complications occur, the lives of mothers and babies can depend on a midwife's ability to recognize and manage a problem while upholding standards of evidence-informed care.

To prepare midwives for dealing with emergencies, I wrote and published *Birth Emergency Skills Training: Manual for Out-of-Hospital Midwives* (*BEST*) in 2008. Thousands of midwives have used *BEST* to develop expertise in recognizing and managing obstetric complications. It is featured on the reference list for the North American Registry of Midwives written examination to become a Certified Professional Midwife. It has been translated into Russian and taught in Spanish. Thousands of students have been certified through the original *BEST* online class and the live workshop codeveloped and taught by Andrea Dixon. In 2020, she and Avril Bowens turned the didactic part of the *BEST* workshop into an online program that participants can attend as prerequisite for in-person instruction or as a free-standing accredited continuing-education program.

To better serve the needs of practicing midwives, *Birth Emergency Skills Training* has expanded into a collection of several related books. This volume, *Birth Emergencies for Community Midwives*, comprehensively explores the recognition and treatment of antepartum, intrapartum, and postpartum complications, bridging the care provided in a community setting to definitive management in a hospital. The second edition of *Birth Emergency Skills Training* will be essentially an abridged version of *Birth Emergencies* similar in format and length to the first edition of *BEST* and complementary to the workshops.

Birth Emergencies for Community Midwives describes assessments and treatments that may not be appropriate for all practices. In some cases, such as a client who calls with severe abdominal pain, an emergency room physician or obstetrician should make the initial assessment. Although many midwives work strictly in community settings, others have hospital privileges and can continue caring for high-risk clients after transfer. Often, I begin a section by discussing the provision of care in community settings, then explain how care will likely be provided once the mother has been transferred to a hospital. It is important for all midwives to understand the basics of downstream care so that they might better educate and prepare their clients and have informed discussions with hospital-based providers. Certain advanced procedures described in the text are part of the standard of care in some areas, though many midwives do not perform them. Midwives seldom use continuous electronic fetal monitoring outside a hospital, but the graphs in this book will help them learn the basics of identifying abnormal heart patterns quickly and accurately, by eye or by ear, in any setting.

Where I have included procedures and treatments that exceed midwives' usual scope of practice, my purpose is to broaden knowledge. For example, even midwives who practice where it is illegal for them to suture lacerations or give medications should be familiar with both and should recognize situations where they are required for optimal care. As always, midwives should function within the applicable standard of care, local protocols, and their own level of training.

In illustrating this volume, I included numerous drawings and engravings from 19th- and early 20th-century textbooks because their unparalleled level of detail can enhance learning. That they are still useful today underscores the timelessness of midwifery and these marvelous works.

A few words on usage: Caring for clients and working successfully with others require an open heart, a reasonable mind, and the ability to communicate clearly.

Biological sex is a physical reality central to obstetrics and gynecology which classifies people by their anatomy and chromosomal makeup, usually as male or female. Sex differences can affect physical, biochemical, and behavioral characteristics of any living creature and influence manifestation of disease and response to treatment. Biological sex, however, is not always strictly binary. Normal human brains, for example, contain a mosaic of female-typical and male-typical features that do not always correspond with chromosomal sex. Some individuals have ambiguous reproductive anatomy or genetic makeup. A few are chimeras (see Chapters 1 and 5). Nonetheless, the terms *male* and *female* are valid for organisms that reproduce sexually, from trees to human beings. *Birth Emergencies* uses these and related words in their scientific senses: *male* and *father* refer to the parent (usually 46 XY) who produces spermatozoa, and *female* and *mother* refer to the parent (usually 46 XX) who produces ova and/or gestates/bears/produces milk for the child.

In contrast to biologic sex, gender is a social construct involving roles, attitudes, feelings, and behaviors associated with identity as a woman, man, girl, boy, or some, all, or none of these. People of all genders, gender identities, and gender expressions deserve compassionate, competent care, the specifics of which differ with circumstances and personal preference. Because there is no universally accepted stock wordage that applies to every individual all the time, each author must choose language that best conveys intended meanings to intended readers. Although gender-neutral language seems more inclusive to some, others find terms such as *pregnant people* and *birth-givers* awkward or alienating. Some point out that replacing *women* and *mothers* with such terms as *pregnant people* risks marginalizing or dehumanizing women and endangering generations of struggle to improve the standing of women in science, politics, culture, and other realms beyond reproduction.

In response to the movement toward greater inclusivity, I use gender-neutral language wherever possible in this book. To prevent confusion, however, I use plural pronouns (*they*, *them*, *their*) only with plural antecedents. When discussing skin color, I routinely capitalize neither *black* nor *white* lest any reader infer bias. Except as noted, people mentioned in the following pages are anonymous, pseudonymous, composite, or invented; they have only the characteristics I gave them. Conversely, when using source materials, I preserve the original wording, assumptions, and identification. The result is a well-intentioned compromise between adopting ever-evolving inclusive language, clarity, and readability. I make a good-faith effort to juggle all three. If I drop one occasionally, I mean no harm.

An expert midwife is not one who knows all the answers. Indeed, not all the answers are truly knowable. Moreover, what we know and what we do are always changing. An expert midwife is one who is constantly learning, adapting, and implementing better practices. Thank you for allowing this book to shape the care you give to your cherished clients. May your hands always be wise.

—Bonnie Gruenberg, MSN, CNM, CRNP

Acknowledgments

The book you hold in your hands represents more than 8 years of research, writing, and editing. *Birth Emergencies* was written not only to convey important information to community midwives, but also to provide the foundation for the second edition of *Birth Emergency Skills Training* and for other works. I am grateful for the many individuals whose time, effort, and support helped bring this project to fruition.

Andrea Dixon has been teaching Birth Emergency Skills Training for more than 15 years in live and virtual workshops. She has a talent for educating both the mind and the hands. She has breathed life into my words in lively lectures, dynamic simulations, and thoughtful discussions. Avril Bowens took Birth Emergency Skills Training to another level by creating an online training program that can be taken independently or combined with the hands-on workshop. Working together, Avril and Andrea have transformed the practices of countless birth professionals. They provided good advice on the needs of my readership, and I am grateful for their contributions.

Nell Tharpe generously agreed to write the foreword and provided in-depth feedback for much of the content. She is a multitalented midwife who has made substantial contributions to her profession, not only through caring for clients in community and hospital settings but also through educational and leadership activities. My copy of her award-winning book, *Clinical Practice Guidelines for Midwifery & Women's Health*, is dog-eared and worn from continual use. I am honored to have her assistance on this project.

Kathleen Nishida, Tonia Moore-Davis, and Suzanne Adkins made valuable contributions to the content of this book. Their sharp minds and clinical expertise improved the clarity and readability of my writing and helped to make it clinically relevant. Suzanne also appears in many of the photographs as a mother and as a midwife. I value her not only as a reviewer but also as a friend.

A vibrant group of midwives provided valuable insights and suggestions that helped to shape this book. I extend heartfelt thanks to Charity Shenk, Debbie Pulley, Kathryn Jones-Stadler, and Lucinda Manges for their support of this project. Thanks also go to Merrylee Morschhauser for allowing me to photograph her births and use the images in this book. I offer thanks to the many teachers, mentors, and colleagues who have imparted wisdom, shared insights, answered questions, provided inspiration, and helped me develop as a midwife over the years.

Alex Gruenberg, my steadfast husband, was invaluable in editing this manuscript as it went through draft after draft. When the project seemed too large for one person to complete, he gave encouragement. Throughout he has given me the space and support to become my best self. We are, in the words of Robert Frost, "together wing to wing and oar to oar."

I hope that this book will help my fellow midwives as my network has helped me. If I have succeeded in paying forward, most of the credit goes to the thousands of clients who have been in my care. Mother by mother, birth by birth, I continue to learn and grow. Thank you for sharing the peak moments of your lives with me. Because of you, I never lose sight of the miracle.

Reviewers

Suzanne Adkins, MSN, CNM
Avril Bowens, BSN, CPM
Amy Desorgher, DNP, CNM
Andrea Dixon, CNM
Kathryn Jones-Stadler, APRN-CNM, CPM, IBCLC
Lucinda Manges, MSN, CNM
Tonia Moore-Davis, MSN, CNM, FACNM
Kathleen Nishida, PhD, CNM
Debbie Pulley, LM, CPM
Charity Shenk, MSN, CNM
Nell Tharpe, MS, CNM, FACNM

Approaches to Maternity Care

1

Objectives

- Discuss reasons for rising maternal mortality in the United States.
- Compare and contrast advantages and disadvantages of birth in a hospital, at home, and in a birth center.
- Describe changes in maternity care that can make birth safer for mothers and babies.
- Name three ways in which researchers' biases can affect their conclusions about the safety of home birth.

Composite Case Study

Mary Ruth L., gravida 5, para 4 (G5 P4), was in labor with what she intended to be her third home birth. She was making slow progress, contracting irregularly, and leaking clear fluid. When she had stalled for a few hours at 7–8 cm/90/0, her midwife, Brooke Richmond, opted to break the forebag of fluid in front of the fetal head. The hope was that amniotomy would bring the head more directly onto the cervix and stimulate more effective contractions. When the forebag was ruptured, however, the previously engaged fetal head unexpectedly ascended out of the pelvis and was now unreachable by Brooke's fingers. Leopold's maneuvers revealed that the fetus was still vertex, and heart tones remained in the 140s with normal variability. Mary Ruth tried deep squats and lunges to bring down the head and then went to the toilet to empty her bladder.

When Mary Ruth returned to bed, Brooke palpated the fetus as transverse lie, head right. She performed a vaginal exam and palpated a pulsing loop of umbilical cord hanging through the cervix in the upper vagina. "We have a cord prolapse," Brooke said calmly to her nurse, Rachel, and quickly helped Mary Ruth to a knee-chest position. She pressed the Doppler to Mary Ruth's abdomen and heard a fetal heart rate (FHR) of 120 bpm. Reinserting her fingers, Brooke felt a hairy scalp at −2 station, indicating that the fetus had moved back to vertex. A loop of cord was loosely coiled in front of the fetal head. As a contraction pressed the fetus lower in the pelvis, the FHR dropped to 70. Brooke pushed firmly on the fetal head and displaced it from the pelvis. She kept her entire hand deep inside the vagina, decreasing cord compression by preventing descent of the fetus.

Immediately after Brooke diagnosed the cord prolapse, Rachel called emergency medical services (EMS) with the cell phone on speaker while giving Mary Ruth a subcutaneous injection of terbutaline 0.25 mg to suppress contractions. She then alerted the triage nurse and physician at the receiving hospital of the impending transport. EMS arrived and brought a stretcher into the room. Mary Ruth, hips modestly covered with a sheet, moved from the bed to the stretcher with Brooke's hand in her vagina. Mary Ruth tried to lie on her side, but the fetal heart rate dropped to 80 until she resumed a knee-chest position. Mary Ruth's husband loaded Brooke's birth bags into the ambulance and jumped into the passenger seat with the prenatal records.

During transport, the paramedic established intravenous access, applied a pulse oximeter, and obtained vital signs while Brooke monitored the FHR and held the head off the cord. The terbutaline escalated the maternal heart rate to the 130s, but the pulse oximeter monitor distinguished it from the FHR. The fetal rate remained 130s–140s en route *and even showed two accelerations into the 160s with no decelerations. Brooke and the paramedic offered emotional support and told Mary Ruth how strong and brave she was.*

Brooke explained to Mary Ruth that upon arrival, things would likely move fast, and she would be taken directly into surgery and receive general anesthesia. The hospital was ready for an emergency cesarean as they rolled into the unit, and staff took Mary Ruth directly to the operating room. The physician walked alongside the stretcher explaining the risks and benefits of surgery to Mary Ruth and her husband. In the OR, staff transferred Mary Ruth to a supine position on the table and hastily prepared her for surgery. The obstetric team splashed skin-preparation solution over the mother's abdomen and layered blue drapes over most of her body. Brooke crouched under the drapes between Mary Ruth's legs with a hand still in her client's vagina as the obstetrician began to cut. She withdrew as the obstetrician brought the baby into the light, a girl with Apgar scores of 7 and 9 and cord-blood pH of 7.3.

The cord prolapse was identified at home at 8:21 a.m. Mary Ruth arrived at the hospital at 8:40 and was in the operating room at 8:42. The physician made the skin incision at 8:48, and the baby was born at 8:52. The home-birth team, EMS team, and hospital team interfaced seamlessly to achieve the best possible outcome for mother and infant, and all professionals involved enjoyed a high level of satisfaction and a feeling of accomplishment

Skeptical readers will undoubtedly roll their eyes. Transport NEVER goes that smoothly. But this account is based on real events. Names and other identifying details have been changed only to protect privacy. The transport was truly seamless, respectful, client-centered, and professional. "Brooke's" colleagues had previously clashed with the same EMS company and hospital to the point of creating unnecessary obstacles that endangered client care. But this time everyone worked together for the good of mother and baby. The providers' professional rapport had grown over many months of bridge-building through meetings, shared educational sessions, and potluck lunches, as discussed in Chapter 16.

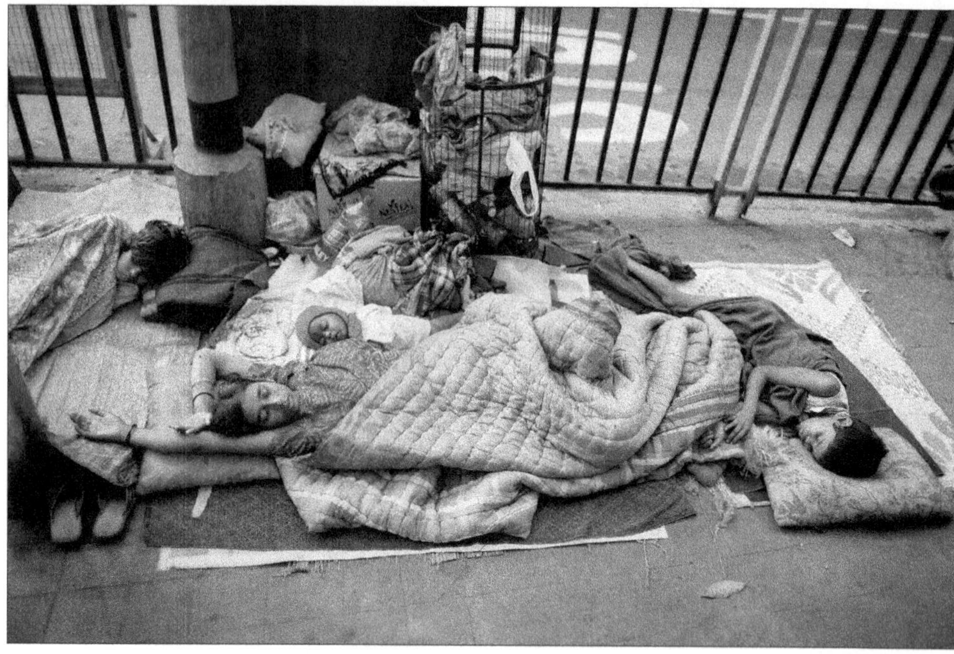

Figure 1-1. A homeless mother and her children sleep on a sidewalk in Kolkata, India. Extreme poverty and lack of nutrition, sanitation, shelter, and health care greatly increase the risk of death for many mothers and babies throughout India. "Kolkata (4131122903)," by Padmanaba01, 2009 [https://commons.wikimedia.org/wiki/File:Kolkata_(4131122903).jpg]. CC BY SA 2.0.

Intrinsic Risks of Childbearing

Each laboring mother is the newest link in a chain of mothers extending to unremembered forebears buried in the dust of time. Normal birth is a well-tuned process best served by nonintervention and watchful waiting. With attentive, supportive care, most mothers and babies will complete this vital journey together with little additional assistance from their providers.

No provider—physician or midwife, in hospital or out—can guarantee a risk-free birth or a good outcome for mother or baby. Any natural process can go awry, and not every problem can be solved. Any obstetrical outcome, good or bad, is influenced by the overall health of mother and baby; the abilities, training, philosophies, and personalities of the birth care providers; laws, regulations, and policies; logistics of transfer to a hospital when transfer is needed; services available there; communication among providers; and many other factors.

Maternal Mortality

In 2020, almost 800 women around the world died every day from preventable causes related to pregnancy and childbirth, about one death every two minutes (World Health Organization [WHO], 2023). Nearly 95% of these deaths occurred in low-income and lower-middle-income countries (WHO, 2023). The maternal mortality ratio (MMR) is the number of mothers per 100,000 live births who die within a given period from pregnancy-related conditions while pregnant or within 42 days after the end of pregnancy (Brown & Small, 2023). MMR is an indicator of the performance of health systems, of the status of women in society, and of the overall health of a population (Douthard, Martin, Chapple-McGruder, Langer, & Chang, 2021).

In industrialized nations, modern obstetric care has dramatically decreased the risks associated with childbirth (Hofmeyr et al., 2009). A mother in a high-resource country is 33 times more likely to survive childbirth than a counterpart in an economically developing country (WHO, 2023). Whereas the lifetime risk of maternal death is 1 in 5,300 in high-income countries, it is 1 in 49 in low-income countries (WHO, 2023). In 2015, about 830 mothers around the globe died each day from largely preventable or treatable obstetric complications; 99% of these deaths occurred in developing countries, 62% in sub-Saharan Africa, and 17% in India (WHO, 2023).

Each year in the United States, about 600–800 mothers die from conditions related to pregnancy and childbirth, and another 50,000–60,000 suffer serious complications that can result in disabilities or other long-term problems (Joseph et al.,

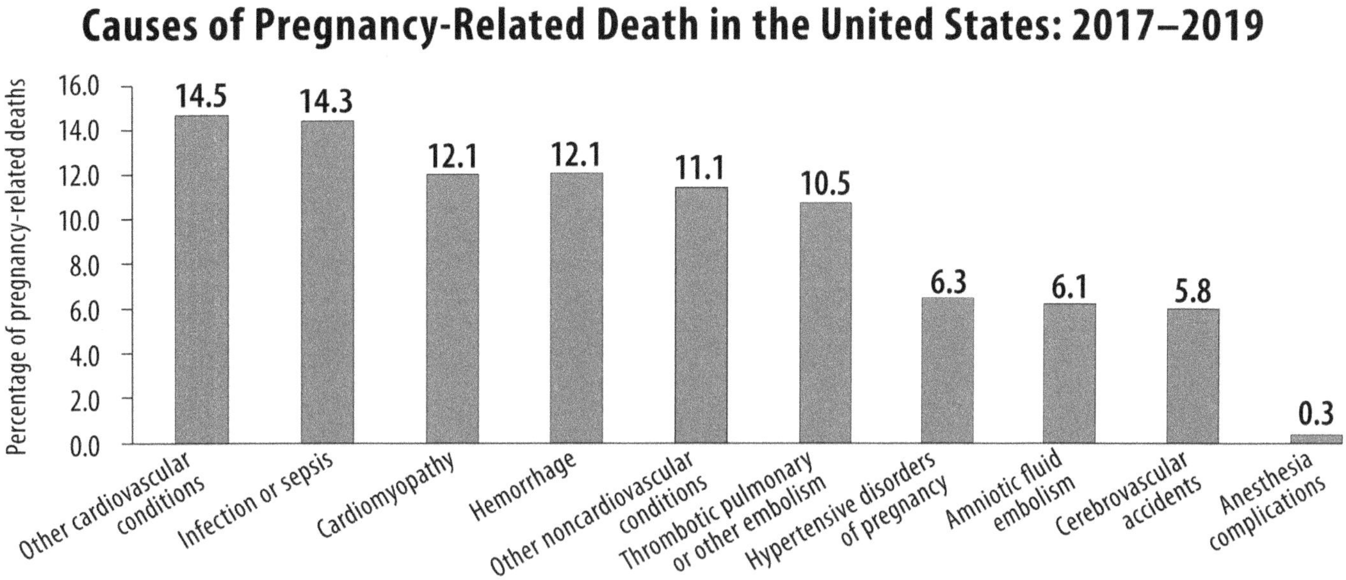

Figure 1-2. Adapted from "Pregnancy Mortality Surveillance System," by Centers for Disease Control and Prevention, 2023b (https://www.cdc.gov/reproductivehealth/maternal-mortality/pregnancy-mortality-surveillance-system.htm). In the public domain.

2021). The national MMR is 17.4 per 100,000 live births (Joseph et al., 2021). Mothers over the age of 40 are much more likely to die in childbirth than mothers in their twenties (Joseph et al., 2021). There has been a rising national trend in maternal mortality from indirect causes such as cardiovascular disease and other chronic conditions (Singh & Lee, 2020). The proportion of maternal deaths in this category increased from 12.0% in 1999 to 26.9% in 2017 (Singh & Lee, 2020).

Pregnancy-related causes of death differ in frequency from region to region and vary from year to year. Worldwide, the leading causes of maternal mortality are obstetric hemorrhage (27%), hypertensive disorders of pregnancy (14%), pregnancy-related sepsis (11%), spontaneous or induced abortion (8%), embolism (3%), other direct causes (e.g., complications of birth, obstructed labor, 10%), and indirect causes (e.g., preexisting medical disorders such as HIV, 28%). In the United States (Petersen et al., 2019), most maternal deaths result from cardiovascular conditions (15.3%), non-cardiovascular medical conditions (14.3%), infection (12.5%), obstetric hemorrhage (11.2%), cardiomyopathy (10.8%), embolism (9.3%), hypertensive disorders of pregnancy (7.1%), cerebrovascular accidents (7.6%), unknown (6.7%), amniotic-fluid embolism (5.8%), and anesthesia complications (0.3%). Since 2006, there has been an increase in maternal deaths from cardiovascular disease, infection, and other medical conditions (including opioid-use disorder) and a decrease in deaths due to hemorrhage, hypertensive disorders of pregnancy, pulmonary embolism, and anesthesia complications (Brown & Small, 2023).

Mothers with multiple or significant medical conditions are at higher risk of complications or death. So are mothers with complex social situations such as poverty, homelessness, abuse, mental illness, drug or alcohol problems, and family separation (Knight et al., 2015). Mothers with comorbidities and social disadvantages are also more likely to die between 6 weeks and 1 year postpartum, but their late deaths are not included in maternal mortality figures (Knight et al., 2015).

Maternal near-miss morbidity occurs when a mother narrowly survives severe complications of pregnancy, childbirth, or the postpartum period (Brown & Small, 2023), either by chance or through appropriate medical intervention. The circumstances surrounding each maternal death are often much like those in cases where mothers come close to death, but ultimately live. Reported maternal severe morbidity and near-miss morbidity in the United States increased by 75% from 1998 to 2009 (Menard et al., 2015).

Racial Disparities

Whether, how long, and how well new mothers and their babies survive can depend on location, who provides their care, and whether they are members of certain minority groups. In the United States, for example, blacks and other minorities are more likely to die in childbirth or experience serious complications than whites. Between 2007 and 2016, the rate of pregnancy-related deaths per 100,000 live births for non-Hispanic black mothers was 40.8; for non-Hispanic Native American mothers, 29.7; and for non-Hispanic white mothers, 12.7 (Kumar, Borders, & Simon, 2021). Maternal mortality and other poor health outcomes are also higher among other minority groups, including Asians/Pacific Islanders and certain subgroups of Hispanic women, e.g., Puerto Ricans (Howell, 2018).

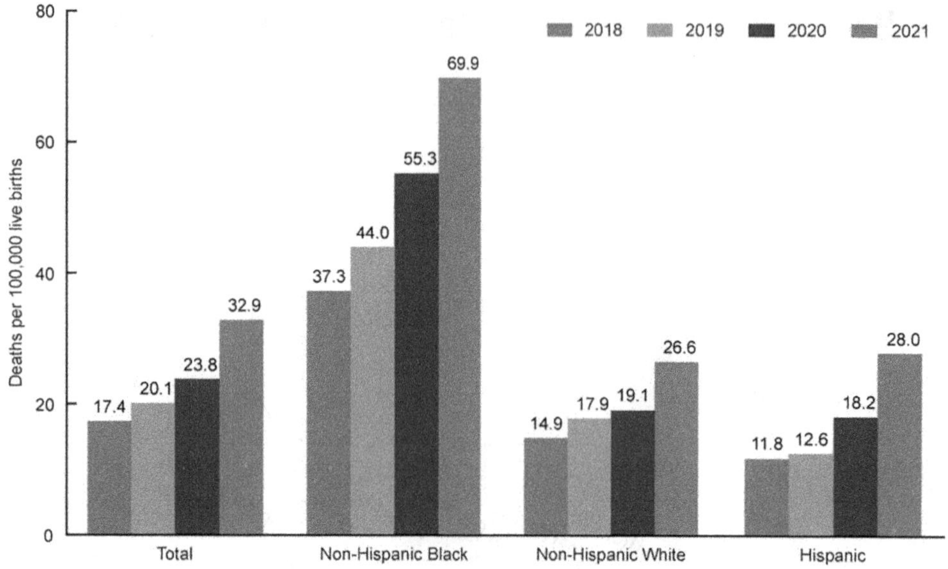

Figure 1-3. U.S. maternal mortality rates (MMRs) by race and Hispanic origin, 2018–2021. Adapted from "Maternal Mortality Rates in the United States, 2021," by D. L. Hoyert, 2023 (https://dx.doi.org/10.15620/cdc:124678). In the public domain.

Black communities experience not only higher maternal morbidity and mortality, but also higher rates of preterm birth, low birthweight, and infant mortality (Dreyer, 2021). Black women are less likely to get proper treatment for sexually transmitted infections; less likely to be vaccinated against the human papilloma virus; and more likely to have cancers of the reproductive system, preterm births, pregnancy complications such as hypertension, and low-birthweight neonates (Sutton, Anachebe, Lee, & Skanes, 2021). Black mothers are more likely to undergo inductions of labor, have episiotomies, and give birth by cesarean section than white mothers (Bingham, Jones, & Howell, 2019). Although black mothers do not develop preeclampsia/eclampsia, placental abruption, placenta previa, or postpartum hemorrhage more frequently, they are 2–3 times more likely to die from these conditions independent of age, parity, or education (Tucker, Berg, Callaghan, & Hsia, 2007). Racial disparities are no less concerning elsewhere. In the United Kingdom, the death rate for black mothers is five times that of white mothers (Joseph et al., 2021).

These disparities are not the result of genetic or constitutional predispositions (Bingham et al., 2019; Treder, White, Woodhams, Pancholi, & Yinusa-Nyahkoon, 2022). Rather, they appear to be the cumulative effect of racism and systemic inequity (Bingham et al., 2019; Treder et al., 2022). Social determinants of health—environmental, material, and conditions in which people live, work, and play—influence wellness, functioning, and quality of life and can contribute to poor health outcomes for certain minority groups (Dagher & Linares, 2022). Structural racism involving public policies, institutional practices, and individual perceptions is a root cause for substandard living conditions and for health care inequities (George, Mitchell, & Stacey, 2022; Treder et al., 2022; Gillispie-Bell, 2021). The health disparities faced by blacks and others in the United States reflect centuries of struggle against social and cultural obstacles, including unequal access to education and employment, housing segregation, economic suppression, and health care inequality (Bingham et al., 2019). Minority mothers are less likely to have access to healthy foods, educational opportunities, and high-paying jobs, and are more likely to live in high-crime areas that increase fear and anxiety.

Minority clients can encounter deeply entrenched prejudice directly or vicariously every day of their lives. Individuals who are repeatedly degraded and dehumanized often come to believe the externally imposed stereotypes and internalize the oppression they experience (Taylor, Guy-Walls, Wilkerson, & Addae, 2019). Through repeated negative interactions with the dominant culture, they can develop mistrust of the attitudes and motivations of others.

Consequently, minority clients may feel uncomfortable or become defensive answering or asking questions because of previous neglect or mistreatment by health care providers (Bingham et al., 2019). When presenting for care, some anticipate maltreatment by becoming guarded and suspicious. Others overstate symptoms to ensure that they are heard or avoid seeking health care entirely (Treder et al., 2022). Some will seek a health care professional of color or bring an advocate to the appointment. Others will self-advocate by overpreparing for their appointments, arriving with an agenda, a list of questions, and research about potential diagnoses or treatments (Treder et al., 2022).

Health care providers are more likely to make negative assumptions about the financial and educational status of minority clients and to direct care rather than use shared decision-making (Treder et al., 2022). Providers tend to spend less time with black clients and dismiss their symptoms and complaints (Treder et al., 2022). Physicians are more likely to prescribe appropriate pain medication, especially opioids, to white clients even though the risk of opioid misuse in the

United States is much higher for whites (Meghani, Byun, & Gallagher, 2012). Racial biases support discriminatory health care systems and practices that lead to worse obstetric outcomes, which then reinforce beliefs, creating a self-sustaining feedback loop (Vela et al., 2022). In many places, unfortunately, racial biases are exacerbated by divisions of ethnicity, religion, class, and even politics.

Too Much Too Soon/Too Little Too Late

More than 80% of pregnancy-related deaths are preventable (Trost, et al., 2022). Contributors to preventable deaths (Joseph et al., 2021) include failing to educate clients about warning signs (38%); misdiagnosis and other provider errors (34%); and systemic factors, which can include poor organization management, insufficient staff, and poor processes for sharing information (22%). Preventable maternal deaths and near misses are associated with either of two opposing conditions: inadequate access to services, resources, or evidence-based care—"too little, too late"—or unnecessary, inappropriate, or excessive use of interventions—"too much, too soon" (Miller et al., 2016).

Too little too late describes the outcomes of obstetric complications in areas with untrained attendants, inadequate hygiene, and minimal resources (Miller et al., 2016). The term can also denote lack of the lifesaving interventions available at a modern medical center, lack of providers, or care withheld until it is no longer beneficial. Better diagnosis and treatment might have prevented 38% of California's 2002–2003 maternal deaths, particularly those resulting from the more common causes—hemorrhage, infection, and preeclampsia (California Dept. of Public Health, 2011).

Too little, too late includes structural health-system deficiencies, such as a lack of equipment, supplies, or drugs, that impede implementation of the most rudimentary evidence-based interventions (Miller et al., 2016). In 2010, an estimated 1.0–3.5 million needed cesareans were not performed in low-income countries, resulting in preventable harm to mothers and infants (Miller et al., 2016). Even where trained providers and adequate equipment are available, substandard care can result if there are no evidence-based guidelines for management. Too little too late disproportionately affects marginalized subpopulations, including migrants; refugees; persons with disabilities; the destitute; and racial, ethnic, or religious minorities

Conversely, providers who intervene too much and too soon also increase risk for mothers and newborns. For example, induction and augmentation, beneficial when clinically indicated, can cause prolonged labor, precipitous labor, uterine hyperstimulation, uterine rupture, fetal asphyxia, or placental

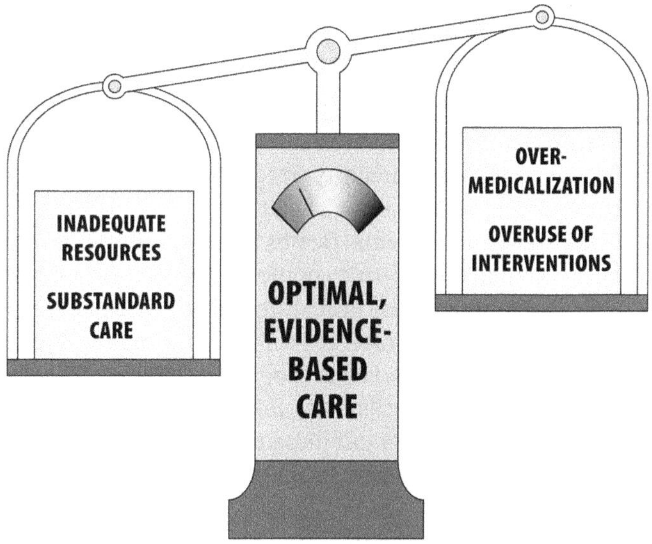

Figure 1-4. Care for mothers and infants is safest when trained providers make prudent use of adequate resources.

abruption when used inappropriately (Miller et al., 2016). Other overused interventions include ultrasound examinations, routine continuous fetal monitoring, routine episiotomy, epidural anesthesia, and amniotomy (Miller et al., 2016). Further, the overuse of interventions tends to increase the need for further interventions, each carrying its own complement of potential risks and negative consequences. In high-resource countries, including the United States, the overmedicalization of uncomplicated birth often leads to substandard outcomes (Kennedy et al., 2020). There are financial incentives to overmedicalize childbirth: people with health insurance, for example, have a higher rate of medical interventions, including cesarean section, than the uninsured (Hoxha, Braha, Syrogiannouli, Goodman, & Jüni, 2019).

As many as half of all deaths from pregnancy complications could be prevented if people had better access to health care, received better care, and were coached by providers to improve their own health and lifestyle (American Congress of Obstetricians & Gynecologists, n.d.). The WHO recommends that care be individualized and mother-centered; that interventions be implemented only if they are of known benefit and there is a clear medical indication; and that providers prioritize a positive experience for the mother, the newborn, and the family (Oladapo et al., 2018). A positive childbirth experience is one that results in a healthy mother and infant; meets or exceeds a client's expectations; and provides a safe environment, emotional support from chosen companions, and kind, competent clinical staff (WHO, 2018).

More Expensive, Less Safe

When compared to other high-resource countries, health care is more expensive in the United States, yet maternal and

Table 1-1

Some Useful Definitions

(Can Differ by Country, State or Province, and Source)

- **Maternal morbidity:** Any health problem that results from pregnancy or birth.
- **Severe maternal morbidity:** Pregnancy-related health problems with significant consequences for a mother's health.
- **Maternal mortality rate:** Deaths from complications of pregnancy or childbirth that occur during the pregnancy or the postpartum period, per 100,000 live births per year. (Some sources use death rate in discussing particular populations or conditions.)
- **Perinatal mortality rate:** The total of fetal deaths beyond 20 (or 28) completed weeks of gestation and early neonatal deaths per 1,000 live births per year.
- **Neonatal morbidity:** Illnesses, injuries, and other health conditions within the first 28 days after birth, not just those that necessitate specialized care.
- **Neonatal mortality rate:** Infant deaths within 28 days after birth per 1,000 live births per year.
- **Infant mortality rate (IMR):** The number of deaths of children under 1 year of age per 1,000 live births per year.
- **Early neonatal mortality:** Infant death within 7 days after birth.

neonatal outcomes are worse than in other countries with similar levels of economic development (Kennedy et al., 2020). For more than a decade, reliable data has indicated that the maternal mortality rate in the United States is more than double that of other high-resource countries and is on the increase (Kennedy et al., 2020; Lothian, 2018). Nichols and Cohen (2021) posited that this high mortality rate is due to a deficit of social policies and programs that support maternal health, low quality of care, inequalities adversely affecting minority and rural mothers, and inadequate monitoring of maternal health issues. Reports published by the National Center for Health Statistics contradicted these assessments, attributing the rising trend to improvements in methods used to record and analyze maternal deaths (Hoyert & Miniño, 2020; Joseph et al., 2021; Rossen, Womack, Hoyert, Anderson, & Uddin, 2020). It appears, however, that this explanation is simplistic; the high rate of maternal mortality is multifactorial and influenced by numerous underlying processes, including broader societal and policy factors.

Implementing strategies to improve the health of mothers can greatly reduce maternal deaths. Kennedy et al. (2020) examined outcome data for four high-resource countries with lower rates of maternal, newborn, and infant mortality and low birthweight than the United States: Australia, Canada, the Netherlands, and the United Kingdom. They found that all four countries, unlike the United States, had universal access to maternity care with a commitment to integration of care across providers and systems, prioritized respectful care and maternal autonomy, and had effective systems for collecting data and evaluating outcome statistics. In three of the four countries, midwives were the primary maternity caregivers across most birth settings.

Although maternal mortality has increased in the United States overall in recent decades, it decreased more than 50% in the state of California from 2006 to 2018, largely because of programs to improve maternal health and expand maternal-health monitoring and surveillance (Nichols & Cohen, 2021). Although disparities remain, maternal mortality for black mothers in California decreased from more than 50 to 26 deaths per 100,000 from 2007 to 2013 (Nichols & Cohen, 2021). These policy changes also decreased maternal morbidity. For example, when the California Pregnancy-Associated Mortality Review Committee implemented consensus-based resources to increase maternal safety (e.g., collaborative research, toolkits, and a Maternal Data Center), participating hospitals achieved a 20.8% reduction in severe maternal morbidity due to hemorrhage (Nichols & Cohen, 2021).

The U.S. Supreme Court 2022 decision in *Dobbs v. Jackson Women's Health Organization*, which overturned its own 1973 ruling in *Roe v. Wade*, returned responsibility for regulating abortion to the states (Espey, Haider, Stone, Gyamfi-Bannerman, & Steinauer, 2023). States that restrict access to abortion have higher rates of maternal and infant mortality, even after adjusting for the general health of the population (Addante et al., 2021; Harper et al., 2022; Pabayo et al., 2020), and certain obstetric complications are more prevalent where legislation prohibits previable abortion in complicated pregnancies (Nambiar, Patel, Santiago-Munoz, Spong, & Nelson, 2022). States, provinces, and countries that enact gestational-age-limit abortion restrictions have higher infant mortality rates than those with no such laws, largely because in these areas fetuses with lethal anomalies die after live birth rather during a pregnancy termination (Karletsos, Stoecker, Vilda, Theall, & Wallace, 2021).

Neonatal Mortality

When mothers are at risk, infants are at much greater risk. The global infant mortality rate (IMR) has decreased from about 63 deaths per 1,000 live births in 1990 to 32 in 2015 (WHO, 2016). Despite this improvement, 2.6 million newborn babies die within the first month of life every year, about half of these in the first 24 hr after birth (Verma & Cleland, 2022; WHO, 2020). In one estimate, the intrapartum deaths of more than 500,000 babies a year could be averted if all laboring individuals had access to comprehensive emergency obstetric care in all birth settings (Lawn et al., 2009). Additionally, it is estimated that more than 100,000 babies per year could be saved if all birth attendants working in health care centers were formally trained in neonatal resuscitation, hand-washing, and placing newborns skin-to-skin with their mothers (Lawn et al., 2009).

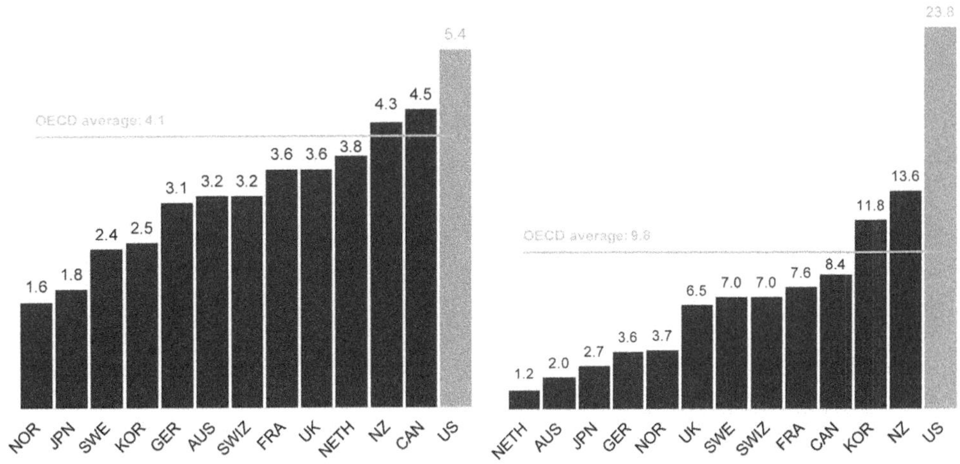

Figure 1-5. Infant mortality rate (IMR) per 1,000 live births (L) and MMR per 100,000 live births (R) for selected countries, 2015–2021. From "U.S. Health Care from a Global Perspective, 2022: Accelerating Spending, Worsening Outcomes," by M. Z. Gunja, E. D. Gumae, and R. D. Williams, II, 2023 (https://doi.org/10.26099/8ejy-yc74). Copyright by the Commonwealth Fund.

It is challenging to compare mortality statistics within or among countries. Definitions differ: in the United States, the minimum gestational age (GA) used to calculate fetal mortality is 20 0/7 weeks of gestation; in European countries, it ranges from 16 0/7 to 28 0/7 weeks of gestation. Some calculations involve birthweight and some use gestational age (which depends on accurate dating). *Perinatal mortality*, for example, can denote newborn deaths that occur in the first 7 (or 28) days after birth. There are also differences in the definition of *live birth* and in registration processes for births and deaths, notably when babies are born very prematurely or die soon after birth (Zacharias, 2023). In economically developing countries, many births are attended by untrained personnel who do not always keep accurate records.

In 2020, the U.S. IMR, 5.4 deaths per 1,000 live births (Centers for Disease Control and Prevention [CDC], 2022b), is higher than that of most other high-resource nations (Ely & Driscoll, 2019). Perinatal mortality differs by state. In 2019, Connecticut reported the lowest rate, 4.11 deaths per 1,000 live births; and Mississippi had the highest, 8.56 per 1,000 (Elflein, 2022). Inequalities persist despite the trend of declining perinatal mortality. There is a fivefold difference in IMR among ethnic groups, from 2.3 deaths per 1,000 live births for Chinese Americans to 11.2 per 1,000 for African Americans (Singh & Stella, 2019).

Preterm birth (PTB) is the leading cause of infant mortality, accounting for up to 35% of all deaths among newborns around the globe (Walani, 2020). Worldwide, about 11% of infants are born preterm (Walani, 2020). The highest rates of PTB occur in low- and middle-income countries such as Southeast Asia and sub-Saharan Africa (Walani, 2020). In 2010, about 39% of infant deaths in the United States were due to PTB (MacDorman, Mathews, Mohangoo, & Zeitlin, 2014). In the United States, rates of PTB (before 37 0/7 weeks of gestation) reached an all-time high of 12.8% of all live births in 2006, primarily caused by a rise in late PTBs, then declined to a rate of 9.9% in 2017 (Barfield, 2018). In 2020, the rate of PTB among non-Hispanic black mothers in the United States was 14.4%, about 50% higher than the 9.1% rate among non-Hispanic white mothers or the 9.8% rate among Hispanic mothers (CDC, 2021).

About 47% of U.S. infant deaths in 2010 occurred among babies born at 37 0/7 weeks of gestation or later, many of them born electively between 37 0/7 and 38 6/7 weeks (MacDorman et al., 2014). Not only do early term births increase risk of newborn death, they also appear to impair brain development, increase risk for long-term neurodevelopmental abnormalities, and increase the likelihood of respiratory and cardiovascular problems that can persist into adulthood (Gutvirtz, Wainstock, Sheiner, Landau, & Walfisch, 2018). Professional organizations for obstetricians, nurses, and midwives; the March of Dimes; task forces such as the California Maternal Quality Care Collaborative and the Joint Commission on Accreditation of Healthcare Organizations; and many other agencies and organizations place strong pressure on providers to end elective births before 39 0/7 weeks of gestation (American College of Obstetricians & Gynecologists [ACOG] & Society for Maternal-Fetal Medicine, 2021/2024; Main et al., 2010).

A Culture of Unnecessary Intervention

A large body of research validates what midwives have known all along: supportive care in labor and birth results in safer, healthier mothers and babies, and routine interventions can create complications (American College of Nurse-Midwives [ACNM], n.d.). Physiologic labor and birth are parts of a finely

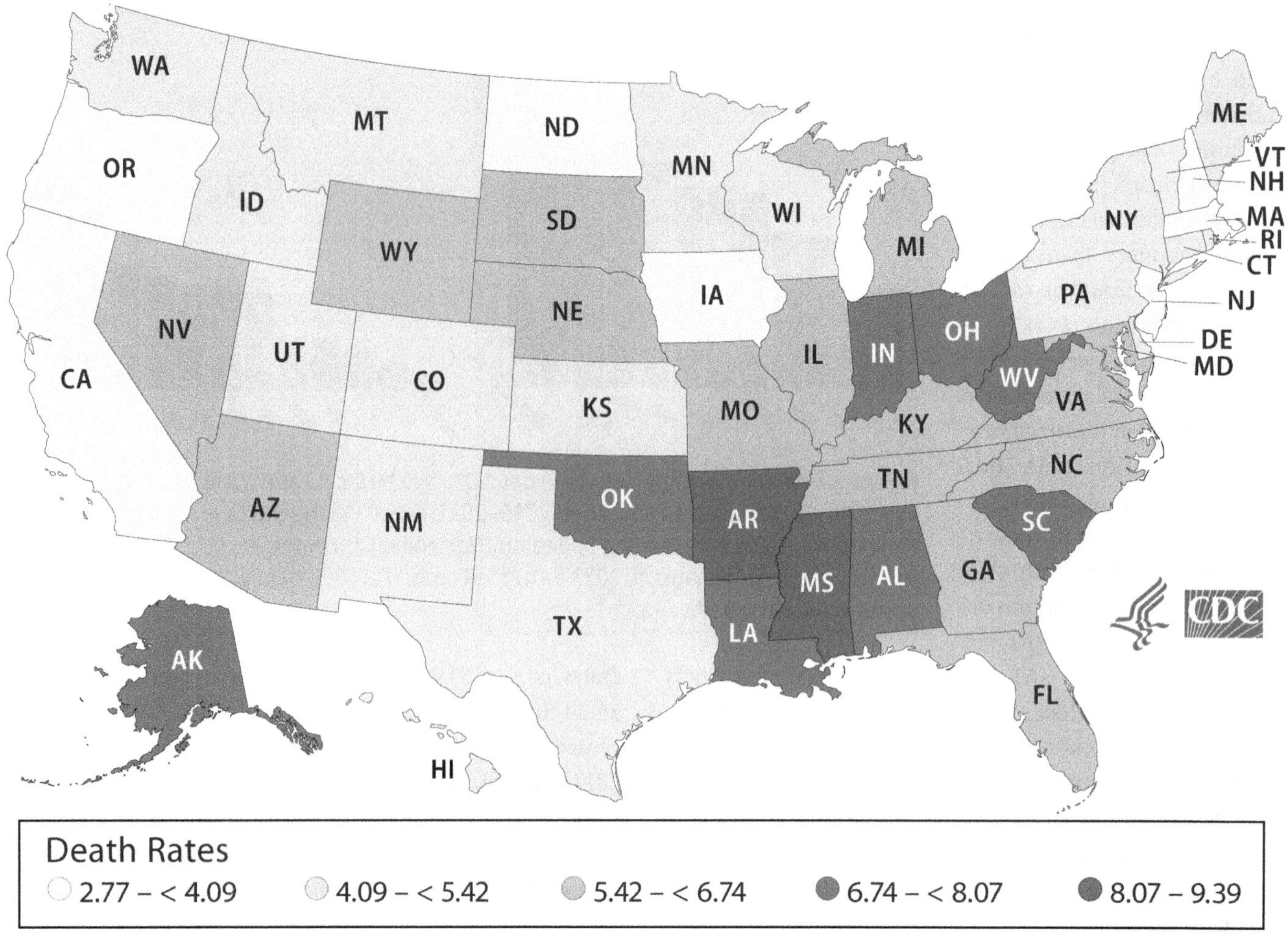

Figure 1-6. Adapted from "Infant Mortality Rates by State [2021]," by Centers for Disease Control and Prevention, 2023a (https://www.cdc.gov/nchs/pressroom/sosmap/infant_mortality_rates/infant_mortality.htm). In the public domain.

tuned biological process natural to our species. With no complications or external disruptions, the birth process is likely to remain safe, healthy, and efficient. When complications occur, access to necessary interventions during pregnancy, childbirth, and the postpartum period can improve outcomes for mother and infant (Zondag, Maas, Beuckens, & Nieuwenhuijze, 2022).

Mainstream obstetrics has seen a dramatic increase in routine interventions, often without evidence of increased safety for low-risk mothers and babies (Chmell, 2012). In the United States in 2017, more than 98% of births occurred in hospitals, and 90% of these were attended by physicians (MacDorman & Declercq, 2019; National Academies of Sciences, Engineering, and Medicine [NASEM], 2020). In their Cochrane review of randomized trials, Olsen and Clausen (2023) note that "It seems increasingly clear that anxiety and easy access to many medical procedures at hospital may lead to increased levels of intervention, which in turn may lead to further interventions and finally to unnecessary complications." A prominent 2007 study of mothers who gave birth in U.S. hospitals revealed that 87% had continuous electronic fetal monitoring, 80% received intravenous (IV) fluids, and 47% had medications to augment labor (Declercq, Sakala, Corry, & Applebaum, 2006). In another study, a whopping 43% of nulliparas underwent induction of labor (Declercq et al., 2006). Of these clients, 60% were not allowed food or drink, 76% were confined to bed, and 92% gave birth in lithotomy position. Yet there is strong evidence that for low-risk mothers, unnecessary interventions can disrupt normal physiologic labor, increase the likelihood of some complications, and decrease maternal satisfaction (Alfirevic, Gyte, Cuthbert, & Devane, 2017; Bugg, Siddiqui, & Thornton, 2013; Coco et al., 2010; Gupta, Sood, Hofmeyr, & Vogel, 2017; Kavitha et al., 2012; Laughon et al., 2012; Lawrence, Lewis, Hofmeyr, & Styles, 2013; NASEM, 2020; Rydahl, Juhl, Declercq, & Maimburg, 2021; Singata, Tranmer, & Gyte, 2013).

The Cesarean Epidemic

For many mothers and babies, cesarean section is clearly beneficial and possibly lifesaving, but it triples the risk for severe maternal morbidities accompanying vaginal birth (Liu et al., 2007). These complications include hemorrhage requiring transfusion or even hysterectomy, anesthetic complications, shock, cardiac arrest, acute renal failure, respiratory failure, venous thromboembolism, major infection, and severe wound compromise (ACOG Cmte. on Clinical Practice Guidelines—Obstetrics, Cahill, Raghuraman, Gandhi, M., & Kaimal, 2024). After a primary cesarean, subsequent pregnancies carry escalating risk of surgical complications, anesthetic complications, infection, bladder injury, thromboembolism, and PTB (ACOG Cmte. on Clinical Practice Guidelines—Obstetrics et al., 2024; Mariani & Vain, 2019). Cesarean birth also causes permanent uterine scarring, which can cause complications in future pregnancies, such as placenta previa, placenta accreta, and uterine rupture (California Dept. of Public Health, 2011). The more cesareans one has, the greater the risk of complications in successive pregnancies (ACOG Cmte. on Clinical Practice Guidelines—Obstetrics et al., 2024). Babies born to a mother after multiple cesareans have a higher rate of adverse outcomes, neonatal intensive care unit (NICU) admission, and perinatal death than babies born to a mother who had only vaginal births (ACOG Cmte. on Clinical Practice Guidelines—Obstetrics et al., 2024). Not only is spontaneous vaginal birth associated with improved short- and long-term mother and infant outcomes, compared to cesarean birth, but most mothers also prefer vaginal birth (Clark & Lake, 2021).

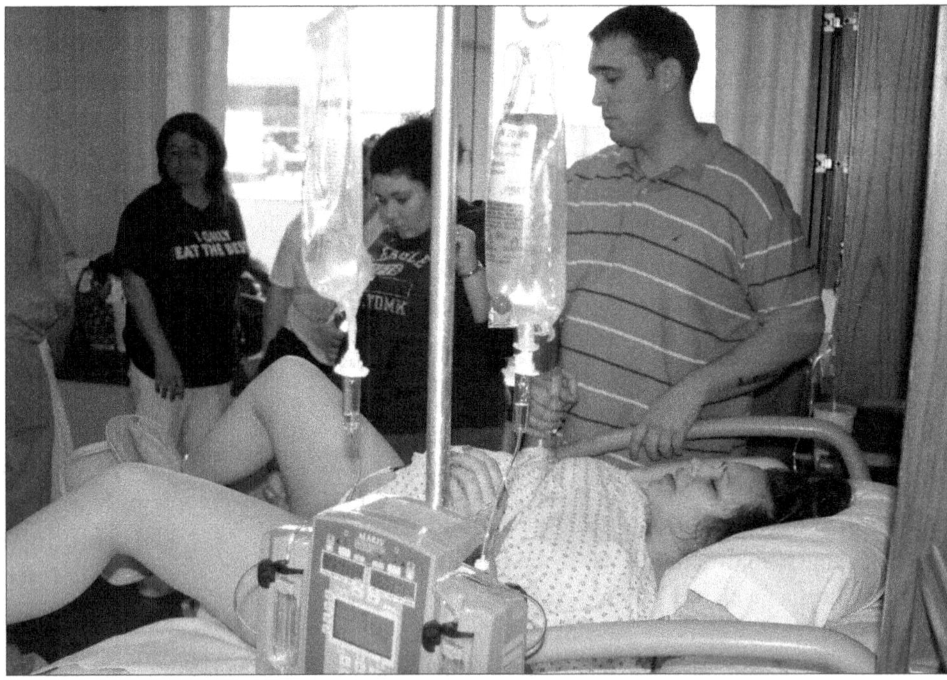

Figure 1-7. In the United States, most births occur in hospitals. In many hospitals, laboring mothers receive many interventions and procedures, and they give birth in lithotomy position attended by a physician who spends minimal time by the bedside. Note that nobody in this room is paying much attention to the laboring woman in the bed.

The rate of cesarean births has skyrocketed in the past half-century without evidence of improvement in maternal or perinatal outcomes, suggesting that the current rate reflects a high number of unnecessary procedures (ACOG Cmte. on Clinical Practice Guidelines—Obstetrics et al., 2024). In the United States, cesarean section is the most common major surgical procedure, accounting for roughly 1 in 3 births (ACOG Cmte. on Clinical Practice Guidelines—Obstetrics et al., 2024; Sakai-Bizmark et al., 2021). The number of cesareans performed in U.S. hospitals has increased 500% since 1970 (Haelle, 2016) even though giving birth today is not 500% riskier (Shah, 2015b). The rate of cesareans in the United States steadily climbed from 5.5% of births in 1970 to 16.5% in 1980 to about 31–32% in 2019 (Antoine & Young, 2021). There is also a racial and ethnic disparity; low-risk nulliparous black and Hispanic individuals have a higher rate of cesarean birth than their non-Hispanic white counterparts (Debbink et al., 2022).

The cesarean epidemic is an issue in other countries as well. Worldwide, the rate of cesarean births nearly doubled from 2000 to 2015 (Bruno, Metz, Grobman, & Silver, 2022). In 2010, providers in high- and middle-income countries performed an estimated 3.5–5.7 million unnecessary cesareans (Miller et al., 2016). In 2016, the cesarean section rate (CSR) was greater than 50% in parts of Europe, China, and South America (Visser et al., 2018).

The percentage of cesarean births can differ within countries and regions, apparently illustrating "provider preferences trumping scientific evidence" (Lincoln, 2015, p. 26). In 2020, the five U.S. states with the highest CSRs (CDC, 2022a) were Mississippi (38.2%), Louisiana (36.8%), Florida (35.9%), Alabama (35.0%), and Texas (34.7%). Those with the lowest rates were Alaska (22.9%), Utah (23.1%), Idaho (23.5%), South Dakota (24.7%) and New Mexico (26.1%). CSRs are considerably lower in community settings for low-risk individuals. One large study showed a rate of 12.3% for birth-center clients (Alliman et al., 2019), and others showed rates of roughly 5% for clients planning home births (George et al., 2022; Nethery et al., 2021; Snowden et al., 2015).

The ideal CSR has not been determined (Bruno et al., 2022). The WHO systematic review, conducted in 1985 at population level, found that CSRs higher than 10–15% are not associated with reductions in maternal and newborn mortality (Betran, Torloni, Zhang, & Gülmezoglu, 2016). Molina et al. (2015) examined CSRs and maternal and neonatal mortality from 54 countries and concluded that a cesarean rate of 19% was associated with the lowest rates of maternal and neonatal death. These studies suggest that a target cesarean rate of 10–20% could reduce maternal and neonatal mortality on a global scale, though it does not necessarily apply to high-resource countries such as the United States because of differences in client risk profiles (Bruno et al., 2022).

Providers often adopt defensive practices in response to the soaring rate of litigation. In 2013, 77% of obstetricians had been sued (ACOG, 2013/2016), and in 2018 about one third of practicing certified nurse-midwives (CNMs) report being named in at least 1 lawsuit at a median of 7 years of practice (K. Page, Aryal, & Guidera, 2022). Providers are most likely to be sued after the birth of a neurologically impaired infant, after a stillbirth or neonatal death, or when a delay in diagnosis or failure to diagnose caused harm to a client (Stiller, 2014). Cesareans can be easily justified: both good and poor outcomes can validate that the procedure was essential and done in time (Shah, 2015b).

Respectful Maternity Care

The care given during labor can affect the physical and emotional health of mother and baby, often for a lifetime (National Institute for Health and Care Excellence in the United Kingdom [NICE], 2023; WHO, 2018). In the United States, about one in six individuals receiving maternity care experiences mistreatment by health care providers (Vedam, Stoll, Taiwo, et al., 2019). Mistreatment can involve physical abuse ("rough touch," hitting, slapping, pinching, being restrained during labor), verbal abuse (harsh or rude language, mocking or belittling, judgmental comments, or threats), discrimination, substandard treatment, sexual abuse, or the performance of procedures without consent (Vedam, Stoll, Taiwo, et al., 2019). Fear of disrespect and abuse by health care providers can prevent individuals from seeking care (Windau-Melmer, 2013). These abuses disproportionately affect

- Mothers giving birth in hospitals (Vedam, Stoll, Taiwo, et al., 2019);
- Mothers of color;
- Mothers with social, economic, or health challenges;
- Mothers who experience unexpected events such as cesareans;
- Mothers transferred from community to hospital care (Vedam, Stoll, Taiwo, et al., 2019); and
- Mothers who disagree with a health care provider (Vedam, Stoll, Taiwo, et al., 2019).

The Seven Rights of Mothers

1. Every mother has the right to be free from harm and ill-treatment.
2. Every mother has the right to information, informed consent and refusal, and respect for personal choices and preferences, including companionship during maternity care.
3. Every mother has the right to privacy and confidentiality.
4. Every mother has the right to be treated with dignity and respect.
5. Every mother has the right to equality, freedom from discrimination, and equitable care.
6. Every mother has the right to health care and to the highest attainable level of health.
7. Every mother has the right to liberty, autonomy, self-determination, and freedom from coercion.

Adapted from *Respectful Maternity Care Charter: Universal Rights of Women & Newborns*, by White Ribbon Alliance, n.d. (https://whiteribbonalliance.org/wp-content/uploads/2022/05/WRA_RMC_Charter_FINAL.pdf).

Giving birth is a culturally and personally significant rite of passage (WHO, 2018). Although every laboring mother has unique needs and expectations, each deserves a calm, supportive birth environment; a choice of birth setting; and considerate care that respects personal autonomy, dignity, feelings, choices, preferences, and choice of companionship (Windau-Melmer, 2013). Respectful maternity care is every mother's birthright.

Birth Settings

Home, birth center, and hospital have unique resources that can benefit mothers and babies as well as unique drawbacks that can increase risk (ACNM, 2015). In the United States, most babies draw their first breaths in a hospital. Community births generally occur in the home or at a birth center and are not suitable for mothers with high-risk pregnancies who are likely to have complicated births (Preis, Mahaffey, & Lobel, 2021).

Community birth is gradually becoming more mainstream in the United States. Although the number of births occurring in community settings increased sharply from 35,578 in 2004 to 62,228 in 2017 (MacDorman & Declercq, 2019), fewer than 2% of babies are born outside a hospital (Preis et al., 2021). Yet, the number of home births increased 22%, from 38,506 in 2019 to 45,646 in 2020—the "highest level since at least 1990"

(Gregory, Osterman, & Valenzuela, 2021, p. 1).

WHO, ACNM, the American Public Health Association, and the National Perinatal Association support a choice of hospital, birth center, or home for carefully screened low-risk mothers with a qualified provider and a backup plan for transfer (Declercq & Stotland, 2023; MacDorman, Declercq, & Mathews, 2011). ACOG and the American Academy of Pediatrics consider hospitals and accredited birth centers the safest settings for healthy mothers to give birth, and oppose home birth while supporting the mother's right to informed choice (ACOG Cmte. on Obstetric Practice, 2017/2023; Watterberg et al., 2020).

Table 1-2

Components of Physiologic Childbirth

Normal physiologic childbirth is one that is powered by the innate human capacity of the woman and fetus, and • Is characterized by spontaneous onset and progression of labor; • Includes biologic and psychologic conditions that promote effective labor; • Results in the vaginal birth of the infant and placenta; • Results in physiologic blood loss; • Facilitates optimal newborn transition through skin-to-skin contact and keeping the mother and infant together during the postpartum period; and • Supports early initiation of breastfeeding.
The following factors disrupt normal physiologic childbirth: • Induction or augmentation of labor; • An unsupportive environment (e.g., bright lights, cold room, lack of privacy, multiple providers, lack of supportive companions); • Time constraints, including those driven by institutional policy and/or staffing; • Nutritional deprivation (e.g., food and drink); • Opiates, regional analgesia, or general anesthesia; • Episiotomy; • Operative vaginal (vacuum, forceps) or abdominal (cesarean) birth; • Immediate cord clamping; and • Separation of mother and infant and/or any situation in which the mother feels threatened or unsupported.
From "Physiologic Childbirth and Active Management of the Third Stage of Labor: A Latent Class Model of Risk for Postpartum Hemorrhage," by E. N. Erickson, C. S. Lee, E. Grose, and C. Emeis, 2019, *Birth*, 46(1), pp. 69–79. Copyright by John Wiley & Sons.

No birth site is completely free of risk (Declercq & Stotland, 2023). Choosing one involves trading some risks for others (Caughey & Cheyney, 2019). In the United States, the safety advantages of birth in a well-equipped hospital include the availability of specialist expertise and technological interventions that can be used if complications develop, including immediate access to imaging studies, laboratory analysis, anesthesia, pharmaceutical pain management, cesarean section, assisted vaginal birth, and a NICU. Often the trade-off is less client autonomy, more interventions, and an unfamiliar, often bewildering environment.

For a low-risk mother, the safety advantage of birth in a community setting is that providers promote physiologic processes and rely on the intrinsic powers of mother and fetus (Declercq & Stotland, 2023). In a planned home birth assisted by an experienced midwife with collaborative medical backup, unnecessary interference is largely avoided, though hospital transfer is available if medical intervention is required (Declercq & Stotland, 2023). Low-risk mothers often choose birth in a community setting because they prefer a familiar, family-friendly environment; greater personal autonomy and control of the birth process; less obstetric intervention; lower cost; or a combination of these incentives (Boucher, Bennett, MacFarlin, & Freeze, 2009; Hildingsson, Rådestad, & Lindgren, 2010; van Haaren-ten Haken et al., 2012; Watterberg et al., 2020). A normal labor tends to remain normal if the provider does not interfere with the natural process. Normal birth provides numerous health benefits for mothers and babies, including a lower risk of postpartum hemorrhage, higher maternal satisfaction, better lactation, and optimal growth of intestinal microbiota in the newborn (Martin-Arribas et al., 2020; Preis et al., 2021). The trade-off is delay in accessing certain therapeutic interventions (such as cesarean section, oxytocin augmentation, or antihypertensive therapy) should a complication occur.

These differences are neither universal nor unchanging, however. Many hospital-based providers support normal physiologic birth, and some community midwives may intervene unilaterally, habitually, or excessively (Caughey & Cheyney, 2019). Some clients experience less anxiety or a greater sense of autonomy relaxing in a tub in a hospital birth suite than in a cramped apartment full of children and pets. A client with complications in an isolated cabin sometimes receives definitive care sooner than one in the same condition laboring in a small hospital where physicians take call from home.

Community birth may have incalculable long-term benefits for the infant. U.S. babies born in homes and birth centers are more likely to breastfeed for at least 6 months than their

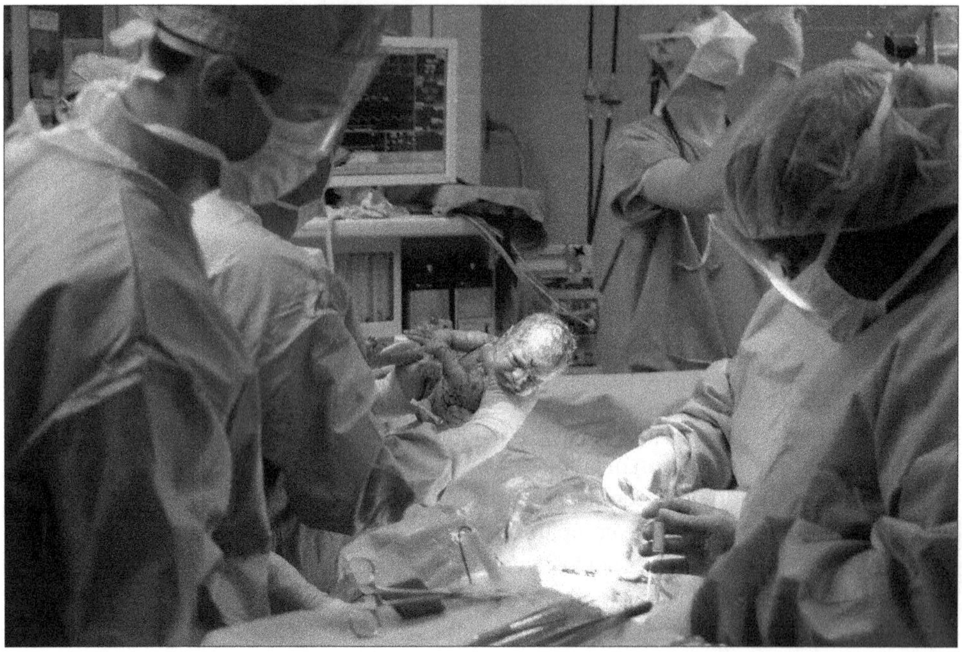

Figure 1-8. Cesarean section is the most common major surgical procedure in the United States, where roughly 1 of every 3 babies is born by cesarean.

hospital-born counterparts. In one study, infants born in a birth center breastfed a median of 44 weeks, versus 17 weeks for hospital-born infants (Börk & Bott, 2015). Infants who breastfeed for at least 6 months have a lower incidence of gastrointestinal disease, otitis media, respiratory illnesses, and allergic conditions (Eidelman et al., 2012) and are 36% less likely to die from sudden infant death syndrome (Ip et al., 2007). Bartick and Reinhold (2010) estimate that the lives of more than 900 U.S. babies a year might be saved if 90% of mothers exclusively breastfed 6 months or longer.

Hospital Birth

Many mothers choose hospital births because they feel safest where physicians can quickly take definitive action if complications develop. Others prefer hospitals because they offer epidural anesthesia and other forms of pain management as well as specialists such as pediatricians, lactation consultants, psychologists, and dietitians. Hospital stays tend to last at least 24 hr, providing greater opportunity for staff to educate families, identify problems, and work out solutions to issues.

Mothers and babies who are at high risk or who develop certain complications such as preeclampsia or fetal growth restriction have better outcomes in a hospital (Lang, Farnell, & Quinlan, 2021). When labor is not normal, intervention is sometimes necessary to help the mother to have a vaginal birth, or even to have a live baby. Oxytocin used to augment an abnormal, nonprogressing labor can help a mother avoid a cesarean. An epidural can relax a tense, exhausted mother and facilitate vaginal birth.

Although hospitals are the ideal birth setting for mothers experiencing medical or obstetrical problems and for those who choose high-intervention births, they do not provide better outcomes for the other 85% (Stapleton, 2023). Hospitals, like any other business, use standardized procedures to increase productivity, efficiency, and cost-effectiveness. These often include interventions in birth, and hospital cultures encourage providers to use them. A study comparing low-risk primigravid hospital and home births attended by the same midwives revealed that the providers were more likely to provide noninterventional, evidence-based care when practicing *outside* a hospital (Miller & Skinner, 2012).

Birth Centers

A birth center is a medical facility with a homelike atmosphere where maternity providers, usually midwives, care for healthy mothers during pregnancy, labor, birth, and the postpartum period (Stapleton, 2023). Most birth centers are freestanding; others are a set of rooms or a wing in a hospital (Alliman & Phillippi, 2016). Forty-two U.S. states license free-standing birth centers or recognize them by statute or regulation (Alliman & Phillippi, 2016). Free-standing birth centers may operate without licensure in seven states. In North Dakota, however, they are not a legal option as a birthplace (Alliman & Phillippi, 2016).

Low-risk mothers who give birth in freestanding birth centers with CNMs, certified professional midwives (CPMs), or certified midwives (CMs) have excellent outcomes and fewer interventions than those in hospitals (Stapleton, Osborne, & Illuzzi, 2013). Because most clients have strong preferences about birth sites, randomized trials that compare birth center outcomes with outcomes of care in hospitals are unfeasible (Stapleton, 2023). There is a large body of evidence, however, suggesting that maternal outcomes in birth centers are at least as good as those in hospitals (Alliman & Phillippi, 2016; Stapleton, 2023). When deaths due to lethal congenital anomalies are excluded, perinatal mortality rates are equivalent or lower in birth centers (Alliman & Phillippi, 2016; Rooks, Weatherby, & Ernst, 1992; Rooks, Weatherby, Ernst, et al., 1989; Stapleton et al., 2013). Rates of episiotomy, elective birth before 39 weeks of gestation, and perineal laceration are lower in birth centers, and rates of exclusive breastfeeding are higher (Alliman & Phillippi, 2016; National Quality Forum, 2012; Stapleton, 2023). Emergent transfers from birth centers are rare; the most common reason for transfer is lack of progress in labor (Alliman & Phillippi, 2016).

Cesarean section rate (CSR) is a quality metric that many hospitals track closely, especially among NTSV clients—Nulliparas with Term Singleton Vertex pregnancies—that is, low-risk new mothers. About 14% of NTSV clients who begin labor at a birth center undergo cesareans; the national CSR for this group is 25.7% (Alliman et al., 2019; George et al., 2022). Birth center clients are much less likely to undergo cesarean section than clients giving birth in hospitals, and severe adverse maternal outcomes are very rare (Alliman & Phillippi, 2016).

Mothers use less pharmacologic pain relief if they begin labor at a birth center, even though their labors are longer (Alliman & Phillippi, 2016). Clients expressed high rates of satisfaction with the birth center environment and providers, even after transfer to a hospital (Alliman & Phillippi, 2016). Birth center clients report increased confidence in themselves in their ability to give birth and as parents; almost 99% would recommend a birth center to a friend (Stapleton, 2023).

The American Association of Birth Centers (AABC) established national standards to assess the services birth centers give their clients and to provide guidelines for ongoing quality improvement (AABC, 2017). State and municipal licensing agencies enhance birth center safety by ensuring compliance with business and health care-related codes, regulations, and ordinances (AABC, 2017). Although state and local standards differ widely, accreditation criteria set uniform benchmarks to encourage optimally safe practices (AABC, 2017). Accreditation is a voluntary program, but its requirements are generally more stringent than those imposed by states or localities. In the United States, three national organizations provide accreditation for birth centers: the Accreditation Association for Ambulatory Health Care, the Joint Commission, and the Commission for the Accreditation of Birth Centers.

Home Birth

Clients who choose home birth often believe that hospital procedures unnecessarily medicalize the natural process of birth and introduce interventions that increase the risk for complications (Declercq & Stotland, 2023; George et al., 2022). Most feel more comfortable giving birth in familiar surroundings and prefer a relaxed environment and the company of family and close friends. Some mothers who have had a traumatic or overly interventive birth in a hospital choose a home birth to exercise greater autonomy. In some cases, home birth is necessary because clients lack financial resources or transportation, or they live a great distance from the nearest birth center or hospital (Declercq & Stotland, 2023). Other clients with breech presentation or a previous cesarean who are good candidates for a trial of labor do not have access to a hospital willing to offer them an attempt at vaginal birth, leaving them caught between a higher-risk home birth and an unnecessary cesarean (Declercq & Stotland, 2023).

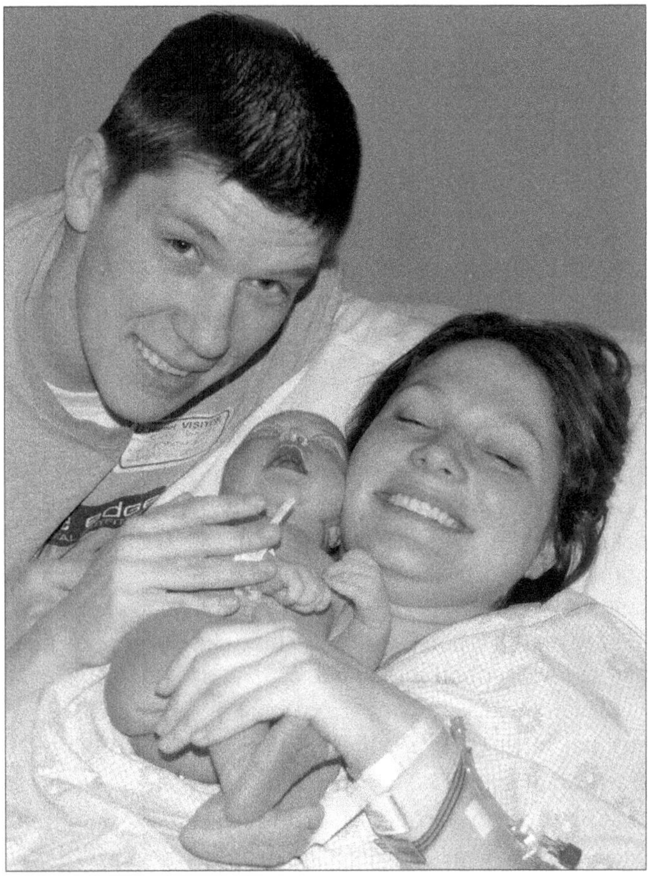

Figure 1-9. Low-risk mothers choose hospital birth for a variety of reasons, including the availability of narcotic and epidural anesthesia, access to physicians, proximity to a surgical suite, and a perception of greater safety. For many, hospital birth is the only available option.

Home birth with a trained, competent midwife and access to reliable transportation and referral systems can be as safe as a hospital birth for healthy mothers with low-risk pregnancies, and it entails fewer interventions and a lower CSR (ACNM, 2003; Catling-Paull, Dahlen, & Homer, 2011; Cheyney, Bovbjerg, et al., 2014; Declercq & Stotland, 2023; Jackson, Dahlen, & Schmied, 2012; Olsen & Clausen, 2023; Rigg, Schmied, Peters, & Dahlen, 2015; Vedam, Stoll, Schummers, & Fulton, 2013). Studies of non-anomalous singleton, term, vertex births have found that the CSR for planned home birth was about 5% compared with about 25% for planned

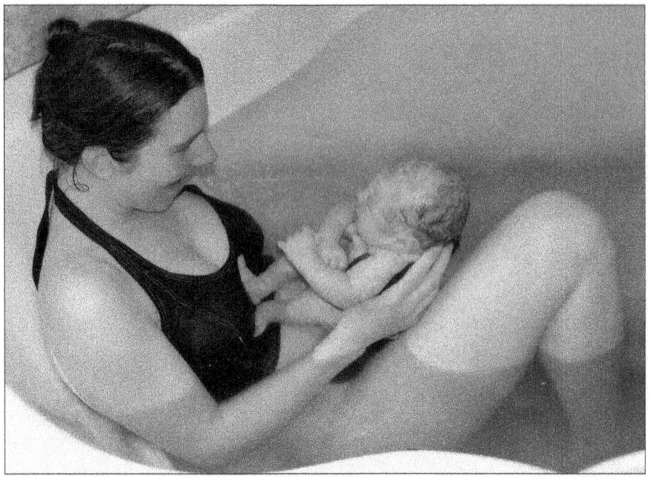

Figure 1-10. Waterbirth at a free-standing birth center. Birth centers are designed and managed to create warm, caring, homelike settings where mothers feel supported, respected, safe, and secure. Birth center midwives and nurses respond to each mother's needs while watching closely for signs that higher-level support is required.

hospital birth (Cheyney, Bovbjerg, et al., 2014; George et al., 2022; Stacey et al., 2017). Studies based on client charts instead of birth certificates (which often lack significant details) show good outcomes for planned home births of low-risk mothers attended by midwives trained to international standards (Daviss, Anderson, & Johnson, 2021).

Although outcomes are usually favorable for mothers, home birth appears to increase perinatal risk, particularly when the mother is nulliparous. Babies born at home in the United States have more than twice the risk of perinatal death and three times the risk of neonatal seizures or other neurologic dysfunction, but the number of babies affected is low: 1–2 of 1,000 babies experience perinatal death, and 0.4–0.6 in 1,000 show signs of neurologic compromise (ACOG Cmte. on Obstetric Practice, 2017/2023). This higher risk of poor neonatal outcomes has been attributed to the lack of hospital resources (including emergency cesarean section, vacuum or forceps assistance, endotracheal intubation, umbilical-vein cannulation), inadequate training of some home-birth providers to identify signs of fetal distress, and intervention delayed by transport (Buchanan et al., 2022).

Studying hypoxic ischemic encephalopathy (HIE), a syndrome of brain injury involving abnormal neurological function in the first few days of life, Buchanan et al. (2022) found that while the overall incidence of HIE is low, neonates born at home in the United States are 2.77 times more likely to develop HIE than infants born in a hospital. HIE develops when poor fetal oxygenation during labor causes brain injury and is more likely to follow births complicated by maternal hypertension, maternal diabetes, chorioamnionitis, or nonvertex presentation (Buchanan et al., 2022). Other studies from the United States found that planned home birth increased the risk for low Apgar scores, neonatal seizures, severe neurologic deficits, and death (Cheng, Snowden, King, & Caughey, 2013; Declercq & Stotland, 2023; Grünebaum et al., 2013; Snowden et al., 2015; Wasden et al., 2017).

Maternal and perinatal outcomes of clients choosing planned home birth appear greatly improved where community midwives are well integrated into the health care system, that is, when they have legal access to necessary emergency medications and equipment, readily available physician consultation, timely safe transportation to the hospital, and respectful hospital-based providers (ACNM, 2015; ACOG Cmte. on Obstetric Practice, 2017/2023; Declercq & Stotland, 2023; Finn et al., 2015; Likis, 2014; Nethery et al., 2021). These essential requirements are met in only a few communities in the United States.

Conversely, planned home birth in the United States is less safe when there is insufficient access to trained and willing providers, when backup systems are fragmented, and where there are inconsistent laws and regulations governing community birth (ACNM, 2015; Likis, 2014; Watterberg et al., 2020). Whereas the European Union sets universal standards for midwifery education and certification, the United States has no uniform standards, licensing some nonphysician birth attendants and ignoring or outlawing others (Snowden et al., 2015). In states where CNMs, CPMs, and CMs are accepted and regulated, outcomes are better for mothers and babies. Rates of spontaneous vaginal birth, vaginal birth after cesarean (VBAC), and breastfeeding are higher, and rates of obstetric interventions, PTB, low birthweight, and neonatal death are lower (Vedam, Stoll, MacDorman, et al., 2018). Lay midwives or traditional midwives are illegal in at least 10 states and unregulated in many others. They practice at various degrees of competence and have not demonstrated that they are able to meet formal training and certification requirements (Cheyney, Olsen, et al., 2015).

Midwifery Care and Home Birth Outside the United States

In many economically developed nations, including the United Kingdom, Iceland, the Netherlands, New Zealand, and parts of Canada, home birth is well-integrated into the health care system (Declercq & Stotland, 2023). Although the Netherlands still has the highest rate of home birth, it has steadily declined by approximately 1% per year from approximately 75% in 1953 to 13% today (Declercq & Stotland, 2023; Visser, 2012). Publicly funded health care systems cover all costs of midwifery care and home births in British Columbia, Iceland, Japan, the Netherlands, New Zealand, and Ontario (Comeau et al., 2018).

United Kingdom: 98% of mothers receive midwifery care from their initial prenatal visit through birth and up to 6 weeks postpartum. Government policy requires that mothers be allowed to choose from a range of birthplaces including those in community settings (Stoll et al., 2020). NICE directs providers to support clients in their choice of birth setting (home, freestanding midwifery unit, in-hospital midwifery unit, or obstetric unit) after discussing risks and benefits of each option (Greene & Ecker, 2015). NICE encourages providers to place control in the hands of the clients, to hear their concerns, to treat them with compassion, and to develop "a culture of respect for each woman as an individual undergoing an important and emotionally intense life experience" in all birth settings (Delgado Nunes, Gholitabar, Sims, & Bewley, 2014, p. 32).

Netherlands: The Dutch health care system birth has always supported community births and has the highest home birth rate of any high-resource country (Bommarito, 2021). The population tends to view the home as a normal and proper place for birth. In The Netherlands, low-risk, term pregnant individuals can choose to give birth at home, in a birth center, or in the hospital. Community midwives work autonomously, usually in group practices with other midwives (Hermus et al., 2017). If complications occur or if pharmacologic pain management is needed, the client is transferred to the hospital via well-integrated emergency services, where the obstetrician assumes care (Verhoeven et al., 2022). Consequently, low-risk clients having planned home birth have low rates of severe maternal complications and there are no significant differences in perinatal or newborn outcomes (Stoll et al., 2020).

Canada: The Canadian midwifery model of care supports informed choice including choice of birthplace; midwives are the lead health care providers for 11% of all births in Canada (Stoll et al., 2020). The government funds maternity care (Stoll et al., 2020). The prevalence of home birth differs by province; British Columbia and Ontario have the highest rates (Murray-Davis et al., 2012). Although the best available evidence confirms the safety of home birth for healthy mothers, a shortage of home-birth providers prevents most clients from choosing this option (Vedam, Schummers, et al., 2012). At the onset of the COVID-19 (SARS-CoV-2) pandemic, the home-birth rate in Ontario rose by up to 20% as mothers sought to avoid contagion (Daviss et al., 2021).

New Zealand: Government-funded maternity care integrates primary, secondary, and tertiary services to meet the needs of each client. In New Zealand, 93% of mothers have midwife-led care; in 2012, 3% of mothers gave birth at home and 9.1% in birth centers (Stoll et al., 2020).

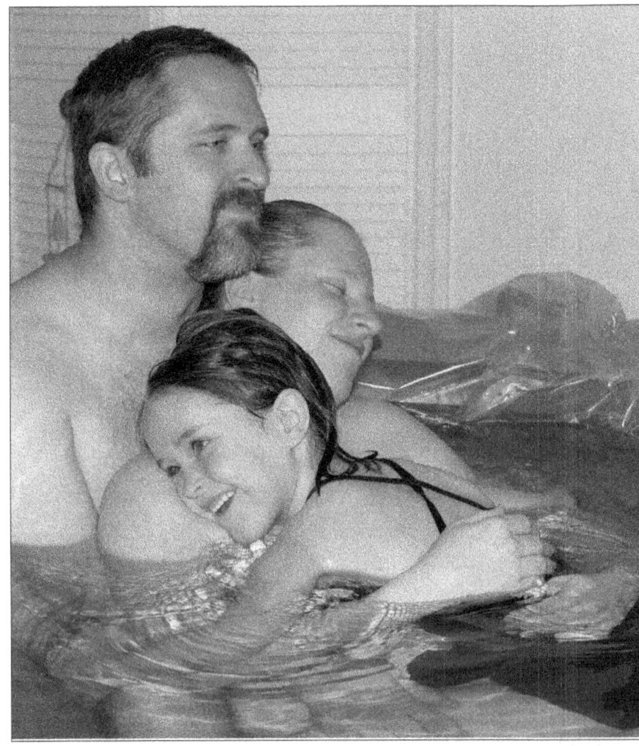

Figure 1-11. Mothers choose home birth for many reasons, including greater family involvement, less obstetric intervention, and lower cost. This mother rented a birth pool and labored with the support of her husband and daughter in the privacy of her bedroom.

Australia: Emergency transfers from home to hospital can be impeded by great distances in rural settings and dense traffic in large cities. Almost 40% of mothers have midwife-led care; 98% give birth in hospitals, 1.8% in birth centers, 0.3% at home (Stoll et al., 2020). Although the Royal Australian and New Zealand College of Obstetricians and Gynaecologists does not endorse home birth, it developed guidelines on home-birth clinical practice, client eligibility, consultation, and transfer of care (Comeau et al., 2018). Malpractice insurance is not available for home birth providers in Australia; midwives who attend home births face professional and financial risk should poor outcomes occur (Comeau et al., 2018).

Germany: Although obstetricians are the primary caregivers for most mothers and more than 98% of births occur in hospitals, federal law mandates that a midwife attend every birth, including cesarean sections (Stoll et al., 2020).

Iceland: Mothers typically have government-funded midwife-led care through the childbearing year; almost every birth is attended by a midwife (Stoll et al., 2020). Healthy mothers have the option of home birth, but only about 2% of Icelandic babies are born at home (Stoll et al., 2020), perhaps because conditions in a sparsely populated country touching the Arctic

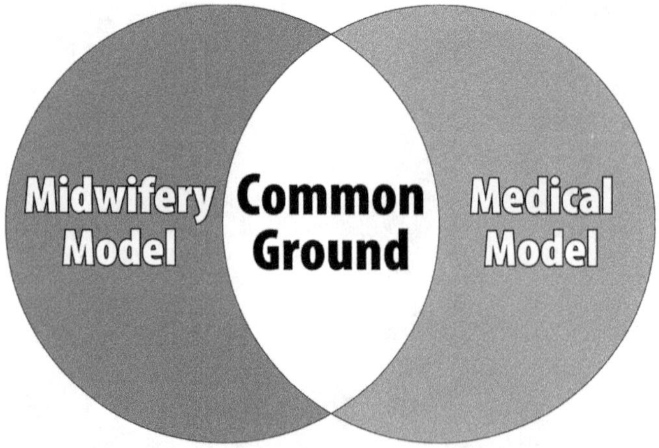

Figure 1-12. The midwifery and medical models overlap to varying degrees. If labor remains normal, care can remain squarely within the midwifery model. If complications occur, management wholly or partly within the medical model often yields the best outcomes.

Circle can interfere with emergency transportation from planned home birth to a hospital (Comeau et al., 2018).

A Clash of Professional Opinions

Whereas the biological processes of pregnancy and birth have not changed over tens of thousands of years, their management has changed radically in the last few decades (Rutherford, Asiodu, & Liese, 2019). All obstetrical providers want to ensure optimal health and wellbeing for mother and baby, but they often disagree on what poses the greatest risks and how to achieve the best outcomes (Shah, 2015a). Home-birth midwives and the clients they serve consider the physiological process of pregnancy, labor, and birth normal and trustworthy, and they tend to believe that interfering makes birth more dangerous for the low-risk mother (Horan, 2013). Providers trained in the medical method tend to assume that risk to any mother or baby is greatly reduced by the use or availability of interventions in a hospital, including continuous or internal monitoring, anesthesia, imaging, laboratory tests, augmentation, vacuum or forceps assistance, and surgery (Healy, Humphreys, & Kennedy, 2016).

Birth in any setting involves risk. Community birth often involves the risk of delayed access to life-saving obstetric and neonatal interventions, but hospital birth can increase the risk of unnecessary interventions and iatrogenic complications (NASEM, 2020). People for and against home birth read current studies and conclude that the evidence validates their own positions (Nove, Berrington, & Matthews, 2012). Research conducted by home-birth advocates concludes that birth in community settings is just as safe, more satisfying, and less expensive compared to hospital birth and that it carries a lower risk of obstetrical interventions (de Melo-Martín & Intemann, 2012). Research by home-birth detractors concludes that home birth is unsafe and increases risks to mother and baby (De Vries & Lemmens, 2006). Although the principal goal for all parents and maternity care professionals is a safe birth and healthy outcome for mother and baby, regardless of birthplace, professional organizations disagree over support of planned home birth (ACNM, 2015). Members of these diverse organizations approach the issue of maternal/child safety and health with the same heartfelt intentions of creating optimal science-based care, but often follow divergent paths and reach very different conclusions.

After a thorough review of evidence, NICE; the United Kingdom's Royal College of Obstetrics and Gynecology and Royal College of Midwives; the International Federation of Midwives; the American Public Health Association; the Australian, New Zealand, and Canadian Colleges of Midwives; and ACNM determined support the choice of home birth for low-risk mothers as a reasonable option that decreases the likelihood of unnecessary interventions (de Melo-Martín & Intemann, 2012; Shah, 2015a). Likewise, the Society of Obstetricians and Gynaecologists of Canada considers a planned home birth within their integrated system attended by a registered midwife or appropriately trained physician a reasonable choice for clients at low risk of complications (Campbell, Carson, Azzam, & Hutton, 2019). ACOG and the American Academy of Pediatrics, however, reviewed the same literature and concluded that hospitals and birth centers are the safest settings for birth while respecting the right of individuals to make *medically informed* decisions about birth setting (ACOG Cmte. on Obstetric Practice, 2017/2023; Watterberg et al., 2020).

Although it can be tempting to choose sides, retreat into echo chambers, or let beliefs manage data, some are working to broaden outlooks and build agreement. The Home Birth Consensus Summits, for example, convene diverse groups of leaders in different fields to improve the care of individuals who plan home births in the United States. Delegates include consumers; physicians; midwives; hospital administrators; legislators; and public health, research, ethics, payor, and liability specialists ("Home Birth Summit," 2022). Together they explore every aspect of the existing system and discuss ways to improve access to safe, culturally competent, and respectful maternity care; to increase collaboration among maternity-care providers; and to integrate community birth into the country's health care system ("Home Birth Summit," 2022).

Midwifery and Medicine

Midwifery and obstetrical medicine are complementary professions with overlapping but distinct purposes and knowledge. The medical model of maternity care tends to focus on complications and on intervening to prevent or mitigate them (Akileswaran & Hutchison, 2016). The midwifery model trusts physiologic pregnancy, labor, and birth as normal processes unless there is indication to suggest otherwise and recognizes that interference with the natural process is likely to *cause* complications (Horan, 2013; Neerland & Skalisky, 2022). A low-touch, high tech approach dominates on the medical side; a high-touch, low-tech approach prevails on the midwifery side. A midwife is more likely than a physician to passively observe clients through labor, getting a sense of their needs and physical and emotional states, remaining attuned to the first signs of abnormal progress, and employing gentle, natural ways of correcting a potential problem in the early stages (Horan, 2013; Lundgren, Berg, Nilsson, & Olafsdottir, 2020).

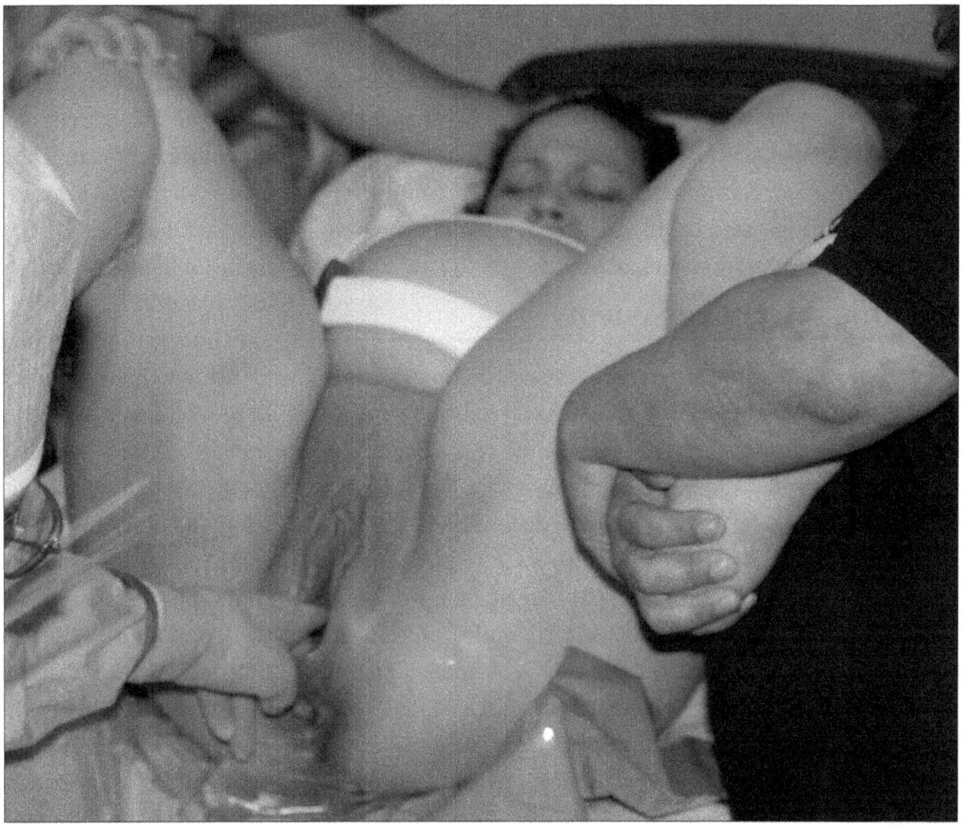

Figure 1-13. Many hospital-based providers, mainly physicians, routinely use unnecessary interventions such as augmentation, immediate cord clamping, antiseptic wash, continuous fetal monitoring, and maternal activity restriction.

The medical model prepares providers to take control of the birth process and actively "correct" it in case it might deviate from the expected course—a practice beneficial in many high-risk pregnancies, but often detrimental to low-risk mothers. Medicalized labors give the provider greater control over the birth process, which can make labor feel more predictable and certain, therefore safer to the provider (M. Page & Mander, 2014). To a provider trained in institutionalized childbirth who has mostly gained experience caring for higher-risk clients with epidural anesthesia, continuous fetal monitoring, labor augmentation, vacuum extraction, artificial rupture of membranes, episiotomy, and other interventions, it can seem that the high-tech approach is always necessary to obtain the best possible outcome, even for low-risk clients. An experienced hospital-based provider who has managed a great number of labors can become comfortable with the usual flow of events and tend to shape each birth to fall neatly into the well-worn groove. These interventions offer little benefit to healthy babies and can cause complications, stress, and discomfort for their mothers (Shah, 2015a). Moreover, the needs of the institution—staffing, budget, case load, etc.—often trump the needs of childbearing individuals and their infants (Lowe, 2015).

In the United States, most families, physicians, nurses, and other professionals tend to view childbirth through the lens of the medical model. They often believe (or profess) that childbirth is safer and more physically comfortable when managed medically in a hospital. Media portrayals show childbirth as dangerous, unpredictable, and fraught with excruciating pain. To hospital-based providers who see the choice between physiologic childbirth and anesthetized childbirth as the choice between agony and comfort, the mother electing to labor without drugs can be as puzzling as one choosing dentistry without anesthetic.

Both midwifery and medical models depend on evidence-based care, timely identification of complications, and access to interventions (Olsen & Clausen, 2023). Many providers, physicians and midwives alike, draw in varying degrees from both, following the midwifery model when a pregnancy is normal and shifting to the medical model when it is not. This blending of modalities occurs most successfully if the culture of the setting encourages it. The midwifery model of care is complementary to the medical model, not an alternative to it (ACNM, Midwives Alliance of North America, & National Association of Certified Professional Midwives,

2012; Choudhary, Jelly, & Mahala, 2020). The midwifery model provides the safest and often the most satisfying mode of management for mothers having a normal pregnancy and physiologic labor (ACNM et al., 2012). When mothers have a high-risk pregnancy or develop complications, the midwifery model overlaps the medical model to provide support, confidence-building, education, and assistance

Building Integrated Systems

Because there will always be individuals who choose to give birth at home, safer home birth should be an indisputable goal for any public health system. Ironically, the resistance of key medical organizations to home birth has obstructed the practices that make it safe. An unsupportive maternity-care system discourages collaborative relationships that would facilitate smoother, safer transfers (Freeze, 2010; Leeman & Goldstein, 2021). Physicians who support home birth philosophically are often fettered by legal, political, cultural, professional, institutional, or insurance limits on collaboration, consultation, or backup care (Freeze, 2010). When physicians are unwilling to provide backup in the event of complications and laws fail to support safe community midwifery, people who choose home birth are at greater risk for catastrophic complications. When complications occur, detractors take them as confirmation that birth is safe only in a hospital (Rigg et al., 2015).

Birth is never completely predictable; labor can shift from healthy to pathological very quickly. About 9–13% of clients planning a home birth will experience transfer to a hospital during labor, usually for nonurgent indications such as failure to progress (ACNM, 2015). Birth in a community setting is safest when midwives have ready access to consultation and transfer and are strongly integrated with capable, responsive hospitals (ACOG Cmte. on Obstetric Practice, 2017/2023). The safest health care systems that accommodate home birth (the United Kingdom, Iceland, the Netherlands, New Zealand, and the Canadian provinces of British Columbia and Ontario) have largely integrated home birth and have demonstrated comparable perinatal outcomes between planned home and hospital birth (ACNM, 2015; Comeau et al., 2018). Unfortunately, in the United States, integrated services are scattered, variable, and sometimes lacking (Levine, Souter, & Sakala, 2021).

A notable exception is Washington State, where community midwifery is regulated and well-integrated into the health care system (Nethery et al., 2021). Community midwives—licensed midwives (LMs), CMs, CPMs, or CNMs—who attend births in homes or state-licensed birth centers generally accept only carefully screened low-risk clients; adhere to national and international standards and guidelines; are authorized to use emergency medication and medical equipment; and have seamless access to consultation, referral, transport, and transfer of care (Nethery et al., 2021). Nethery et al. (2021) found no significant differences in adverse maternal or perinatal outcomes by birth setting and found complication rates comparable to those in high-income countries with integrated community birth and community midwifery. They also found that community-setting births in Washington State had a low CSR (4.7%), a high rate of physiologic birth (85%), a high breastfeeding rate (93%), and low rates of complications overall (Nethery et al., 2021). This success story gives hope that safe home birth can be integrated into the health care systems of other states and, ultimately, the whole country.

Topics for Discussion

1. Amber says that because childbirth is a natural process, every mother is safer giving birth at home. Explain to her the risks and benefits of home birth.
2. The midwifery model overlaps the medical model. Describe a situation that would fall in the area where the two overlap.
3. Name two factors of the high rate of neonatal mortality in the United States.
4. In community settings, birth is safest when midwives have legal access to necessary emergency medications and equipment, readily available physician consultation, access to timely safe transportation to the hospital, and respectful hospital-based health care providers. Pick one of these and discuss how risks to mother an infant increase when it is lacking.

References

Addante, A. N., Eisenberg, D. L., Valentine, M. C., Leonard, J., Maddox, K. E. J., Hoofnagle, M. H. (2021). The association between state-level abortion restrictions and maternal mortality in the United States, 1995–2017. *Contraception, 104*(5), 496–501. https://doi.org/10.1016/j.contraception.2021.03.018

Akileswaran, C. P., & Hutchison, M. S. (2016). Making room at the table for obstetrics, midwifery, and a culture of normalcy within maternity care. *Obstetrics & Gynecology, 128*(1), 176–180. https://doi.org/10.1097/AOG.0000000000001493

Alfirevic, Z., Gyte, G. M. L., Cuthbert, A., & Devane, D. (2017). Continuous cardiotocography (CTG) as a form of electronic fetal monitoring (EFM) for fetal assessment during labour. *Cochrane Database of Systematic Reviews*. https://doi.org/10.1002/14651858.CD006066.pub3

Alliman, J., & Phillippi, J. C. (2016). Maternal outcomes in birth centers: An integrative review of the literature. *Journal of Midwifery & Women's Health, 61*(1), 21–51. https://doi.org/10.1111/jmwh.12356

Alliman, J., Stapleton, S. R., Wright, J., Bauer, K., Slider, K., & Jolles, D. (2019). Strong Start in birth centers: Socio-demographic characteristics, care processes, and outcomes for mothers and newborns. *Birth, 46*(2), 234–243. https://doi.org/10.1111/birt.12433

American Association of Birth Centers. (2017). *Standards for birth centers* (12th ed.). Perkiomenville, PA: Author. Retrieved from https://cdn.ymaws.com/www.birthcenters.org/resource/resmgr/AABC-STANDARDS-RV2017.pdf

American College of Nurse-Midwives. (n.d.). *What is physiologic birth?* Retrieved from http://www.birthtools.org/What-Is-Physiologic-Birth

American College of Nurse-Midwives. (2003). Criteria for provision of home birth services (Clinical Bulletin 7). *Journal of Midwifery & Women's Health, 48*(4), 299–301. https://doi.org/10.1016/S1526-9523(03)00159-4

American College of Nurse-Midwives. (2015). Midwifery provision of home birth services (Clinical Bulletin 14). *Journal of Midwifery & Women's Health, 61*(1), 127–133. https://doi.org/10.1111/jmwh.12431

American College of Nurse-Midwives, Midwives Alliance of North America, & National Association of Certified Professional Midwives. (2012). *Supporting healthy and normal physiologic childbirth: A consensus statement by ACNM, MANA, and NACPM.* Retrieved from https://www.midwife.org/ACNM/files/ACNMLibraryData/UPLOADFILENAME/000000000272/Physiological Birth Consensus Statement- FINAL May 18 2012 FINAL.pdf

American College of Obstetricians and Gynecologists. (2013, reaffirmed 2016). *Coping with the stress of medical professional liability litigation* (Committee Opinion 551). Retrieved from https://www.acog.org/clinical/clinical-guidance/committee-opinion/articles/2013/01/coping-with-the-stress-of-medical-professional-liability-litigation

American College of Obstetricians and Gynecologists & Society for Maternal-Fetal Medicine. (2021, reaffirmed 2024). *Medically indicated late-preterm and early-term deliveries* (Committee Opinion 831). Retrieved from https://www.acog.org/Clinical/Clinical-Guidance/Committee-Opinion/Articles/2021/07/Medically-Indicated-Late-Preterm-and-Early-Term-Deliveries

American College of Obstetricians and Gynecologists Committee on Clinical Practice Guidelines—Obstetrics, Cahill, A. G., Raghuraman, N., Gandhi, M., & Kaimal, A. J. (2024). *First and second stage labor management* (Clinical Practice Guideline 8). *Obstetrics & Gynecology, 143*(1), 144–162.

American College of Obstetricians and Gynecologists Committee on Obstetric Practice. (2017, reaffirmed 2023). *Planned home birth* (Committee Opinion 697, interim update). Retrieved from https://www.acog.org/clinical/clinical-guidance/committee-opinion/articles/2017/04/planned-home-birth

American Congress of Obstetricians and Gynecologists. (n.d.). *Women's Health Stats & Facts 2011.* Washington, DC: Author. Retrieved from https://www.acog.org/-/media/NewsRoom/MediaKit.pdf

Antoine, C., & Young, B. K. (2021). Cesarean section one hundred years 1920–2020: The good, the bad and the ugly. *Journal of Perinatal Medicine, 49*(1), 5–16. https://doi.org/10.1515/jpm-2020-0305

Barfield, W. D. (2018). Public health implications of very preterm birth. *Clinics in Perinatology, 45*(3), 565–577. https://doi.org/10.1016/j.clp.2018.05.007

Bartick, M., & Reinhold, A. (2010). The burden of suboptimal breastfeeding in the United States: A pediatric cost analysis. *Pediatrics, 125*(5), e1048–e1056. https://doi.org/10.1542/peds.2009-1616

Berg, M. (2005). A midwifery model of care for childbearing women at high risk: Genuine caring in caring for the genuine. *Journal of Perinatal Education, 14*(1), 9–21. https://doi.org/10.1624/105812405X23577

Betran, A. P., Torloni, M. R., Zhang, J. J., & Gülmezoglu, A. M. (2016). WHO statement on caesarean section rates. *BJOG, 123*(5), 667–670. https://doi.org/10.1111/1471-0528.13526

Bingham, D., Jones, D. K., & Howell, E. A. (2019). Quality improvement approach to eliminate disparities in perinatal morbidity and mortality. *Obstetrics and Gynecology Clinics of North America, 46*(2), 227–238.

Bommarito, R. K. (2021). Structures for sustainable collaboration between midwives and obstetricians in the Netherlands: The obstetric and midwifery manual and perinatal care partnerships. In Gutschow, K., Davis-Floyd, R., & Daviss, B.-A. (Eds.), *Sustainable birth in disruptive times* (pp. 73–84). Cham, Switzerland: Springer.

Börk, L. & Bott, M. J. (2015). Maternal/infant characteristics and birth location: Impact on breastfeeding initiation and duration. *Journal of BSN Honors Research, 8*(1), 2–31. Retrieved from https://kuscholarworks.ku.edu/handle/2271/1334

Boucher, D., Bennett, C., MacFarlin, B., & Freeze, R. S. (2009). Staying home to give birth: Why women in the United States choose home birth. *Journal of Midwifery & Women's Health, 54*(2), 119–126. https://doi.org/10.1016/j.jmwh.2008.09.006

Brown, H. L., & Small, M. J. (2023). Overview of maternal mortality. In A. Chakrabarti (Ed.), *UpToDate.* Retrieved September 30, 2023, from http://www.uptodate.com/contents/overview-of-maternal-mortality

Bruno, A. M., Metz, T. D., Grobman, W. A., & Silver, R. M. (2022). Defining a cesarean delivery rate for optimizing maternal and neonatal outcomes. *Obstetrics & Gynecology 140*(3), 399–407. https://doi.org/10.1097/AOG.0000000000004876

Buchanan, C., Kuo, S., Minton, L., Lee, M.-J., Choi, S. Y., & Soon, R. (2022). Neonatal hypoxic ischemic encephalopathy and planned home birth. *Journal of Midwifery & Women's Health, 67*(1), 69–74. https://doi.org/10.1111/jmwh.13309

Bugg, G. J., Siddiqui, F., & Thornton, J. G. (2013). Oxytocin versus no treatment or delayed treatment for slow progress in the first stage of spontaneous labour. *Cochrane Database of Systematic Reviews.* https://doi.org/10.1002/14651858.CD007123.pub3

California Department of Public Health, Maternal, Child and Adolescent Health Division. (2011). *The California pregnancy-associated mortality review: Report from 2002 and 2003 maternal death reviews.* Sacramento, CA: Author. Retrieved from https://www.cdph.ca.gov/Programs/CFH/DMCAH/CDPH%20Document%20Library/PAMR/CA-PAMR-Report.pdf

Campbell, K., Carson, G., Azzam, H., & Hutton, E. (2019). Statement on planned homebirth (Practice Guideline 372). *Journal of Obstetrics and Gynaecology Canada, 41*(2), 223–227. https://doi.org/10.1016/j.jogc.2018.08.008

Catling-Paull, C., Dahlen, H., & Homer, C. C. S. E. (2011). Multiparous women's confidence to have a publicly-funded homebirth: A qualitative study. *Women and Birth, 24*(3), 122–128. https://doi.org/10.1016/j.wombi.2010.09.001

Caughey, A. B., & Cheyney, M. (2019). Home and birth center birth in the United States: Time for greater collaboration across models of care. *Obstetrics & Gynecology, 133*(5), 1033–1050. https://doi.org/10.1097/AOG.0000000000003215

Centers for Disease Control and Prevention. (2021). *Premature birth.* Retrieved from https://www.cdc.gov/reproductivehealth/features/premature-birth/index.html

Centers for Disease Control and Prevention. (2022a). *Cesarean delivery rate by state,* Retrieved from https://www.cdc.gov/nchs/pressroom/sosmap/cesarean_births/cesareans.htm

Centers for Disease Control and Prevention. (2022b). *Infant mortality.* Retrieved from https://www.cdc.gov/reproductivehealth/maternalinfanthealth/infantmortality.htm

Centers for Disease Control and Prevention. (2023a). *Infant mortality rates by state* [2021]. Retrieved from https://www.cdc.gov/nchs/pressroom/sosmap/infant_mortality_rates/infant_mortality.htm

Centers for Disease Control and Prevention. (2023b). *Pregnancy mortality surveillance system.* Retrieved from https://www.cdc.gov/reproductivehealth/maternalinfanthealth/pmss.html

Cheng, Y. W., Snowden J. M., King, T. L., & Caughey, A. B. (2013). Selected perinatal outcomes associated with planned home births in the United States. *American*

Journal of Obstetrics & Gynecology, 209(4), 325.e1–325.e8. https://doi.org/10.1016/j.ajog.2013.06.022

Cheyney, M., Bovbjerg, M., Everson, C., Gordon, W., Hannibal, D., & Vedam, S. (2014). Outcomes of care for 16,924 planned home births in the United States: The Midwives Alliance of North America Statistics Project, 2004 to 2009. *Journal of Midwifery & Women's Health, 59*(1), 17–27. https://doi.org/10.1111/jmwh.12172

Cheyney, M., Olsen, C., Bovbjerg, M., Everson, C., Darragh, I., & Potter, B. (2015). Practitioner and practice characteristics of certified professional midwives in the United States: Results of the 2011 North American Registry of Midwives survey. *Journal of Midwifery & Women's Health, 60*(5), 534–545. https://doi.org/10.1111/jmwh.12367

Chmell, A. (2012). Home sweet home: A place to deliver, care for, and raise our children. *Journal of Legal Medicine, 33*(1), 137–148. https://doi.org/10.1080/01947648.2012.657949

Choudhary, S., Jelly, P., & Mahala, P. (2020). Models of maternity care: A continuity of midwifery care. *International Journal of Reproduction, Contraception, Obstetrics and Gynecology, 9*(6), 2666–2670. https://doi.org/10.18203/2320-1770.ijrcog20202373

Clark, R. R. S., & Lake, E. T. (2021). Spontaneous vaginal birth varies significantly across US hospitals. *Birth, 48*(1), 44–51. https://doi.org/10.1111/birt.12508

Coco, A., Derksen-Schrock, A., Coco, K., Raff, T., Horst, M. & Hussar, E. (2010). A randomized trial of increased intravenous hydration in labor when oral fluid is unrestricted. *Family Medicine, 42*(1), 52–56. Retrieved from http://www.stfm.org/Portals/49/Documents/FMPDF/FamilyMedicineVol42Issue1Coco52.pdf

Comeau, A., Hutton, E. K., Simioni, J., Anvari, E., Bowen, M., Kruegar, S., & Darling, E. K. (2018). Home birth integration into the health care systems of eleven international jurisdictions. *Birth, 45*(3), 311–321. https://doi.org/10.1111/birt.12339

Dagher, R. K., & Linares, D. E. (2022). A critical review on the complex interplay between social determinants of health and maternal and infant mortality. *Children, 9*(3), 394. https://doi.org/10.3390/children9030394

Daviss, B. A., Anderson, D. A., & Johnson, K. C. (2021). Pivoting to childbirth at home or in freestanding birth centers in the US during COVID-19: Safety, economics and logistics. *Frontiers in Sociology, 6*. https://doi.org/10.3389/fsoc.2021.618210

De Vries, R., & Lemmens, T. (2006). The social and cultural shaping of medical evidence: Case studies from pharmaceutical research and obstetric science. *Social Science & Medicine, 62*(11), 2694–2706. https://doi.org/10.1016/j.socscimed.2005.11.026

de Melo-Martín, I., & Intemann, K. (2012). Interpreting evidence: Why values can matter as much as science. *Perspectives in Biology and Medicine, 55*(1), 59–70. http://doi.org/10.1353/pbm.2012.0007

Debbink, M. P., Ugwu, L. G., Grobman, W. A., Reddy, U. M., Tita, A. T. N., El-Sayed, Y. Y., . . . Simhan, H. N. (2022). Racial and ethnic inequities in cesarean birth and maternal morbidity in a low-risk, nulliparous cohort. *Obstetrics & Gynecology, 139*(1), 73–82. https://doi.org/10.1097/AOG.0000000000004620

Declercq, E. R., Sakala, C., Corry, M. P., & Applebaum, S. (2006). *Listening to mothers II: Report of the second national U.S. Survey of women's childbearing experiences*. New York, NY: Childbirth Connection. Retrieved from http://www.nationalpartnership.org/research-library/maternal-health/listening-to-mothers-ii-2006.pdf

Declercq, E., & Stotland, N. E. (2023). *Planned home birth.* In V. A. Barss (Ed.), *UpToDate.* Retrieved September 30, 2023, from http://www.uptodate.com/contents/planned-home-birth

Delgado Nunes, V., Gholitabar, M., Sims, J. M., & Bewley, S. (2014). Intrapartum care of healthy women and their babies: Summary of updated NICE guidance. *BMJ, 32, 349*, g6886. Retrieved from https://www.ncbi.nlm.nih.gov/pmc/articles/PMC4707719/

Douthard, R. A., Martin, I. K., Chapple-McGruder, T., Langer, A., & Chang, S. (2021). U.S. maternal mortality within a global context: Historical trends, current state, and future directions. *Journal of Women's Health, 30*(2), 168–177. https://doi.org/10.1089/jwh.2020.8863

Dreyer, B. P. (2021). The toll of racism on African American mothers and their infants. *JAMA Network Open, 4*(12), e2138828. https://doi.org/10.1001/jamanetworkopen.2021.38828

Eidelman, A. I., Schanler, R. J., Johnston, M., Landers, S., Noble, L., . . . Viehmann, L. (2012). Breastfeeding and the use of human milk. *Pediatrics, 129*(3), e827–e841. https://doi.org/10.1542/peds.2011-3552

Elflein, J. (2022). *Perinatal mortality rates in the United State in 2019, by state*. Retrieved from https://www.statista.com/statistics/1310169/perinatal-mortality-rates-by-state-us/

Ely, D. M., & Driscoll, A. K. (2019). Infant mortality in the United States, 2017: Data from the period linked birth/infant death file. *National Vital Statistics Reports, 68*(10), 1–20. retrieved from https://www.cdc.gov/nchs/data/nvsr/nvsr68/nvsr68_10-508.pdf

Erickson, E. N., Lee, C. S., Grose, E., & Emeis, C. (2019). Physiologic childbirth and active management of the third stage of labor: A latent class model of risk for postpartum hemorrhage. *Birth, 46*(1), 69–79. https://doi.org/10.1111/birt.12384

Espey, E., Haider, S., Stone, J., Gyamfi-Bannerman, C., & Steinauer, J. (2023). Now is the time to stand up for reproductive justice and abortion access. *American Journal of Obstetrics & Gynecology, 228*(1), 48–52. https://doi.org/10.1016/j.ajog.2022.07.033

Finn, K. T., Condon, S., Doyle, K. M., Hernandez, E. M., Kieltyka, C., Jefferson, K., & Ritter, R. (2015). *Planned home birth in New York State: New York State Association of Licensed Midwives guidelines for best practice*. (n.p.): New York State Association of Licensed Midwives. Retrieved from http://nysalm.org/wp-content/uploads/2016/10/HomeBirthGuidelines.pdf

Freeze, R. A. S. (2010). Attitudes towards home birth in the USA. *Expert Review of Obstetrics & Gynecology, 5*(3), 283–99. https://doi.org/10.1586/eog.10.22

George, E. K., Mitchell, S. & Stacey, D. (2022), Choosing a birth setting: A shared decision-making approach. *Journal of Midwifery & Women's Health, 67*(4), 510–514. https://doi.org/10.1111/jmwh.13377

Gillispie-Bell, V. (2021). The contrast of color: Why the Black community continues to suffer health disparities. *Obstetrics & Gynecology, 137*(2), 220–224. https://doi.org/10.1097/AOG.0000000000004226

Greene, M. F., & Ecker, J. L. (2015). Choosing benefits while balancing risks. *New England Journal of Medicine, 373*(27), 2681–2682. https://doi.org/10.1056/NEJMe1511068

Gregory, E. C. W., Osterman, M. J. K., & Valenzuela, C. P. (2021). Changes in home births by race and Hispanic origin and state of residence of mother: United States, 2018–2019 and 2019–2020. *National Vital Statistics Reports, 70*(15), 1–10. https://doi.org/10.15620/cdc:110853

Grünebaum, A., McCullough, L. B., Sapra, K. J., Brent, R. L., Levene, M. I., Arabin, B., & Chervenak, F. A. (2013). Apgar score of 0 at 5 minutes and neonatal seizures or serious neurologic dysfunction in relation to birth setting. *American Journal of Obstetrics & Gynecology, 209*(4), 323.e1–323.e6. https://doi.org/10.1016/j.ajog.2013.06.025

Gunja, M. Z., Gumae, E. D., & Williams, R. D., II. (2023). *U.S. health care from a global perspective, 2022: Accelerating spending, worsening outcomes*. https://doi.org/10.26099/8ejy-yc74

Gupta, J. K., Sood, A., Hofmeyr, G. J., & Vogel, J. P. (2017). Position in the second stage of labour for women without epidural anaesthesia. *Cochrane Database of Systematic Reviews*. https://doi.org/10.1002/14651858.CD002006.pub4

Gutvirtz, G., Wainstock, T., Sheiner, E., Landau, D., & Walfisch, A. (2018). Pediatric cardiovascular morbidity of the early term newborn. *Journal of Pediatrics, 194*, 81–86.e2. https://doi.org/10.1016/j.jpeds.2017.09.060

Haelle, T. (2016). Your biggest c-section risk may be your hospital. *Consumer Reports*. Retrieved from http://www.consumerreports.org/doctors-hospitals/your-biggest-c-section-risk-may-be-your-hospital/

Harper, L. M., Leach, J. M., Robbins, L., Blanchard, C., Metz, T. D., Mazzoni, S., . . . Szychowski, J. (2022). All-cause mortality in reproductive-aged females by state: An analysis of the effects of abortion legislation. *Obstetrics & Gynecology, 141*(2), 236–242. https://doi.org/10.1097/AOG.0000000000005035

Healy, S., Humphreys, E., & Kennedy, C. (2016). Midwives' and obstetricians' perceptions of risk and its impact on clinical practice and decision-making in labour: An integrative review. *Women and Birth, 29*(2), 107–116. https://doi.org/10.1016/j.wombi.2015.08.010

Hermus, M. A. A., Hitzert, M., Boesveld, I. C., van den Akker-van Marie, M. E., van Dommelen, P., Franx, A., . . . van der Pal-de Bruin, K. M. (2017). Differences in optimality index between planned place of birth in a birth centre and alternative planned places of birth, a nationwide prospective cohort study in the Netherlands: Results of the Dutch Birth Centre Study. *BMJ Open, 7*(11), e016958. https://doi.org/10.1136/bmjopen-2017-016958

Hildingsson, I., Rådestad, I., & Lindgren, H. (2010). Birth preferences that deviate from the norm in Sweden: Planned home birth versus planned cesarean section. *Birth, 37*(4), 288–295. https://doi.org/10.1111/j.1523-536X.2010.00423.x

Hofmeyr, G. J., Haws, R. A., Bergström, S., Lee, A. C. C., Okong, P., Darmstadt, G. L., . . . Lawn, J. E. (2009). Obstetric care in low-resource settings: What, who, and how to overcome challenges to scale up? *International Journal of Gynecology & Obstetrics, 107*, S21–S45. https://doi.org/10.1016/j.ijgo.2009.07.017

Home Birth Summit. (2022). Retrieved from https://www.homebirthsummit.org/

Horan, A. R. (2013). *Risking it: An examination of risk perception amongst obstetricians and certified professional midwives in Missouri* (Undergraduate Research Symposium Posters & Abstracts, Paper 10). Retrieved from http://openscholarship.wustl.edu/undergrad_research/10

Howell, E. A. (2018). Reducing disparities in severe maternal morbidity and mortality. *Clinical Obstetrics and Gynecology, 61*(2), 387–399. https://doi.org/10.1097/GRF.0000000000000349

Hoxha, I., Braha, M., Syrogiannouli, L., Goodman, D. C., & Jüni, P. (2019). Caesarean section in uninsured women in the USA: Systematic review and meta-analysis. *BMJ Open, 9*(3), e025356. https://doi.org/10.1136/bmjopen-2018-025356

Hoyert, D. L. (2023). *Maternal mortality rates in the United States, 2021*. https://dx.doi.org/10.15620/cdc:124678

Hoyert, D. L., & Miniño, A. M. (2020). Maternal mortality in the United States: Changes in coding, publication, and data release. *National Vital Statistics Reports, 69*(2),1–18. Retrieved from https://www.cdc.gov/nchs/data/nvsr/nvsr69/nvsr69-02-508.pdf

Ip, S., Chung, M., Raman, G., Chew, P., Magula, N., DeVine, D., . . . Lau, J. (2007). *Breastfeeding and maternal and infant health outcomes in developed countries* (Evidence Report/Technology Assessment 153; AHRQ Publication 07-E0007). Rockville, MD: Agency for Healthcare Research and Quality. Retrieved from https://archive.ahrq.gov/downloads/pub/evidence/pdf/brfout/brfout.pdf

Jackson, M., Dahlen, H., & Schmied, V. (2012). Birthing outside the system: Perception of risk amongst Australian women who have freebirths and high risk homebirths. *Midwifery, 28*(5), 561–567. https://doi.org/10.1016/j.midw.2011.11.002

Joseph, K. S., Boutin, A., Lisonkova, S., Muraca, G. M., Razaz, N., John, S., . . . Schisterman, E. (2021). Maternal mortality in the United States: Recent trends, current status, and future considerations. *Obstetrics & Gynecology, 137*(5), 763–771. https://doi.org/10.1097/AOG.0000000000004361

Karletsos, D., Stoecker, C., Vilda, D., Theall, K. P., & Wallace, M. E. (2021). Association of state gestational age limit abortion laws with infant mortality. *American Journal of Preventive Medicine, 61*(6), 787–794. https://doi.org/10.1016/j.amepre.2021.05.022

Kavitha, A., Chacko, K. P., Thomas, E., Rathore, S., Christoper, S., Biswas, B., & Mathews, J. E. (2012). A randomized controlled trial to study the effect of IV hydration on the duration of labor in nulliparous women. *Archives of Gynecology and Obstetrics, 285*(2), 343–346. https://doi.org/10.1007/s00404-011-1978-7

Kennedy, H. P., Balaam, M.-C., Dahlen, H., Declercq, E., de Jonge, A., Downe, S., . . . Wolfe, I. (2020). The role of midwifery and other international insights for maternity care in the United States: An analysis of four countries. *Birth, 47*(4), 332–345. https://doi.org/10.1111/birt.12504

Knight, M., Tuffnell, D., Kenyon, S., Shakespeare, J., Gray, R., & Kurinczuk, J. J. (Eds.), on behalf of MBRRACE-UK. (2015). *Saving lives, improving mothers' care: Surveillance of maternal deaths in the UK 2011–13 and lessons learned to inform maternity care from the UK and Ireland confidential enquiries into maternal deaths and morbidity 2009–13*. Oxford, United Kingdom: National Perinatal Epidemiology Unit.

Kumar, N. R., Borders, A., & Simon, M. A. (2021). Postpartum Medicaid extension to address racial inequity in maternal mortality. *American Journal of Public Health, 111*(2), 202–204. https://doi.org/10.2105/AJPH.2020.306060

Lang, G., Farnell, IV, E. A., & Quinlan, J. D. (2021). Out-of-hospital birth. *American Family Physician, 103*(11), 672–679. Retrieved from https://www.aafp.org/pubs/afp/issues/2021/0601/p672.html

Laughon, S. K., Zhang, J., Grewal, J., Sundaram, R., Beaver, J., & Reddy, U. M. (2012). Induction of labor in a contemporary obstetric cohort. *American Journal of Obstetrics & Gynecology, 206*(6), 486.e1–486.e9. https://doi.org/10.1016/j.ajog.2012.03.014

Lawn, J. E., Kinney, M., Lee, A. C. C., Donnay, F., Paul, V. K., . . . Darmstadt, G. L. (2009). Reducing intrapartum-related deaths and disability: Can the health system deliver? *International Journal of Gynecology & Obstetrics, 107*(Suppl.), S123–S142. https://doi.org/10.1016/j.ijgo.2009.07.021

Lawrence, A., Lewis, L., Hofmeyr, G. J., & Styles, T. (2013). Maternal positions and mobility during first stage labour. *Cochrane Database of Systematic Reviews*. https://doi.org/10.1002/14651858.CD003934.pub4

Leeman, L., & Goldstein, J. T. (2021). Promoting safety in community-based birth settings. *American Family Physician, 103*(11), 650–652. Retrieved from https://www.aafp.org/pubs/afp/issues/2021/0601/p650.html

Levine, A., Souter, V., & Sakala, C. (2021). Are perinatal quality collaboratives collaborating enough? How including all birth settings can drive needed improvement in the United States maternity care system. *Birth, 49*(1), 3–10. https://doi.org/10.1111/birt.12600

Likis, F. E. (2014). Home birth: Moving toward shared goals. *Journal of Midwifery & Women's Health, 59*(6), 567–568. https://doi.org/10.1111/jmwh.12277

Lincoln, T. (2015). *Solutions in sight: Safety initiatives have dramatically reduced harms during childbirth but are unevenly implemented*. Washington, DC: Public Citizen. Retrieved from http://www.citizen.org/documents/obstetrics-healthcare-safety-report.pdf

Liu, S., Liston, R. M., Joseph, K. S., Heaman, M., Sauve, R., & Kramer, M. S. (2007). Maternal mortality and severe morbidity associated with low-risk planned cesarean delivery versus planned vaginal delivery at term. *Canadian Medical Association Journal, 176*(4), 455–60. https://doi.org/10.1503/cmaj.060870

Lothian, J. A. (2018). Transforming maternity care in the United States. *Journal of Perinatal Education, 27*(3), 123–126. https://doi.org/10.1891/1058-1243.27.3.123

Lowe, N. (2015). The myth of women's choices in U.S. maternity care. *Journal of Obstetric, Gynecologic, & Neonatal Nursing, 44*(6), 691–692. https://doi.org/10.1111/1552-6909.12757

Lundgren, I., Berg, M., Nilsson, C., & Olafsdottir, O. A. (2020). Health professionals' perceptions of a midwifery model of woman-centered care implemented on a hospital labour ward. *Women and Birth, 33*(1), 60–69. https://doi.org/10.1016/j.wombi.2019.01.004

MacDorman, M. F., & Declercq, E. (2019). Trends and state variations in out-of-hospital births in the United States, 2004–2017. *Birth, 46*(2), 279–288. https://doi.org/10.1111/birt.12411

MacDorman, M. F., Declercq, E., & Mathews, T. J. (2011). United States home births increase 20 percent from 2004 to 2008. *Birth, 38*(3), 185–190. https://doi.org/10.1111/j.1523-536X.2011.00481.x

MacDorman, M. F., Mathews, T. J., Mohangoo, A. D., & Zeitlin, J. (2014). International comparisons of infant mortality and related factors: United States and Europe, 2010. *National Vital Statistics Reports, 63*(5). Retrieved from http://www.cdc.gov/nchs/data/nvsr/nvsr63/nvsr63_05.pdf

Main, E., Oshiro, B., Chagolla, B., Bingham, D., Dang-Kilduff, L., & Kowalewski, L. (2010). *Elimination of non-medically indicated (elective) deliveries before 39 weeks gestational age. California maternal quality care collaborative toolkit to transform maternity care.* Retrieved from http://health.usf.edu/NR/rdonlyres/B74F2943-B3C4-42FD-A889-61FEB381FD64/47839/MODLessThan39WeeksToolkit_Reduced.pdf

Mariani, G. L., & Vain, N. E. (2019). The rising incidence and impact of non-medically indicated pre-labour cesarean section in Latin America. *Seminars in Fetal & Neonatal Medicine, 24*(1), 11–17. https://doi.org/10.1016/j.siny.2018.09.002

Martin-Arribas, A., Canet-Velez, O., Casañas Sanchez, R., Salgado Poveda, I., Espada-Trespalacios, X., Rodriguez Coll, P., . . . Escuriet, R. (2020). Midwives' experiences of the factors that facilitate normal birth among low risk women in public hospitals in Catalonia (Spain). *Midwifery, 88*. https://doi.org/10.1016/j.midw.2020.102752

Meghani, S. H., Byun, E., & Gallagher, R. M. (2012). Time to take stock: A meta-analysis and systematic review of analgesic treatment disparities for pain in the United States. *Pain Medicine, 13*(2), 150–174. https://doi.org/10.1111/j.1526-4637.2011.01310.x

Menard, M. K., Kilpatrick, S., Saade, G., Hollier, L. M., Joseph, G. F., Jr., Barfield, . . . Conry, J. (2015). Levels of maternal care. *American Journal of Obstetrics & Gynecology, 212*(3), 259–271. https://doi.org/10.1016/j.ajog.2014.12.030

Miller, S., Abalos, E., Chamillard, M., Ciappponi, A., Colaci, D., Comandé, D., . . . Althabe, F. (2016). Beyond too little, too late and too much, too soon: A pathway towards evidence-based, respectful maternity care worldwide. *Lancet, 388*(10056), 2176–2192. https://doi.org/10.1016/S0140-6736(16)31472-6

Miller, S., & Skinner, J. (2012). Are first-time mothers who plan home birth more likely to receive evidence-based care? A comparative study of home and hospital care provided by the same midwives. *Birth, 39*(2), 135-144. https://doi.org/10.1111/j.1523-536X.2012.00534.x

Molina, G., Weiser, T. G., Lipsitz, S. R., Esquivel, M. M., Uribe-Leitz, T., Azad, T., . . . Haynes, A. B. (2015). Relationship between cesarean delivery rate and maternal and neonatal mortality. *JAMA, 314*(21), 2263–2270. https://doi.org/10.1001/jama.2015.15553

Murray-Davis, B., McNiven, P., McDonald, H., Malott, A., Elarar, L., & Hutton, E. (2012). Why home birth? A qualitative study exploring women's decision making about place of birth in two Canadian provinces. *Midwifery, 28*(5), 576–581. https://doi.org/10.1016/j.midw.2012.01.013

Nambiar, A., Patel, S., Santiago-Munoz, P., Spong, C. Y., & Nelson, D. B. (2022). Maternal morbidity and fetal outcomes among pregnant women at 22 weeks' gestation or less with complications in 2 Texas hospitals after legislation on abortion. *American Journal of Obstetrics & Gynecology, 227*(4), 648–650.e1. https://doi.org/10.1016/j.ajog.2022.06.060

National Academies of Sciences, Engineering, and Medicine. (2020). *Birth settings in America: Outcomes, quality, access, and choice.* Washington, DC: National Academies Press. https://doi.org/10.17226/25636

National Quality Forum. (2012, April 2). *NQF endorses perinatal measures.* Retrieved from https://www.qualityforum.org/News_And_Resources/Press_Releases/2012/NQF_Endorses_Perinatal_Measures.aspx

Neerland, C. E. & Skalisky, A. E. (2022), A qualitative study of US women's perspectives on confidence for physiologic birth in the birth center model of prenatal care. *Journal of Midwifery & Women's Health, 67*(4), 435–441. https://doi.org/10.1111/jmwh.13349

Nethery, E., Schummers, L., Levine, A., Caughey, A. B., Souter, V., & Gordon, W. (2021). Birth outcomes for planned home and licensed freestanding birth center births in Washington State. *Obstetrics & Gynecology, 138*(5), 693–702. https://doi.org/10.1097/AOG.0000000000004578

[NICE] National Institute for Health and Care Excellence. (2023). *Intrapartum care* (NICE Guideline NG235). Retrieved from https://www.nice.org.uk/guidance/ng235

Nichols, C. R., & Cohen, A. K. (2021). Preventing maternal mortality in the United States: Lessons from California and policy recommendations. *Journal of Public Health Policy, 42*(1), 127–144. https://doi.org/10.1057/s41271-020-00264-9

Nove, A., Berrington, A., & Matthews, Z. (2012). The methodological challenges of attempting to compare the safety of home and hospital birth in terms of the risk of perinatal death. *Midwifery, 28*(5), 619–626. https://doi.org/10.1016/j.midw.2012.07.009

Oladapo, O. T., Tunçalp, Ö., Bonet, M., Lawrie, T. A., Portela, A., Downe, S., & Gülmezoglu, A. M. (2018). WHO model of intrapartum care for a positive childbirth experience: Transforming care of women and babies for improved health and wellbeing. *BJOG, 125*(8), 918–922. https://doi.org/10.1111/1471-0528.15237

Olsen, O., & Clausen, J. A. (2023). Planned hospital birth compared with planned home birth for pregnant women at low risk of complications. *Cochrane Database of Systematic Reviews.* https://doi.org/10.1002/14651858.CD000352.pub3

Pabayo, R., Ehntholt, A., Cook, D. M., Reynolds, M., Muennig, P., & Liu, S. Y. (2020). Laws restricting access to abortion services and infant mortality risk in the United States. *International Journal of Environmental Research and Public Health,17*(11), 3773. https://doi.org/10.3390/ijerph17113773

Padmanaba01 [Screen name]. (2009, November 16). *Kolkata (4131122903)* [Photograph]. Retrieved from https://commons.wikimedia.org/wiki/File:-Kolkata_(4131122903).jpg

Page, K., Aryal, S., & Guidera, M. (2022). Midwives and liability: Results of the 2018 National Midwives and Liability Survey. *Journal of Midwifery & Women's Health, 67*(2), 226–234. https://doi.org/10.1111/jmwh.13355

Page, M., & Mander, R. (2014). Intrapartum uncertainty: A feature of normal birth, as experienced by midwives in Scotland. *Midwifery, 30*(1), 28–35. https://doi.org/10.1016/j.midw.2013.01.012

Petersen, E. E., Davis, N. L., Goodman, D., Cox, S., Mayes, N., Johnston, E., . . . Barfield, W. (2019). Vital signs: Pregnancy-related deaths, United States, 2011–2015, and strategies for prevention, 13 states, 2013–2017. *Morbidity and Mortality Weekly Report, 68*(18), 423–429. https://doi.org/10.15585/mmwr.mm6818e1

Preis, H., Mahaffey, B., & Lobel, M. (2021). The role of pandemic-related pregnancy stress in preference for community birth during the beginning of the COVID-19 pandemic in the United States. *Birth, 48*(2), 242–250. https://doi.org/10.1111/birt.12533

Rigg, E., Schmied, V., Peters, K., & Dahlen, H. (2015). Not addressing the root cause: An analysis of submissions made to the South Australian government on a proposal to protect midwifery practice. *Women and Birth, 28*(2), 121–128. https://doi.org/10.1016/j.wombi.2014.12.005

Rooks. J. P., Weatherby, N. L., & Ernst, E. K. (1992). The National Birth Center Study. Part III—Intrapartum and immediate postpartum and neonatal complications and transfers, postpartum and neonatal care, outcomes, and client satisfaction. *Journal of Nurse-Midwifery, 37*(6), 361–397. https://doi.org/10.1016/0091-2182(92)90122-j

Rooks. J. P., Weatherby, N. L., Ernst, E. K., Stapleton, S., Rosen, D., & Rosenfield, A. (1989). Outcomes of care in birth centers. The National Birth Center Study. *New England Journal of Medicine, 321*,1804–1811. https://doi.org/10.1056/NEJM198912283212606

Rossen, L. M., Womack, L. S., Hoyert, D. L., Anderson, R. N., & Uddin, S. F. G. (2020). The impact of the pregnancy checkbox and misclassification on maternal mortality trends in the United States, 1999–2017. *Vital and Health Statistics, 3*(44), 1–61. Retrieved from https://www.cdc.gov/nchs/data/series/sr_03/sr03_044-508.pdf

Rutherford, J. N., Asiodu, I. V., & Liese, K. L. (2019). Reintegrating modern birth practice within ancient birth process: What high cesarean rates ignore about physiologic birth. *American Journal of Human Biology., 31*(2), e23229. https://doi.org/10.1002/ajhb.23229

Rydahl, E., Juhl, M., Declercq, E., & Maimburg, R. D. (2021). Disruption of physiological labour;—A population register-based study among nulliparous women at term. *Sexual & Reproductive Healthcare, 27.* https://doi.org/10.1016/j.srhc.2020.100571

Sakai-Bizmark, R., Ross, M. G., Estevez, D., Bedel, L. E. M., Marr, E. H., & Tsugawa, Y. (2021). Evaluation of hospital cesarean delivery–related profits and rates in the United States. *JAMA Network Open, 4*(3), e212235. https://doi.org/10.1001/jamanetworkopen.2021.2235

Shah, N. (2015a). A NICE delivery—The cross-Atlantic divide over treatment intensity in childbirth. *New England Journal of Medicine, 372*(23), 2181–2183. https://doi.org/10.1056/NEJMp1501461

Shah, N. (2015b). Are hospitals the safest place for healthy women to have babies? An obstetrician thinks twice. *The Conversation*. Retrieved from https://theconversation.com/are-hospitals-the-safest-place-for-healthy-women-to-have-babies-an-obstetrician-thinks-twice-42654

Singata, M., Tranmer, J., & Gyte, G. M. L. (2013). Restricting oral fluid and food intake during labour. *Cochrane Database of Systematic Reviews*. https://doi.org/10.1002/14651858.CD003930.pub3

Singh, G. K., & Lee, H. (2020). Trends and racial/ethnic, socioeconomic, and geographic disparities in maternal mortality from indirect obstetric causes in the United States, 1999–2017. *International Journal of Maternal and Child Health and AIDS, 10*(1), 43–54. https://doi.org/10.21106/ijma.448

Singh, G. K., & Stella, M. Y. (2019). Infant mortality in the United States, 1915–2017: Large social inequalities have persisted for over a century. *International Journal of Maternal and Child Health and AIDS, 8*(1), 19–31. https://doi.org/10.21106/ijma.271

Snowden, J. M., Tilden, E. L., Snyder, J., Quigley, B., Caughey, A. B., & Cheng, Y. W. (2015). Planned out-of-hospital birth and birth outcomes. *New England Journal of Medicine, 373*(27), 2642–2653. https://doi.org/10.1056/NEJMsa1501738

Stacey, D., Légaré, F., Lewis, K., Barry, M. J., Bennett, C. L., Eden, K. B., . . . Trevena, L. (2017). Decision aids for people facing health treatment or screening decisions. *Cochrane Database of Systematic Reviews*. https://doi.org/10.1002/14651858.CD001431.pub5

Stapleton, S. (2023). Birth centers. In V. A. Barss (Ed.), *UpToDate*. Retrieved September 30, 2023, from http://www.uptodate.com/contents/birth-centers

Stapleton, S. R., Osborne, C., & Illuzzi, J. (2013). Outcomes of care in birth centers: Demonstration of a durable model. *Journal of Midwifery & Women's Health, 58*(1), 3–14. https://doi.org/10.1111/jmwh.12003

Stiller, R. J. (2014). 4 ways to lower your risk of an obstetric malpractice suit. *Contemporary OB/GYN*. Retrieved from http://contemporaryobgyn.modernmedicine.com/contemporary-obgyn/content/tags/lawsuits/4-ways-lower-your-risk-obstetric-malpractice-suit?page=full

Stoll, K. H., Downe, S., Edmonds, J., Gross, M. M., Malott, A., McAra-Couper, J., . . . ICAPP Study Team. (2020). A survey of university students' preferences for midwifery care and community birth options in 8 high-income countries. *Journal of Midwifery & Women's Health, 65*(1), 131–141. https://doi.org/10.1111/jmwh.13069

Sutton, M. Y., Anachebe, N. F., Lee, R., & Skanes, H. (2021). Racial and ethnic disparities in reproductive health services and outcomes, 2020. *Obstetrics & Gynecology, 137*(2), 225–233. https://doi.org/10.1097/AOG.0000000000004224

Taylor, E., Guy-Walls, P., Wilkerson, P., & Addae, R. (2019). The historical perspectives of stereotypes on African-American males. *Journal of Human Rights and Social Work, 4*, 213–225. https://doi.org/10.1007/s41134-019-00096-y

Treder, K., White, K. O., Woodhams, E., Pancholi, R., & Yinusa-Nyahkoon, L. (2022). Racism and the reproductive health experiences of U.S.-born black women. *Obstetrics & Gynecology, 139*(3), 407–416 https://doi.org/10.1097/AOG.0000000000004675

Trost, S., Beauregard, J., Chandra, G., Njie, F., Berry, J., Harvey, A., & Goodman, D. A. (2022). *Pregnancy-related deaths: Data from maternal mortality review committees in 36 US states, 2017–2019.* Atlanta, GA: Centers for Disease Control and Prevention. Retrieved from https://www.cdc.gov/reproductivehealth/maternal-mortality/erase-mm/data-mmrc.html

Tucker, M. J., Berg, C. J., Callaghan, W. M., & Hsia, J. (2007). The black–white disparity in pregnancy-related mortality from 5 conditions: Differences in prevalence and case-fatality rates. *American Journal of Public Health, 97*(2), 247–251. https://doi.org/10.2105/AJPH.2005.072975

van Haaren-ten Haken, T., Hendrix, M., Nieuwenhuijze, M., Budé, L., de Vries, R., & Nijhuis, J. (2012). Preferred place of birth: Characteristics and motives of low-risk nulliparous women in the Netherlands. *Midwifery, 28*(5),609-618. https://doi.org/10.1016/j.midw.2012.07.010

Vedam, S., Schummers, L., Stoll, K., Rogers, J., Klein, M. C., Fairbrother, N., . . . Kaczorowski. J. (2012). The Canadian Birth Place Study: Describing maternity practice and providers' exposure to home birth. *Midwifery, 28*(5), 600–608. https://doi.org/10.1016/j.midw.2012.06.011

Vedam, S., Stoll, K., MacDorman, M., Declercq, E., Cramer, R., Cheyney, M., . . . Kennedy, H. P. (2018). Mapping integration of midwives across the United States: Impact on access, equity, and outcomes. *PloS ONE 13*(2), e0192523. https://doi.org/10.1371/journal.pone.0192523

Vedam, S., Stoll, K., Schummers, L., & Fulton, C. (2013). *Home birth: An annotated guide to the literature.* Vancouver, Canada: University of British Columbia Midwifery Program. Retrieved from http://midwifery.ubc.ca/files/2013/11/HomeBirth_AnnotatedGuideToTheLiterature.pdf

Vedam, S., Stoll, K., Taiwo, T. K., Rubashkin, N., Cheyney, M., Strauss, N., . . . GVtM-US Steering Council. (2019). The Giving Voice to Mothers study: Inequity and mistreatment during pregnancy and childbirth in the United States. *Reproductive Health, 16*(1), 1–18. https://doi.org/10.1186/s12978-019-0729-2

Vela, M. B., Erondu, A. I., Smith, N. A., Peek, M. E., Woodruff, J. N., & Chin, M. H. (2022). Eliminating explicit and implicit biases in health care: Evidence and research needs. *Annual Review of Public Health, 43*, 477–501. https://doi.org/10.1146/annurev-publhealth-052620-103528

Verhoeven, C. J., Boer, J., Kok, M., Nieuwenhuijze, M., de Jonge, A., & Peters, L. L. (2022). More home births during the COVID-19 pandemic in the Netherlands. *Birth, 49*(4), 792–804. https://doi.org/10.1111/birt.12646

Verma, A., & Cleland, J. (2022). Is newborn survival influenced by place of delivery? A comparison of home, public sector and private sector deliveries in India. *Journal of Biosocial Science, 54*(2), 184–198. https://doi.org/10.1017/S0021932021000080

Visser, G. H. A. (2012). Obstetric care in the Netherlands: Relic or example? *Journal of Obstetrics and Gynaecology Canada, 34*(10), 971–975. https://doi.org/10.1016/S1701-2163(16)35410-X

Visser, G. H. A., Ayres-de-Campos, D., Barnea, E. R., de Bernis, L., Di Renzo, G. C., Vidarte, M. F. E., . . . Walani, S. (2018). FIGO position paper: How to stop the caesarean section epidemic. *Lancet, 392*(10155), 1286-1287. https://doi.org/10.1016/S0140-6736(18)32113-5

Walani, S. R. (2020). Global burden of preterm birth. *International Journal of Gynecology & Obstetrics, 150*(1), 31–33. https://doi.org/10.1002/ijgo.13195

Wasden, S. W., Chasen, S. T., Perlman, J. M., Illuzzi, J. L., Chervenak, F. A., & Lipkind, H. S. (2017). Planned home birth and the association with neonatal hypoxic ischemic encephalopathy. *Journal of Perinatal Medicine, 45*(9), 1055–1060. https://doi.org/10.1515/jpm-2016-0292

Watterberg, K., Cummings, J. J., Adams-Chapman, I. S., Aucott, S. W., Goldsmith, J. P., Hand, I. L., . . . Barfield, W. D. (2020). Providing care for infants born at home. *Pediatrics, 145*(5), e202000626. https://doi.org/10.1542/peds.2020-0626

White Ribbon Alliance. (n.d.). *Respectful maternity care: The universal rights of women & newborns.* Retrieved from https://whiteribbonalliance.org/wp-content/uploads/2022/05/WRA_RMC_Charter_FINAL.pdf

Windau-Melmer, T. (2013). *A guide for advocating for respectful maternity care.* Washington, DC: Futures Group, Health Policy Project. Retrieved from http://www.healthpolicyproject.com/pubs/189_RMCGuideFINAL.pdf

World Health Organization. (2016). *Infant mortality: Situations and trends.* Retrieved from http://www.who.int/gho/child_health/mortality/neonatal_infant_text/en/

World Health Organization. (2018). *WHO recommendations: Intrapartum care for a positive childbirth experience.* Geneva, Switzerland: author. Retrieved from https://apps.who.int/iris/bitstream/handle/10665/260178/9789241550215-eng.pdf

World Health Organization. (2020). *Children: Improving survival and well-being.* Retrieved from http://www.who.int/en/news-room/fact-sheets/detail/children-reducing-mortality

World Health Organization. (2023, February 22). *Maternal mortality.* Retrieved from https://www.who.int/news-room/fact-sheets/detail/maternal-mortality

Zacharias, N. (2023). Perinatal mortality. In C. Armsby (Ed.), *UpToDate.* Retrieved September 30, 2023, from https://www.uptodate.com/contents/perinatal-mortality

Zondag, L. D., Maas, V. Y., Beuckens, A., & Nieuwenhuijze, M. J. (2022). Experiences, beliefs, and values influencing midwives' attitudes toward the use of childbirth interventions. *Journal of Midwifery & Women's Health, 67*(5), 618–625. https://doi.org/10.1111/jmwh.13392

Healthy Pregnancy and Deviations from Normal

2

Objectives

- Describe four uterine anomalies and discuss the associated risks they pose to pregnancy.
- Discuss how pregnancy-related changes in cardiovascular function can be mistaken for pathology.
- Discuss the signs and symptoms of hyperemesis gravidarum.
- Discuss how changes in carbohydrate metabolism during pregnancy can affect serum glucose levels.
- Explain how pregnancy related changes to the urinary tract can predispose to urinary tract infection (UTI).

Composite Case Study

Erin Sensenig was near the end of her midwifery course of study and was looking forward to finally assuming independent practice. She felt confident in the skills she required to be a safe provider, and her preceptors frequently complimented her on her gentle manner and capable hands. Midwifery was her calling, and she found her greatest joy in supporting mothers through the challenges of physiologic labor.

Marcella A., an 18-year-old primigravida at 38 weeks of gestation, came into the birth center breathing hard and trembling with every contraction. She had previously declined any intervention beyond basic bloodwork and had not undergone ultrasound evaluation or a pelvic exam. Erin explained the need for cervical assessment and provided reassurance. She positioned Marcella on the bed, slipped a glove over her left hand, and performed a cervical exam. Her cervix was only 2 cm dilated and thick, a finding that surprised Erin; Marcella's long, hard, frequent contractions and her dramatic response to them gave the impression that she was in transition. Karolina, Erin's seasoned preceptor, was also surprised at the assessment. Although she trusted Erin's judgment, she donned a glove on her right hand and, with Marcella's permission, performed a second cervical exam. "Actually, Erin, she is 8 cm, thin and stretchy," she said. Erin was shocked and devastated. How could she mistake a thin, stretchy 8 cm cervix for a thick, 2 cm one? It made no sense.

Together, preceptor and student performed a thorough examination of Marcella's genitals. They discovered that their client had a septate vagina and two cervixes. The baby was making its exit through the right-side cervix, which was dilated to 8 cm and more easily accessible to right-handed Karolina. The left-sided cervix, most accessible to left-handed Erin, was not subjected to the pressures of a descending baby but had dilated to 2 cm in response to the hormones of labor.

As Erin and Karolina pondered this unexpected turn of events, Marcella began to push and the baby's head distended the perineum in a gush of blood. The birth was rapid, and Marcella sustained complex lacerations involving the vaginal septum, both vaginal sidewalls, the periclitoral area, and the perineum, necessitating hospital transport for repair. It also seemed likely that there were retained placental fragments. The midwife and her student controlled the bleeding from the lacerations with tranexamic acid and hemostatic gauze en route. *An ultrasound examination at the hospital revealed that Marcella had a double uterus* (uterus didelphys).

Maternal Adaptations to Pregnancy

Normal changes of pregnancy can mask or mimic pathology, and pathology can mask or mimic normal changes. The midwife who has a good understanding of anatomy, physiology, and pathophysiology can be better able to solve such clinical puzzles. This knowledge also helps the midwife to determine when to stand back and observe, when to intervene to shift a situation back to normal, and when to decisively take control.

For pregnancy to be successful, a mother's body must undergo profound alterations in structure and function in nearly every organ system (Cunningham et al., 2022, ch. 4). Most of the physical changes are progressive and relate to either hormonal or physical changes wrought by the developing fetus. Each organ transforms and recovers at its own rate, and some organs never return to their prepregnant condition. With practice, the body becomes more efficient at maintaining pregnancy; for example, firstborn children have lower average birthweights than subsequent children (Howe et al., 2014).

The healthy client who conceives with a body mass index (BMI) in the optimal range should gain roughly 22–37 lb

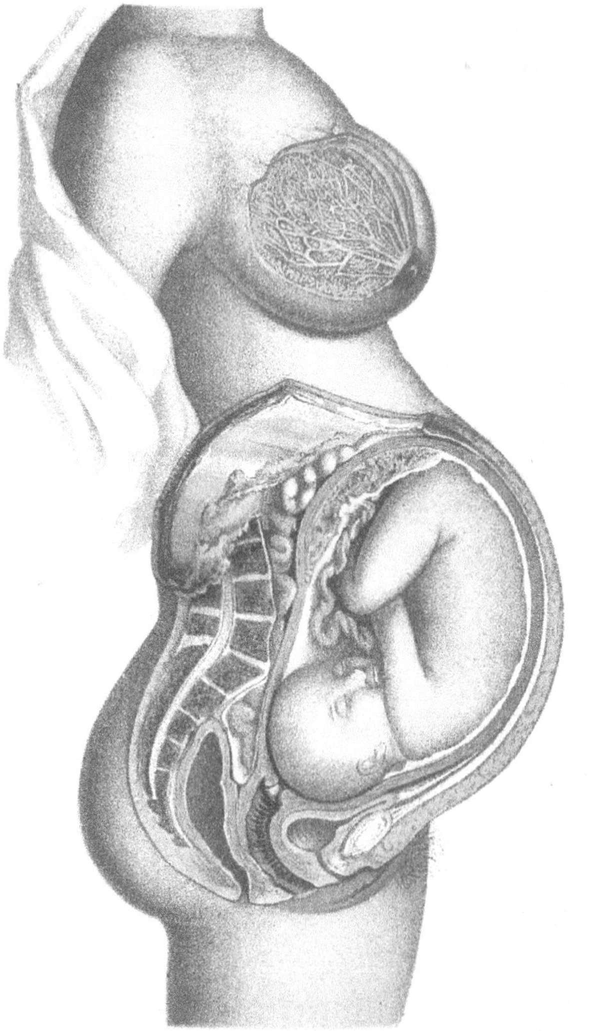

Figure 2-1. Pregnancy causes major changes in all body systems. From *Handbook of Obstetric Nursing* (frontispiece), by F. W. N. Haultain and J. H. Ferguson, 1898, Edinburgh, United Kingdom: Y. J. Pentland. In the public domain.

(10.0–16.8 kg) during pregnancy (Antony, Racusin, Aagard, & Dildy, 2021). Weight gain includes not only the fetus, but also the increased mass of the uterus and breasts, amniotic fluid, placenta, extravascular and extracellular fluid, enlarged maternal vital organs, and fat deposits. Total body water and fat increase throughout pregnancy; the mothers who have the greatest gains tend to grow the largest babies, larger still if the mothers were overweight or obese at conception (Cunningham et al., 2022, ch. 4).

The maternal immune system must change radically to tolerate the fetus while continuing to protect the mother from infection. Depressed leukocyte function during pregnancy reduces the mother's resistance to infection but can cause improvement in autoimmune disease (Mattson & Smith, 2016). It is thought that the fetal immune system undertakes similar adaptations to "tolerate" the mother (Mattson & Smith, 2016).

Interestingly, although mother and fetus are unique and separate organisms, during pregnancy they exchange cells, each incorporating a bit of the other into their bodies. In a condition called microchimerism, fetal cells move through the placenta and establish lineages within the mother while the cells of the mother move into the body of the child, often persisting for decades after birth. They integrate into tissue and proliferate, becoming liver, heart, bone marrow (O'Donoghue et al., 2004)—even neurons in the brain (Chan et al., 2012; Zeng et al., 2010). Fetal cells remain in the maternal circulation after a spontaneous abortion and can remain in greater quantities after an elective abortion (Miech, 2010). Even more astonishing, cells from older siblings and even cells from the maternal grandmother can be transferred to the fetus (Boddy, Fortunato, Wilson Sayres, & Aktipis, 2015). It is possible that our bodies carry living bits of our recent ancestors or even our ancient foremothers.

Microchimerism seems to have benefits and drawbacks. For example, fetal cells appear to migrate to the site of a maternal wound and aid in healing (Mahmood & O'Donoghue, 2014), and they are thought to protect against breast cancer and possibly other kinds of malignancy (Kallenbach, Johnson, & Bianchi, 2011). But they have also been associated with pregnancy complications, such as preeclampsia, miscarriage, and premature birth (Boddy et al., 2015) and with autoimmune conditions such as scleroderma (Miech, 2010).

Reproductive System

Uterine enlargement is one of the most obvious changes in pregnancy. The nonpregnant uterus weighs about 2 oz (70 g) and is mostly solid except for a small central hollow of 10 ml or less (Cunningham et al., 2022, ch. 4). At term, it weighs about 2.4 lb (1,100 g) and has a total volume that averages 5 L but can exceed 20 L (Cunningham et al., 2022, ch. 4). Uterine enlargement is not due solely to the growing fetus and surrounding fluid; it also reflects a hormonally influenced increase in myometrial muscle mass. Uterine walls thicken in early pregnancy, but then thin to about 0.6 in. (1.5 cm) or less at term, transforming the organ from a nearly solid globe to a hollow vessel (Mattson & Smith, 2016).

The uterus outgrows the confines of the pelvis at about 12 weeks of gestation and modifies the position of many organs as it enlarges. At 5 weeks of gestation, the uterus is the size of a small, unripe pear; by 8 weeks of gestation, it is the size of a large navel orange; by 10 weeks of gestation, it is the size of a grapefruit; and by 12 weeks of gestation, it is about the size of a cantaloupe (Murray & Hendley, 2020). It rotates to the mother's right as it grows, displaced by the sigmoid colon on the left side of the abdomen. The stomach shifts upward, and the intestines move to the side (Danhausen & King, 2024). At term, the uterus nearly reaches the liver. The appendix can be displaced as far as the right costal margin, which can distort the classic presentation of appendicitis (Blackburn, 2021).

Throughout pregnancy, uterine blood flow increases to perfuse the growing placenta. By term, the blood flow to the uterus has increased from 50 ml/min to approximately 750 ml/min (Danhausen & King, 2024); 80% of this flow perfuses the placental bed (Blackburn, 2021). Uterine blood flow is affected by maternal position, maternal arterial pressure, and presence or absence of contractions.

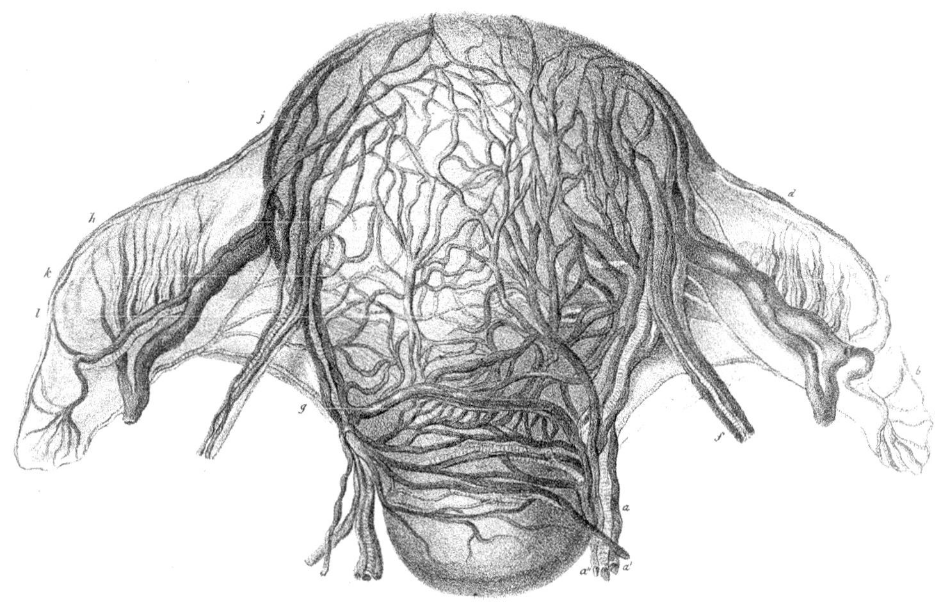

Figure 2-2. Uterine blood supply. The pregnant uterus is a highly vascular organ. From *A Practical Treatise on Midwifery*... (plate XXII, fig, 2), by F. J. Moreau (T. F. Betton, Trans.), 1844, Philadelphia, PA: Carey and Hart. In the public domain.

At least 30–60 uterine spiral arteries supply the intervillous space of the placenta and maintain perfusion during pregnancy (Staff et al., 2020). Upon implantation, fetal cytotrophoblast cells migrate out of the placenta and modify parts of the maternal spiral arteries, remodeling them into the low-pressure, high-volume channels needed to meet fetal demands (Blackburn, 2021). This process occurs twice. The first alteration, occurring in the first weeks after implantation, involves arteries in the decidua, increasing blood flow and rendering the arteries incapable of constriction (Danhausen & King, 2024). With the second modification, occurring between 12 and 20 weeks of gestation, the cytotrophoblast extends into the myometrial part of the spiral arteries and makes further changes (Danhausen & King, 2024).

In preeclampsia, this second remodeling wave does not occur (Staff et al., 2020). The vessels remain narrow and limit placental perfusion. Abnormal placental perfusion generates free radicals and causes the release of inflammatory placental factors. These substances can cause widespread maternal inflammatory response involving inflammation and dysfunction of the vascular endothelium (lining of the blood vessels) and generalized vascular inflammation. These changes begin early in pregnancy, but do not cause clinical signs and symptoms until mid-second or third trimester, when they can manifest as the clinical signs of preeclampsia—e.g., hypertension; generalized edema; and abnormal function of the kidneys, liver, and central nervous system (Staff et al., 2020). Abnormal placentation is also associated with fetal growth restriction (FGR), preterm rupture of membranes, and preterm labor (Danhausen & King, 2024).

Through the first part of pregnancy, the uterus remains largely quiescent because of the interaction of numerous hormones, prostacyclin, and nitric oxide and because of complex signals between fetus and mother (Murray & Hendley, 2020). Progesterone, produced first by the corpus luteum and later by the placenta, relaxes the uterus by blocking the myometrial response to oxytocin. Electrical conduction between uterine muscle cells is poor through most of the pregnancy, and estrogen and progesterone dampen electrical activity within the uterus by influencing calcium and potassium channels (Murray & Hendley, 2020).

Braxton Hicks contractions, initially described by John Braxton Hicks in 1872, are fragmented bursts of irregular, poorly coordinated, low-amplitude contractions present throughout pregnancy (Cunningham et al., 2022, ch. 4). It can be difficult to differentiate among Braxton Hicks contractions, false labor, and labor. Runs of painful Braxton Hicks contractions can mimic labor in the third trimester, but the contractions of progressing preterm labor can be painless.

In early pregnancy, the cervix is a closed, rigid structure that maintains the pregnancy, but by the end of pregnancy it transforms to soft, elastic, paper-thin ring of tissue capable of dilating 10 cm or more to accommodate the passage of a term fetus. Whereas the body of the uterus is mostly comprised of smooth muscle, cervical tissue is mostly formed from connective tissue, which consists of collagen, elastin, and proteins. The endocervical mucosal cells seal the cervical canal with thick mucus that is rich in immunoglobulins and cytokines that appear to act as a physical and immunological

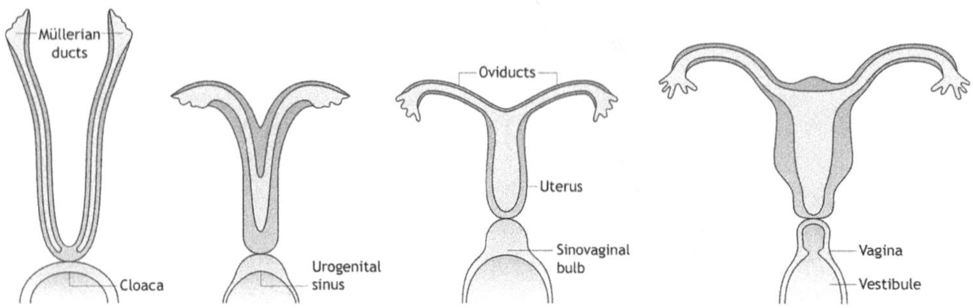

Figure 2-3. During human embryonic development, the Müllerian ducts begin as two separate tubes that undergo midline fusion. The septum resorbs, and the structure develops into the female reproductive tract. From "Studying Müllerian Duct Anomalies—From Cataloguing Phenotypes to Discovering Causation," by L. S. González, M. Artibani, and A. A. Ahmed, 2021, *Disease Models & Mechanisms, 14*(6), fig. 1. CC BY 4.0.

barrier to protect the pregnancy from infection (Cunningham et al., 2022, ch. 4).

The vagina, vulva, and cervix can become so vascular and blood-engorged that they turn purplish or bluish. The connective tissue beneath the vaginal epithelium relaxes, muscle cells hypertrophy, and the vaginal mucosa thickens in preparation for tremendous distension in second stage labor. Because progesterone makes veins more distensible, varicosities can appear or worsen in the vulva and vagina and even in the legs (Antony et al., 2021).

Reproductive Tract Anomalies and Pregnancy

Müllerian duct anomalies (MDAs) are congenital anomalies of the female reproductive tract related to lack of development, failure of fusion, or failure of resorption. Early embryos of most vertebrates from sharks to primates have two systems of paired ducts that develop into reproductive organs (Major, Estermann, Roly, & Smith, 2021). Müllerian ducts (paramesonephric ducts) can develop into a female reproductive tract, and Wolffian ducts can develop into a male reproductive tract (Roly et al., 2020). If an embryo is 46 XY male, the testes secrete androgens that cause Müllerian ducts to regress and Wolffian ducts to develop into male reproductive structures—epididymis, vas deferens, and seminal vesicles (Hannema & Hughes, 2007). If the embryo is 46 XX female and produces no testosterone, the Müllerian ducts develop, and the Wolffian ducts regress.

When this process goes awry, the embryo can develop a unicornuate uterus—one uterine horn, one fallopian tube; uterus didelphys—usually two uteruses, two cervixes, and two vaginas; septate uterus—uterus divided by a partition of myometrium covered by endometrium; arcuate uterus—heart-shaped uterine chamber; or bicornuate uterus—two uterine chambers, usually with one cervix and a single lower uterine segment (Laufer & DeCherney, 2023). Because the urinary tract forms in conjunction with the genital tract, up to 30% of individuals with congenital uterine defects also have renal anomalies such as renal agenesis, pelvic kidney, or horseshoe kidney (Kim, Wirth, & Templeman, 2020).

MDAs can be caused by lack of development, failure of fusion, or failure of resorption.

Failure of development: Müllerian agenesis occurs when part or all of the Müllerian duct fails to develop (Goyal, Dhaliwal, Singh, Ganjoo, & Goyal, 2020). It can result in complete absence of the vagina and uterus or rudimentary structures that are sometimes fused. Fallopian tubes and ovaries are usually present (Trad & Palmer, 2013). Urinary tract, skeletal, and middle-ear malformations are sometimes associated with the syndrome.

If only one Müllerian duct develops, the individual will have a vagina, a cervix, and a banana-shaped unicornuate uterus. Despite lacking a fallopian tube and half of the uterus, individuals with a unicornuate uterus usually have two ovaries, although they can fail to descend into the pelvis or remain higher in the abdomen (Pereira et al., 2021). A unicornuate uterus correlates with higher risk for recurrent pregnancy loss, ectopic pregnancy, fetal demise, preterm birth (PTB), and malpresentation.

Failure of fusion: If the Müllerian ducts develop but fail to fuse, a didelphys uterus will develop, usually resulting in two uteruses and two cervixes, although other variations exist (Smith, Brown, Carter, & Famuyide, 2014). A double cervix can also develop in a septate uterus, bicornuate uterus, or normal uterus (Smith et al., 2014). Up to 75% of individuals with a didelphys uterus will have two vaginas or a vaginal septum (Lovelace, 2016). A longitudinal vaginal septum can be thin and stretchy or thick and inelastic (Rezai, et al, 2015).

Didelphys uterus is uncommon, occurring in 1 in 1,000 female individuals (Post, Templeman, & Benoit, 2019), and is often detected at puberty when clients complain about heavy menstrual bleeding that cannot be stopped with tampons (Trad & Palmer, 2013). If there is a thick, obstructing vaginal septum, sexual intercourse can be difficult and painful (Rezai et al, 2015). In pregnancy, didelphys uterus carries a higher risk of PTB, malpresentation, FGR, retained placenta, and postpartum hemorrhage. A vaginal septum can tear during birth, causing excessive bleeding. Unicornuate and didelphys uteruses create higher risk for vasa previa, placenta previa, and placenta accreta spectrum disorders (Anderson, Lekovic, Niemasik, & Chasen, 2013).

If the Müllerian ducts partially fuse, the result is a bicornuate uterus, the most common uterine malformation. This usually involves a normal cervix and lower uterine segment with two separate uterine fundi (Lovelace, 2016). The tissue of the septum is often different from that of the normal myometrium and is sometimes thinner toward the cervix (Osazuwa & Ejenobo, 2012). The fundus can be convex, flat, or heart-shaped. A bicornuate uterus confers a greater risk of spontaneous abortion, PTB, and malpresentation. The unfused medial walls of the uterine horns can produce a wider, structurally abnormal cervix that is at risk for cervical insufficiency.

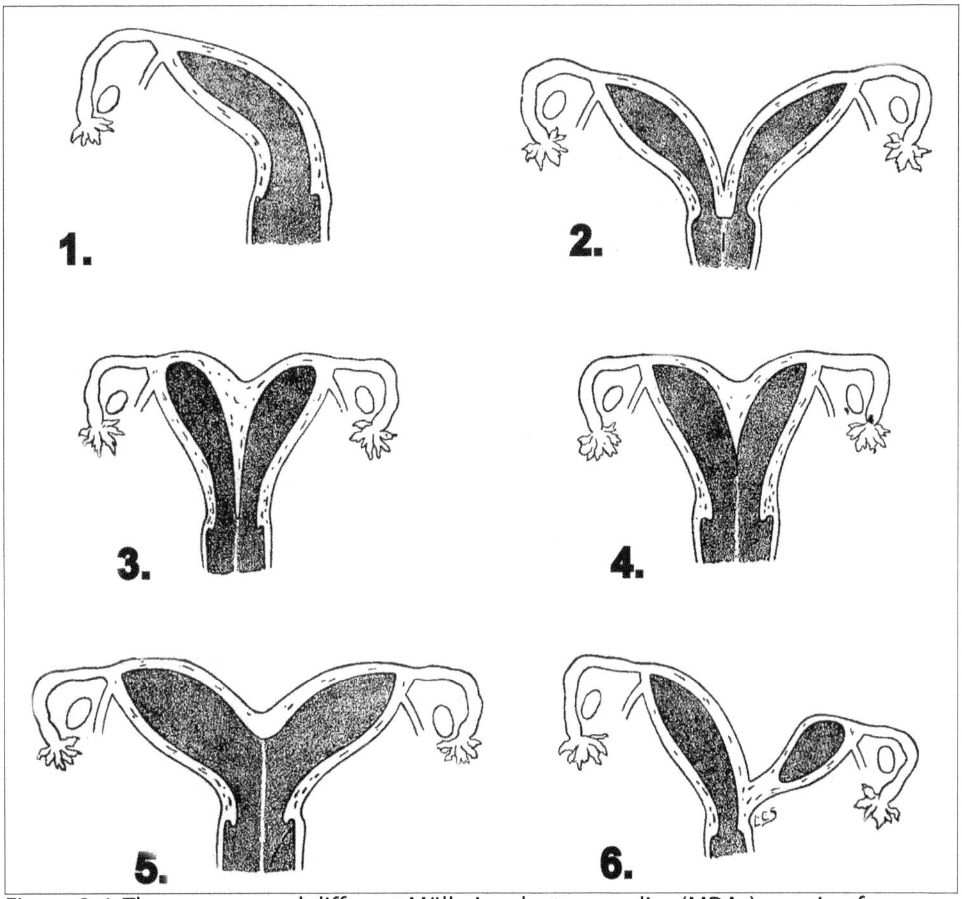

Figure 2-4. There are several different Müllerian duct anomalies (MDAs), ranging from no uterus to a double uterus. The cervix and vagina can also be affected. 1. Unicornuate uterus. 2. Uterus didelphys. 3. Septate uterus. 4. Arcuate uterus. 5. Bicornuate uterus. 6. Unicornuate uterus with rudimentary noncommunicating horn. Adapted from *Obstetrics: A Text-Book for the Use of Students and Practitioners* (3rd ed., p. 569, fig. 458–463), by J. W. Williams, 1912, New York, NY: Appleton. In the public domain.

Failure of resorption: The last step in uterine formation is degeneration of the central septum. Disruption of this process results in a septate uterus, which carries the highest risk of poor pregnancy outcomes of all MDAs (Lovelace, 2016). Individuals with a septate uterus are at high risk for recurrent first- and second-trimester pregnancy loss, FGR, and PTB. In labor, they are at risk for stillbirth, malpresentation, labor dystocia, and placental abruption. There is also greater risk of primary infertility.

An arcuate uterus forms when some of a uterine septum remains at the fundus, leaving a heart-shaped uterine chamber. An arcuate uterus doubles the risk of second-trimester spontaneous abortion, malpresentation, and placental abruption (Lovelace, 2016).

MDAs were once thought to be rare. Ogilvie's 1957 review of literature found no rate higher than 1%. Recent research suggests that defects occur in more than 6% of female individuals, almost 8% of people with female infertility, and almost 17% of people with repeated pregnancy loss (González, Artibani, & Ahmed, 2021). Although this difference in reported incidence can be related to improved imaging techniques, it has been proposed that environmental toxins that cause reproductive malformations in animals affect humans similarly (National Institute of Environmental Health Sciences, 2022). Evidence suggests that most MDAs are multifactorial, however, and genetics cannot account for them all (Laufer & DeCherney, 2023). Most people with congenital uterine anomalies are 46 XX karyotype (Laufer & DeCherney, 2023).

Pregnancy complications related to congenital uterine defects appear related to lower uterine muscle mass, abnormal placentation, and lower uterine blood flow. The abnormal shape and reduced size of the uterine cavity predisposes to malpresentation and preterm labor (PTL). The uterus with a congenital anomaly can have abnormal myometrial contractility and demonstrate asymmetric stretching and thinning during labor, predisposing to dystocia and uterine rupture (Lovelace, 2016). Abnormal endometrium can predispose to placenta accreta. About 80% of individuals with congenital uterine anomalies have greater resistance to blood flow through the uterine artery (Lovelace, 2016).

Uterine anomalies are often missed on ultrasound, particularly late in gestation. Even with comprehensive obstetric care, a mother can have several pregnancies and remain

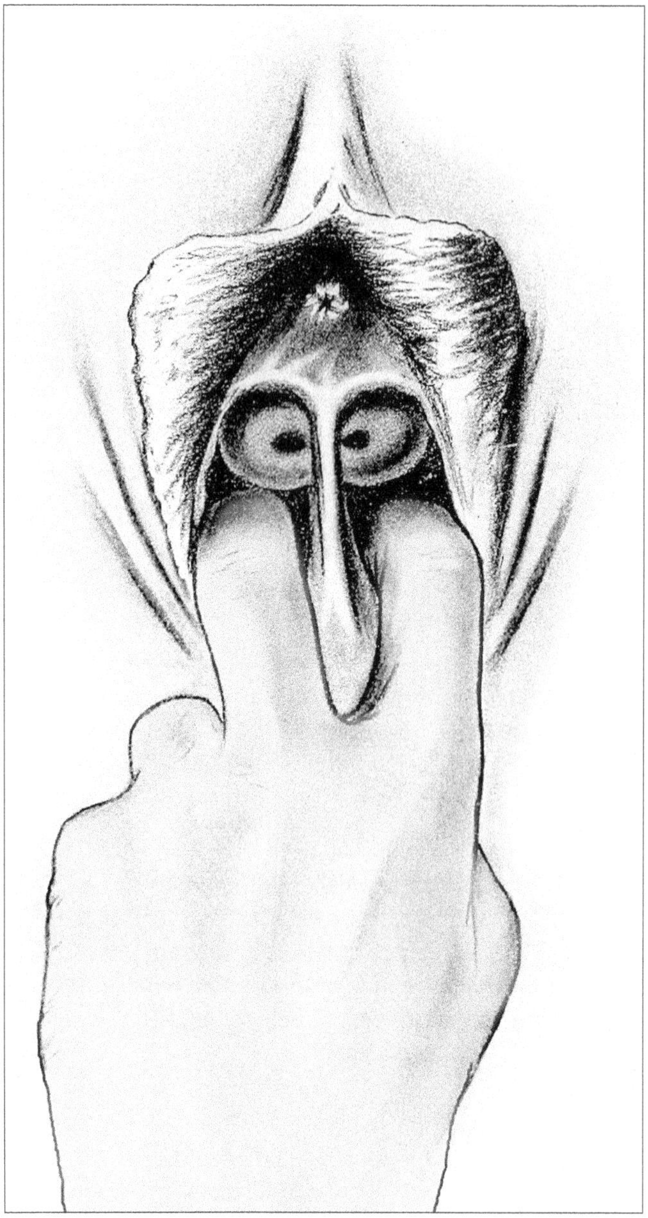

Figure 2-5. A didelphys uterus is usually accompanied by two vaginas and two cervixes. Adapted from *The Principles and Practice of Obstetrics* (p. 510, fig. 439), by J. B. De Lee, 1914, Philadelphia, PA: W. B. Saunders. In the public domain.

unaware of the presence of a significant uterine anomaly. The accuracy of sonographic studies is influenced by hardware and software, the experience and skill of the sonographer and radiologist, the habitus of the client, and the quality of the images. Magnetic-resonance imaging is the standard for accurately diagnosing uterine anomalies and identifying related anomalies in the urinary tract.

Surgical resection of a uterine septum can decrease the risk of spontaneous abortion and PTB in individuals with recurrent pregnancy loss. Surgery does not seem to improve reproductive outcomes for those with didelphys or bicornuate uteruses. Cerclage is also sometimes used to reduce the risk of recurrent pregnancy loss and PTB due to a bicornuate uterus. Uterine anomalies are a contraindication for the use of the Bakri® uterine tamponade balloon and the Jada suction device for control of postpartum hemorrhage (Alydia Health, 2022; Cook Medical, 2020).

Metabolism

During pregnancy, maternal body temperature rises not only because basal metabolic rate increases by 20–25% (Danhausen & King, 2024), but also because of the effects of progesterone and heat generated by the metabolically active fetus. The mother compensates by sending more blood to the skin for cooling and by sweating more; but despite these mechanisms, the body temperature remains elevated by an average of 0.2–0.4F° (0.36–0.72C°). A pregnant mother's resting oxygen consumption is 20–30% greater than that of a nonpregnant counterpart (Murray & Hendley, 2020).

Protein and Lipid Metabolism

Maternal serum cholesterol and triglyceride levels increase markedly through the last months of pregnancy to build fetal cell membranes and steroid hormones, and fasting plasma triglycerides rise to levels two to four times higher than before pregnancy (Murray & Hendley, 2020). Lipolysis (fat-burning) increases, allowing the mother to burn free fatty acids, triglycerides, and ketone bodies for fuel and reserve more glucose and amino acids for fetal use.

The placenta actively transports amino acids to the fetus for use in protein synthesis and as fuel (Antony et al., 2021) and is also involved in protein synthesis (Cunningham et al., 2022, ch. 4). Amino acid concentrations are higher in the fetus (Cunningham et al., 2022, ch. 4). In late pregnancy, about half the protein consumed by a pregnant mother is deposited in the fetus to be used for growth, and the remainder accumulates in the placenta, uterine muscle, breast, and other maternal tissues (Cunningham et al., 2022, ch. 4).

Drug Metabolism

Pharmacokinetics (the movement of drugs into, through, and out of the body) includes the processes of drug absorption, distribution, metabolism, and excretion. *Pharmacodynamics* refers to the effects of the drug on the body (Kazma, van den Anker, Allegaert, Dallmann, & Ahmadzia, 2020). These mechanisms change significantly during pregnancy because of an increase in plasma volume, a decrease in plasma proteins, weight gain, change in fat composition, and changes in renal, cardiovascular, and gastrointestinal function (Kazma et al., 2020). The gastrointestinal tract moves more slowly during pregnancy, potentially altering

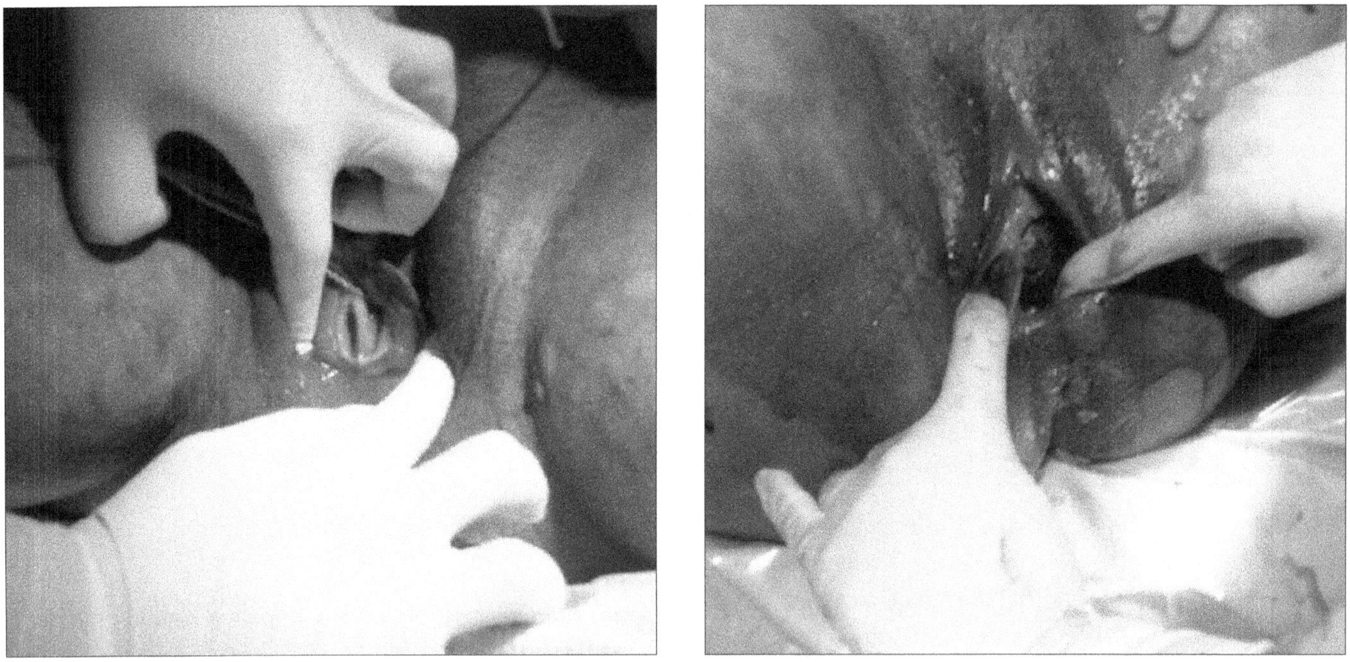

Figure 2-6. A 29-year-old gravida 2, para 0 (G2 P0) woman in Bangladesh at 38 4/7 weeks of gestation with didelphys uterus. She presented with rupture of membranes and bloody show but no contractions. Her left cervix was 1/50/−3, and her right cervix was closed. She was induced with misoprostol and augmented with oxytocin. She received epidural anesthesia and progressed to full cervical dilation of the left cervix with the right cervix dilated to 4–5 cm. As the baby descended in second stage, the vaginal septum tore completely. She had a vaginal birth of a boy weighing 5 lb 6 oz (2,660 g) but was transferred to the operating room for removal of a retained placenta. From "Didelphys Uterus: A Case Report and Review of the Literature," by S. Rezai et al., 2015, *Case Reports in Obstetrics and Gynecology*. CC BY 3.0.

drug absorption. Renal filtration rates increase and accelerate excretion of some medications. The second-trimester drop in maternal blood pressure (BP) can increase the orthostatic hypotension associated with certain medications such as antipsychotics, tricyclic antidepressants, and antihypertensives. Some medications, such as gentamicin and cefazolin, require higher doses to achieve therapeutic serum levels during pregnancy, creating the potential for toxicity after birth. Pregnant clients can require higher doses of ampicillin but lower doses of theophylline, for example, than nonpregnant ones (Brucker & King, 2019).

Carbohydrate Metabolism

The growing fetus requires glucose as a primary source of energy for cellular metabolism. To support continuous transport of glucose to the fetus and placenta, placental hormones cause dramatic physiologic changes in maternal carbohydrate metabolism (Antony et al., 2021). Maternal blood glucose is generally 10–20% higher than that of the fetus to ensure uninterrupted flow of glucose across the placenta into the fetus by facilitated diffusion (King, Brucker et al., 2015; Murray & Hendley, 2020). Maternal fasting glucose levels can be lower than those of the nonpregnant, and postprandial (after-meal) levels can be higher; but the fetus is not generally affected by these extremes in maternal serum glucose levels (Murray & Hendley, 2020).

Insulin-secreting pancreatic beta cells enlarge to produce more insulin (Antony et al., 2021). The body of a healthy pregnant mother develops increased insulin sensitivity early in gestation, encouraging the uptake of glucose into fat stores to prepare for the energy requirements of later pregnancy. As pregnancy progresses, however, maternal and placental hormones (including estrogen, progesterone, leptin, cortisol, placental lactogen, and placental growth hormone) promote a state of mild insulin resistance to facilitate easy transport of glucose across the placenta to support fetal growth. Endogenous glucose production and the breakdown of fat stores increase, further raising blood-glucose and free fatty-acid concentrations. Transient maternal hyperglycemia (high blood glucose), often noted after meals, is due to increasing insulin resistance, and transient hypoglycemia before meals and overnight is due to the unrelenting fetal requirements.

Gestational Diabetes

Gestational diabetes mellitus (GDM) develops when pregnancy-related changes in glucose metabolism are excessive and the mother develops persistent hyperglycemia. The term *diabetes mellitus* derives from the Greek *diabetes*, meaning to

Table 2-1
Distribution of Weight Gain in Pregnancy

- Fetus: 7–8 lb (3,200–3,600 g)
- Fat stores: 6–8 lb (2,700–3,600 g)
- Increased blood volume: 3–4 lb (1,400–1,800 g)
- Increased extravascular fluid volume: 2–3 lb (900–1,400 g)
- Amniotic fluid: 2 lb (900 g)
- Breast enlargement: 1–3 lb (450–1, 400g)
- Uterine hypertrophy: 2 lb (900 g)
- Placenta: 1 lb 8 oz (700 g)

Adapted from "Gestational Weight Gain," by L. Poston, 2023, in V. A. Barss (Ed.), *UpToDate*. Copyright by UpToDate.

siphon or pass through (a reference to frequent urination), and the Latin *mellitus*, meaning sweet, a reference to the sweet-tasting urine voided by people with this condition (Sapra & Bhandari, 2023). GDM is defined as diabetes diagnosed in the second or third trimester of pregnancy that was not evident before gestation (Durnwald, 2023b). GDM is common, affecting about 14–16% of pregnancies globally (Plows, Stanley, Baker, Reynolds, & Vickers, 2018).

There is no clear threshold of higher risk for poor obstetric outcomes (Durnwald, 2023b). Poorly controlled GDM increases risk for (Durnwald, 2023b)

- Hypertensive disorders of pregnancy (which can carry a risk of iatrogenic PTB);
- Large for gestational age or macrosomic newborn (which increases risk for shoulder dystocia and maternal and/or newborn birth trauma);
- Operative delivery (vacuum, forceps, or cesarean);
- Stillbirth;
- Fetal/neonatal hypertrophic cardiomyopathy;
- Neonatal respiratory problems and metabolic complications (e.g., hypoglycemia, hyperbilirubinemia, hypocalcemia, polycythemia); and
- Polyhydramnios.

The client with impaired glucose tolerance is typically referred to a medical nutritional therapist, who formulates an individualized dietary plan and teaches the client to monitor blood-glucose levels. Glucose readings are usually assessed before breakfast (fasting) and 1 or 2 hr after the beginning of a meal. Target antepartum glucose readings (Caughey, 2023) are typically

- Fasting blood-glucose concentration: less than 95 mg/dl (5.3 mmol/L);
- 1-hr postprandial blood-glucose concentration: less than 140 mg/dl (7.8 mmol/L); and
- 2-hr postprandial blood-glucose concentration: less than 120 mg/dl (6.7 mmol/L).

Table 2-2
Risk Factors for Gestational Diabetes Mellitus (GDM)

- Physical inactivity.
- First-degree relative with diabetes.
- Membership in a high-risk population (e.g., African American, Hispanic, Native American, Asian American, Pacific Islander).
- Previous birth of an infant weighing 8 lb 13 oz (4,000 g) or more.
- Previous GDM.
- Hypertension (140/90 mm Hg) or therapy for hypertension.
- Significantly elevated triglycerides or low high-density lipoprotein cholesterol level.
- Polycystic ovarian syndrome.
- Hemoglobin A1C ≥5.7%.
- Impaired glucose tolerance or impaired fasting glucose on previous testing.
- Prepregnancy BMI >40 kg/m^2.
- History of cardiovascular disease.

Adapted from "Gestational Diabetes Mellitus," by American College of Obstetricians and Gynecologists, 2018/2019. Copyright by ACOG.

Up to 85% of individuals with gestational diabetes can achieve target glucose levels with lifestyle changes alone (Durnwald, 2023a). A meal plan for clients with GDM usually includes three small- to moderate-sized meals and two to four snacks and is adjusted in response to glucose monitoring values, appetite, weight changes, maternal dietary preferences, exercise programs, and personal schedules (Durnwald, 2023a). A program of moderate exercise can reduce both fasting and postprandial blood-glucose concentrations. Exercise that increases muscle mass, such as cycling, walking or circuit training is especially effective (Cremona, O'Gorman, Cotter, Saunders, & Donnelly, 2018). Although glucose readings generally normalize postpartum, clients with GDM are at high risk for recurrent GDM and for developing impaired glucose tolerance or overt diabetes within five years (Durnwald, 2023a). GDM has also been associated with higher long-term maternal risks for cardiovascular disease and obesity, abnormal glucose tolerance, hypertension, and metabolic syndrome in the offspring (Caughey, 2023).

Cardiovascular System

In pregnancy the heart is pushed up and to the left by displacement of the diaphragm and pregnancy-related flaring of the rib cage. It also rotates along its long axis, causing it to appear enlarged on imaging studies (Antony et al., 2021). The growing uterus raises the diaphragm about 1.6 in. (4 cm), which pushes the heart up and to the left into a more horizontal position (Blackburn, 2021). The chambers of the heart dilate and the heart muscle thickens, enlarging the ventricular wall muscle by 10–15% and lengthening of myocardial fibers in a process like the reversible cardiac remodeling caused by athletic training (Antony et al., 2021; Murray & Hendley, 2020).

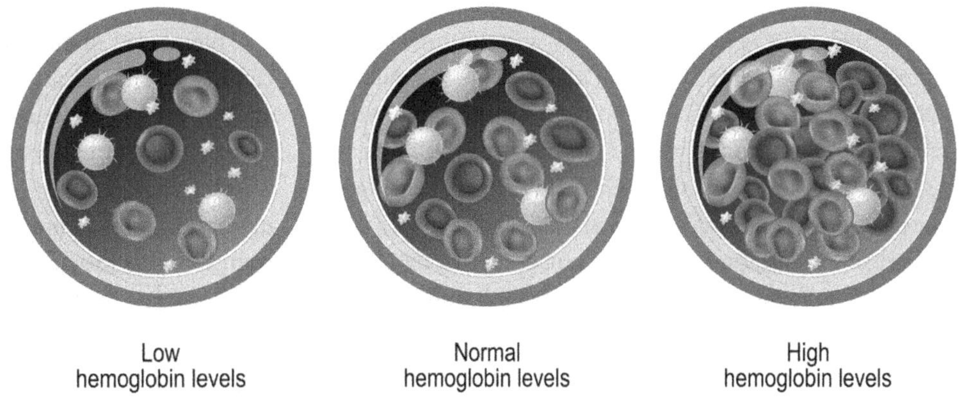

Figure 2-7. Levels of hemoglobin. Low hemoglobin levels reduce the ability of the blood to carry oxygen and can be associated with inadequate intake of iron. High hemoglobin levels increase the viscosity of maternal blood, potentially impeding uteroplacental circulation (©designua/Adobe Stock).

During pregnancy, changes to the maternal cardiovascular system maximize oxygen delivery to mother and fetus. Red blood cell (RBC) mass—the mass of all red cells in circulation, not of individual cells—begins to increase around 10 weeks of gestation in response to the higher metabolic requirement for oxygen. During pregnancy, the number of RBCs increases by as much as 20–30% (Gersh, 2022). RBC mass typically increases about 18% by the end of pregnancy, but iron supplementation can raise RBC mass by an additional 30% and create a corresponding improvement in hemoglobin levels (Antony et al., 2021).

White blood cell (WBC) count rises in response to the physiologic stress of pregnancy (Chandra, Tripathi, Mishra, Amzarul, & Vaish, 2012). The additional stress of childbirth can elevate WBC counts markedly—healthy mothers can have a WBC count as high as 25,000–30,000/mm^3 in labor and for a few hours postpartum (Antony et al., 2021). A mother who has received betamethasone to accelerate lung maturation of a preterm fetus will have a transient elevation in WBCs after the injections, as well as an elevation in blood-glucose levels.

Within 5 weeks of conception, maternal blood vessels throughout the body have begun to soften and enlarge (Murray & Hendley, 2020). This vasodilation causes underfilling of the maternal vasculature, which triggers increased fluid and electrolyte retention, causing the plasma and extracellular fluid volumes to expand (Murray & Hendley, 2020). Pregnant individuals retain about 1000 mEq of sodium and 6–8 L of water (Gersh, 2022).

Blood volume increases by 40–50% over prepregnant levels, beginning as early as 6 weeks of gestation, peaking at 30–34 weeks of gestation, then stabilizing until the baby is born (Antony et al., 2021). On average, pregnancy increases intravascular volume about 1.5 L (Chandra et al., 2012). This increase in blood volume is necessary to perfuse the placenta and the enlarged reproductive organs; protect against orthostatic and supine hypotension; support the metabolic needs of the fetus; improve perfusion of other maternal organs; compensate for the increased capacity of dilated maternal arteries and veins; dissipate excess body heat; and serve as a hemodynamic safeguard against excessive blood loss during birth (Murray & Hendley, 2020).

Plasma volume increases 30–50%, outpacing the production of new RBCs and thus creating a physiologic dilutional anemia that reaches a nadir at 30–34 weeks of gestation (Antony et al., 2021; Gersh, 2022). This decrease in the proportion of RBCs decreases blood viscosity, facilitating tissue perfusion and reducing cardiac workload. Mild anemia is therefore an indicator of good health in pregnancy, suggesting an expanding plasma volume (Saleem, Muhammed, Al-Hetty, & Salman, 2022). Lack of this hemodilution, as evidenced by a hemoglobin concentration of 14.6 g/dl or higher at the first prenatal visit, increases risk of stillbirth (Gersh, 2022) and can be an early warning sign of preeclampsia. Hemoglobin greater than 13 g/dl in the second trimester is associated with FGR, low birthweight, stillbirth, PTL, and pregnancy-induced hypertension (Mattson & Smith, 2016). In the United States, iron deficiency anemia is most likely to develop in mothers who are multiparous, socioeconomically disadvantaged, and/or of African or Hispanic descent.

Heart rate increases approximately 15–20 beats per min, and BP decreases from prepregnancy values as early as 7 weeks of gestation (Gersh, 2022). In healthy mothers, this decrease reaches a nadir in the second trimester. Second-trimester readings as low as 90/60 are common due to vasodilation, especially in small, young mothers and those who exercise regularly. Persistently low BP carries a small increased risk of stillbirth (Warland, 2012). BP that fails to decrease during the second trimester can indicate chronic hypertension or a higher risk for developing pregnancy-induced hypertension (Danhausen & King, 2024).

Elevated blood-pressure is always a cause for concern in pregnancy. A reading of 140/90 can indicate the onset of a serious hypertensive disorder, if accompanied by generalized edema and symptoms such as malaise, headache, or epigastric pain. Readings higher than 160/110 are considered severe-range hypertension and are managed acutely with antihypertensive medications to prevent congestive heart failure, myocardial ischemia, renal injury or failure, and ischemic or hemorrhagic stroke (American College of Obstetricians & Gynecologists [ACOG], 2020). BP elevations occurring before 20 weeks of gestation are generally diagnosed as chronic hypertension; those occurring afterwards are usually diagnosed as gestational hypertension or preeclampsia.

Beginning early in the first trimester, cardiac output increases up to 50%, aided by elevated heart rate, lower systemic vascular resistance, and greater blood volume. By weeks 25–30, total blood volume reaches about 5,000–6,000 ml (Danhausen & King, 2024). Most of this increase is directed to the uterus, placenta, and breasts; by term, the uterus receives 17% (450–650 ml/min) of the mother's cardiac output (Antony et al., 2021).

During labor, cardiac output becomes even more robust, increasing an additional 15% in early labor, 25% in active labor, and about 50% while pushing (Gersh, 2022). To protect against excessive blood loss, the uterus contracts immediately after birth, returning as much as 500–750 ml of blood from the placental bed and uterine vasculature to the maternal circulation and relieving pressure on the vena cava (Gersh, 2022). In the first 10–30 min postpartum, maternal heart rate often decreases, probably because of this increase in blood volume (Antony et al., 2021). Postpartum cardiac output increases by 80% above prelabor values despite postpartum blood loss (Gersh, 2022).

Activity, anxiety, or slight changes of posture can greatly influence cardiac output, pulse rate, BP, and regional blood flow (Murray & Hendley, 2020). Postural hypotension, evidenced by dizziness and fainting when standing, can become pronounced during pregnancy because of low peripheral vascular resistance and pooling of blood in the legs. Pressure from the gravid uterus can compress the aorta and vena cava, reducing cardiac output when the mother lies supine. About 10% of pregnant individuals will show symptoms of supine hypotensive syndrome within 3–10 min of lying flat (Gersh, 2022; Murray & Hendley, 2020). The client can become bradycardic, hypotensive, lightheaded, short of breath, panicky, or nauseated and can even lose consciousness because of reduced blood flow to the brain. Aortic and vena caval compression can also reduce blood flow to the uterus, placenta, and fetus. Circulation can be restored by placing the client on the left side or creating a 30° tilt by placing a pillow or wedge under one hip.

Blood clots more easily in pregnancy because of increased clotting factors, decreased fibrinolysis, and decreased anticoagulant activity, lowering the mother's risk of hemorrhage but raising the risk of venous thrombosis (Danhausen & King, 2024). Compression of the inferior vena cava by the pregnant uterus increases venous stasis in the lower extremities and contributes to the development of varicose veins in the legs, rectum, vulva, and pelvis. This combination of dilated veins, sluggish venous return, and a propensity to clot increases the risk of thromboembolic disease (e.g., deep-vein thrombosis, pulmonary embolism) five- to sixfold (Antony et al., 2021). About 85% of venous thrombosis in pregnancy develops in the left leg because of compression of the left iliac vein by the overlying iliac and ovarian arteries (Murray & Hendley, 2020). These clots can break free and migrate to the lungs to become a pulmonary embolus—a leading cause of maternal death. Pulmonary embolism can occur at any stage of pregnancy but is most common during the postpartum period.

Normal maternal cardiovascular adaptations to pregnancy often mimic pathological processes, and symptoms of cardiac disease can masquerade as normal changes of pregnancy. Dyspnea (difficulty breathing) occurs in normal pregnancy but also with cardiac and lung disease. Pregnancy-related dyspnea usually occurs before 20 weeks of gestation and does not worsen with advancing gestation (Antony et al., 2021). Physiologic dyspnea, thought to be secondary to the increased effort of inspiratory muscles, is usually mild, does interfere with daily activities, and does not occur at rest (Antony et al., 2021). Normal pregnancy can also involve fatigue, lower exercise tolerance, orthopnea (dyspnea when supine), occasional syncope, and chest discomfort that can mimic cardiac disease. A normal pregnant mother can have peripheral edema, mild tachycardia, a new-onset systolic murmur, and jugular venous distension that could indicate cardiac disease in the nonpregnant (Antony et al., 2021). Chest pain with exertion, worsening orthopnea, coughing up blood, or waking in the night with difficulty breathing is not normal and warrants investigation by a cardiologist (Antony et al., 2021).

From the first trimester, the first heart sound becomes louder on auscultation due to increased blood flow across the pulmonic and aortic valves, and a subtle third heart sound can be due to rapid diastolic filling (Antony et al., 2021; Gersh, 2022). The provider sometimes hears exaggerated splitting of S-1 and a systolic ejection murmur up to grade 2/4 over the pulmonary and tricuspid areas. Although systolic murmurs are almost universal in pregnancy, diastolic murmurs are unusual and can suggest a pathological process. Arrhythmias such as supraventricular tachycardia and premature ventricular contractions are frequently noted in healthy pregnant individuals, but the client with persistent symptomatic palpitations should be referred to a cardiologist (Antony et al., 2021).

In pregnancy, platelet count typically decreases slightly, but platelet function increases to maintain hemostasis. Roughly 8% of pregnant individuals develop gestational thrombocytopenia with platelet counts between 70,000 and 150,000/mm3 (Antony et al., 2021). Gestational thrombocytopenia does not increase the risk of pregnancy complications, and platelet counts normalize by 1–2 weeks postpartum. Low platelets can also indicate disease processes that can be serious or life-threatening, including preeclampsia, HELLP (**H**emolysis, **E**levated **L**iver enzymes, **L**ow **P**latelets) syndrome, disseminated intravascular coagulation, acute fatty liver of pregnancy, immune thrombocytopenia, hereditary thrombocytopenia, antiphospholipid syndrome, or thrombotic thrombocytopenic purpura (Park, 2022).

Respiratory System

The respiratory system must change dramatically to meet maternal and fetal metabolic needs. Numerous modifications in form and function allow the mother's body to meet these demands. In the first trimester, long before the gravid uterus rises into the abdomen, the ribs flare, changing the subcostal angle from 68° to as much as 103° (Weinberger, 2023). As pregnancy progresses, the diaphragm rises as much as 1.6 in. (4 cm), decreasing the length of the lungs, but the chest diameter increases 0.8 in. (2 cm), or more, growing wider front to back and becoming more barrel-shaped (Weinberger, 2023).

Pregnant individuals require 20–40% more oxygen to meet the demands of the placenta, fetus, and maternal organs (Antony et al., 2021). The amount of air held by the lungs at maximal inspiration decreases 5%, but from 8 weeks of gestation, tidal volume (amount of air moved with each breath) increases 30–40% (Blackburn, 2021). Arterial oxygen levels rise. Arterial carbon dioxide levels decline during pregnancy, making the blood more alkaline and presumably helping the fetus to eliminate carbon dioxide across the placenta (Weinberger, 2023). To correct this physiologic respiratory alkalosis, the kidneys excrete bicarbonate, shifting a pregnant client's pH to the alkalotic end of the normal range and creating mild compensated respiratory alkalosis. Healthy gravidas carrying twins have similar respiratory function to those carrying a single fetus (Weinberger, 2023).

In labor, demand increases another 40–60% (Blackburn, 2021). Oxygen consumption can triple during a contraction (Antony et al., 2021). Thus, maternal oxygen reserves decrease during labor. Pregnant individuals become hypoxic more quickly than their nonpregnant counterparts. If a laboring mother becomes apneic for only 3 min, life-threatening hypoxia, hypercapnia, and respiratory acidosis can develop (Antony et al., 2021).

Because of these changes in respiratory physiology, up to 70% of pregnant people feel short of breath at times, even when they are apparently breathing normally and oxygen saturations are optimal (Blackburn, 2021). Breathlessness seems to result from the mother's perception of overbreathing, effects of progesterone, greater need for oxygen, a decrease in (and altered sensitivity to) CO_2 levels (Murray & Hendley, 2020), and later in pregnancy by pressure on the diaphragm from the growing uterus (Blackburn, 2021). Sitting or standing tall and holding the hands high above the head while taking deep breaths can lessen the sensation of breathlessness (Murray & Hendley, 2020). Shortness of breath in pregnancy can also be a sign of cardiac or pulmonary disease, so any complaint of difficulty breathing should be evaluated carefully.

The mucosa of the nasal passages develop vascular congestion and edema during pregnancy. There is an increase in mucus secretion caused by increased estrogen. These changes can cause nasal congestion and rhinitis. Epistaxis (nosebleed) is common. The mother with nasal congestion should avoid using nasal decongestants because of the risk for hypertension and rebound congestion (Antony et al., 2021); saline sprays or use of a neti pot can safely clear mucus and provide some relief. Humidifying a dry bedroom can also improve symptoms.

Snoring is two to three times more common during pregnancy and indicates upper airway restriction or obstruction. Sleep-disordered breathing (SDB) is a serious disorder involving repeated episodes of hypopnea or apnea (partial or complete airway obstruction during sleep), intermittent hypoxia, and sleep fragmentation (Laposky & Pemberton, 2021). SDB leads to elevated sympathetic tone, oxidative stress, systemic inflammation, endothelial dysfunction, and glucose dysregulation, and it is associated with hypertension, diabetes, and other serious conditions (Laposky & Pemberton, 2021). Mucosal edema, nasal congestion, increased blood volume, diaphragm elevation, a more compressible airway, and increased fat deposition in the upper airway predispose the gravida to SDB. The incidence of SDB is two to three times higher during pregnancy and carries an increased risk of preeclampsia and gestational diabetes (Laposky & Pemberton, 2021). If a pregnant client reports snoring or significant sleep disturbance, refer to a specialist in sleep disorders for evaluation. Although sleep-clinic polysomnography is the standard for diagnosing sleep disorders, home testing with U.S. Food and Drug Administration–approved devices is reliable, convenient, and relatively inexpensive.

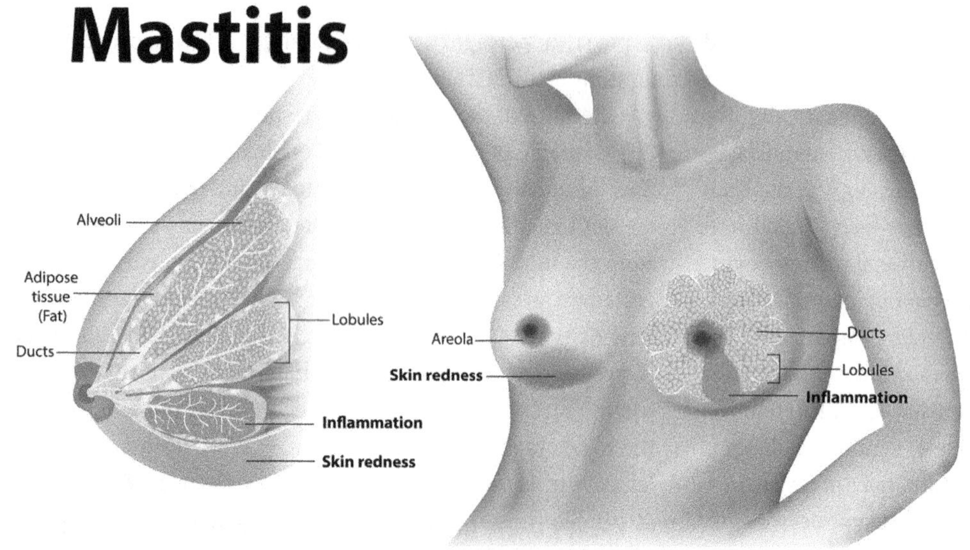

Figure 2-8. Mastitis involves inflammation and/or infection within the glandular breast tissue. Infective mastitis is usually caused by *Staphylococcus aureus* (including methicillin-resistant *S. aureus*, a.k.a. MRSA), *S. epidermidis*, streptococci, and sometimes gram-negative rods (©sakurra/Adobe Stock).

Breasts

In pregnancy, progesterone, estrogen, human growth hormone, thyroxine, prolactin, and human placental lactogen prepare the breasts for lactating by *hypertrophy*, enlarging the cells of the breast, and *hyperplasia*, increasing the number of breast cells (Danhausen & King, 2024). The mature breast weighs an average of 200 g in the nonpregnant state, 500 g during pregnancy, and 600–800 g when lactating (Antony et al., 2021). Toward the end of pregnancy, the alveoli begin to secrete colostrum, but high levels of progesterone largely suppress milk production.

The areolas enlarge and darken; the contrast between the dark areola and the lighter surrounding skin provides a visual cue for an infant attempting to nurse (Antony et al., 2021). Sebaceous and sweat glands (Montgomery tubercles) enlarge during pregnancy and lactation, and they secrete lubricating and anti-infective substances that protect the nipple and areola during lactation. A nursing mother should avoid washing the nipples with soap, which will wash away these substances and predispose to cracking and infection.

Humans, like all mammals, have the potential to develop mammary-gland or nipple tissue anywhere along a milk line that extends from the axilla and inner upper arm down the abdomen and along the midclavicular line to the upper lateral mons and upper inner thigh (Antony et al., 2021). Accessory breast tissue is most commonly found in the axilla; it can swell painfully during pregnancy or with the onset of lactation. About 11% of people with supernumerary nipples also have renal abnormalities (Antony et al., 2021).

Mastitis

Lactational mastitis affects one in seven nursing mothers (Barker, Peters, Adelson, & Steen, 2020). This condition develops when blocked milk ducts cause inflammation and infection of the breast. Mastitis most commonly develops within the first four weeks postpartum and is associated with maternal fatigue, poor nursing technique, nipple trauma, rapid reduction in nursing frequency, and constrictive clothing. Symptoms can include localized pain; redness; and flu-like symptoms, such as fever, shaking chills, nausea, and vomiting (Barker et al., 2020). Antibiotic therapy should be started upon diagnosis to avoid progression to a breast abscess or even to septic shock. Mastitis is usually treated with a regimen of dicloxacillin 500 mg every 6 hr for 10–14 days; cephalexin or clindamycin can be used if the mother has a penicillin allergy. Management of mastitis includes (Antony et al., 2021)

- A supportive bra;
- Appropriate fluid intake;
- Evaluation of nursing technique;
- Nursing on the uninfected side first to establish let-down, taking care to completely empty the infected breast with each feeding. Use a breast pump if the baby does not empty the breast; and
- Analgesia with a nonsteroidal anti-inflammatory medication such as ibuprofen.

Breast abscess will occur in approximately 10% of mothers who develop infective mastitis (Antony et al., 2021). The client will usually feel quite ill, have a high fever of 102.2°F (39°C) or more, and have a red, firm, tender area on the breast that can be softer in the center. Abscesses are most likely to develop in the upper outer quadrant of the breast.

Gastrointestinal System

In pregnancy, hormonal and mechanical changes alter the functioning of many organs and structures along the alimentary canal. Late in pregnancy, the stomach and intestines are displaced upward, and the diaphragm is raised. The appendix can be displaced upward and laterally, sometimes reaching the right flank (Antony et al., 2021). The motility of the small intestines and colon can change, causing constipation in some gravidas and loose stools in others.

The normal reference ranges for many liver-function tests change during pregnancy. Placental metabolism causes marked elevations in serum alkaline phosphatase values, and hemodilution from increased plasma volume causes a decrease in serum albumin. There is an increase in many proteins produced by the liver, including fibrinogen.

In pregnancy, gallbladder volume increases about 50% and gallbladder contractility declines (Cunningham et al., 2022, ch. 4). The composition of the bile becomes more favorable to the formation of cholesterol crystals. This concentrated, cholesterol-rich bile pools within the gallbladder and can become stones and sludge (Antony et al., 2021).

Because progesterone and estrogen reduce muscle tone and strength in the lower esophageal sphincter, acidic gastric secretions are more likely to reflux into the lower esophagus. Up to 85% of pregnant individuals experience heartburn (pyrosis) and reflux (Murray & Hendley, 2020). Although pregnancy does not appear to directly affect antepartum gastric emptying, food can remain in the stomach for a prolonged time during labor at term (Antony et al., 2021). Consequently, the mother who requires general anesthesia for cesarean birth is at greater risk of aspirating gastric contents. Increased levels of progesterone and compression by the fetus prolong the transit of food through the intestines as well (Bianco, 2023).

Intrahepatic Cholestasis of Pregnancy (ICP)

Intrahepatic cholestasis of pregnancy is a condition involving a decrease in bile flow from the liver, resulting in the accumulation of bile components in the liver and in the blood. Signs and symptoms include severe pruritus (itching) that typically worsens at night (particularly on the palms and on the soles of the feet); an elevation in levels of serum bile acids; and often elevations in bilirubin, alkaline phosphatase, and serum transaminase levels (Cunningham et al., 2022, ch. 58). The cause is unclear, but susceptibility is probably related to a combination of genetic, hormonal, and environmental influences (Lindor & Lee, 2023). It most commonly develops in the later part of the second or third trimester and resolves quickly postpartum. ICP increases the risk for intrauterine demise, PTB, and neonatal respiratory distress syndrome, particularly when bile acid levels are very high.

Nausea and Vomiting

About 70–85% of pregnant individuals experience nausea and vomiting during pregnancy, often called "morning sickness" (Murray & Hendley, 2020). Typically, nausea first occurs in the 4th week of pregnancy, worsens as human chorionic gonadotropin (hCG) levels peak at 5–10 weeks of gestation, then disappears by 20 weeks of gestation (Murray & Hendley, 2020). Symptoms linger through 20–22 weeks of gestation for 10–25% of gravidas, and some have symptoms throughout gestation (Antony et al., 2021). Although persistent nausea and vomiting can greatly interfere with daily activities, increase health care costs, and necessitate time off work, simple morning sickness does not usually cause significant weight loss or electrolyte disturbance (Antony et al., 2021). The condition is influenced by genetic, cultural, endocrine, environmental, and psychosocial factors and tends to be more troublesome for younger mothers, multigravidas, and mothers carrying more than one fetus (Murray & Hendley, 2020). Except in the case of molar pregnancies, pregnancies complicated by nausea and vomiting are less likely to end in miscarriage than those that are not (Cunningham et al., 2022, ch. 4).

Supportive care includes reassurance that the condition is common and not usually detrimental to the pregnancy as well as dietary modifications such as small frequent meals, increasing protein intake, and avoiding foods that trigger nausea. Nausea and vomiting of pregnancy is sometimes related to deficiency of vitamin B_6 and is less likely to occur if the mother takes prenatal vitamins for a month before conception (ACOG, 2018/2021). Vitamin B_6 therapy, alone or in combination with doxylamine (Unisom® et al.), is well studied and shown to be safe and effective (ACOG, 2018/2021; Antony et al., 2021). Acupuncture, acupressure, acupressure wristbands, or supplementation with ginger root can be beneficial.

Hyperemesis Gravidarum

Hyperemesis gravidarum is the most severe form of nausea and vomiting in pregnancy and affects about 0.3–3% of gestations (ACOG, 2018/2021). Definitions differ, but clinical criteria for diagnosis usually include persistent vomiting unrelated to other causes, evidence of acute starvation (usually large ketones in the urine), and weight loss (usually at least 5% of prepregnancy weight). Sometimes severe dehydration and electrolyte, thyroid, or liver abnormalities are present. Nausea and vomiting are not always attributable to pregnancy alone, especially when symptoms are severe or when onset occurs after 9 weeks of gestation (Antony et al., 2021). Consider other conditions, including COVID-19 (SARS-CoV-2), hepatitis, gallbladder disease, appendicitis, intestinal obstruction, pyelonephritis, or, in the second half of pregnancy, preeclampsia (Cunningham et al., 2022, ch. 4).

Endocrine System

The placenta serves as an important endocrine gland for mother and fetus, secreting hormones, growth factors, and other substances (Blackburn, 2021). The most significant of these hormones are hCG, human placental lactogen (hPL), estrogen, and progesterone. To support the dramatic metabolic changes of pregnancy, the placenta also produces hormones similar to those made by many other glands (Blackburn, 2021; Simmonds, Karsenty, Karaplis, & Kovacs, 2010). It plays a role in the metabolism of glycogen, cholesterol, and protein and produces peptide hormones (hCG, hPL, cytokines, growth hormone, insulin-like growth factors, corticotropin releasing hormone, vascular endothelial growth factor, placental growth factor) and steroid hormones such as estrogens, progesterone, and glucocorticoids (Roberts & Myatt, 2023).

The placenta secretes hCG largely to ensure that the corpus luteum maintains production of progesterone and estrogen until the placenta takes over production about 10 weeks of gestation (Blackburn, 2021). The presence of hCG can inhibit contractions, support uterine growth, and benefit maternal immune function. It can also play a part in fetal testosterone and corticosteroid production and the development of fetal blood vessels. Estrogens, initially secreted by the ovaries and thereafter by the placenta, inhibit the development of ovarian follicles during pregnancy, increase production of hormone-binding globulins in the liver, prepare the breasts for lactation, and influence the contractility of the uterus (Blackburn, 2021). Progesterone, first produced by the corpus luteum and later chiefly by the placenta, primes the decidua for implantation and impedes uterine contractions by inhibiting prostaglandins (PGs) and decreasing contraction-associated proteins (Blackburn, 2021). Progesterone relaxes the smooth muscle in the gastrointestinal and renal systems, promotes systemic vasodilation to accommodate the expanded volume of blood, changes respiratory-center sensitivity to carbon dioxide, promotes breast development for lactation, and helps reprogram the immune system to stop it from attacking the genetically foreign fetus and placenta (Blackburn, 2021).

Relaxin is secreted first by the corpus luteum, then by the myometrium and placenta. It helps to inhibit contractions, can help suppress oxytocin release during pregnancy, and plays a role in cervical ripening at term (Blackburn, 2021). During pregnancy, large concentrations of PGs and similar substances are found in the reproductive organs, decidua, and fetal membranes. PGs affect smooth-muscle contractility, vascular tone, myometrial contractility, and cervical ripening, and they can play a role in hypertensive disorders in pregnancy. Near term, the influence of corticotropin-releasing hormone, fetal cortisol, and uterine stretch increase the responsiveness of PG receptors. PGs help to initiate labor by forming gap junctions, which allow ions and electrical impulses to flow between cells; developing oxytocin receptors in the uterine muscle; and increasing the strength and number of uterine contractions (Blackburn, 2021).

The fetus needs maternal thyroid hormones for normal central nervous system development, most acutely in early pregnancy (Blackburn, 2021). Thyroid stimulating hormone (TSH) levels can be lower through the first trimester and slightly elevated at term. High levels of estrogen and hCG, which has mild thyroid-stimulating activity, and increased urinary excretion of iodide stimulate production of thyroxine, T4, and triiodothyronine, T3 (Ross, 2023). Total T4 and T3 peak by 10–15 weeks of gestation and remain 40%–100% higher than before pregnancy (Blackburn, 2021).

Because TSH and hCG are structurally similar, hCG can bind to a TSH receptor on thyroid epithelial cells and signal the thyroid to increase production, causing about 15% of gravidas to develop transient hyperthyroidism (Blackburn, 2021; Bowen, 2012). The clinical signs of hyperthyroidism can be easily mistaken for the normal changes of pregnancy—heat intolerance, tachycardia, and increased sweating (Ross, 2022). Untreated maternal hypothyroidism increases the risk of spontaneous abortion and abnormal fetal brain development (Antony et al., 2021).

The hypothalamus regulates and coordinates much of maternal endocrine function and sends releasing hormones to the pituitary. The anterior lobe of the pituitary gland enlarges up to threefold during pregnancy as the hormonal milieu changes: growth hormone production declines; adrenocorticotropic hormone increases; prolactin increases throughout pregnancy and rises further during lactation. The intermediate lobe of the pituitary also grows larger during pregnancy. It increases production of melanocyte-stimulating hormone (MSH), which is responsible for the hyperpigmentation (linea nigra, chloasma) common in pregnancy.

The posterior lobe of the pituitary gland stores antidiuretic hormone (ADH) and oxytocin, both of which are important to pregnancy. ADH influences plasma osmolality and sodium concentration. Maternal plasma concentrations rise continuously across gestation, and the uterus becomes more sensitive to its effects around the time of labor. Oxytocin causes uterine contractions and the "let down" of milk during lactation. Nipple stimulation stimulates oxytocin release, which in turn causes contraction of myoepithelial cells in ductal smooth muscle and milk ejection.

Renal and Urinary System

Kidneys enlarge by 0.4–0.6 in. (1.0–1.5 cm) during pregnancy, and kidney volume increases up to 30% (Thadhani & Maynard, 2022). Increased cardiac output, plasma volume expansion, and vasodilation increase renal perfusion and filtration. During pregnancy, blood flow to the kidneys increases 80%, and glomerular filtration rate (GFR) increases by 50% by the end of the first trimester (Antony et al., 2021).

Blood urea nitrogen levels are also lower in pregnancy at 8–10 mg/dl (Thadhani & Maynard, 2022). Serum creatinine concentration decreases to a normal range of 0.4–0.8 mg/dl in pregnancy. A serum creatinine of 0.9 mg/dl or higher, normal in the nonpregnant, indicates renal impairment during pregnancy and warrants prompt evaluation (Cunningham et al., 2022, ch. 4).

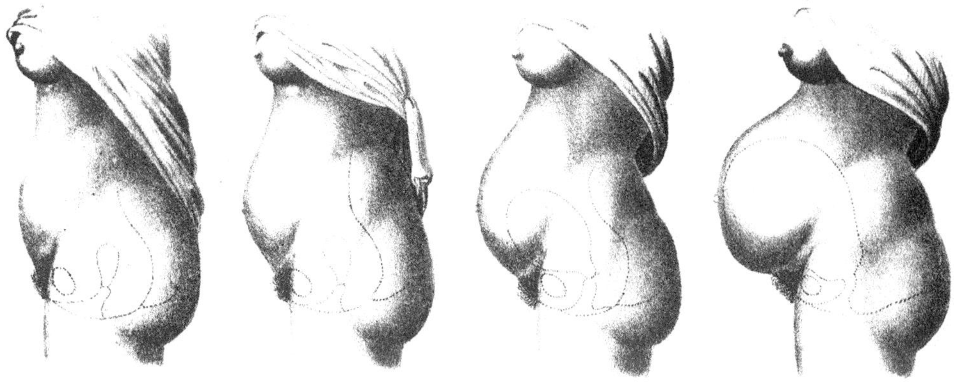

Figure 2-9. Posture and balance change markedly as gestation advances. The lumbar curve exaggerates into pronounced lordosis. From *Midwifery Illustrated* (plate 62), by J. P. Maygrier (A. S. Doane, Trans.), 1834, New York, NY: Harper & Brothers. In the public domain.

Progesterone relaxes the tone and decreases peristalsis of the ureters, and pressure from the gravid uterus and other structures can cause them to become displaced, elongated, or winding. Hydronephrosis (dilation and distension of the renal calyces) and hydroureter (distension of the upper two-thirds of the ureters) develop in up to 90% of pregnancies and are usually asymptomatic (Weerakkody & El-Feky, 2022). These conditions are thought to result from compression of the ureter between the gravid uterus and iliopsoas muscle (Weerakkody & El-Feky, 2022). These changes appear by the second trimester and can persist until 6–12 weeks postpartum (Thadhani & Maynard, 2022). A dilated renal collecting system can hold 200–300 ml of slow-moving urine, which can encourage bacterial growth and lead to pyelonephritis (Thadhani & Maynard, 2022). Urinary glucose excretion increases 100-fold because of the increased GFR (Danhausen & King, 2024). Alkaline urine with a higher glucose content, an increase in bladder volume, immune suppression, and inefficient ureteral valves also predispose the gravida toward UTI (Danhausen & King, 2024).

During pregnancy, nutrients such as amino acids and water-soluble vitamins are excreted through the urine in much greater amounts (Cunningham et al., 2022, ch. 4). Urinary protein excretion can be twice as high as in the nonpregnant, often reaching 180–200 mg per 24 hr in the third trimester, enough to result in a positive dipstick if the urine is concentrated (Thadhani & Maynard, 2022). Total urine protein excretion of more than 300 mg in 24 hr indicates abnormal kidney function and/or preeclampsia (Mattson & Smith, 2016). Healthy gravidas carrying multiples, however, appear to excrete more protein in the urine than those carrying singletons (Thadhani & Maynard, 2022).

Posture late in pregnancy greatly influences certain aspects of renal function. The kidneys excrete twice as much sodium when the mother assumes a lateral recumbent position as they do when the mother is lying supine (Cunningham et al., 2022, ch. 4). In pregnancy, urine calcium excretion increases substantially while excretion of urine citrate and magnesium (substances that protect against stone formation) increases only slightly (Preminger & Curhan, 2021). The urinary stasis of pregnancy can encourage excess calcium to form renal calculi (kidney stones), which can obstruct flow and cause or worsen ureteral dilation (Preminger & Curhan, 2021). Urinary stones are also extremely painful and increase the risk for pyelonephritis.

The mucosa of the bladder, like mucosae elsewhere in the body, becomes increasingly vascular and edematous during pregnancy (Thadhani & Maynard, 2022). Progesterone relaxes the bladder muscle and increases its capacity until the enlarging uterus squeezes it flat. Urinary frequency, nocturia (waking at night to void), dysuria (painful urination), urgency, and stress incontinence are common during pregnancy. Urinary incontinence occurs in response to uterine pressure on the bladder, hormonally influenced changes to the suspensory ligaments of the urethra, and altered function of the urethral sphincter (Thadhani & Maynard, 2022). Weak pelvic floor tone from previous pregnancies and high BMI can also play a role.

Total body water increases 6.5–8.5 L by the end of gestation, including an expansion of maternal blood volume by 1,500–1,600 ml and plasma volume by 1,200–1,300 ml (Antony et al., 2021). Urinary output increases 25% during pregnancy, and most gravidas experience urinary frequency and nocturia (Cunningham et al., 2022, ch. 4). Pregnant individuals can void more than seven times a day and more than twice overnight. They tend to develop dependent edema during the day and then mobilize this fluid through diuresis when recumbent at night, necessitating nocturnal urination.

Nervous System

Difficulties with attention, concentration, and memory are reported by many pregnant individuals; but systematic studies

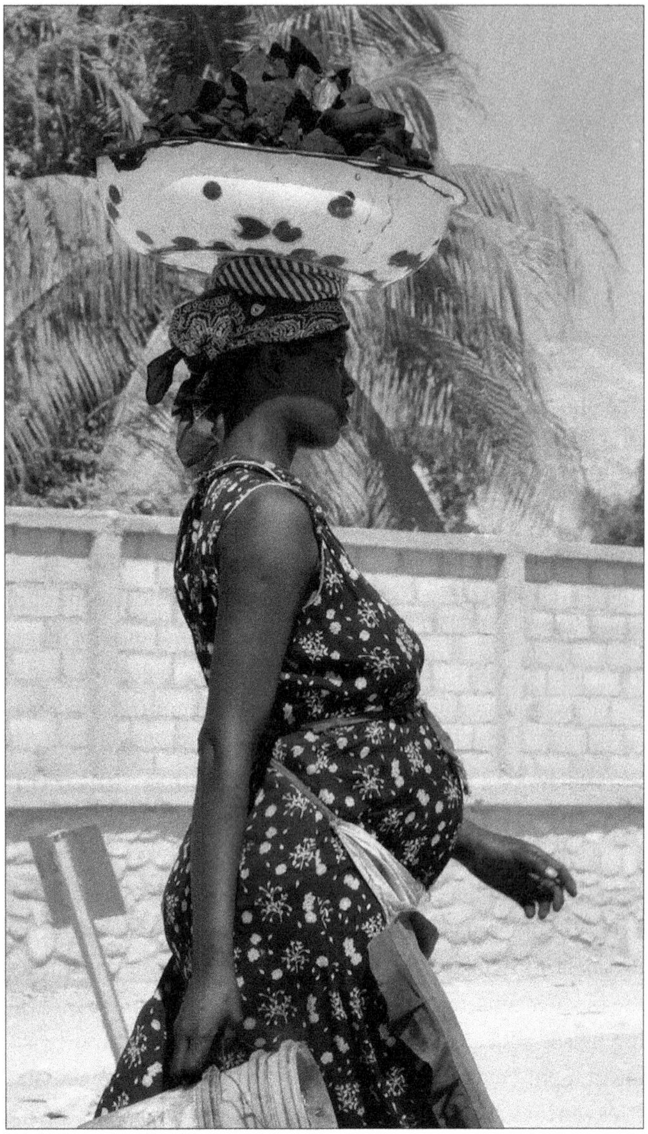

Figure 2-10. A pregnant woman carries a load of charcoal to be used for cooking food after a 7.0-magnitude earthquake in Haiti in 2010. Although remaining physically fit and active is beneficial to pregnancy and overall health, strenuous work appears to increase the risk of preterm birth (PTB). "Haiti relief efforts continue [Image 1 of 44]," by R. J. Fluegel, 2012 (https://www.dvidshub.net/image/251591/haiti-relief-efforts-continue). In the public domain.

of memory in pregnancy are limited, and reports are often anecdotal (Cunningham et al., 2022, ch. 4). Pregnancy-related memory decline appears to be worst in the third trimester and does not seem attributable to depression, anxiety, sleep deprivation, or physical changes of pregnancy (Cunningham et al., 2022, ch. 4; Davies, Lum, Skouteris, Byrne, & Hayden, 2018). These memory changes resolve quickly after pregnancy.

Mechanical and hormonal influences, such as nocturia, dyspnea, nasal congestion, stress, and anxiety as well as muscular aches and pains, leg cramps, and fetal activity can affect the sleep during pregnancy (Murray & Hendley, 2020). Sleep disturbances such as delayed sleep onset, frequent awakenings, and reduced sleep efficiency and duration begin as early as 12 weeks of gestation and continue through the first 2 months postpartum (Laposky & Pemberton, 2021). Sleep disturbance has been associated with longer labors, higher cesarean rates, anxiety, and depression (Murray & Hendley, 2020).

Integumentary System

To dissipate heat, blood flow to the skin increases to 300–400% of nonpregnant rates (Blackburn, 2021). Mucous membranes become very vascular, swollen, and prone to capillary rupture. Increased estrogen levels cause vascular congestion of mucous membranes in the upper respiratory system, causing nasal stuffiness, rhinitis, and nosebleeds (Blackburn, 2021). Slight bleeding can occur with tooth brushing or sexual intercourse.

About 90% of pregnant individuals develop hyperpigmentation due to higher levels of MSH and estrogen (Antony et al., 2021). The gravida can develop a dark line (linea nigra) on the midline of the abdomen, deeply pigmented nipples, and facial blotching (chloasma). Stretch marks can occur on abdomen and breast, and increased estrogen levels can encourage the development of telangiectasia (spider veins). Many mothers experience a thickening of scalp hair during pregnancy due to a large proportion of follicles entering a prolonged anagen (growth) phase; this new growth typically enters a telogen (resting) phase between 1 and 5 months postpartum, resulting in significant hair loss (Antony et al., 2021).

Musculoskeletal System

During pregnancy, weight gain and hormonal changes cause profound alterations in the structure and function of the musculoskeletal system. An active individual who gains 20% of prepregnant weight can increase the force on a joint by as much as 100% (Noon & Hoch, 2012). Healthy joints can become painful, and unstable or arthritic joints can suffer further damage.

Pregnant mothers gain an average of 25–35 lb (11.4–15.9 kg) over the course of gestation, experience a shift in their center of gravity, and undergo major biomechanical alterations that burden the axial skeleton and pelvis (Bermas, 2022), including

- Profound postural changes such as lordosis of the lumbar spine, kyphosis of the cervical spine, lowering of the shoulder girdle, and anterior tilting of pelvis;
- Stretching, weakening, and separation of abdominal muscles;
- Instability in the lumbar spine, sacroiliac joints, pubic symphysis, and weight-bearing joints from the pelvis to the foot;
- Increased use of hip extensor, abductor, and ankle plantar flexor muscles; and

- Increased reversible bone loss during both pregnancy and lactation which is greater with longer duration of breastfeeding (Antony et al., 2021).

Laxity of joint articulations can develop as early as 10–12 weeks of gestation (Murray & Hendley, 2020). The sacroiliac joints and pubic symphysis become wider, relaxed, and more mobile to facilitate pelvic expansion during birth, when an extra centimeter can be crucial. These changes affect balance and gait, increasing the likelihood of falls.

Back Pain

The most common musculoskeletal complaint during pregnancy is back pain. About 75% of pregnant individuals in the United States report low-back pain, which largely results from altered posture, muscle weakness, joint laxity, and vertebral facet joint irritation (Noon & Hoch, 2012; Tharpe, Farley, & Jordan, 2022). It can be challenging to distinguish pregnancy-related pain from other pathologies (Bermas, 2022). Renal stones, UTI, placental abruption, cholecystitis, and other medical conditions can present with a complaint of back pain, and lumbar disc herniation and bone cancer can (rarely) occur in pregnancy. Clients with the following alarm findings should be referred for further evaluation by a primary care physician, emergency care physician, obstetrician, orthopedic surgeon, or neurologist (Bermas, 2022):

- Severe back pain that interferes with normal activities;
- Persistent back pain at night unrelated to position or movement;
- Pain when coughing, sneezing, or bearing down;
- New-onset bladder incontinence other than pregnancy-related stress incontinence;
- Urinary retention;
- Bowel incontinence;
- Systemic symptoms such as fever, vomiting, diaphoresis, or weight loss;
- Severe back pain following recent epidural anesthesia;
- Back pain accompanied by weakness, abnormal sensations or abnormal reflexes involving one or more extremities; or
- Severe back pain in individuals at risk for compression fracture (e.g., from trauma or chronic glucocorticoid use).

Carpal Tunnel Syndrome

Second only to low-back pain in prevalence, carpal tunnel syndrome (CTS) is one of the most common musculoskeletal problems experienced by pregnant individuals (Afshar & Tabrizi, 2021). It is characterized by numbness and paresthesia along the distribution of the median nerve, wrist pain that can interfere with sleep, and difficulty grasping (Afshar & Tabrizi, 2021). CTS develops when the median nerve is compressed at the level of the carpal tunnel in the wrist producing paresthesia, disability, and pain in the first three fingers and the radial side of the ring finger (Ayhan, Ayhan, Çaglar, & Sahin, 2022). CTS is more common in clients with greater fluid retention related to gestational hypertension and preeclampsia (Afshar & Tabrizi, 2021). It is also partially attributable to lordosis and associated anterior neck flexion and shoulder girdle slumping, which can produce traction on the ulnar and median nerves (Afshar & Tabrizi, 2021).

CTS is prevalent in clients with a higher pregravid BMI, a history of smoking and alcohol consumption, non-Caucasian ethnicity, abnormal glucose metabolism, older maternal age, and history of CTS in a previous pregnancy. Symptoms typically resolve during the postpartum period. Symptomatic relief of pregnancy-related CTS is usually achieved by activity modification, edema control, and splints that hold the wrist in a neutral position. Sometimes steroid injections are used to achieve temporary pain relief (Afshar & Tabrizi, 2021). Surgery is seldom indicated.

Topics for Discussion

1. Yuliya R. has been struggling with nausea and vomiting for much of the first trimester of her pregnancy. She called today because she has vomited five times in 4 hr, has had almost no food or fluid intake in the past 24 hr, and is passing very little urine. What is your clinical impression? What is your management plan? Why?
2. Jamila J. presented for her appointment groggy and yawning with a complaint of feeling tired "all the time." Her husband, Jason, complained that she has been "snoring like a lawnmower" for the last couple of months. What condition do you suspect, and what referral do you make?
3. Indigo Y., the proud mother of a 4-month-old nursing infant, called to report a 102°F (39°C) fever with chills and rigors and a hot red spot on her left breast. What is your clinical impression and what is your plan of care?
4. Tanya S., a G1 P0 at 35 weeks of gestation, was awake all night with severe itching, which was worse on the palms and soles. There are no lesions visible. What is your clinical impression? What blood test results would confirm your suspicion?
5. Robbie K. had an ultrasound examination which showed a fetus at 16 weeks of gestation in a unicornuate uterus. What would you tell Robbie about the risks associated with this anatomical abnormality?

References

Afshar, A., & Tabrizi, A. (2021). Pregnancy-related hand and wrist problems. *Archives of Bone and Joint Surgery, 9*(3), 345–349. https://doi.org/10.22038/abjs.2020.50995.2531

[Alydia Health]. (2022). *Vacuum-induced hemorrhage control system: Instructions for use*. Retrieved from https://www.organon.com/product/usa/pi_circulars/j/jada/jada_system_ifu_blue_seal.pdf

American College of Obstetricians and Gynecologists. (2018, reaffirmed 2019). *Gestational diabetes mellitus* (Practice Bulletin 190). Retrieved from https://www.acog.org/clinical/clinical-guidance/practice-bulletin/articles/2018/02/gestational-diabetes-mellitus

American College of Obstetricians and Gynecologists. (2018, reaffirmed 2021). *Nausea and vomiting of pregnancy* (Practice Bulletin 189). Retrieved from https://www.acog.org/clinical/clinical-guidance/practice-bulletin/articles/2018/01/nausea-and-vomiting-of-pregnancy

Anderson, S., Lekovic, J., Niemasik, E., & Chasen, S. T. (2013). Patients with uterine anomalies may have increased risk of placenta accreta. *Fertility and Sterility, 100*(3, Suppl.), S379. https://doi.org/10.1016/j.fertnstert.2013.07.744

Antony, K. M., Racusin, D. A., Aagard, K., & Dildy, II, G. A. (2021). Maternal physiology. In M. B. Landon, H. L. Galan, E. R. M. Jauniaux, D. A. Driscoll, V. Berghella, W. A. Grobman, . . . A. G. Cahill (Eds.), *Gabbe's obstetrics: Normal and problem pregnancies* (8th ed., Kindle version, ch. 3). Philadelphia, PA: Elsevier.

Ayhan, S. G., Ayhan, E., Çaglar, A. T., & Sahin, D. (2022). Ultrasonography for carpal tunnel syndrome in pregnancy: a prospective cross-sectional study. *Journal of Obstetrics and Gynaecology, 42*(6), 1769–1774. https://doi.org/10.1080/01443615.2022.2036970

Barker, M., Peters, M. D. J., Adelson, P., & Steen, M. (2020). Probiotics and human lactational mastitis: A scoping review protocol. *JBI Evidence Synthesis, 18*(6), 1341–1348. https://doi.org/10.11124/JBISRIR-D-19-00190

Bermas, B. L. (2022). Maternal adaptations to pregnancy: Musculoskeletal changes and pain. In A. Chakrabarti (Ed.), *UpToDate*. Retrieved October 1, 2023, from https://www.uptodate.com/contents/maternal-adaptations-to-pregnancy-musculoskeletal-changes-and-pain

Bianco, A. (2023). Maternal adaptations to pregnancy: Gastrointestinal tract. In V. A. Barss (Ed.), *UpToDate*. Retrieved November 13, 2023, from https://www.uptodate.com/contents/maternal-adaptations-to-pregnancy-gastrointestinal-tract

Blackburn, S. T. (2021). Physiologic changes of pregnancy. In K. R. Simpson, P. Creehan, N. O'Brien-Abel, C. K. Roth, & A. J. Rohan (Eds.), *Perinatal nursing* (5th ed., pp. 71–88). Philadelphia, PA: Wolters Kluwer/Lippincott Williams & Wilkins Health.

Boddy, A. M., Fortunato, A., Wilson Sayres, M. and Aktipis, A. (2015). Fetal microchimerism and maternal health: A review and evolutionary analysis of cooperation and conflict beyond the womb. *BioEssays, 37*(10), 1106–1118. https://doi.org/10.1002/bies.201500059

Bowen, R. (2012). Thyroid hormones: Pregnancy and fetal development. *Hypertexts for Biomedical Sciences*. Retrieved from http://www.vivo.colostate.edu/hbooks/pathphys/endocrine/thyroid/thyroid_preg.html

Brucker, M. C., & King, T. L. (2019). Pharmacotherapeutics. In T. L. King, M. C. Brucker, K. Osborne, & C. M. Jevitt (Eds.), *Varney's midwifery* (6th ed., Kindle version, ch. 9). Burlington, MA: Jones & Bartlett Learning.

Caughey, A. B. (2023). Gestational diabetes mellitus: Obstetric issues and management. In V. A. Barss (Ed.), *UpToDate*. Retrieved October 1, 2023, from https://www.uptodate.com/contents/gestational-diabetes-mellitus-obstetric-issues-and-management

Chan, W. F. N., Gurnot, C., Montine, T. J., Sonnen, J. A., Guthrie, K. A., & Nelson, J. L. (2012). Male microchimerism in the human female brain. *PloS ONE, 7*(9), e45592. https://doi.org/10.1371/journal.pone.0045592

Chandra, S., Tripathi, A. K., Mishra, S., Amzarul, M., & Vaish, A. K. (2012). Physiological changes in hematological parameters during pregnancy. *Indian Journal of Hematology and Blood Transfusion, 28*(3), 144–146. https://doi.org/10.1007/s12288-012-0175-6

[Cook Medical]. (2020). *Bakri® postpartum balloon: Instructions for use*. Retrieved from https://www.cookmedical.com/data/IFU_PDF/T_J-SOSR_REV4.PDF

Cremona, A., O'Gorman, C., Cotter, A., Saunders, J., & Donnelly, A. (2018). Effect of exercise modality on markers of insulin sensitivity and blood glucose control in pregnancies complicated with gestational diabetes mellitus: A systematic review. *Obesity Science and Practice, 4*(5), 455–467. https://doi.org/10.1002/osp4.283

Cunningham, F. G., Leveno, K. J., Dashe, J. S., Hoffman, B. L., Spong, C. Y., & Casey, B. M. (Eds.). (2022). *Williams obstetrics* (26th ed., Kindle version). New York, NY: McGraw-Hill.

Danhausen, K., & King, T. L. (2024). In J. Phillippi & I. Kantrowitz-Gordon (Eds.), *Varney's midwifery* (7th ed., Kindle version, ch. 19). Burlington, MA: Jones & Bartlett Learning.

Davies, S. J., Lum, J. A., Skouteris, H., Byrne, L. K., & Hayden, M. J. (2018). Cognitive impairment during pregnancy: A meta-analysis. *Medical Journal of Australia, 208*(1), 35–40. https://doi.org/10.5694/mja17.00131

De Lee, J. B. (1914). *The principles and practice of obstetrics*. Philadelphia, PA: W. B. Saunders. Retrieved from https://archive.org/details/principlespracti00dele

Durnwald, C. (2023a). Gestational diabetes mellitus: Glucose management and maternal prognosis. In V. A. Barss (Ed.), *UpToDate*. Retrieved October 1, 2023, from https://www.uptodate.com/contents/gestational-diabetes-mellitus-glucose-management-and-maternal-prognosis

Durnwald, C. (2023b). Gestational diabetes mellitus: Screening, diagnosis, and prevention. In V. A. Barss (Ed.), *UpToDate*. Retrieved October 1, 2023, from https://www.uptodate.com/contents/gestational-diabetes-mellitus-screening-diagnosis-and-prevention

Fluegel, R. J. [Photographer]. (2010, February 12). *Haiti relief efforts continue [Image 1 of 44]*. Retrieved from https://www.dvidshub.net/image/251591/haiti-relief-efforts-continue

Gersh, B. J. (2022). Maternal adaptations to pregnancy: Cardiovascular and hemodynamic changes. In V. A. Barss (Ed.), *UpToDate*. Retrieved October 1, 2023, from https://www.uptodate.com/contents/maternal-adaptations-to-pregnancy-cardiovascular-and-hemodynamic-changes

González, L. S., Artibani, M., & Ahmed, A. A. (2021). Studying Müllerian duct anomalies—From cataloguing phenotypes to discovering causation. *Disease Models & Mechanisms, 14* (6). https://doi.org/10.1242/dmm.047977

Goyal, L. D., Dhaliwal, B., Singh, P., Ganjoo, S., & Goyal, V. (2020). Management of Mullerian development anomalies: 9 years' experience of a tertiary care center. *Gynecology and Minimally Invasive Therapy, 9*(2), 81–87. https://doi.org/10.4103/GMIT.GMIT_13_19

Hannema, S. E., & Hughes, I. A. (2007). Regulation of Wolffian duct development. *Hormone Research in Paediatrics, 67*(3), 142–151. https://doi.org/10.1159/000096644

Haultain, F. W. N., & Ferguson, J. H. (1898). *Handbook of obstetric nursing*. Edinburgh, United Kingdom: Y. J. Pentland. Retrieved from https://archive.org/details/b20387362

Howe, L. D., Hallal, P. C., Matijasevich, A., Well, J. C., Santos, I. S., Barros, A. J. D., . . . Smith, G. D. (2014). The association of birth order with later body mass index and blood pressure: A comparison between prospective cohort studies from the United Kingdom and Brazil. *International Journal of Obesity, 38*(7), 973-979. https://doi.org/10.1038/ijo.2013.189

Kallenbach, L. R., Johnson, K. L., & Bianchi, D. W. (2011). Fetal cell microchimerism and cancer: A nexus of reproduction, immunology, and tumor biology. *Cancer Research, 71*(1), 8–12. https://doi.org/10.1158/0008-5472.CAN-10-0618

Kazma, J. M., van den Anker, J., Allegaert, K., Dallmann, A., & Ahmadzia, H. K. (2020). Anatomical and physiological alterations of pregnancy. *Journal of Pharmacokinetics and Pharmacodynamics, 47*(4), 271–285. https://doi.org/10.1007/s10928-020-09677-1

Kim, A., Wirth, H., & Templeman, C. (2020). Is unilateral renal agenesis a useful screening tool to diagnose Mullerian anomalies? *Journal of Pediatric and Adolescent Gynecology, 33*(2), 198. https://doi.org/10.1016/j.jpag.2020.01.122

Laposky, A. D., & Pemberton, V. L. (2021). Sleep-disordered breathing and pregnancy-related cardiovascular disease. *Journal of Women's Health, 30*(2), 194-198. https://doi.org/10.1089/jwh.2020.8869

Laufer, M. R., & DeCherney, A. H. (2023). Congenital uterine anomalies: Clinical manifestations and diagnosis. In A. Chakrabarti (Ed.), *UpToDate*. Retrieved October 1, 2023, from https://www.uptodate.com/contents/congenital-uterine-anomalies-clinical-manifestations-and-diagnosis

Lindor, K. D., & Lee, R. H. (2023). Intrahepatic cholestasis of pregnancy. In K. M. Robson & V. A. Barss (Eds.), *UpToDate*. Retrieved October 1, 2023, from https://www.uptodate.com/contents/intrahepatic-cholestasis-of-pregnancy

Lovelace, D. (2016). Congenital uterine anomalies and uterine rupture. *Journal of Midwifery & Women's Health, 61(4), 501–506*. https://doi.org/10.1111/jmwh.12423

Mahmood, U., & O'Donoghue, K. (2014). Microchimeric fetal cells play a role in maternal wound healing after pregnancy. *Chimerism, 5*(2), 40–52. https://doi.org/10.4161/chim.28746

Major, A. T., Estermann, M. A., Roly, Z. Y., & Smith, C. A. (2021). An evo-devo perspective of the female reproductive tract. *Biology of Reproduction, 2021*, ioab166. https://doi.org/10.1093/biolre/ioab166

Mattson, S., & Smith, J. (2016). *Core curriculum for maternal-newborn nursing* (5th ed., e-book). St. Louis, MO: Elsevier.

Maygrier, J. P. (1834). *Midwifery illustrated*. (A. S. Doane, Trans.). New York, NY: Harper & Brothers. Retrieved from https://collections.nlm.nih.gov/bookviewer?PID=nlm:nlmuid-67310750R-bk

Miech, R. P. (2010). The role of fetal microchimerism in autoimmune disease. *International Journal of Clinical and Experimental Medicine, 3*(2), 164–168. Retrieved from https://www.ncbi.nlm.nih.gov/pmc/articles/PMC2894651/

Moreau, F. J., (1844). *A practical treatise on midwifery: Exhibiting the present advanced state of the science*. (T. F. Betton, Trans.). Philadelphia, PA: Carey and Hart. Retrieved from https://archive.org/stream/b28270253

Murray, I., & Hendley, J. (2020). Change and adaptation in pregnancy. In J. E. Marshall & M. D. Raynor (Eds.), *Myles' textbook for midwives* (17th ed., pp. 197–245). London, United Kingdom: Elsevier Health Sciences UK.

National Institute of Environmental Health Sciences. (2022). *Endocrine disruptors*. Retrieved from https://www.niehs.nih.gov/health/topics/agents/endocrine/index.cfm

Noon, M. L., & Hoch, A. Z. (2012). Challenges of the pregnant athlete and low back pain. *Current Sports Medicine Reports, 11*(1), 43-8. https://doi.org/10.1249/JSR.0b013e31824330b6

O'Donoghue, K., Chan, J., de la Fuente, J., Kennea, N., Sandison, A., Anderson, J. R., . . . Fisk, N. M. (2004). Microchimerism in female bone marrow and bone decades after fetal mesenchymal stem-cell trafficking in pregnancy. *Lancet, 364*(9429), 179–182. https://doi.org/10.1016/S0140-6736(04)16631-2

Ogilvie, L. A. (1957). True unicornate uterus: Report of a case with a review of the literature. *BJOG, 64*(3), 407-412. https://doi.org/10.1111/j.1471-0528.1957.tb02662.x

Osazuwa, H., & Ejenobo, D. (2012). Twin gestation in a septate bicornuate uterus. *Case Reports in Obstetrics and Gynecology, 2012*. https://doi.org/10.1155/2012/563085

Park, Y. H. (2022). Diagnosis and management of thrombocytopenia in pregnancy. *Blood Research, 57*(Suppl. 1), 79–85. https://doi.org/10.5045/br.2022.2022068

Pereira, N., Willson, S., McCarter, K., Chung, P. H., Kligman, I., & Rosenwaks, Z. (2021). Combined transvaginal and transabdominal oocyte retrieval in a patient with an ectopic ovary and unicornuate uterus. *Fertility and Sterility, 115*(5), 1347–1349. https://doi.org/10.1016/j.fertnstert.2020.12.006

Plows, J. F., Stanley, J. L., Baker, P. N., Reynolds, C. M., & Vickers, M. H. (2018). The pathophysiology of gestational diabetes mellitus. *International Journal of Molecular Sciences, 19*(11), 3342. https://doi.org/10.3390/ijms19113342

Post, R. J., Templeman, C. L., & Benoit, R. M. (2019). Twin gestation in a uterus didelphys with only one functional cervix: A case report. *Case Reports in Women's Health, 22*, e00118. https://doi.org/10.1016/j.crwh.2019.e00118

Poston, L. (2023). Gestational weight gain. In V. A. Barss (Ed.), *UpToDate*. Retrieved October 1, 2023, from https://www.uptodate.com/contents/gestational-weight-gain

Preminger, G. M., & Curhan, G. C. (2021). Kidney stones in adults: Kidney stones during pregnancy. In A. Q. Lam (Ed.), *UpToDate*. October 1, 2023, from https://www.uptodate.com/contents/kidney-stones-in-adults-kidney-stones-during-pregnancy

Rezai, S., Bisram, P., Lora Alcantara, I., Upadhyay, R., Lara, C., & Elmadjian, M. (2015). Didelphys uterus: A case report and review of the literature. *Case Reports in Obstetrics and Gynecology, 2015*. https://doi.org/10.1155/2015/865821

Roberts, V., & Myatt, L. (2023). Placental development and physiology. In V. A. Barss (Ed.), *UpToDate*. Retrieved October 1, 2023, from https://www.uptodate.com/contents/placental-development-and-physiology

Roly, Z. Y., Godini, R., Estermann, M. A., Major, A. T., Pocock, R., & Smith, C. A. (2020). Transcriptional landscape of the embryonic chicken Müllerian duct. *BMC Genomics, 21*, 688. https://doi.org/10.1186/s12864-020-07106-8

Ross, D. S. (2022). Hyperthyroidism during pregnancy: Clinical manifestations, diagnosis, and causes. In J. E. Mulder (Ed.), *UpToDate*. Retrieved October 1, 2023, from https://www.uptodate.com/contents/hyperthyroidism-during-pregnancy-clinical-manifestations-diagnosis-and-causes

Ross, D. S. (2023). Overview of thyroid disease and pregnancy. In J. E. Mulder (Ed.), *UpToDate*. Retrieved October 1, 2023, from https://www.uptodate.com/contents/overview-of-thyroid-disease-and-pregnancy

Saleem, H. M., Muhammed, T. M., Al-Hetty, H. R. A. K., & Salman, D. A. (2022). Physiological, hematological and some biochemical alterations during pregnancy. *International Journal of Health Sciences 6*(Special Issue 6), 7156–7169. https://doi.org/10.53730/ijhs.v6nS6.12017

Sapra, A., & Bhandari, P. (2023). Diabetes mellitus. In *StatPearls*. Treasure Island, FL: StatPearls Publishing. Retrieved September 30, 2023, from https://www.ncbi.nlm.nih.gov/books/NBK551501/

Simmonds, C. S., Karsenty, G., Karaplis, A. C., & Kovacs, C. S. (2010). Parathyroid hormone regulates fetal-placental mineral homeostasis. *Journal of Bone and Mineral Research, 25*(3), 594–605. https://doi.org/10.1359/jbmr.090825

Smith, B. C., Brown, D. L., Carter, R. E., & Famuyide, A. O. (2014). Double cervix: Clarifying a diagnostic dilemma. *American Journal of Obstetrics & Gynecology, 211*(1), 26.e1–26.e5. https://doi.org/10.1016/j.ajog.2014.03.014

Staff, A. C., Fjeldstad, H. E., Fosheim, I. K., Moe, K., Turowski, G., Johnsen, G. M., . . . Sugulle, M. (2020). Failure of physiological transformation and spiral artery atherosis: Their roles in preeclampsia. *American Journal of Obstetrics & Gynecology, 226*(2, Suppl.), S895–S906. https://doi.org/10.1016/j.ajog.2020.09.026

Thadhani, R. I., & Maynard, S. E. (2022). Maternal adaptations to pregnancy: Renal and urinary tract physiology. In A. Chakrabarti (Ed.), *UpToDate*. Retrieved October 1, 2023, from https://www.uptodate.com/contents/maternal-adaptations-to-pregnancy-renal-and-urinary-tract-physiology

Tharpe, N. L., Farley, C. L., & Jordan, R. G. (2022). *Clinical practice guidelines for midwifery & women's health* (6th ed., Kindle version). Burlington, MA: Jones & Bartlett Learning.

Trad, M., & Palmer, S. (2013). Müllerian duct anomalies and a case study of unicornuate uterus. *Radiologic Technology, 84*(6), 571–576. Retrieved from http://www.radiologictechnology.org/content/84/6/571.abstract

Warland, J. (2012). Low blood pressure. *BMC Pregnancy and Childbirth, 12*(Suppl. 1), A9. https://doi.org/10.1186/1471-2393-12-S1-A9

Weerakkody, Y., & El-Feky, M. (2022). Maternal hydronephrosis in pregnancy. *Radiopaedia*. https://doi.org/10.53347/rID-13274

Weinberger, S. E. (2023). Maternal adaptations to pregnancy: Dyspnea and other physiologic respiratory changes. In V. A. Barss (Ed.), *UpToDate*. Retrieved October 1, 2023, from https://www.uptodate.com/contents/maternal-adaptations-to-pregnancy-dyspnea-and-other-physiologic-respiratory-changes

Williams, J. W. (1912). *Obstetrics: A text-book for the use of students and practitioners* (3rd ed.). New York: Appleton. Retrieved from https://archive.org/details/obstetricstextbo1912will

Zeng, X. X., Tan, K. H., Yeo, A., Sasajala, P., Tan, X., Xiao, Z. C., . . . Udolph, G. (2010). Pregnancy-associated progenitor cells differentiate and mature into neurons in the maternal brain. *Stem Cells and Development, 19*(12), 1819–1830. https://doi.org/10.1089/scd.2010.0046

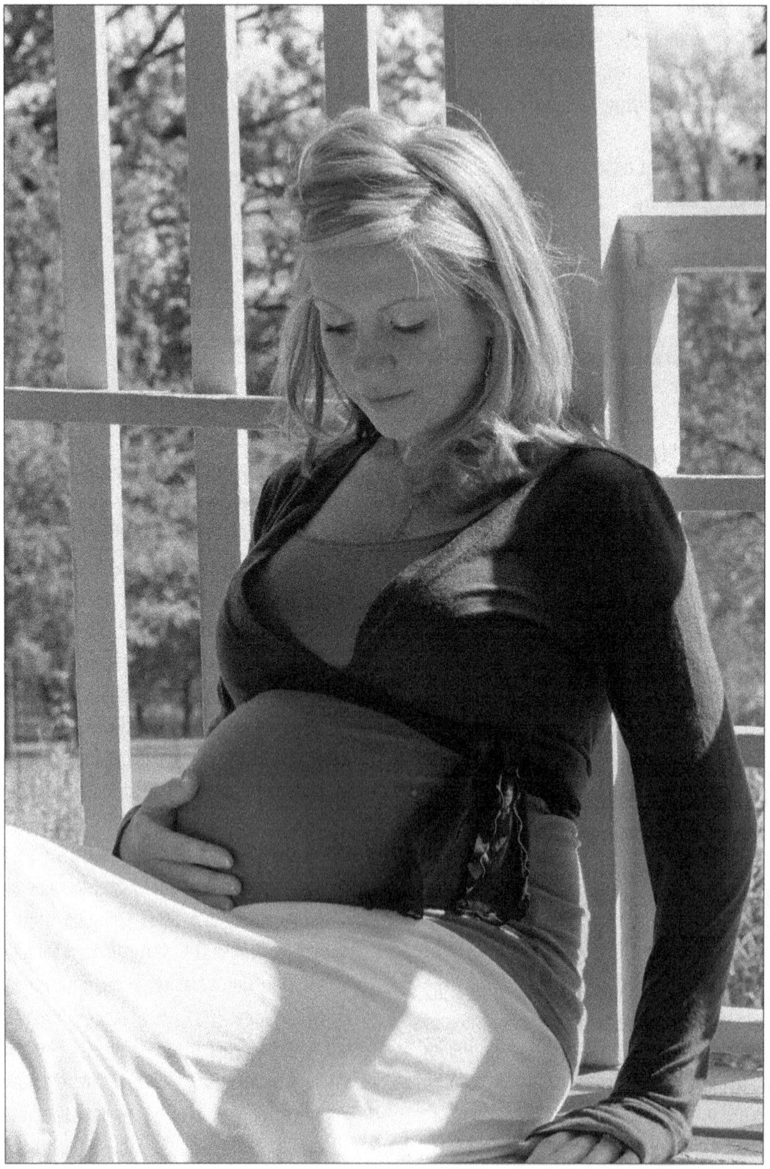

Critical Thinking and Risk Assessment 3

Objectives

- Explain how the beginning provider processes information differently from the expert.
- Describe three processes used by midwives to make clinical decisions.
- Describe a situation in which home birth would decrease risk to mother and child and one in which it would increase risk.
- List three antepartal conditions that would necessitate comanagement with a physician or transfer of care.
- Discuss why the process of risk assessment is critical to the safety of community birth.

Composite Case Study

The spring snowstorm was worse than expected. The governor declared a snow emergency and closed the roads. Pamela Whitlock, a CPM at the Mayapple Hollow Birth Center, placed the center on divert until the roads were reopened. A client in labor called, and Pamela instructed her to call emergency medical services (EMS) for transport to the nearest hospital. The ambulance was unable to reach her, and the fire department took her by snowmobile from the house to the highway, where the ambulance intercepted and took her to the hospital in plenty of time for a safe birth.

Two days later, Pamela began her shift taking call from home. The main roads were cleared, but some local lanes were still clogged with snow. The birth center manager instructed her to call the fire department to determine the status of road closures if there were any labor calls.

Melvin K. called at 10 p.m. to report that his wife, Linda Sue, at term with her second baby, had been contracting every 2–3 minutes for the past hour. They had planned a home birth. Melvin, an Amishman, did not have a phone and was calling from a phone shed beside a recently plowed road. Pamela told Melvin to stay by the phone and she would call him back in a couple of minutes with instructions. Pamela called the fire department but reached a recording. She presented the problem to her manager, who determined the main roads were clear enough for safe passage and reopened the center for births. Because local roads and driveways were not predictably accessible, the manager decided that laboring clients planning a home birth should come to the birth center.

Pamela called Melvin back to tell him to proceed to the birth center, but Melvin had just checked in on Linda Sue, and she had said that she was almost ready to push. The birth center was 9 minutes from their home; but because they were Amish, they needed to hire a driver to get there, and it would take time to find one. Pamela lived 7 minutes from the client's house and 7 minutes from the birth center. Pamela decided to attend Linda Sue's birth at the residence. Neither she nor the birth assistant had trouble reaching the house, and the baby was born 15 minutes after Pamela's arrival—a girl, 7 lb 15 oz (3,600 g), Apgars 9/10.

Pamela felt secure with her decision to attend the birth at home. Her manager, however, had a different perspective. "Pamela, you were very lucky," she said. "You had no way of knowing the condition of the roads. If mother or baby had a complication, you might not have been able to get them to the hospital quickly or at all."

Pamela and her manager discussed other ways Pamela could have handled this situation. Ultimately, they agreed that Pamela could have called EMS to send an ambulance to Linda Sue's home while driving there herself. In the past, the local responders had been willing to stand by in the next room during a birth and leave if not needed. Pamela would have had access to emergency transportation but could have provided care independently if all went well. At another birth center, providers and staff might have reached a different conclusion and made different plans.

Optimal Midwifery Management

A midwife relies on not only heart and hands, but also on intelligence and intuition. Without scientific knowledge and reasoning skills, the art of midwifery has no integrity or substance. Critical thinking—forming judgments by systematically analyzing knowledge, evidence, and arguments—is the frame on which the midwife builds a storm-resistant structure of insight, wisdom, compassion, and commitment.

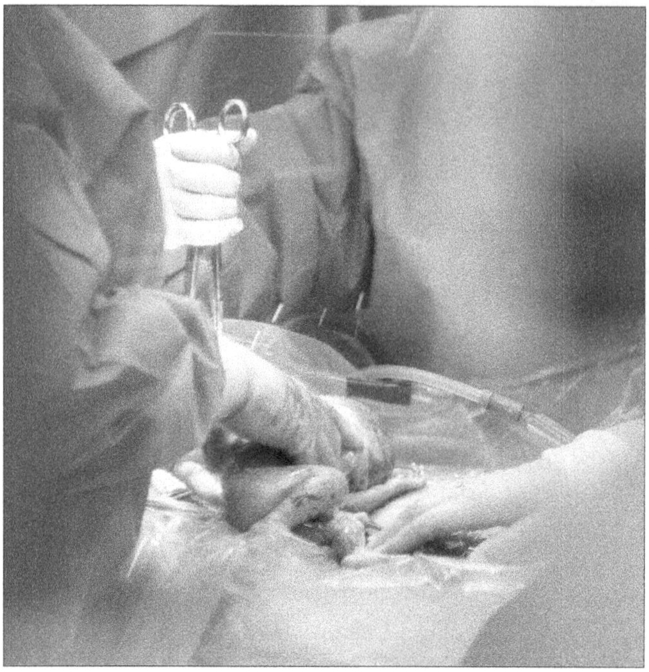

Figure 3-1. Unanticipated emergencies can occur in healthy clients and can take the client and midwife by surprise. This woman was enjoying a low-risk pregnancy until her water broke at 30 weeks of gestation, precipitating active labor with a fetus in transverse lie. Before she had a chance to process the sudden turn of events, she was rushed into the operating room to give birth to a preterm infant by cesarean section.

The Inevitability of Complications

Although most low-risk mothers have normal, healthy, and physiological births, any natural process can go awry. Inevitably some mothers and babies develop complications despite good health and good care. Community midwifery practices that accept only low-risk clients have a much lower rate of complications than obstetrical practices that care for high-risk individuals. Almost every midwife, however, encounters emergencies. Sometimes the midwife will feel like a hero, saving the day with proficiency and fast thinking. Other times, complications will spiral into crisis despite the best management. Midwifery and life are like that.

When pregnancy and labor are normal, it is tempting to assume that they will remain normal. This assumption is true most of the time and is so comforting that it is easy to discount early signs of an evolving problem. Serious complications, however, can present unexpectedly, requiring decisive intervention until the problem is resolved or the client is under a physician's care. The delay in treatment that can occur when moving a client from home to hospital can increase the risks of morbidity and mortality for mothers and babies with certain complications. The outcomes of these kinds of emergency can depend on the midwife's expertise, training, skill level, and quick action.

The community midwife can unwittingly manage clients who are at risk for complications. Some apparently healthy mothers who choose not to use a primary care physician can have undiagnosed problems such as heart defects, diabetes, or hypothyroidism. When the mother opts out of routine fetal anatomical scans, a fetal anomaly might not be recognized until after birth. Certain insular groups such as the Amish have a high incidence of genetic disorders, and midwives who serve them may sometimes see infants with catastrophic conditions such as Amish lethal microcephaly or newborns with abnormalities requiring immediate treatment, such as severe combined immunodeficiency.

Clinical judgment and decision-making are affected by the context of a situation. Often when mothers and babies develop unexpected problems, their symptoms do not match any textbook, and clinical signs will present with various degrees of ambiguity. Knowledge of pathophysiology is important; but to recognize a problem from its earliest presentation, a provider must become a detective who pieces together a story or a pattern to form a diagnosis.

Clinical Reasoning

When midwives become aware of how they arrive at the choices they make, they can make better decisions and have better outcomes. Good clinical reasoning skills help to ensure that diagnostic and treatment decisions are grounded (Jefford, Fahy, & Sundin, 2011). Critical thinking raises questions about the strength of evidence for a given conclusion and can generate creative solutions. Even seemingly incontrovertible data must be examined critically.

Although watchful waiting and noninterference with physiologic processes are the foundation of midwifery care, they are not passive activities. The savvy midwife constantly assesses and reassesses clients, takes preventative measures to avoid difficulties, tunes in to abnormal findings or subtle indications of developing complications and prepares to intervene as necessary. Clinical decision-making is a continuous process that involves gathering and evaluating data, prioritizing issues, forming a hypothesis, weighing options, considering their consequences, choosing an evidence-informed course of action, and reevaluating by repeating the process at intervals (Tiffen, Corbridge, & Slimmer, 2014). In emergencies, all this must be done quickly, but not at the expense of accuracy.

The human brain has long- and short-term memory, and these two are as different as the RAM and the hard drive in a computer. Short-term memory, like RAM, is the processing

Table 3-1
Steps to Clinical Reasoning

Step	Example
Acquire information.	Client is 36 weeks pregnant and is complaining of a severe headache. She had preeclampsia without severe features in a previous pregnancy.
Cluster pieces of information that are possibly related and discard information that is clearly unrelated.	On questioning, the client is also experiencing nausea and vomiting and visual disturbances—symptoms that suggest preeclampsia—and pain in the sacroiliac and pubic region when climbing stairs—symptoms probably unrelated to preeclampsia or other serious conditions.
Generate multiple hypotheses.	Your first thought is preeclampsia, but you consider other causes of headache, visual changes, and vomiting (migraine, carbon monoxide poisoning, head trauma).
Collect new information to support or refute your hypotheses.	You find that the client has a blood pressure (BP) of 172/96 and elevated liver transaminases and serum creatinine. Protein/creatinine ratio is also elevated. Platelets are 80,000. The fetus has a category I electronic fetal monitor tracing.
Interpret information and select the working diagnosis with the most empirical support.	The client's signs, symptoms, and laboratory data are consistent with HELLP syndrome (Hemolysis, Elevated Liver enzymes, Low Platelets).
Implement a treatment plan.	The client undergoes induction of labor in a hospital with continuous fetal monitoring, oxytocin titration, magnesium sulfate for seizure prophylaxis, and intravenous labetalol to reduce her severe-range BP.
Evaluate treatment. Remain vigilant for information that might refute the diagnosis or call for a different course of treatment. If need be, begin the steps of clinical reasoning again.	An hour after starting magnesium sulfate and labetalol, the client's BP normalized to 130s/80s. After 12 hr of labor, the client gave birth to a small but healthy daughter. Her condition quickly improved during the postpartum period.

space where current information is managed. Long-term memory is stored on the biological equivalent of a hard drive, often for a lifetime. Like a file on a computer, this data is more easily retrieved if it is stored systematically. Unlike a computer, people filter information through emotions, intuition, and empathy, a tendency that can either clarify or obscure the truth of the matter in a way a computer cannot. Further, misunderstood or misremembered information can masquerade as unassailable truth.

Information processing theory holds that information is coded as symbols when stored within memory (Jefford et al., 2011). Symbols are clustered into patterns in the brain associated with external stimuli (Jefford et al., 2011). These groups of symbols and experiences are stored in long-term memory and retrieved when a person encounters similar stimuli, creating the opportunity to repeat or avoid an action (Jefford et al., 2011). Information that is frequently reviewed or used is easier to retrieve. Mnemonic tricks also improve retrieval. The provider's ability to integrate, interpret, and analyze information and learn from experience can improve decision-making and lead to appropriate action.

Reason is usually held as the standard for gathering knowledge, and emotion is often dismissed as a hindrance. In truth, when providers attune emotionally to a situation, meaningful aspects can stand out as important and guide their reasoning. Unease about a diagnosis can mean that key elements are missing or that the original impression was inaccurate. Reason, emotion, and intuition are complementary, not mutually exclusive, and can be combined to enhance the practitioner's ability to care for a client during labor and birth.

Clinical decision-making is a process that encompasses clinical reasoning; intuition; awareness of psychological, social, spiritual, and environmental influences; and what the midwife thinks, feels, and does within a clinical encounter (Jefford et al., 2010). A provider's personal experience can strongly influence clinical decision-making. For example, a midwife in practice for a year who has managed two severe

Tune in to every laboring mother. If you feel uneasy, ask yourself why.

postpartum hemorrhages can find that these experiences have informed her beliefs about *all* postpartum hemorrhages, including relative frequency, techniques for effective control, likely outcome, and her ability to manage this complication. To her, those two cases can be more influential than the thousands of cases underpinning textbook recommendations or the experiences of other midwives.

Forming a Clinical Impression

The client's own impression of what is wrong often supplies vital information that aids diagnosis. Clients can misinterpret signs, however, or focus on emotionally charged aspects of the issue rather than their cause—which can distract the midwife from addressing the underlying problem. The midwife must place the client's impression into context by asking the right questions and investigating potential sources of symptoms. For example, a client can request treatment for a urinary tract infection (UTI) when in fact the presenting symptoms are caused by chlamydia, which necessitates appropriate antibiotic therapy, treatment of the partner(s), counseling, and testing for sexually transmitted coinfections.

The first step in managing an obstetric complication is anticipation and early identification of deviations from the natural and usually trustworthy process of birth. The second is to consider possible explanations for what is occurring, taking care not to overcommit to any of them. Systematically analyze and incorporate new data and note whether it supports one hypothesis or eliminates others. The next step is to make a plan that will correct or improve the situation. With experience, you will learn to find patterns and to determine what information is relevant, then rapidly compare key features to your knowledge base to generate a clinical impression. But even an experienced provider can develop a blind spot in judgment, commonly when resonating emotionally with a client. For example, a community midwife sometimes delays transfer for a retained placenta, increasing the risk for hemorrhage, because of reluctance to uproot the client from the home environment and disrupt bonding with the infant.

Pattern recognition is a conscious judgment based on experience of similar situations (Barber, 2012). The seasoned clinician who has seen many unusual presentations and rare conditions can compare the complaints of the present client with those previously encountered and form an impression. When a third-trimester client presents with dysuria, urinary frequency, and foul-smelling bloody or cloudy urine, the cluster of signs and symptoms points to a probable bladder infection. But if this same client is also having abdominal tightening, fever, and increased vaginal discharge, the clinical picture gets murkier. Is the client in preterm labor (PTL)? Is the cause pyelonephritis (kidney inflammation/infection) or intraamniotic infection—or several problems simultaneously?

Four Fundamental Patterns of Clinical Knowing

Empirical (knowledge from science)

Personal (knowledge from personal understanding)

Ethical (knowledge from an ethical framework)

Aesthetic (awareness of unique client situation)

Adapted from "Fundamental Patterns of Knowing in Nursing," by B. A. Carper, 1978, Advances in Nursing Science, 1(1), pp. 13–24. Copyright by Aspen Publishers.

Intuition

Most experienced health care providers find intuition an important source of knowledge, but midwives are more likely than obstetricians to acknowledge its role in their practice (Davis-Floyd & Davis, 1996). Intuition has been described as subconscious recognition of patterns that seems to burst into consciousness effortlessly or from an external source (Barber, 2012). All features, obvious and subtle, come together in a synergy of experience, knowledge, and expertise, emerging as a whole concept (Barber, 2012; Noon, 2014). Intuition has also been described as gut feeling, sixth sense, and the ability to acquire understanding without interpretation or the use of reason (Anwar & Razzak, 2015). Because the processing is unconscious, the provider who relies on intuition often has trouble pointing to specific data that support convictions though they tend to be highly accurate.

Maternity care providers often use intuition in forming clinical impressions, and more experienced and competent providers rely on it to a greater degree (Noon, 2014). Although an experienced midwife sometimes cannot describe what is concerning about a baby's breathing pattern, the subconscious mind recalls that the last baby that presented similarly stopped breathing shortly thereafter and rings the alarm bell. Intuitive management includes honoring the sense of uneasiness that manifests while triaging a client's vague complaints over the telephone or validating the perception that there is "something wrong" even when the signs do not point to a serious issue (Barnes & Dossey, 1999).

Forming a Clinical Impression

- Guard against tunnel vision by periodically considering alternative viewpoints.
- Periodically reflect on the big picture. Have all possibilities have been explored? Does the most likely explanation still make sense? Are my conclusions based on evidence?
- Remain alert to clues that contradict your working diagnosis and listen when your instincts reveal that something is not adding up. "You cannot dig a hole in a different place by digging the same hole deeper" (de Bono, 1970, p. 13).
- Avoid inflating the importance of clues that support your clinical impression—or ignoring those that do not support it.

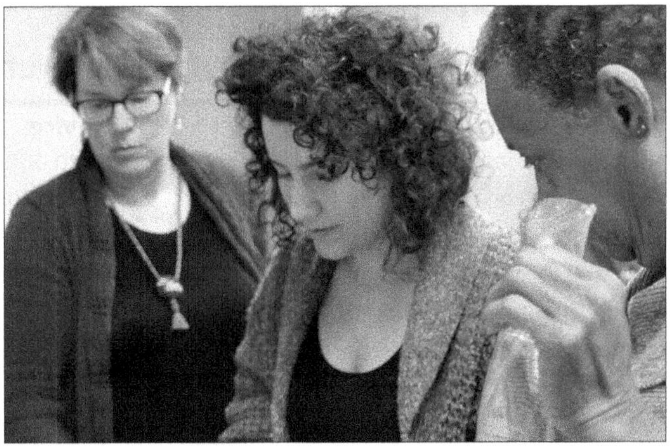

Figure 3-2. Expert midwives process information so rapidly, sometimes subconsciously, that insights and conclusions flash into their minds as fully formed concepts. Novices tend to organize data using an internal checklist. When people of differing backgrounds and experience are together in a class like Birth Emergency Skills Training, they learn as much from one another as they do from the curriculum.

Intuition can be hard to distinguish from other unconscious currents, especially for providers new to practice. Sometimes the vague unease that a midwife feels about a variation in a client's labor is simply free-floating anxiety about present surroundings (perhaps a remote farmhouse in a blizzard), office politics, or other personal dramas. Sometimes it is based on an old memory of some unpleasant event.

Intuition should complement analytical reasoning. Both are valid and, used together, they expose a larger part of the picture than either can separately. Evidence-based care and professional accountability are essential to safe practice, so midwives must be able to provide reasonable rationales for all decisions (Steinhauer, 2015). Communicating rationales for treatment decisions tends to reassure colleagues, clients, and anxious bystanders.

Experienced midwives who rely on intuitive decision-making without reflection on existing evidence are more likely to have poor outcomes and have more difficulty defending the reasons for their decisions in a court of law (Barber, 2012). Likewise, a midwife who lacks the skills to make an analytical decision sometimes relies on intuition to form a clinical judgment and makes errors related to lack of experience. The best midwives use a combination of intuition and critical thinking (Barber, 2012).

Novice to Expert

Midwives process clinical information differently at each level of expertise. Inexperienced providers tend to reason step by step and can usually explain their rational cognitive processes. Expert providers cannot always explain how they know what they know and often attribute their judgments to "gut feeling," "hunch," or "sixth sense" (Noon, 2014).

Novice providers tend to make logical decisions drawn from principles and rules, moving through an internal or external checklist with little awareness of context (Benner, 2001; Noon, 2014). They often feel overwhelmed and can suffer incapacitating anxiety when faced with something new. They are also susceptible to tunnel vision, focusing on the task rather than the client. A beginner who can pass a test on clinical manifestations of disease sometimes struggles to apply this knowledge. The advanced beginner is more sensitive to the nuances of the situation at hand and understands underlying principles but needs help setting priorities.

Competent providers feel a sense of mastery based on experience and plan goals purposefully. They have a strong grasp of clinical knowledge and understand the "why" of what they do (Benner, 2001). Proficient providers develop a more holistic perspective. They recognize immediately when situations deviate from normal and can grasp the long-term implications of problems and possible solutions (Benner, 2001).

The expert provider transcends rules and trusts the intuition that arises from deep internal wellsprings of knowledge. The expert is flexible, inventing workable solutions through leaps of creativity and improvisation. Expert midwives attune to clinical information that is difficult to quantify or describe;

they fit new situations into old frameworks to formulate innovative solutions. Experts do not often think consciously about reasons for choosing actions and are usually unaware that they are processing knowledge at all. The salient facts just jump out. Intuition melds the clues into a whole that flashes intact into the conscious mind without an obvious linear progression. Often the flash of clinical insight occurs before perceptible cues are identified (Benner, 2001).

These levels of expertise are neither rigid nor permanent. An advanced beginner can show flashes of proficiency in some areas, or an expert can have an off day and backslide into proficiency. Although providers tend to climb this theoretical framework as they develop, not all reach or remain at the top (Mortimore, Reynolds, Forman, Brannigan, & Mitchell, 2021). Providers who excel in critical thinking and clinical decision-making are most likely to become experts (Mortimore et al., 2021).

Table 3-2
Dreyfus Model of Skill Acquisition

Level 1	**Novice** Rigid adherence to rules or plans. Little situational perception. No discretionary judgment.
Level 2	**Advanced Beginner** Guidelines for action based on attributes or aspects. Situational perception still limited. Treats all attributes and aspects separately and gives them equal importance.
Level 3	**Competent** Can see big picture. Considers long-term goals. Conscious deliberate planning.
Level 4	**Proficient** Sees situations holistically rather than focusing on components. Sees what is most important in a situation. Perceives deviations from normal patterns. Decision-making is less labored. Takes guidance from maxims with meanings that vary with the situation.
Level 5	**Expert** No longer relies on rules, guidelines, or maxims. Intuitive grasp of situations based on deep tacit understanding. Uses analytic approaches only in novel situations or when problems occur. Sees what is possible.

Adapted from *Simulations and Drills: Educational Tool #6* (pp. 16–17), by L. Casper, 2010. Copyright by California Dept. of Public Health.

Manage, Comanage, or Refer?

Midwife-led care supports childbirth as a normal physiologic process, but no midwife can independently manage every contingency that nature and other forces offer. Midwives improve safety when they select clients wisely, remain vigilant for deviations from normal, establish whether the increased risk is temporary or correctable, refer judiciously, and stand ready to manage emergencies (American College of Nurse-Midwives [ACNM], 2015). All models of safe, effective midwifery care include a mechanism for consultation with and referral to other care providers (Martijn, Jacobs, Maassen, Buitendijk, & Wensing, 2013).

Midwives continually assess risks to a client's wellbeing while promoting normal physiologic function (Peterwerth, Halek, & Schäfers, 2022). This process includes rigorous screening based on current knowledge and standards to determine whether the client is a good candidate for community birth (Hofmeyr et al., 2009). The experience level of the midwife, the local standard of care, the distance from a hospital able to handle obstetrical complications, and the prevailing legal climate of the midwife's location of practice can influence the decision to "risk out" a client or comanage with another provider. Community birth centers and home-birth practices are "distinguished by a high tolerance for the unusual and a low threshold for the truly abnormal" (Barnes & Dossey, 1999, p. 458). Although community birth is usually safe for low-risk mothers and their babies, risk increases significantly in the presence of certain maternal conditions such as hypertension, preterm birth (PTB), postdates beyond 41–42 weeks of gestation, multiple gestation, and breech (American College of Obstetricians & Gynecologists [ACOG], 2017/2023; Bastian, Keirse, & Lancaster, 1998; Cheyney et al., 2014; Cox, Bovbjerg, Cheyney, & Leeman, 2015; Kennare, Keirse, Tucker, & Chan, 2010; Mehl-Madrona & Madrona, 1997; Midwives Alliance of North America [MANA], 2014).

Safe, effective midwifery care includes a mechanism for consultation with and referral to other care providers.

The Nature of Risk

Level of risk is expressed as a probability calculated when the number of subjects studied is divided by the number that experienced the effect, usually expressed as a fraction, ratio, or percentage. Probabilities do not always fit reality. A 50% chance of rain in a city rises to 100% where rain falls and drops to 0% in dry spots. Risk assessment estimates whether certain outcomes are more likely or less, but in most cases cannot foretell the outcome for a particular client.

Because everything we do in life involves risk, it can never be eliminated. People can be injured or killed by a fall from a roof, a horse, or a toilet. An athlete with a healthy lifestyle can die suddenly from an arrhythmia or ruptured aneurysm. A nonsmoker can develop lung cancer. Because everyone eventually dies, the odds of dying from *something* are 100%, or 1:1, regardless of risk status. Everyone takes risks; risk management involves balancing risks and rewards (Adams, 1998). Some people have greater risk tolerance than others and willingly take bigger risks in hope of a greater reward or in ignorance of, or indifference to, potential negative outcomes.

Risk perception is the judgment that we form about the characteristics and severity of risks (Grima, Hamarat, Özen, Girlando, & Dalli-Gonzi, 2021). Many laypeople gauge risk within the context of their own limited personal experience and draw conclusions from small samples that seem meaningful. Those who have had serious motor vehicle crashes (MVCs) on distant highways can feel much safer driving around their own familiar cities even though most vehicular crashes occur on slow urban streets close to home (Burdett, Starkey & Charlton, 2018). People generally do not have an intuitive grasp of large numbers or probabilities of events. Because it seems inevitable that *someone* will win a lottery, it is tempting to believe that *anyone* can, so people buy tickets though the chance of hitting a jackpot may be 1 in hundreds of millions.

Mass media skew our perceptions of risk by emphasizing rare occurrences and playing on our sympathies and fears. Reporters headline extraordinary deaths by fire, flood, and violence, but ignore commonplace mortality from strokes, heart attacks, and influenza. The odds of dying in an airline crash are small, 1 in 4.7 million flights (Dresang & Rochin, 2020; Ornato & Peberdy, 2014), but 24/7 newscasts, sensational reporting, and social media exaggerate the dangers of flying. After watching domestic news broadcasts, viewers in the United States might think that they are much more likely to die in an attack by foreign-born terrorists or in a mass

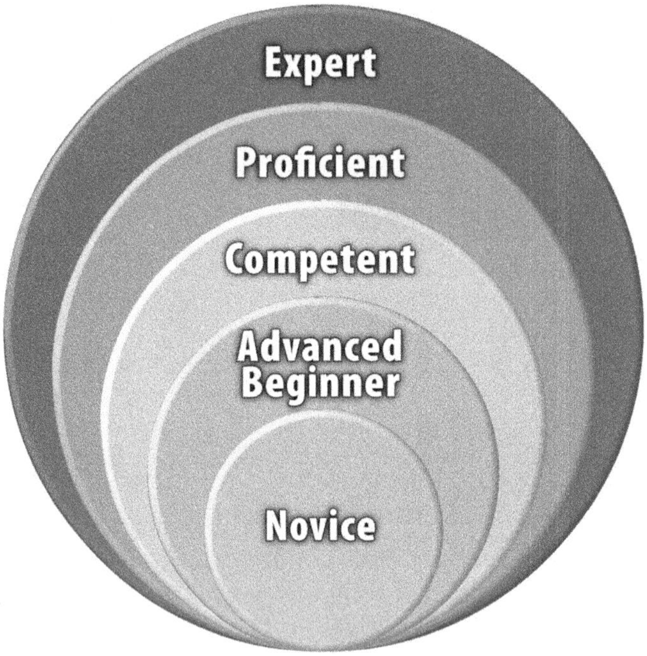

Figure 3-3. With time and experience, most providers grow in clinical skill and ability to think critically. Not all providers will become experts.

shooting than in a traffic accident. The estimated lifetime odds, however, are 1:45,785, 1:11,125, and 1:491, respectively (Mosher & Gould, 2018).

Emotionally, people perceive a risk as greater when it is uncontrollable, unfair, involuntary, or potentially catastrophic or when it is imposed on them by others, for example, the risk of violent crime or the risk of illness from pesticide residues on food (Wilson, Zwickle, & Walpole, 2019). People may attempt to control inherently risky situations by taking steps to reduce risk and uncertainty (Lothian, 2012). They wear sunscreen, install safety gates on staircases when a toddler is afoot, and get regular Pap tests. They avoid talking to strangers in dark parking lots and keep their children close while shopping.

Prudence becomes paternalism when people in positions of authority or influence restrict the freedoms and responsibilities of others with the actual or stated intention of acting in their best interests. Lawmakers, regulators, health care practitioners, and others often must choose between upholding people's right to make their own choices and acting to promote their wellbeing (Andre & Velasquez, 2013). The practice of public health is based on addressing population outcomes rather than personal outcomes. The District of Columbia and every state except New Hampshire have mandatory seat belt laws that restrict individual freedoms but sharply reduce death from MVCs (Insurance Institute for Highway Safety & Highway Loss Data Institute, 2023). From 2004 to 2008, seat belts saved more than 75,000 lives and minimized or prevented uncountable injuries

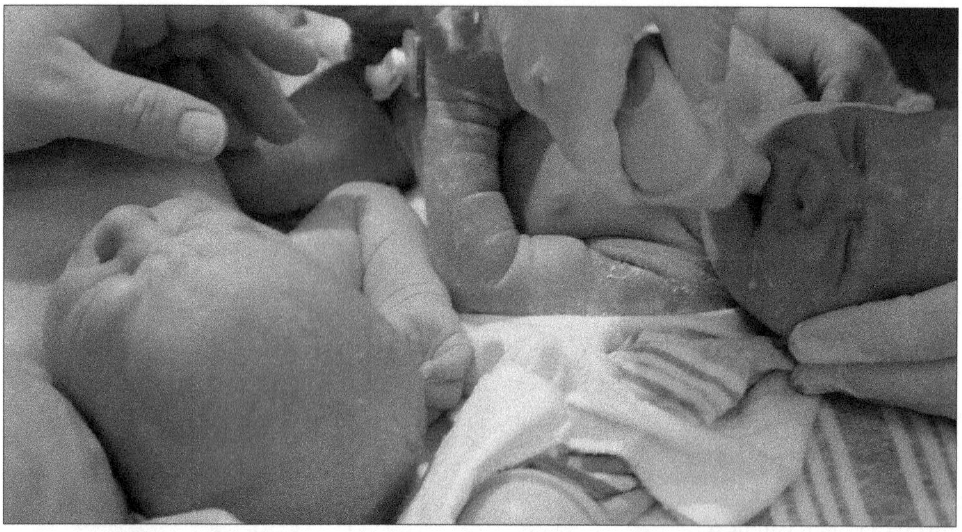

Figure 3-4. Normal childbirth is widely defined as healthy, uncomplicated term singleton pregnancy in a cephalic position with spontaneous onset and progress of labor. Among mothers not fitting this definition of normal who are accepted for community birth, the risk of adverse outcomes can be significantly greater. Whether to plan the birth of twins in a community setting remains a controversial topic.

(National Safety Council, 2016). Some, however, contend that seatbelt laws are unconstitutional or too restrictive and should be repealed.

Denying people choices deprives them of the fundamental right to self-determination (World Health Organization, 2019). In the United States and many other countries, a competent adult has the freedom to choose lawful activities that carry significant risk to health or life, such as motorcycle racing, bull riding, chain smoking, or swapping body fluids with strangers. But we often feel justified in preventing children, people with limited cognitive capacities, and people impaired by drugs or alcohol from making risky decisions and in punishing those who exploit them.

Competent pregnant individuals have the right to weigh risks and benefits and make decisions based on what they think is best for themselves and their families. Pregnant mothers may choose to body surf, climb rock faces, bounce on trampolines, play rugby, smoke cigarettes, or scuba dive even though these activities entail risk of injury to themselves and their fetuses. They drive cars, though the risk of a healthy pregnant mother having a traffic accident is higher than that of having a life-threatening emergency in childbirth (Redelmeier, May, Thiruchelvam, & Barrett, 2014; Vladiutu, et al, 2013). In fact, one study showed thata driver's risk of having an automobile accident increases by 42% during pregnancy to a rate of about 1 in 50, regardless of socioeconomic status, age, or obstetrical complications—the reason is unclear (Redelmeier et al., 2014). Life is fraught with great risks and small, and everyone must decide how best to navigate them.

During pregnancy, a mother's risk perception is shaped by experience and the perceptions of others as well as information conveyed by providers and the media. Entertainment, news, and social media typically amplify the risks of childbirth for the sake of a good story, distorting public perception of what is normal and typical, and what is not. One study evaluated 85 "reality-based" birth television programs, depicting 123 births, aired in the United States on Discovery Health and The Learning Channel in November 2007 (Morris & McInerney, 2010). These episodes highlighted danger and complications (including abnormal fetal positions, hypertension, postpartum bleeding, cervical cancer, bicornuate uterus, and PTL) in their titles and in advertising "teasers," painting pregnancy and birth as dramatic and perilous (Morris & McInerney, 2010). To increase entertainment value, complications are managed to happy resolutions by physicians, nurses, and midwives who save the day with skills and technology.

Many primigravidas who regularly watch "reality-based" programs about pregnancy and childbirth expect education and encouragement (Morris & McInerney, 2010), yet almost one third reported feeling more worried about giving birth afterwards (Declercq, Sakala, Corry, & Applebaum, 2006). Greater awareness of what can go wrong in childbirth can create the perception that complications occur more often than they do. Healthy pregnant mothers *can* experience a critical intrapartum event, but most do not, and the likelihood of serious harm or death for mother or baby is low, especially in the presence of a skilled birth attendant.

Perception of Risk for Planned Home Birth

In the United States, the home-birth debate is contentious and emotionally charged. Whereas a conversation about the risks of dengue fever is likely to remain respectful and rational, discussion of home birth often opens seemingly unbridgeable rifts (Vedam et al., 2014). Although the dispute seems to hinge on authoritative evidence of the safety of home birth, the real issues can be related to social and ethical values including what risks are relevant, how to weigh them, how much risk is acceptable, what might be lost or compromised when an alternative approach is chosen, and who is entitled to make such decisions (de Melo-Martín & Intemann, 2012).

Table 3-3
Incidence of Selected Events

Event	Incidence
Death from lightning strike (U.S.A., 2020)	0.0000001/1,000 inhabitants (Insurance Information Institute, 2022; U.S. Census Bureau, n.d.)
Amniotic fluid embolism	0.02–0.06/1,000 births (Baldisseri & Clark, 2023)
Acute fatty liver of pregnancy	0.05–0.14/1,000 birth (Lee & Reau, 2023)
Death by homicide (U.S.A., 2019)	0.06/1,000 inhabitants (Xu, Murphy, Kochanek, & Arias, 2021)
Quadruple nuchal cord at birth	<0.1/1,000 births (Schaffer & Zimmerman, 2022)
Eclampsia	0.15–1/1,000 births in high-resource countries, 1.96–14.2/1,000 births in low- and middle-resource countries (Norwitz, 2023)
Death from influenza and pneumonia (U.S.A., 2019)	0.15/1,000 inhabitants (Xu et al., 2021)
HELLP syndrome	1–10/1,000 births (Sibai, 2022)
Shoulder dystocia	1–11/1,000 pregnancies without maternal diabetes, birthweight <4,000 g 200–500/1,000 pregnancies with maternal diabetes, birthweight >4,000 g (Rodis, 2023)
Placental abruption	3–10/1,000 births (Ananth & Kinzler, 2022)
Preeclampsia	46/1,000 pregnancies, worldwide 50/1,000 pregnancies, U.S.A. (August & Sibai, 2023)
Gestational diabetes	78/1,000 births, U.S.A. 20–380/1,000 pregnancies, elsewhere (Durnwald, 2023)

Since the 1800s, physicians and midwives have tended to view the inescapable risks of childbirth differently and to have different interpretations of what it means for mothers and fetuses to be safe. All providers want to ensure optimal health and wellbeing for mother and baby, but midwives and physicians often disagree on what poses the greatest risk and how to achieve the best outcomes. Obstetric providers—physicians and midwives alike—are poor at estimating risk, and they frequently exaggerate the likelihood of rare events (Page & Mander, 2014). All providers filter their perceptions through emotion and assess risk in the context of their knowledge, education, personal experiences, and culture (Horan, 2013). Because standards of care are partially defined by how peers would manage the situation at hand, midwives and obstetricians alike tend to define risk within the framework of guidelines, practice guidelines, and recommendations issued by regulators and professional organizations (Horan, 2013).

Within the medical model, obstetrical providers tend to determine the course they deem most likely to reduce risk and guide the client along it. Because these providers' perceptions are based on an interpretation of science and the prevailing standard of care, the courses they chart are often viewed as authoritative, objective, and in everyone's best interest (Horan, 2013). From this perspective, alternative health care options that run counter to the medical standard can be viewed as substandard, unacceptably risky, or irresponsible (Horan, 2013).

To many hospital-based providers operating squarely within the medical model, home birth appears uncontrolled, unpredictable, and dangerous. Most have never witnessed a home birth and know little about the knowledge base and capabilities of home-birth midwives, partly because of lack of contact (Davis-Floyd, 2003), and frequently have no experience with an uninterrupted labor and birth. Physicians are more likely to hold negative attitudes toward home birth if it is illegal in their state or if they or their colleagues have had personal experience with home-birth transports that were stressful, placed physicians in a high-liability situations, or resulted in poor outcomes (Vedam et al., 2014).

A physician whose only experience with home birth is in receiving emergent or poorly managed transfers can come to view home birth as reckless or community midwives as incompetent. Physicians who assume that the immediate availability of lifesaving interventions in the hospital greatly reduces risk to any mother and baby can fail to consider that a low-risk mother is unlikely to need intervention. Further, there are risks and consequences to routine interventions used in hospitals, such as continuous electronic fetal monitoring, elective induction, epidurals, immediate cord cutting, and early separation of mother and baby, and physicians often fail to inform clients about these risks (Lothian, 2012).

Midwives are more likely than physicians to view home birth as safe, feel confident as home-birth providers, and incorporate low-intervention approaches to labor and birth (Vedam et al., 2014). Nurse-midwives exposed to home birth during professional education or practice are more likely to support

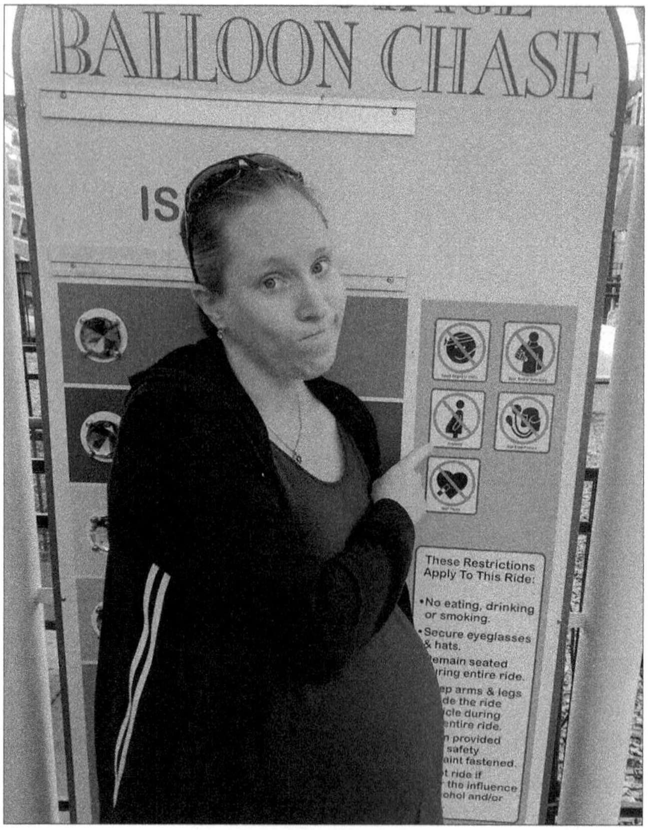

Figure 3-5. Sometimes a pregnant individual can choose what risks to take. Sometimes others make the choice. Photograph by Eric Adkins.

and attend home births (Vedam, Stoll, White, Aaker, & Schummers, 2009). Collaboration with other health care providers can influence a midwife's attitude toward the use of interventions (Zondag, Maas, Beuckens, & Nieuwenhuijze, 2022). Midwives who collaborate with obstetricians are more likely to perform unnecessary interventions to uphold the physician-dictated standard of care (Zondag et al., 2022).

Because mothers must understand the risks and benefits of their chosen birthplaces in relation to their own unique circumstances, the midwife must raise the subject at each visit to deepen their understanding. Discussions should include the possibility of transfer from a planned home birth if complications arise and the presentation of a realistic but positively-framed assessment of the likely receiving hospital so that mothers will feel prepared if they are to give birth there; complications that can arise; how place of birth can affect outcomes; and how transport can affect the timing of treatment (College of Midwives of Manitoba [CMM], 2011). Clients should be reminded that they may change their decisions about place of birth at any time and that the midwife may conclude at any time that they are no longer good candidates for community birth. Because memory is imperfect and some people are litigious, the midwife should document each discussion.

A client with multiple risk factors can be at higher risk for complications than a client with a single risk factor.

Defining *Low Risk*

There is no standard definition of low perinatal risk, but the term usually denotes the absence of medical or obstetric complications in pregnancy, childbirth, or postpartum (George, Mitchell, & Stacey, 2022). "Normal" childbirth is defined by most resources as a healthy, uncomplicated term singleton pregnancy in a cephalic position with spontaneous onset and progress of labor without a history of uterine incision (Bovbjerg, Cheyney, Brown, Cox, & Leeman, 2017; Cheyney et al., 2014; Grünebaum et al., 2015; Lang, Farnell, & Quinlan, 2021; Nethery et al., 2021). The healthy mother experiencing a normal pregnancy, intrapartum, postpartum, and newborn course can give birth safely in any birth setting, including home, birth center, and hospital (ACNM, 2005/2016).

It can be difficult to apply the concept of normality to pregnancy because what is commonplace or insignificant for one client can indicate a problem for another. The process of physiologic birth is variable, unpredictable, and often surprising even to seasoned providers. Every client is an individual, and physiologic labor encompasses a broad range of variations.

The judgments and decisions made by midwives are influenced by their individual definitions of *normal*, which are often imprecise and changeable and usually shaped by personal experience, the experiences of others, academic knowledge, and practice guidelines (Page & Mander, 2014). When midwives care for healthy clients in a variety of circumstances and repeatedly experience good outcomes, they become comfortable with a broad range of normality (Page & Mander, 2014).

In the United States, there are no national guidelines that identify characteristics of clients that are inappropriate candidates for home birth (Likis, 2014). It is accepted, however, that in the presence of certain conditions or risk factors, a client will have better outcomes in a hospital than at home. For example, a client with a transverse lie or a complete placenta previa requires a cesarean section to achieve a good outcome.

Risk Assessment and Analysis

Midwives perform risk assessments by collecting historical and clinical data and comparing those findings with known factors for risk (Tharpe, Farley, & Jordan, 2022). Then they interpret these risks in the context of each client's unique circumstances to form a clinical impression on which to make

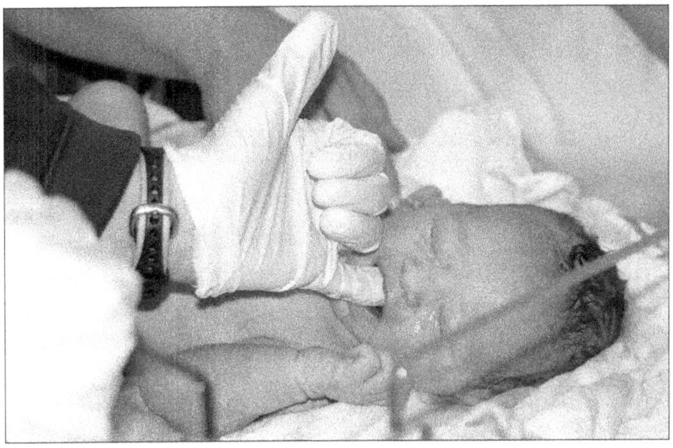

Figure 3-6. In many hospitals, newborns are routinely moved from a provider's hands to the radiant warmer. As the mother watches from across the room, the baby is dried, weighed, measured, examined, footprinted, and medicated. As part of a routine assessment immediately after birth, this nurse tested the suck reflex with a finger before the baby had breastfed or even felt his mother's touch. In the background, a grandmother hesitantly touches the baby's hand. In the midwifery model, a healthy baby and healthy mother have uninterrupted skin contact at least until successful breastfeeding. Comprehensive assessments can wait until bonding is well underway, and the midwife can usually perform many of them with baby and mother skin-to-skin.

Table 3-4
Relative Frequency of Obstetrical Complications in Community Midwifery Practice in the United States

High frequency—complications most encountered
- Postpartum hemorrhage
- Neonatal resuscitation, briefly supporting respirations with bag and mask
- Preeclampsia necessitating hospital birth
- Preterm labor (PTL)
- Persistent fetal heart rate (FHR) abnormalities

Moderate frequency—complications encountered infrequently
- Newborn with a symptomatic congenital heart defect
- Abnormal intrapartum bleeding
- Ectopic pregnancy
- Intraamniotic infection
- Shoulder dystocia

Low frequency—complications encountered rarely
- Full newborn resuscitation with chest compressions
- Umbilical cord prolapse
- Eclampsia
- Unexpected breech
- Undiagnosed twins

Extremely rare catastrophic event
- Amniotic fluid embolism
- Maternal heart attack or stroke
- Maternal death
- Postpartum hemorrhage requiring hysterectomy

recommendations. On average, 10–20% of potential home-birth clients are "risked out" for antepartum complications such as hypertension, twins, placenta previa, fetal growth restriction (FGR), or PTL (Brown & Small, 2023; Vedam, Goff, & Marnin, 2007). Of the remainder, 5–10% require intrapartum referrals (most commonly for failure to progress), 1% need postpartum referrals, and 1% need neonatal referrals (Brown & Small, 2023; Vedam, Goff, et al., 2007).

Risk analysis can identify a given client's likelihood of developing a particular adverse outcome and allow the midwife to suggest interventions that can ameliorate this risk. For example, a client who develops iron deficiency anemia in the second trimester is more likely to develop complications if postpartum hemorrhage occurs after childbirth. The midwife can discuss iron-rich food options, recommend iron supplements, or prescribe intravenous (IV) iron infusions with the goal of normalizing hemoglobin and hematocrit levels by term.

Midwives must consider each client as an individual with a complex life and a dynamic state of health (Tharpe et al., 2022). They must consider whether the client has a *potential* problem or an *actual* condition affecting the client. For example, a client with blood pressure (BP) in the severe range (≥160/90) is at much higher risk for a poor outcome than one who has a *history* of severe hypertension. When a client is classified as high-risk, the likelihood of having a poor obstetrical outcome is higher, but it does not mean that every client considered high-risk will have a poor outcome (Mehl-Madrona & Madrona, 1997). In fact, a client with a 25% chance of developing preeclampsia, which is considered high risk for the disorder, also has a 75% chance of *not* developing preeclampsia. Moreover, even low-risk clients can develop preeclampsia.

Sometimes a procedure or treatment can reduce risk in the short term but increase risk in the long term. For example, cesarean birth for breech can sometimes decrease the risk of death or injury to the fetus in the current pregnancy. But it also *increases* the risk of complications for the mother in the current pregnancy *and* elevates risk in future pregnancies for both the mother and all future infants (ACOG Cmte. on Clinical Practice Guidelines—Obstetrics, Cahill, Raghuraman, Gandhi, & Kaimal, 2024).

One method of protecting people against rare but severe adverse outcomes is to take precautions with everyone,

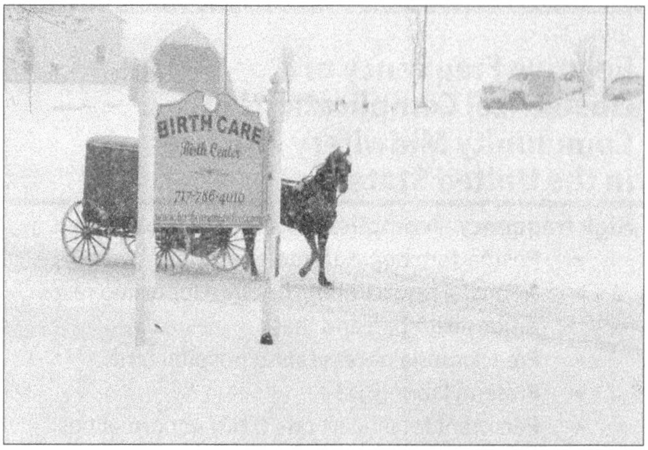

Figure 3-7. An Amish couple arrives at a birth center for a labor check on a snowy afternoon. Weather can affect the client's ability to reach the birth center and the midwife's ability to transport the client to the hospital in an emergency.

regardless of apparent risk level, as in Group B *Streptococcus* (GBS) testing and prophylaxis. GBS disease remains the leading cause of newborn infection in the United States (ACOG, 2020/2022). GBS can be found in the vagina, intestines, and/or rectum of about 10–30% of mothers at term (Verani, McGee, & Schrag, 2010). Half of babies born to untreated mothers become colonized with GBS (ACOG, 2020/2022). About 1–2% of them develop invasive early-onset GBS disease, which is always serious and can cause sepsis, pneumonia, meningitis, brain damage, blindness, hearing loss, or death (Seedat et al., 2017).

After implementation of national guidelines for intrapartum antibiotic prophylaxis, the incidence of early-onset GBS disease declined by 87%, from 1.8 newborns per 1,000 live births in the 1990s to 0.23 per 1,000 in 2015 (ACOG, 2020/2022). Most babies born to untreated mothers, however, remain healthy. Antibiotic treatment can increase antibiotic resistance, derange the microbiome of mother and baby, and encourage the proliferation of fungi, which can cause infant thrush, maternal vaginitis, and other problems. Asthma, obesity, and diabetes in children have been associated with microbiota changes from antibiotics (Seedat et al., 2017). Rarely, a mother has an anaphylactic reaction to an antibiotic.

ACOG (2020) recommends universal antepartum GBS screening between 36 0/7 and 37 6/7 weeks of gestation regardless of planned mode of birth, and prophylactic antibiotic treatment for those who test positive, those with a history of a previous GBS-infected newborn, and those with antepartum GBS bacteriuria. These recommendations remain controversial, however, and the harms of overusing antibiotics have not been fully explored. Some question whether reducing the risk to the health or life of some babies justifies treating many, many healthy fetuses and mothers needlessly.

Conditions that Increase Client Risk

The following is a list of some situations that can require consultation, comanagement, or referral (ACNM, 2015; CMM, 2011; Declercq & Stotland, 2023; Delgado Nunes, Gholitabar, Sims, & Bewley, 2014; Finn et al., 2015; Midwives' Assn. of Washington State, 2008; National Institute for Health and Care Excellence [NICE], 2023). As always, follow your own local guidelines and laws. Many of these conditions do not automatically risk a mother or baby out of home or birth center care, but all should be considered in evaluating overall risk status.

Lifestyle and History

- Adverse socioeconomic conditions.
- Age under 17 years or over 40 years.
- Late presentation to care.
- Uncertain due date.
- Complications with prior pregnancy that are likely to reoccur (such as preeclampsia and gestational diabetes).
- Grand multipara (five or more previous births).
- Body mass index (BMI) less than 18 or greater than 35.
- Poor nutrition.
- Rubella during first trimester of pregnancy.
- Significant use of drugs, alcohol, tobacco, or other toxic substances.
- History of infant(s) over 4,500 g.
- History of late miscarriage (after 14 weeks of gestation) or PTB.
- History of low-birthweight infant(s).
- Prior infant(s) with abnormalities (e.g., cardiac anomalies and Ellis-van Creveld dwarfism).
- Less than 12 months from last childbirth to present due date.
- Previous severe postpartum hemorrhage.
- History of severe hypertension or preeclampsia.
- Repeated elective abortions.
- History of long, difficult labor.
- High risk for genetic disorders, hereditary disease, or anomalies.
- History of cervical cerclage or incompetent cervix.
- History of repeated spontaneous abortions.
- History of significant medical illness.
- History of 3rd- or 4th-degree perineal trauma.
- Previous myomectomy, hysterotomy, or cesarean section.
- Previous neonatal mortality or stillbirth.
- History of pelvic fracture.

Maternal Disease

- Blood disorders such as thrombophilias, thrombocytopenia, or certain anemias.
- Any serious medical condition, such as cardiac disease, renal disease, neurological disorders, severe gastrointestinal disease, or cancer.
- Chronic lung disease requiring medications or treatments, such as asthma.
- Deep-vein thrombosis—current or past.
- Diabetes (especially concerning if the client is on insulin or oral hypoglycemic medications or if the condition is poorly controlled).
- Hepatitis.
- HIV.
- Tuberculosis.
- Persistent anemia, hemoglobinopathies, or blood disease.
- Hypertension.
- Cervical surgery—e.g., LEEP, cone biopsy.
- Lupus or other autoimmune disorder.
- Marfan syndrome, Ehlers-Danlos syndrome, or other connective-tissue disease.
- Renal disease or recurrent pyelonephritis.
- Seizure disorder.
- Syphilis.
- Thyroid disorder.
- UTI unresponsive to treatment.
- Significant psychiatric illness.
- Known uterine malformations or fibroids.
- MRSA carrier or other communicable disease at term.
- Significant abnormal Pap test or breast lump.
- Morbid obesity.

Present Obstetrical Conditions

- Inappropriate uterine growth.
- Significant placental abnormalities.
- Medical conditions arising during pregnancy.
- Placenta previa.
- Polyhydramnios or oligohydramnios.
- Repeated or significant vaginal bleeding.
- Abnormal antepartum fetal assessment.
- Thromboembolism or thrombophlebitis.
- Abnormal fetal growth—suspected FGR or fetal macrosomia.
- IUD in uterus.
- Intraamniotic infection.
- Fetal anomaly.
- Intrauterine fetal death.
- Incompetent cervix.
- Malpresentation at term, such as breech or transverse lie.
- Positive screen for antibody capable of causing fetal hemolytic anemia.
- Maternal trauma.
- Multifetal gestation.
- Preeclampsia or chronic hypertension.
- PTL before 37 0/7 weeks of gestation.
- Preterm rupture of the membranes.
- Postdates by more than 1–2 weeks of gestation.
- Active genital herpes.
- Uterine malformations (unicornuate, bicornuate, et al.).
- Suspected or diagnosed fetal anomaly.
- Acute infection such as varicella, parvovirus, toxoplasmosis, cytomegalovirus, herpes, or rubella.
- Second or third trimester bleeding.

Maternal Assessment Abnormalities

- Pulse over 120 beats per min on 2 occasions 30 min apart.
- Systolic blood pressure (SBP) of 140 mm Hg or more, or diastolic blood pressure (DBP) of 90 mm Hg or more on two consecutive readings 4 hr apart.
- A reading of either SBP of 160 mm Hg or more, or DBP of 110 mm Hg or more, confirmed within a few minutes.
- Sustained maternal fever, over 100.4°F (38°C), or other evidence of maternal infection.
- Proteinuria.

Intrapartum Complications

- Abnormal fetal heart rate (FHR) patterns unresponsive to position changes and fluid bolus.
- Arrested active phase of labor (over 4–6 hr of regular, strong contractions without significant change in cervix and/or station and/or dilation).
- Arrested 2nd stage of labor (multipara with more than 1 hr of active pushing without significant change, primigravida with more than 2 hr of pushing without significant change).
- Prolonged rupture of membranes (more than 24–48 hr); especially risky if GBS is unknown or positive.
- Maternal exhaustion unresponsive to rest/hydration.
- Fetal demise.
- Moderate or thick meconium-stained fluid.
- Prolapsed umbilical cord.
- Bleeding more than bloody show.
- Sustained maternal vital-sign instability or shock.
- Maternal seizure.
- GBS+ and no prophylactic antibiotics; especially concerning with prolonged rupture of membranes.
- Shoulder dystocia.

> Midwives must consider applicable laws, regulations, and professional standards in all matters concerning refusal to provide requested care or discharging a client from practice. They should seek legal counsel in either situation.

- Active genital herpes in vaginal, perineal, or vulvar area in labor or after ROM.
- Client's decision to transport for pain management or other concerns.
- Client requesting care outside the standards of practice.

Postpartum Complications

- Hemorrhage unresponsive to treatment.
- Blood loss greater than 1,000 ml or any blood loss that produces symptoms (tachycardia, faintness, hypotension).
- Laceration beyond the midwife's ability to repair.
- Unstable vital signs.
- Persistent fainting.
- Thrombophlebitis.
- SBP of 140 mm Hg or more, or DBP of 90 mm Hg or more on 2 consecutive readings.
- SBP of 160 mm Hg or more, or DBP of 110 mm Hg or more, confirmed within a few minutes.
- Sustained maternal fever of over 100.4°F (38°C) or other evidence of maternal infection.
- Uterine inversion.
- Retained placenta or membranes.
- Subinvolution.
- Mastitis unresponsive to treatment, breast abscess.
- Wound infection, abnormal healing, dehiscence.
- Endometritis (uterine infection).
- Significant postpartum depression or psychosis.

Newborn

These conditions can warrant immediate or prompt referral to the appropriate pediatric provider:

- Apgar score lower than 7 at 5 min of age.
- Heart rate irregular, below 100, or persistently above 160; persistent cardiac arrhythmias or murmurs, abnormal critical congenital heart disease (CCHD) screen.
- Seizures.
- Significant congenital anomaly.
- Persistent hypoglycemia.
- Persistent temperature instability.
- Less than 37 0/7 weeks of gestation or significant clinical evidence of prematurity.
- Low birthweight.
- Cephalohematoma; other significant trauma or injury.
- Poor suck, hypotonia, abnormal cry.
- Respiratory distress, abnormal respiratory rate or pattern, persistent grunting, and retractions.
- Persistent central cyanosis or pallor.
- Jaundice in first 24 hr or pathologic jaundice at any time.
- Vomiting or diarrhea.
- Infection of umbilical stump site.
- Failure to pass urine or meconium within 24 hr of birth.
- Excessive weight loss, inadequate weight gain.

Other Considerations Relative to the Safety of Community Birth

- Distance and travel time to specialized care (can vary with location, topography, road conditions, traffic, time of day, day of the week, season of the year).
- Access to telephone or availability of cellular service.
- Weather: ice, snow, flooding, wind, downed power lines, etc.
- Availability of emergency medical services.
- Condition of the client's birth environment.

Standard of Care

Standards of practice specify the requisite knowledge and actions of midwives at each level of education, certification, and licensure (Tharpe et al., 2022). ACNM, MANA, the National Association of Certified Professional Midwives, and the International Confederation of Midwives define the professional standards of midwifery practice in the United States. Standards of care are the same whether the client is self-pay or insured, conservative or liberal, wealthy or destitute, black or white, urban or rural, academic or uneducated. Midwives are expected to follow applicable professional standards, national and state laws, local standards, and rules that govern their midwifery practices and to provide care within these boundaries (Tharpe et al., 2022).

Midwives are accountable not only to mothers and their families, but also to the profession, to regulatory bodies, to local health agencies, and to their own consciences to provide proficient, ethical care. Their actions should serve the best interests of the mothers and babies they serve, enhance the reputation of the profession, and inspire public confidence. They should avoid actions that expose them to unacceptable risk or liability or that make them uncomfortable or uneasy.

At intake into the practice and in every subsequent encounter, the midwife should evaluate and discuss risk factors with the client and work out a plan within the bounds of safe, evidence-based care (Clinical Excellence Queensland, 2020). Sometimes the midwife may deviate from the standard of care to meet the client's needs, for example, by agreeing to longer intervals between appointments for a healthy client with transportation problems. The midwife may deem it reasonable for a client to decline a test or treatment, such as when a monogamous mother with an Rh-negative partner declines an antenatal dose of RhD immune globulin. At other times, the client requests or simply exercises options that are below the standard of care, as when a mother with severe hypothyroidism declines medication that would reduce the risk of damage to her fetus.

When the midwife or client deviates from the standard of care, the risk of complications can increase. Potential consequences range from none or minor issues to crises resulting in damage or death. For example, the client with longer-interval office visits can develop severe hypertension between evaluations. The mother who declines glucose testing can have a stillbirth related to uncontrolled gestational diabetes. These extreme outcomes are uncommon, but they happen. When they do, they can expose the midwife to liability.

Clinician-Client Relationship

State and national definitions differ, but a client-provider relationship is usually established when a provider examines, diagnoses, or treats someone or agrees to do so (Blake, 2012). Once this relationship is formed, the clinician has a legal and ethical duty to provide care until one party ends the relationship. With this relationship comes an expectation of mutual trust and loyalty and an understanding that the clinician will act in the client's best interest (Schorn, 2007). A provider who wishes to discharge a client from care must give reasonable notice and must arrange for another provider to assume responsibility for care. A midwife can be legally charged with abandonment or negligence or sued for breach of contract for failing to discharge a client in an orderly, humane manner (Schorn, 2007). Become familiar with local and national laws and regulations regarding clinician-client relations.

Worldwide, professional organizations acknowledge that pregnant clients have the right to self-determination and affirm their right to decline any treatment or care plan (ACOG, 2016/2019, 2017/2023; Childbirth Connection, 2006; Clinical Excellence Queensland, 2020; NICE, 2023; White Ribbon Alliance, n.d.). Clients have medical decision-making capacity if they can show understanding of the situation, demonstrate reasoning in their thought process, appreciate the consequences of their decisions, and can communicate their wishes (Barstow, Shahan, & Roberts, 2018). In the United States, pregnant individuals with medical decision-making capacity have almost complete autonomy when deciding for themselves, even if their fetuses may be adversely affected (ACOG, 2016/2019). Yet at the moment of birth, parents lose some of their power to make decisions about a baby's medical treatment (Vedam et al., 2014). The care of a baby born in a hospital can follow more restrictive guidelines than would apply elsewhere. For example, some hospitals mandate a 24–48-hr stay for babies born to mothers with positive or unknown GBS carrier status and mothers who did not receive a full course of antibiotics before giving birth. In a birth center, the same baby might be discharged home a few hours after birth. Some parental decisions, such as not vaccinating children, are seen as medical neglect by some health care providers. If providers have significant

Table 3-5

Some Conditions Requiring Immediate Transport

Maternal/Fetal
Cardiac arrest.
Seizures.
Significant bleeding.
Persistent or worsening FHR abnormalities.
Meconium-stained amniotic fluid (if birth not imminent).
Cord prolapse.
Maternal fever.
Foul-smelling amniotic fluid.
Respiratory difficulty, poor oxygen saturation.
Labor with malpresentation incompatible with home birth.
Shoulder dystocia unresolved by initial maneuvers.
Postpartum hemorrhage unresponsive to treatment.
Shock.
Laceration beyond the midwife's ability to repair.
Persistent fainting.
Persistently abnormal or unstable vital signs.
Retained placenta.
Inability to void.
Chest pain, cardiac abnormalities.
Uterine inversion.
Newborn
Persistent newborn pallor or central cyanosis.
Poor suck, hypotonia, abnormal cry.
Respiratory distress, abnormal rate or pattern, persistent grunting and retractions, poor oxygen saturation.
Seizures.
Heart rate irregular, below 100, or above 170; abnormal murmurs; abnormal critical congenital heart disease (CCHD) screen.
Persistent hypoglycemia.
Significant birth injury.
Significantly abnormal feeding, voiding, or stooling.
Temperature instability.
Significant congenital anomaly.
Prematurity or very low birthweight.
Pathological or severe jaundice.

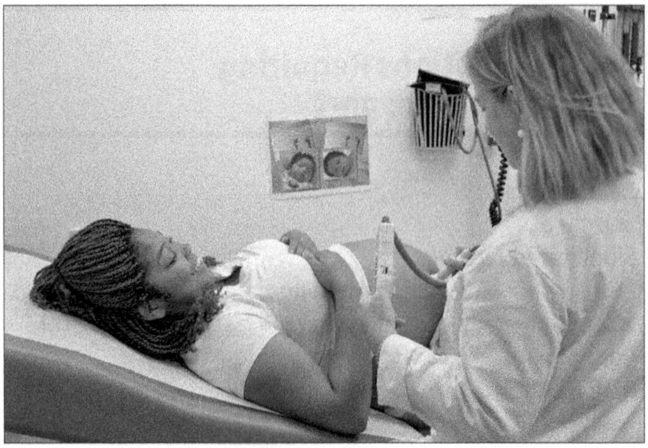

Figure 3-8. Although clients have the right to make choices regarding their care, midwives need to observe their own personal boundaries of safe practice and feel comfortable with the degree of risk they assume with a client.

concerns for a baby's wellbeing, they can seek a court order or contact child protective services to ensure treatment according to medical standards (Vedam et al., 2014).

The midwife is responsible for informing the client of the benefits and drawbacks of available options, but ultimately it is the client who accepts or rejects the recommendations (ACNM, 2015). Sometimes clients make choices for themselves that fall outside the scope or standards of safe midwifery practice or decline care that the midwife considers essential to safety. Many clients who resist procedures or processes within the standard of care do so while making well-considered choices. Clients are more likely to opt out when the benefits of an intervention seem theoretical or irrelevant to their situation. For example, healthy, well-nourished clients without risk factors may decline antepartum glucose testing, feeling that their individual risk for gestational diabetes is minimal. When a client does not consent to the standard of care, explain the rationale for your recommendations and discuss the possible consequences of alternatives while maintaining an atmosphere of respect and support. Document the conversation and have the client sign to acknowledge understanding.

When a client chooses potentially unsafe options and things go badly, the attending midwife may encounter a life-threatening emergency, face malpractice or even criminal charges, and suffer loss of licensure or reputation. For example, parents who refuse auscultation of FHR during labor increase the risk for an adverse outcome that can devastate everyone involved. In most non-emergent situations, a provider who believes that a client's wishes are dangerous is not obliged to follow them (Schorn, 2007). ACNM (2015) advises that when a client declines the provider's recommendation in urgent circumstances—for example, a malpresentation in labor—the provider is obliged continue providing care until another appropriate provider assumes responsibility. The following is a general guideline illustrating possible courses of action when a client requests nonstandard care. *It is not to be considered legal advice.*

1. Explain to the client and family why you cannot comply. Be clear about the standard of care and your scope of practice, education and training, and limitations. Explain the rationale for the standard, the evidence supporting it, and your own clinical judgment of the situation. Inform client and family about risks, benefits, and alternate approaches (College of Midwives of British Columbia [CMBC], 2016a, 2016b).
2. Share your clinical concerns for the wellbeing of client or baby likely to result from the requested deviation from standards. Be explicit. If the risk of breech head entrapment can lead to death or serious damage to the baby, say so clearly. Offer compromises that can satisfy the client's wishes, fears, or concerns while upholding an acceptable standard of midwifery practice. Let the client respond. Throughout the informed-choice and consultation process, clearly document every step in the client's health record. Record when the conversation takes place; who is present; and explicit details of topics covered, including harm that can occur. Quote the client's responses exactly whenever possible. Document the clinical assessment.
3. If you and your client are still at an impasse, seek help. The most appropriate consultant may be a physician, another midwife, a peer review group, an ethicist, or a combination. Discuss options and solutions that would honor the client's needs while remaining within midwifery standards. Continue documenting all interactions. Consider how to proceed if the client declines alternatives (CMBC, 2016a, 2016b).
4. If a generally acceptable solution cannot be found, the midwife should either continue care or discharge the client from the practice in accordance with local standards, laws, and regulations.

Continuing care: Respect the client's choices but continue to make recommendations for safe care. As appropriate, involve other providers who can be called on to participate in caregiving, such as hospital staff and midwife colleagues (CMBC, 2016a, 2016b). Thoroughly document all discussions and decisions involving the client.

Discontinuing care: *To minimize liability and ensure that you comply with local laws, regulations, and standards—which can change unpredictably or have conflicting interpretations—consult a lawyer before terminating a client's care.* This book supplies broad ideas that have been used by some midwifery practices; your own situation will be unique. Most termination-of-care guidelines involve giving the provider time to help the client find a replacement and allowing the client reasonable time to establish a relationship with another practice (Willis & Zerr, 2005).

Documentation is crucial, and it is often the only evidence that a task was or was not performed. It should provide an accurate record of events that occurred while the client was in your care. Not only does careful and complete documentation help protect the health professional against litigation, it also paints a picture of the client's health care experience that can shape the care provided by others (Brass, 2012).

Decision-Making Conflicts

Practicing midwives around the world differ in legal scope of practice and the risk levels they are willing or obliged to assume. Clinicians and authorities alike debate whether frank breech, single previous cesarean section with prior vaginal birth, and vertex full-term twins should be considered normal variations of parturition or unacceptably risky for community birth (Fischbein & Freeze, 2018; Freeze, 2010). Even in hospitals, authorities disagree over appropriate management of these clients and whether it is safer to attempt vaginal birth or to proceed directly to cesarean. As always, mothers must be fully informed of the absolute and relative risks and benefits of their options concerning where and how to give birth (Fischbein & Freeze, 2018).

How much risk is too much? The answer varies. Many authorities consider a small increase in risk of poor outcomes acceptable if most mothers or babies reap significant benefits. For example, in the United Kingdom, the NICE guidelines recommend that providers offer low-risk nulliparous clients the option of home birth. Home birth for these clients, however, is associated with slightly higher risk for adverse neonatal outcomes, 9/1,000 newborns born at home vs. 4/1,000 newborns born in a hospital (NICE, 2023). The authors analyzed the potential benefits and the degree of risk involved with home birth and deemed home birth an appropriate option for those who understand the higher risks. On the other hand, NICE guidelines consider breech and multiple gestation conditions "indicating increased risk and suggesting planned birth at an obstetric unit" (NICE, 2023, table 7). Also in the United Kingdom, the Royal College of Obstetricians and Gynaecologists unequivocally asserts that vaginal breech birth should occur in a hospital with facilities for emergency cesarean section (Hofmeyr & Impey, 2006).

Some believe that twins, breech presentations, and VBAC can be safely managed outside a hospital (Fischbein & Freeze, 2018). It is common to find articles (usually not in peer-reviewed research journals) promoting the planned community

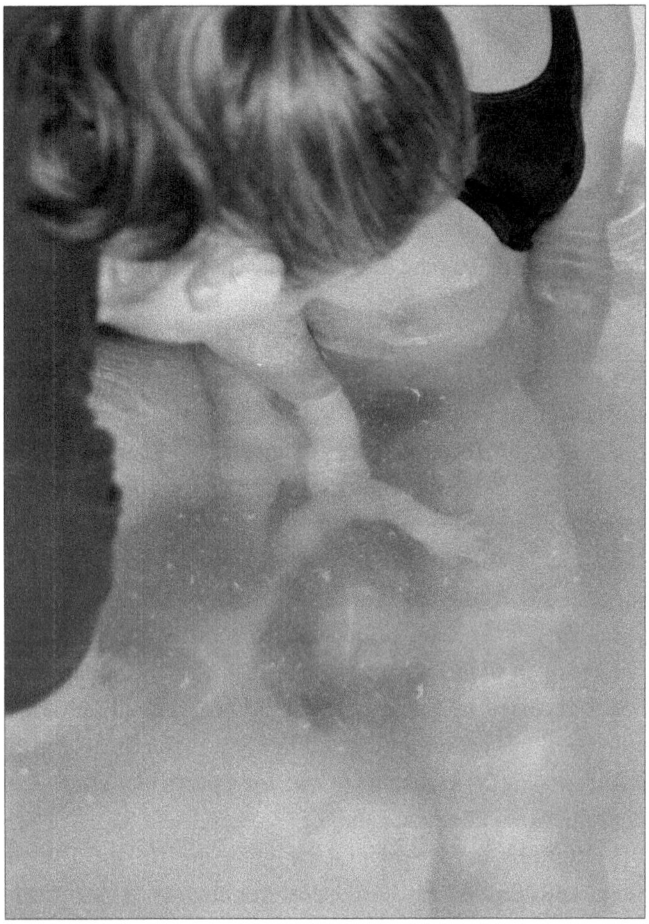

Figure 3-9. A healthy boy is born into the tub at a birth center. All births contain an element of risk. How much risk should a provider or parent accept? Answers to this question depend on circumstances, degrees of risk, ratios of risks to benefits, and potential consequences.

birth of twins, VBACs, and significantly postdate pregnancies. An Internet search with the words *breech home birth* or *twin home birth* yields thousands of stories of these births, including unattended births; births with CNMs, certified professional midwives (CPMs), and lay midwives; waterbirths; footling breech births; and double-breech twins. Most of these births are accomplished with no damage to mother or baby, leading one midwifery magazine article to ask, "Why aren't more breech babies born at home?" (Peacock, 2014, p. 51).

Although breech and twin pregnancies have higher perinatal mortality rates regardless of the mode and setting of birth, risks are greater for such babies born vaginally at home (Bastian et al., 1998; Bovbjerg et al., 2017; Caughey & Cheyney, 2019; Lang et al., 2021; Zielinski, Ackerson, & Low, 2015). In the United States, Cheyney et al. (2014) found significantly higher rates of perinatal death when certain high-risk births occurred at home: 5 deaths in 222 breech presentations, 5 deaths in 1,052 trials of labor after cesarean (TOLACs), 1 death out of 120 clients with multiple gestation, 2 of 131 with GDM, and 1 of 28 with preeclampsia. The same study found that the planned home birth of a fetus who starts labor in a breech presentation is associated with an intrapartum mortality rate of 13.5/1,000 and a neonatal mortality rate of 9.2/1,000 (Cheyney et al., 2014). Low-risk vertex babies in the same study had intrapartum, early-neonatal, and late-neonatal mortality rates of 1.30, 0.41, and 0.35 per 1,000, respectively, if lethal anomalies were excluded (Cheyney et al., 2014). Because of the small sample size, however, the authors were unsure whether the data indicated correlation or causation and were unable to reach firm conclusions about the differences in mortality (Cheyney et al., 2014). Conversely, one study showed good outcomes for frank breech births at an Amish birth center in Wisconsin (Deline et al., 2012). Another study by Fischbein and Freeze (2018) suggested that vaginal breech birth in community settings under specific practice guidelines and with a skilled provider can result in high rates of vaginal birth (84%, compared to 57.2% reported by Cheyney et al., 2014) and good maternal outcomes, but the authors noted that whether a breech birth in this setting is reasonable or safe for a particular client is a multifactorial judgment call.

Although obstetrical practice guidelines in the United States and United Kingdom oppose community vaginal birth after cesarean (VBAC), TOLAC at home is increasing in the United States (ACNM, 2015; ACOG, 2019; Cmte. on Fetus and Newborn et al., 2013; Gupta, Smith, & Chodankar, 2015; MacDorman, Mathews, & Declercq, 2014; NICE, 2023; Niemczyk, 2016). Successful VBAC benefits mother, baby, and future babies by avoiding the risks associated with repeat cesarean births, which increase with every operation (Bayrampour et al., 2021; Metz, 2023). Most research indicates that mothers attempting TOLAC have an average vaginal birth rate of 60–80%. Most maternal morbidity associated with TOLAC occurs if the trial is unsuccessful and the client requires a cesarean (Metz, 2023). Conversely, the benefit of elective repeat cesarean birth without TOLAC is derived from avoiding the risks associated with TOLAC, such as uterine rupture (Metz, 2023). A failed TOLAC, however, carries a higher risk of complications than a successful TOLAC or elective repeat cesarean, and it increases the risk of uterine rupture, which can be life-threatening for mother and baby (Lazarou, Oestergaard, Netzl, Siedentopf, & Henrich, 2021; Metz, 2023).

The rate of uterine rupture for mothers at term who enter labor after one prior cesarean birth is 4.7/1,000 at home and in the hospital (ACNM, 1992/2017). Among those who suffer uterine rupture during TOLAC, the risk of postpartum hysterectomy is 14–33% and the rate of perinatal death is as high as 2.8% (Metz, 2023). Mothers attempting TOLAC at home are more likely to give birth vaginally and have similarly good maternal-infant outcomes when compared to mothers attempting TOLAC in a hospital (Bayrampour et al., 2021; Cox et al., 2015; Niemczyk, 2016; Rowe, Li, Knight, Brocklehurst, & Hollowell, 2016). When complications do occur, however, mothers and babies are more likely to have poor outcomes at home (Cox et al., 2015; Niemczyk, 2016; Rowe et al., 2016). One U.S. study of planned home births found a higher rate of intrapartum fetal death associated with TOLAC, about 1 in 210 (Cheyney et al., 2014). Another found the combined intrapartum and neonatal mortality rates for home TOLAC to be 3.02/1,000 (Cox et al., 2015), considerably higher than for planned hospital TOLAC, 0.13/1,000 (Cox et al., 2015; Landon & Grobman, 2021). These differences are the central argument against TOLAC in community settings.

Community midwives who accept mothers carrying twins or breech fetuses typically manage only a handful of such births in their careers. Many CPMs work in low-volume solo practices and are assisted at births by students, apprentices, or fellow midwives. Of CPM respondents to the 2011 North American Registry of Midwives Survey, 86.9% reported that they attend VBACs, at a rate of roughly 1 a year; 36.4% attend multiple-gestation births, at a rate of about 1 every 3 years; and 34.7% attend planned vaginal breech births, at a rate of about 1 a year (Cheyney et al., 2014). Any high-level skill requires frequent practice to develop and maintain. The low volume of mostly low-risk clients offers most community midwives little opportunity to acquire and keep the specialized competencies needed to safely manage higher-risk vaginal births (Cheyney et al., 2014).

The guidelines of many professional organizations in the United States, United Kingdom, and Canada maintain that breech presentation and multiple gestation increase risk, and they encourage mothers to give birth in a hospital (ACNM, 2015). ACOG considers both absolute contraindications to home birth (ACOG, 2017/2023). To receive accreditation from the Commission for the Accreditation of Birth Centers (CABC), a birth center must prohibit planned multiple and breech births, though in some cases it may allow a mother meeting certain criteria to choose TOLAC (CABC, 2023). These include having only one prior cesarean birth, a documented low-transverse incision, and ultrasound confirmation that the placenta is not anterior and low-lying (CABC, 2023). The informed-consent process for this option includes a comprehensive discussion of the specific risks associated with TOLAC in community settings, resources at the birth center and at area hospitals for managing emergencies that can occur during TOLAC, and time considerations for emergency transport from onset of complication to the time of treatment at the hospital (CABC, 2023).

Topics for Discussion

1. Cassandra J., 28-year-old gravida 4, para 3 (G4 P3), is in labor at 41 0/7 weeks of gestation. She had been making slow but steady progress, averaging about 1 cm of dilation and 0.5 cm of descent every 2.5 hr. She has been at 9 cm dilation for 3 hr, however. She is tired and discouraged because all her prior labors were fast and easy. Discuss how a seasoned midwife with 15 years of experience and 1,000 births might evaluate this situation differently from one who has been a midwife for a year and attended 60 births.
2. How does a midwife know when labor is "normal"? How does perception of "normal" change as a midwife moves from beginner to expert?
3. What shapes a pregnant mother's perception of risk in childbirth? What shapes the midwife's and physician's perception of risk? Can all three have differing perspectives and be correct?
4. A client at 32 0/7 weeks of gestation carrying breech triplets wants to transfer into your practice because she wants her husband to catch the babies in a backyard pool with a midwife standing by. Her prior provider is an obstetrician at a tertiary medical center who would require her to have a cesarean birth. Discuss how you would counsel this individual.
5. You are a licensed CPM in a solo home-birth practice. Martha R., a client in your care planning a home birth, had preeclampsia in a prior pregnancy. She has been normotensive throughout pregnancy until yesterday, when she had a BP of 142/90 at her antenatal visit at 34 weeks of gestation. Today her BP is 154/94. Your practice guidelines require any client with elevated BP to have a complete metabolic panel, a complete blood count, a urine protein/creatinine ratio, a nonstress test, and a consultation with an obstetrician. You spend 45 min discussing the reasons you believe that it is important for her to have these tests and possible consequences if she does not. Martha refuses all these, stating she has the right to choose what tests she will have. Discuss how you would manage this client. Would you discharge her from your practice? If so, what issues should you consider?

References

Adams, J. (1998). *Risk, freedom and responsibility.* Paper for conference on The Risk of Freedom, Institute of United States Studies, University of London. Retrieved from http://john-adams.co.uk/wp-content/uploads/2006/risk, freedom & responsibility.pdf

American College of Nurse-Midwives. (1992, revised 2017). *Vaginal birth after cesarean* (Position Statement). Retrieved from https://www.midwife.org/acnm/files/ACNMLibraryData/UPLOADFILENAME/000000000090/VBAC-PS-FINAL-10-10-17.pdf

American College of Nurse-Midwives. (2005, revised 2016). *Planned home birth* (Position Statement). Retrieved from https://www.midwife.org/acnm/files/ACNMLibraryData/UPLOADFILENAME/000000000251/Planned-Home-Birth-Dec-2016.pdf

American College of Nurse-Midwives. (2015). Midwifery provision of home birth services (Clinical Bulletin 14). *Journal of Midwifery & Women's Health, 61*(1), 127–133. https://doi.org/10.1111/jmwh.12431

American College of Obstetricians and Gynecologists. (2016, reaffirmed 2019). *Refusal of medically recommended treatment during pregnancy* (Committee Opinion 664). Retrieved from https://www.acog.org/clinical/clinical-guidance/committee-opinion/articles/2016/06/refusal-of-medically-recommended-treatment-during-pregnancy

American College of Obstetricians and Gynecologists. (2019). *Vaginal birth after cesarean delivery* (Practice Bulletin 205). Retrieved from https://www.acog.org/clinical/clinical-guidance/practice-bulletin/articles/2019/02/vaginal-birth-after-cesarean-delivery

American College of Obstetricians and Gynecologists. (2020, reaffirmed 2022). *Prevention of Group B streptococcal early-onset disease in newborns* (Committee Opinion 797, interim update). Retrieved from https://www.acog.org/clinical/clinical-guidance/committee-opinion/articles/2020/02/prevention-of-group-b-streptococcal-early-onset-disease-in-newborns

American College of Obstetricians and Gynecologists Committee on Clinical Practice Guidelines—Obstetrics, Cahill, A. G., Raghuraman, N., Gandhi, M., & Kaimal, A. J. (2024). *First and second stage labor management* (Clinical Practice Guideline 8). *Obstetrics & Gynecology, 143*(1), 144–162.

American College of Obstetricians and Gynecologists Committee on Obstetric Practice. (2017, reaffirmed 2023). *Planned home birth* (Committee Opinion 697, interim update). Retrieved from https://www.acog.org/clinical/clinical-guidance/committee-opinion/articles/2017/04/planned-home-birth

Ananth, C. V., & Kinzler, W. L. (2022). Acute placental abruption: Pathophysiology, clinical features, diagnosis, and consequences. In V. A. Barss (Ed.), *UpToDate*. Retrieved November 13, 2023, from https://www.uptodate.com/contents/acute-placental-abruption-pathophysiology-clinical-features-diagnosis-and-consequences

Andre, C., & Velasquez, M. (2013). *For your own good*. Retrieved from https://www.scu.edu/ethics/ethics-resources/ethical-decision-making/for-your-own-good/

Anwar, S., & Razzak, A. A. (2015). Intuition and care. *Journal of Nursing and Care, 2015* (Special Issue 1). Retrieved from https://www.hilarispublisher.com/open-access/intuition-and-care-2167-1168-S1-002.pdf

August, P., & Sibai, B. M. (2023). Preeclampsia: Clinical features and diagnosis. In V. A. Barss (Ed.), *UpToDate*. Retrieved November 13, 2023, from https://www.uptodate.com/contents/preeclampsia-clinical-features-and-diagnosis

Baldisseri, M. R., & Clark, S. L. (2023). Amniotic fluid embolism. In G. Finlay & V. A. Barss (Eds.), *UpToDate*. Retrieved November 13, 2023, from http://www.uptodate.com/contents/amniotic-fluid-embolism

Barber, K. (2012). The complexity of decision-making in midwifery: A case study. *British Journal of Midwifery, 20*(4), 289–294. https://doi.org/10.12968/bjom.2012.20.4.289

Barnes, P. M., & Dossey, M. S. (1999). Triage issues in an out-of-hospital birth center. *Journal of Midwifery & Women's Health, 44*(5), 458–470. https://doi.org/10.1016/S0091-2182(99)00081-6

Barstow, C., Shahan, B., & Roberts, R. (2018). Evaluating medical decision-making capacity in practice. *American Family Physician, 98*(1), 40–46. Retrieved from https://www.aafp.org/pubs/afp/issues/2018/0701/p40.html

Bastian, H., Keirse, M. J. N. C., & Lancaster, P. A. L. (1998). Perinatal death associated with planned home birth in Australia: Population based study. *BMJ, 317*(7155), 384–388. https://doi.org/10.1136/bmj.317.7155.384

Bayrampour, H., Lisonkova, S., Tamana, S., Wines, J., Vedam, S., & Janssen, P. (2021). Perinatal outcomes of planned home birth after cesarean and planned hospital vaginal birth after cesarean at term gestation in British Columbia, Canada: A retrospective population-based cohort study. *Birth, 48*(3), 301–308. https://doi.org/10.1111/birt.12539

Benner, P. (2001). *From novice to expert: Excellence and power in clinical nursing practice* (commemorative ed.). Upper Saddle River, NJ: Prentice Hall.

Blake, V. (2012). When is a patient-physician relationship established? *Virtual Mentor, 14*(5), 403–406. https://doi.org/10.1001/virtualmentor.2012.14.5.hlaw1-1205

Bovbjerg, M. L., Cheyney, M., Brown, J., Cox, K. J., & Leeman, L. (2017). Perspectives on risk: Assessment of risk profiles and outcomes among women planning community birth in the United States. *Birth, 44*(3), 209–221. https://doi.org/10.1111/birt.12288

Brass, R. (2012). Caring for the woman who goes against conventional medical advice. *British Journal of Midwifery, 20*(12), 898–901. https://doi.org/10.12968/bjom.2012.20.12.898

Brown, H. L., & Small, M. J. (2023). Overview of maternal mortality. In A. Chakrabarti (Ed.), *UpToDate*. Retrieved September 30, from http://www.uptodate.com/contents/overview-of-maternal-mortality

Burdett, B. R. D., Starkey, N. J., & Charlton, S. G. (2018). Characteristics of the close to home crash. *Safety Science, 105*, 222–227. https://doi.org/10.1016/j.ssci.2018.02.020

Carper, B. A. (1978). Fundamental patterns of knowing in nursing. *Advances in Nursing Science, 1*(1), 13–24. https://doi.org/10.1097/00012272-197810000-00004

Casper, L. (2010). *Simulations and drills: Educational tool #6*. Retrieved from https://www.cmqcc.org/resource/1328/download

Caughey, A. B. & Cheyney, M. (2019). Home and birth center birth in the United States: Time for greater collaboration across models of care. *Obstetrics & Gynecology, 133*(5), 1033–1050 https://doi.org/10.1097/AOG.0000000000003215

Cheyney, M., Bovbjerg, M., Everson, C., Gordon, W., Hannibal, D., & Vedam, S. (2014). Outcomes of care for 16,924 planned home births in the United States: The Midwives Alliance of North America Statistics Project, 2004 to 2009. *Journal of Midwifery & Women's Health, 59*(1), 17–27. https://doi.org/10.1111/jmwh.12172

Childbirth Connection. (2006). *The rights of childbearing women*. Retrieved from https://www.nationalpartnership.org/our-work/resources/health-care/maternity/the-rights-of-childbearing-women.pdf

Clinical Excellence Queensland. (2020). *Guideline: Partnering with the woman who declines recommended maternity care*. Brisbane, Australia: Queensland Health. Retrieved from https://www.health.qld.gov.au/__data/assets/pdf_file/0022/736213/maternity-decline-guide.pdf

College of Midwives of British Columbia. (2016a). *Policy for client requests outside midwifery standards of practice and required procedures for midwife-initiated termination of care*. Retrieved from http://cmbc.bc.ca/wp-content/uploads/2016/03/Policy-for-Client-Requests-Outside-Midwifery-Standards-of-Practice.pdf

College of Midwives of British Columbia. (2016b). *Policy for required procedures for midwife or client-initiated termination of care*. Retrieved from http://cmbc.bc.ca/wp-content/uploads/2016/03/Policy-for-Required-Procedures-for-Midwife-or-Client-Initiated-Termination-of-Care.pdf

College of Midwives of Manitoba. (2011). *Standard for planned out of hospital birth*. Retrieved from http://www.midwives.mb.ca/policies_and_standards/standard-planned-out-of-hospital-birth-july2011.pdf

Commission for the Accreditation of Birth Centers. (2023). *CABC indicators of compliance with standards for birth centers* (reference ed. 2.3). Hamburg, PA: Author. Retrieved from https://www.birthcenteraccreditation.org/wp-content/uploads/2023/09/CABC_IndicatorsRefEd-2.3_2023-0915.pdf

Committee on Fetus and Newborn, Watterberg, K., Papile, L. A., Baley, J. E., Benitz, W., Cummings, J., . . . Tan, R. C. (2013). Planned home birth. *Pediatrics, 131*(5), 1016–1020. https://doi.org/10.1542/peds.2013-0575

Cox, K. J., Bovbjerg, M. L., Cheyney, M., & Leeman, L. M. (2015). Planned home VBAC in the United States, 2004–2009: Outcomes, maternity care practices, and implications for shared decision making. *Birth, 42*(4), 299–308. https://doi.org/10.1111/birt.12188

Davis-Floyd, R. (2003). Home-birth emergencies in the US and Mexico: The trouble with transport. *Social Science & Medicine, 56*(9), 1911–1931. https://doi.org/10.1016/S0277-9536(02)00213-7

Davis-Floyd, R., & Davis, E. (1996). Intuition as authoritative knowledge in midwifery and homebirth. *Medical Anthropology Quarterly, 10*(2), 237–269. https://doi.org/10.1525/maq.1996.10.2.02a00080

de Bono, E. (1970). *Lateral thinking: Creativity step by step*. New York, NY: Harper & Row.

de Melo-Martín, I., & Intemann, K. (2012). Interpreting evidence: Why values can matter as much as science. *Perspectives in Biology and Medicine, 55*(1), 59–70. http://doi.org/10.1353/pbm.2012.0007

Declercq, E., & Stotland, N. E. (2023). *Planned home birth*. In K. Eckler (Ed.), *UpToDate*. Retrieved September 30, 2023, from http://www.uptodate.com/contents/planned-home-birth

Declercq, E. R., Sakala, C., Corry, M. P., & Applebaum, S. (2006). *Listening to mothers II: Report of the second national U.S. Survey of women's childbearing experiences*. New York, NY: Childbirth Connection. Retrieved from http://www.nationalpartnership.org/research-library/maternal-health/listening-to-mothers-ii-2006.pdf

Delgado Nunes, V., Gholitabar, M., Sims, J. M., & Bewley, S. (2014). Intrapartum care of healthy women and their babies: Summary of updated NICE guidance. *BMJ, 349*, g6886. https://doi.org/10.1136/bmj.g6886 Retrieved from https://www.ncbi.nlm.nih.gov/pmc/articles/PMC4707719/

Deline, J., Varnes-Epstein, L., Dresang, L. T., Gideonsen, M., Lynch, L., & Frey, J. J. (2012). Low primary cesarean rate and high VBAC rate with good outcomes in an Amish birthing center. *Annals of Family Medicine, 10*(6), 530–537. https://doi.org/10.1370/afm.1403

Dresang, L., & Rochin, E. (2020). Safety in maternity care. In L. Leeman, L. Dresang, J. S. Quinlan, & S. R. Magee (Eds.), *Advanced life support in obstetrics: Provider manual* (9th ed., pp. 1–17). Leawood, KS: American Academy of Family Physicians.

Durnwald, C. (2023). Diabetes mellitus in pregnancy: Screening, diagnosis, and prevention. In V. A. Barss (Ed.), *UpToDate*. Retrieved October 1, 2023, from https://www.uptodate.com/contents/gestational-diabetes-mellitus-screening-diagnosis-and-prevention

Finn, K. T., Condon, S., Doyle, K. M., Hernandez, E. M., Kieltyka, C., Jefferson, K., & Ritter, R. (2015). *Planned home birth in New York State: New York State Association of Licensed Midwives guidelines for best practice*. (n.p.): New York State Association of Licensed Midwives. Retrieved from http://nysalm.org/wp-content/uploads/2016/10/HomeBirthGuidelines.pdf

Fischbein, S. J., & Freeze, R. (2018). Breech birth at home: Outcomes of 60 breech and 109 cephalic planned home and birth center births. *BMC Pregnancy and Childbirth, 18*(1), 1–12. https://doi.org/10.1186/s12884-018-2033-5

Freeze, R. A. S. (2010). Attitudes towards home birth in the USA. *Expert Review of Obstetrics & Gynecology, 5*(3), 283–299. https://doi.org/10.1586/eog.10.22

George, E. K., Mitchell, S. & Stacey, D. (2022), Choosing a birth setting: A shared decision-making approach. *Journal of Midwifery & Women's Health, 67*(4), 510–514. https://doi.org/10.1111/jmwh.13377

Grima, S., Hamarat, B., Özen, E., Girlando, A., & Dalli-Gonzi, R. (2021). The relationship between risk perception and risk definition and risk-addressing behaviour during the early COVID-19 stages. *Journal of Risk and Financial Management, 14*(6), 272. https://doi.org/10.3390/jrfm14060272

Grünebaum, A., McCullough, L. B., Brent, R. L., Arabin, B., Levene, M. I., & Chervenak, F. A. (2015). Perinatal risks of planned home births in the United States. *American Journal of Obstetrics & Gynecology, 212*(3), 350.e1–350.e6. https://doi.org/10.1016/j.ajog.2014.10.021

Gupta, J. K., Smith, G. C. S., & Chodankar, R. R. (2015). *Birth after previous caesarian birth* (Green-top Guideline 45). Retrieved from https://www.rcog.org.uk/globalassets/documents/guidelines/gtg_45.pdf

Hofmeyr, G. J., Haws, R. A., Bergström, S., Lee, A. C. C., Okong, P., Darmstadt, G. L., . . . Lawn, J. E. (2009). Obstetric care in low-resource settings: what, who, and how to overcome challenges to scale up? *International Journal of Gynecology & Obstetrics, 107*, S21–S45. https://doi.org/10.1016/j.ijgo.2009.07.017

Hofmeyr, G. J., & Impey, L. W. M. (2006). *The management of breech presentation* (RCOG Guideline 20b). Retrieved from https://www.rcog.org.uk/globalassets/documents/guidelines/gtg-no-20b-breech-presentation.pdf

Horan, A. R. (2013). *Risking it: An examination of risk perception amongst obstetricians and certified professional midwives in Missouri* (Undergraduate Research Symposium Posters & Abstracts, Paper 10). Retrieved from http://openscholarship.wustl.edu/undergrad_research/10

Insurance Information Institute. (2022). *Facts + statistics: Mortality risk. Retrieved from* https://www.iii.org/fact-statistic/facts-statistics-mortality-risk

Insurance Institute for Highway Safety & Highway Loss Data Institute. (2023). *Seat belt and child seat laws by state.* Retrieved from https://www.iihs.org/topics/seat-belts/seat-belt-law-table

Jefford, E., Fahy, K., & Sundin, D. (2010). A review of the literature: Midwifery decision-making and birth. *Women and Birth, 23*(4), 127–134. https://doi.org/10.1016/j.wombi.2010.02.001

Jefford, E., Fahy, K., & Sundin, D. (2011). Decision-making theories and their usefulness to the midwifery profession both in terms of midwifery practice and the education of midwives. *International Journal of Nursing Practice, 17*(3), 246–253. https://doi.org/10.1111/j.1440-172X.2010.01900.x

Kennare, R. M., Keirse, M. J. N. C., Tucker, G. R., & Chan, A. C. (2010). Planned home and hospital births in South Australia, 1991–2006: Differences in outcomes. *Medical Journal of Australia, 192*(2), 76–80. Retrieved from https://www.mja.com.au/journal/2010/192/2/planned-home-and-hospital-births-south-australia-1991-2006-differences-outcomes

Landon, M. B., & Grobman, W. A. (2021). Vaginal birth after cesarean delivery. In M. B. Landon, H. L. Galan, E. R. M. Jauniaux, D. A. Driscoll, V. Berghella, W. A. Grobman, . . . A. G. Cahill (Eds.), *Gabbe's obstetrics: Normal and problem pregnancies* (8th ed., Kindle version, ch. 20). Philadelphia, PA: Elsevier.

Lang, G., Farnell, IV, E. A., & Quinlan, J. D. (2021). Out-of-hospital birth. *American Family Physician, 103*(11), 672–679. Retrieved from https://www.aafp.org/pubs/afp/issues/2021/0601/p672.html

Lazarou, A., Oestergaard, M., Netzl, J., Siedentopf, J. P., & Henrich, W. (2021). Vaginal birth after cesarean (VBAC): Fear it or dare it? An evaluation of potential risk factors. *Journal of Perinatal Medicine, 49*(7), 773–782. https://doi.org/10.1515/jpm-2020-0222

Lee, R. H., & Reau, N. (2023). Acute fatty liver of pregnancy. In K. M. Robson & V. A. Barss (Eds.), *UpToDate*. Retrieved October 1, 2023, from https://www.uptodate.com/contents/acute-fatty-liver-of-pregnancy

Likis, F. E. (2014). Home birth: Moving toward shared goals. *Journal of Midwifery & Women's Health, 59*(6), 567–568. https://doi.org/10.1111/jmwh.12277

Lothian, J. A. (2012). Risk, safety, and choice in childbirth. *Journal of Perinatal Education, 21*(1), 45–47. https://doi.org/10.1891/1058-1243.21.1.45

MacDorman, M. F., Mathews, T. J., & Declercq, E. (2014). *Trends in out-of-hospital births in the United States, 1990–2012* (NCHS Data Brief 124). Hyattsville, MD: National Center for Health Statistics. Retrieved from http://www.cdc.gov/nchs/data/databriefs/db144.pdf

Martijn, L. L. M., Jacobs, A. J. E., Maassen, I. I. M., Buitendijk, S. S. E., & Wensing, M. M. (2013). Patient safety in midwifery-led care in the Netherlands. *Midwifery, 29*(1), 60–66. https://doi.org/10.1016/j.midw.2011.10.013

Mehl-Madrona, L., & Madrona, M. M. (1997). Physician- and midwife-attended home births: Effects of breech, twin, and post-dates outcome data on mortality rates, *Journal of Nurse-Midwifery, 42*(2), 91–98. Retrieved from http://www.azdhs.org/documents/licensing/special/midwives/committees/mspac/additional-resources/physician-midwife-attended-home-births.pdf

Metz, T. D. (2023). Choosing the route of delivery after cesarean birth. In V. A. Barss (Ed.), *UpToDate*. Retrieved October 1, 2023, from http://www.uptodate.com/contents/choosing-the-route-of-delivery-after-cesarean-birth

Midwives Alliance of North America. (2014). *Fact Sheet: What new research says about the benefits and risks of home birth.* Retrieved from http://mana.org/pdfs/DOR-Outcomes-Paper-Fact-Sheet-on-Risk.pdf

Midwives' Association of Washington State. (2008). *Indications for discussion, consultation, and transfer of care in an out-of-hospital midwifery practice.* Retrieved from http://www.washingtonmidwives.org/assets/MAWSindications-4.24.08.pdf

Morris, T., & McInerney, K., (2010). Media representations of pregnancy and childbirth: An analysis of reality television programs in the United States. *Birth, 37*(2), 134–140. https://doi.org/10.1111/j.1523-536X.2010.00393.x

Mortimore, G., Reynolds, J., Forman, D., Brannigan, C., & Mitchell, K. (2021). From expert to advanced clinical practitioner and beyond. *British Journal of Nursing, 30*(11), 656–659. https://doi.org/10.12968/bjon.2021.30.11.656

Mosher, D., & Gould, S. (2018, October 29). The odds that a gun will kill the average American may surprise you. *Business Insider.* Retrieved from https://www.businessinsider.com/us-gun-death-murder-risk-statistics-2018-3?op=1

National Highway Traffic Safety Administration. (2010). *Seat belts save over 13,000 lives every year. One of them could be yours . . .* [Flyer]. Retrieved from https://www.trafficsafetymarketing.gov/campaign-search?keyword=seat belt top 5&topic=All

Nethery, E., Schummers, L., Levine, A., Caughey, A. B., Souter, V., & Gordon, W. (2021). Birth outcomes for planned home and licensed freestanding birth center births in Washington State. *Obstetrics & Gynecology, 138*(5), 693–702. https://doi.org/10.1097/AOG.0000000000004578

[NICE] National Institute for Health and Care Excellence. (2023). *Intrapartum care* (NICE Guideline NG235). Retrieved from https://www.nice.org.uk/guidance/ng235

Niemczyk, N. A. (2016). Planned home vaginal birth after cesarean. *Journal of Midwifery & Women's Health, 61*(2), 276–277. https://doi.org/10.1111/jmwh.12444_1

Noon, A. J. (2014). The cognitive processes underpinning clinical decision in triage assessment: A theoretical conundrum? *International Emergency Nursing, 22*(1), 40–46. https://doi.org/10.1016/j.ienj.2013.01.003

Norwitz, E. R. (2023). Eclampsia. In V. A. Barss (Ed.), *UpToDate.* Retrieved October 1, 2023, from https://www.uptodate.com/contents/eclampsia

Ornato, J. P., & Peberdy, M. A. (2014). Applying lessons from commercial aviation safety and operations to resuscitation. *Resuscitation; 85*(2), 173–176. https://doi.org/10.1016/j.resuscitation.2013.10.029

Page, M., & Mander, R. (2014). Intrapartum uncertainty: A feature of normal birth, as experienced by midwives in Scotland. *Midwifery, 30*(1), 28–35. https://doi.org/10.1016/j.midw.2013.01.012

Peacock, K. (2014). *Why aren't more breech babies born at home? A student midwife's perspective.* Retrieved from https://www.midwiferytoday.com/articles/breechbabieshome.asp

Peterwerth, N. H., Halek, M., & Schäfers, R. (2022). Intrapartum risk perception—A qualitative exploration of factors affecting the risk perception of midwives and obstetricians in the clinical setting. *Midwifery, 106*. https://doi.org/10.1016/j.midw.2021.103234

Redelmeier, D. A., May, S. C., Thiruchelvam, D., & Barrett, J. F. (2014). Pregnancy and the risk of a traffic crash. *Canadian Medical Association Journal, 186*(10). https://doi.org/10.1503/cmaj.131650

Rodis, J. F. (2023). Shoulder dystocia: Risk factors and planning birth of high-risk pregnancies. In V. A. Barss (Ed.), *UpToDate*. Retrieved October 1, 2023, from https://www.uptodate.com/contents/shoulder-dystocia-risk-factors-and-planning-birth-of-high-risk-pregnancies

Rowe, R., Li, Y., Knight, M., Brocklehurst, P., & Hollowell, J. (2016). Maternal and perinatal outcomes in women planning vaginal birth after caesarean (VBAC) at home in England: Secondary analysis of the Birthplace national prospective cohort study. *BJOG, 123*(7), 1123–1132. https://doi.org/10.1111/1471-0528.13546

Schaffer, L., & Zimmermann, R. (2022). Nuchal cord. In A. Chakrabarti (Ed.), *UpToDate*. Retrieved October 1, 2023, from https://www.uptodate.com/contents/nuchal-cord

Schorn, M. N. (2007). Midwives' practices and beliefs about discharging clients from their practice. *Journal of Midwifery & Women's Health, 52*(5), 465–472. https://doi.org/10.1016/j.jmwh.2007.03.012

Seedat, F., Stinton, C., Patterson, J., Geppert, J., Tan, B., Robinson, E. R., . . . Taylor-Phillips, S. (2017). Adverse events in women and children who have received intrapartum antibiotic prophylaxis treatment: A systematic review. *BMC Pregnancy and Childbirth, 17*(1), 247. https://doi.org/10.1186/s12884-017-1432-3

Steinhauer, S. (2015). Decision making in midwifery: Rationality and intuition. *Practising Midwife, 18*(4), 14–18.

Tharpe, N. L., Farley, C. L., & Jordan, R. G. (2022). *Clinical practice guidelines for midwifery & women's health* (6th ed., Kindle version). Burlington, MA: Jones & Bartlett Learning.

Tiffen, J., Corbridge, S. J., & Slimmer, L. (2014). Enhancing clinical decision making: Development of a contiguous definition and conceptual framework. *Journal of Professional Nursing, 30*(5), 399–405. https://doi.org/10.1016/j.profnurs.2014.01.006

Vedam, S., Goff, M., & Marnin, V. N. (2007). Closing the theory-practice gap: Intrapartum midwifery management of planned homebirths. *Journal of Midwifery & Women's Health, 52*(3), 291–300. https://doi.org/10.1016/j.jmwh.2007.02.013

Vedam, S., Leeman, L., Cheyney, M., Fisher, T. J., Myers, S., Low, L. K., & Ruhl, C. (2014). Transfer from planned home birth to hospital: Improving interprofessional collaboration. *Journal of Midwifery & Women's Health, 59*(6), 624–634. https://doi.org/10.1111/jmwh.12251

Vedam, S., Stoll, K., White, S., Aaker, J., & Schummers, L. (2009). Nurse-midwives' experiences with planned home birth: impact on attitudes and practice. *Birth, 36*(4), 274–282. https://doi.org/10.1111/j.1523-536X.2009.00354.x

Verani, J. R., McGee, L., & Schrag, S. J. (2010). Prevention of perinatal Group B streptococcal disease: Revised guidelines from CDC, 2010. *Morbidity and Mortality Weekly Report, 59*(RR-10). Retrieved from http://www.cdc.gov/mmwr/pdf/rr/rr5910.pdf

Vladiutu, C. J., Poole, C., Marshall, S. W., Casteel, C., Menard, M. K., & Weiss, H. B. (2013). Pregnant driver-associated motor vehicle crashes in North Carolina, 2001–2008. *Accident Analysis & Prevention, 55*, 165–171. https://doi.org/10.1016/j.aap.2013.03.004

White Ribbon Alliance. (n.d.). *Respectful maternity care: The universal rights of women & newborns.* Retrieved from https://whiteribbonalliance.org/wp-content/uploads/2022/05/WRA_RMC_Charter_FINAL.pdf

Willis, D. R., & Zerr, A. D. (2005). Terminating a patient: Is it time to part ways? *Family Practice Management, 12*(8), 34–38. Retrieved from https://www.aafp.org/pubs/fpm/issues/2005/0900/p34.html

Wilson, R. S., Zwickle, A., & Walpole, H. (2019). Developing a broadly applicable measure of risk perception. *Risk Analysis, 39*(4), 777–791. https://doi.org/10.1111/risa.13207

World Health Organization. (2019). *Legal capacity and the right to decide: WHO Quality Rights core training: mental health and social services: Course guide.* Geneva, Switzerland: Author. Retrieved from https://apps.who.int/iris/bitstream/handle/10665/329539/9789241516716-eng.pdf

Xu, J., Murphy, S. L., Kochanek, K. D., & Arias, E. (2021). Deaths: Final Data for 2019. *National Vital Statistics Reports, 70*(8). https://doi.org/10.15620/cdc:106058

Yan, Q., Qiu, D., Liu, X., Xing, Q., Liu, R., & Hu, Y. (2022). The incidence of gestational diabetes mellitus among women with polycystic ovary syndrome: a meta-analysis of longitudinal studies. *BMC Pregnancy and Childbirth, 22*(1), 370. https://doi.org/10.1186/s12884-022-04690-3

Zielinski, R., Ackerson, K., & Low, L. K. (2015). Planned home birth: Benefits, risks, and opportunities. *International Journal of Women's Health, 7*, 361–377. https://doi.org/10.2147/IJWH.S55561

Zondag, L. D., Maas, V. Y., Beuckens, A., & Nieuwenhuijze, M. J. (2022). Experiences, beliefs, and values influencing midwives' attitudes toward the use of childbirth interventions. *Journal of Midwifery & Women's Health, 67*(5), 618–625. https://doi.org/10.1111/jmwh.13392

Recognizing and Managing Emergencies 4

Objectives

- Give an example of how an intervention used inappropriately can negatively affect a normal labor.
- Give an example of how an intervention used appropriately can help a dysfunctional labor normalize.
- Describe the Intervention Staircase and how it can be applied to a mother with postpartum hemorrhage.
- Discuss how to systematically assess a client with a pregnancy complication.
- Explain the CAPED mnemonic and the Midwifery Management Cycle.
- Explain how to use GOLDCART to assess pain in a pregnant client.
- Discuss how to manage an intrapartum transport from home to hospital.

Composite Case Study

Tamika Thomas, a CPM in a rural home-birth practice, was returning from a birth when she received a phone call from a client's sister. "Willow has been acting weird. She used to be on anxiety medicine, and I think she needs to start taking it again." The sister went on to say that for about a week and a half, Willow had been highly emotional and had many angry and tearful outbursts. She also had episodes of severe headache and vomiting, and she dragged her right leg a little when she walked. "Today," said the sister, "I stopped by to check on her and she refuses to talk to me at all!"

Tamika knew Willow and her sister well and found these signs and symptoms potentially concerning. Willow had appeared healthy at her 16-week prenatal visit the week before. Mothers sometimes report headaches, vomiting, mood swings, and musculoskeletal problems as normal parts of pregnancy, but Tamika always took these complaints seriously until she could be sure they were benign. Headaches and vomiting, she knew, are present in many conditions, including migraine, preeclampsia with severe features, COVID-19 (SARS-CoV-2), brain cancer, and carbon monoxide poisoning. Angry and tearful outbursts and reluctance to talk or socialize suggest extreme emotional stress, anxiety, or even psychosis. And why did Willow have trouble walking?

Because Tamika was within a half mile of Willow's house, she stopped in to assess her. She found Willow alert and making good eye contact. Her vital signs and the fetal heart rate (FHR) were normal, and she seemed relieved to see Tamika. However, it seemed to Tamika that Willow was unable to speak. When Tamika asked a question, Willow would grunt as if she were trying to form words, then give up with a look of frustration. She had difficulty lifting her right leg and her hand grip was weaker on the right than the left.

Tamika, quickly concluding that her client was having a stroke, called emergency medical services, which transported Willow to the emergency department of a large teaching hospital. With some investigation, the neurosurgeon unraveled the mystery. Apparently, Willow's abusive ex-boyfriend had come for a visit 9 days earlier and had punched Willow in the left side of the head. At first, she complained of headaches and mood swings; but as time went on, she experienced vomiting, aphasia (inability to speak), and right-sided weakness (hemiparesis).

The punch to the head had caused a subdural hematoma (bleeding between the surface of the brain and the dura mater), which slowly enlarged until it caused hemiparesis and compromised Broca's area, the part of the frontal lobe associated with speech production. This injury could have been fatal for Willow, but she underwent emergency surgery to evacuate the blood clot and alleviate the pressure on her brain. The emergency physician commended Tamika on her quick action and noted that she probably saved Willow's life. Some months later, she gave birth to a healthy baby girl. Willow ended her relationship with the abuser and with counseling eventually made a full recovery.

Timely Intervention

In general, the midwife's goal is to support the mother and baby in achieving the greatest health and wellbeing by physiologically optimal means. The initial assessment sets the course for management, whether upon presentation in labor, office visit, or when another midwife assumes care of the client. Ongoing management involves ongoing reassessment: the midwife considers whether the original clinical impression is still correct, and, if it is not, forms a new one and starts down

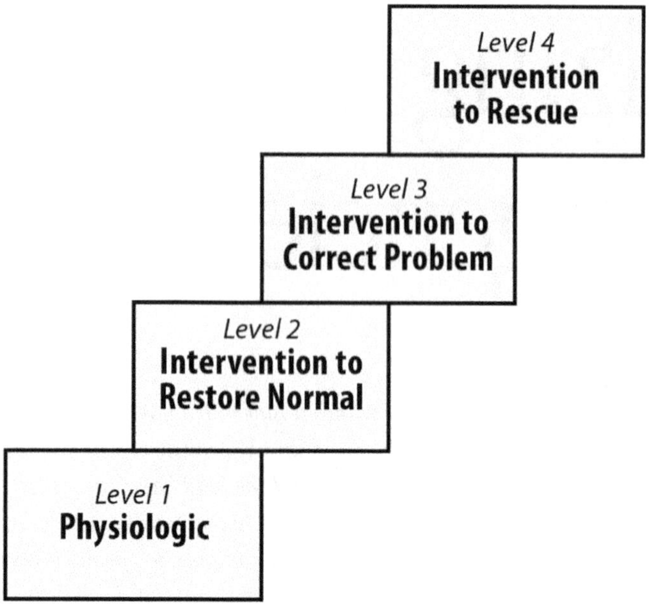

Figure 4-1. The Intervention Staircase. The midwife moves up the staircase from level 1, Physiologic Support when complications occur and back down if complications resolve.

> **The Intervention Contention**
>
> Unnecessary intervention can be life-threatening.
> Necessary intervention can be life-saving.

a new management path. The process is much like navigating wilderness with a map and compass. In unfamiliar territory, hikers must stop periodically, take stock of where they are in relation to where they want to be, and ensure they are on the most direct route to their destination.

Nonintervention Versus Action

Appropriate antepartum, intrapartum, and postpartum interventions can prevent maternal and perinatal morbidity and mortality (Zondag, Maas, Beuckens, & Nieuwenhuijze, 2022). Provider preparedness, timely detection, and appropriate response to early signs of severe maternal morbidity can dramatically affect maternal and perinatal outcomes and prevent the decline from serious illness to death (Guglielminotti, Wong, Friedman, & Li, 2021). To identify complications at their earliest presentation, the midwife must understand the potential for risk and closely monitor the client with eyes, ears, heart, intuition, and common sense. Failure to rescue occurs when a provider does not recognize or manage a complication, causing harm to the client (Dahlen & Caplice, 2014). In the United States, the failure-to-rescue rate for pregnant people is lowest for white mothers, higher for minority mothers, and highest for black mothers (Guglielminotti et al., 2021; Renfrew, 2021).

Midwives are geared philosophically to nonintervention in the natural processes of pregnancy and birth, knowing that normal labor treated as normal tends to stay normal, and every disruption to the physiologic process is likely to create new problems that require more intervention. When labor deviates from normal, however, intervention during the early stages of a problem with the right level of action can shift the client back within the boundaries of normality. If the problem resolves, in many cases the midwife can return to watchful waiting and nonintervention. If not, aggressive treatment and/or transport may become necessary.

When the labor is no longer normal, interventions often become necessary to prevent or manage maternal or perinatal complications or to avoid cesarean birth. Common interventions include oxytocin augmentation, antibiotic therapy, continuous fetal monitoring, and epidural anesthesia. Often, implementing small interventions early in the process can prevent major interventions later. Knowing when to intervene, when to back off, and when to transport is extremely subjective, but it is the essential art of midwifery (Renfrew, 2021).

The Intervention Staircase (Figure 4-1) illustrates the four ascending steps of intervention used by maternity providers.

Level 1, physiologic support, is a baseline of watchful waiting and supportive care for normal labor.

Level 2, intervention to restore natural processes, involves minimally intrusive corrections intended to shift the problem back to normal.

Level 3, intervention to correct problem, involves more assertive action to rectify or stabilize a problem that is unlikely to resolve without assistance.

Level 4, intervention to rescue, involves taking focused, determined action to prevent serious harm or death for client or infant.

Let us consider postpartum bleeding in relation to the Intervention Staircase. Most low-risk clients will remain at *level 1*, the physiologic baseline. A healthy mother is unlikely to have a postpartum hemorrhage after a physiologic birth in a supportive environment when the newborn remains skin-to-skin and is nuzzling at the breast. If bleeding is more than expected, the midwife moves to *level 2*, intervening to massage the uterus to optimal firmness and express clots. If the bleeding continues, the midwife moves to *level 3*, using more assertive interventions to achieve hemostasis, including giving additional uterotonics and performing an internal examination to remove clots from the uterus. If blood loss is excessive or ongoing, the midwife should move to *level 4*, Intervention to Rescue, calling for an ambulance and holding

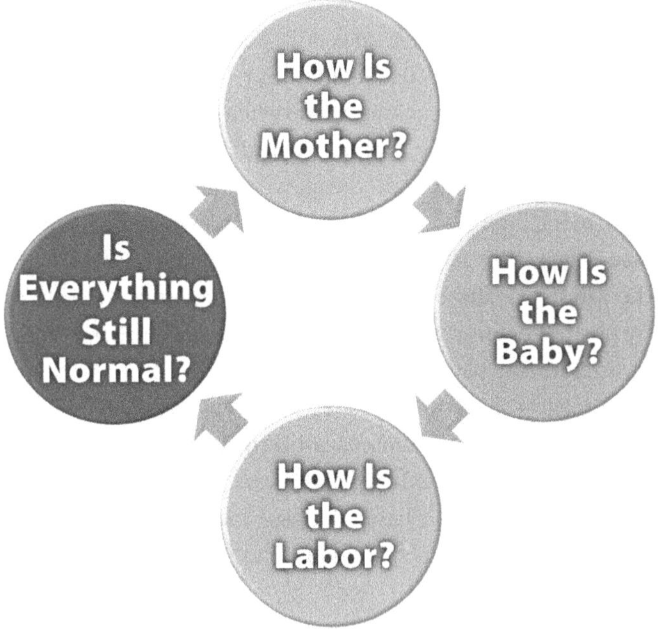

Figure 4-2. Intentional periodic assessment is essential to timely recognition of problems. Throughout every labor, consider the Four Key Questions: How is the mother? (Vital signs, comfort level, state, positioning, nutrition, hydration, etc.) How is the baby? (Fetal heart rate [FHR] pattern, position, presentation, attitude, movement patterns, etc.). How is the labor? (Spacing, duration, strength of contractions; labor progress; etc.) Is everything still normal? (Consider the big picture and decide whether to intervene or allow physiologic birth to proceed.) Cycle through these questions regularly to identify the earliest signs of deviation from normal.

bimanual compression or packing the uterus while an assistant obtains intravenous (IV) access and starts a fluid bolus. At the hospital, the physician will likely continue level 4 interventions which may include administering blood products, using an intrauterine balloon tamponade or intrauterine vacuum device, performing a dilation and evacuation (D&E) procedure, or placing B-Lynch sutures.

Consultation, Collaboration, and Transfer of Care

Research has demonstrated that optimal outcomes can be achieved when midwives work collaboratively with other providers to manage maternity care (Freytsis, Phillippi, Cox, Romano, & Cragin, 2017). Because midwives are specialists in the supervision of low-risk pregnancies, seamless collaboration with providers in other health care disciplines, physicians above all, is essential to client safety (King, 2015). Referral is the process by which the midwife sends the client to a physician or another health care professional for management of a condition or aspect of care (American College of Nurse-Midwives [ACNM], 2014). Collaborative practice between midwives and physicians can increase access to care, decrease costs, and improve efficiency (D. C. Smith, 2015).

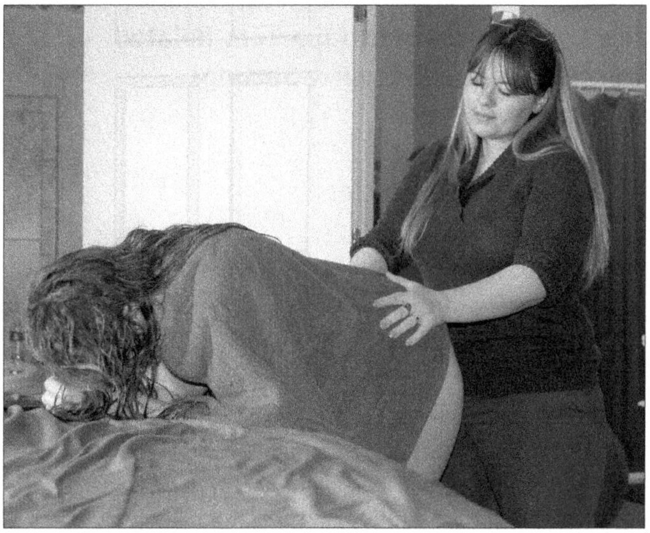

Figure 4-3. Sometimes a client benefits from minimal intrusions and passive support. Other times, active involvement can improve outcomes or save lives. The essential art of midwifery is knowing the difference between unnecessary and beneficial intervention.

There are four levels of relationship between midwives and physicians or other team members:

Autonomy: The midwife works independently, without physician input. A totally autonomous midwifery practice would have worse outcomes for clients with complications because the midwives would be unable or unauthorized to independently perform advanced procedures such as cesarean section and hysterectomy. Example: An international midwife tending mothers in a remote low-resource region is a 5-hr mule ride from the nearest hospital. A mother with a placenta accreta hemorrhages to death.

Consultation: The midwife who maintains primary management responsibility for the client's care seeks the advice of a physician or another health care provider (ACNM, 2014). Example: A client's initial prenatal laboratory tests include a positive screen for anti-M antibody. The midwife consults the physician to determine whether this antibody could harm the fetus, what follow-up and testing is recommended, and whether the client should plan to give birth at home.

Collaboration: The midwife and physician jointly manage the care of a client with issues or complications (ACNM, 2014; King, 2015). Example: A client is noted to have a moderately shortened cervix on routine ultrasound examination at 24 0/7 weeks of gestation. She is referred to a maternal-fetal medicine (MFM) specialist, who evaluates carefully for risk of PTL and finds no signs of imminent birth. The client continues to obtain

The Top 7 Causes of Intrapartum-Related Mortality in Low-Resource Settings

- Obstructed labor
- Breech position
- Suspected fetal distress
- Hemorrhage
- Severe hypertension/preeclampsia
- Postterm pregnancy
- Intraamniotic infection

Adapted from "Obstetric Care in Low-Resource Settings: What, Who, and How to Overcome Challenges to Scale Up?" by G. J. Hofmeyr et al., 2009, *International Journal of Gynecology and Obstetrics, 107* (Suppl.), pp. S21–S45. Copyright by International Federation of Gynecology and Obstetrics.

routine midwifery care from her midwife and is reevaluated by MFM every month. At 37 0/7 weeks of gestation, the client is still pregnant, and MFM sees no contraindications for a home birth. The client sees only the midwife for the rest of her pregnancy and gives birth safely at home.

Transfer of care: When the client falls out of the midwife's scope of practice or comfort level, the client should be transferred to a higher level of care. Example: The midwife performs a cervical examination on a client in labor and finds that the fetus is a face presentation, mentum posterior. Knowing that a fetus in this presentation is unlikely to fit through the birth canal, the midwife initiates transport to the hospital via ambulance and transfers care to the physician for urgent cesarean section.

Informed Consent and Shared Decision-making

Competent adults are entitled to make informed, voluntary decisions about their own health care. Informed consent requires a clinician to provide individualized counseling about proposed courses of action and how they relate to a client's unique circumstances, whether in writing or in person. The clinician should explain the proposed treatments; cover their risks, benefits, alternatives; make recommendations; assess the client's understanding; elicit the client's preference; and document the conversation (American College of Obstetricians & Gynecologists [ACOG], 2021; Shah, Thornton, Turrin, & Hipskind, 2023). The informed consent process can be informal, for example a conversation that occurs before the birth attendant gives an injection of oxytocin to control bleeding, or formal, for example a discussion that occurs when signing documents before surgery. In an emergency, informed consent can be waived if there is no time for discussion or if the client is unable to communicate and a surrogate decision maker is not available (American Medical Association, 2022, opinion 2.1.1).

Shared decision-making occurs when clients and clinicians work together to make health care decisions aligned with the best available evidence and the client's values and preferences while being informed by the provider's knowledge and experience (Agency for Healthcare Research & Quality, 2016/2020). The process of shared decision-making encourages clients to express preferences and personal beliefs and to provide input on a treatment plan that incorporates their values, interpersonal relationships, and broader social environment (ACOG, 2021). The result is a consensus-based decision with mutual responsibility (Nieuwenhuijze, Korstjens, de Jonge, de Vries, & Lagro-Janssen, 2014). Shared decision-making supports client autonomy and improves outcomes and satisfaction with care (ACOG, 2021).

Responding to Emergencies

Perinatal complications requiring emergent transfer occur in fewer than 2% of birth center births (Olvera, Smith, Prater, & Hastings-Tolsma, 2020) and are similarly uncommon in home births. The community midwife can avoid many emergencies through thoughtful preventative care, careful management, close observation, referral of high-risk clients, and adherence to clinical guidelines. Some crises, however, arise unexpectedly despite optimal care and monitoring. Every midwife should maintain competency with cardiopulmonary resuscitation (CPR) and neonatal resuscitation, participate in emergency drills, and remain current with recommendations for managing complications frequently encountered in practice.

Triage

Early detection of complications generally yields better outcomes. Triage—from the French word *trier*, meaning to separate or sort—involves a dynamic decision-making process which prioritizes clients by their immediate need for care (Noon, 2014). The term was first used on battlefields in the 1800s, when medical personnel determined which soldiers had treatable injuries and could return to battle, which were so seriously injured that they could no longer fight, and which would die regardless of treatment. Triage is used on disaster scenes and in emergency departments to discover the acuity of illness or injury, assign treatment order, and initiate appropriate interventions, often in chaotic and emotionally charged environments.

Midwives use triage skills to ascertain whether a client is a good candidate to give birth in a community setting, whether a complaint is serious or benign, and whether a client is in labor. For example, a client complaining of abdominal pain can have round-ligament pain, Braxton Hicks contractions, contractions of active labor, appendicitis, or something else. The midwife obtains a history and performs a physical assessment, gathering information quickly, processing it logically, then acting decisively. Findings determine whether intervention, referral to another provider, or watchful waiting is necessary at that time of assessment.

Obstetric complications can be categorized using the Priority Pyramid triage system.

- **Priority 1, "Code Red"—Critical Emergencies**
  Very uncommon but life-threatening; require immediate action.
- **Priority 2, "Code Orange"—Urgent Problems**
  Fairly uncommon but potentially life-threatening; must be treated as soon as possible.
- **Priority 3, "Code Yellow"—Concerning Problems**
  Common but with the potential for progression to significant problems, but the client is currently stable.
- **Priority 4, "Code Green"—Normal**
  Most low-risk clients will remain normal throughout labor and birth.

Recognizing the signs of clinical deterioration in pregnant clients can be challenging. The physiological adaptations of healthy pregnancy render a mother susceptible to rapid disease progression and alter the reference ranges of laboratory and imaging assessments (V. Smith, Kenny, Sandall, Devane, & Noonan, 2021). The astute midwife, however, often notes subtle changes in vital signs, skin color and temperature, labor pattern, mental status, or other indicators at the earliest stages of compromise. Upon recognizing these changes, the midwife can respond with a timely intervention or escalation of care to physician management (V. Smith, O'Malley, & Cithambaram, 2022). The cumulative effects of two or more conditions may place the client at greater risk than a single issue (N. Tharpe, personal communication, February 24, 2018). It is up to the midwife to synthesize the collective effect of all factors and gauge the severity and urgency of the client's unique circumstances (N. Tharpe, personal communication, February 24, 2018).

Initial Assessment

Sometimes the unexpected happens. The intrapartum client can suddenly start bleeding heavily and go into shock. It is possible that you will hear a crash and find a client twitching on the bathroom floor; witness a mass shooting; encounter an unconscious pregnant client, family member, or total stranger; or be the first to encounter a motor vehicle crash.

Most midwives are strongly motivated to help people in need, but some do not know what actions are appropriate or

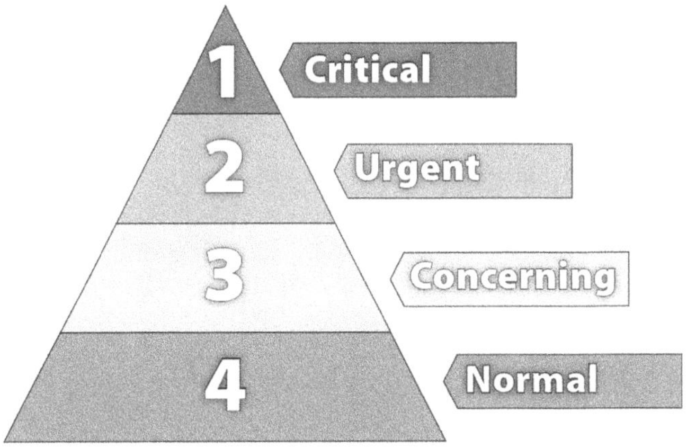

Figure 4-4. The Priority Pyramid. Most labors will be normal throughout, and critical incidents are uncommon.

necessary. Emergency medical training is beneficial to community midwives. It is beyond the scope of this book to provide in-depth instruction in emergency medicine. All midwives, however, should master the basic skills to assist with any emergency while concentrating on obstetrical ones. They should also be aware of where they and their skills fit in the larger picture.

Community midwives are proficient in supervising normal pregnancy and birth and in recognizing abnormal conditions that can be best managed by other professionals. Obstetrical complications can require consultation or transfer of care to an obstetrician or evaluation in a hospital maternity unit. Nonobstetrical problems (for example chest pain, worsening asthma, or leg pain) can necessitate referral to the client's primary care physician or a hospital emergency department (Pearlman & Desmond, 2005).

When a problem is detected, calmly take charge or designate a leader. A single leader helps avoid confusion. If you are not the only responder, find out who is in charge. If a physician, a fire captain, or someone else is in charge, cooperate and coordinate with them. If extra hands are needed or transport is required, get help early on. Avoid leaving the victim unattended.

Midwives assisting at disaster scenes and in low-resource locations may be assigned to help a wide range of clients, not just mothers and babies. The Federal Emergency Management Agency uses and promotes an incident command system model to organize the response of agencies and individuals to large-scale disasters such as floods, tornadoes, and bombings (Farcas et al., 2021). This approach is also used by responders to smaller-scale incidents such as fires, road traffic accidents, train crashes, and pandemics. There is a predetermined chain of command under an incident commander in charge of response and coordination of resources and agencies (Farcas et al., 2021). Self-directed volunteers can interfere with the coordinated efforts of response teams and can place themselves

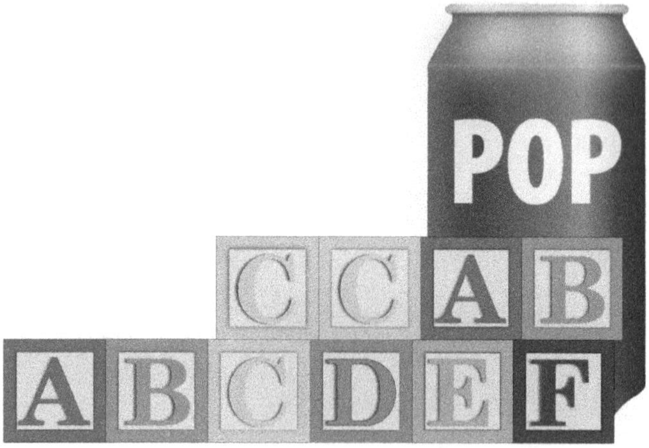

Figure 4-5. Airway first or circulation first? Authorities disagree. The Advanced Trauma Life Support® program advocates the ABCDE approach (American College of Surgeons Cmte. on Trauma [ACS], 2018). Birth Emergency Skills Training adds F for Fetal and uterine assessment. Another mnemonic is CCAB, beginning with consideration of Cervical spine motion restriction and Control of bleeding then proceeding to opening the Airway and evaluating Breathing (American Academy of Orthopedic Surgeons [AAOS], 2018). Any method of stabilizing a pregnant individual should involve taking measures to ensure that the placenta is optimally perfused (POP).

and others at greater risk (Persson & Uhnoo, 2021). People who wish to volunteer their services should obtain permission from the incident commander and take direction from the response team (Johansson, Danielsson, Kvarnlöf, Eriksson, & Karlsson, 2018).

Approaching the Victim

Whether the issue at hand is a postpartum hemorrhage, a vehicular accident, or a health crisis involving your client's support person, your priorities are the same, and you should move through the initial steps of assessment and management in the same sequence. Get help: contact emergency medical services (EMS) or ask someone to make the call. Ensure that the scene is safe for you before you attempt to provide care. Evaluate the potential for contracting infectious disease. Minimize exposure to body fluids and potentially harmful substances at the scene by using personal protective equipment when approaching the victim. Ensure that the victim's environment poses no threat to you or others. For example, if it seems that an unconscious individual received an electrical shock in the bathtub, do not move or touch the victim until you have dealt with the shock hazard. When in doubt, stay out. If you become injured, you will be less able to render assistance. If the scene becomes unsafe, attempt to remove yourself and the victim from danger, if possible. Consider that if the injury occurred through violence, the perpetrator could still be present and pose a risk to rescuers (World Health Organization [WHO] & International Cmte. of the Red Cross [ICRC], 2018).

The goal of the initial assessment is to quickly identify and correct potentially life-threatening conditions such as airway compromise, inadequate breathing, and hemorrhage before considering complex conditions and causes. Medical issues can present with a well-defined onset and a clear cause or with overlapping symptoms and multiple concerns distorting the clinical picture. In any case, capture important information quickly to determine the source and severity of the problem (Johnson, Boyd, Grantham, & Eastwood, 2015).

A midwife can glean information from the victim's history, physical assessment, environment, and mechanism of injury and gut instinct. Ask yourself

- What is going on here?
- Is this a trauma? Do I need to stabilize the cervical spine?
- What is the level of consciousness?
- Are vital signs stable or unstable?
- What are my priorities?

Using a checklist can reduce a complex task to an orderly sequence of steps (Johnson et al., 2015). Even though the mnemonics in this chapter are presented as step-by-step sequences, American Heart Association (AHA) guidelines encourage fast, simultaneous assessment and response (Panchal et al., 2020). As providers gain experience, they tend to move from simply following the usual steps to providing comprehensive assessment and treatment.

As you move through the initial assessment, correct critical problems as you find them. If the client appears to be in cardiac arrest, use the **CAB** mnemonic—**C**irculation, **A**irway, **B**reathing—which recommends starting chest compressions before giving rescue breaths (Panchal et al., 2020). The **CCAB** mnemonic (developed for Birth Emergency Skills Training) adds a **C** to **CAB** to limit **C**ervical spine motion in trauma victims. Otherwise, the **ABCDE** approach to assessment—**A**irway, **B**reathing, **C**irculation, **D**isability, **E**xposure—guides the provider to assess the most important problems in order (Thim, Krarup, Grove, Rohde, & Løfgren, 2012; WHO & ICRC, 2018). For pregnant mothers, continue with **F** to assess **F**etal status. Include the mnemonic **POP**—**P**lacenta **O**ptimally **P**erfused—to address maternal position and oxygenation. The following is an overview of maternal assessment.

Primary Survey with Placenta Optimally Perfused (POP)

The primary survey is a rapid assessment to identify life-threatening issues. Although it is presented here as discrete steps in order of importance, ideally several rescuers will perform multiple actions simultaneously. Form a general impression by looking at the client and the surroundings and rapidly assessing the basic vital signs. If the mechanism of injury suggests the possibility of cervical spine damage, have an assistant gently hold the head and neck in neutral alignment.

Ask the victim/client to tell you his or her name and what happened. An appropriate response indicates that the airway is patent, air is moving sufficiently to allow speech, and the client is reasonably alert. An alert victim is also usually the best source of information about issues that require attention and events that led to the present situation. If the victim cannot provide the information, ask witnesses and bystanders. Form a general impression by looking at the client and the surroundings and rapidly assess the basic vital signs.

Placenta Optimally Perfused—Unless contraindicated by maternal injuries, place pregnant victims beyond 20 weeks of gestation (uterine fundus at or above the umbilicus) in a side-lying position or a left lateral tilt of 15–30° to improve cardiac output and optimally perfuse the placenta (Refa, Ali, & Gomaa, 2019). A wedge, a pillow, towels, or other items can be placed under the client's right hip to achieve a left lateral tilt. Supine positioning can compress the inferior vena cava and the aorta between the spine and the gravid uterus, reducing cardiac output by as much as 30% and producing symptoms of shock (Refa et al., 2019). The position that optimizes circulation to the fetus usually does the same for the mother. Pregnant trauma victims requiring immobilization on a spine board should be secured in the left lateral position (WHO & ICRC, 2018).

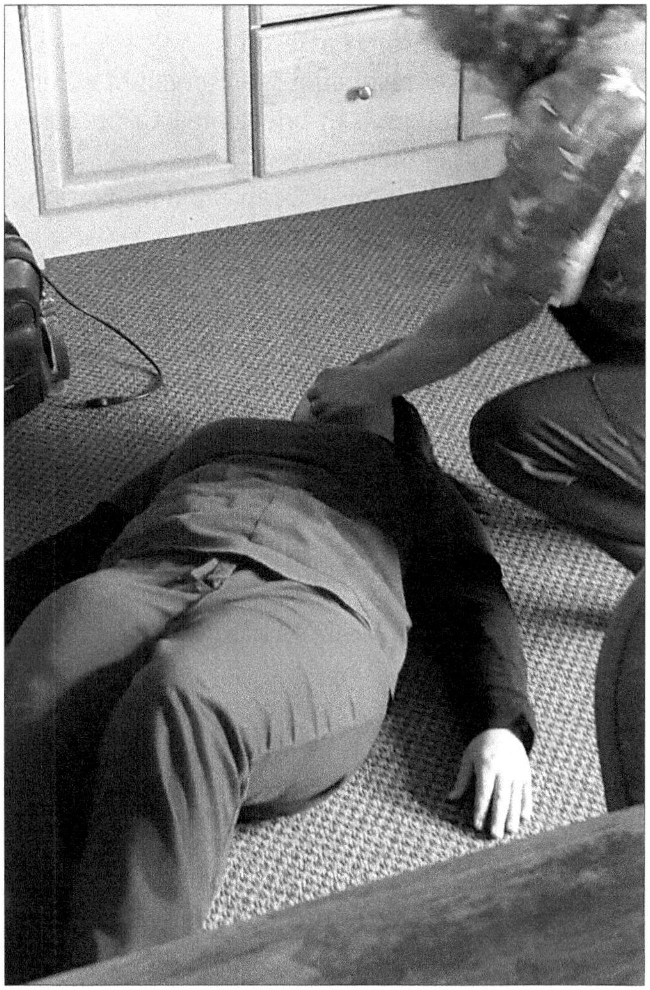

Figure 4-6. If the victim appears to be in cardiac arrest, use the CCAB (Cervical spine, Circulation, Airway, Breathing) mnemonic, which recommends starting chest compressions before giving rescue breaths. If not, use the ABCDEF-POP approach to assessment—Airway, Breathing, Circulation, Disability, Exposure, and Fetal status with Placenta Optimally Perfused—to assess the most important problems first.

A—Airway with Restriction of Cervical Spine Motion

Cervical spine: Cervical spine trauma can lead to spinal cord injury, which can affect many bodily functions and cause severe disability or death. The most common mechanisms for cervical spine injuries are traffic accidents, falls, and violence such as gunshots (Zileli et al., 2020). Presume cervical spine injury in the victim of head or facial trauma. If the cervical spine has been fractured, unintentional movement of the neck by a rescuer can sever the spinal cord (Zileli et al., 2020). A spinal-cord injury above the 5th cervical vertebra typically causes respiratory failure because the nerves supplying the diaphragm are compromised (Rabinstein, 2020). In this case, immediate respiratory support can be lifesaving.

Airway: Airway compromise can result from head trauma, aspiration of a foreign object, smoke inhalation, anaphylaxis, or direct physical trauma to the airway (American College of Surgeons Cmte. on Trauma [ACS], 2018). If the client is talking, the airway is open. When the airway is completely obstructed, air does not move.

In the unconscious client, the tongue can shift backwards and block the flow of air (WHO & ICRC, 2018). Untreated airway obstruction can lead to cardiac arrest. If a spinal injury is suspected in an unconscious client, stabilize the cervical spine (ACS, 2018). Perform the jaw-thrust maneuver by placing your hands on the client's cheeks and lifting on the angle of the jaw with your fingers (Mastenbjörk & Meloni, 2021). Do not turn the client's head to the side to drain secretions or vomit.

If trauma is not a concern, open the airway of the unconscious client by using the head-tilt chin-lift maneuver and repositioning the head (Peate & Brent, 2021). Place one hand on the client's forehead and lift the chin with the fingers of your

Abnormal Respiratory Patterns

- Cheyne-Stokes respirations—Intervals of waxing, then waning deep full breaths followed by brief apnea. Can occur with heart failure or with stroke or other brain injuries.
- Kussmaul respirations—Deep, rapid respirations seen in people with diabetic ketoacidosis.
- Biot's (ataxic) respirations—Irregular rate, depth, and pattern of breathing with periods of apnea, usually from increased intracranial pressure.
- Agonal respirations—Slow, shallow, irregular, or occasional ineffective breaths. Often seen shortly after cardiac arrest.

other hand. Inspect for foreign bodies that threaten the airway (such as food or broken teeth) and wipe or suction blood and secretions. Identify facial, tracheal, and other injuries that can obstruct air flow. It is important to anticipate vomiting in all injured clients and be prepared to manage the situation.

Look for chest rise and listen to the flow of air. Clients who are unresponsive or in an altered level of consciousness cannot protect their own airways, so providers must ensure that airways remain patent with suctioning, positioning, and airway adjuncts if available. A client who cannot move air is in respiratory arrest. If a foreign body obstructs the airway and the client is moving minimal air or losing consciousness, employ the Heimlich maneuver in accordance with AHA guidelines (Panchal et al., 2020).

Snoring occurs when the tongue partially blocks the airway. Gurgling indicates secretions or foreign material. High-pitched stridor indicates an upper-airway obstruction that can become lethal if not rapidly resolved. A foreign body lodged in the airway, swelling, anaphylaxis, or respiratory burns can cause stridor (WHO & ICRC, 2018). Crowing is a high-pitched upper airway sound resulting from a partial airway obstruction, most often heard in children with croup or epiglottitis.

Airway obstruction can be partial or complete, and it is more likely to occur above the vocal cords (Johnson et al., 2015). An unconscious client can require an oropharyngeal or nasopharyngeal airway or a cuffed airway such as a laryngeal mask airway or endotracheal tube to maintain an open airway.

B—Breathing

After opening the airway, assess for evidence of ineffective breathing such as labored respirations, speaking in broken sentences, retractions, use of accessory muscles of the neck and abdomen, audibly noisy breaths, and nasal flaring. Count the rate of respirations. The normal rate is 12–20 respirations per min. A rate of over 25/min or less than 10/min is abnormal and can presage imminent deterioration (Resuscitation Council UK [RCUK], 2022).

If the victim is breathing ineffectively, assist ventilation with any method available—mouth-to-mouth, mouth-to-mask, or a bag-valve-mask device. Watch for chest rise. If the chest does not rise, adjust the airway and reattempt ventilation. When ventilating a client who has a pulse, use a ventilation rate of one breath every 6 sec or 10 breaths/min (Panchal et al., 2020).

Reduced oxygen reserve and increased oxygen consumption put the pregnant client and the fetus at higher risk for hypoxemia. The hypoxic client will often be confused, restless, or agitated. Pulse oximetry provides valuable information about the adequacy of breathing by measuring the percentage of hemoglobin saturated by oxygen. Administer oxygen as needed to maintain saturations over 95% (Neuman & Promes, 2021). If the oxygen saturation does not improve with supplementary oxygen, consider the effectiveness of respirations and make corrections to improve effectiveness of breathing, such as using an airway adjunct or changing the client's position.

Auscultate breath sounds and note abnormalities such as wheezing or crackles. During severe bronchoconstriction, as in an acute asthma exacerbation or anaphylaxis, the airway can be so narrow that what little air passes produces greatly diminished or absent breath sounds with no audible wheezing. Unequal breath sounds can point to a pneumothorax or hemothorax. If trauma is suspected, quickly expose the chest and look for signs of injury (including asymmetric or paradoxical movement) and palpate for crepitus and deformity (Raja & Zane, 2023).

Observe the respiratory pattern. Abnormal breathing patterns often develop with pathologic conditions as the body attempts to correct or compensate for the disease state. For example, a client with metabolic acidosis, such as diabetic ketoacidosis, tends to have deep, frequent respirations as the body converts acids to carbon dioxide and water and expels them through the respiratory system (de Moraes & Surani, 2019). A client with elevated intracranial pressure due to head trauma can have a higher-than-usual respiratory rate (Chourpiliadis & Bhardwaj, 2022). A client in pain can also have rapid respirations. A client unconscious from an opioid overdose will have very slow respirations or apnea (Chourpiliadis & Bhardwaj, 2022). Cheyne-Stokes respirations—a pattern of cyclical episodes of apnea and hyperventilation—can indicate congestive heart failure or stroke (Rudrappa, Modi, & Bollu, 2023). Biot's respirations (irregular, short, and gasping) indicate acute neurological disease or brain injury (Wijdicks, 2007). Agonal respirations are the last slow gasps before total apnea.

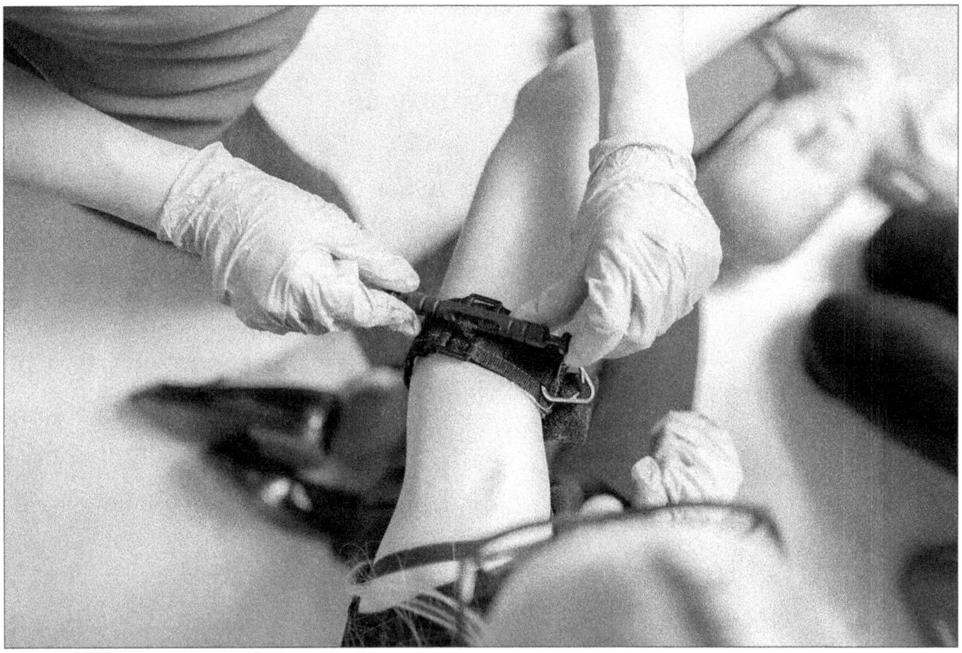

Figure 4-7. A tourniquet can effectively stop life-threatening hemorrhage from a limb injury. In response to the recent upsurge in mass shootings and other mass-casualty incidents, rescuers have developed public-education programs to teach bystanders basic hemorrhage-control techniques. Someday laypeople may learn hemorrhage-control methods alongside CPR training, and supplies of tourniquets and hemostatic dressings may be available in public places alongside automated external defibrillators (©rh2010/Adobe Stock).

C—Circulation

Assessing circulation involves assessing for a beating heart, restoring circulation in the case of absent or inadequate cardiac function, and controlling active bleeding. In the case of the unresponsive client who is not breathing or who is breathing ineffectively, AHA urges immediate activation of the emergency response system and initiation of CPR (Panchal et al., 2020). The lone health care provider should first call EMS, then provide chest compressions and ventilations if possible.

Client With a Pulse

If the client has a pulse, assess it for strength, rate, and regularity. If the client is breathing, the heart is beating; but if the blood pressure (BP) is low, a pulse is not always palpable. If a pulse is present but adequate respirations are absent, continue to ventilate the lungs.

The rate and rhythm of the pulse can give clues to the source of compromise. People with certain cardiac problems, such as heart block, medication overdose, head injury, or vasovagal syncope, can present with severe bradycardia (fewer than 50 beats per min [bpm]). Some causes of tachycardia (over 110 bpm) include shock, exposure to chemicals such as caffeine or medications, dehydration, sepsis, hypothermia, lung problems, thyroid disorders, hypoglycemia, cardiovascular problems (e.g., arrhythmia or pulmonary embolism), panic disorder, pain, or fear. An irregular pulse can indicate cardiac arrhythmia such as atrial fibrillation, heart block, or ectopic beats.

A rapid, thready pulse can indicate a rate too fast to allow for adequate cardiac filling or hypovolemia due to hemorrhage. Because the mother's blood volume increases during pregnancy, signs of hypovolemia sometimes do not appear until 40% of blood volume is lost (American Academy of Orthopedic Surgeons, 2018). Trauma victims with a weak radial pulse are 15 times more likely to die than people with a normal pulse (National Assn. of Emergency Medical Technicians [NAEMT] & ACS, 2020).

Evaluate skin color—pallor indicates poor perfusion, and cyanosis indicates hypoxia. Flushed, red skin can indicate hyperthermia, adverse reaction to IV vancomycin, or, rarely, advanced carbon monoxide poisoning. Clammy, cool, pale skin indicates sympathetic stimulation is causing vasoconstriction, often in response to hypotension or shock (Casey, 2002).

Client Without a Pulse

If the client is in cardiac arrest, start CPR. Surprisingly, survival rates from adult cardiac arrests caused by cardiac issues are similar whether CPR is performed with or without rescue breaths before EMS arrives (Panchal et al., 2020). Because chest compressions are the single most important intervention for the client in cardiac arrest, it is acceptable for lay rescuers to provide them without rescue breathing if they are unable or unwilling to give mouth-to-mouth resuscitation (Mastenbjörk & Meloni, 2021, p. 13; Panchal et al., 2020). Health care providers should perform both compressions

AVPU

Alert—Awake; eyes open. Can be oriented or disoriented.

Verbal stimuli—Appears asleep, but rouses when spoken to. Take note of any confusion or disorientation.

Painful stimuli—Not responsive to verbal stimulation but responds to painful stimuli. Test the client's responsiveness to pain by rubbing the sternum in adults, pinching the sole of the foot in children, or pinching the bridge of nose if spinal injury is suspected (WHO & ICRC, 2018). Purposeful responses include awakening, moaning, pushing the rescuer away, or withdrawing. Nonpurposeful responses to painful stimuli include decorticate posturing (arms flexed, legs extended) and decerebrate posturing (arms and legs extended), both of which can indicate grave neurological damage.

Unresponsive—Comatose, no response to any stimulus.

and ventilation and can tailor interventions to the most likely cause of arrest (Panchal et al., 2020).

If the uterus of a pregnant individual is palpable at or above the umbilicus, displace it to the left before initiating chest compressions to improve cardiac filling and output (Panchal et al., 2020). Start chest compressions before giving rescue breaths (CAB rather than ABC) by giving 30 chest compressions followed by 2 breaths (Panchal et al., 2020). Focus on making the rate of compressions, 100–120/min, and their depth, 2.0–2.4 in. (5–6 cm), as effective as possible, permitting complete chest recoil after each compression, reducing interruptions in compressions, and avoiding excessive ventilation (Mastenbjörk & Meloni, 2021, p. 13; Panchal et al., 2020).

The rescuer should continue CPR until an automated external defibrillator (AED) is available for use, EMS providers assume care, or the victim starts to move (Panchal et al., 2020). CPR and early defibrillation are crucial to survival when cardiac arrest is caused by ventricular fibrillation (VF) or pulseless ventricular tachycardia (VT). Defibrillation is most likely to succeed when begun as soon as possible after onset of VF/VT. When VF/VT persists, the heart's energy reserves become depleted, and defibrillation becomes less effective. Minimize disruptions in CPR while setting up the AED and preparing to shock the victim. Trained teams of rescuers can perform multiple tasks simultaneously: one person calls EMS, another starts chest compressions, a third ventilates the client, and a fourth manages the AED.

FETAL Mnemonic

Assess for

Fetal heart rate or presence of fetal movement.

Estimated gestational age based on maternal or family report, abdominal measurement, or proximity of the uterus to the umbilicus. Is there only one fetus?

Trauma—observe for evidence of direct injury or penetrating trauma to uterus.

Abdominal palpation for tenderness and presence of uterine contractions.

Loss of amniotic fluid or vaginal bleeding.

The most common causes of maternal cardiac arrest are hemorrhage, heart failure, amniotic fluid embolism, sepsis, aspiration pneumonia, venous thromboembolism, preeclampsia/eclampsia, or complications of anesthesia (Panchal et al., 2020). In the hospital, resuscitative hysterotomy (perimortem cesarean section) should be considered at 4 min after onset of maternal cardiac arrest if there is no return of spontaneous circulation (Cullinan, 2020). Resuscitative hysterotomy allows for resuscitating a potentially viable fetus and resolving aortocaval compression which can improve the likelihood of the mother's survival (Panchal et al., 2020). See Chapter 9 for an in-depth discussion of maternal cardiac arrest.

C—Control Bleeding

Evaluating circulation also involves identifying external and internal bleeding, including vaginal bleeding. Around the world, postpartum hemorrhage is a leading cause of maternal morbidity and mortality (Rath, 2011). See Chapter 7 for a comprehensive discussion of managing postpartum hemorrhage. Miscarriage, ectopic pregnancy, placenta previa, uterine rupture, and placental abruption can be accompanied by severe bleeding that can cause maternal compromise or death (see Chapters 5 and 6).

Most preventable deaths due to trauma involve uncontrolled hemorrhage (ACS, 2018). Shootings, stabbings, motor vehicle crashes, falls, and other traumatic events have the potential to cause life-threatening bleeding. The most critical sites of traumatic internal hemorrhage are the chest, abdomen, retroperitoneum, pelvis, and long bones (ACS, 2018). Bleeding that is entirely internal requires surgical management.

Controlling external bleeding, however, saves lives. Potentially life-threatening situations include

- Wounds that spurt arterial blood;
- Intractable bleeding;
- Blood loss large enough to form a pool;
- Blood that soaks through clothing or bandages;
- Loss of all or part of a limb; and/or
- Altered mental status in a bleeding client (Pons & Jacobs, 2016).

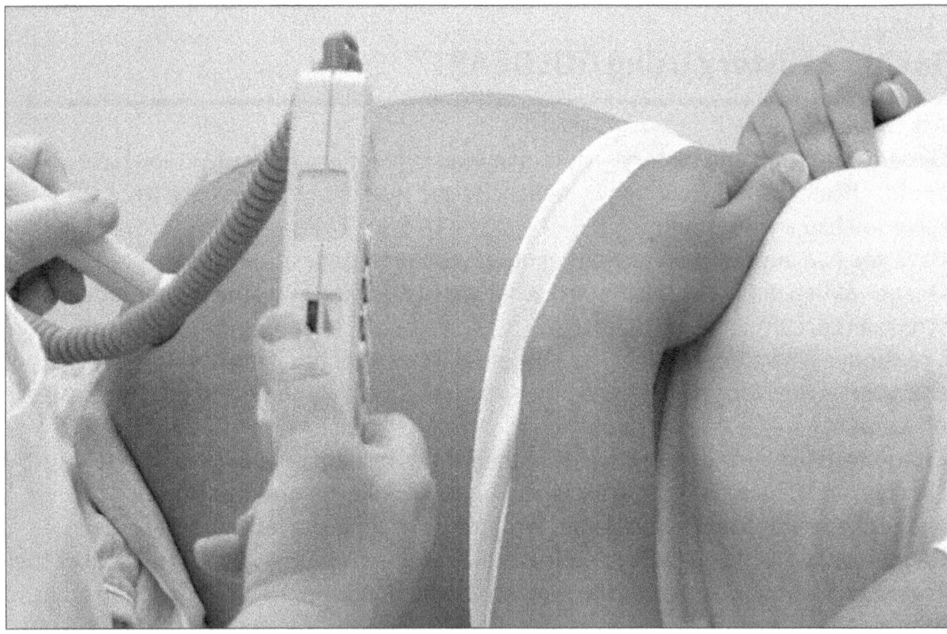

Figure 4-8. Auscultating the FHR is the last step of the ABCDEF approach to assessment. Maternal wellbeing is always assessed first because the mother is the life-support system for the fetus. If the mother is compromised, the fetus is often compromised as well.

Find the source of bleeding by opening or removing clothing. Using pressure points or elevation to control bleeding is not supported by evidence (NAEMT & ACS, 2020). Immediately compress bleeding vessels by using one or more of the following methods:

Direct pressure: Direct pressure and hemostatic packing and dressings should be used for all nonarterial severe bleeding in the extremities and in all severe bleeding from the victim's trunk (NAEMT & ACS, 2020). Expose the bleeding wound and wipe away pooled blood. Try to identify the precise site of bleeding. Cover the wound with gauze or a clean cloth and press hard with both hands. If there is critical bleeding from a large, deep injury, stuff the dressing down into the wound and press hard (WHO & ICRC, 2018). Hemostatic gauze is the preferred dressing, but plain gauze, a clean cloth, or even a shirt will suffice (NAEMT & ACS, 2020). Apply continuous pressure as hard as you can with both hands directly over the injury. Continue the pressure until emergency responders assume care of the victim, or at least 3 min for hemostatic gauze and 10 min for plain gauze (NAEMT & ACS, 2020). Do not remove the gauze to check bleeding; this disturbance can disrupt the clot and restart the bleeding. If the dressing soaks through, add another on top without removing the first (WHO & ICRC, 2018).

Tourniquet: A tourniquet is a simple, efficient tool for managing uncontrolled arterial bleeding unresponsive to direct pressure, such as that from mangled extremities, penetrating or blast injuries, or traumatic amputations (Pons & Jacobs, 2016). All commercial brands are equally effective. A tourniquet can be improvised from available materials, such as a strip of cloth at least 24 in. (61 cm) wide or a tee-shirt (Galante, 2017). Use the widest bandage possible, never a belt, rope, or wire. Most tourniquets require a windlass (a stick, screwdriver, or rod used to tighten the bandage by twisting). Inflatable tourniquets work without a windlass and resemble a blood-pressure cuff.

Apply the tourniquet directly against the skin on the affected limb, taking care to avoid joints (NAEMT & ACS, 2020). It should be between the injury and the heart and as high as possible, near the groin or axilla. Pull the free end to make it as tight as possible and secure it. Turn the windlass until bleeding stops and the distal pulse is no longer palpable, then secure the windlass to keep the tourniquet tight. Document the time the tourniquet was applied. If the bleeding does not stop, do not remove the tourniquet. Apply a second tourniquet between the first one and the heart. A tourniquet should be left in place until a surgeon removes it in the operating room, but the time of use should be as short as possible. Improper or prolonged application of a tourniquet can rarely lead to nerve paralysis and limb ischemia (Rossaint et al., 2016).

D—Disability and Neurologic Status

Disability refers to the client's level of consciousness and neurologic function. Use the mnemonic AVPU to categorize whether the client is **A**lert, responds to **V**erbal or **P**ainful stimuli, or is **U**nresponsive (WHO & ICRC, 2018; see below). Rapidly assess the victim's pupil size, reaction to light and the ability to move all extremities equally. One-sided paralysis or weakness can indicate a stroke or injury to that area. If consciousness is altered, immediately reassess the victim's oxygenation,

Table 4-1

Taking a History Using GOLDCART™

Ask the client about

General situation and history—How many weeks pregnant are you? Do you have any pregnancy complications or other health issues? How many pregnancies and how many babies have you had? Is the baby moving?
Have you had an ultrasound?
Have you had any cesarean sections or other uterine surgeries?

Onset—When did the problem start? What were you doing? Was the onset gradual or rapid? In what order did the symptoms occur?

Location—Where does it hurt? Did the pain start there or has it moved? Is it localized, or does it radiate?

Duration—How long have you had the symptoms? Do they come and go? Have you experienced them before? Frequency of the pains?

Characteristics—What is the quality of the pain? Is it sharp or dull? On a scale of 0–10, with 10 being the worst pain you ever had and 0 being no pain at all, what number would you give this pain?

Associated symptoms—What other symptoms are you experiencing?

Relieving/aggravating factors—What makes your symptoms better? What makes them worse?

Treatment—Have you treated the symptoms (with medications, herbs, remedies, hot soaks, etc.)? Did the treatment help or make things worse?

ventilation, and perfusion and consider other causes such as hypoglycemia or the use of alcohol or drugs.

Confusion or erratic behavior can have a wide range of etiologies, from head injury to heatstroke, brain hemorrhage, drug ingestion, or hypoglycemia. If consciousness is impaired, check the blood glucose (RCUK, 2022). Altered level of consciousness due to hypoglycemia in people with diabetes is easily corrected by administering oral or IV glucose (Thim et al., 2012).

E—Exposure and Environment (Temperature Control)

Exposure refers to removing or rearranging the clothing of a suspected trauma victim to examine the body for injury while preserving dignity and warmth. Seek clues to the client's underlying problem and/or present condition. Is there a laceration on the face and broken eyeglasses with no trauma to the hands, suggesting loss of consciousness before falling? Is there evidence of tongue biting or incontinence, suggesting seizure activity? Is there a medical-alert bracelet indicating a preexisting condition such as diabetes or cardiac arrhythmia? Are there track marks on the arms implying IV drug use or finger bruises suggesting assault?

F—Fetal and Uterine Assessment

Consider potentially life-threatening conditions in the mother before turning attention to the fetus. Because the mother is the life-support system for the fetus, the best way to care for the fetus is usually to stabilize the mother (Aggarwal, Soni, & Trikha, 2018). Determine approximate gestational age; the fetus is potentially viable if the fundal height is at or above the level of the umbilicus (Neuman & Promes, 2021). If the mother is compromised to the point where iatrogenic preterm birth is required—for example, by a placental abruption at 26 weeks of gestation—the client should be urgently transported to a facility with a neonatal intensive care unit (NICU) capable of managing an infant of that gestational age.

Quickly scan for visible or palpable fetal movement. If a Doppler device or fetoscope is available, listen to heart tones. Assess for pain, abdominal trauma, and the presence of vaginal bleeding or leaking of amniotic fluid. Gently palpate the mother's abdomen to check for guarding or tenderness. Note the strength and frequency of uterine contractions or abnormal uterine tone. If the pregnancy is advanced, note the size and presentation of the fetus.

In trauma cases, maternal shock and death are the leading causes of fetal death. Again, the fetus is best served by making maternal stabilization your priority (MacArthur, Foley, Gray, & Sisley, 2019). Pregnant victims of major trauma should be treated generally like other trauma victims, but with accommodations for the physiological and anatomic changes of pregnancy. Because gestational age and trauma to the pregnant abdomen can have a profound impact on the stability of the pregnant victim, assess the gravid abdomen after the primary survey and before the secondary survey. Contusions and abrasions on the skin of the abdomen can indicate blunt uterine trauma (ACS, 2018). The mnemonic FETAL is used to quickly perform a targeted history and physical examination of the pregnant abdomen.

Secondary Survey

The secondary survey is a head-to-toe assessment of the trauma victim, including a GOLDCART history (see below), consideration of the clinical impression or mechanism of injury, physical examination, and reassessment of vital signs. Begin the secondary survey after the primary survey (ABCDEF) is completed, resuscitative efforts have been started, and the victim's vital functions have begun to improve (ACS, 2018). If there are several rescuers, one can perform the secondary survey while the other(s) manage the primary survey and begin resuscitation (ACS, 2018). If the victim's condition worsens during the secondary survey, go back and reassess using the primary survey.

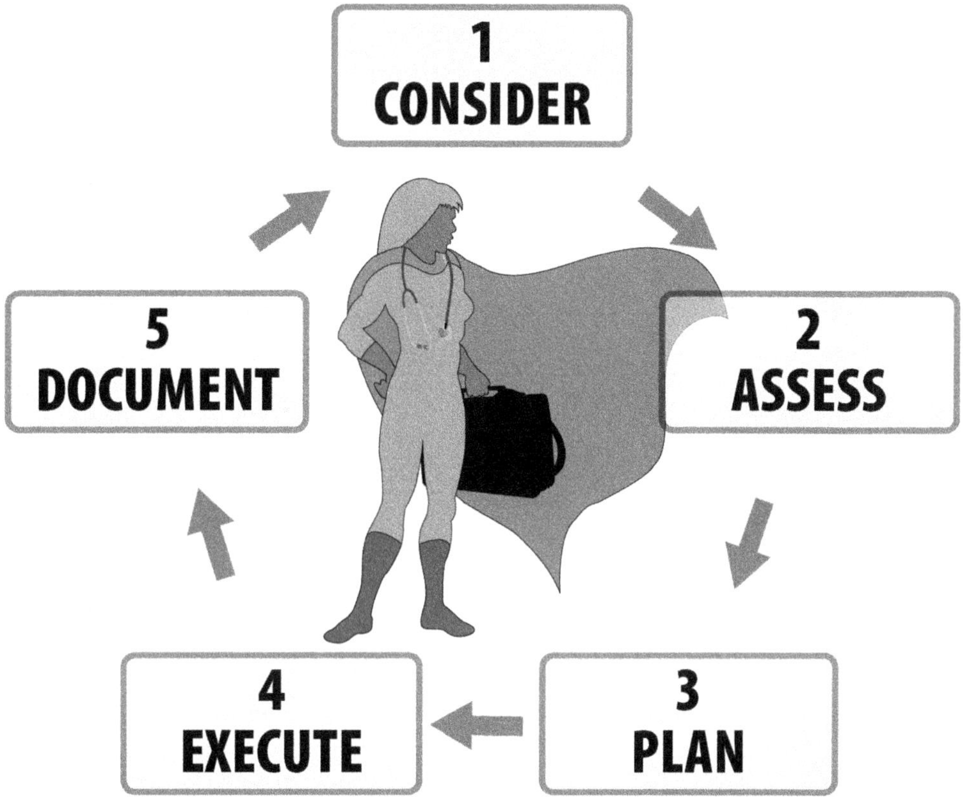

Figure 4-9. The mnemonic CAPED (Consider, Assess, Plan, Execute, and Document) provides a framework for the midwifery management process that helps the midwife perform like a superhero. The midwife should cycle through the sequence repeatedly while caring for any client.

Taking a History

Take the client's history by asking specific questions. The chief complaint is the reason for the visit or the primary problem at hand, for example, abdominal pain at 36 0/7 weeks of gestation. While taking a history, the midwife casts a wide net for relevant information, then collects the most important facts. Some clients will have a straightforward complaint; others will focus on a minor concern instead of the real issue. A single fact or finding seldom uncovers the true nature of the problem, but a cluster of relevant clues can clinch a diagnosis.

Often several possible conditions fit the clinical presentation, and the correct diagnosis emerges only as the provider solicits further clues, processes information, and reformulates treatment. A provider can evaluate most complaints and pains using the GOLDCART mnemonic. See Table 4-1. GOLDCART is a systematic method of gathering information that will help you to understand the nature of the problem. GOLDCART is a mnemonic for

- **G**eneral situation and history,
- **O**nset,
- **L**ocation,
- **D**uration,
- **C**haracteristics,
- **A**ssociated symptoms,
- **R**elieving/aggravating factors, and
- **T**reatment.

With any client, midwifery management involves an orderly process that includes gathering information, determining a course of action, implementing a plan, documenting, and reassessing. This process is ongoing throughout the course of client care. The mnemonic CAPED provides a memorable framework for this process as follows:

Consider: Consider differential diagnoses. Using GOLDCART, collect information about the situation at hand and form a fluid clinical impression that can be modified as new information emerges. View the client holistically, considering the physical, emotional, and spiritual dimensions.

Assess: Perform an examination or otherwise take measure of the client's physical condition, such as listening to the client's breathing over the telephone during a contraction to determine the approximate stage of labor. Use the information to form, solidify, or refute your clinical impression.

Plan: Formulate a course of action with the client using shared decision-making while discussing the risks, benefits, and alternatives of each option.

Execute: Execute the plan and monitor effectiveness.

Document: Evaluate the effectiveness of the plan and record your actions and your client's response.

Organize your initial impressions using
FIRST THOUGHT, WORST THOUGHT:
What is the most likely cause?
What is the worst it could be?

The CAPED process is ongoing. After completing the initial management cycle, reassess and work through the process again, over and over, changing your impressions as the client's circumstances change.

The CAPED Mnemonic and the Midwifery Management Cycle

Evaluating the Present Complaint

Human bodies and disease presentations are highly variable, and clinical situations can take unexpected turns. Clients can convey distorted impressions of their condition due to fear, pain, anxiety, or lack of understanding. Provider and client can have differing perceptions of the issue at hand and can disagree about what is relevant and important (Johnson et al., 2015). It is important to inquire about and address the client's stated concerns (N. Tharpe, personal communication, February 25, 2018).

When seeking the cause of an obstetrical complication or health complaint, organize your initial impressions by using the "First Thought, Worst Thought" technique. Ask yourself, "What is the most likely cause?" and "What is the worst it could be?" Identify the problem that is most likely to explain the symptoms while asking "Could this problem be life-threatening?" Using this technique, you will give your initial attention to the most important aspects—identifying the most likely and most dangerous diagnoses—while keeping your mind open to other explanations as you gather data.

Determine the sequence of events: did the client faint and then fall, or fall and then lose consciousness? Even when the problem is obvious, such as cord prolapse, consider the presence of other issues that might be important to the clinical picture. Is the fetus term? Is there more than one fetus? Is there a malpresentation?

Because pregnant mothers experience many conditions and concerns, it can be difficult to determine which symptoms are normal and which are worrisome. Preconceived ideas about the nature of the problem can cause the clinician to decide on a diagnosis prematurely and miss the true problem. If you simply answer a question about whether ibuprofen is safe during pregnancy and move along, the client is less likely mention abdominal pain from a fall down stairs.

Give your client the opportunity to explain what is happening and to tell the whole story. Research involving physician-client interactions show that 77% of the time, physicians assessing a client interrupt within 12–23 sec to ask about specific issues (Johnson et al., 2015). Male physicians interrupt clients more often than female physicians, and physicians of either sex interrupt female clients more often than male clients (Rhoades, McFarland, Finch, & Johnson, 2001). It is understandable that providers tend to focus on what seems important in order to identify the true problem quickly and make better use of limited appointment time. Clients who can complete their opening statements uninterrupted, however, will speak only 10 sec longer on average than those who are redirected. Even clients with complex complaints can usually fully describe their conditions in less than 2 min (Johnson et al., 2015).

The client expects you to be engaged psychologically, socially, and emotionally and determines whether you are listening largely by your body language (Johnson et al., 2015). Every client wants a "good" provider and feels safer and more confident if the midwife's expertise and judgment are perceived as trustworthy. But clients often determine whether a provider is "good" with little information. The client does not usually know the standards for safe maternity care or whether a provider adheres to them, what a provider's strengths and weaknesses are, or how other providers compare. In the absence of hard data, a client often judges a provider on displays of empathy, honesty, kindness, and respect (Johnson et al., 2015). Eye contact is helpful when communicating with people from most cultural backgrounds. If you take notes, glance down to write, and then immediately resume eye contact. After the client provides information, summarize what you have learned to verify the accuracy of your understanding. For example, "So, yesterday you had headaches and pain in your right upper abdomen all afternoon, and when you stepped on the scale this morning, you noticed you gained 10 pounds in 4 days. Is that right?"

Winnow the list of possible diagnoses as you integrate new data, excluding conditions that are not consistent with the facts and retaining those that are (Hirsch, 2020). Likely diagnoses are ranked in order of probability; as the aphorism goes: "If you hear hoofbeats, think horses, not zebras" (Hirsch, 2020). Occam's Razor, a classic problem-solving principle, maintains that if there are several explanations for an occurrence, the simplest is most likely to be accurate. In other words, more assumptions or additional hypotheses can make your impressions less accurate.

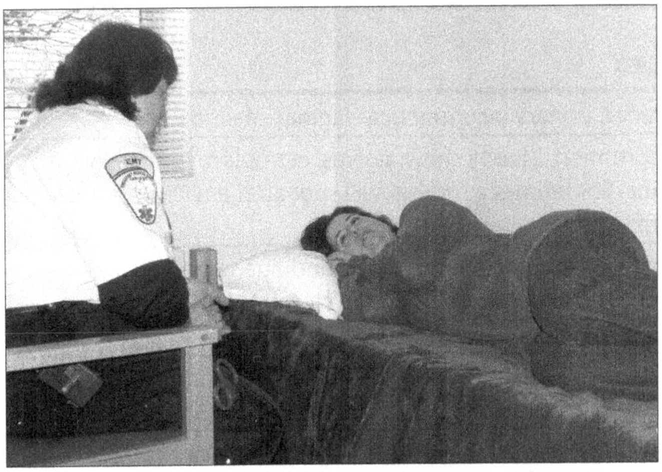

Figure 4-10. Emergency transfer to a hospital is smoother when everyone involved is prepared for the possibility.

Transfer and Referral

In the United States, about 9–13% of mothers planning a home birth are transferred to a hospital after the onset of labor (ACNM, 2015; Davis-Floyd, 2003). About 2% of these transfers occur for critical conditions (Olvera et al., 2020). The most common reasons for transfer are failure to progress in labor and prolonged rupture of membranes (ACNM, 2015; Cox, Schlegel, Payne, Teaf, & Albers, 2013; Vedam et al., 2014). Multiparas are five times more likely than nulliparas to transfer from birth center care in the antepartum period; nulliparas are 5 times more likely to transfer intrapartum (ACNM, 2015; Alliman & Phillippi, 2016). In a large prospective study of mothers planning to have their babies at birth centers in the United States, 4.5% of subjects were referred to a hospital before admission to the birth center; 11.9% were transferred during labor (82% of them were nulliparous); and 2% were transferred postpartum, most commonly for hemorrhage (Stapleton, Osborne, & Illuzzi, 2013). In addition, 2.2% of newborns were transferred, mostly for respiratory issues (Stapleton et al., 2013).

The Chain of Support

Hospital transfer is not a failure, but a change of plans necessitated by a change of condition. Although hospital transfer is often disappointing and anxiety-provoking for the mother, the family, and the midwife, it should not be an unanticipated event. Upon intake into a practice that offers community birth, the mother and any support people should be informed of the possibility of transfer and what the process might involve (Home Birth Summit, 2014). Seamless coordination of care during both routine and critical obstetric transfers improves outcomes and reduces stress for clients and providers alike.

Ideally, all participants in the birth form a chain of support which includes the mother and any support people, the midwife and any assistants, emergency medical personnel, local hospital personnel, and tertiary hospital personnel (Figure 4-11). Community birth involves the first two links in the chain. Participants should be prepared to access other links if complications arise.

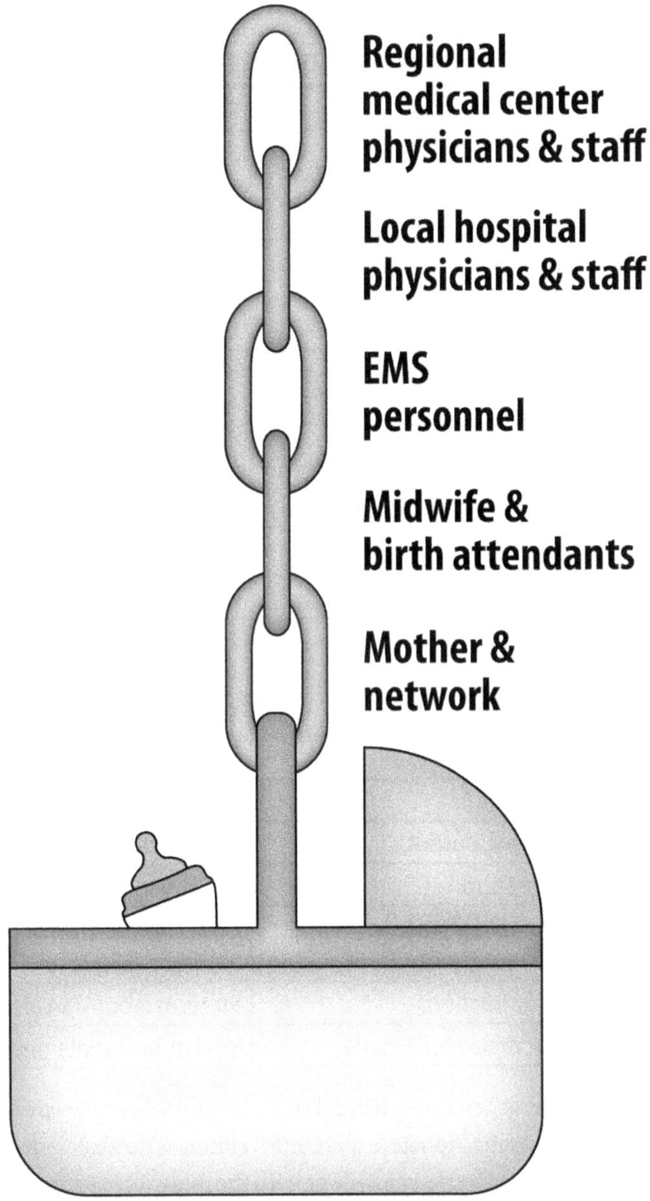

Figure 4-11. Chain of support for safe community birth.

A strong chain is comprised of strong links. Good candidates for community birth strive to keep themselves healthy and comply with recommendations from their providers. They are knowledgeable about their options as well as the risks and benefits of each choice. The midwife's team forms the second link in the chain by bringing knowledge, support, perspective, and experience to the family. If a significant complication occurs, EMS can transport the mother and/or infant in a controlled environment with medical supervision—ideally, accompanied by the midwife. The local hospital stands ready to

Table 4-2
Danger Signs in Pregnancy and Possible Causes

Sudden gush of fluid	Prelabor rupture of membranes, urinary incontinence, vaginal infection.
Vaginal bleeding	Placenta previa, placental abruption, bloody show, polyps, ectropion, trauma, or lesions of the cervix or vagina. Sometimes a mother will spot after a recent vaginal examination or sexual intercourse.
Abdominal pain	Preterm labor (PTL), placental abruption, appendicitis, round-ligament pain, gall-bladder inflammation, urinary tract infection (UTI), renal calculi, hydronephrosis, or pancreatitis.
Dizziness	Hypotension or hypertension, medications, hypoglycemia, hot environment, inner ear issues, or generalized illness..
Visual disturbances	Preeclampsia, stroke, retinal detachment, presyncope, migraine, ocular disorder.
Severe vomiting	Gastroenteritis, appendicitis, pyelonephritis, COVID-19 or other infective disorder; hyperemesis gravidarum head injury; anxiety; medication reaction; or other condition.
Edema of hands, feet, or face	Preeclampsia. (Mild pedal edema is often normal in pregnancy.)
Severe headache	Can be related to preeclampsia or can result from tension, migraine, head injury, brain tumor, or other causes.
Severe leg pain	Thrombophlebitis, leg cramps, or trauma.
Seizure	Eclampsia, preexisting seizure disorder, or head injury.
Epigastric pain	Preeclampsia, gallbladder inflammation, or heartburn.
Reduced urine output	Preeclampsia, poor fluid intake, or renal dysfunction.
Painful urination	UTI or vaginal or vulvar infection.
Absence of or decrease in fetal movement	Fetal compromise or death, maternal distraction, drug effects, or abnormalities in amniotic fluid level.
Preterm contractions	Preterm labor; can also be triggered by UTI, dehydration, or uterine irritability.
Elevated temperature, chills	Viral or bacterial infection.

receive emergencies with helpful staff and physicians prepared to provide compassionate, expert intervention as needed—ideally, comanaged by the midwife or with the midwife present for support and advice. In the case of an emergency beyond the capabilities of the local hospital, a regional medical center provides the highest-level and most definitive medical interventions as needed. Good outcomes are more likely if all mothers and their support people are treated with respect, regardless of choice of birthplace, and the providers who manage their care work together in an atmosphere of professionalism, collaboration, and mutual regard (Davis-Floyd, 2003).

Communication in an Emergency

There is never a good time to give bad news. Critical information must be communicated immediately, regardless of the circumstances, but certain details and noncrucial decision-making can be deferred or discussed after the family has processed the initial emotional blow. Communicate sensitive information directly to the client, ideally in a private location without interruptions. Position yourself at the client's level and make eye contact, giving nonverbal cues that communicate respect, concern, and empathy. Avoid discussing sensitive or emotionally charged matters when the client is undressed or otherwise in a physically or emotionally vulnerable situation.

In most cases, clear, empathetic communication and underlying trust increase the client's acceptance of an often disappointing and unsettling change of plans. When preparing for transport, explain to the client why you think transfer is necessary, and discuss the risks, benefits, and alternatives to your proposed management options. Answer any questions, and, if time permits, allow the family to discuss the matter privately. Discuss the expected course of events that will occur upon arrival at the hospital. For example, if the client is being transferred for a mentum-posterior face presentation, explain that a cesarean section will be required for birth and discuss the usual process, which can include having blood drawn, continuous fetal monitoring, IV fluids, an infusion of antibiotics, insertion of a bladder catheter, and spinal anesthesia. Although shared decision-making is the optimal model in most circumstances, in emergencies the focus is on providing care first and discussing it afterwards (N. Tharpe, personal communication, February 25, 2018).

In a crisis, your words and actions will leave an indelible imprint. What you say and how you say it can remain with the client for life. Use clear language and assess for understanding. Be honest and direct, but do not overwhelm the client with too much information. Offer hope if there is any, but not false hope lest you undermine your credibility and set the client up for a harder fall later. You can tailor your discussion to the client's knowledge gaps by asking open-ended questions, such as, "What do you know about high blood pressure in pregnancy?"

A crisis occurs when a client is overwhelmed by a critical or stressful event (Kavan, Guck, & Barone, 2006). When the event is not inherently traumatic, the client's perception that it is serious, uncontrollable, or difficult to manage can make it so and trigger a crisis response (Kavan et al., 2006). For example, the experience of a cesarean birth can be fulfilling for a mother who anticipates it or calamitous for a mother who had planned for a low-intervention birth or who fears hospitals. Clients in crisis can become emotionally numb and have difficulty processing information. If they do not understand your explanations, you need to repeat them several different ways. Some people cope with crisis by focusing on data, identifying and solving problems, and forming a plan of action. Others process information emotionally and seek solutions that "feel" right.

Families involved in emergencies often experience various stages of grief (Baker, 2020; Collini, Parker, & Oliver, 2021). Initially they can have trouble believing that there is truly an emergency. They can feel guilty and assume they are somehow responsible or seek to blame others. They can attempt to take control of the situation by bargaining or feel that they have somehow failed. Sometimes anger, depression, or harsh self-judgment set in. They can feel cheated. Often, they feel as if they were the only ones who ever had to face this circumstance. Sometimes the family will hold the provider responsible for the outcome or harbor justified or unjustified resentment and hostility. Often clients become bitter toward themselves, family members, God, the universe, or Fate.

It can be difficult when angry clients reject emotionally invested midwives, and it can be difficult to remain kind and supportive in the face of hostility. In this situation, your response should be an authentic expression of who you want to be in that moment, not a reflexive reaction to anger or ejection (N. Tharpe, personal communication, February 25, 2018). Antepartum discussions can be instrumental in helping families understand that adverse outcomes can occur and can cultivate adaptability in working with unexpected situations (N. Tharpe, personal communication, February 25, 2018).

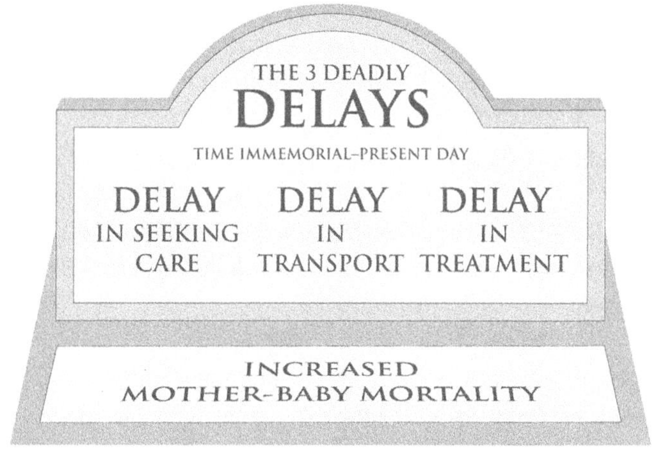

Figure 4-12. The Three Deadly Delays. Adapted from (1) "Overview of Maternal Mortality," by H. L. Brown and M. J. Small, 2022, in A. Chakrabarti (Ed.), *UpToDate*. Copyright by UpToDate. (2) "The Role of Delays in Severe Maternal Morbidity and Mortality: Expanding the Conceptual Framework," by R. C. Pacagnella, J. G. Cecatti, M. J. Osis, and J. P. Souza, 2012, *Reproductive Health Matters, 20*(39), pp. 155–163. Copyright by Reproductive Health Matters.

Timely Transport

Whenever a client is transferred from a community setting to definitive care, time is lost through transportation and initiating care in the hospital. If transfer is emergent, delays can (rarely) be deadly. Delays can occur at any of three stages in transfer: in the client's seeking care, in reaching an appropriate facility, and in receiving adequate care at that facility (Pacagnella, Cecatti, Osis, & Souza, 2012). Delays can also occur if a midwife fails to recognize a problem or delays initiating an intervention (N. Tharpe, personal communication, February 25, 2018).

Getting the client to the hospital often involves arranging transportation or stabilizing the client in an ambulance. Travel time can be affected by distance, traffic, weather, and law-enforcement operations. At the hospital, certain procedures and processes can delay definitive care. For example, preparing a client for an urgent cesarean section usually includes gowning, signing consent forms, starting electronic fetal monitoring, placing IV and bladder catheters, taking blood samples, readying the operating suite, convening a multidisciplinary surgical team, initiating anesthesia, giving medications, and disinfecting and draping the abdomen. Personnel who take call from home can cause further delays. The interval from problem onset to birth can also depend on obstetricians' willingness to act on the information conveyed by midwives.

The time delay between decision to transport and obtaining definitive care at the hospital can be significant and varies by location. In most cases, these delays do not appear to affect

Hospital transfer is not a failure, but a change of plans necessitated by a change of condition.

outcomes (Grigg, Tracy, Tracy, Schmied, & Monk, 2015). A study of 11,869 planned home births in Ontario, Canada, found no increased risk of adverse outcomes when births occurred more than 30 min from a hospital (Darling, Lawford, Wilson, Kryzanauskas, & Bourgeault, 2019).

Certain rare, time-sensitive emergencies can have worse outcomes when they occur in a community setting (Grünebaum et al., 2019). An emergency involving anoxia (such as umbilical cord prolapse with compromised oxygenation) can result in irreversible damage or death with even a short delay before cesarean birth (Boehm, 2012; Caughey & Cheyney, 2019). Wong and colleagues (2021) found that when cord prolapse results in fetal bradycardia, cord arterial pH deteriorates rapidly (0.009/min): the risk of significant acidosis (pH less than 7) is 80% when bradycardia-to-birth interval is longer than 20 min, and 17.2% when the interval is shorter.

Guidelines for care in a hospital typically recommend 30-min decision-to-incision intervals for emergent cesarean births—but this standard is unsupported by evidence and was arbitrary in origin (Grobman et al., 2018; Mooney, Ogrinc, & Steadman, 2007; Nageotte, 2014; Nasrallah et al., 2004). In fact, Bousleiman et al. (2022) found that overall, the best outcomes for emergent cesarean births occurred over a wide range of intervals from 21 to longer than 50 min. Some obstetric emergencies, such as ruptured vasa previa, can unavoidably result in adverse outcomes regardless of the interval (de Regt, Marks, Joseph, & Malmgren, 2009). Some fetuses with abnormal heart rate tracings appear to benefit from delays in decision-to-incision; these delays can provide time for the implementation of intrauterine resuscitation measures which allow the fetus to stabilize before birth (Boehm, 2012). With other problems, such as a fetal malpresentation in latent labor, moderate delays sometimes neither increase nor decrease risk. Some hospitals, such as small rural ones with surgical teams that take call from home, have difficulty meeting the 30-min standard (de Regt et al., 2009; Mooney et al., 2007).

A midwife attending a healthy client two blocks from a tertiary hospital can feel justified in adopting a wait-and-see attitude when minor deviations from normal arise. The same midwife may opt to transfer at the earliest sign of a problem if the hospital is more than 15–20 min from the planned birthplace, if environmental conditions such as flooding or snowfall increase transport time, or if the client's issues hold the potential for severe compromise. When roads are impassible, as in a blizzard or flood, the midwife may divert all labors to a hospital rather than risk encountering an emergency with no ability to transfer (Declercq & Stotland, 2023).

Levels of Maternal and Neonatal Care Facilities

Mothers who experience major medical or obstetric complications and infants that are extremely preterm or otherwise compromised have better outcomes when they are born at a hospital with clinical expertise and specialized care (California Dept. of Public Health, 2011). In the 1970s, most U.S. states developed coordinated regional systems for perinatal care facilities wherein regional or tertiary-care centers provided the highest levels of neonatal care and accepted transfers from lower-level facilities (Menard et al., 2015). A hospital with level I neonatal care facilities can provide a basic level of care to neonates who are low-risk, perform neonatal resuscitation, care for stable preterm infants at 35 0/7–37 0/7 weeks of gestation who are physiologically stable, and stabilize newborns that are ill or who are less than 35 0/7 weeks of gestation until they can be transferred to a facility capable of specialty neonatal care (Cmte. on Fetus and Newborn [COFAN] et al., 2012). A hospital with level II neonatal care facilities can generally provide care to stable or moderately ill neonates who are born at 32 0/7 weeks of gestation or greater or who weigh at least 4 lb 5 oz (1,500 g) at birth (COFAN et al., 2012). A level III facility offers the full range of maternal and neonatal services and can provide care for certain critically ill infants. Level IV units include the additional capabilities for managing the most complex and critically ill newborn infants, have pediatric specialty consultants always available, and have the capability for surgical repair of complex conditions (COFAN et al., 2012). Newborns can be transported to a higher-level facility if they require care beyond the capabilities of the local hospital.

Expanding these systems to include regionalized *maternal* care increases safety and access to services (ACOG, 2019/2021). In 2015, the ACOG and the Society for Maternal-Fetal Medicine jointly developed a consensus document, *Levels of Maternal Care*, and introduced a classification system that defines and standardizes maternal care across the United States (Menard et al., 2015). Stakeholders developed a five-tier system of maternal care ranging from local birth centers capable of managing low-risk mothers to regional perinatal hospitals that can meet the needs of those at highest risk (Menard et al., 2015). *Levels of Maternal Care* was endorsed by the American Association of Birth Centers, ACNM, the Association of Women's Health, Obstetric and Neonatal Nurses, the Commission for the Accreditation of Birth Centers, AAP, the American Society of Anesthesiologists, and the Society for Obstetric Anesthesia and Perinatology (ACOG,

2019/2021). This system omits home birth, however. The attending midwife and the consulting physician can determine together which local and regional hospitals offer the services each client requires.

The following lists the levels for maternal care facilities, from low to high acuity (ACOG, 2019/2021):

Accredited birth center: Able to care for low-risk clients with uncomplicated singleton term vertex pregnancies who are expected to have uncomplicated births.

Level I facility: Can manage uncomplicated pregnancies and clients with higher risk conditions such as uncomplicated twin gestation, trial of labor after cesarean, uncomplicated cesarean birth, preeclampsia, or well-controlled gestational diabetes. Can also stabilize clients for transfer to a higher level of care.

Level II facility: Has all capabilities of a level I facility but can also manage moderate-to-high-risk antepartum, postpartum, or newborn conditions such as placenta previa with no prior uterine surgery, anticipated complicated cesarean birth, and maternal medical conditions that require additional monitoring (e.g., pregestational diabetes, poorly controlled asthma, poorly controlled or complicated chronic hypertension).

Level III facility: Has all capabilities of a level II facility but can also manage more complex maternal conditions, obstetric complications, and fetal conditions such as moderate maternal heart disease, suspected placenta accreta or percreta, placenta previa with previous uterine surgery, acute respiratory distress syndrome or other conditions that require ventilatory support, acute fatty liver of pregnancy, coagulation disorders, complex hematologic or autoimmune disorders, or expectant management of preeclampsia with severe features remote from term.

Level IV facility: Has all capabilities of a level III facility, but also provides onsite medical and surgical care for the most complex maternal conditions and critically ill mothers and fetuses throughout the antepartum, intrapartum, and postpartum period such as severe maternal cardiac conditions, severe pulmonary hypertension, clients who require neurosurgery or cardiac surgery, or clients in unstable condition and in need of an organ transplant.

Initiating a Transfer

All midwives should know whom to call and how to send client records in the case of hospital transfer. Ideally, the midwife accompanies the client during transport and provides skilled care *en route* within local EMS standards (ACNM, 2015). Failure to accompany the mother during transfer can constitute client abandonment (ACNM, 2015). If EMS guidelines prohibit midwives from accompanying the client, they should travel to the hospital by other means to transfer care and support the client (ACNM, 2015).

Ineffective care transitions can result in misunderstandings that can harm the client. Research has shown that more than two thirds of adverse events and serious errors involve poor communication during the handoff between health care providers (Barry, 2014; Joint Commission, 2012). Miscommunication is especially likely when the client transfers from one setting to another, such as from home to hospital.

The SBAR Tool

The SBAR (**S**ituation, **B**ackground, **A**ssessment, **R**ecommendation) report is a standardized framework to guide the transfer of care from one provider to the next (Maine Center for Disease Control & Prevention, 2014). Originally developed by the United States Navy to improve communication on nuclear submarines, the SBAR format allows the provider to organize thoughts quickly and focus on key information (Stewart, 2016). To give an SBAR report, quickly organize the information into four elements: situation, background, assessment, and recommendations. In 8–12 sec, convey the level of urgency, stating the most serious problem first and your client's immediate needs. Fill in the relevant background and the events leading to the current issue. Conclude by making a recommendation for ongoing care to serve as a starting point to discuss solutions. Give the receiver the opportunity to ask questions and clarify information.

In many localities, the midwife will take the following steps to initiate transport (ACNM, 2015; Finn, et al, 2015; Home Birth Summit, 2014; Midwives' Assn. of Washington State [MAWS], 2011; Vedam et al., 2014):

1. If the transfer is an emergency, call EMS, give a concise synopsis of the situation or SBAR report, and provide detailed instructions on how to reach your location. You can have a birth assistant or family member place the call. If the telephone is on speaker, you can give information while taking care of the client. Transfers for emergencies are usually to the nearest hospital with the capacity to manage an obstetrical or neonatal emergency. Other transfers may bypass the nearest hospital to reach one with a level 4 NICU or a maternity department appropriate for managing high-risk clients, one where the referring midwife has privileges, or one of the client's choosing. Whenever possible, the midwife should collaborate with the EMS team to manage the client *en route* and address any emotional and social needs during transport (Finn et al., 2015).
2. Call the receiving practitioner and state that you would like to transfer your client to their facility. If you do not

Table 4-3

Template for SBAR Report Call to Activate EMS

Situation
Identify yourself and give a concise statement of the problem.
This is (name and credential or relationship).
Calling for (emergency or non-emergency) transport of a (mother/baby/mother and baby).
From a (planned home birth or freestanding birth center birth).
Reason for transport:
Client's name and date of birth:
My call-back number:
The client's location (street address and information on how to find it):
Client will be accompanied by:
Background
What has happened and what is important about the clinical picture?
Briefly, these are the events leading up to my call:
Significant history includes vital signs and FHR (usually "stable" or "unstable" will suffice):
I have initiated these interventions:
Assessment
Your clinical impression.
The problem is (or) I think the problem is (or) I don't know what the problem is, but...
The client is stable/unstable.
Recommendation/Request
What you think should be done.
I recommend you send (basic life support/advanced life support) EMS providers.
Do you have questions or need clarification?

know who the accepting provider will be, call the labor and delivery (L&D) unit and ask who is on duty and how to make contact. Some hospitals put all involved parties (community midwife, physician, charge nurse, neonatologist, hospital midwife, et al.) together on a conference call. Give an SBAR report, which includes the reason for transport, mode of transport, the client's condition, brief obstetrical history, brief medical and surgical history, ETA, and any other significant information that would help the hospital prepare for the transfer (Home Birth Summit, 2014). Identify what services might be required, for example neonatal intensive care or a medical translator. You can offer an anticipated management plan, for example, "She will probably need an epidural for pain management and exhaustion and oxytocin augmentation to strengthen ineffective contractions, but I believe she is still a good candidate for a vaginal birth." Ask whether the provider requires any more information before ending the call.

3. If not already addressed via conference call, contact the L&D department of the receiving hospital, state your name and that you have a client who will transfer, and ask whom you should give report to—usually a triage or charge nurse. Give clear information about the client, including date of birth, reason for transfer, and ETA. Provide a concise overview of the situation and ask whether more information is required. If possible, fax prenatal and labor records to the receiving hospital.
4. The midwife should accompany the client into the hospital, records in hand, and give a professional, face-to-face report to the receiving providers. Sometimes midwives who have hospital privileges continue as primary maternity care providers in collaboration with the receiving physician. If the midwife does not have privileges or if the client's condition exceeds the midwife's scope of practice, care is transferred to the receiving provider and the hospital staff. Thereafter, the midwife's role changes from primary provider to companion or support person who may remain at the bedside if the mother chooses (Home Birth Summit, 2014; Washington State Perinatal Collaborative [WSPC], 2015).
5. Facilitate good communication by helping the receiving provider understand the client's unique situation and concerns and deflect any negative comments by refocusing on the immediate care needs of the client (N. Tharpe, personal communication, February 25, 2018). Help your client to comprehend and accept the plan of care. When you cultivate an attitude of respect, you increase the likelihood that every member of the hospital staff will view you as trustworthy, capable, and professional and will be more inclined to collaborate. Ideally, the receiving provider and staff share the decision-making process with the client and agree upon a plan that incorporates the client's values, beliefs, and preferences (Home Birth Summit, 2014).
6. Coordinate postpartum follow-up with the hospital providers. Make sure your client signs a records release

allowing you to obtain updates and documentation for the chart. Request copies of relevant medical records, which can be faxed, mailed, or hand-carried by the client to the next appointment. Follow up to clarify outcomes and strengthen your relationship with the hospital providers. Arrange a fact-focused debriefing session to examine the transport process: determine what went well and what could be improved, and assess the family's perception of interprofessional relations (N. Tharpe, personal communication, February 25, 2018; see Chapter 16, "Debriefing").

Table 4-4

Template for SBAR Report to Receiving Provider

Situation *Identify yourself and give a concise statement of the problem.* This is (name and credential or relationship). I am calling because I am transporting a (mother/baby/mother and baby) to your hospital. From a (planned home birth or freestanding birth center birth). • Reason for transport. • Client's name and date of birth. • Who will accompany the client. • Mode of Transportation, ETA.
Background *What has happened and what is important about the clinical picture?* Briefly, these are the events leading up to my call: Significant history (may include): • Gravida, para • Gestational weeks • Significant medical and prenatal history or labs • Dilation and station • Ruptured membranes, time of rupture • Fluid color: clear, meconium • Group B *Streptococcus* status • Previous cesarean • Estimated blood loss • Medications • Therapies administered to mother or baby • Time of birth • Apgar score • Newborn resuscitation • Estimated gestational age I have initiated these interventions: Vital signs and fetal heart rate are:
Assessment *Your clinical impression.* The problem is (or) I think the problem is (or) I don't know what the problem is, but . . . The client is stable/unstable.
Recommendation/Request What you think should be done. I am recommending . . . (or) I think the client needs . . . (or) I think you should consider . . . or I intend to . . . Do you have questions or need clarification? Is there anyone else I should notify? Do you need any more information?

Respect and Professionalism

Although most home-birth transfers are low-acuity, emergency transfers are often dramatic and frightening, not only for mother, family, and midwife, but also for hospital staff. If every transport involves an emergency or abnormal situation, hospital-based providers can develop the impression that home birth is unsafe. After witnessing adrenaline-charged emergencies or hearing stories about them, it is natural for hospital providers to experience anxiety when assuming responsibility for a client who has transferred from home (Cheyney, Everson, & Burcher, 2014). For these providers, achieving a positive outcome does not ameliorate the anxiety that sparks whenever a midwife calls with a transfer (Cheyney et al., 2014).

Unfortunately, community midwives and their clients are sometimes treated punitively or disrespectfully by hospital staff after transfer (Declercq & Stotland, 2023). Maltreatment, or the perception or expectation of maltreatment, can make midwives reluctant to transfer when the client develops a complication (Cheyney et al., 2014). If physicians and nurses assume that midwives are likely to mismanage a client, they can perceive shortcomings despite evidence of high-quality care (Cheyney et al., 2014).

Disrespectful behavior can occur among providers of every kind within and among disciplines (Joint Commission, 2021). It can occur in a hospital, on an ambulance,

Table 4-5
Sample SBAR Report to Physician for Transfer from Home to Hospital

Situation This is Hannah Meacham. I am a certified nurse-midwife with Birch Valley Midwifery. I am transferring a client to your hospital from a home birth in Haverton for evaluation of hypertension with active labor. The client is Flora Powers, DOB 9/4/99. She will be transporting by ambulance. I will be accompanying her as a support person. You can expect us in about 30 minutes.
Background Flora is a gravida 2, para 1 at 38 2/7 weeks who started spontaneous labor about 8 a.m. When I arrived at around noon, she was 5 cm/80/-2 and her blood pressure was 150/90. On retake her BP was 156/100, so we are transporting to labor and delivery. Fetal heart tones are 140 with accelerations to 160. Contractions are every 2–3 min and palpate moderate. She has been healthy and normotensive through this pregnancy and her last. No headaches, no visual changes, no right upper quadrant pain, but hands and face are edematous, and she hasn't felt well the last few days. Her patellar reflexes are brisk, +3 bilaterally, and there was one beat of clonus on the left. I have a saline well in place. Pulse, respiration, and temp are normal.
Assessment It appears that she has preeclampsia versus gestational hypertension. She seems to be laboring well and will probably have a vaginal birth in a few hours. The fetus is very active and has many accelerations.
Recommendation Flora will require assessment and treatment of hypertension and labor management.

or at a birth center. Disrespectful behaviors include overt aggression such as verbal abuse, intimidation or threats, and passive aggression such as lack of cooperation, reluctance to complete tasks or return telephone calls or pages, condescending tones of voice, or impatience (Joint Commission, 2021).

Intimidating and disruptive behaviors can lead to medical errors, preventable adverse outcomes, costlier care, poor client satisfaction, and higher staff turnover (Joint Commission, 2021). Clients feel embarrassed, insecure, and unsafe when they witness power struggles, arguments, or intimidation among caregivers. Bullying, disrespect, and intimidation frequently go unchallenged and unreported by those who fear retaliation or whistle-blower stigma, avoid confrontation, or believe that perpetrators will escape accountability (Joint Commission, 2021). The Joint Commission, a nonprofit organization that accredits health care organizations and programs in the United States, recommends a zero-tolerance policy for unprofessional behavior upheld by all members of the team, in and out of the hospital. As a condition of accreditation, the Joint Commission (2021) requires healthcare facilities to have a code of conduct that defines what are unacceptable, disruptive, or inappropriate behaviors and sets guidelines for actively addressing them.

You cannot always change another person's behavior, but you can protect your own boundaries. Respectful communication means showing unconditional honor, acceptance, and civility toward others. Be honest and direct, but polite, even when others are not. Be open to new viewpoints and information. Accept negative feedback with neutral emotions, thank the person for sharing, and calmly state whether you agree (Preston, 2005). Stand firm for evidence-informed care and what you believe to be true. Do not allow others to mistreat you or your clients. If you receive or witness disrespectful treatment, consider lodging a complaint with the appropriate authority after the situation has ended, and propose that all parties take steps to improve interactions (Gephart & Cholette, 2012). Because hospital reputation and reimbursement often depend on client satisfaction, the client is often best situated to file a complaint or report an unsafe situation.

Interprofessional communication can serve either to solidify divisions or promote mutual respect, accommodation, and bridge-building (Vedam et al., 2014). Community midwifery practices should facilitate transfer of care by developing positive relationships with the receiving facility (ACOG, 2019/2021; WSPC, 2015). Some community midwives have privileges that allow them to continue caring for clients in a professional capacity at a hospital. The receiving hospital should support the midwife without privileges to remain in the capacity of doula, advisor, and friend. When midwives and staff maintain helpful client-centered attitudes, clear and respectful communication, continuity, and appropriate, timely care, mothers have a greater sense of security and outcomes improve (MAWS, 2011).

Topics for Discussion

1. Your client has presented to your birth center with ruptured membranes (SROM 10 hr ago), thick meconium fluid, and no contractions. You have decided to initiate

transport to the nearest hospital. Give a report to the receiving physician in SBAR format.

2. Hermione G. is in active labor at home, and has developed hypertension, headache, and swelling consistent with pre-eclampsia. Discuss the Three Deadly Delays and how they might lead to a poor outcome for Hermione and her baby.
3. The steps of rapid assessment are followed stepwise, ABCDEF. The last letter, *F* stands for *fetal*. Why does the fetal assessment come only after a lengthy chain of maternal assessments? What might happen if the fetus were assessed first and maternal management were based on fetal status?
4. Physicians sometimes resist collaboration with home-birth midwives. Name some strategies midwives can use to build professional relationships with hospital physicians for the good of their clients.
5. Failure to rescue occurs when a provider does not recognize and manage a problem, causing harm to the client. Describe a situation in which a midwife's failure to rescue results in harm to mother or baby.

References

Agency for Healthcare Research and Quality. (2016, reviewed 2020). *The SHARE approach: A model for shared decisionmaking—Fact sheet*. Rockville, MD: Author. Retrieved from https://www.ahrq.gov/health-literacy/professional-training/shared-decision/tools/factsheet.html

Aggarwal, R., Soni, K. D., & Trikha, A. (2018). Initial management of a pregnant woman with trauma. *Journal of Obstetric Anaesthesia and Critical Care, 8*(2), 66–72. https://doi.org/10.4103/joacc.JOACC_4_18

Alliman, J., & Phillippi, J. C. (2016). Maternal outcomes in birth centers: An integrative review of the literature. *Journal of Midwifery & Women's Health, 61*(1), 21–51. Https://doi.org/10.1111/jmwh.12356

American Academy of Orthopedic Surgeons. (2018). *Nancy Caroline's emergency care in the streets* (8th ed.). Burlington, MA: Jones & Bartlett Learning.

American College of Nurse-Midwives. (2014). *Collaborative management in midwifery practice for medical, gynecologic and obstetric conditions* (Position Statement). Retrieved from https://midwife.org/ACNM/files/ACNMLibraryData/UPLOADFILENAME/000000000058/Collaborative-Mgmt-in-Midwifery-Practice-Sept-2014.pdf

American College of Nurse-Midwives. (2015). Midwifery provision of home birth services (Clinical Bulletin 14). *Journal of Midwifery & Women's Health, 61*(1), 127–133. Https://doi.org/10.1111/jmwh.12431

American College of Obstetricians and Gynecologists. (2019, reaffirmed 2021). *Levels of maternal care* (Obstetric Care Consensus 9). Retrieved from https://www.acog.org/clinical/clinical-guidance/obstetric-care-consensus/articles/2019/08/levels-of-maternal-care

American College of Obstetricians and Gynecologists. (2021). *Informed consent and shared decision making in obstetrics and gynecology* (Committee Opinion 819). Retrieved from https://www.acog.org/clinical/clinical-guidance/committee-opinion/articles/2021/02/informed-consent-and-shared-decision-making-in-obstetrics-and-gynecology

American College of Surgeons Committee on Trauma. (2018). *Advanced Trauma Life Support® student course manual* (10th ed.). Chicago, IL: American College of Surgeons.

American Medical Association. (2022). Informed consent. In *American Medical Association code of medical ethics*. Retrieved January 31, 2023, from https://code-medical-ethics.ama-assn.org/ethics-opinions/informed-consent

Baker, M. J. (2020). Nurses, patients, and families: Caring at the intersection of health, illness, and culture. In B. P. Black (Ed.), *Professional nursing: Concepts & challenges* (9th ed., Kindle version, ch. 13). St. Louis, MO: Elsevier.

Barry, M. E. (2014). Hand-off communication: Assuring the transfer of accurate patient information. *American Nurse Today, 9*(1), 30–34. Retrieved from http://www.nursingworld.org/MainMenuCategories/ANAMarketplace/ANAPeriodicals/AmericanNurseToday/Archive/2014-ANT/Jan14-ANT/Issues-up-close-Jan14.pdf

Boehm, F. (2012). Decision to incision: Time to reconsider. *American Journal of Obstetrics & Gynecology, 206*(2), 97–98. Https://doi.org/10.1016/j.ajog.2011.09.009

Bousleiman, S., Rouse, D. J., Gyamfi-Bannerman, C., Huang, Y., D'Alton, M. E., Siddiq, Z., . . . Friedman, A. M. (2022). Decision to incision and risk for fetal acidemia, low Apgar Scores, and hypoxic ischemic encephalopathy. *American Journal of Perinatology, 39*(4), 416–424. Https://doi.org/10.1055/s-0040-1717068

Brown, H. L., & Small, M. J. (2023). Overview of maternal mortality. In A. Chakrabarti (Ed.), *UpToDate*. Retrieved September 30, 2023, from http://www.uptodate.com/contents/overview-of-maternal-mortality

California Department of Public Health, Maternal, Child and Adolescent Health Division. (2011). *The California pregnancy-associated mortality review: Report from 2002 and 2003 maternal death reviews*. Sacramento, CA: Author. Retrieved from https://www.cdph.ca.gov/Programs/CFH/DMCAH/CDPH%20Document%20Library/PAMR/CA-PAMR-Report.pdf

Casey, G. (2002). Physiology of the skin. *Nursing Standard, 16*(34), 47–51. https://doi.org/10.7748/ns2002.05.16.34.47.c3193

Caughey, A. B., & Cheyney, M. (2019). Home and birth center birth in the United States: Time for greater collaboration across models of care. *Obstetrics & Gynecology, 133*(5)1033–1050. Https://doi.org/10.1097/AOG.0000000000003215

Cheyney, M., Everson, C., & Burcher, P. (2014). Homebirth transfers in the United States: Narratives of risk, fear, and mutual accommodation. *Qualitative Health Research, 24*(4),443–456. Https://doi.org/10.1177/1049732314524028

Chourpiliadis, C., & Bhardwaj, A. (2022). Physiology, respiratory rate. *StatPearls*. Treasure Island, FL: StatPearls Publishing. Retrieved September 30, 2023, from https://www.ncbi.nlm.nih.gov/books/NBK537306/

Collini, A., Parker, H., & Oliver, A. (2021). Training for difficult conversations and breaking bad news over the phone in the emergency department. *Emergency Medicine Journal, 38*(2), 151–154. https://doi.org/10.1136/emermed-2020-210141

Committee on Fetus and Newborn, Barfield, W. D., Papile, L.-A., Baley, J. E., Benitz, W., Cummings, J., . . . Watterberg, K. L. (2012). Levels of neonatal care. *Pediatrics, 130*(3), 587–597. https://doi.org/10.1542/peds.2012-1999

Cox, K. J., Schlegel, R., Payne, P., Teaf, D., & Albers, L. (2013). Outcomes of planned home births attended by certified nurse-midwives in Southeastern Pennsylvania, 1983–2008. *Journal of Midwifery & Women's Health, 58*(2), 145–149. Https://doi.org/10.1111/j.1542-2011.2012.00217.x

Cullinan, B. (2020). Maternal resuscitation and trauma. In L. Leeman, L. Dresang, J. S. Quinlan, & S. R. Magee (Eds.), *Advanced life support in obstetrics: Provider manual* (9th ed., pp. 205–227). Leawood, KS: American Academy of Family Physicians.

Dahlen, H. G., & Caplice, S. (2014). What do midwives fear? *Women and Birth, 27*(4), 266–270. Https://doi.org/10.1016/j.wombi.2014.06.008

Darling, E. K., Lawford, K. M. O., Wilson, K., Kryzanauskas, M., & Bourgeault, I. L. (2019). Distance from home birth to emergency obstetric services and neonatal outcomes: A cohort study. *Journal of Midwifery & Women's Health, 64*(2), 170–178. Https://doi.org/10.1111/jmwh.12896

Davis-Floyd, R. (2003). Home-birth emergencies in the US and Mexico: The trouble with transport. *Social Science & Medicine, 56*(9), 1911–1931. Https://doi.org/10.1016/S0277-9536(02)00213-7

de Moraes, A. G., & Surani, S. (2019). Effects of diabetic ketoacidosis in the respiratory system. *World Journal of Diabetes, 10*(1), 16–22. https://doi.org/10.4239/wjd.v10.i1.16

de Regt, R. H., Marks, K., Joseph, D. L., & Malmgren, J. A. (2009). Time from decision to incision for cesarean deliveries at a community hospital. *Obstetrics & Gynecology, 113*(3), 625–629. Https://doi.org/10.1097/AOG.0b013e31819970b8 Retrieved from http://journals.lww.com/greenjournal/Fulltext/2009/03000/Time_From_Decision_to_Incision_for_Cesarean.9.aspx

Declercq, E., & Stotland, N. E. (2023). *Planned home birth.* In K. Eckler (Ed.), *UpToDate.* Retrieved September 30, 2023, from http://www.uptodate.com/contents/planned-home-birth

Farcas, A., Ko, J., Chan, J., Malik, S., Nono, L., & Chiampas, G. (2021). Use of incident command system for disaster preparedness: A model for an emergency department COVID-19 response. *Disaster Medicine and Public Health Preparedness, 15*(3), e31–e36. https://doi.org/10.1017/dmp.2020.210

Finn, K. T., Condon, S., Doyle, K. M., Hernandez, E. M., Kieltyka, C., Jefferson, K., & Ritter, R. (2015). *Planned home birth in New York State: New York State Association of Licensed Midwives guidelines for best practice.* (n.p.): New York State Association of Licensed Midwives. Retrieved from http://nysalm.org/wp-content/uploads/2016/10/HomeBirthGuidelines.pdf

Freytsis, M., Phillippi, J. C., Cox, K. J., Romano, A., & Cragin, L. (2017), The American College of Nurse-Midwives Clarity in Collaboration Project: Describing midwifery care in interprofessional collaborative care models. *Journal of Midwifery & Women's Health, 62*(1), 101–108. Https://doi.org/10.1111/jmwh.12521

Galante, J. M. (2017). Using tourniquets to stop bleeding. *JAMA, 317*(14), 1490. https://doi.org/10.1001/jama.2015.8581

Gephart, S., & Cholette, M. (2012). PURE communication: A strategy to improve care coordination for high-risk birth. *Newborn and Infant Nursing Reviews, 12*(2), 109–114. https://doi.org/10.1053/j.nainr.2012.03.007

Grigg, C. P., Tracy, S. K., Tracy, M., Schmied, V., & Monk, A. (2015). Transfer from primary maternity unit to tertiary hospital in New Zealand—Timing, frequency, reasons, urgency and outcomes: Part of the Evaluating Maternity Units study. *Midwifery, 31*(9), 879-887. https://doi.org/10.1016/j.midw.2015.04.018

Grobman, W. A., Bailit, J., Sandoval, G., Reddy, U. M., Wapner, R. J., Varner, M. W., . . . Tolosa, J. E. (2018). The association of decision-to-incision time for cesarean delivery with maternal and neonatal outcomes. *American Journal of Perinatology, 35*(3), 247–253. https://doi.org/10.1055/s-0037-1606641

Guglielminotti, J., Wong, C. A., Friedman, A. M., & Li, G. (2021). Racial and ethnic disparities in death associated with severe maternal morbidity in the United States: Failure to rescue. *Obstetrics & Gynecology, 137*(5), 791–800. https://doi.org/10.1097/AOG.0000000000004362

Hirsch, E. (2020). Horses and zebras: Probabilities, uncertainty, and cognitive bias in clinical diagnosis. *American Journal of Obstetrics & Gynecology, 222*(5), 469.e1–469.e3. https://doi.org/10.1016/j.ajog.2020.01.010

Hofmeyr, G. J., Haws, R. A., Bergström, S., Lee, A. C. C., Okong, P., Darmstadt, G. L., . . . Lawn, J. E. (2009). Obstetric care in low-resource settings: What, who, and how to overcome challenges to scale up? *International Journal of Gynecology & Obstetrics, 107,* S21–S45. https://doi.org/10.1016/j.ijgo.2009.07.017

Home Birth Summit. (2014). *Best practice guidelines: Transfer from planned home birth to hospital.* Retrieved from http://www.homebirthsummit.org/wp-content/uploads/2014/03/HomeBirthSummit_BestPracticeTransferGuidelines.pdf

Johansson, R., Danielsson, E., Kvarnlöf, L., Eriksson, K., & Karlsson, R. (2018). At the external boundary of a disaster response operation: The dynamics of volunteer inclusion. *Journal of Contingencies and Crisis Management, 26*(4), 519–529. https://doi.org/10.1111/1468-5973.12228

Johnson, M., Boyd, L., Grantham, L., & Eastwood, K. (2015). *Paramedic principles and practice ANZ: A clinical reasoning approach.* Chatswood, NSW, Australia: Elsevier Australia.

Joint Commission. (2012). *Transitions of care: The need for a more effective approach to continuing patient care* (Hot Topics in Health Care). Retrieved from https://web.archive.org/web/20130612011942/http://www.jointcommission.org/assets/1/18/hot_topics_transitions_of_care.pdf

Joint Commission. (2021). *Behaviors that undermine a culture of safety* (Sentinel Event Alert 40). Retrieved from https://www.jointcommission.org/resources/sentinel-event/sentinel-event-alert-newsletters/sentinel-event-alert-issue-40-behaviors-that-undermine-a-culture-of-safety/

Kavan, M. G., Guck, T. P., & Barone, E. J. (2006). A practical guide to crisis management. *American Family Physician, 74*(7), 1159–1164. Retrieved from https://www.aafp.org/pubs/afp/issues/2006/1001/p1159.html

King, T. L. (2015), Interprofessional collaboration: Changing the future. *Journal of Midwifery & Women's Health, 60*(2), 117–119. https://doi.org/10.1111/jmwh.12318

MacArthur, B., Foley, M., Gray, K., & Sisley, A. (2019). Trauma in pregnancy: A comprehensive approach to the mother and fetus. *American Journal of Obstetrics & Gynecology, 220*(5), 465–468e1. https://doi.org/0.1016/j.ajog.2019.01.209

Maine Center for Disease Control and Prevention. (2014). *Best practice recommendations for handoff communication during transport from a home or freestanding birth center to a hospital setting.* Retrieved from http://www.maine.gov/dhhs/mecdc/population-health/mch/documents/01-2014-Maine-CDC-Transport-Guidelines-FINAL.pdf

Mastenbjörk, M., & Meloni, S. (2021). *Basic life support (BLS) provider manual: A comprehensive guide covering the latest guidelines* (Kindle version). [Las Vegas, NV]: Medical Creations.

Menard, M. K., Kilpatrick, S., Saade, G., Hollier, L. M., Joseph, G. F., Jr., Barfield, . . . Conry, J. (2015). Levels of maternal care. *American Journal of Obstetrics & Gynecology, 212*(3), 259–271. https://doi.org/10.1016/j.ajog.2014.12.030

Midwives' Association of Washington State. (2011). *Planned out-of-hospital birth transport guideline.* Retrieved from http://www.washingtonmidwives.org/documents/MAWS-OOH-transport-policy0211.pdf

Mooney, S. E., Ogrinc, G., & Steadman, W. (2007). Improving emergency caesarean delivery response times at a rural community hospital. *Quality & Safety in Health Care, 16*(1), 60–66. https://doi.org/10.1136/qshc.2006.019976

Nageotte, M. P. (2014). The 30-minute standard: How fast is fast enough? *American Journal of Obstetrics & Gynecology, 210*(3), 177–178. https://doi.org/10.1016/j.ajog.2014.01.017

Nasrallah, F. K., Harirah, H. M., Vadhera, R., Jain, V., Franklin, L. T., & Hankins, G. D. (2004). The 30 minute decision-to-incision interval for emergency cesarean delivery: Fact or fiction? *American Journal of Perinatology, 21*(2), 63–68. https://doi.org/10.1055/s-2004-820513

National Association of Emergency Medical Technicians & American College of Surgeons, Committee on Trauma. (2020). *PHTLS: Prehospital trauma life support for first responders* (9th ed.). Burlington, MA: Jones & Bartlett Learning,

Neuman, J. E., & Promes, S. B. (2021). Trauma in pregnancy. In A. B. Wolfson et al. (Eds.), *Harwood-Nuss' clinical practice of emergency medicine* (7th ed., pp. 329–332). Philadelphia, PA: Wolters Kluwer.

Nieuwenhuijze, M. J., Korstjens, I., de Jonge, A., de Vries, R., & Lagro-Janssen, A. (2014). On speaking terms: A Delphi study on shared decision-making in maternity care. *BMC Pregnancy and Childbirth, 14*(1), 1–11. https://doi.org/10.1186/1471-2393-14-223

Noon, A. J. (2014). The cognitive processes underpinning clinical decision in triage assessment: A theoretical conundrum? *International Emergency Nursing, 22*(1), 40–46. https://doi.org/10.1016/j.ienj.2013.01.003

Olvera, L., Smith, J. S., Prater, L. & Hastings-Tolsma, M. (2020), Interprofessional communication and collaboration during emergent birth center transfers: A quality improvement project. *Journal of Midwifery & Women's Health, 65*(4), 555–561. https://doi.org/10.1111/jmwh.13076

Pacagnella, R. C., Cecatti, J. G., Osis, M. J., & Souza, J. P. (2012). The role of delays in severe maternal morbidity and mortality: Expanding the conceptual framework. *Reproductive Health Matters, 20*(39), 155–163. https://doi.org/10.1016/S0968-8080(12)39601-8

Panchal, A. R., Bartos, J. A., Cabañas, J. G., Donnino, M. W., Drennan, I. R., Hirsch, K. G., . . . Adult Basic and Advanced Life Support Writing Group. (2020). Adult basic and advanced life support: 2020 American Heart Association guidelines for cardiopulmonary resuscitation and emergency cardiovascular care, part 3. *Circulation, 142*(16, Suppl. 2), S366–S468. https://doi.org/10.1161/CIR.0000000000000916

Pearlman, M. D., & Desmond, J. S. (2005, May). Pregnant with danger. *WebM&M Case Studies*. Retrieved from https://psnet.ahrq.gov/web-mm/pregnant-danger

Peate, I., & Brent, D. (2021). Using the ABCDE approach for all critically unwell patients. *British Journal of Healthcare Assistants, 15*(2), 84–89. https://doi.org/10.12968/bjha.2021.15.2.84

Persson, S., & Uhnoo, S. (2021). Dilemmas and discretion in complex organizations: Professionals in collaboration with spontaneous volunteers during disasters. *Professions and Professionalism, 11*(2), e3961. https://doi.org/10.7577/pp.3961

Pons, P. T., & Jacobs, L. (2016). *Save a life: What everyone should know to stop bleeding after an injury*. Chicago, IL: American College of Surgeons.

Preston, P. (2005). Dealing with "difficult" people. *Journal of Healthcare Management, 50*(6), 367–370. Retrieved from https://journals.lww.com/jhmonline/citation/2005/11000/dealing_with__difficult__people.4.aspx

Rabinstein, A. A. (2020). Traumatic spinal cord injury. In A. A. Rabinstein (Ed.), *Neurological emergencies: A practical approach*, pp. 271–280. Cham, Switzerland: Springer.

Raja, A., & Zane, R. D. (2023). Initial management of trauma in adults. In J. Grayzel (Ed.), *UpToDate*. Retrieved October 1, 2023, from https://www.uptodate.com/contents/initial-management-of-trauma-in-adults

Rath, W. H. (2011). Postpartum hemorrhage—Update on problems of definitions and diagnosis. *Acta Obstetricia et Gynecologica Scandinavica, 90*(5), 421–428. https://doi.org/10.1111/j.1600-0412.2011.01107.x

Refa, N., Ali, R. A. R., & Gomaa, H. (2019). Update in obstetric trauma management. *Update in Obstetric Anaesthesia, 14*, 63–70. Retrieved from https://resources.wfsahq.org/wp-content/uploads/uia34-Update-in-obstetric-trauma-management.pdf

Renfrew, M. J. (2021). Scaling up care by midwives must now be a global priority. *Lancet Global Health, 9*(1), e2–e3. https://doi.org/10.1016/S2214-109X(20)30478-2

Resuscitation Council UK. (2022). *The ABCDE approach*. Retrieved from https://www.resus.org.uk/library/abcde-approach

Rhoades, D. R., McFarland, K. F., Finch, W. H., & Johnson, A. O. (2001). Speaking and interruptions during primary care office visits. *Family Medicine, 33*(7), 528–532. Retrieved from http://www.interruptions.net/literature/Rhoades-FM01.pdf

Rossaint, R., Bouillon, B., Cerny, V., Coats, T. J., Duranteau, J., Fernández-Mondéjar, E., . . . Spahn, D. R. (2016). The European guideline on management of major bleeding and coagulopathy following trauma. *Critical Care, 20*, 100. https://doi.org/10.1186/s13054-016-1265-x

Rudrappa, M., Modi, P., & Bollu, P. C. (2023). Cheyne Stokes respirations. *StatPearls*. Treasure Island, FL: StatPearls Publishing. Retrieved September 30, 2023, from https://www.ncbi.nlm.nih.gov/books/NBK448165/

Shah, P., Thornton, I., Turrin, D., & Hipskind, J. E. (2023). Informed consent. *StatPearls*. Treasure Island, FL: StatPearls Publishing. Retrieved September 30, 2023, from https://www.ncbi.nlm.nih.gov/books/NBK430827/

Smith, D. C. (2015). Midwife–physician collaboration: A conceptual framework for interprofessional collaborative practice. *Journal of Midwifery & Women's Health, 60*(2), 128–139. https://doi.org/10.1111/jmwh.12204

Smith, V., Kenny, L. C., Sandall, J., Devane, D., & Noonan, M. (2021). Physiological track-and-trigger/early warning systems for use in maternity care. *Cochrane Database of Systematic Reviews*. https://doi.org/10.1002/14651858.CD013276.pub2

Smith, V., O'Malley, D., & Cithambaram, K. (2022). Early warning systems in maternity care: A qualitative evidence synthesis of maternity care providers' views and experiences. *Midwifery, 112*. https://doi.org/10.1016/j.midw.2022.103402

Stapleton, S. R., Osborne, C., & Illuzzi, J. (2013). Outcomes of care in birth centers: Demonstration of a durable model. *Journal of Midwifery & Women's Health, 58*(1), 3–14. https://doi.org/10.1111/jmwh.12003

Stewart, K. R. (2016). *SBAR, communication, and patient safety: An integrated literature review* (Honors thesis). Retrieved from http://scholar.utc.edu/cgi/viewcontent.cgi?article=1070&context=honors-theses

Thim, T., Krarup, N. H. V., Grove, E. L., Rohde, C. V., & Løfgren, B. (2012). Initial assessment and treatment with the Airway, Breathing, Circulation, Disability, Exposure (ABCDE) approach. *International Journal of General Medicine. 2012*(5), 117–121. https://doi.org/10.2147/IJGM.S28478

Vedam, S., Leeman, L., Cheyney, M., Fisher, T. J., Myers, S., Low, L. K., & Ruhl, C. (2014). Transfer from planned home birth to hospital: Improving interprofessional collaboration. *Journal of Midwifery & Women's Health, 59*(6), 624–634. https://doi.org/10.1111/jmwh.12251

Washington State Perinatal Collaborative. (2015). *Smooth transitions: Enhancing the safety of planned out-of-hospital transports*. Retrieved from http://www.washingtonmidwives.org/documents/Smooth-Transitions-Hospital-Transport-QI-Project.pdf

Wijdicks, E. F. M. (2007). Biot's breathing. *Journal of Neurology, Neurosurgery & Psychiatry, 78*(5), 512–513. https://doi.org/10.1136/jnnp.2006.104919

Wong, L., Tse, W. T., Lai, C. Y., Hui, A. S. Y., Chaemsaithong, P., Sahota, D. S., . . . Leung, T. Y. (2021). Bradycardia-to-delivery interval and fetal outcomes in umbilical cord prolapse. *Acta Obstetricia et Gynecologica Scandinavica, 100*(1), 170–177. https://doi.org/10.1111/aogs.13985

World Health Organization & International Committee of the Red Cross. (2018). *Basic emergency care: Approach to the acutely ill and injured*. Geneva, Switzerland: Authors. Retrieved from https://apps.who.int/iris/rest/bitstreams/1159117/retrieve

Zileli, M., Osorio-Fonseca, E., Konovalov, N., Cardenas-Jalabe, C., Kaprovoy, S., Mlyavykh, S., & Pogosyan, A. (2020). Early management of cervical spine trauma: WFNS Spine Committee recommendations. *Neurospine, 17*(4), 710–722. https://doi.org/10.14245/ns.2040282.141

Zondag, L. D., Maas, V. Y., Beuckens, A., & Nieuwenhuijze, M. J. (2022). Experiences, beliefs, and values influencing midwives' attitudes toward the use of childbirth interventions. *Journal of Midwifery & Women's Health, 67*(5), 618–625. https://doi.org/10.1111/jmwh.13392

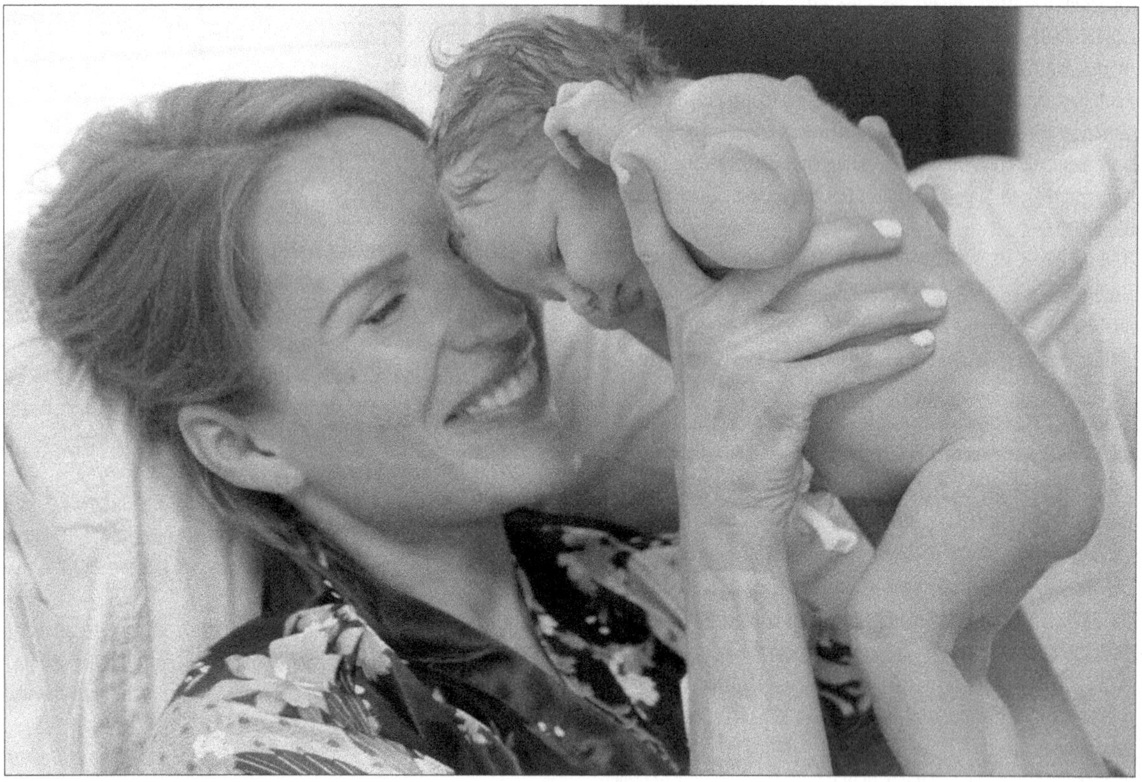

Antepartum Bleeding—First Half of Pregnancy 5

Objectives

- Discuss how a provider might distinguish an impending miscarriage from an ectopic pregnancy.
- Name two signs/symptoms associated with hydatidiform mole.
- Discuss risk factors for ectopic pregnancy.
- List 3 conditions of the cervix that can cause early pregnancy bleeding.

Composite Case Study

Tasha Lake, CPM, received a call from her client Maria C., a 30-year-old mother of three who reported vaginal bleeding in early pregnancy. Maria stated that she had her menses on schedule 5 weeks ago and flowed for 5 days. For several weeks, she has experienced early pregnancy symptoms: fatigue, frequent urination, and breast tenderness. A week ago, she took two over-the-counter urine pregnancy tests. The first was negative, but a few days later the second was positive. Since then, she has been spotting unpredictably, some days bright red, some days brownish, some days not at all. For the past 2 days, the bleeding has been heavier and redder. She had "uncomfortable but not terrible" pain in her right lower quadrant and occasional sharp cramps. When she coughed, her entire abdomen hurt.

Tasha immediately considered the possibility of ectopic pregnancy and recommended that Maria go directly to the emergency department. She called the triage nurse to give a report and faxed records. In the emergency department, Maria's ultrasound evaluation showed a 2 cm right adnexal mass and an empty uterus. The emergency department resident physician concluded that she had recently miscarried and diagnosed the adnexal mass as a corpus luteum cyst. Maria's pain decreased after she took ibuprofen, and the physician sent her home without recommendations for follow-up.

Three weeks later, Maria called Tasha to say her abdomen felt "sensitive." She had continued to bleed daily since her visit to the emergency department, some days heavier than others, with occasional cramping. Suspecting retained products of conception, Tasha recommended a quantitative β-hCG level and an ultrasound, followed by an office visit. Maria declined the blood work and ultrasound because they were expensive and she did not think they were necessary. At Maria's office visit, Tasha felt a tender mass in the right adnexa, a nontender nonpregnant-sized uterus, and a closed cervix with positive cervical motion tenderness.

Suspecting the emergency department physician had missed an ectopic pregnancy at her initial visit, Tanya recommended that Maria return to the hospital for evaluation as soon as possible. Upon arrival, Maria's pain had increased significantly. Ultrasound showed an empty uterus, a complex right adnexal mass measuring 6.2 cm x 3.8 cm x 4.9 cm, and a moderate amount of complex free fluid, presumably blood, in the right adnexa. The emergency department physician consulted the obstetrician, who recommended emergency surgery to remove what appeared to be a ruptured ectopic pregnancy. Maria was taken to the operating room and placed under general anesthesia. Through laparoscopic surgery the obstetrician visualized a very dilated right fallopian tube, which was bleeding actively from the fimbriated end. There was about 800 ml of free blood in her abdomen. The physician removed the fallopian tube, drained the pooled blood from her abdomen, and copiously irrigated her pelvis. Maria tolerated the procedure well. Eight months later, she conceived a healthy pregnancy.

Causes of Early Pregnancy Bleeding

About 25% of pregnant individuals experience bleeding during the first trimester (Norwitz & Park, 2023). Antepartum bleeding can be benign or catastrophic, depending on etiology, gestational age, and clinical context. Although most mothers who experience vaginal bleeding in the first trimester go on to have healthy pregnancies, this complication is associated with higher risk for adverse outcomes, including preterm labor (PTL), preterm prelabor rupture of membranes (PPROM), and placental abruption (John, Sreedevi, & John, 2022). Most bleeding in early pregnancy results from one of the five causes listed in the TEMPT mnemonic in Table 5-1

Table 5-1
Possible Causes of Early Pregnancy Bleeding: The TEMPT Mnemonic

Threatened/inevitable abortion
- Incomplete or missed abortion
- Subchorionic/retroplacental bleeding
- Anembryonic pregnancy
- Loss of one fetus in multiple pregnancy
- Hydatidiform mole

Ectopic pregnancy

Maternal conditions
- Polyp
- Cervical ectropion
- Cervical carcinoma
- Cervical hemangioma
- Condyloma, herpetic lesion, foreign body, ulceration
- Cervicitis—trichomonas, chlamydia, gonorrhea, yeast

Physiologic bleeding
- Implantation bleeding
- Anteroposterior placenta

Trauma
- Vaginal, cervical, or vulvar laceration or abrasion

Threatened or Inevitable Early Pregnancy Loss

The American College of Obstetricians and Gynecologists (ACOG) defines early pregnancy loss as the presence of a nonviable intrauterine pregnancy (IUP) at less than 13 weeks of gestation (ACOG, 2018/2021). Miscarriage is the most common complications of early pregnancy and one of the most serious. Clearly, demise is the worst possible outcome for a fetus, and the process of expulsion can result in maternal hemorrhage or sepsis. Moreover, individuals who experience pregnancy loss can experience severe emotional stress, trauma, and grief, sometimes for a lifetime.

It is estimated that as many as 30% of spontaneous conceptions miscarry by the end of the first trimester (Jauniaux & Simpson, 2022). Most miscarriages occur before 8 weeks, typically before implantation or during the first few weeks of gestation (Jauniaux & Simpson, 2022). Often the individual is unaware of pregnancy. After pregnancy has been clinically recognized, the loss rate decreases to 10–15% (Jauniaux & Simpson, 2022). Mothers who experience bleeding early in the first trimester are more likely to suffer pregnancy loss than mothers who bleed late in the first trimester (Ellsworth Bowers & Kitzman, 2024). The rate of fetal loss is less than 11% when bleeding occurs at 10–13 gestational weeks, even when blood loss is heavy (Ellsworth Bowers & Kitzman, 2024).

Risk Factors and Etiologies

Clients suffering miscarriage want to know why the loss occurred and what they can do to prevent reoccurrence. Although the cause of most miscarriages remains unknown, potential etiologies include chromosomal abnormalities, maternal conditions, medication or substance use, environmental exposures, and trauma. Often pregnancy loss is multifactorial.

Chromosomal abnormality. Chromosomal abnormalities account for at least 50% of clinically recognized miscarriages (Jauniaux & Simpson, 2022). Even normal-appearing fetuses lost to miscarriage have a 25%–50% incidence of chromosomal abnormalities (Jauniaux & Simpson, 2022). These abnormalities can involve too many or too few chromosomes, defective or missing genes, or missing chromosomal segments. One or both parents can carry a balanced rearrangement of chromosomes (usually a translocation or inversion), or each parent can carry a harmless single copy of problematic gene that can be lethal if the embryo inherits one from each parent.

Abnormalities in placental perfusion. A normal human conceptus develops in a comparatively low-oxygen environment during the early weeks of gestation because it requires this environment to optimally balance the chemical activity of free oxygen radicals inside the placenta with protective antioxidant activity during its critical early development. To protect the embryo from the comparatively oxygen-rich maternal circulation during this vulnerable period, specialized cells plug the tips of the uteroplacental arteries and limit the flow of blood into the intervillous space (Jauniaux, Johns, & Burton, 2005; Jauniaux & Simpson, 2022). Between 10 and 12 weeks of gestation, these plugs break up, increasing the flow of maternal blood into the intervillous space and more than doubling the oxygen concentration within the placenta (Jauniaux et al., 2005; Jauniaux & Simpson, 2022; Nguyen, Chang, & Bendikson, 2019). Abnormal implantation that lets too much maternal blood reach the placenta early in gestation increases the formation of free radicals, leading to complications ranging from miscarriage in the short term to PPROM and preeclampsia later in pregnancy (Jauniaux et al., 2005). On transvaginal ultrasound, about two thirds of early pregnancy losses show signs of defective placentation (Jauniaux et al., 2005).

Increasing maternal age increases the risk of pregnancy loss due to poor egg quality, a less-receptive endometrium, and endocrine dysfunction. Individuals toward the end of their reproductive years are more likely to miscarry; a 40-year-old has double the risk of miscarriage of a 20-year-old, regardless of whether the embryo has normal chromosomes (Prager, Micks, & Dalton, 2023d). In one study, the risk of miscarriage was 8.9% in individuals aged 20–24 years and 74.7% in those aged 45 years or more (Nybo Andersen, Wohlfahrt, Christens, Olsen, & Melbye, 2000). Advanced paternal age can also increase the likelihood of pregnancy loss.

Maternal conditions. Mothers with endocrine problems such as hyper- and hypothyroidism, cardiovascular disease, and metabolic disorders are at higher risk of pregnancy loss (Magnus, Morken, Wensaas, Wilcox, & Håberg, 2021). Antiphospholipid syndrome, an autoimmune disease that can cause clotting in the veins, arteries, and microvasculature, increases the risk for pregnancy loss, stillbirth, early and severe preeclampsia, and premature birth due to placental dysfunction (Alijotas-Reig et al., 2019). Infection with bacterial, protozoan, or viral agents (e.g., parvovirus, Zika virus, cytomegalovirus, and untreated syphilis) can greatly increase the risk of miscarriage and stillbirth (Giakoumelou et al., 2016).

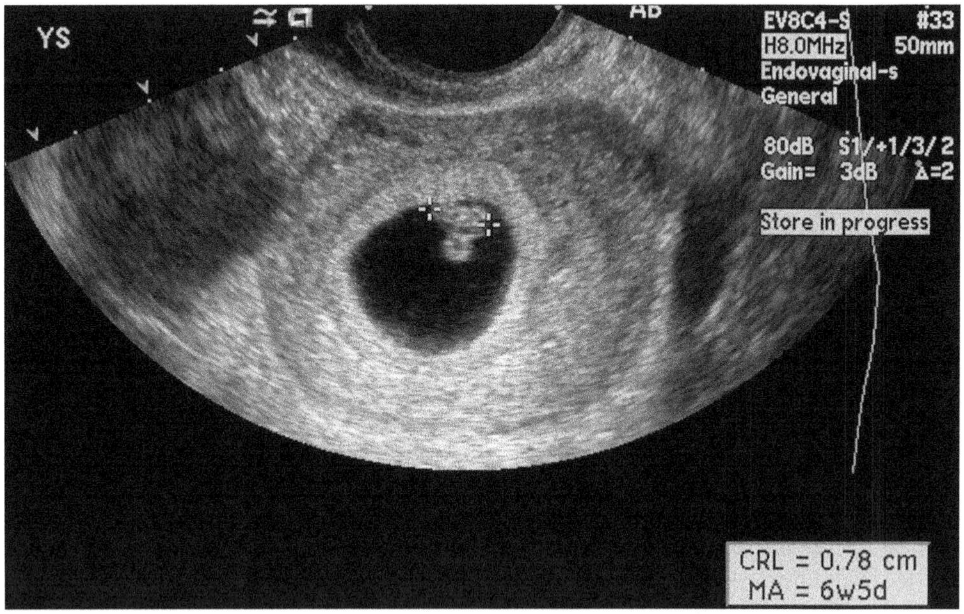

Figure 5-1. Healthy pregnancy at 6 5/7 weeks gestational age on transvaginal ultrasound. This embryo had a normal crown-rump length, yolk sac, gestational sac, and heartbeat.

Uterine conditions. Congenital uterine anomalies and other conditions that distort the uterine cavity (e.g., intrauterine adhesions, polyps, or submucosal myomas) can increase the risk of miscarriage. Individuals with an abnormally thin endometrium or with cervical insufficiency are also at higher risk of pregnancy loss (Deng, Liao, & Zhu, 2022). Müllerian duct anomalies (MDAs), a group of congenital abnormalities of the uterus, cervix and/or vagina, can affect uterine muscle mass, blood flow, contractility, and internal dimensions, increasing the risk of abnormal placentation, PTL, dysfunctional labor, and miscarriage (Lovelace, 2016). See Chapter 2.

Prior pregnancy loss. For individuals who have never experienced a loss, the overall likelihood of miscarriage is 5% for primigravidas and 4% for multigravidas (Jauniaux & Simpson, 2022). After one loss, the risk of another increases, after further losses the risk continues to escalate until a person with three or more losses has a 30–40% chance of miscarriage (Jauniaux & Simpson, 2022).

Medications and drug exposure. Many medications are considered teratogenic. Therapeutic radiation and antineoplastic (anticancer) medications can increase the risk of not only miscarriage, but also premature birth, abortion, fetal/neonatal death, and congenital anomalies (Abdel-Rahman & Ghosh, 2022). The use of certain antibiotics (quinolones, tetracyclines, sulfonamides, metronidazole, and some macrolides) and certain antidepressants (mirtazapine, venlafaxine, and duloxetine) in early pregnancy has been associated with a slightly higher risk of miscarriage (Kjaersgaard et al., 2013; Muanda, Sheehy, & Bérard, 2017). Conversely, there is strong evidence that the administration of an mRNA COVID-19 (SARS-CoV-2) vaccine either before conception or during pregnancy *does not* increase the risk of pregnancy loss (Bleicher, Kadour-Peero, Sagi-Dain, & Sagi, 2021; Fu et al., 2022; Vitiello, Ferrara, Zovi, Trama, & Boccellino, 2022; Zauche et al., 2021).

Substance use. One large meta-analysis found that each 100 mg/day increment in daily maternal caffeine intake (~1 cup of coffee) was associated with a 7% higher risk of pregnancy loss (L.-W. Chen et al., 2016). Tobacco smoking, both active and passive, floods maternal systems with toxins that affect placental and fetal cell proliferation and differentiation, increasing the risk for stillbirth, preterm birth (PTB), and placental abruption (Jauniaux & Simpson, 2022). *Any* active smoking increases the risk for miscarriage, and that risk increases by 1% for each additional cigarette smoked per day. Exposure to secondhand smoke increases the risk of miscarriage by 11% (Jauniaux & Simpson, 2022). Heavy or chronic alcohol use increases the risk of miscarriage and fetal damage (Cunningham et al., 2022, ch. 11). Cocaine and methamphetamine use appear to increase the risk of miscarriage (Prager et al., 2023d).

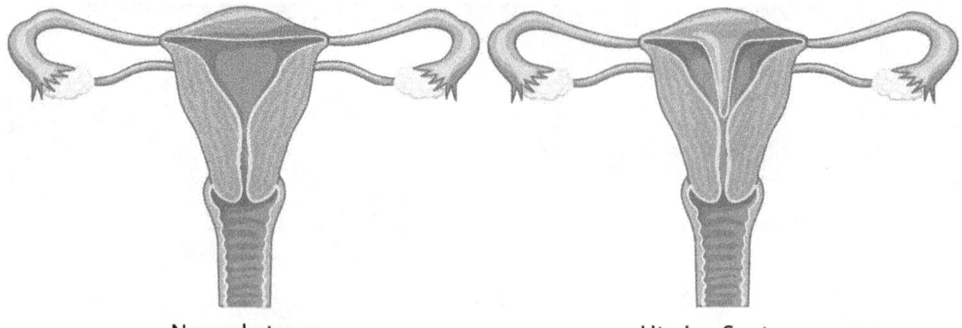

Figure 5-2. A normal uterus compared with a septate uterus. Individuals with a septate uterus are at high risk for recurrent first- and second-trimester pregnancy loss, fetal growth restriction (FGR), and preterm birth (PTB). In labor, they are at risk for stillbirth, malpresentation, labor dystocia, and placental abruption (©Vectoressa/Adobe Stock)

Lifestyle influences. Obesity is the most common health problem of female individuals of reproductive age. Clients with obesity have a higher risk of miscarriage and recurrent miscarriage, and their babies are more likely to suffer neural-tube defects, hydrocephaly, and other congenital anomalies (ACOG, 2021; Creanga, Catalano, & Bateman, 2022). Emotional stress can increase the risk of pregnancy loss alone or exacerbated by racial/ethnic or financial disparities in health care, threat of violence, housing or food insecurity, or other long-term life stressors (Prager et al., 2023d). Consistent night-shift work and working more than 40 hr/week appears to increase the risk of miscarriage (Cai et al., 2019; Quenby et al., 2021; Rangel et al., 2021; Zhu, Hjollund, Andersen, & Olsen).

Environmental exposures. Cleaners, pesticides, pollutants, anesthetics, radiation, and other agents can increase the risk of pregnancy loss by causing cell death or chromosomal damage, altering growth of tissues, or interfering with normal processes (Prager et al., 2023d). Because pregnant individuals encounter countless agents every day, it is usually impossible to attribute any adverse effect to a single exposure (Jauniaux & Simpson, 2022).

Race and ethnicity. Black, indigenous, and other people of color have higher rates of pregnancy loss than white people. In one study, black American mothers had almost twice the risk of pregnancy loss between 10 and 20 weeks of gestation than white American mothers (Mukherjee, Velez Edwards, Baird, Savitz, & Hartmann, 2013). The authors attribute this difference to cumulative stressors of systemic racism, social determinants of health, and occupational or environmental exposure to potential toxins.

Trauma. Although the bony pelvis protects the embryo from trauma in early pregnancy, penetrating trauma (stabbing or gunshot wounds), and iatrogenic trauma such as chorionic villus sampling or amniocentesis can cause pregnancy loss (Prager et al., 2023d).

Definition of Terms

The terms *miscarriage*, *spontaneous abortion*, and *early pregnancy loss* are used interchangeably in the literature and encompass the conditions of threatened abortion, incomplete abortion, complete abortion, and anembryonic pregnancy (ACOG, 2018/2021; Jackson & Watkins, 2021). More specific terms are commonly used to describe nonviable pregnancies, but usage varies, leading to confusion and misunderstanding for providers and clients alike (Shaker & Smith, 2022). Although spontaneous abortion is a clinically correct term, the word *abortion* can be upsetting to mothers experiencing pregnancy loss. Words such as *miscarriage* and *pregnancy loss* can be preferable (Prager et al., 2023d; Shaker & Smith, 2022; Thorstensen, 2000).

Threatened abortion is defined as bleeding through a closed cervix in the first 20 weeks of gestation with a live embryo or fetus (Cunningham et al., 2022, ch. 11; Hendriks, MacNaughton, & MacKenzie, 2019). It can herald miscarriage, or it can be associated with benign conditions such as conceptus implantation. Ectopic pregnancy, cervical infection, cervical or vaginal trauma, and dysplastic or malignant cervical lesions can cause bleeding that can be mistaken for threatened abortion (Cunningham et al., 2022, ch. 11). A placenta that covers the cervix (placenta previa) can cause (usually painless) bleeding in the second and third trimester (Anderson-Bagga & Sze, 2023). The bleeding or spotting associated with threatened abortion can continue for weeks and can be accompanied by suprapubic discomfort, mild cramps, pelvic pressure, or low back ache (Cunningham et al., 2022, ch. 11).

Missed abortion. When pregnancy loss occurs in the first trimester, the death of the embryo or fetus nearly always occurs before spontaneous expulsion (Cunningham et al., 2022, ch. 11). Death typically is accompanied by hemorrhage into the decidua basalis, which leads to necrosis of the adjacent tissue that stimulates uterine contractions and expulsion (Cunningham et al., 2022, ch. 11). Fetal heart activity can cease weeks before the mother experiences signs or symptoms of impending miscarriage. The nausea, breast tenderness, and urinary frequency of pregnancy can subside, and vaginal spotting can occur, though the cervix usually remains closed.

Anembryonic pregnancy. Anembryonic miscarriage or pre-embryonic loss describes a pregnancy without an identifiable embryo or yolk sac (Prager et al., 2023d). It occurs when an early embryo forms but is resorbed after death or when embryonic development fails at an early stage or does not occur at all (Prager et al., 2023d). The use of *blighted ovum* is outdated (Farquharson, Jauniaux, & Exalto, 2005). These pregnancies are often chromosomally abnormal. An anembryonic pregnancy can be indistinguishable from a very early viable pregnancy on an initial ultrasound evaluation. The diagnosis can be made if there is no change on ultrasound two or more weeks later (Cunningham et al., 2022, ch. 11).

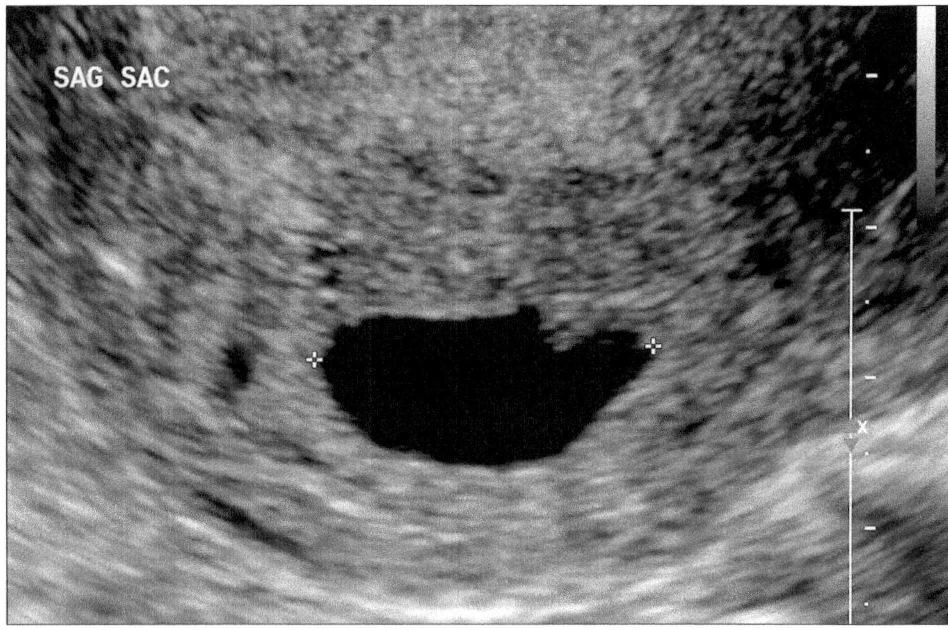

Figure 5-3. An anembryonic pregnancy does not contain an identifiable embryo or a yolk sac. This condition may be first recognized as an unanticipated finding on ultrasound examination.

Complete abortion. When all products of conception have been expelled and the uterus is empty, a complete abortion has occurred.

Incomplete abortion. When some products of conception are expelled (usually the embryo and amniotic sac), but others (usually all or parts of the placenta) are retained in the uterus, an incomplete abortion has occurred.

Inevitable abortion. When cervical dilation or rupture of the membranes are present without passage of tissue, pregnancy loss is inevitable (Ellsworth Bowers & Kitzman, 2024).

Septic abortion. Pregnancy loss accompanied by severe intrauterine infection is termed a septic abortion. This condition can be life-threatening. It can follow spontaneous pregnancy loss or elective termination procedures. Signs and symptoms include fever, malaise, abdominal pain, tachycardia, hypotension, vaginal bleeding, and foul-smelling discharge that can be bloody or purulent (Prager et al., 2023c). On examination, the uterus can be boggy and tender, rebound and cervical-motion tenderness can be present, and the cervix can be open or closed. Ultrasound scan can show thickened endometrium or retained products of conception. The microorganisms responsible are most often part of the vaginal flora (Cunningham et al., 2022, ch. 11).

Clinical Presentation of Threatened Pregnancy Loss

About 25% of mothers experience bleeding in the first trimester (Hendriks, MacNaughton, et al., 2019). Vaginal bleeding and cramping, the hallmark symptoms of impending miscarriage, also occur in many healthy gestations and in molar and ectopic pregnancies. Pregnancy loss usually involves bleeding equal to or heavier than a menstrual period. Vaginal bleeding can present as spotting, clotting, or gushing. Although heavy bleeding and a client's report of passing clots and tissue is concerning for pregnancy loss, miscarriage cannot be confirmed with certainty without physical examination, laboratory assessments, and/or ultrasound examination, alone or in combination (Prager et al., 2023a). A viable gestation can persist after episodes of heavy bleeding, and a multiple pregnancy can continue after the loss of a fetus.

The pain associated with pregnancy loss is usually crampy and can be mild to intense and constant or intermittent. During passage of gestational tissue, the pain is usually severe and the bleeding becomes heavy. The client may pass an embryo or fetus, membranes, or placenta, which can be integrated into blood clots and not readily identifiable as tissue. In very early pregnancies, the products of conception can be encased within a decidual cast, a solid mass of thickened endometrium in the shape of the uterine cavity (Cunningham et al., 2022, ch. 13). With completion of the miscarriage, bleeding slows, pain diminishes, and the cervix closes.

Clients with nonviable pregnancies can be asymptomatic or present with bleeding, cramping, ruptured membranes, or signs of infection. Clients with threatened abortion are managed expectantly until their symptoms resolve or they suffer pregnancy loss (Prager et al., 2023c). Miscarriage is more likely to have a complicated course with increasing gestational age, especially beyond 13 weeks of gestation (Prager et al., 2023a).

The most common complications associated with early pregnancy loss are hemorrhage and infection. Severe hemorrhage can require surgical management, and about 1% of individuals with miscarriage develop hypovolemia, severe anemia, and shock (Prager et al., 2023a).

Management of Miscarriage

Individuals experiencing pregnancy loss may be candidates for expectant management, medical treatment (misoprostol), or surgical uterine evacuation. Unless there is a compelling reason to recommend one option over the others, the plan is usually the result of shared decision-making between the provider and client (Prager et al., 2023b). Individuals managed according to their own preferences tend to have better outcomes (Wieringa-De Waard et al., 2002).

Expectant management. Because most early miscarriages resolve spontaneously without medical involvement, expectant management is an option for clients less than 14 weeks of gestation who have stable vital signs and no evidence of infection (Prager et al., 2023c). It is a safe option only if emergency care and surgical intervention are readily available because if hemorrhage occurs, a delay in receiving care can be life-threatening. Expectant management carries a higher risk of hemorrhage than surgical management, higher still for clients with anemia, cardiovascular disease, or clotting abnormalities (Shaker & Smith, 2022).

About 90% of clients with incomplete miscarriage (those who have passed tissue or have ultrasound findings suggesting incomplete expulsion) complete the loss spontaneously within 4 weeks (Hendriks, MacNaughton, et al., 2019). Consequently, many providers wait up to 2 weeks before offering medical or surgical intervention for nonviable pregnancy (Ellsworth Bowers & Kitzman, 2024). After 4 weeks, anembryonic gestation and embryonic demise are less likely to resolve with expectant management; their completion rates are 66% and 76%, respectively.

Counsel the client about what to expect during the process of miscarriage. While actively miscarrying, the client should always have a support person present to summon help in case of hemorrhage. Although all losses are unique, the individual typically experiences spotting or light vaginal bleeding and mild cramping, which grow worse. Around the time tissue is expelled, moderate-to-heavy bleeding and very painful cramps or contractions are to be expected, and bleeding usually increases for 2–4 hr. Pain should be managed with nonsteroidal anti-inflammatory medications (Shaker & Smith, 2022).

The midwife may ask the client to place a strainer in the toilet to catch any tissue for later inspection. Although it is not necessary to send the products of conception to a pathology laboratory with every miscarriage, histopathological examination of the tissue is recommended when clients are considered at high risk for trophoblastic disease (Alsibiani, 2014), and genetic studies can be useful if the client has had two or more miscarriages (Dahdouh & Kutteh, 2021). Often the fetus passes first and slips out easily, sometimes in an intact gestational sac. The embryo or fetus is usually gray, tan, or pinkish and smooth, and can pass unnoticed in early gestation. An 8-week fetus is about the size of a lima bean. Fresh clots are soft, loose, and red; older clots are firmer and darker. A fresh clot breaks apart easily. Older clots can contain tough strands of fibrin and can resemble placenta. The placenta can be slower to detach and may appear after hours of cramps. Placental tissue may be pink or white and may look like gristle. It has feathery chorionic villi; when floated in water with a light source behind, these look like seaweed (Univ. of Chicago Dept. of Pathology, 2019). Membranes look like cellophane. Maternal endometrial tissue is a firm, pale, gray-white sheet with a smooth side and a rough side (Ravishankar, 2022). Clusters of grapelike vesicles appearing like currant jam in prune juice can indicate molar or partial molar pregnancy. Pus or foul-smelling material can indicate infection.

Instruct the client to call with fever; pain outside the pelvis; and symptoms of excessive blood loss, such as dizziness, syncope, weakness, or rapid heart rate. Soaking two maxi pads per hr for two or more consecutive hr is an indication to go to the hospital (ACOG, 2018/2021; Shaker & Smith, 2022). After the uterus is emptied, pain and bleeding usually decrease or subside. The client can have spotting and mild cramps for up to 2 weeks after the loss.

Medical (pharmacological) management. Administration of misoprostol or other prostaglandin (PG) analogs can expedite the expulsion of a pregnancy loss before 13 weeks of gestation without the need for surgical intervention (ACOG, 2018/2021). Used judiciously, misoprostol is well-studied, safe, and inexpensive. It has few serious side effects, is stable at room temperature, and can be taken at home by the client. Consult a physician before administering misoprostol to manage a miscarriage—a significant number of clients will subsequently hemorrhage or otherwise require surgical evacuation of the uterus, especially in the second trimester. The standard protocol is misoprostol 800 mcg vaginally with one repeat dose as needed, no earlier than 3 hr after the first dose but within 7 days if there is no response to the initial dose (ACOG, 2018/2021). Administration of one dose of 800 mcg of vaginal misoprostol has been shown to complete the expulsion of a first-trimester pregnancy loss by day three in 71% of clients; a second dose 24–48 hr later increases the success rate to 84% (ACOG, 2018/2021; Zhang et al., 2005).

Mifepristone (200 mg orally) may be used with misoprostol to shorten the process and reduce pain (ACOG, 2018/2021; Prager et al., 2023b; Schreiber et al., 2005). Mifepristone competitively blocks progesterone receptors, increasing cervical dilation, decidual necrosis, and endogenous PG production. Mifepristone gradually makes the uterus five times more sensitive to PGs 24–48 hr after dosing, increasing the effectiveness of misoprostol and potentially decreasing side effects (Hammond, 2023). In many areas, mifepristone is available only from a physician or is prohibited by local restrictions (N. Tharpe, personal communication, February 25, 2018).

Close follow-up is essential. The provider can obtain serial measurements of the β subunit of human chorionic gonadotropin (β-hCG) until they reach nonpregnant levels (Shaker & Smith, 2022). Surgical management may be necessary if pharmacological therapy is ineffective.

Surgical management. Early pregnancy loss can be effectively managed with a suction curettage procedure in which the provider aspirates the uterine contents using either a manual or electric vacuum device (ACOG, 2018/2021). Suction curettage can be undertaken in an office under local anesthesia with or without sedation or in an operating suite under regional or general anesthesia. Individuals who present with hemorrhage, unstable vital signs, or signs of infection require urgent treatment with surgical uterine evacuation (ACOG, 2018/2021). Surgical evacuation may also be the safest option for clients with severe anemia, bleeding disorders, or cardiovascular disease and for those without ready access to emergency care. Many individuals choose surgical evacuation rather than expectant or medical treatment because it brings the ordeal of pregnancy loss to an immediate, safe conclusion.

Follow-Up After Miscarriage

Clients should be advised to put nothing in the vagina for 2 weeks after the loss and to call if heavy bleeding, fever, or abdominal pain develops. The individual should follow up with the provider after the loss to confirm by examination that the cervix is closed and the uterus is involuting and to evaluate for ongoing bleeding. If an empty uterus has not been documented on ultrasound, perform a quantitative β-hCG weekly until levels are undetectable, which can take as long as 3–4 weeks (ACOG, 2018/2021). Clients who continue to bleed or who have pelvic or abdominal pain require ultrasound examination and physician consultation for suspicion of retained products, infection, or both. Mild uterine tenderness with an empty uterus on ultrasound examination, with or without fever, can indicate endometritis necessitating treatment with oral broad-spectrum antibiotics.

Ectopic pregnancy often presents with the classic triad of amenorrhea, vaginal bleeding, and abdominal/pelvic pain, but any or all of these findings can be absent.

An individual may resume ovulation days or weeks after early pregnancy loss (Prager et al., 2023b). Menses usually resume within 4–6 weeks. If the client does not want to try to achieve another pregnancy, discuss contraception options. Although individuals have traditionally been cautioned to avoid pregnancy for three months after a miscarriage, evidence favors trying again immediately. People who attempt conception immediately after the loss have a shorter interval to pregnancy than those who wait more than 3 months to conceive, and they are more likely to achieve a live birth (53% versus 36%) without higher risk of pregnancy complications (Prager et al., 2023b; Schliep et al., 2016). Miscarriages are unfortunately very common, but clients who have had one or two pregnancy losses are likely to have live births in the future (Quenby et al., 2021). Clients should be encouraged to assess their emotional readiness before attempting to conceive again.

Losing a pregnancy is emotionally challenging for most families. One quarter to one third of individuals with pregnancy loss experience high levels of depression, anxiety, and symptoms of posttraumatic stress (Prager et al., 2023b). Grief reactions do not follow an orderly timeline and can be prolonged or delayed (Grauerholz, Berry, Capuano, & Early, 2021). Although intense grief symptoms tend to decline over time (Mergl, Quaatz, Edeler, & Allgaier, 2022), parents can have significant levels of emotional distress 9 months (Farren et al., 2020) or even 10 years later (Kokou-Kpolou, Megalakaki, & Nieuviarts, 2018). Individuals having recurrent miscarriages may find that levels of grief peak months or years after a loss (Mergl et al., 2022). Often feelings of anxiety and depression increase around the due date of the lost child, on the anniversary of the loss, over holidays, and during the next pregnancy (especially around the gestational age when the loss occurred).

Provide empathy and support and acknowledge and validate the bereaved family's grief. At the time of diagnosis, treatment, and/or follow-up visit, people experiencing pregnancy loss should be screened for depression with a validated screening tool, such as the Edinburgh Postpartum Depression Scale (Prager et al., 2023b). The client with a positive depression screen or symptoms of distress or depression should be referred to the primary care provider or mental health care provider and introduced to helpful community resources. Grief counseling may also be helpful.

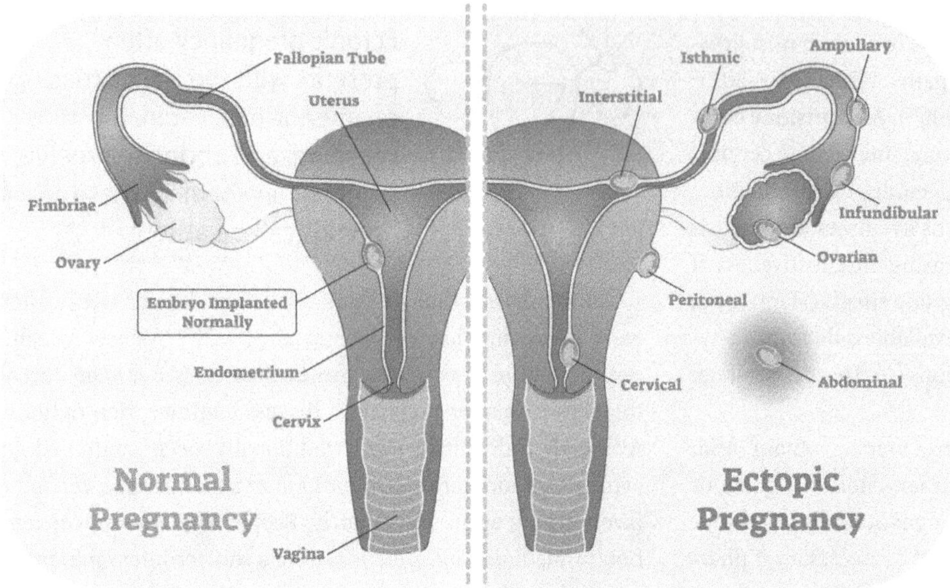

Figure 5-4. Although most ectopic pregnancies implant in the ampullary (middle) part of the fallopian tube, they can also occur in the interstitial or infundibular parts, in the cervix, on the ovary, in the maternal abdomen, or elsewhere (©Vectormine/Adobe Stock)

Ectopic Pregnancy

Ectopic pregnancy (from Greek *ektopos*, "out of place") occurs when the developing embryo embeds somewhere other than the uterine endometrium (Ellsworth Bowers & Kitzman, 2024). The fallopian tubes are the site of implantation in 96% of all ectopic gestations (Tulandi, 2023b). Ectopic pregnancies are both fairly common and potentially lethal in the United States, occurring in at least 2% of all reported pregnancies and responsible for nearly 3% of pregnancy-related deaths (ACOG, 2018/2022).

Risk Factors

Ectopic pregnancies are thought to result from conditions that delay or block the embryo from entering the uterine cavity, including salpingitis, maternal physiologic issues, or issues with the embryo itself that encourage premature implantation (Tulandi, 2023b). Risk factors for ectopic pregnancy include previous pelvic or tubal surgery, history of infertility, smoking, maternal age over 35, maternal douching, abnormal maternal hormone levels, and congenital anomalies of the fallopian tubes (Tulandi, 2023b). Use of an intrauterine device (IUD) or estrogen/progestin oral contraceptives greatly reduces the likelihood of pregnancy, but any conceptions that occur are at high risk for ectopic implantation. Chlamydia or gonorrhea infection can damage the intrafallopian cilia, encouraging ectopic implantation—one episode of salpingitis precedes ectopic pregnancy in up to 9% of individuals (Cunningham et al., 2022, ch. 12). Prior ectopic pregnancy increases the risk of reoccurrence to nearly 10% (Cunningham et al., 2022, ch. 12).

Individuals who undergo tubal sterilization surgery have a risk of ectopic pregnancy approaching 0.3% within 15 years of the procedure (Malacova, Kemp, Hart, Jama-Alol, & Preen, 2014). These clients might not realize that they are pregnant. People who undergo tubal reconstructive surgery to repair tubal damage or to reverse tubal ligation have a 3–30% chance of ectopic pregnancy (Tulandi, 2023b).

Implantation Sites

Ectopic pregnancies can implant not only in a fallopian tube but also into the cervix, an ovary, the peritoneal cavity, a cesarean scar, a rudimentary uterine horn, or elsewhere.

Tubal pregnancy. The most common site of ectopic pregnancy is a fallopian tube, and most of these implantations (70%) occur in the ampullary section (Cunningham et al., 2022, ch. 12). The narrow lumen of the tube cannot expand to contain a growing pregnancy, and in most cases it will eventually rupture. Rupture is usually spontaneous but can occasionally follow coitus or bimanual examination. The ensuing hemorrhage can be life-threatening.

Interstitial and cornual pregnancy. The terms are often used interchangeably for ectopic implantations located eccentrically within the uterine cavity (Finlinson, Bollig, & Schust, 2020). More specifically, an interstitial pregnancy occurs when the conceptus implants within the part of the fallopian tube that is embedded within the muscular wall of the uterus and closest to the uterine cavity (Tulandi, 2023b). Interstitial ectopic pregnancies can cause uterine rupture and have a higher rate of maternal mortality (2–3%) than most other forms of ectopic pregnancy (Finlinson et al., 2020). The term *cornual pregnancy* is used specifically for implantation in a horn of a bicornuate uterus, a rudimentary horn of a unicornuate uterus, or in the lateral aspect of a septated or partially septated uterus (Tulandi, 2023b).

Rudimentary horn pregnancy. Almost 75% of individuals with a unicornuate uterus also have a rudimentary uterine horn (Lovelace, 2016); 85% of rudimentary horns do not communicate with the rest of the genital tract (Tesemma, 2019). Very rarely (1 in 76,000 cases), a pregnancy can implant in a noncommunicating horn. The origin of noncommunicating rudimentary horn pregnancies is unclear; proposed mechanisms include the migration of sperm or relocation of a fertilized ovum from the opposite fallopian tube or through a microscopic fistulous tract that connects to the unicornuate uterus (Herchelroath, Miller, & Wang, 2018).

Most rudimentary horns are too small and poorly vascularized to carry a fetus to term (Trad & Palmer, 2013). Only 13 documented cases of term live birth from a rudimentary horn occurred from 1960 to 2000 (Iyoke, Okafor, Ugwu, & Oforbuike, 2014). If a pregnancy implants in a rudimentary horn, there is a 70% chance of uterine rupture, usually in the second trimester (Lovelace, 2016). In the absence of imaging studies, a rudimentary-horn pregnancy can remain undetected until the client presents with vaginal bleeding, lower abdominal pain, dizziness, fainting, or cardiovascular collapse (Iyoke et al., 2014).

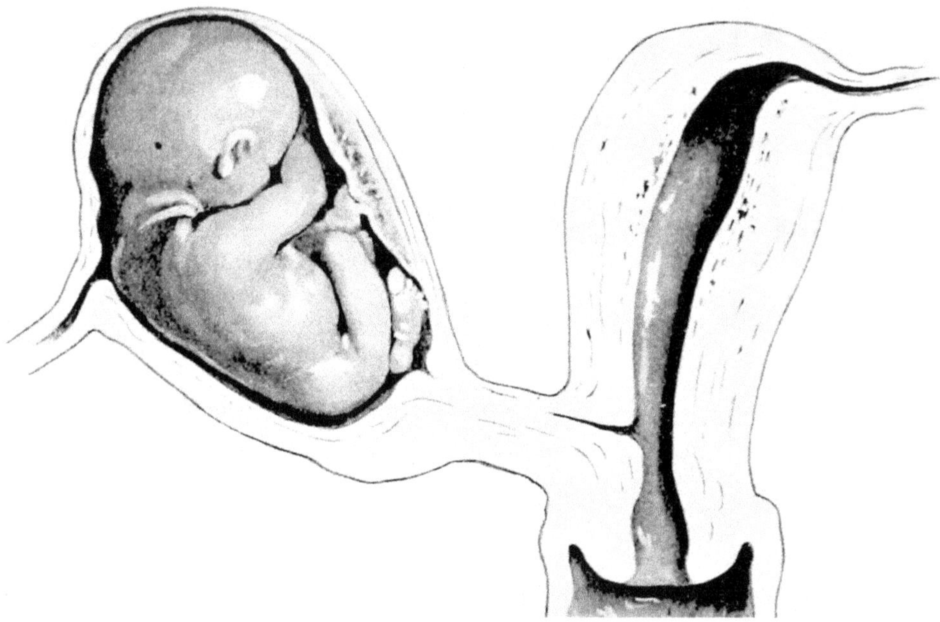

Figure 5-5. Pregnancy can occur in a small, rudimentary uterine horn with no obvious entryway accompanying a functional unicornuate uterus. In the very unlikely event that an embryo implants in a rudimentary horn, it is likely to rupture during the first or second trimester, causing torrential internal bleeding. From *Operative Midwifery: A Guide to the Difficulties and Complications of Midwifery Practice* (2nd ed., p. 574, fig. 266), by J. M. Munro Kerr, 1911, New York, NY: William Wood. In the public domain.

Cervical pregnancy is a rare condition with an incidence of about 1 in 9,000 gestations and comprising 1% of ectopic pregnancies (Tulandi, 2023a). The entire gestational sac, sometimes with an embryo and yolk sac, is located within the dilated cervix below the internal os. Profuse, painless bleeding is a common finding. On speculum examination the cervix may be congested and bulging, and the external os may be open. Fetal membranes or placental tissue is sometimes visible at the external cervical os. If cervical pregnancy is suspected, bimanual examination should be omitted to avoid causing hemorrhage.

Cesarean-scar pregnancy (CSP) involves ectopic implantation into the defect of uterine muscle at the site of a previous uterine incision (Asif, Aijawi, & Agten, 2021). The estimated prevalence of CSP is 1.7 per 1,000 pregnancies (Panaitescu, Ciobanu, Gică, Peltecu, & Botezatu, 2021), comprising 1–3% of ectopic gestations (ACOG, 2018/2022) overall and 6.1% of ectopic pregnancies among individuals with a previous cesarean section (Gull, Klerelid, Jormeus, & Strandell, 2021). Categories of CSP are based on the level of implantation (Timor-Tritsch, 2022):

- "On-the-scar" (type 1)—Implantation of the CSP on the well-healed scar of a hysterotomy incision.
- "In-the-niche" (type 2)—Implantation of the CSP within the defect or "niche" of a dehiscent or incompletely healed scar. Type 2 implantations appear to confer higher risk of poor pregnancy outcomes (Timor-Tritsch, 2022).

In contrast to other kinds of ectopic pregnancy, CSP occurs within the uterine cavity and can result in a viable infant (Timor-Tritsch, 2022). The placenta invades ever more deeply as pregnancy progresses, however, putting the mother at increasing risk for uterine rupture, damage to adjacent organs (such as bowel and bladder), severe hemorrhage necessitating hysterectomy, and death. The risk of severe maternal morbidity is 100% (Panaitescu et al., 2021). The risk of first or second trimester uterine rupture is 9.9–13.4% (Timor-Tritsch, 2022). Clients who continue their pregnancies are best managed in a regional hospital offering interventional radiology, a blood bank, and experienced surgeons able to perform urgent peripartum hysterectomy (Asif et al., 2021).

Intramural pregnancy becomes established within the muscular uterine wall, surrounded by myometrium and separated from the uterine cavity and fallopian tube. Some CSPs can fit this description. Untreated intramural pregnancy will almost inevitably cause catastrophic uterine rupture between 11 and 22 weeks of gestation (Moumna, El Ghorfi, El Haddad, Allali, & Chat, 2020). Predisposing conditions include prior hysterotomy, uterine procedures such as dilation and curettage (D&C), previous myomectomy, and

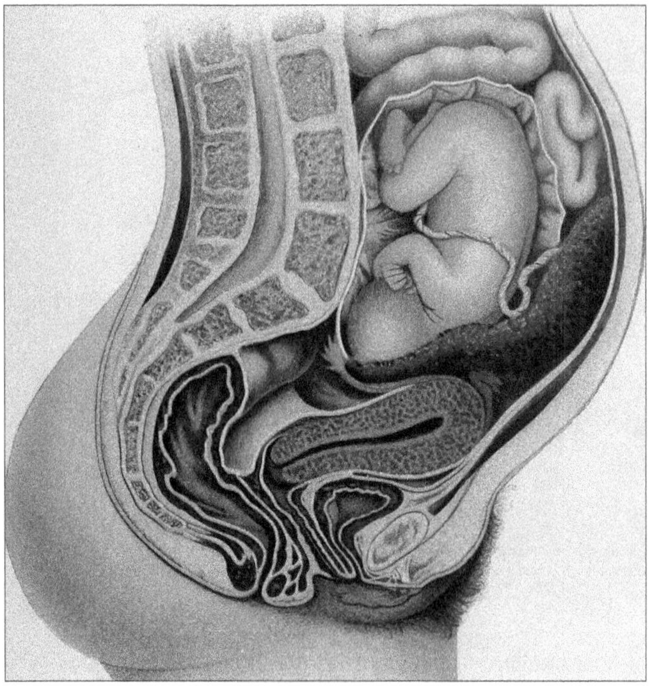

Figure 5-6. Abdominal pregnancy. Advanced abdominal pregnancy with a live fetus is exceedingly rare. In this case, the conceptus implanted in a fallopian tube, which subsequently ruptured. The fetus was expelled into the abdominal cavity where it continued to grow for 8 months. After the rupture, the placenta became attached to a large surface on the anterior abdominal wall and continued to grow. The child was born through a retrouterine vaginal incision. From *The Diagnosis of Diseases of Women: A Treatise for Students and Practitioners* (2nd ed., plate XXI), by P. Findley, 1905, Philadelphia, PA: Lea Brothers. In the public domain.

myometrial pathology such as adenomyosis (Kashi, Welch, Presti, Tabbarah, & Dengler, 2022).

Ovarian pregnancy (implantation on or within the ovary) appears to occur at random and without risk factors (Tulandi, 2023b). Because of the robust vascularity of the ovary, a ruptured ovarian pregnancy is associated with massive hemorrhage, even greater than that of a ruptured tubal pregnancy (Melcer et al., 2016). Ovarian pregnancies can be difficult to differentiate from hemorrhagic ovarian cysts or pregnancy in the distal tube, and they are usually treated surgically.

Heterotopic pregnancy involves simultaneous pregnancies at two different implantation sites, usually one intrauterine and one extrauterine. Dual ectopic implantations are rare. Among spontaneous pregnancies, the incidence of heterotopic gestation is about 1 in 10,000–50,000 pregnancies. When assisted reproductive technologies are used, the incidence ranges from 1 in 100–3,600 (Na et al., 2018).

Abdominal pregnancy. A primary abdominal pregnancy occurs when the blastocyst implants in the peritoneal cavity. A secondary abdominal pregnancy occurs when a pregnancy that was previously located elsewhere, e.g., a ruptured tubal pregnancy, reimplants within the peritoneal cavity (Chauhan & Bhalwal, 2022). The placenta can invade the surface of the uterus, the omentum, the peritoneum, pelvic sidewall, the broad ligament, the spleen, the bowel, the liver, the diaphragm, large blood vessels in the abdominal cavity, or other tissue (Y. Chen et al., 2022). The growing placenta can rupture the structure to which it is attached or tear away at any time during pregnancy, causing uncontrollable hemorrhage.

Abdominal pregnancy is a very rare condition comprising about 1% of all ectopic pregnancies (George, Powers, & Gunby, 2021). In settings without routine ultrasound examinations, it can remain undetected until the pregnancy is advanced. During the first 20 weeks of gestation there are typically no physical signs or symptoms. Beyond 20 weeks, the individual may have severe gastrointestinal issues, unusual abdominal pain, painful fetal movements, vaginal bleeding (from a decidual reaction in the uterus) or signs of massive intraabdominal hemorrhage (Chauhan & Bhalwal, 2022). Physical findings include abnormal fetal lie, easily palpable fetal parts, fetal growth restriction (FGR), fetal demise, absence of labor at term, or failed induction of labor (Chauhan & Bhalwal, 2022). The classic sonographic features of abdominal pregnancy—oligohydramnios, poor placental definition, placenta and fetus outside the uterine cavity, abnormal fetal lie, empty uterus low in the pelvis—are diagnostic, but even when ultrasound is used, up to 50% of abdominal pregnancies are misdiagnosed as intrauterine, particularly in the second and third trimesters (Chauhan & Bhalwal, 2022; Worley, Hnat, & Cunningham, 2008).

Clinical Presentation

Ectopic pregnancy is rare but potentially life-threatening. Hemorrhage from ectopic pregnancy is the leading cause of pregnancy-related maternal death in the first trimester (Tulandi, 2023c). Rupture of a tubal pregnancy can initially present as a small defect in the tube with minimal pain and bleeding or as massive hemorrhage that rapidly spills liters of blood into the abdominal cavity. Consider this diagnosis when a client of reproductive age presents with lower abdominal pain or vaginal bleeding and any of the following (Norwitz & Park, 2023):

- Pregnant, but IUP has not been confirmed;
- Pregnant and conceived with assisted reproduction technology;
- Pregnancy status uncertain; suspect possible ectopic if the current episode of bleeding follows more than 4 weeks of amenorrhea;
- Client is in shock with an acute abdomen not attributable to another diagnosis.

Remember this axiom: "You have only one chance to miss an ectopic" (Ellsworth Bowers & Kitzman, 2024). Consider ectopic pregnancy even if the individual has not missed a period, has undergone tubal ligation, or believes that pregnancy is not possible. More than 50% of clients with ectopic pregnancy have no symptoms before tubal rupture and have no known risk factors (Cunningham et al., 2022, ch. 12; Tulandi, 2023c).

Ectopic pregnancy begins as clinically indistinguishable from an IUP. Pain and bleeding usually appear by 6–8 weeks of gestation, but symptoms can occur as early as 5 weeks of gestation or may appear later. Early and late symptoms are especially likely if the ectopic pregnancy is not in the fallopian tube (Tulandi, 2023c). Among individuals presenting to the emergency department with first-trimester vaginal bleeding, abdominal pain, or both, the rate of ectopic pregnancy is as high as 18% (ACOG, 2018/2022). Possible signs and symptoms include

- Amenorrhea;
- Positive pregnancy test;
- Abdominal/pelvic pain—may be diffuse or unilateral, mild or severe, sudden or gradual, continuous or intermittent, dull or sharp. Tubal rupture can be accompanied by sudden, severe pain that is sharp, stabbing, or tearing. Pain is usually located in the lower abdomen or pelvic area although free blood in the abdomen or (rarely) abdominal pregnancy can cause pain in the middle or upper abdomen (Tulandi, 2023c). Free blood in the abdomen irritating the diaphragm can cause referred pain in the neck or shoulder, especially on inspiration;
- Vaginal bleeding/spotting;
- Presumptive signs of pregnancy, such as breast tenderness, frequent urination, or nausea;
- Palpable adnexal mass;
- Cervical motion tenderness;
- Vomiting;
- Diarrhea;
- Rectal pressure. Blood collecting in the posterior cul-de-sac (pouch of Douglas) can cause rectal pressure (Tulandi, 2023c);
- Tachycardia;
- Pallor and clammy skin;
- Confusion and restlessness;
- Hypotension;
- Dizziness; and/or
- Loss of consciousness.

In high-resource areas, advanced sonography, sensitive assays for β-hCG concentrations, and laparoscopy allow detection of 85% of ectopic pregnancies before catastrophic tubal rupture (Dvash et al., 2021). An ultrasound evaluation that excludes ectopic pregnancy makes that diagnosis less likely, but not impossible. Very early ectopic pregnancies, heterotopic pregnancies, and cornual pregnancies are easily missed, even at respected medical centers (Norwitz & Park, 2023).

Table 5-2
Risk Factors for Ectopic Pregnancy

Risk level	Risk factors
Lower risk	Previous pelvic/abdominal surgery Vaginal douching Intercourse before 18 years of age
Moderate risk	Infertility Previous gonorrhea, chlamydia, puerperal sepsis, ruptured appendix, pelvic inflammatory disease Multiple sexual partners Smoking
Higher risk	Previous ectopic pregnancy Previous tubal surgery Tubal ligation Tubal reanastomosis Tubal pathology Current IUD use

Management of Ectopic Pregnancy

Timely intervention in the form of pharmacological or surgical treatment can avert the catastrophic outcomes associated with ruptured ectopic pregnancy. Care should be transferred to a physician. After confirmation of ectopic pregnancy, the physician will determine whether expectant management, laparoscopic or open surgery, or medical management is indicated. Emergency surgery is necessary for clients who are hemodynamically unstable or who show indications of impending or actual rupture of the ectopic mass.

Medical (pharmacologic) management. Clients with a probable or confirmed early ectopic pregnancy who are hemodynamically stable, who have an unruptured mass, and who do not have absolute contraindications to methotrexate generally have the option of either pharmacologic management with methotrexate or surgical management (ACOG, 2018/2022). Methotrexate is a folic acid antagonist that inhibits DNA synthesis and cell reproduction in actively multiplying cells, including malignancies, trophoblasts, and fetal cells (Cunningham et al., 2022, ch. 12). The ideal candidate for methotrexate is asymptomatic, has a low initial serum β-hCG, has a small ectopic mass without fetal cardiac activity, and can be relied upon to return for follow-up after treatment (Cunningham et al., 2022, ch. 12).

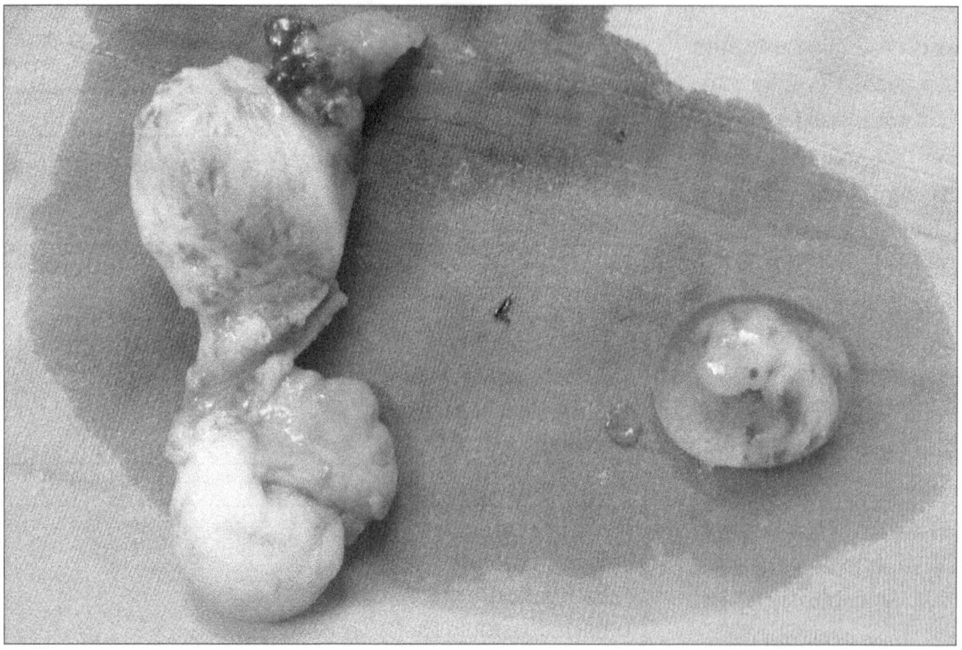

Figure 5-7. Ruptured tubal-cornual pregnancy of 8-week gestational-age embryo with intact embryonic sac. "Ruptured Ectopic Pregnancy," by Drvgaikwad, 2010 (https://commons.wikimedia.org/wiki/File:Ruptured_ectopic_pregnancy.jpg).

Emotional Aftercare

In one study, 23% of individuals who had ectopic pregnancies met the criteria for posttraumatic stress 1 month after resolution; 28% met the criteria at 3 months, and 21% met the criteria at 9 months (Farren et al., 2020). Similar percentages of individuals were diagnosed with moderate to severe anxiety and depression at those same time points (Farren et al., 2020). Anyone experiencing pregnancy loss should be screened for emotional distress and referred to appropriate providers or resources.

Surgical management. Indications include hemodynamic instability, risk of (or actual) rupture, contraindications to methotrexate, failed medical therapy, or client preference. Although some cases necessitate laparotomy, most surgeries for ectopic pregnancy are performed laparoscopically because of shorter operation time, less perioperative blood loss, shorter hospital stay, lower costs, and faster recovery (ACOG, 2018/2022). Salpingectomy (removal of the fallopian tube) or salpingostomy (opening the tube and removing the pregnancy, then repairing the tube) are often used to treat tubal pregnancy.

Expectant management can be an option in some circumstances for clients who have been counseled about the clinical implications and risks of ectopic pregnancy (Tulandi, 2022d). Clients with ectopic pregnancy and an initial β-hCG level less than 200 mIU/ml will experience spontaneous resolution in 88% of cases (ACOG, 2018/2022). Candidates must be asymptomatic, have no evidence of extrauterine gestational sac or mass consistent with ectopic pregnancy on transvaginal ultrasound, have β-hCG levels ≤200 mIU/ml and declining, and be compliant with close follow-up (ACOG, 2018/2022). One protocol is to follow the β-hCG level every 48 hr for three measurements to confirm that it is declining, and then weekly until it is undetectable (Tulandi, 2022d). If a client experiences abdominal pain, if the tube ruptures, or if the serum β-hCG increases or fails to decrease, medical or surgical management is indicated (ACOG, 2018/2022).

DIFFERENTIAL DIAGNOSES

Differential diagnoses include spontaneous abortion, ruptured ovarian cyst, appendicitis, salpingitis (infection of the fallopian tube), torsion (twisting) of the ovary, round-ligament pain, torsion or degeneration of a uterine fibroid, kidney stone, abscess, and urinary tract infection.

Hydatidiform Mole

A molar pregnancy (from Latin *moles*, "mass" or "lump"), is one of a group of gestational trophoblastic diseases. (*Hydatidiform* comes from Greek for "water drop.") A hydatidiform mole consists of rapidly growing, fluid-filled vesicles that can pack the uterine cavity, invade the uterine lining, and metastasize. Those who have had a molar pregnancy are at higher risk for aggressive cancer of the uterus. About 15–20% of complete molar pregnancies and 1–5% of partial molar pregnancies transform into malignant gestational trophoblastic neoplasia (GTN): choriocarcinoma, placental-site trophoblastic tumor, epithelioid trophoblastic tumor, or invasive mole (Baergen, 2021; Berkowitz, Horowitz, & Elias, 2023a). Molar pregnancies are uncommon, occurring in 66–121 per 100,000 pregnancies in the United States and Europe (Berkowitz et al., 2023a).

A molar pregnancy can be complete or partial. A complete molar pregnancy occurs when a sperm fertilizes a defective egg that lacks a nucleus and duplicates its own chromosomes; these conceptions are diploid (46XX or 46XY) and contain only paternal genes (Soper, 2021). Complete molar pregnancies occur in about 1 per 1,000 pregnancies, and partial molar pregnancies occur in about 3 per 1,000 pregnancies (Kalogiannidis et al.,

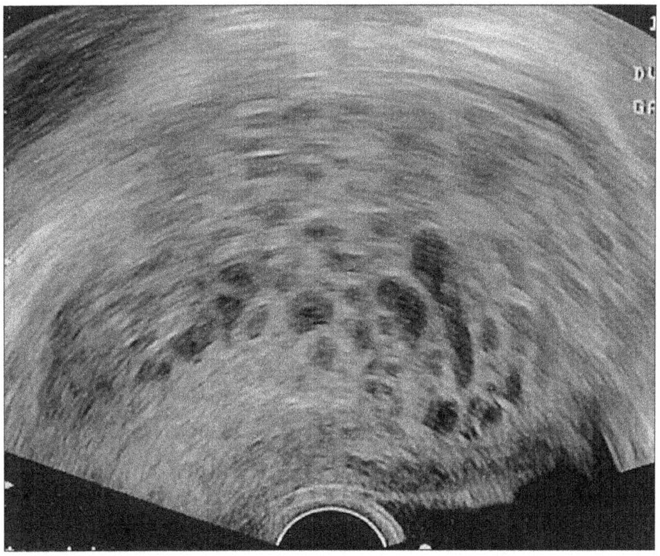

Figure 5-8. Molar pregnancy. On ultrasound, a molar pregnancy often has a snowstorm or Swiss-cheese appearance. "Molar Pregnancy" [sonogram], in "Medical Gallery of Mikael Häggström 2014," by M. Häggström, 2014, *WikiJournal of Medicine, 1*(2). CC0 1.0.

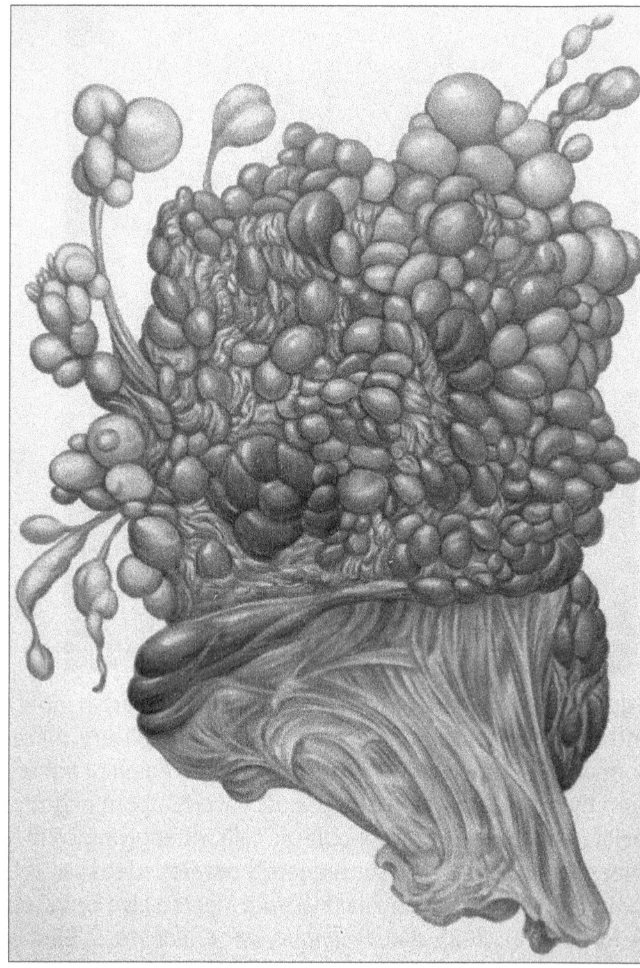

Figure 5-9. A hydatidiform mole is a malformed, rapidly growing mass of placental tissue containing many grapelike fluid-filled vesicles. From *Anatomical Atlas of Obstetrics with Special Reference to Diagnosis and Treatment* (fig. 89), by O. Schaeffer, 1901, Philadelphia, PA: W. B. Saunders. In the public domain.

2018). Partial molar pregnancies can be recurrent in some individuals, either as an autosomal recessive condition with both maternal and paternal components or without obvious cause (Kalogiannidis et al., 2018).

A partial mole consists of a thick, multicystic placenta and a fetus or fetal tissue (Cunningham et al., 2022, ch. 13). Partial moles occur when a normal ovum is fertilized by two sperm or a sperm with double the usual chromosomes, resulting in triploid conceptions that are usually 69XXX, 69XXY, or 69XYY (Berkowitz et al., 2023a; Kalogiannidis et al., 2018). Affected embryos typically die in the first trimester, and those that survive usually show growth restriction, oligohydramnios, and multiple anomalies including limb or central nervous system defects (Cunningham et al., 2022, ch. 13). The abnormal placental tissue fills and distends the uterus as with a complete mole.

Uncommonly, molar pregnancy occurs within a twin gestation in which one chromosomally normal fetus is paired with a complete diploid molar pregnancy (Cunningham et al., 2022, ch. 13). These conceptions are rare, occurring in 20,000–100,000 pregnancies (Ciebiera, Wojtyła, Jakiel, & Roszkowski, 2018). They can be difficult to distinguish from a single partial molar pregnancy, with its accompanying abnormal fetus, or from mosaicism, a discrepancy between the chromosomal makeup of the fetus and the placenta (Zilberman Sharon, Maymon, Melcer, & Jauniaux, 2020). Hyperthyroidism, preeclampsia, stillbirth, hemorrhage, oligohydramnios, and FGR frequently complicate these pregnancies (Cunningham et al., 2022, ch. 13). There is also the potential that the mother will develop subsequent malignancy from gestational trophoblastic disease; terminating the pregnancy does not appear to reduce this risk (Cunningham et al., 2022, ch. 13).

Consider the possibility of hydatidiform mole when any reproductive-age individual presents with abnormal vaginal bleeding. Hydatidiform moles are usually diagnosed during the first half of gestation. Often the condition is recognized on first trimester ultrasound before signs and symptoms develop. The initial clinical presentation is sometimes indistinguishable from that of threatened abortion or the discomforts that accompany normal pregnancy. Common features of molar pregnancies include

- Abnormal bleeding, sometimes with expulsion of hydropic villi. When a complete mole is identified later in gestation, bleeding can be heavy and prolonged. Often, bloody discharge undergoes oxidation and liquefaction before passing out of the vagina, giving it a distinctive "prune juice" appearance (Berkowitz et al., 2023a);

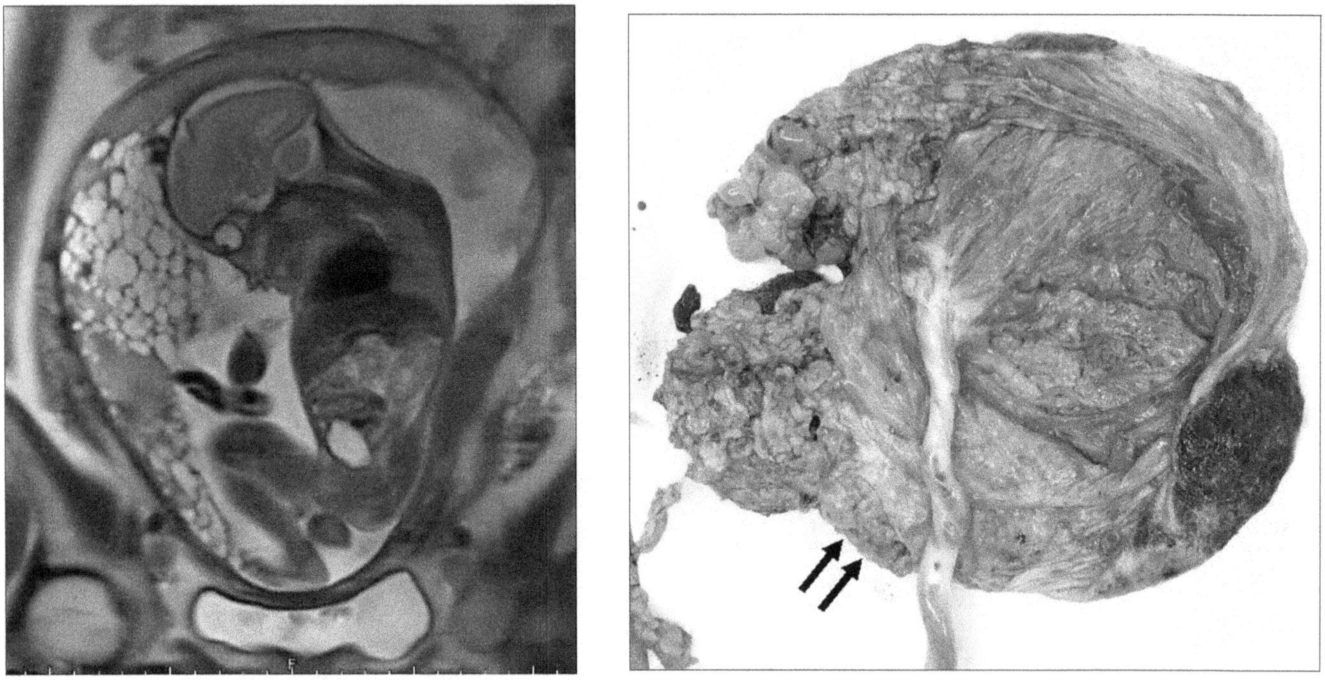

Figure 5-10. Rare case of twin pregnancy with a partial mole and a normal fetus. Left: a placenta with a normal-appearing area and an attached multicystic mass. Right: After delivery, placental examination showed that most of the placenta appeared normal, but there was a 10 cm x 7 cm x 1 cm region of adherent edematous cysts. At 41 2/7 weeks of gestation, the baby was born by cesarean section because of concerns about oligohydramnios and FGR and the risk that uterine contractions would facilitate metastasis of trophoblastic cells. After giving birth, the mother developed choriocarcinoma. She achieved remission after chemotherapy, but subsequently developed suspected metastasis to her lungs, necessitating a partial pulmonary lobectomy. From "When a Vesicular Placenta Meets a Live Fetus: Case Report of Twin Pregnancy with a Partial Hydatidiform Mole," by M. Lin et al., 2021, *BMC Pregnancy and Childbirth 21*, 694, fig. 1. b. (left), 3. b. (right). CC BY 4.0.

- Uterine size greater than expected for gestational dates;
- Absent fetal heart tones;
- An abnormally high level of beta human chorionic gonadotropin (β-hCG) for dates;
- Enlargement of the ovaries. Theca lutein cysts develop when high levels of β-hCG hyperstimulate the ovaries;
- Pelvic pressure and pain;
- Hyperemesis gravidarum;
- Hyperthyroidism, which can present with tachycardia, warm skin, weight loss, and tremor;
- Preeclampsia during the first half of pregnancy. Individuals with preeclampsia before 20 weeks of gestation should be assumed to have gestational trophoblastic disease unless proven otherwise (Berkowitz et al., 2023a);
- On ultrasound, a molar pregnancy can have a characteristic "snowstorm" or "Swiss cheese" pattern with a central heterogeneous mass containing many discrete anechoic spaces.

In any case of suspected hydatidiform mole, refer the client to an obstetrician for management and follow-up. Pregnancy is usually evacuated by suction curettage. Hydatidiform mole is a histologic diagnosis based on analysis of products removed from the uterus. Partial molar pregnancy can be identified as a surprise finding when the pathologist examines a uterine curettage sample after a spontaneous abortion.

Serial measurement of serum β-hCG levels is essential to management after a molar pregnancy (Cunningham et al., 2022, ch. 13). If β-hCG levels plateau or rise, GTN is diagnosed and is treated with chemotherapy (Berkowitz et al., 2023b). Before sensitive assays for β-hCG and chemotherapy were developed, individuals with malignant GTN often died (Soper, 2021). Most individuals with GTN can be cured and future reproductive function can be preserved if initial management and follow-up are timely and appropriate (Soper, 2021). A person who has had a molar pregnancy requires vigilant first-trimester screening to detect a reoccurrence (Ellsworth Bowers & Kitzman, 2024). The risk of reoccurrence is about 1–2% after one molar pregnancy and 15–17.5% after two (Berkowitz et al., 2023b).

Choriocarcinoma is rare, highly aggressive epithelial tumor. Gestational choriocarcinoma can follow any kind of pregnancy (e.g., molar pregnancy, spontaneous or induced abortion, ectopic pregnancy, preterm or term IUP) or can be nongestational, arising in people of either sex as part of a mixed germ-cell tumor (Baergen, 2021). Choriocarcinoma is most strongly associated with molar pregnancies, following 1 in 40 molar pregnancies in Europe and North America but only 1 in

30,000–40,000 pregnancies overall (Smith et al., 2003). Choriocarcinoma usually originates in the uterus but can metastasize to the lung, brain, liver, pelvis, vagina, spleen, intestine, kidney, or elsewhere and cause bleeding in those locations (Baergen, 2021). Any client with abnormal uterine bleeding after pregnancy should be evaluated with β-hCG testing to exclude the diagnosis. Consider gestational choriocarcinoma in any nonpregnant premenopausal client with metastatic disease from an unknown primary site (Soper, 2021). Most people with gestational choriocarcinoma can be cured and their reproductive function can be preserved if initial management and follow-up are timely and appropriate (Soper, 2021).

Other Conditions that Cause Antepartum Bleeding

Often, early pregnancy bleeding is maternal in origin, arising from conditions affecting the lower genital tract. Vaginal trauma is an important and sometimes overlooked cause of early pregnancy bleeding. Implantation bleeding and an anteroposterior placenta can cause physiologic bleeding.

Lesions of the Lower Genital Tract

Lesions of the cervix and vagina are common causes of early pregnancy bleeding. They are usually benign and can be identified on speculum examination. Lesions of the lower genital tract can be asymptomatic or present with spotting, abnormal discharge, or odor.

Cervicitis refers to acute or chronic inflammation of the cervical stroma, which can cause bleeding and spotting. The most common causes of cervicitis are sexually transmitted infections, including gonorrhea (*Neisseria gonorrhoeae*), chlamydia (*Chlamydia trachomatis*), trichomonas (*Trichomonas vaginalis*), mycoplasma (*Mycoplasma genitalium*), and herpes simplex virus (Powell & Nyirjesy, 2022). Other infectious etiologies include bacterial vaginosis, candida vulvovaginitis, and Group A streptococci. Chronic cervicitis is not usually related to infection (Tarney & Han, 2014).

Cervical ectropion is a nonpathological condition in which the cervix partially everts, exposing the friable columnar (glandular) epithelium of the endocervix to the vaginal environment. The exposed columnar epithelium can bleed how about insertion of a speculum, digital examination, or cellular sampling for a Pap test. Cervical ectropion is a common finding, affecting 37% of female individuals of childbearing years and higher percentages in pregnancy (Isoardi, 2009).

Cervical polyps are the most common benign growths on the cervix, occurring most frequently in multiparous individuals in their 40s and 50s. The etiology is unknown, but chronic inflammation of the cervical canal may contribute. Cervical polyps are tear-shaped or lobular structures that can appear red, purple, or flesh-colored. They vary in size from very small to (very rarely) large enough to fill the vagina and present at the introitus (Laufer, 2023). They can bleed when inflamed or when traumatized by intercourse.

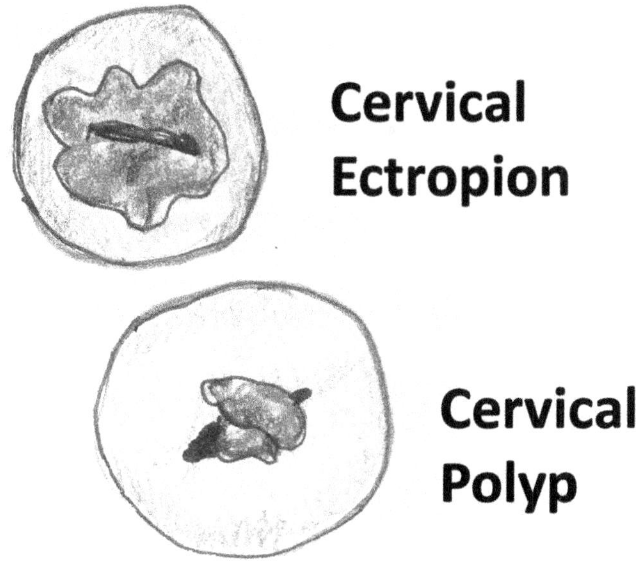

Figure 5-11. Cervical ectropion and cervical polyps can cause vaginal bleeding, especially when infection causes inflammation or coitus causes friction.

Leiomyomas (fibroids) are common tumors of the uterus and occasionally develop on the cervix. Cervical leiomyomas can be subserosal, intramural, or submucosal and may not be visible on speculum examination (Laufer, 2023). Upon bimanual examination, a very firm, solid mass may be felt. A cervical fibroid can also present as a pedunculated lesion (one that hangs from a stalk) that can originate in the uterine cavity or the cervix itself. Pedunculated leiomyomas can twist and infarct or bleed (Laufer, 2023).

Cervical intraepithelial neoplasia is a precancerous, premalignant condition of the squamous epithelium covering the outer surface of the uterine cervix. Glandular cervical neoplasia involves premalignant changes to the columnar epithelium lining the cervical canal (endocervix). Either condition can cause abnormal bleeding, as can neoplasia of the vagina or vulva. In the United States, 2–7% of pregnant individuals have an abnormal Papanicolaou (Pap) test during pregnancy (Hunter, Monk, & Tewari, 2008). The most advanced forms of cervical neoplasia, carcinoma *in situ* and invasive carcinoma, are rare but very serious in pregnancy (McCormick & Peterson, 2018).

Trauma of Genital Tract

Severe vaginal lacerations unrelated to childbirth are seldom reported in the literature but are frequently encountered by emergency department providers (Sloin, Karimian, &

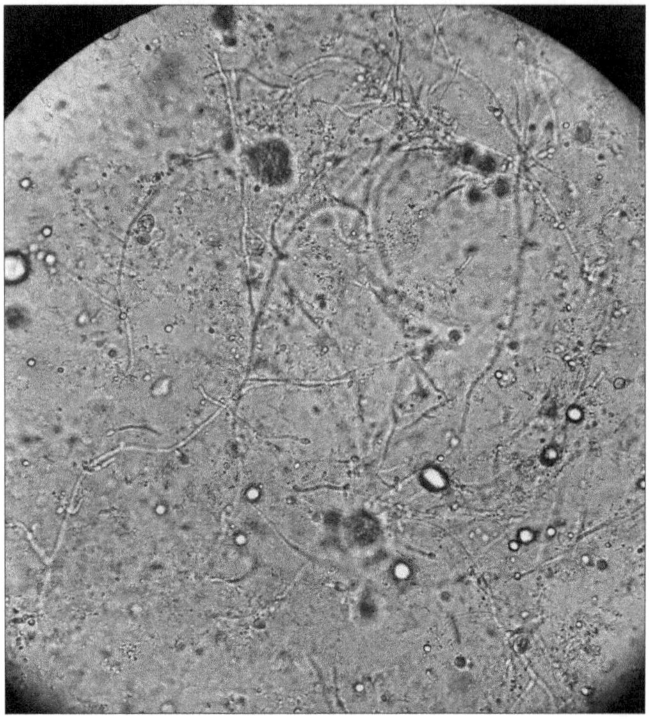

Figure 5-12. A vaginal infection, such as the one evidenced by the candida (yeast) hyphae on this wet mount, can trigger inflammation that causes vaginal bleeding. "Vaginal Wet Mount of Candidal Vulvovaginitis" [photograph], in "Medical Gallery of Mikael Häggström 2014," by M. Häggström, 2014, *WikiJournal of Medicine, 1*(2). CC0 1.0.

Ilbeigi, 2006). Vaginal trauma can present as a minor abrasion or as a gushing wound that leads to hypovolemic shock. Up to 75% of people who present to the emergency department with vaginal lacerations, including those who are not pregnant, require suturing of the wound (Sloin et al., 2006).

Aside from childbirth, coitus is the most common mechanism for vaginal injury (Jana, Santra, Das, Das, & Dasgupta, 2008). Precipitating events may include rough and violent penile thrusting, inserting, or forcing foreign bodies into the vagina, and sexual assault. The external genitalia can be bruised or lacerated by straddle injuries, such as a fall onto the frame of a bicycle (Lopez, Focseneanu, & Merritt, 2018). Water can fill the vagina to the point of rupture in a water-sports accident (Laufer & Makai, 2022). Vaginal lacerations can be caused by major blunt or penetrating abdominal trauma such as that sustained in a motor vehicle crash, especially if the pelvis has been fractured. The client may not disclose the true mechanism of injury (especially if the trauma is related to sex or violence) fearing judgment, embarrassment, or reprisal from an abusive partner. Individuals with significant vaginal injuries may seek care late and experience significant blood loss. Always consider the possibility of sexual assault (Laufer & Makai, 2022).

People in some cultures may encounter mechanisms for vaginal injury not commonly seen in the United States. Of 52 individuals (none of whom was pregnant) who presented to a rural hospital in India with genital-tract injury, 17 had suffered coital trauma, 10 had experienced bicycle or automobile accidents, 7 had fallen from a height, 7 had been gored by cattle, 6 had sustained straddle injuries, 3 had leech bites, and 2 had foreign bodies in their vaginas (Jana et al., 2008). Of these, 15 required blood transfusions, but none died (Jana et al., 2008).

Physiologic Bleeding

Implantation bleeding occurs about 10–14 days after fertilization (around the time of the missed menstrual period) and is thought to result from vascular disruption occurring when an embryo implants in the uterine lining (Norwitz & Park, 2023). Implantation bleeding is usually scant and pink but occasionally is heavier. It is benign.

Anteroposterior placenta is a benign cause of bleeding in the first half of pregnancy (Poureisa et al., 2014). A placenta attached to both the anterior and posterior walls of the uterus in early pregnancy can partially detach as the uterus grows, causing bleeding (Poureisa et al., 2014). Succenturiate or bilobed placentas can also result from this mechanism (Poureisa et al., 2014).

Assessment of Early Pregnancy Bleeding

History and Primary Survey

Begin your assessment by doing a primary survey (see Chapter 4, Primary Survey with Placenta Optimally Perfused) and taking a GOLDCART history. The goal of the assessment is to identify or exclude serious or life-threatening conditions and to form a clinical impression. If the client is bleeding heavily or appears to have a serious problem, call for an ambulance and transfer to the nearest hospital. If the client's signs and symptoms do not indicate an emergency, conduct an examination. Even with excellent clinical skills and access to imaging and laboratory technologies, a provider cannot always determine the exact etiology of first-trimester uterine bleeding.

Assess for Risk Factors and Findings

Assess for risk factors and findings that would make a clinical impression more or less likely. *Always* consider ectopic pregnancy when clients of childbearing age present with lower abdominal pain or vaginal bleeding, even when they deny the possibility of pregnancy, have not missed a period, or have undergone tubal ligation. A client with a history of

Ask yourself, Is the client stable or unstable? Is this a normal intrauterine pregnancy (IUP), an abnormal IUP, or an extrauterine pregnancy?

pelvic inflammatory disease, previous ectopic pregnancy, or tubal reanastomosis is at higher risk for ectopic pregnancy. A client with a history of two or more consecutive pregnancy losses, bicornuate uterus, or antiphospholipid antibodies is at higher risk for spontaneous abortion. A client with profuse, frothy, malodorous discharge is likely to have cervicitis due to a trichomonas infection. Keep your mind open. A client's signs and symptoms may point to a clearcut diagnosis or confound you with an atypical presentation. Some clients will present with multiple concurrent problems, for example, postcoital spotting from cervicitis and a preclinical ectopic pregnancy.

Pain and Bleeding

The amount and pattern of pain and bleeding reported by the client can aid diagnosis. Fresh bleeding is usually bright red and may contain loose gelatinous clots. Brown bleeding and firm, formed clots indicate older bleeding (Aggarwal, 2020).

Consider how the client's signs and symptoms fit with potential diagnoses. As discussed previously, the first sign of pregnancy loss is usually light bleeding. Pain may follow a few hours or days later. It can begin as a low backache or pelvic discomfort and progress to an intense rhythmic suprapubic cramping much like the contractions of term labor. Over time, bleeding usually becomes heavy and the individual passes clots and tissue. The heaviest bleeding typically lasts only 1–2 hr. After the uterus is empty, bleeding and pain quickly improve. If miscarriage is incomplete, pain and heavy bleeding persist.

Bleeding from polyps, implantation, cervicitis, or ectropion is usually light, intermittent, and painless. Clients with a complete or partial molar pregnancy can pass blood that looks like prune juice (and may contain tissue with grapelike vesicles), sometimes with pelvic cramping and pressure. Clients with ectopic pregnancies can experience bleeding, due to sloughing of decidual endometrium, that can range from scant spotting to bleeding that is like a heavy menstrual flow (Hendriks, Rosenberg, & Prine, 2020). Ectopic pregnancy can be painless or mildly uncomfortable until tubal rupture (impending or actual), at which point severe unilateral pelvic or abdominal pain is typical.

Excessive blood loss can present with a large amount of bleeding over a short time or moderate bleeding over a longer interval. Blood volume and red blood cell (RBC) mass increase significantly in the first trimester and continue increasing through pregnancy; a pregnant individual has almost 150% of prepregnant blood volume by the third trimester (Gersh, 2022).

Physical Assessment for Early Pregnancy Bleeding

- **Vital signs.** Assess vital signs and auscultate heart and lungs. Measure temperature and oxygen saturation.
- **Abdominal examination.** Correlate gestational age with fundal height. Evaluate for distension, rigidity, and tenderness. Check costovertebral-angle tenderness. Obtain fetal heart rate (FHR) if appropriate.
- **Pelvic examination.** Note quality and characteristics of bleeding. Look for vaginal and cervical lesions and evidence of trauma. Observe whether the cervix appears to be open or closed and if clots or tissue is present in the os. Perform bimanual examination to assess for adnexal mass or tenderness. Assess for cervical motion tenderness.

Consequently, gravidas at term can tolerate the loss of up to 35–40% of their circulating blood without becoming symptomatic (Hancock, Weeks, & Tina, 2019). Because blood volume increases less in early pregnancy, losing 1,500 ml of blood through miscarriage or ruptured ectopic pregnancy is more likely to cause shock than losing the same amount through postpartum hemorrhage. Blood volume also increases with body mass index (Sharma & Sharma, 2023). Anyone with anemia or dehydration is at greater risk for hemodynamic instability.

Clients and providers often have differing ideas about how much blood loss constitutes an emergency. Assess the amount of blood loss by asking questions that provide specific answers, for example, "How many super-absorbency pads have you soaked in the past 2 hr?" "Was the toilet so full of blood you could not see the bottom?" "Was the clot you passed the size of a walnut or a lemon?"

Sometimes a client reports vaginal bleeding when the actual source is in the gastrointestinal or urinary tract. Hemorrhoids are common in pregnancy, especially late in gestation, and can be associated with bleeding. An anal fissure, a tear in the skin of the anal canal that can be exquisitely painful during a bowel movement, can produce bright-red bleeding.

Targeted Physical Examination

Vital Signs

Assess the client's vital signs and auscultate heart and lungs. Tachycardia or hypotension can indicate hypovolemia due to internal or external hemorrhage (Lyons, 2020; see also

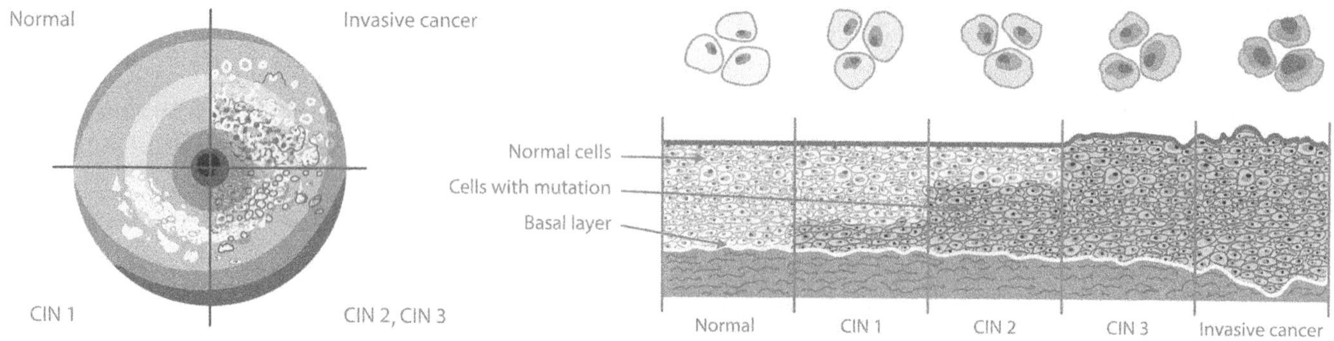

Figure 5-13. Cervical intraepithelial neoplasia (CIN) is a premalignant condition of the squamous epithelium covering the outer surface of the uterine cervix (©Vectoressa/Adobe Stock)

Chapter 9, "Hypovolemic Shock"). Fever can indicate infection/sepsis. Hyperthyroidism associated with molar pregnancy can cause tachycardia. Fear and pain can cause tachycardia or hypertension.

Orthostatic hypotension, a postural drop in blood pressure, can indicate hypovolemia, dysfunction of the autonomic nervous system, decreased venous return, or inability to increase cardiac output in response to changes in posture (Kim & Farrell, 2020). In nonpregnant people, orthostatic hypotension is indicated by a drop in systolic pressure of 20 mm Hg or more, a decrease in diastolic pressure of 10 mm Hg or more, and/or a pulse elevation of 30 or more beats per min (bpm) within 3 min of standing (Kim & Farrell, 2020). Test for orthostatic hypotension by evaluating vital signs in a supine or left lateral position, then reassess when the client is standing. (If the client is dizzy or faint, assess for orthostatic hypotension by raising the head of the bed.) Peripheral vascular resistance decreases during pregnancy, however, and a healthy gravida can demonstrate orthostatic hypotension upon standing, particularly in the later months.

Abdominal Examination

If the fundus is palpable, estimate gestational age and note whether it correlates with the date of the last menstrual period (LMP). Evaluate the client's abdomen by first observing for bruising or discoloration. Cullen's sign, a blue tint beneath the umbilicus indicating free blood in the abdomen, is a rare sign of ruptured ectopic pregnancy. Gently palpate the client's abdomen to assess whether the abdomen is rigid or distended. Assess for pain by gently palpating at the area of least pain and examining the painful area last. Because kidney conditions such as pyelonephritis and renal calculi can refer pain to the pelvis, check for costovertebral angle tenderness; (Ellsworth Bowers & Kitzman, 2024).

Spontaneous abortion usually presents with midline suprapubic pain and lower-back pain. Ectopic pregnancy typically involves unilateral pain in the right or left lower quadrant that can radiate to the back, the shoulder, or elsewhere. A ruptured ectopic pregnancy can evidence abdominal rigidity, distension, and rebound tenderness. The pain of cystitis usually worsens with voiding, and there can be urinary frequency, burning, or unusual smell to the urine. Ovarian torsion or rupture of an ovarian cyst can present similarly to ectopic pregnancy.

Rebound tenderness (Blumberg's sign) may be elicited by pressing slowly and deeply into the abdomen for approximately 15–30 sec, then suddenly removing the palpating hand. When the client has peritonitis from infection (such as appendicitis) or free blood in the abdomen (as with a ruptured ectopic pregnancy), the release will be much more painful than the gradual pressure. Rebound tenderness can also be detected with gentle percussion of the abdomen, by having the client cough, or by having the client rise onto the toes, then drop weight onto the heels (Macaluso & McNamara, 2012). Clients with peritonitis tend to have worse pain with walking or with bumps in the road during transport.

A fetal heartbeat may be auscultated with a Doppler device after 9–12 weeks of gestation. Failure to hear heart tones does not necessarily indicate fetal loss. A fetal heartbeat may be difficult to find if the uterus is retroverted, the fetus is active, the placenta is anterior, and/or the mother is overweight. It can be easier to find a fetal heart rate (FHR) if the uterus is elevated by the examining fingers during a bimanual examination while the other hand holds the Doppler suprapubically. You might also try putting the client in left lateral or Sims' position to encourage her uterus to move toward her abdominal wall. The presence of normal heart tones by Doppler eliminates the possibility of missed abortion and makes ectopic pregnancy unlikely, but the presence of a fetal heartbeat does not guarantee a viable pregnancy.

Speculum Examination

After examining the external abdomen, proceed to the pelvic examination. Examine the external genitalia and anus for lesions or injuries. Gently insert a speculum and

If ectopic pregnancy is suspected, do not delay care by monitoring β-hCG levels; refer the client to the obstetrician or the emergency department.

Decreasing β-hCG levels indicate a nonviable pregnancy, but cannot distinguish whether the pregnancy is intrauterine or ectopic.

inspect the vaginal vault, sidewalls, and cervix for signs of vaginitis, trauma, vaginal varicosities, herpetic lesions, vaginal or cervical neoplasia, warts, or polyps (Norwitz & Park, 2023). A ruptured ectopic pregnancy with bleeding into the abdomen and pelvis can cause bulging of the posterior vaginal fornix (Ellsworth Bowers & Kitzman, 2024). Use sponge sticks or gauze sponges on ring forceps to remove pooled blood and clots for better visibility.

Note the quality and characteristics of bleeding, including location (pooling in the vagina, flowing through the cervical os, oozing from an abrasion on the vaginal wall), character (serous, bright red, clotted, brown), and quantity (scant spotting, active bleeding, blood-tinged mucus). Look for vaginal and cervical lesions and evidence of trauma. Bleeding that originates from the cervix or vagina is not usually associated with pregnancy loss. Evaluate for infection, especially gonorrhea, chlamydia, and trichomoniasis, and obtain cultures as appropriate (Ellsworth Bowers & Kitzman, 2024).

Observe whether the cervix appears open or closed and whether clots or membranes are present in the os. If a miscarriage is complete, the cervix can be open or closed, the uterus will feel small and tightly contracted, and bleeding and cramping will become minimal. The cervix may be open if the client is actively miscarrying or has just completed a miscarriage or if there are retained products of conception. Remove tissue that has wedged in the os with ring forceps by grasping and gently pulling it straight out. Often its removal will control the bleeding of an incomplete abortion. Within minutes of removing the tissue from the os, the pain and cramping typically improve dramatically.

Bimanual Examination

If the cervix appears closed and there are no bleeding lesions, perform a gentle bimanual examination (Norwitz & Park, 2022). Use caution: even the gentlest examination can (rarely) rupture an ectopic pregnancy (N. Tharpe, personal communication, February 25, 2018). Check for cervical dilation and cervical motion tenderness. Evaluate the size, shape, position, consistency, and any tenderness of the pelvic organs. Note any adnexal mass.

When the uterus palpates small for dates, consider the presence of a completed miscarriage, ectopic pregnancy, incorrect dates, or missed abortion. In ectopic pregnancy, the hormones of early pregnancy can cause the uterus to enlarge to the same size and consistency as would be palpated with an IUP (Ellsworth Bowers & Kitzman, 2024). When the uterus is larger than expected, consider multiple gestation (possibly with loss of one of the fetuses) molar pregnancy, uterine fibroids, adenomyosis, or incorrect dates. Whereas a uterus enlarged by fibroids is irregularly shaped, multiple pregnancy or hydatidiform mole causes uniform enlargement. A uterus with a Müllerian duct anomaly (e.g., bicornuate, arcuate, didelphys) can also feel asymmetrical and irregular. See Chapter 2, "Reproductive Tract Anomalies and Pregnancy."

FIRST THOUGHT, WORST THOUGHT:

What is the most likely cause of first-trimester pain and bleeding?

Threatened abortion.

What is the worst it could be?

Ectopic pregnancy. Miscarriage. Hemorrhagic shock.

If an ectopic pregnancy is present, you may palpate a unilateral adnexal mass or fullness to the right or left of the uterus. Ectopic pregnancy can also displace the uterus away from the midline (Ellsworth Bowers & Kitzman, 2024). Cervical motion or adnexal palpation may elicit pain. Pain from a prominent corpus luteum cyst can also cause unilateral low-abdominal pain and a palpable mass or adnexal fullness (Institute of Obstetricians & Gynaecologists, 2014).

Ovarian torsion (rotation of the ovary resulting in partial or complete obstruction of its blood supply) and adnexal torsion (twisting of fallopian tube and ovary) are gynecologic emergencies requiring immediate surgery (Krishnan, Kaur, Bali, & Rao, 2011). Although these are unusual causes of abdominal pain in pregnancy, 12–25% of clients with ovarian or adnexal torsion are pregnant. The incidence is higher for clients who have used assisted reproductive technologies (Hasson et al., 2020). Symptoms are nonspecific but can include severe right or left lower abdominal pain, a palpable mass, and rebound tenderness.

Imaging and Laboratory Tests

Often, early pregnancy bleeding is associated with either an IUP of uncertain viability or a pregnancy in an uncertain location. Distinguishing between these two clinical entities is often a "wait and see" situation in which the client is clinically stable: with repeated testing, the diagnosis forms over days or weeks. Anyone with excessive bleeding or pain, abnormal vital signs,

Table 5-3

Sample GOLDCART History for Bleeding in the First Half of Pregnancy

General situation and history—How many weeks pregnant are you? When was your last menstrual period (LMP)? What kind of contraception had you been using, if any? Did you take a pregnancy test—if yes did it require urine or blood? Do you feel movement? Do you have any health issues or pregnancy complications? How many pregnancies have you had—how many pregnancy losses and how many live births? Any previous ectopic pregnancies? Have you had any cesarean sections or other uterine surgeries? Have you had ultrasound imaging? If so, how many weeks pregnant were you then? Was a heartbeat detected? Was the fetus visualized in the uterus or was ectopic pregnancy a concern?
Onset—When did you first start to bleed? What were you doing? Was the onset gradual or rapid? Which came first, pain or bleeding? Did you have recent intercourse or put anything inside your vagina before the bleeding started?
Location—Are you sure the blood is coming from your vagina? Could it be from your bladder or rectum? Where do you feel the pain? Is it on one side or right in the middle? Does it start in one place and radiate to somewhere else? Where?
Duration—How long have you been bleeding? Has it been steady or does it come and go?
Characteristics—Was the blood brown, red, or pink? How long does it take to soak a pad? How many pads have you soaked since the bleeding began? Large pads or small? Is the blood on the tissue when you wipe, soaking through your underwear, or turning the toilet water red? Are you passing clots? Did you pass any tissue? Is the pain sharp, dull, or crampy? How would you rate the pain on a scale of 0–10, with 10 being the worst pain imaginable?
Associated symptoms—Any nausea, vomiting, fever, dizziness, or fainting? Any abnormal vaginal discharge? Any diarrhea or constipation? Any pain or burning with urination?
Relieving/aggravating factors—Do you get a fresh gush of blood or clots when you have been lying down for a while? Does your pain increase when you empty your bladder?
Treatment—Have providers evaluated your bleeding? What did they recommend? Have you been following the recommendations? Have you been using alternative remedies? Has your condition changed since these treatments?

significant anemia, or possible ectopic pregnancy requires immediate physician evaluation (Ellsworth Bowers & Kitzman, 2024).

Laboratory and imaging tests can refute or confirm the clinical impression but are not always diagnostic. Often the cause of bleeding is never discovered. In the absence of an unequivocal diagnosis, the provider must focus on determining whether the bleeding indicates serious underlying pathology. Ectopic pregnancy must always be a consideration until definitively excluded (N. Tharpe, personal communication, February 25, 2018).

Human Chorionic Gonadotropin (hCG)

The syncytiotrophoblast cells of the blastocyst (which later form the placenta) secrete the β subunit of hCG (β-hCG) after the conceptus implants in the uterine lining. This glycoprotein hormone acts as a chemical communication from the embryo to the mother that pregnancy has occurred. It signals the corpus luteum to continue progesterone production until the placenta is mature enough to take over the task. A single β-hCG measurement is of little value in assessing viability, but serial measurements taken 48 hr apart during the first 5–6 weeks of gestation can aid in differentiating a healthy pregnancy from an abnormal one (Bastian & Brown, 2023). After about 6 weeks of gestation, sonography can be used to determine the location and viability of the pregnancy. There is rarely a reason to monitor β-hCG levels once an IUP is confirmed on ultrasound (ACOG, 2018/2022; Barnhart et al., 2016; Norwitz & Park, 2022).

Serum β-hCG rises most rapidly until about 41 days of gestation. It is first detectable upon implantation at approximately 6–12 days after ovulation and doubles every 1.6 days during the 5th week of gestation, every 2 days during the 6th week, and every 2.5 days during the 7th week (Ellsworth Bowers & Kitzman, 2024). After week 7, the rate of rise slows. Levels peak at 8–10 weeks of gestation at about 60,000–90,000 mIU/ml and decline to a plateau of approximately 10,000–20,000 mIU/ml in the second and third trimesters (Hendriks, Rosenberg, et al., 2020). Although adequately rising β-hCG levels are most likely to indicate viable IUP, they also rise at a normal rate in some ectopic gestations, especially in the early weeks (ACOG, 2018/2022). Four to six weeks after pregnancy loss or childbirth, serum β-hCG should be undetectable (Harvey, 2023).

Whereas serum pregnancy tests measure β-hCG, urine pregnancy tests measure hCG beta core fragment (hCGβcf), the end metabolite of β-hCG degradation. The most sensitive urine tests have a minimum detection threshold of about 20 mIU/ml. Quantitative serum blood tests can detect β-hCG

Table 5-4
Differential Diagnoses of Vaginal Bleeding in Early Pregnancy

Condition	Usual Presentation	Atypical Presentation
Threatened abortion	Bleeding, light or heavy Closed cervix Uterine size appropriate for dates	Cramping and pain in lower abdomen
Ectopic pregnancy	Light bleeding Abdominal pain Closed cervix Empty uterus on ultrasound Complex adnexal mass β-hCG slow to rise, plateaued, or slowly dropping Free blood in *cul de sac*	Fainting Tender adnexal mass Hypovolemic shock Cervical motion tenderness Peritoneal irritation
Inevitable abortion	Heavy bleeding, clots Dilated cervix Cramping and pain in lower abdomen, can be severe β-hCG dropping	No expulsion of products of conception
Incomplete abortion	Heavy bleeding Dilated cervix Partial expulsion of products of conception Cramping and pain in lower abdomen	Uterine tenderness Fever and foul discharge if infection present
Molar pregnancy	Bleeding—often the color of prune juice Dilated cervix Uterus large for dates and unusually soft Passage of grapelike vesicles β-hCG elevated and rising faster than normal Molar tissue visualized on ultrasound Nausea/vomiting Spontaneous abortion if partial molar pregnancy Cramping and pain in lower abdomen Large cystic ovaries No evidence of a fetus if complete molar pregnancy	Early-onset preeclampsia

levels as low as 1 mIU/ml. A serum level of less than 5 mIU/ml (5 IU/L) can be considered negative and anything above 25 mIU/ml (25 IU/L) positive for pregnancy. Values that fall between these thresholds are equivocal and necessitate repeat testing. The normal β-hCG concentration varies widely from person to person and pregnancy to pregnancy, and measurements differ from laboratory to laboratory (Bastian & Brown, 2023). Because results processed by different labs may not reflect a true change in β-hCG values, the client should use same laboratory for all measurements.

Although home urine tests are highly accurate, false negative results can occur when the test is performed too soon after conception, usually because of a delay in ovulation. Often, a home urine test will not read positive until 5 or 6 weeks of gestation (Bastian & Brown, 2023). False negatives can also occur, most commonly between 7 and 12 weeks of gestation when urine hCGβcf levels are so high that they can overwhelm the binding capacity of the test (Harvey, 2023). False positives are very rare and can indicate gestational trophoblastic disease, malignancy, a pituitary issue, or a defective test (Bastian & Brown, 2023).

Decreasing β-hCG levels indicate a nonviable pregnancy but cannot distinguish whether the pregnancy is intrauterine or ectopic. A decrease by 21% or more over 48 hr suggests failed IUP; a decrease below this threshold is concerning for ectopic pregnancy (Hendriks, Rosenberg et al., 2020). If β-hCG levels rise very slowly or plateau, suspect an ectopic pregnancy or an abnormal IUP that will eventually miscarry.

Because every pregnancy takes a unique interval to establish itself in the uterus, dating a pregnancy by LMP is not always accurate. In a 28-day menstrual cycle, ovulation usually occurs around day 14; but individuals with shorter cycles may ovulate as early as day 8 and those with longer cycles may ovulate on day 21 or later. The conceptus typically

Table 5-5
Management of β-hCG Results in Early Pregnancy

When β-hCG is **increasing normally** by at least 53% in 48 hr OR doubling in 72 hr, perform transvaginal ultrasound when the β-hCG levels reach the discriminatory zone (3,500 mIU/ml or per institutional guidelines) to confirm viable IUP.
When β-hCG is **increasing abnormally** or plateaus from baseline through two serial measurements, the pregnancy is probably either ectopic or an otherwise abnormal pregnancy that will eventually miscarry. Consult with your collaborating physician.
When β-hCG is **decreasing**, the pregnancy is probably a spontaneous abortion, a tubal abortion (ectopic pregnancy expelled into abdominal cavity), or a spontaneously resolving ectopic pregnancy. Follow β-hCG levels weekly until undetectable and manage based on clinical symptoms.
When β-hCG is **above the discriminatory zone**, results of transvaginal ultrasound guide management. Manage as ectopic pregnancy when definitive IUP is absent or ultrasound shows a complex adnexal mass.
From "Ectopic Pregnancy: Methotrexate Therapy," by T. Tulandi, 2023d, in A. Chakrabarti (Ed.), *UpToDate*. Copyright by UpToDate.

implants in the uterus 8–10 days after ovulation but can take 12 or more; this is one reason that even sensitive pregnancy tests may be slow to recognize a viable pregnancy (Wilcox, Baird, & Weinberg, 1999). The risk of miscarriage is higher with later implantation (Wilcox et al., 1999). β-hCG levels can be used to estimate gestational age in the first 1–3 weeks of pregnancy but are not useful afterwards because the range of normal values widens. For example, a healthy pregnancy of 8–10 weeks can have β-hCG levels as low as 5,000 or as high as 150,000 mIU/ml (Bastian & Brown, 2023).

Discriminatory Zone

The serum β-hCG discriminatory zone is a threshold above which transvaginal ultrasound should show a gestational sac when an IUP is present (Dawodu, Wu, Gallop, & Barnhart, 2022). The threshold differs among institutions and measurement methods. Because pregnancies develop uniquely, the value for the discriminatory zone is set high, up to 3,500 mIU/ml, to reduce the potential for misdiagnosis (ACOG, 2018/2022). Multiple gestations might require a higher threshold to be visualized on ultrasound. Improvements in sonographic technology may enable the sonographer to visualize a pregnancy much sooner. Under research conditions, a gestational sac has been consistently identified with β-hCG values as low as 390 mIU/ml, a yolk sac with values as low as 1,094 mIU/ml, and a fetal pole with values as low as 1,394 mIU/ml (Connolly, Ryan, Stuebe, & Wolfe, 2013).

Progesterone

Progesterone plays a key role in the menstrual cycle, implantation, and pregnancy maintenance. In very early pregnancy, the corpus luteum in the ovary produces progesterone to sustain the pregnancy. As the placenta develops, it produces increasing quantities of progesterone and becomes the dominant source by 12 weeks of gestation (Coomarasamy et al., 2019).

When a client presents with early pregnancy bleeding and an inconclusive ultrasound report, a single progesterone measurement can provide information on the viability of the pregnancy. In clients with early pregnancy bleeding, serum progesterone levels of less than 5 ng/ml reliably exclude viable pregnancy (99% negative predictive value) but cannot determine whether the gestation is intrauterine or ectopic (Verhaegen et al., 2012). More than 90% of clients with a level ≥20–25 ng/ml have a viable pregnancy (Ghaedi et al., 2022).

Ultrasound Examination

Sonography is the preferred means of distinguishing a viable IUP from pregnancy loss or ectopic gestation. In some cases, a diagnosis of early pregnancy loss is straightforward. For example, early pregnancy loss is evident in a client who presents with significant vaginal bleeding and an empty uterus on ultrasound examination when prior ultrasound imaging documented an IUP. Early transvaginal ultrasound can also identify gestational age, multiple gestation, ovarian cysts, subchorionic hemorrhage, hydatidiform mole, fibroids, and uterine anomalies.

The embryologic events of early gestation are predictable and occur in a stepwise fashion. Deviations from the expected progression suggest impending early pregnancy loss or ectopic gestation (Hendriks, MacNaughton, et al., 2019). Key developmental milestones observable by sonographic examination include the following:

Gestational sac, a small, fluid-filled sac with an echogenic rim situated within the endometrium. It should be evident by 4 5/7–5 0/7 weeks of gestation and is the first sonographic sign of an IUP (MacKenzie, Stephenson, & Funai, 2023). An abnormally small gestational sac is associated with higher risk of pregnancy loss (Abd Ellatif, Ahmad, & Halawa, 2018). An empty intrauterine gestational sac visualized on ultrasound does not always indicate an IUP. Importantly, in 20% of ectopic pregnancies, a collection of fluid (pseudosac) can be visualized within the uterine cavity (Norwitz & Park, 2023). If more than 5 5/7–6 0/7 weeks have elapsed since the first day of the client's LMP, absence of a gestational sac suggests that either ovulation was delayed and the gestational age is earlier than expected or the pregnancy is ectopic (Norwitz & Park, 2023).

Yolk sac, a vital structure that attaches to the embryo, serving to exchange gases, absorb nutrients, initiate hematopoiesis (manufacture of blood cells), and perform other endocrine and metabolic functions until these tasks are assumed by the fetus and/or the placenta. The yolk sac is visible as a round, echogenic structure within the gestational sac, becoming identifiable at 5 0/7 weeks of gestation and persisting until about 10 0/7–12 0/7 weeks of gestation. A misshapen, enlarged, free-floating, duplicated, or calcified yolk sac is associated with a poor prognosis (Abd Ellatif et al., 2018).

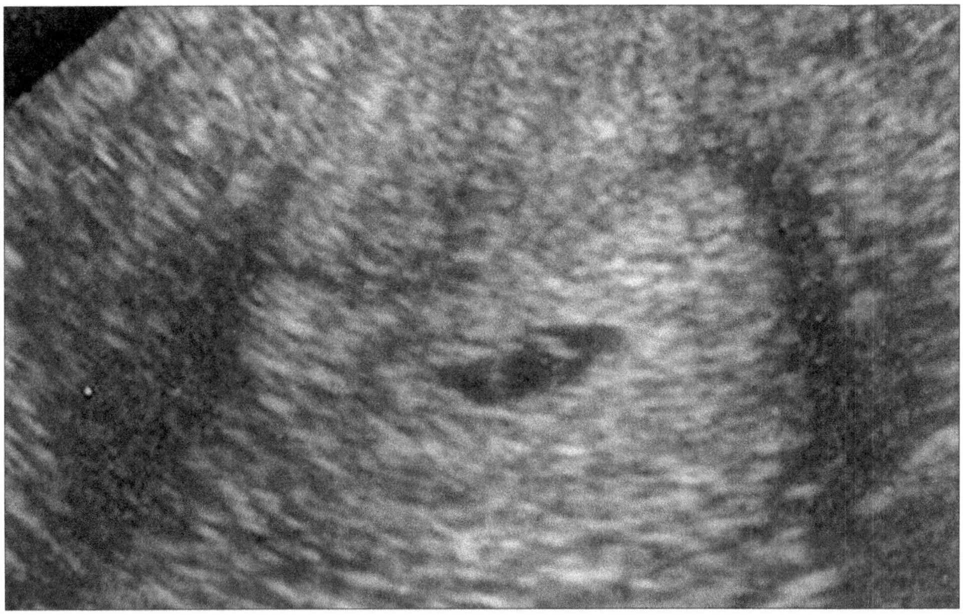

Figure 5-14. The gestational sac is visible within the uterus via transvaginal ultrasound by about 4 4/7–5 0/7 weeks of gestation or when β-hCG levels reach about 1,500–3,500 mIU/ml.

Fetal Pole. The embryo first appears as an echogenic thickening along the bright outer edge of the yolk sac known as the fetal pole. It is visible on transvaginal ultrasound from about 5 0/7 weeks of gestation by menstrual dates (Phillips & Saxby, 2019). A fetal pole is measured from one end to the other (crown-rump length).

Heart rate. Cardiac activity may be first detected by transvaginal ultrasound at a gestational age of 5 5/7–6 0/7 weeks (Bastian & Brown, 2023). Heart rate can be obtained transabdominally with a Doppler device at 10 0/7–12 0/7 weeks of gestation or earlier (Bastian & Brown, 2023). First-trimester heart rates vary with gestational age (Poornima, Vijayalakshmi, Anuradha, & Sailatha, 2020). Before 6 0/7 weeks of gestation, the heart rate averages 100–115 bpm, then rises to an average of 137–144 bpm after 9 0/7 weeks of gestation (Poornima et al., 2020). Slow embryonic heart rates are strongly associated with nonviable pregnancies. Virtually no embryo with a heart rate below 70 bpm at 6 0/7–8 0/7 weeks of gestation survives (Doubilet & Benson, 2005). About 62% of embryos with heart rates less than 100 bpm by 6 2/7 weeks of gestation or less than 120 bpm at 6 3/7–7 0/7 weeks of gestation miscarry, but only 8% with normal heart rates are lost (Doubilet, Benson, & Chow, 1999). Embryos with slow heart rates early in gestation that later rise to the normal range remain at higher risk for demise (Doubilet, Benson, Bourne, & Blaivas, 2013).

Ectopic Pregnancy

Extrauterine pregnancies can be difficult to detect by history and physical examination. *As many as 40% of ectopic pregnancies are undiagnosed on initial presentation* (Baker & dela Cruz, 2023). Timely sonography, however, can identify findings that are concerning for or diagnostic of ectopic pregnancy, such as masses in the adnexa or abdomen, fluid in the abdomen, or an identifiable pregnancy outside the uterus (Baker & dela Cruz, 2023). The accuracy of transvaginal ultrasound for diagnosing an extrauterine pregnancy ranges from 73% to 93%, depending on gestational age, the kind and condition of the equipment, and the expertise of the sonographer and radiologist (Angelini & LaFontaine, 2013). Extrauterine pregnancy can be mistakenly identified on ultrasound as an adjacent bowel, a cyst, an endometrioma, or the corpus luteum (Angelini & LaFontaine, 2013; N. Tharpe, personal communication, March 3, 2018).

Because fluid or blood in the uterus can be mistaken for a gestational sac, visualization of a gestational sac with a yolk sac or embryo within the uterus is considered definitive evidence of an IUP (ACOG, 2018/2022). Rarely, a twin gestation can include both an ectopic and an intrauterine pregnancy (heterotopic pregnancy). If the client has a serum β-hCG greater than 2,000 mIU/ml and there is no intrauterine gestation identified on transvaginal ultrasound, the client should be considered to have an ectopic pregnancy until proven otherwise (Baker & dela Cruz, 2023). Unequivocal evidence of

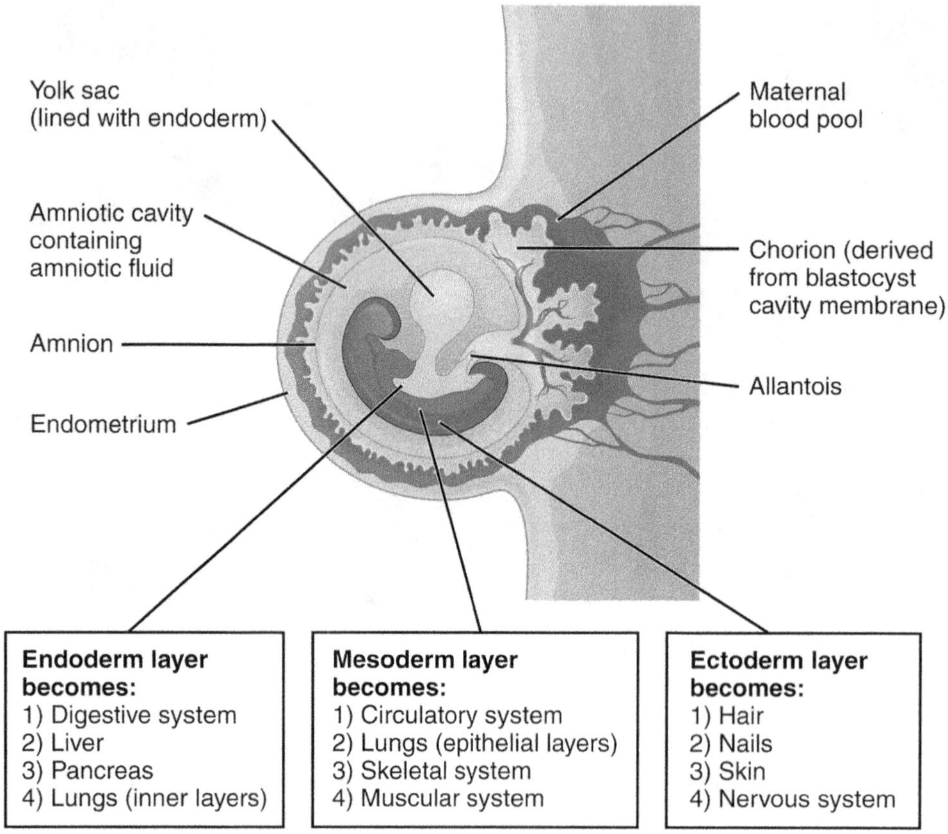

Figure 5-15. Human embryo, 3 weeks after conception, 5 weeks by menstrual dates. The three primary layers of embryonic cells—endoderm, mesoderm, and ectoderm—will organize to form the structures and tissues of the body. The embryo does not yet have a heartbeat. The yolk sac exchanges gases, absorbs nutrients, initiates hematopoiesis, and performs other endocrine and metabolic functions. From *Anatomy and Physiology* (fig. 28.10), by J. G. Betts et al., 2013, Houston, TX: OpenStax. Copyright 2022 by OpenStax. Access for free at https://openstax.org/books/anatomy-and-physiology/pages/1-introduction

ectopic pregnancy includes visualization of a gestational sac with a yolk sac, embryo, or both in the adnexa or elsewhere in the abdomen; but most ectopic gestations do not progress to this stage (ACOG, 2018/2022). Fluid with debris (consistent with blood) in the pelvic cul-de-sac or abdomen or a blood clot near the uterus and adnexa suggests rupture of an ectopic pregnancy (Tulandi, 2023c).

Vanishing Twin / Fetus Papyraceous

Vanishing twin syndrome (VTS) refers to multifetal pregnancy that results in the birth of a singleton infant (McNamara, Kane, Craig, Short, & Umstad, 2016). One of the embryos dies and is resorbed, thus becoming clinically undetectable, leaving behind an empty sac, which is absorbed over time. VTS is common, occurring in 7–36% of twin pregnancies resulting from use of assisted reproduction technology and an unknowable percentage of spontaneous conceptions (Chasen, 2023). Up to 80% occur before 9 weeks of gestation (McNamara et al., 2016). Resorption of the demised twin has been observed from 6 to 11 weeks of gestation (Zamani & Parekh, 2023). When a twin dies in the first 6–8 weeks of gestation, it may regress to a subtle lesion on the placenta such as a cyst or fibrin deposit (Anderson-Berry, 2016). The surviving fetus is at risk for adverse outcomes, especially cerebral palsy and PTB (Blickstein, 2021). Sometimes a surviving twin incorporates genetic material from the lost twin in a process known as chimerism, confounding cell-free DNA tests, chorionic villi samples, and even tissue matching for organ donation.

Often the empty sac of the lost twin is noted as an incidental finding in a routine first-trimester ultrasound. Most cases are asymptomatic, but some present with vaginal bleeding. An anechoic oval representing a subchorionic hemorrhage can sometimes be mistaken for a vanishing twin.

Fetus papyraceous occurs when a twin greater than 8 weeks of gestation is retained *in utero* for a minimum of 10 weeks, becoming mummified and compressed. The amniotic fluid and placental tissue are reabsorbed, and the fetus is flattened between the membranes beside the surviving twin (Usharani, Joshi, & Veena, 2015). It occurs in about 1 in 200 twin pregnancies and is more commonly found in monochorionic pregnancies and those with velamentous cord insertion (McNamara et al., 2016). Fetus papyraceous is also associated with chromosomal abnormalities, especially triploidy, in the demised twin.

Subchorionic Hemorrhage (Subchorionic Hematoma)

A subchorionic hemorrhage (subchorionic hematoma) is a collection of blood between the chorionic membrane surrounding the fetus and the uterine wall. It is caused by the separation of the chorion from the endometrium (Günay & Yardımcı, 2022; Maso et al., 2005) and is the most common cause of vaginal bleeding between 10 and 20 weeks of gestation

(Bondick, Das, & Fertal, 2023). Subchorionic hematoma can also be an incidental finding of ultrasound examination in an otherwise normal pregnancy. On ultrasound imaging, a chorionic hematoma appears as a hypoechoic (snowstorm appearance) or anechoic (dark) crescent-shaped area. Fresh blood is usually anechoic. After clotting, it becomes more echogenic (bright). As the clot begins to break down, it becomes anechoic again (Benavides-Reyes et al., 2015).

Many studies have examined the relationship between subchorionic hematoma and adverse pregnancy outcomes, but findings are inconsistent. Whereas some authors correlate subchorionic hemorrhage with higher risk of first-trimester pregnancy loss (Ali & Ismail, 2021; Günay & Yardımcı, 2022; Maso et al., 2005; Norwitz & Park, 2023), others do not (Johns, Hyett, & Jauniaux, 2003; Naert, Khadraoui, Muniz Rodriguez, Naqvi, & Fox, 2019; Naert, Muniz Rodriguez, Khadraoui, Naqvi, & Fox, 2019; Özkaya, Altay, & Gelişen, 2011; Özler & Güler, 2019; Pedersen & Mantoni, 1990). Likewise, some authors found that subchorionic hematoma is associated with higher risk for placental abruption, late pregnancy loss, PPROM, and PTB (Thakkar et al., 2022); others found no association with adverse outcomes (Naert, Muniz, Rodriguez et al., 2019).

Table 5-6

Timeline of Normal Fetal Development

Time in weeks from LMP	Developmental milestone
4 5/7	Gestational sac
5 0/7–5 5/7	Yolk sac
6 0/7	Embryo with cardiac activity
6 1/7	Amniotic membrane
7 0/7–8 0/7	Fetal spine
8 0/7–8 5/7	Noticeable fetal motion

Adapted from "Role of Ultrasound in the Evaluation of First-Trimester Pregnancies in the Acute Setting," by V. A. Murugan, B. O. Murphy, C. Dupuis, A. Goldstein, and Y. H. Kim, 2020, *Ultrasonography, 39*(2), pp. 178–189, Table 1. Copyright by Korean Society of Ultrasound in Medicine.

Management of Severe Early Pregnancy Bleeding

In some cases, light early pregnancy bleeding can be managed outside the hospital by a midwife. In others, physician collaboration or referral is necessary. The person with severe bleeding or a symptomatic suspected ectopic pregnancy requires immediate transport to the nearest hospital. Ambulance transport is often the most appropriate mode of transfer.

If you can establish venous access, start an infusion of crystalloid intravenous (IV) solution—normal saline (NS) or lactated Ringer's (LR)—if it does not delay care. See Chapter 9 for a comprehensive discussion of managing shock. Ideally, any hemodynamically unstable client should be transported by an advanced life support (ALS) ambulance with care provided by a paramedic (U.S.) or equivalent. Some basic life support (BLS) ambulance services are prohibited from transporting a client who is receiving an IV infusion of fluids or medication. In this case, infusions may be discontinued for transport. Upon arrival at the hospital, a physician should evaluate laboratory results and perform an examination and an ultrasound to arrive at a diagnosis.

Anti-D Prophylaxis

The International Society of Blood Transfusion recognizes 33 unique human blood group systems, which include more than 300 antigens (Calhoun & Bahr, 2023). The Rh blood group system (named for the rhesus monkeys used in the original research) comprises more than 50 antigen proteins attached to the surface of RBCs (Huszti, Gica, Botezatu, Peltecu, & Panaitescu, 2022). In North America, about 85% of people have the RhD antigen and are considered RhD-positive; the 15% lacking this antigen are RhD-negative (ACOG, 2017/2021).

RhD-negative individuals exposed to RhD-positive RBCs can develop anti-D antibodies in a process called isoimmunization or alloimmunization. If the father is Rh positive, the fetus can also be Rh positive. Isoimmunization can develop in an Rh-negative mother carrying an Rh-positive fetus if fetal blood enters the maternal circulation. The maternal immune system can respond to the fetal blood cells as intruders and produce antibodies against the RhD antigen on their surface. Hemolytic disease of the fetus and newborn (HDFN) can develop when these anti-D antibodies cross the placenta and destroy fetal RBCs, causing severe anemia and hydrops. In subsequent pregnancies, hemolytic disease tends to occur earlier and with greater severity.

Although mother and fetus have separate circulatory systems, the mixing of maternal and fetal blood is common, especially during placental separation in third stage labor. RhD alloimmunization can be caused by a fetal-maternal hemorrhage as small as 0.1 ml (ACOG, 2017/2021). The RhD antigen is present on the red cells of the embryo by 38 days after conception (7 3/7 weeks by menstrual dates). Fetomaternal bleeding (fetal blood entering maternal circulation) after this threshold can cause alloimmunization (ACOG, 2017/2021; Moise, 2022). Miscarriage, ectopic pregnancy, amniocentesis, chorionic villus sampling, and placenta abruption can also cause fetal cells to enter maternal circulation.

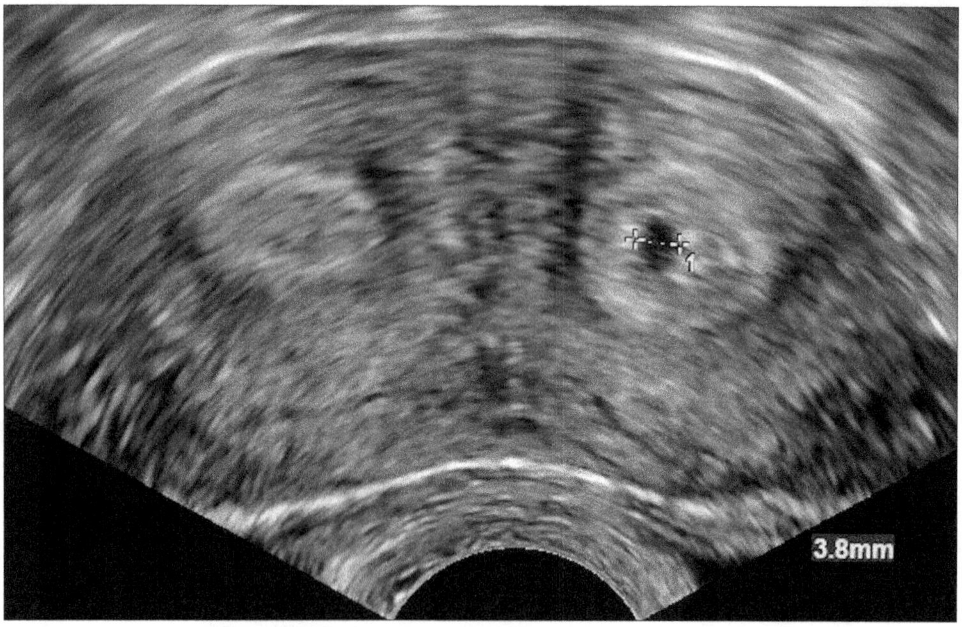

Figure 5-16. Transvaginal ultrasound clearly shows both horns of this bicornuate uterus. A gestational sac indicating a 4–5-week pregnancy lies in the horn to the right. This woman sought care because she had a positive pregnancy test with a copper-wire IUD in place, which was situated in the opposite horn and visible on other images during this evaluation. "Bicornuate uterus with pregnancy" [sonogram], in "Medical Gallery of Mikael Häggström 2014," by M. Häggström, 2014, *WikiJournal of Medicine, 1*(2). CC0 1.0.

Maternal sensitization to RhD can be prevented by administering an RhD immune globulin (RhIg) injection in the early third trimester, immediately postpartum, and after any event that may result in fetal blood entering the maternal circulation. The high levels of passively acquired antibodies provided by the RhIg injection bind to fetal RBCs expressing D-antigen within the mother and destroy them before the maternal system can mount an immune response (Hamilton, 1991). In about 9% of cases, RhIg crosses the placenta, but does not cause clinically significant hemolysis in the fetus or newborn (Maayan-Metzger, Schwartz, Sulkes, & Merlob, 2001). Before this treatment was introduced in the 1970s, isoimmunization developed in 13–16% of at-risk pregnancies, carrying a stillbirth rate of 14% and a 50% rate of neonatal brain injury or death. The administration of postpartum RhIg decreases the rate of hemolytic anemia to 0.5–1.8%, and administering a prophylactic dose at about 28 weeks of gestation further reduces the risk to 0.14–0.2% (ACOG, 2017/2021). Low-resource regions without access to RhIg still suffer high mortality from HDNF (ACOG, 2017/2021).

RhIg should be administered within 72 hr after vaginal or cesarean birth; spontaneous abortion; abdominal trauma; ectopic pregnancy; an episode of antepartum bleeding; or an invasive prenatal procedure such as chorionic villus sampling or amniocentesis. Research, however, has demonstrated partial to complete benefit when RhIg was delayed by as much as 13 days after exposure (ACOG, 2017/2021). Although effectiveness decreases with longer intervals between exposure and administration, the client can derive some benefit from RhIg given as late as 28 days postpartum (ACOG, 2017/2021). The provider should not give RhIg in response to an incidental ultrasound finding of subchorionic hematoma (Moise, 2022).

Because the early embryo contains very little blood, emerging data suggests that RhIg may not be necessary for some RhD-negative clients with early pregnancy loss. The World Health Organization (WHO) and certain other organizations do not recommend Rh testing or RhIg administration for pregnancy bleeding or miscarriage before 12 weeks of gestation (Horvath, Goyal, Traxler, & Prager, 2022; National Abortion Federation, 2022; Prager et al., 2023c; Royal College of Obstetricians & Gynaecologists, 2022; WHO, 2022). ACOG maintains that while there is insufficient evidence to support or oppose administering RhIg for a pregnancy loss before 12 weeks of gestation, providers should consider administering at least 50 mcg of RhIg in cases of spontaneous first-trimester miscarriage, especially those occurring toward the end of the first trimester (ACOG, 2017/2021). Although the risk of alloimmunization is low in the first trimester, it is not zero, and the consequences of maternal sensitization can be significant (ACOG, 2017/2021). After the first trimester, the Society of Family Planning committee consensus on Rh testing in early pregnancy recommends administering RhIg (one 100-mcg dose or two 50-mcg doses) after bleeding or pregnancy loss between 12 and 18 weeks of gestation (Horvath et al., 2022). *Always follow local guidelines and consult with your collaborating physician if you are uncertain about which dose to give.*

A standard dose of RhIg (300 mcg) can protect clients exposed to as much as 15 ml of fetal RBCs (30 ml D-positive fetal whole blood) from sensitization and should be given to clients ≥18 weeks of gestation (ACOG, 2017/2021). About 2–3 individuals per 1,000 experiencing pregnancy loss beyond the first half of pregnancy have a fetomaternal hemorrhage exceeding this amount and require multiple doses of RhIg for protection. For this reason, ACOG recommends that Rh-negative clients with Rh-positive infants undergo a qualitative screening test and, if indicated, a Kleihauer–Betke test to quantify the percentage of fetal red cells in the maternal circulation to determine the appropriate dose (ACOG, 2017/2021).

Table 5-7

Guidelines for Transvaginal Sonographic Diagnosis in a Client with IUP of Uncertain Viability

Findings Diagnostic of Pregnancy Loss	Findings Suspicious for Pregnancy Loss
• Crown-rump length 7 mm or greater and no heartbeat • Mean sac diameter 25 mm or greater and no embryo • Absence of embryo with a heartbeat 2 weeks or more after a scan that showed a gestational sac without a yolk sac • Absence of embryo with a heartbeat 11 days or more after a scan that showed a gestational sac with a yolk sac	• Crown-rump length <7 mm and no heartbeat • Mean sac diameter 16–24 mm and no embryo • Absence of embryo with heartbeat 7–13 days after a scan that showed a gestational sac without a yolk sac • Absence of embryo with a heartbeat 7–10 days after a scan that showed a gestational sac with a yolk sac • Absence of embryo for ≥6 weeks after LMP • Empty amnion adjacent to yolk sac with no visible embryo • Yolk sac measuring >7 mm • Small gestational sac in relation to the size of the embryo (<5mm difference between mean sac diameter and crown-rump length) • Slow FHR (<100 bpm) • Significant subchorionic hemorrhage
When findings are suspicious for pregnancy loss, consider a repeat ultrasound at 7–10 days to reassess for viability.	

From "Diagnostic Criteria for Nonviable Pregnancy Early in the First Trimester," by P. M. Doubilet, C. B. Benson, T. Bourne, and M. Blaivas, 2013, *New England Journal of Medicine, 369*, pp. 1443–1451. Copyright 2022 by Massachusetts Medical Society.

Hemolytic disease of the newborn and fetus is most associated with maternal/fetal incompatibilities involving the major Rhesus blood groups, A, B, AB, and O. Less commonly, it can involve minor blood groups such as Kell, Duffy, MNS, P, and Diego (Calhoun & Bahr, 2023). Antibodies targeting the C, c, E, and e antigens and others can cause HDNF by destroying fetal RBCs (Healsmith, Savoia, & Kane, 2019). Antibodies targeting Kell blood group antigens (named for Mrs. Kelleher, a mother in whom anti-Kell antibodies had caused HDNF) can also suppress the fetal production of RBCs (Dean, 2005, ch. 8). Duffy antibodies also hold the potential for causing HDNF, but Lewis antibodies do not. One mnemonic advises, "Duffy dies, Kell kills, and Lewis lives."

Considerations for Limited-Resource Settings

Hemorrhage, infection, and shock are much greater concerns for clients with complicated miscarriage or ectopic pregnancy in low-resource settings. Where skilled staff, antibiotics, or equipment for uterine curettage or vacuum aspiration are not available, a mother's only hope for survival may be immediate transfer to a facility able to provide appropriate treatment. Early diagnosis is critical.

Low cost, high efficacy, and long shelf life make misoprostol a first-line therapy for uncomplicated first-trimester incomplete miscarriage in low-resource settings (Gemzell-Danielsson, Fiala, & Weeks, 2007). In communities without access to ultrasound to confirm a nonviable pregnancy, misoprostol should be given only to clients with an open cervical os (denoting an inevitable abortion) lest it end a viable pregnancy. Manual vacuum aspiration may be used for surgical evacuation of a failed IUP, but it is often unavailable or unaffordable in low-resource settings (Almahabrish, Abdelhafez, Taman, & Allakany, 2021). It is the treatment of choice for clients with complicated miscarriage and those unable to adhere to follow-up care (Almahabrish et al., 2021).

Unsafe Abortion

In some settings, "miscarriages" with poor outcomes are the result of ineffective attempts to terminate a pregnancy (Gemzell-Danielsson et al., 2007). An "unsafe" abortion is one performed by an unqualified person with inappropriate materials and techniques or in an environment below minimal standards for safe medical care (WHO, 2019). Complications of unsafe induced abortion remain among the leading causes of maternal mortality (WHO, 2019). Worldwide, between 4.7% and 13.2% of all maternal deaths follow unsafe abortions—as many as 38,940 maternal deaths every year (WHO, 2022, pp. 1–2). These deaths

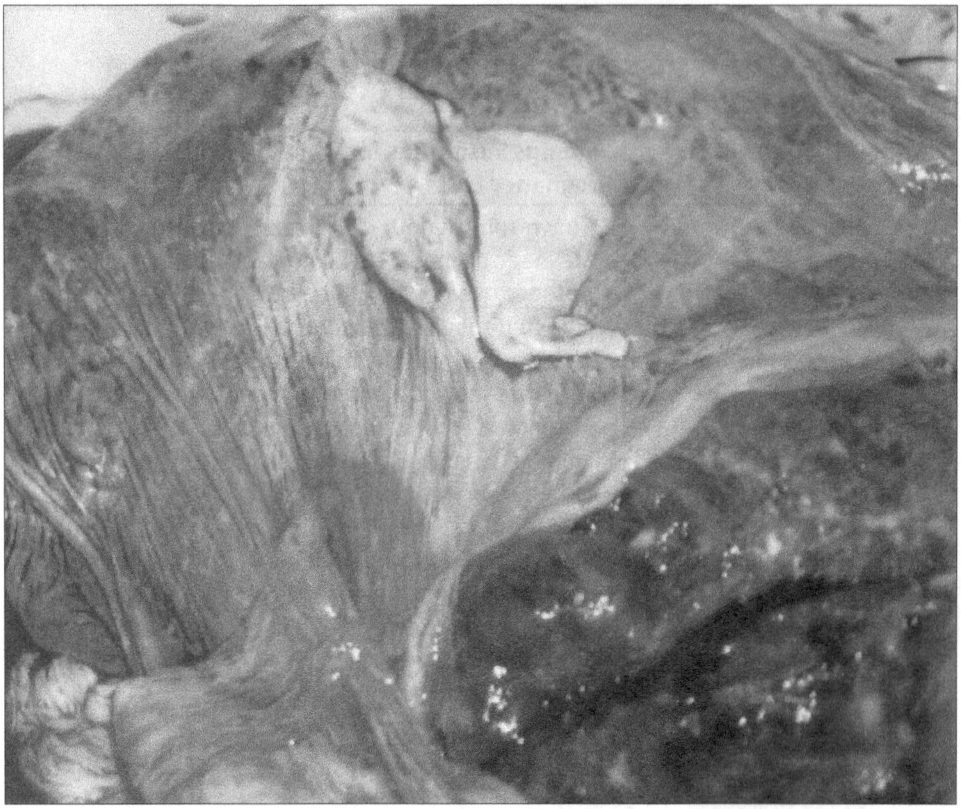

Figure 5-17. Fetus papyraceous. This fetus died in utero at 11 0/7 weeks of gestation, but its twin was born full term. At birth, the barely recognizable fetus was found attached to the chorionic membrane.

are mostly preventable (Namagembe et al., 2022). An additional 5 million individuals each year suffer complications such as hemorrhage or sepsis associated with the procedure (Schwartz, 2013). Globally, about 45% of all elective abortions are performed in unsafe conditions. The majority occurring in Asia (53.8%) fit this description, but Africa (24.8%), Latin America and the Caribbean (19.5%) fall below the world average (WHO, 2022, pp. 1–2). Countries with highly restrictive abortion laws have a significantly higher incidence of unsafe abortions than in those with less restrictive laws (WHO, 2022, pp. 1–2).

Some lay abortionists concoct toxic mixtures of turpentine, bleach, pesticides, quinine, and manure for the gravida to drink (Grimes, 2003). Others attempt to insert a twig, knitting needle, coat hanger, or chicken bone into the uterus or place herbs or inappropriate medications in the vagina or rectum (Polgar & Fried, 1976; Schwartz, 2013). Caustic or toxic liquids such as chloroquine, detergents, hormones, kerosene, lead, metal salts, and phosphorus are sometimes swallowed, placed in the rectum, or infused in the form of a douche (Bridwell, Long, Montrief, & Gottlieb, 2022). Some abortionists attempt dilation and curettage (D&C) without sterile instruments in unhygienic settings, blow air into the uterus with a syringe, or inflict blunt trauma to the abdomen (Schwartz, 2013).

Clients presenting with complications resulting from unsafe abortion may deny that they have undergone the procedure, especially where it is illegal. They may delay seeking care (Namagembe et al., 2022) and can present with life-threatening infection; retained products of conception; cervical or vaginal laceration; perforation of the uterus, bladder, or bowel; uterine atony; shock; severe anemia; or coagulopathy (Bridwell et al., 2022). Traumatic injuries contaminated by dirt or feces carry the risk of tetanus. Infection by toxin-producing bacteria such as *Clostridium* species or Group A *Streptococcus* can cause life-threatening sepsis (Eschenbach, 2015). There have been cases of uterine perforation that allowed the intestines to protrude through the vagina, often with accompanying intestinal obstruction or gangrene of the uterus or bowel (Olofinbiyi et al., 2019; Tchuenkam et al., 2021). Although most clients with abortion-related symptoms are in stable condition, hemodynamically unstable clients require rapid evaluation; simultaneous resuscitation, stabilization, and treatment; and immediate referral to a gynecologic surgeon (Harris & Grossman, 2020). All clients, including those experiencing complications related to abortion, must be managed with kindness, empathy, and compassion, regardless of the provider's personal beliefs about abortion.

Early Second-Trimester Bleeding

Vaginal bleeding is less common in the second and third trimesters. Like bleeding in the first trimester, second trimester bleeding can involve cervical inflammation, trauma, or fetal demise. Like bleeding in the first trimester, second-trimester bleeding can involve the bloody show of labor, placental abruption, or placenta previa (Norwitz & Park, 2023). See Chapter 6 for assessment and management of third-trimester bleeding.

Vaginal bleeding is assessed similarly in the first or early second trimester. Use GOLDCART to determine the characteristics and amount of bleeding and pain, then follow with a primary and secondary survey. Light, irregular, painless bleeding may indicate bloody show from cervical insufficiency, a small marginal placental abruption, or a cervical or vaginal lesion (Norwitz & Park, 2023). Heavier bleeding associated with pain is suggestive of impending pregnancy loss or a large placental abruption.

As with first-trimester bleeding, speculum examination may reveal localized bleeding from cervical ectropion, laceration, infection, or other issue unrelated to the pregnancy. Pregnancy loss is usually imminent if the internal os is dilated or fetal membranes are presenting (Norwitz & Park, 2023). A sonographic scan can sometimes reveal the reason for bleeding and determine whether the fetus is still alive. Transfer clients with heavy bleeding or signs of hemodynamic instability (fever, fainting, dizziness, tachycardia, etc.) immediately to emergency hospital care.

Table 5-8

Management of Severe Early Pregnancy Bleeding in Community Settings

(Order of steps may vary)
• Airway, breathing, circulation, vital signs.
• Explain concerns to the client and family.
• Call for ambulance and implement emergency transport plan.
• If the client is hypotensive or tachycardic, start two large-bore intravenous (IV) lines of NS or Lactated Ringer's (LR), run wide.
• Administer high-flow oxygen if oxygen saturation is low.
• Consult with collaborating physician.
• Remove any tissue from the cervical os and take cultures as indicated.
• If gestation is beyond the first trimester, massage uterus to control bleeding.
• Consider oxytocin infusion or misoprostol if the client has a nonviable IUP which has been confirmed on ultrasound and the collaborating physician recommends this treatment.
• Transport rapidly to a facility with the capacity for immediate surgery.
• Chart essential data and history for the receiving facility. Fax, transmit, or hand-carry the chart to the receiving provider.

Second-trimester bleeding is associated with higher risk for PTB, preterm rupture of membranes, gestational diabetes mellitus, and polyhydramnios (Norwitz & Park, 2023). The risk of placental abruption also appears higher (Akkaya & Uysal, 2018; Ananth, Oyelese, Prasad, Getahun, & Smulian, 2006). Consequently, pregnancies complicated by second-trimester bleeding require close follow-up.

Second Trimester Fetal Demise

Second-trimester pregnancy loss is uncommon. For chromosomally and structurally normal singleton fetuses with healthy mothers, the miscarriage rate from 16–20 weeks of gestation is only about 0.6%. In individuals with first-trimester bleeding, the rate of second-trimester pregnancy loss is as high as 4.5% (Gollapalli & Gunda, 2020). Mid-trimester spontaneous pregnancy losses may be related to

- Chromosomal or structural fetal anomalies;
- Congenital uterine defects;
- Uterine fibroids;
- Cervical insufficiency;
- Placental abruption;
- Defective spiral-artery transformation;
- Chorioamnionitis;
- Maternal autoimmune or metabolic disorders; and/or
- Maternal infections.

After the diagnosis of fetal demise, many families need time to process the information before deciding on a plan. Some physicians are comfortable with performing surgical evacuation for early second-trimester losses. Surgical evacuation quickly brings the pregnancy to an end and may be

Table 5-9

Common Etiologies of Second-Trimester Bleeding

Bloody show associated with labor Cervical insufficiency Miscarriage Placenta previa Placental abruption Nontubal ectopic pregnancy (abdominal, cervical, cesarean scar, or cornual or heterotopic) Gestational trophoblastic disease Vasa previa (rare) Cervical, vaginal, or uterine polyps, inflammation, infection, or neoplasm
From "Overview of the Etiology and Evaluation of Vaginal Bleeding in Pregnancy," by E. R. Norwitz and J. S. Park, 2023, in V. A. Barss (Ed.), *UpToDate*. Copyright by UpToDate.

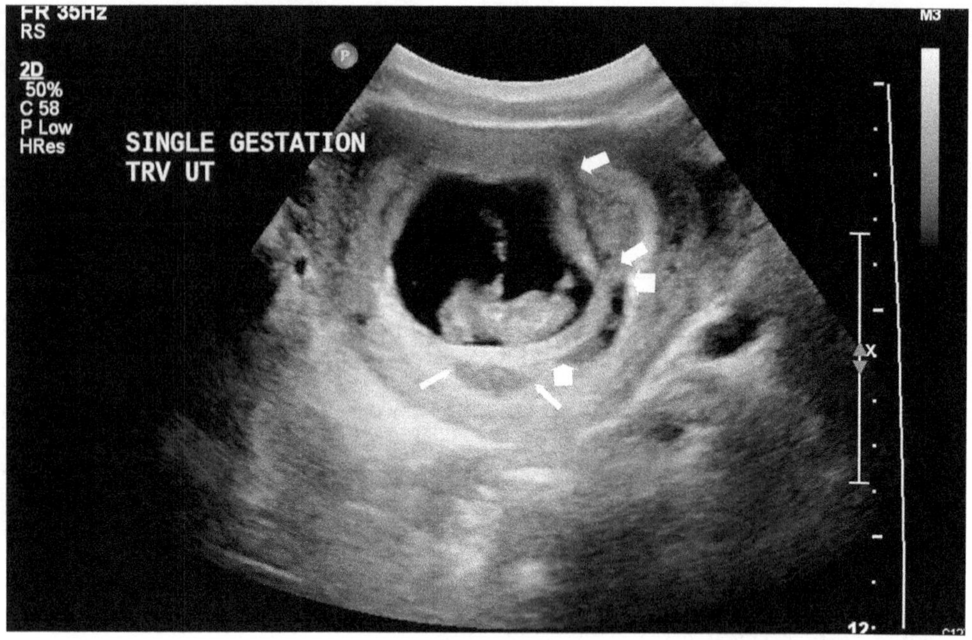

Figure 5-18. Early pregnancy ultrasound with subchorionic hematomas. The three separate collections of differing echogenicity indicate that there were three episodes of bleeding. This client presented to the midwife with bleeding several times; but the problem resolved, and the client gave birth to a healthy baby.

favored by mothers who do not wish to experience labor. It also eliminates the risk of retained placenta. Because the fetus is not intact after this procedure, induction of labor is preferred for mothers who wish to see and hold their babies.

Mothers who are stable with no medical contraindications may choose to proceed with induction of labor right away or wait days or even weeks. In most cases, clients with second-trimester demise are induced with misoprostol, with or without mifepristone, in a hospital. To induce labor for a fetal demise up to 28 weeks of gestation, ACOG suggests giving 400–600 mcg of misoprostol vaginally every 3–6 hr; lower doses are less effective (ACOG et al., 2020/2021). Potential side-effects of misoprostol include nausea, vomiting, diarrhea, fever, and shivering.

Contraindications to induction of a client with fetal demise with misoprostol include suspected or confirmed ectopic pregnancy, gestational trophoblastic disease, IUD present in the uterus (it must be removed before misoprostol is given), allergy to PGs, coagulopathy, and hemodynamic instability (Dragoman, Shannon, & Winikoff, 2023). Rarely, second-trimester induction with misoprostol causes uterine rupture, mostly in clients with more than one hysterotomy scar, a classical (vertical) or T-shaped uterine incision, or myomectomy involving incision through the fundus to the uterine cavity (Dragoman et al., 2023). Retained placenta is a common complication with second-trimester miscarriage, affecting about 25% of cases (Gómez Ponce de León, Wing, & Fiala, 2007). Placental delivery with an uncomplicated second-trimester loss can take 2 hr or more (Behrens et al., 2019). An injection of 10 units of intramuscular oxytocin (not oxytocin infusion) during the third stage of labor may decrease the likelihood of placenta retention (Kolp, Eberlein, & Kelly, 2014). Clients with fever or blood loss of 500 ml or more require prompt surgical removal of retained products (Behrens et al., 2019).

Some midwifery services have practice agreements with collaborating physicians that allow midwives to induce labor with misoprostol for first- and second-trimester losses in community settings. Because of the risk for hemorrhage, infection, and retained products of conception, these inductions should not be undertaken without first discussing the case with a collaborating physician. As always, follow the guidelines, regulations, and laws applicable to your practice.

Topics for Discussion

1. What is a molar pregnancy? How is it diagnosed, and what follow-up is necessary?
2. Katie Lynn H. had an ectopic pregnancy 3 years ago and a normal vaginal birth last year. She is pregnant again, about 5 weeks of gestation, and everything seems normal. What testing and evaluation should be considered?
3. Anyanka V. was diagnosed with a 10-week fetal demise almost 2 weeks ago and opted for expectant management. She started to bleed this morning. When the bleeding and pain grew worse this afternoon, she decided to stop by your office so you could examine her. On examination, her cervix is open, there are pieces of tissue coming through the os, and she is bleeding briskly. She is not faint or dizzy, her BP is 110/70, and her pulse is 88. How would you proceed?
4. Discuss which laboratory and/or imaging evaluations would be appropriate for a client with spotting at 8 0/7 weeks of gestation. Would these evaluations be appropriate if the client were at 5 0/7 weeks of gestation?

References

Abd Ellatif, E. M., Ahmad, A. K., & Halawa, M. A. A. (2018). Yolk sac size and shape, gestational sac diameter and embryonic heart rate as prognostic factors for first trimesteric outcome. *Egyptian Journal of Hospital Medicine, 73*(9), 7418–7428. https://doi.org/10.21608/ejhm.2018.18649

Abdel-Rahman, O., & Ghosh, S. (2022). Pregnancy and perinatal outcomes following exposure to antineoplastic agents around pregnancy within the US FDA Adverse Event Reporting System. *Future Oncology, 18*(21), 2635–2642. https://doi.org/10.2217/fon-2021-1255

Aggarwal, K. (2020). Vaginal bleeding in early pregnancy. In A. Sharma (Ed.), *Labour room emergencies* (pp. 155–161). Singapore: Springer. https://doi.org/10.1007/978-981-10-4953-8_18

Akkaya, H., & Uysal, G. (2018). Relationship between first trimester vaginal bleeding and the risk of placental abruption. *Medicine Science International Medical Journal, 7*(3), 660–683. https://doi.org/10.5455/medscience.2018.07.8776

Ali, H. Z., & Ismail, S. K. (2021). First trimester subchorionic hematoma and outcome of pregnancy. *Scholars International Journal of Obstetrics and Gynecology, 4*(7), 297–303. Retrieved from m https://saudijournals.com/media/articles/SIJOG_47_297-303_FT_8nQmfgs.pdf

Alijotas-Reig, J., Esteve-Valverde, E., Ferrer-Oliveras, R., Sáez-Comet, L., Lefkou, E., Mekinian, A., . . . Farran-Codina, I. (2019). The European Registry on Obstetric Antiphospholipid Syndrome (EUROAPS): A survey of 1000 consecutive cases. *Autoimmunity Reviews, 18*(4), 406–414. https://doi.org/10.1016/j.autrev.2018.12.006

Almahabrish, O. M., Abdelhafez, M. S., Taman, M. E., & Allakany, N. M. S. (2021). Misoprostol versus manual vacuum aspiration in treatment of missed miscarriage in first trimester. *Medical Journal of Cairo University, 89*, 1195–1200. https://doi.org/10.21608/mjcu.2021.185010

Alsibiani, S. A. (2014). Value of histopathologic examination of uterine products after first-trimester miscarriage. *BioMed Research International, 2014*. https://doi.org/10.1155/2014/863482

American College of Obstetricians and Gynecologists. (2017, reaffirmed 2021). *Prevention of Rh D alloimmunization* (Practice Bulletin 181). Retrieved from https://www.acog.org/clinical/clinical-guidance/practice-bulletin/articles/2017/08/prevention-of-rh-d-alloimmunization

American College of Obstetricians and Gynecologists. (2018, reaffirmed 2021). *Early pregnancy loss* (Practice Bulletin 200). Retrieved from https://www.acog.org/clinical/clinical-guidance/practice-bulletin/articles/2018/11/early-pregnancy-loss

American College of Obstetricians and Gynecologists. (2018, reaffirmed 2022). *Tubal ectopic pregnancy* (Practice Bulletin 193). Retrieved *from* https://www.*acog.org/clinical/clinical-guidance/practice-bulletin/articles/2018/03/tubal-ectopic-pregnancy*

American College of Obstetricians and Gynecologists. (2021, reaffirmed 2021). *Obesity in pregnancy* (Practice Bulletin 230). Retrieved from https://www.acog.org/clinical/clinical-guidance/practice-bulletin/articles/2021/06/obesity-in-pregnancy

Ananth, C. V., Oyelese, Y., Prasad, V., Getahun, D., & Smulian, J. C. (2006). Evidence of placental abruption as a chronic process: Associations with vaginal bleeding early in pregnancy and placental lesions. *European Journal of Obstetrics & Gynecology and Reproductive Biology, 128*(1–2), 15–21. https://doi.org/10.1016/j.ejogrb.2006.01.016

Anderson-Bagga, F. M., & Sze, A. (2023). Placenta previa. In *StatPearls*. Treasure Island, FL: StatPearls Publishing. Retrieved September 30, 2023, from https://www.ncbi.nlm.nih.gov/books/NBK539818/

Anderson-Berry, A. L. (2016). Vanishing twin syndrome. *Medscape*. Retrieved from http://emedicine.medscape.com/article/271818-overview

Angelini, D. J., & LaFontaine, D. (Eds.). (2013). *Obstetric triage and emergency care protocols*. New York, NY: Springer Publishing.

Asif, S., Aijawi, S., & Agten, A. K. (2021). Caesarean scar pregnancy: Diagnosis and management. *Obstetrics, Gynaecology and Reproductive Medicine, 31*(10), 271–274. https://doi.org/10.1016/j.ogrm.2021.08.001

Baergen, R. N. (2021). Gestational trophoblastic disease: Pathology. In A. Chakrabarti (Ed.), *UpToDate*. Retrieved October 1, 2023, from https://www.uptodate.com/contents/gestational-trophoblastic-disease-pathology

Baker, M., & dela Cruz, J. (2023). Ectopic pregnancy, ultrasound. In *StatPearls*. Treasure Island, FL: StatPearls Publishing. Retrieved September 30, 2023, from https://www.ncbi.nlm.nih.gov/books/NBK482192/

Barnhart, K. T., Guo, W., Cary, M. S., Morse, C., Chung, K., Takacs, P., . . . Sammel, M. D. (2016). Differences in serum human chorionic gonadotrophin rise in early pregnancy by race and value at presentation. *Obstetrics & Gynecology, 128*(3), 504–511. https://doi.org/10.1097/AOG.0000000000001568

Bastian, L. A., & Brown, H. L. (2023). Clinical manifestations and diagnosis of early pregnancy. In V. A. Barss (Ed.), *UpToDate*. Retrieved November 13, 2023, from https://www.uptodate.com/contents/clinical-manifestations-and-diagnosis-of-early-pregnancy

Behrens, J. A., Greer, D. M., Kram, J. J. F., Schmit, E., Forgie, M. M., & Salvo, N. P. (2019). Management of the third stage of labor in second-trimester deliveries: How long is too long? *European Journal of Obstetrics & Gynecology and Reproductive Biology, 232*, 22–29. https://doi.org/10.1016/j.ejogrb.2018.10.038

Benavides-Reyes, I., Reyna-Villasmi, E., Mejia-Montilla, J., Torres-Cepeda, D., Navarro-Briceño, Y., Santos-Bolívar, J., . . . Cerda, M. (2015). Subchorionic hematoma volume in the first trimester and risk of spontaneous abortion. *Revista Latinoamericana de Hipertensión, 10*(3), 56–60. Retrieved from http://saber.ucv.ve/ojs/index.php/rev_lh/article/view/11929/11639

Berkowitz, R. S., & Horowitz, N. S., & Elias, K. M. (2023a). Hydatidiform mole: Epidemiology, clinical features, and diagnosis. In A. Chakrabarti (Ed.), *UpToDate*. Retrieved October 1, 2023, from https://www.uptodate.com/contents/hydatidiform-mole-epidemiology-clinical-features-and-diagnosis

Berkowitz, R. S., & Horowitz, N. S., & Elias, K. M. (2023b). Hydatidiform mole: Treatment and follow-up. In A. Chakrabarti & S. R. Vora (Eds.), *UpToDate*. Retrieved October 1, 2023, from https://www.uptodate.com/contents/hydatidiform-mole-treatment-and-follow-up

Betts, J. G., Young, K. A., Wise, J. A., Johnson, E. Poe, B., Kruse, D. H., . . . Desaix, P. (2013). *Anatomy and physiology*. Houston, TX: OpenStax. Access for free at https://openstax.org/books/anatomy-and-physiology/pages/1-introduction

Bleicher, I., Kadour-Peero, E., Sagi-Dain, L., & Sagi, S. (2021). Early exploration of COVID-19 vaccination safety and effectiveness during pregnancy: Interim descriptive data from a prospective observational study. *Vaccine, 39*(44), 6535–6538. https://doi.org/10.1016/j.vaccine.2021.09.043

Blickstein, I. (2021). The vanishing twin syndrome. In A. Khalil, L. Lewi, & E. Lopriore (Eds.), *Twin and higher-order pregnancies* (pp. 3–9). Cham, Switzerland: Springer Nature. https://doi.org/10.1007/978-3-030-47652-6_1

Bondick, C. P., Das, J. M., & Fertel, H. (2023). Subchorionic hemorrhage. In *StatPearls*. Treasure Island, FL: StatPearls Publishing. Retrieved September 30, 2023, from https://pubmed.ncbi.nlm.nih.gov/32644443/

Bridwell, R. E., Long, B., Montrief, T., & Gottlieb, M. (2022). Post-abortion complications: A narrative review for emergency clinicians. *Western Journal of Emergency Medicine, 23*(6), 919–925. https://doi.org/0.5811/westjem.2022.8.57929

Cai, C., Vandermeer, B., Khurana, R., Nerenberg, K., Featherstone, R., Sebastianski, M., & Davenport, M. H. (2019). The impact of occupational shift work and working hours during pregnancy on health outcomes: A systematic review and meta-analysis. *American Journal of Obstetrics & Gynecology, 221*(6), 563–576. https://doi.org/10.1016/j.ajog.2019.06.051

Calhoun, D. A., & Bahr, T. (2023). Alloimmune hemolytic disease of the newborn: Postnatal diagnosis and management. In C. Armsby (Ed.), *UpToDate*. Retrieved October 1, 2023, from https://www.uptodate.com/contents/alloimmune-hemolytic-disease-of-the-newborn-postnatal-diagnosis-and-management

Chasen, S. T. (2023). Twin pregnancy: Overview. In V. A. Barss (Ed.), *UpToDate*. Retrieved October 30, 2023, from https://www.uptodate.com/contents/twin-pregnancy-overview

Chauhan, S. P., & Bhalwal, A. B. (2022). Abdominal pregnancy. In A. Chakrabarti (Ed.), *UpToDate*. Retrieved October 1, 2023, from https://www.uptodate.com/contents/abdominal-pregnancy

Chen, L.-W., Wu, Y., Neelakantan, N., Chong, M. F.-F., Pan, A., & van Dam, R. M. (2016). Maternal caffeine intake during pregnancy and risk of pregnancy loss: A categorical and dose–response meta-analysis of prospective studies. *Public Health Nutrition, 19*(7), 1233–1244. https://doi.org/10.1017/S1368980015002463

Chen, Y., Peng, P., Li, C., Teng, L., Liu, X., Liu, J., . . . Lang, J. (2023). Abdominal pregnancy: A case report and review of 17 cases. *Archives of Gynecology and Obstetrics, 307*(1), 263–274. https://doi.org/10.1007%2Fs00404-022-06570-9

Ciebiera, M., Wojtyła, C., Jakiel, G., & Roszkowski, T. (2018). Molar pregnancy with a coexisting live fetus as a challenge for perinatology: A mini-review with two case reports. *Journal of Health Inequalities, 4*(1), 39–45. https://doi.org/10.5114/jhi.2018.77649

Connolly, A., Ryan, D. H., Stuebe, A. M., & Wolfe, H. M. (2013). Reevaluation of discriminatory and threshold levels for serum β-hCG in early pregnancy. *Obstetrics & Gynecology, 121*(1), 65–70. https://doi.org/10.1097/aog.0b013e318278f421

Coomarasamy, A., Devall, A. J., Cheed, V., Harb, H., Middleton, L. J., Gallos, I. D., . . . Jurkovic, D. (2019). A randomized trial of progesterone in women with bleeding in early pregnancy. *New England Journal of Medicine, 380*(19), 1815–1824. https://doi.org/10.1056/NEJMoa1813730

Creanga, A. A., Catalano, P. M., & Bateman, B. T. (2022). Obesity in pregnancy. *New England Journal of Medicine, 387*(3), 248–259. https://doi.org/10.1056/NEJMra1801040

Cunningham, F. G., Leveno, K. J., Dashe, J. S., Hoffman, B. L., Spong, C. Y., & Casey, B. M. (Eds.). (2022). *Williams obstetrics* (26th ed., Kindle version). New York, NY: McGraw-Hill.

Dahdouh, E. M., & Kutteh, W. H. (2021). Genetic testing of products of conception in recurrent pregnancy loss evaluation. *Reproductive BioMedicine Online, 43*(1), 120–126. https://doi.org/10.1016/j.rbmo.2021.03.015

Dawodu, O., Wu, J. B. S.; Gallop, R., & Barnhart, K. T. (2022). Perinatal outcomes of pregnancies of unknown location with human chorionic gonadotropin concentration above the discriminatory zone. *Obstetrics & Gynecology, 140*(5), 793–795. https://doi.org/10.1097/AOG.0000000000004939

Dean, L. (2005). *Blood groups and red cell antigens*. Bethesda, MD: National Center for Biotechnology Information. Retrieved from https://www.ncbi.nlm.nih.gov/books/NBK2270/

Deng, T., Liao, X., & Zhu, S. (2022). Recent advances in treatment of recurrent spontaneous abortion. *Obstetrical & Gynecological Survey, 77*(6), 355–366. https://doi.org/10.1097/OGX.0000000000001033

Doubilet, P. M., & Benson, C. B. (2005). Outcome of first-trimester pregnancies with slow embryonic heart rate at 6–7 weeks gestation and normal heart rate by 8 weeks at US. *Radiology, 236*(2), 643–646. https://doi.org/10.1148/radiol.2362040880

Doubilet, P. M., Benson, C. B., Bourne, T., & Blaivas, M. (2013). Diagnostic criteria for nonviable pregnancy early in the first trimester. *New England Journal of Medicine, 369*, 1443–1451. https://doi.org/10.1056/NEJMra1302417

Doubilet, P. M., Benson, C. B., & Chow, J. S. (1999). Long-term prognosis of pregnancies complicated by slow embryonic heart rates in the early first trimester. *Journal of Ultrasound in Medicine, 18*(8), 537–541. https://doi.org/10.7863/jum.1999.18.8.537

Dragoman, M., Shannon, C., & Winikoff, B. (2023). Misoprostol as a single agent for medical termination of pregnancy. In A. Chakrabarti (Ed.), *UpToDate*. Retrieved October 1, 2023, from https://www.uptodate.com/contents/misoprostol-as-a-single-agent-for-medical-termination-of-pregnancy

Drvgaikwad [Vilas Gayakwad]. (2010, February 26). *Ruptured ectopic pregnancy* [Photograph]. Retrieved from https://commons.wikimedia.org/wiki/File:Ruptured_ectopic_pregnancy.jpg

Dvash, S., Cuckle, H., Smorgick, N., Vaknin, Z., Padoa, A., & Maymon, R. (2021). Increase rate of ruptured tubal ectopic pregnancy during the COVID-19 pandemic. *European Journal of Obstetrics & Gynecology and Reproductive Biology, 259*, 95–99. https://doi.org/10.1016/j.ejogrb.2021.01.054

Ellsworth Bowers, E. R., & Kitzman, M. E. (2024). Pregnancy-related conditions. In J. Phillippi & I. Kantrowitz-Gordon (Eds.), *Varney's midwifery* (7th ed., Kindle version, ch. 23). Burlington, MA: Jones & Bartlett Learning.

Eschenbach, D. A. (2015). Treating spontaneous and induced septic abortions. *Obstetrics & Gynecology, 125*(5), 1042–1048. https://doi.org/10.1097/AOG.0000000000000795

Farquharson, R. G., Jauniaux, E., & Exalto, N. (2005). Updated and revised nomenclature for description of early pregnancy events. *Human Reproduction, 20*(11), 3008–3011. https://doi.org/10.1093/humrep/dei167

Farren, J., Jalmbrant, M., Falconieri, N., Mitchell-Jones, N., Bobdiwala, S., Al-Memar, M., . . . Bourne, T. (2020). Posttraumatic stress, anxiety and depression following miscarriage and ectopic pregnancy: A multicenter, prospective, cohort study. *American Journal of Obstetrics & Gynecology, 222*(4), 367.e1–367.e22. https://doi.org/10.1016/j.ajog.2019.10.102

Findley, P. (1905). *The diagnosis of diseases of women: A treatise for students and practitioners* (2nd ed.). Philadelphia, PA: Lea Brothers. Retrieved from https://books.google.com/books/about/The_Diagnosis_of_Diseases_of_Women.html?id=yxM1AQAAMAAJ

Finlinson, A. R., Bollig, K. J., & Schust, D. J. (2020). Differentiating pregnancies near the uterotubal junction (angular, cornual, and interstitial): A review and recommendations. *Fertility Research and Practice, 6*, 8. https://doi.org/10.1186/s40738-020-00077-0

Fu, W., Sivajohan, B., McClymont, E., Albert, A., Elwood, C., Ogilvie, G., & Money, D. (2022). Systematic review of the safety, immunogenicity, and effectiveness of COVID-19 vaccines in pregnant and lactating individuals and their infants. *International Journal of Gynecology & Obstetrics, 156*(3), 406–417. https://doi.org/10.1002/ijgo.14008

Gemzell-Danielsson, K., Fiala, C., & Weeks, A. (2007). Misoprostol: First-line therapy for incomplete miscarriage in the developing world. *BJOG, 114*(11), 1337–1339. https://doi.org/10.1111/j.1471-0528.2007.01491.x

George, R., Powers, E., & Gunby, R. (2021). Abdominal ectopic pregnancy. *Baylor University Medical Center Proceedings, 34*(4), 530–531. https://doi.org/10.1080/08998280.2021.1884932

Gersh, B. J. (2022). Maternal adaptations to pregnancy: Cardiovascular and hemodynamic changes. In V. A. Barss (Ed.), *UpToDate*. Retrieved October 1, 2023, from https://www.uptodate.com/contents/maternal-adaptations-to-pregnancy-cardiovascular-and-hemodynamic-changes/print

Ghaedi, B., Cheng, W., Ameri, S., Abdulkarim, K., Costain, N., Zia, A., & Thiruganasambandamoorthy, V. (2022). Performance of single serum progesterone in the evaluation of symptomatic first-trimester pregnant patients: a systematic review and meta-analysis. *Canadian Journal of Emergency Medicine, 24*(6), 1–11. https://doi.org/10.1007/s43678-022-00332-x

Giakoumelou, S., Wheelhouse, N., Cuschieri, K., Entrican, G., Howie, S. E. M., & Horne, A. W. (2016). The role of infection in miscarriage. *Human Reproduction Update, 22*(1), 116–133. https://doi.org/10.1093/humupd/dmv041

Gollapalli, S., & Gunda, J. (2020). Pregnancy outcome in women with first-trimester bleeding per vaginum. *International Journal of Clinical Obstetrics and Gynaecology, 4*(2), 321–323. https://doi.org/10.33545/gynae.2020.v4.i2f.544

Gómez Ponce de León, R., Wing, D., & Fiala, C. (2007). Misoprostol for intrauterine fetal death. *International Journal of Gynecology & Obstetrics, 99*(Suppl. 2), S190–193. https://doi.org/10.1016/j.ijgo.2007.09.010

Grauerholz, K. R., Berry, S. N., Capuano, R. M., & Early, J. M. (2021). Uncovering prolonged grief reactions subsequent to a reproductive loss: Implications for the primary care provider. *Frontiers in Psychology, 12*. https://doi.org/10.3389/fpsyg.2021.673050

Grimes, D. A. (2003). Unsafe abortion: The silent scourge. *British Medical Bulletin, 67*(1), 99–113. https://doi.org/10.1093/bmb/ldg002

Gull, B., Klerelid, V., Jormeus, A., & Strandell, A. (2021). Potential risk factors for caesarean scar pregnancy: A retrospective case–control study. *Human Reproduction Open, 2021*(2). https://doi.org/10.1093/hropen/hoab019

Günay, T., & Yardımcı, O. D. (2022). How does subchorionic hematoma in the first trimester affect pregnancy outcomes? *Archives of Medical Science, 18*(3), 639–646. https://doi.org/10.5114/aoms/113645

Häggström, M. (2014). Medical gallery of Mikael Häggström 2014. *WikiJournal of Medicine, 1* (2). https://doi.org/10.15347/wjm/2014.008

Hamilton, E. G. (1991). Rh° (D) immunoglobulin (Rh°Gam): How it came into being. *Obstetrics & Gynecology, 77*(6), 957–958. Retrieved from https://journals.lww.com/greenjournal/Citation/1991/06000/RH___D___IMMUNOGLOBULIN__RHOGAM___HOW_IT_CAME_INTO.34.aspx

Hammond, C. (2023). Second trimester pregnancy termination: Induction (medication) termination. In A Chakrabarti (Ed.), *UpToDate*. Retrieved October 1, 2023, from http://www.uptodate.com/contents/second-trimester-pregnancy-termination-induction-medication-termination

Hancock, A., Weeks, A. D., & Tina, L. D. (2019). Assessing blood loss in clinical practice. *Best Practice & Research Clinical Obstetrics & Gynaecology, 61*, 28–40. https://doi.org/10.1016/j.bpobgyn.2019.04.004

Harris, L. H., & Grossman, D. (2020). Complications of unsafe and self-managed abortion. *New England Journal of Medicine, 382*(11), 1029–1040. https://doi.org/10.1056/NEJMra1908412

Harvey, R. A. (2023). Human chorionic gonadotropin: Biochemistry and measurement in pregnancy and disease. In A. Chakrabarti (Ed.), *UpToDate*. Retrieved October 1, 2023, from https://www.uptodate.com/contents/human-chorionic-gonadotropin-biochemistry-and-measurement-in-pregnancy-and-disease

Hasson, J., Tsafrir, Z., Azem, F., Bar-On, S., Almog, B., Mashiach, R., . . . Grisaru, D. (2010). Comparison of adnexal torsion between pregnant and nonpregnant women. *American Journal of Obstetrics & Gynecology, 202*(6), 536.e1–536.e6. https://doi.org/10.1016/j.ajog.2009.11.028

Healsmith, S., Savoia, H., & Kane, S. C. (2019). How clinically important are non-D Rh antibodies? *Acta Obstetricia et Gynecologica Scandinavica, 98*(7), 877–884.https://doi.org/10.1111/aogs.13555

Hendriks, E., MacNaughton, H., & MacKenzie, M. C. (2019). First trimester bleeding: Evaluation and management. *American Family Physician, 99*(3), 166–174. Retrieved from https://www.aafp.org/pubs/afp/issues/2019/0201/p166.html

Hendriks, E., Rosenberg, R., & Prine, L. (2020). Ectopic pregnancy: diagnosis and management. *American Family Physician, 101*(10), 599–606. https://doi.org/https://www.aafp.org/pubs/afp/issues/2020/0515/p599.html

Herchelroath, D., Miller, J. L., & Wang, K. C. (2018). Novel management of ectopic pregnancy in a noncommunicating rudimentary horn of a unicornuate uterus. *Journal of Osteopathic Medicine, 118*(9), 623–626. https://doi.org/10.7556/jaoa.2018.137

Horvath, S., Goyal, V., Traxler, S., & Prager, S. (2022). Society of Family Planning committee consensus on Rh testing in early pregnancy. *Contraception, 114*, 1–5. https://doi.org/10.1016/j.contraception.2022.07.002

Hunter, M. I., Monk, B. J., & Tewari, K. S. (2008). Cervical neoplasia in pregnancy. Part 1: Screening and management of preinvasive disease. *American Journal of Obstetrics & Gynecology, 199*(1), 3–9. https://doi.org/10.1016/j.ajog.2008.04.010

Huszti, A. M., Gica, N., Botezatu, R., Peltecu, G., & Panaitescu, A. M. (2022). Hemolytic disease of the newborn, beyond the Rhesus disease. *Romanian Medical Journal, 69*(2), 45–49. https://doi.org/10.37897/RMJ.2022.2.1

Isoardi, K. (2009). The use of pelvic examination within the emergency department in the assessment of early pregnancy bleeding. *Emergency Medicine Australasia, 21*(6), 440–448. https://doi.org/10.1111/j.1742-6723.2009.01227.x

Iyoke, C. A., Okafor, C. N., Ugwu, G. O., & Oforbuike, C. (2014). Live birth following a term pregnancy in a non-communicating rudimentary horn of a unicornuate uterus. *Annals of Medical and Health Sciences Research, 4*(1), 126–128. Retrieved from https://www.amhsr.org/articles/live-birth-following-a-term-pregnancy-in-a-noncommunicating-rudimentary-horn-of-a-unicornuate-uterus.html

Jackson, T., & Watkins, E. (2021). Early pregnancy loss. *Journal of the American Academy of Physician Assistants, 34* (3), 22–27. https://doi.org/10.1097/01.JAA.0000733216.66078.ac

Jana, N., Santra, D., Das, D., Das, A. K., & Dasgupta, S. (2008). Nonobstetric lower genital tract injuries in rural India. *International Journal of Gynecology & Obstetrics, 103*(1), 26–29. https://doi.org/10.1016/j.ijgo.2008.04.026

Jauniaux, E., Johns, J., & Burton, G. J. (2005). The role of ultrasound imaging in diagnosing and investigating early pregnancy failure. *Ultrasound in Obstetrics & Gynecology, 25*(6), 613–624. https://doi.org/10.1002/uog.1892

Jauniaux, E. R. M., & Simpson, J. L. (2022). Pregnancy loss. In D. A. Driscoll, V. Berghella, W. A. Grobman, . . . A. G. Cahill (Eds.), *Gabbe's obstetrics: Normal and problem pregnancies* (8th ed., Kindle version, ch. 33). Philadelphia, PA: Elsevier.

John, S., Sreedevi, N. P. S. B., & John, R. (2022). Threatened miscarriage and adverse fetomaternal outcome late in pregnancy—A prospective study. *Journal of South Asian Federation of Obstetrics and Gynaecology, 14*(4), 387–392.

Johns, J., Hyett, J., & Jauniaux, E. (2003). Obstetric outcome after threatened miscarriage with and without a hematoma on ultrasound. *Obstetrics & Gynecology, 102*(3), 483–487. https://doi.org/10.1016/s0029-7844(03)00580-5

Kalogiannidis, I., Kalinderi, K., Kalinderis, M., Miliaras, D., Tarlatzis, B., & Athanasiadis, A. (2018). Recurrent complete hydatidiform mole: Where we are, is there a safe gestational horizon? *Journal of Assisted Reproduction and Genetics, 35*(6), 967–973. https://doi.org/10.1007/s10815-018-1202-9

Kashi, P. K., Welch, E., Presti, C. L., Tabbarah, R., & Dengler, K. L. (2022). Minimally invasive abdominal curettage for an intramural twin pregnancy: A new twist to the traditional D&C. *American Journal of Obstetrics & Gynecology, 226*(3, Suppl.), S1362. https://doi.org/10.1016/j.ajog.2021.12.204

Kim, M. J., & Farrell, J. (2022). Orthostatic hypotension: A practical approach. *American Family Physician, 105*(1), 39–49. Retrieved from https://www.aafp.org/pubs/afp/issues/2022/0100/p39.html

Kjaersgaard, M. I. S., Parner, E. T., Vestergaard, M., Sørensen, M. J., Olsen, J., Christensen, J., . . . Pedersen, L. H. (2013). Prenatal antidepressant exposure and risk of spontaneous abortion—A population-based study. *PloS ONE, 8*(8), e72095. https://doi.org/10.1371/journal.pone.0072095

Kokou-Kpolou, K., Megalakaki, O., & Nieuviarts, N. (2018). Persistent depressive and grief symptoms for up to 10 years following perinatal loss: Involvement of negative cognitions. *Journal of Affective Disorders, 241*, 360–366. https://doi.org/10.1016/j.jad.2018.08.063

Kolp, C. Z., Eberlein, D., & Kelly, R. B. (2014). In patients undergoing induction for a second-trimester fetal demise, does the use of high-dose oxytocin reduce the incidence of retained placenta? *Evidence-Based Practice, 17*(10), 11. https://doi.org/10.1097/01.EBP.0000540795.87671.08

Krishnan, S., Kaur, H., Bali, J., & Rao, K. (2011). Ovarian torsion in infertility management—Missing the diagnosis means losing the ovary: A high price to pay. *Journal of Human Reproductive Sciences, 4*(1), 39–42. https://doi.org/10.4103/0974-1208.82359

Laufer, M. R. (2023). Benign cervical lesions and congenital anomalies of the cervix. In A. Chakrabarti (Ed.), *UpToDate*. Retrieved October 1, 2023, from https://www.uptodate.com/contents/benign-cervical-lesions-and-congenital-anomalies-of-the-cervix

Laufer, M. R., & Makai, G. (2023). Evaluation and management of female lower genital tract trauma. In A. Chakrabarti (Ed.), *UpToDate*. Retrieved October 1, 2023, from https://www.uptodate.com/contents/evaluation-and-management-of-female-lower-genital-tract-trauma

Lin, M., Chen, J., Liao, B., He, Z., Lin, S., & Luo, Y. (2021). When a vesicular placenta meets a live fetus: case report of twin pregnancy with a partial hydatidiform mole. *BMC Pregnancy and Childbirth, 21*, 694. https://doi.org/10.1186/s12884-021-04160-2

Lopez, H. N., Focseneanu, M. A., & Merritt, D. F. (2018). Genital injuries acute evaluation and management. *Best Practice & Research Clinical Obstetrics & Gynaecology, 48*, 28–39. https://doi.org/10.1016/j.bpobgyn.2017.09.009

Lovelace, D. (2016). Congenital uterine anomalies and uterine rupture. *Journal of Midwifery & Women's Health, 61(4), 501–506.* https://doi.org/10.1111/jmwh.12423

Lyons, P. (2020). Early pregnancy bleeding. In P. Lyons & N. McLaughlin (Eds.), *Obstetrics in family medicine: A practical guide* (3rd ed., ch. 10). Cham, Switzerland: Humana Press. https://doi.org/10.1007/978-3-030-39888-0_10

Maayan-Metzger, A., Schwartz, T., Sulkes, J., & Merlob, P. (2001). Maternal anti-D prophylaxis during pregnancy does not cause neonatal haemolysis. *Archives of Disease in Childhood—Fetal and Neonatal Edition, 84*(1), F60-F62. https://doi.org/10.1136/fn.84.1.f60

Macaluso, C. R., & McNamara, R. M. (2012). Evaluation and management of acute abdominal pain in the emergency department. *International Journal of General Medicine, 5*, 789–797. https://doi.org/10.2147/IJGM.S25936

MacKenzie, A. P., Stephenson, C. D., & Funai, E. F. (2023). Prenatal assessment of gestational age, date of delivery, and fetal weight. In V. A. Barss (Ed.), *UpToDate*. Retrieved October 1, 2023, from https://www.uptodate.com/contents/prenatal-assessment-of-gestational-age-date-of-delivery-and-fetal-weight

Magnus, M. C., Morken, N.-H., Wensaas, K.-A., Wilcox, A. J., & Håberg, S. E. (2021). Risk of miscarriage in women with chronic diseases in Norway: A registry linkage study. *PloS Medicine, 18*(5), e1003603. https://doi.org/10.1371/journal.pmed.1003603

Malacova, E., Kemp, A., Hart, R., Jama-Alol, K., & Preen, D. B. (2014). Long-term risk of ectopic pregnancy varies by method of tubal sterilization: A whole-population study. *Fertility and Sterility, 101*(3), 728–734. https://doi.org/10.1016/j.fertnstert.2013.11.127

Maso, G., D'Ottavio, G., De Seta, F., Sartore, A., Piccoli, M., & Mandruzzato, G. (2005). First-trimester intrauterine hematoma and outcome of pregnancy. *Obstetrics & Gynecology, 105*(2), 339–344. https://doi.org/10.1097/01.AOG.0000152000.71369.bd

McCormick, A., & Peterson, E. (2018). Cancer in pregnancy. *Obstetrics and Gynecology Clinics of North America, 45*(2), 187–200. https://doi.org/10.1016/j.ogc.2018.01.009

McNamara, H. C., Kane, S. C., Craig, J. M., Short, R. V., & Umstad, M. P. (2016). A review of the mechanisms and evidence for typical and atypical twinning. *American Journal of Obstetrics & Gynecology, 214*(2), 172–191. https://doi.org/10.1016/j.ajog.2015.10.930

Melcer, Y., Maymon, R., Vaknin, Z., Pansky, M., Mendlovic, S., Barel, O., & Smorgick, N. (2016). Primary ovarian ectopic pregnancy: Still a medical challenge. *Journal of Reproductive Medicine, 61*(1–2), 58–62. Retrieved from https://pubmed.ncbi.nlm.nih.gov/26995890/

Mergl, R., Quaatz, S. M., Edeler, L.-M., & Allgaier, A.-K. (2022). Grief in women with previous miscarriage or stillbirth: A systematic review of cross-sectional and longitudinal prospective studies. *European Journal of Psychotraumatology, 13*(2), 2108578. https://doi.org/10.1080/20008066.2022.2108578

Moise, K. J., Jr. (2022). RhD alloimmunization: Prevention in pregnant and postpartum patients. In V. A. Barss (Ed.), *UpToDate*. Retrieved October 1, 2023, from https://www.uptodate.com/contents/rhd-alloimmunization-prevention-in-pregnant-and-postpartum-patients

Moumna, S., El Ghorfi, S., El Haddad, S., Allali, N., & Chat, L. (2020). Intramural gestation: A rare localization of ectopic pregnancy. *International Journal of Case Reports and Images, 11*. https://doi.org/10.5348/101087z01sm2020cr

Muanda, F. T., Sheehy, O., & Bérard, A. (2017). Use of antibiotics during pregnancy and risk of spontaneous abortion. *CMAJ,189*(17), E625–E633. https://doi.org/10.1503/cmaj.161020

Mukherjee, S., Velez Edwards, D. R., Baird, D. D., Savitz, D. A., & Hartmann, K. E. (2013). Risk of miscarriage among black women and white women in a US prospective cohort study. *American Journal of Epidemiology, 177*(11), 1271–1278. https://doi.org/10.1093/aje/kws393

Munro Kerr, J. M. (1911). *Operative midwifery: A guide to the difficulties and complications of midwifery practice* (2nd ed.). New York, NY: William Wood. Retrieved from https://archive.org/details/operativemidwife00munr

Murugan, V. A., Murphy, B. O., Dupuis, C., Goldstein, A., & Kim, Y. H. (2020). Role of ultrasound in the evaluation of first-trimester pregnancies in the acute setting. *Ultrasonography, 39*(2), 178–189. https://doi.org/10.14366/usg.19043

Na, E. D., Jung, I., Choi, D. H., Kwon, H., Heo, S. J., Kim, H. C., . . . Cho, H. (2018). The risk factors of miscarriage and obstetrical outcomes of intrauterine normal pregnancy following heterotopic pregnancy management. *Medicine, 97*(37), e12233. https://doi.org/10.1097/MD.0000000000012233

Naert, M. N., Khadraoui, H., Muniz Rodriguez, A., Naqvi, M., & Fox, N. S. (2019). Association between first-trimester subchorionic hematomas and pregnancy loss in singleton pregnancies. *Obstetrics & Gynecology, 134*(2). 276–281. https://doi.org/10.1097/AOG.0000000000003360

Naert, M. N., Muniz Rodriguez, A., Khadraoui, H., Naqvi, M., & Fox, N. S. (2019). Association between first-trimester subchorionic hematomas and adverse pregnancy outcomes after 20 weeks of gestation in singleton pregnancies. *Obstetrics & Gynecology, 134*(4), 863–868. https://doi.org/10.1097/AOG.0000000000003487

Namagembe, I., Nakimuli, A., Byamugisha, J., Moffett, A., Aiken, A., & Aiken, C. (2022). Preventing death following unsafe abortion: A case series from urban Uganda. *AJOG Global Reports, 2*(1), 100039. https://doi.org/10.1016/j.xagr.2021.100039

National Abortion Federation. (2022). 2022 *Clinical policy guidelines for abortion care*. n.p.: Author. Retrieved from https://prochoice.org/providers/quality-standards/

Nguyen, B. T., Chang, E. J., & Bendikson, K. A. (2019). Advanced paternal age and the risk of spontaneous abortion: An analysis of the combined 2011–2013 and 2013–2015 National Survey of Family Growth. *American Journal of Obstetrics & Gynecology, 221*(5), 476.e1–476.e7. https://doi.org/10.1016/j.ajog.2019.05.028

Norwitz, E. R., & Park, J. S. (2023). Evaluation and differential diagnosis of vaginal bleeding before 20 weeks of gestation. In V. A. Barss (Ed.), *UpToDate*.

Retrieved October 1, 2023, from https://www.uptodate.com/contents/evaluation-and-differential-diagnosis-of-vaginal-bleeding-before-20-weeks-of-gestation

Nybo Andersen, A. M., Wohlfahrt, J., Christens, P., Olsen, J., & Melbye, M. (2000). Maternal age and fetal loss: Population based register linkage study. *BMJ, 320*(1751), 1708–1712. https://doi.org/10.1136/bmj.320.7251.1708

Olofinbiyi, B. A., Ige, J. T., Olaogun, O. D., Alao, O. O., Adewumi, O. A., & Olofinbiyi, R. O. (2019). A stone age conduct of unsafe abortion in adolescent: Complicated by gangrenous uterus and bowel. *Tropical Journal of Obstetrics and Gynaecology, 36*(2), 315–318. https://doi.org/10.4103/TJOG.TJOG_15_19

Özkaya, E., Altay, M., & Gelişen, O. (2011). Significance of subchorionic haemorrhage and pregnancy outcome in threatened miscarriage to predict miscarriage, pre-term labour and intrauterine growth restriction. *Journal of Obstetrics and Gynaecology, 31*(3), 210–212. https://doi.org/10.3109/01443615.2010.545899

Özler, S., & Güler, B. G. (2019). Does the measurement of the size of the first trimester subchorionic hematoma by 2D and 3D ultrasonographic techniques have any effect on adverse pregnancy outcomes? *Archives of Clinical and Experimental Medicine, 4*(3), 122–126. https://doi.org/10.25000/acem.586513

Panaitescu, A. M., Ciobanu, A. M., Gică, N., Peltecu, G., & Botezatu, R. (2021). Diagnosis and management of cesarean scar pregnancy and placenta accreta spectrum. *Journal of Ultrasound in Medicine, 40*(9), 1975–1986. https://doi.org/10.1002/jum.15574

Pedersen, J. F., & Mantoni, M. (1990). Large intrauterine haematomata in threatened miscarriage: Frequency and clinical consequences. *BJOG, 97*(1), 552–553. https://doi.org/10.1111/j.1471-0528.1990.tb01720.x

Phillips, F., Saxby, F. (2019). Complications in Early Pregnancy. In D. Holloway (Ed.), *Nursing management of women's health* (pp. 127–152). Cham, Switzerland: Springer Nature. https://doi.org/10.1007/978-3-030-16115-6_7

Polgar, S., & Fried, E. S. (1976). The bad old days: Clandestine abortions among the poor in New York City before liberalization of the abortion law. *Family Planning Perspectives, 8*(3), 125–127. Retrieved from https://www.jstor.org/stable/2133634

Poornima, J. K., Vijayalakshmi, K., Anuradha, C. R., & Sailatha, R. (2020). Efficacy of first trimester sonographic parameters—Yolk sac diameter and embryonic heart rate in predicting pregnancy outcome till mid pregnancy. *Annals of Tropical Medicine and Public Health, 23*(20). Retrieved from https://web.archive.org/web/20210504022034id_/https://www.journal.atmph-specialissues.org/uploads/179/8788_pdf.pdf

Poureisa, M., Ajiri, A. H., Fouladi, D. F., Sayah Melli, M., Ghojazadeh, M., & Hagigi, A. (2014). 'Anteroposterior placenta': A novel, simple sonographic feature indicating benign vaginal bleeding in early pregnancy. *Journal of Obstetrics and Gynaecology, 34*(4), 305–308. https://doi.org/10.3109/01443615.2013.870139

Powell, A. M., & Nyirjesy, P. (2022). Acute cervicitis. In K. Eckler (Ed.), *UpToDate*. Retrieved October 1, 2023, from https://www.uptodate.com/contents/acute-cervicitis

Prager, S., Micks, E., & Dalton V. K. (2023a). Pregnancy loss (miscarriage): Clinical presentations, diagnosis, and initial evaluation. In K. Eckler (Ed.), *UpToDate*. Retrieved October 1, 2023, from https://www.uptodate.com/contents/pregnancy-loss-miscarriage-clinical-presentations-diagnosis-and-initial-evaluation

Prager, S., Micks, E., & Dalton V. K. (2023b). Pregnancy loss (miscarriage): Counseling and comparison of treatment options and discussion of related care. In K. Eckler (Ed.), *UpToDate*. Retrieved October 1, 2023, from https://www.uptodate.com/contents/pregnancy-loss-miscarriage-counseling-and-comparison-of-treatment-options-and-discussion-of-related-care

Prager, S., Micks, E., & Dalton V. K. (2023c). Pregnancy loss (miscarriage): Description of management techniques. In K. Eckler (Ed.), *UpToDate*. Retrieved October 1, 2023, from https://www.uptodate.com/contents/pregnancy-loss-miscarriage-description-of-management-techniques

Prager, S., Micks, E., & Dalton V. K. (2023d). Pregnancy loss (miscarriage): Terminology, risk factors, and etiology. In K. Eckler (Ed.), *UpToDate*. Retrieved October 1, 2023, from https://www.uptodate.com/contents/pregnancy-loss-miscarriage-terminology-risk-factors-and-etiology

Quenby, S., Gallos, I. D., Dhillon-Smith, R. K., Podesek, M., Stephenson, M. D., Fisher, J., . . . Coomarasamy, A. (2021). Miscarriage matters: The epidemiological, physical, psychological, and economic costs of early pregnancy loss. *Lancet, 397*(10285), 1658–1667. https://doi.org/10.1016/S0140-6736(21)00682-6

Rangel, E. L., Castillo-Angeles, M., Easter, S. R., Atkinson, R. B., Gosain, A., Hu, Y. Y., . . . Kim, E. (2021). Incidence of infertility and pregnancy complications in US female surgeons. *JAMA Surgery, 156*(10), 905–915. https://doi.org/10.1001/jamasurg.2021.3301

Ravishankar, S. (2022). *Grossing—products of conception*. Retrieved from https://www.pathologyoutlines.com/topic/placentagrossingPOC.html

Royal College of Obstetricians and Gynaecologists. (2022). *Best practice in abortion care*. London, United Kingdom: Author. Retrieved from www.rcog.org.uk/media/geify5bx/abortion-care-best-practice-paper-april-2022.pdf

Schaeffer, O. (1901). *Anatomical atlas of obstetrics with special reference to diagnosis and treatment*. Philadephia, PA: W. B. Saunders. Retrieved from https://babel.hathitrust.org/cgi/pt?id=uc1.b3717762

Schliep, K. C., Mitchell, E. M., Mumford, S. L., Radin, R. G., Zarek, S. M., Sjaarda, L., & Schisterman, E. F. (2016). Trying to conceive after an early pregnancy loss: An assessment on how long couples should wait. *Obstetrics & Gynecology, 127*(2), 204–212. https://doi.org/10.1097/AOG.0000000000001159

Schreiber, C. A., Creinin, M. D., Atrio, J., Sonalkar, S., Ratcliffe, S. J., & Barnhart, K. T. (2018). Mifepristone pretreatment for the medical management of early pregnancy loss. *New England Journal of Medicine, 378*(23), 2161–2170. https://doi.org/10.1056/NEJMoa1715726

Schwartz, D. A. (2013). Challenges in improvement of perinatal health in developing nations: Role of perinatal pathology. *Archives of Pathology & Laboratory Medicine, 137*(6), 742–746. https://doi.org/10.5858/arpa.2012-0089-ED

Shaker, M., & Smith, A. (2022). First trimester miscarriage. *Obstetrics and Gynecology Clinics of North America, 49*(3), 623–635. https://doi.org/10.1016/j.ogc.2022.04.004

Sharma, R., & Sharma, S. (2023). Physiology, blood volume. In *StatPearls*. Treasure Island, FL: StatPearls Publishing. Retrieved September 30, 2023, from https://www.ncbi.nlm.nih.gov/books/NBK526077/

Sloin, M. M., Karimian, M., & Ilbeigi, P. (2006). *Journal of the American Osteopathic Association, 106*(5), 271–273. Retrieved from http://jaoa.org/article.aspx?articleid=2093273

Smith, H. O., Qualls, C. R., Prairie, B. A., Padilla, L. A., Rayburn, W. F., & Key, C. R. (2003). Trends in gestational choriocarcinoma: A 27-year perspective. *Obstetrics & Gynecology, 102*(5, Pt. 1), 978–987. https://doi.org/10.1016/s0029-7844(03)00669-0

Soper, J. T. (2021). Gestational trophoblastic disease: Current evaluation and management. *Obstetrics & Gynecology, 137*(2), 355–370. https://doi.org/10.1097/AOG.0000000000004240

Tarney, C. M., & Han, J. (2014). Postcoital bleeding: A review on etiology, diagnosis, and management. *Obstetrics and Gynecology International, 2014*. https://doi.org/10.1155/2014/192087

Tchuenkam, L. W., Mbonda, A. N., Tochie, J. N., Mbem-Ngos, P. P., Noah-Ndzie, H. G., & Bang, G. A. (2021). Transvaginal strangulated bowel evisceration through uterine perforation due to unsafe abortion: A case report and literature review. *BMC Women's Health, 21*, 98. https://doi.org/10.1186/s12905-021-01247-y

Tesemma, M. G. (2019). Pregnancy in noncommunicating rudimentary horn of unicornuate uterus: A case report and review of the literature. *Case Reports in Obstetrics and Gynecology, 2019.* https://doi.org/10.1155/2019/1489751

Thakkar, M., Dinglas, C., & Rosner, J. (2022). Does vaginal bleeding in the presence of a subchorionic hematoma increase adverse pregnancy outcomes? *Obstetrics & Gynecology, 139* (Suppl.), 82S. https://doi.org/10.1097/01.AOG.0000825692.64605.a1

Thorstensen, K. A. (2000). Midwifery management of first trimester bleeding and early pregnancy loss. *Journal of Midwifery & Women's Health, 45*(6), 481–497. https://doi.org/10.1016/S1526-9523(00)00071-4

Timor-Tritsch, I. E. (2023). Cesarean scar pregnancy. In A. Chakrabarti (Ed.), *UpToDate*. Retrieved October 1, 2023, from https://www.uptodate.com/contents/cesarean-scar-pregnancy

Trad, M., & Palmer, S. (2013). Müllerian duct anomalies and a case study of unicornuate uterus. *Radiologic Technology, 84*(6), 571–576. Retrieved from http://www.radiologictechnology.org/content/84/6/571.abstract

Tulandi, T. (2023a). Cervical pregnancy: Diagnosis and management. In A. Chakrabarti (Ed.), *UpToDate*. Retrieved October 1, 2023, from https://www.uptodate.com/contents/cervical-pregnancy-diagnosis-and-management

Tulandi, T. (2023b). Ectopic pregnancy: Epidemiology, risk factors, and anatomic sites. In A. Chakrabarti (Ed.), *UpToDate*. Retrieved October 1, 2023, from https://www.uptodate.com/contents/ectopic-pregnancy-epidemiology-risk-factors-and-anatomic-sites

Tulandi, T. (2023c). Ectopic pregnancy: Expectant management of tubal pregnancy. In A. Chakrabarti (Ed.), *UpToDate*. Retrieved October 1, 2023, from https://www.uptodate.com/contents/ectopic-pregnancy-expectant-management-of-tubal-pregnancy

Tulandi, T. (2023d). Ectopic pregnancy: Methotrexate therapy. In A. Chakrabarti (Ed.), *UpToDate*. Retrieved October 1, 2023, from https://www.uptodate.com/contents/ectopic-pregnancy-methotrexate-therapy

University of Chicago Department of Pathology. (2019). Products of conception. In *Gross pathology manual*. Retrieved from https://voices.uchicago.edu/grosspathology/peds-perinatal/products-of-conception/

Usharani, N., Joshi, S. D., & Veena, D. (2015). Fetus papyraceous: A rare case report and review of literature. *International Journal of Scientific Study, 3*(4), 183–186. Retrieved from http://www.ijss-sn.com/uploads/2/0/1/5/20153321/ijss_jul_cr06.pdf

Verhaegen, J., Gallos, I. D., van Mello, N. M., Abdel-Aziz, M., Takwoingi, Y., Harb, H., . . . Coomarasamy, A. (2012). Accuracy of single progesterone test to predict early pregnancy outcome in women with pain or bleeding: Meta-analysis of cohort studies. *BMJ, 345*, e6077. https://doi.org/10.1136/bmj.e6077

Vitiello, A., Ferrara, F., Zovi, A., Trama, U., & Boccellino, M. (2022). Pregnancy and COVID-19, focus on vaccine and pharmacological treatment. *Journal of Reproductive Immunology, 151.* https://doi.org/10.1016/j.jri.2022.103630

Wieringa-De Waard, M., Hartman, E. E., Ankum, W. M., Reitsma, J. B., Bindels, P. J. E., & Bonsel, G. J. (2002). Expectant management versus surgical evacuation in first trimester miscarriage: Health-related quality of life in randomized and non-randomized patients. *Human Reproduction, 17*(6), 1638–1642. https://doi.org/10.1093/humrep/17.6.1638

Wilcox, A. J., Baird, D. D., & Weinberg, C. R. (1999). Time of implantation of the conceptus and loss of pregnancy. *New England Journal of Medicine, 340*(23), 1796–1799. https://doi.org/10.1056/NEJM199906103402304

World Health Organization. (2019). *Preventing unsafe abortion: Evidence brief.* Retrieved from https://apps.who.int/iris/bitstream/handle/10665/329887/WHO-RHR-19.21-eng.pdf

World Health Organization. (2022). *Abortion care guideline*. Geneva, Switzerland: Author. Retrieved from https://apps.who.int/iris/rest/bitstreams/1394380/retrieve

Worley, K. C., Hnat, M. D., & Cunningham, F. G. (2008). Advanced extrauterine pregnancy: Diagnostic and therapeutic challenges. *American Journal of Obstetrics & Gynecology, 198*(3), 297.e1–297.e7. https://doi.org/10.1016/j.ajog.2007.09.044

Zamani, Z., & Parekh, U. (2023). Vanishing twin syndrome. In *StatPearls*. Treasure Island, FL: StatPearls Publishing. Retrieved September 30, 2023, from https://www.ncbi.nlm.nih.gov/books/NBK563220/

Zauche, L. H., Wallace, B., Smoots, A. N., Olson, C. K., Oduyebo, T., Kim, S. Y., . . . Ellington, S. R. (2021). Receipt of mRNA Covid-19 vaccines and risk of spontaneous abortion. *New England Journal of Medicine, 385*(16), 1533–1535. https://doi.org/10.1056/NEJMc2113891

Zhang, J., Gilles, J. M., Barnhart, K., Creinin, M. D., Westhoff, C., & Frederick, M. M. (2005). A comparison of medical management with misoprostol and surgical management for early pregnancy failure. *New England Journal of Medicine, 353*(8), 761–769. https://doi.org/10.1056/NEJMoa044064

Zhu, J. L., Hjollund, N. H., Andersen, A.-M. N., & Olsen, J. (2004). Shift work, job stress, and late fetal loss: The National Birth Cohort in Denmark. *Journal of Occupational and Environmental Medicine, 46*(11),1144–1149. https://doi.org/10.1097/01.jom.0000145168.21614.21

Zilberman Sharon, N., Maymon, R., Melcer, Y., & Jauniaux, E. (2020). Obstetric outcomes of twin pregnancies presenting with a complete hydatidiform mole and coexistent normal fetus: A systematic review and meta-analysis. *BJOG, 127*(12), 1450–1457. https://doi.org/10.1111/1471-0528.16283

Antepartum Bleeding—Second Half of Pregnancy 6

Objectives

- Compare and contrast the presentation of placental abruption and placenta previa, including
  - Predisposing conditions;
  - Signs and symptoms;
  - Pathophysiology;
  - Indicated diagnostic workup; and
  - Maternal and fetal complications.
- Discuss the signs, symptoms, and risk factors for uterine rupture.
- Use the BLEEDERS mnemonic to describe how you would respond to a client with heavy vaginal bleeding.
- Discuss when immediate cesarean birth might be recommended for bleeding with placenta previa and when expectant management could be considered.

Composite Case Study

Hannah Rinehart, CNM, a midwife in practice at an accredited birth center, was brewing a much-needed cup of coffee when she received a phone call from her client. Mary M., a 24-year-old gravida 3, para 1 (G3 P1) at 36 weeks of gestation, was eating supper when she felt a gush of fluid. She ran to the bathroom and was horrified to find a moderate amount of bright-red blood flowing from her vagina.

Mary had not had an ultrasound examination during this pregnancy. Her blood type was A negative. Hannah told Mary to call emergency medical services (EMS) and said that she would meet her at Rural Community Hospital, where she had provider privileges. Hannah informed her collaborating obstetrician and the maternity unit charge nurse, then faxed Mary's records before she rushed to the hospital.

Hannah arrived at the hospital before the obstetrician, who took call from home. The nursing staff had opened the operating suite and alerted the anesthesiologist that an emergency cesarean section might be necessary. Hannah quickly assessed Mary and noted that her membranes had ruptured. Grossly bloody fluid the color of cranberry juice flowed onto the bed. Mary said she had lost at least a cup of this fluid on the way to the hospital and another half cup in the toilet. Fearing vasa previa, but considering placenta previa or abruption, Hannah quickly surveyed her client. Continuous electronic fetal monitoring showed a reassuring category I fetal heart rate on the screen. Mary was alert and oriented, with pink lips and dry, well-perfused skin. She experienced no tachycardia or dizziness when she stood. She was in no pain, and her blood pressure was 110/70, which was typical for her. Her abdomen was soft and not tender to palpation, and Leopold's maneuvers indicated that the fetus was in vertex presentation and of appropriate size for the gestational age. Mary was having contractions every 5–8 min on the monitor, but she did not feel them.

Hannah was relieved for the moment. Ruptured vasa previa was unlikely with a category I fetal heart pattern. There were no clots, just copious gushes of watery red fluid. Hannah did not perform a vaginal exam because of the possibility of placenta previa, but ordered a stat ultrasound, complete blood count, coagulation studies, type and crossmatch, and Kleihauer-Betke test. She typed and crossed two units of packed red blood cells and alerted the blood bank that Mary was at risk for severe hemorrhage. Because the fetus was preterm and Mary had not yet been cultured for GBS, she ordered penicillin for GBS prophylaxis. The nurses obtained intravenous access and withheld food and oral fluids because a cesarean section might be imminently necessary.

The ultrasound was performed at the bedside. The placenta was fundal, and the edges were echoic and curved oddly upward. There were no definite signs of abruption on the placenta, but a heterogeneous mass near the fetal neck changed position and shape when the fetus moved. The radiologist's report stated that the placenta was abnormal, and the mass in question was probably a free-floating blood clot.

Hannah updated her collaborating physician, who by now was in-house, and added that all laboratory studies had come back normal. Mary's cervical exam was 3 cm dilated, 90% effaced, and -2 station, and her cervix was soft and stretchy. The fetal heart tracing remained category I, and Mary was having mild contractions every 2 min. The physician explained that it was likely that there was a placenta abruption but at this time she and the fetus were stable, and she seemed to be starting labor. Using shared decision-making, he offered Mary a cesarean section, which would reduce the risk of severe bleeding in labor, versus a trial of labor with continuous monitoring, which could result in an emergency cesarean if she began to hemorrhage. Mary chose to attempt a vaginal birth.

Mary's labor spontaneously accelerated, and her baby girl was born about 2 hr later, weighing 5 lb (2,300 g), which was the 8th percentile for gestational age. The neonatologist present at birth assigned 8/9 Apgar scores. When the baby's head emerged, an 8 cm purple blood clot slipped out onto the bed. Mary then delivered a stiff, fibrous circumvallate placenta with a thick ring of membranes on the fetal surface. A dark, fresh clot about the size of Hannah's thumb was adherent to the maternal side of the placenta, marking the site of an abruption comprising about 10% of the maternal interface.

Mother and baby were released from the hospital after a 48-hr stay. The baby was a poor feeder because of prematurity and required formula supplementation to maintain her weight. She was readmitted for phototherapy for jaundice at the age of 5 days. She was closely monitored by a pediatrician for her first months of life but ultimately did well.

Antepartum Bleeding

About 2–5% of pregnant individuals experience bleeding in the second half of pregnancy (Baeseman, 2022). Antepartum hemorrhage is a factor in one fifth of early preterm births (PTB) and increases the risk of cerebral palsy, developmental delays, blindness, and other long-term issues related to PTB (Royal College of Obstetricians & Gynaecologists [RCOG], 2011). Although definitions vary, antepartum hemorrhage is usually described as significant bleeding from the genital tract that occurs after 20 weeks of gestation (Society for Maternal-Fetal Medicine [SMFM] & Gyamfi-Bannerman, 2018). RCOG (2011) classifies antepartum hemorrhage as follows:

- Spotting—staining, streaking, or blood-spotting noted on underwear or sanitary protection;
- Minor hemorrhage—blood loss less than 50 ml that has resolved;
- Major hemorrhage—blood loss of 50–1,000 ml with no signs of clinical shock; or
- Massive hemorrhage—blood loss greater than 1,000 ml and/or signs of clinical shock.

The origin of antepartum bleeding can be

- *Uterine*: Placenta previa, placental abruption;
- *Cervical or vaginal*: Cervical ectropion or polyps, vaginal inflammation, cervical hemangioma, cervical or vaginal varix, genital tract neoplasm;
- *Fetal*: Vasa previa;
- *Hematological*: Coagulation disorders;
- *Traumatic*: Uterine rupture, vaginal injury, cervical bleeding following intercourse or digital examination; or
- *Physiologic*: Bloody show.

The sources of late-pregnancy hemorrhage most associated with poor maternal and perinatal outcomes are the "Big Four"—placenta previa, placental abruption, vasa previa, and uterine rupture. Placenta previa and placental abruption are the most common causes for antepartum hemorrhage in the second half of pregnancy (Mhyre & Khan, 2022). Common sources of minor bleeding include minor cervical trauma secondary to a pelvic examination or sexual intercourse, irritation from genital tract infection, cervical ectropion or polyps, or, when labor has begun, bloody show (Young & White, 2019). Very rarely, cervical hemangioma, cervical or vaginal varix, or genital-tract neoplasm can cause serious bleeding that can be difficult to control. Early recognition and appropriate intervention can reduce maternal and perinatal morbidity and mortality (Young & White, 2019).

Placenta Previa

Placenta previa denotes a placenta implanted in the lower uterine segment that overlaps the cervical os to any degree (Francois & Foley, 2021). When the edge of the placenta is within 2 cm of the internal os but does not overlap it, it is described as a low-lying placenta (Heinrichs, 2020). The terms *complete*, *total*, *partial*, and *marginal placenta previa* are outdated (Heinrichs, 2020).

Placenta previa carries a high risk for uncontrolled bleeding that increases late in gestation. In the third trimester, uterine contractions, lower uterine segment remodeling, and cervical ripening can cause the inflexible placental attachment site to shear and partially detach, causing small amounts of bleeding (Cunningham et al., 2022, ch. 43; Oyelese & Smulian, 2006). This bleeding can stimulate more uterine contractions, which result in more placental separation and bleeding (Oyelese & Smulian, 2006). Digital examination or coitus can also potentially damage the placental interface and cause bleeding (Lockwood & Russo-Stieglitz, 2023a, 2023b). Although bleeding associated with placenta previa is primarily maternal, fetal hemorrhage can occur if fetal vessels are damaged (Lockwood & Russo-Stieglitz, 2023a, 2023b). Individuals with placenta previa who have acute vaginal bleeding require immediate evaluation in a hospital (Francois & Foley, 2021).

With placenta previa, blood loss at cesarean birth is often excessive, even when performed non-emergently under optimal conditions with a stable mother and fetus. Because myometrial fibers in the lower uterine segment do not contract well, they can be less effective at constricting torn vessels to control bleeding. Consequently, it can be difficult to gain control of bleeding from a placenta previa in the antepartum

Table 6-1

Differential Diagnoses for Antepartum/Intrapartum Bleeding

Bleeding	Uterine Tone	Abdominal Pain	Fetal Status
Placenta previa (usually in the third trimester)			
Scant, moderate, or profuse. Typically bright red. Shock can be present.	Normal resting tone, or can have contractions.	Usually painless unless labor contractions are present.	Usually normal unless mother is compromised. Presenting part might be high and nonvertex.
Placental abruption			
Can be absent, scant, moderate, or heavy. May be purplish, dark, or bright red. Shock can be present.	Can be firm or rigid, with frequent low amplitude contractions.	Abdominal or back pain can be severe or absent.	Can be normal in small abruption. In moderate abruption, typically category II or III fetal heart patterns. In large abruption, heart tones can be absent.
Vasa previa			
Variable, bright red, usually after rupture of membranes. No maternal shock.	Normal resting tone, or labor contractions.	Usually painless unless contractions are present.	Typically category III within minutes of onset of bleeding. Bradycardia or sinusoidal pattern common.
Uterine rupture			
Can be light, moderate, or heavy.	Normal or soft uterine tone. Contractions can stop.	Usually sudden onset of severe, sharp pain in abdomen or back. Rebound tenderness.	Typically quickly deteriorates from category II to category III. Fetal parts might be easily palpable through abdominal wall. Presenting part can be high.
Preterm or term labor			
Bloody show involves light bleeding that may be mixed with mucus or amniotic fluid.	Contractions.	Suprapubic or low back pain.	Usually normal.
Genital tract trauma (can follow vigorous coitus or sexual assault)			
Bright red.	Normal uterine tone.	Sometimes vaginal or perineal discomfort.	Usually normal.
Ruptured varicosity			
Copious, dark red.	Normal uterine tone unless in labor.	Usually painless.	Usually normal unless mother is compromised.

period as well as after birth. Additionally, if the placenta covers the anterior wall of the uterus where the incision is made, the surgeon sometimes needs to cut through the placenta to remove the baby, causing brisk bleeding.

Incidence and Pathogenesis

The incidence of placenta previa is about 1 in 200–250 births but varies globally (Francois & Foley, 2021; Lockwood & Russo-Stieglitz, 2023a; Oyelese & Canterino, 2011). Sinclair and colleagues (2021) found that 10.6% of pregnant individuals undergoing routine cervical-length screening between 16 and 24 weeks of gestation are diagnosed with either placenta previa or low-lying placenta. Some of these diagnoses prove incorrect. By the third trimester, most resolve. Several authors give a rate of resolution greater than 90% by term (Lockwood & Russo-Stieglitz, 2023a; Oyelese & Smulian, 2006; Sinclair et al., 2021). Placenta previa is more likely to persist until birth if it is located on the posterior uterine wall, if it extends over the os by more than 25 mm, or if it is still present on follow-up ultrasound in the third trimester (Lockwood & Russo-Stieglitz, 2023a). Importantly, a low-lying placenta or placenta previa is more likely to persist if there is a prior cesarean scar on the uterus (Lockwood & Russo-Stieglitz, 2023a).

Placenta previa is less prevalent late in pregnancy because of normal changes in the relationship between placental location and the cervix with advancing gestation. The

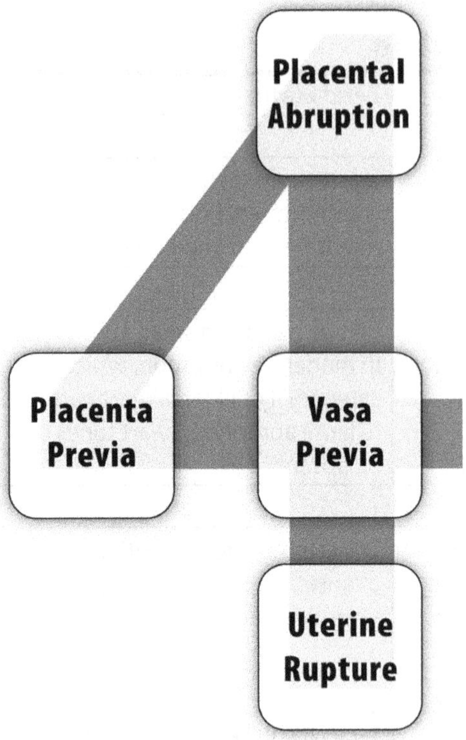

Figure 6-1. The Big Four are the most serious causes of antepartum bleeding: Placental abruption, placenta previa, vasa previa, and uterine rupture.

lower uterine segment, undeveloped and short in the first half of gestation, thins and lengthens over time, relocating the lower edge of the (stationary) placenta farther away from the internal os (Lockwood & Russo-Stieglitz, 2023a). It also appears that the placenta preferentially grows and expands into the well-perfused upper uterus in a "migration" termed *trophotropism* while the placenta overlying the poorly vascularized cervix atrophies. Occasionally, this remodeling of placental tissue leaves fetal vessels unsupported in the membranes between the umbilical cord and the placenta, resulting in velamentous umbilical cord insertion or vasa previa (Lockwood & Russo-Stieglitz, 2023b).

Risk Factors

Endometrial damage and uterine scarring increase the risk for placenta previa (Francois & Foley, 2021). Previous placenta previa is a major risk factor for reoccurrence affecting 4–8% of subsequent pregnancies (Lockwood & Russo-Stieglitz, 2023a). Previous uterine curettage during miscarriage or induced abortion and surgery involving lower uterine incision are also risk factors for placenta previa (Francois & Foley, 2021). Cesarean birth increases the risk for subsequent placenta previa by 47–60% (Lockwood & Russo-Stieglitz, 2023a). Risk increases with prelabor cesarean birth and with increasing numbers of cesarean sections (Lockwood & Russo-Stieglitz, 2023a).

Table 6-2

Potential Maternal Complications of Antepartum Hemorrhage

- Consequences of blood loss such as hypovolemia, coagulopathy, hypoxemia, organ damage or failure.
- Blood transfusion sequelae such as transfusion reactions, infection, antibody sensitization, and transfusion associated acute lung injury.
- Peripartum hysterectomy.
- Intensive care treatment.
- Delayed bonding with baby.
- Posttraumatic stress disorder (PTSD).
- Cardiac arrest.
- Death.

From "Management of Massive Obstetric Haemorrhage: Antepartum, Intrapartum and Postpartum," by A. P. Carillo and E. Chandraharan, in E. Chandraharan and S. Arulkumaran (Eds.), *Obstetric and Intrapartum Emergencies: A Practical Guide to Management* (2nd ed., ch. 5, Kindle version), 2021, Cambridge, United Kingdom: Cambridge University Press. Copyright by publisher.

Risk of placenta previa is 40% higher in twin births (even higher in dichorionic twins) than with singletons (Lockwood & Russo-Stieglitz, 2023a). Risk is also elevated with grand multiparity, advanced maternal age, prior induced or spontaneous abortion, endometriosis, fibroid uterus, and use of assisted reproductive technologies (Jenabi, Salimi, Bashirian, Khazaei, & Ayubi, 2022). Tobacco or cocaine use and living at high altitudes increase the risk of placenta previa, presumably because greater placental surface area is necessary to compensate for lower uteroplacental oxygenation (Cashion, 2016). Interestingly, a male fetus is more likely to have a placenta previa than a female fetus, probably because males tend to have larger placentas.

Maternal and Perinatal Risks

Individuals with placenta previa are at high risk for hemorrhage before, during, or after giving birth, and it is especially high for those with previa-accreta (see below). More than half of individuals with placenta previa experience antepartum hemorrhage (Kuribayashi et al., 2021); 12% require blood transfusion; and 5.3% require postpartum hysterectomy, uterine/iliac artery ligation, or embolization of the pelvic vessels to control bleeding (Kuribayashi et al., 2021). Mothers with placenta previa are at higher risk for amniotic fluid embolism syndrome (Lockwood & Russo-Stieglitz, 2023a). In the United States from 2006 to 2013, 3% of maternal deaths from hemorrhage were related to placenta previa (Cunningham et al., 2022).

Placenta previa also increases risk for the infant, often through complications related to PTB. About 44% of mothers

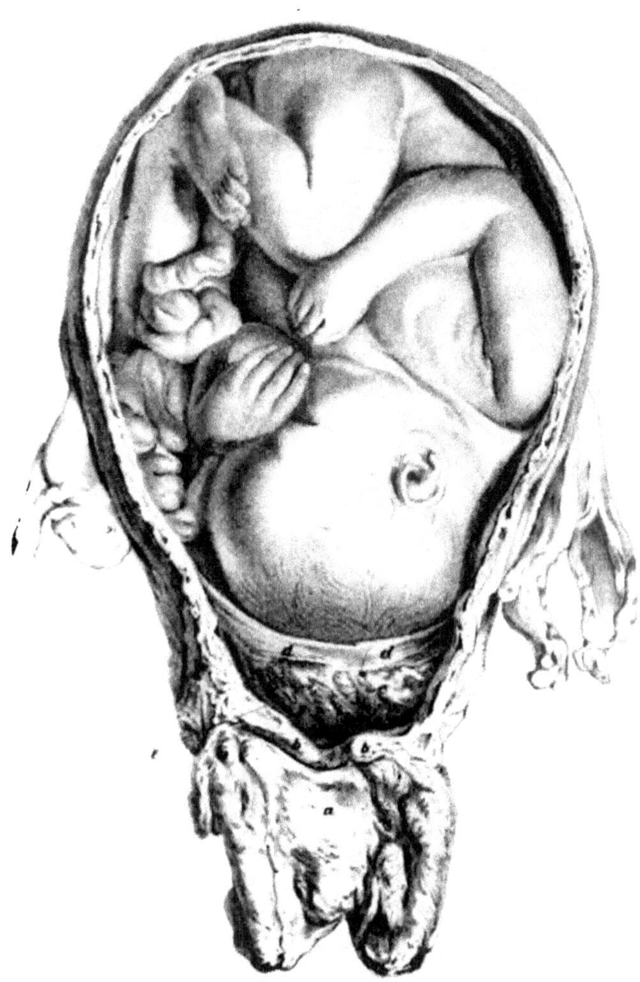

Figure 6-2. Placenta previa occurs when the placenta covers the cervical os. From *An American Text-Book of Obstetrics for Practitioners and Students* (fig. 388, p. 588), by J. C. Cameron et al., 1897, Philadelphia, PA: W. B. Saunders. In the public domain.

with placenta previa give birth preterm, most of them between 34 and 37 weeks of gestation (Lockwood & Russo-Stieglitz, 2023a). PTB increases the need for admission to a neonatal intensive care unit (NICU) and the risk of perinatal and neonatal mortality (Lockwood & Russo-Stieglitz, 2023a). Vasa previa and velamentous umbilical cord insertion are more common in pregnancies with placenta previa, and there is a slightly higher risk for fetal growth restriction, or FGR (Balayla, Desilets, & Shrem, 2019). The rate of fetal anomalies is two to three times higher in pregnancies with placenta previa (Cunningham et al., 2022, ch. 43; Silver, 2022). Neonatal anemia often follows antepartum hemorrhage due to placenta previa (Lockwood & Russo-Stieglitz, 2023a). Because placenta previa tends to prevent fetal descent onto the pelvis, malpresentation is common.

Placenta Accreta Spectrum (PAS)

The placenta accreta spectrum (PAS), which includes placenta accreta (63%), increta (15%), and percreta (22%), is

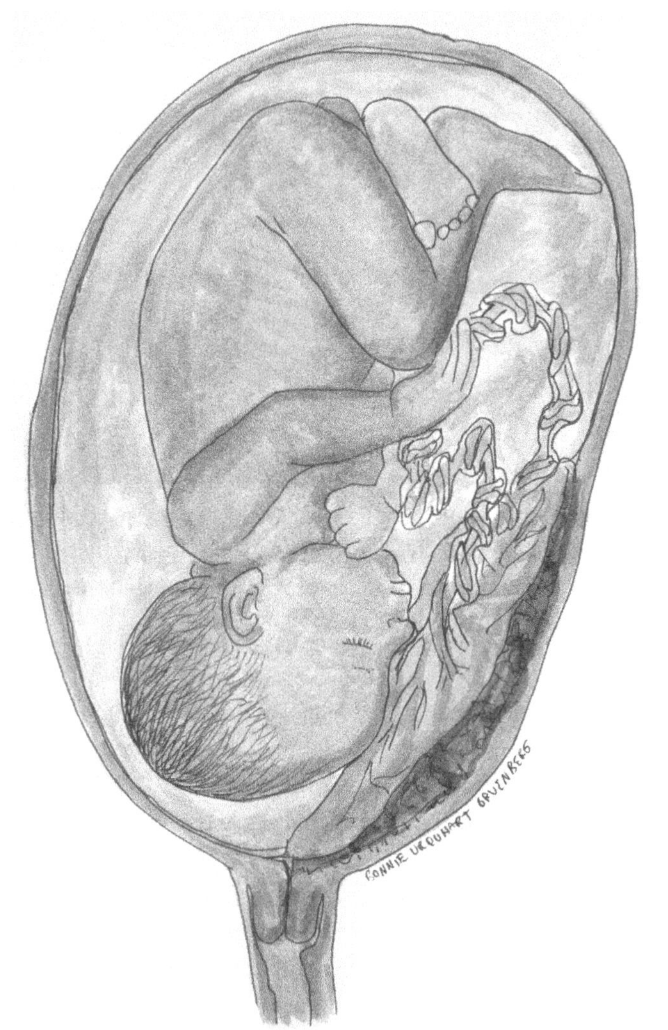

Figure 6-3. A low-lying placenta is diagnosed when the placenta edge is within 2 cm of the internal cervical os but does not cover it. Most low-lying placentas diagnosed in the second trimester resolve by the third trimester.

commonly associated with placenta previa (Silver, 2022). PAS develops when the decidua basalis and Nitabuch's layer are totally or partially absent in the region where the conceptus implants, causing the placenta to develop with no physiological line of cleavage between the uterus and all or part of the placenta (Cunningham et al., 2022, ch. 43). In placenta accreta, chorionic villi attach directly to the uterine myometrium; in placenta increta, the villi invade deeply through the myometrium into the uterine serosa; and in placenta percreta, the villi pass through the entire uterus to invade other organs such as the bladder (Varouxaki, Gnanasambanthan, Datta, & Amokrane, 2018). These grades of PAS can coexist in the same pregnancy and can involve a small area or most of the placental bed (Jauniaux, Grønbeck, Bunce, Langhoff-Roos, & Collins, 2019). This topic is discussed more fully in Chapter 7, "Placenta Accreta Spectrum."

PAS is a major cause of life-threatening obstetric hemorrhage. Up to 90% of afflicted mothers require blood transfusion,

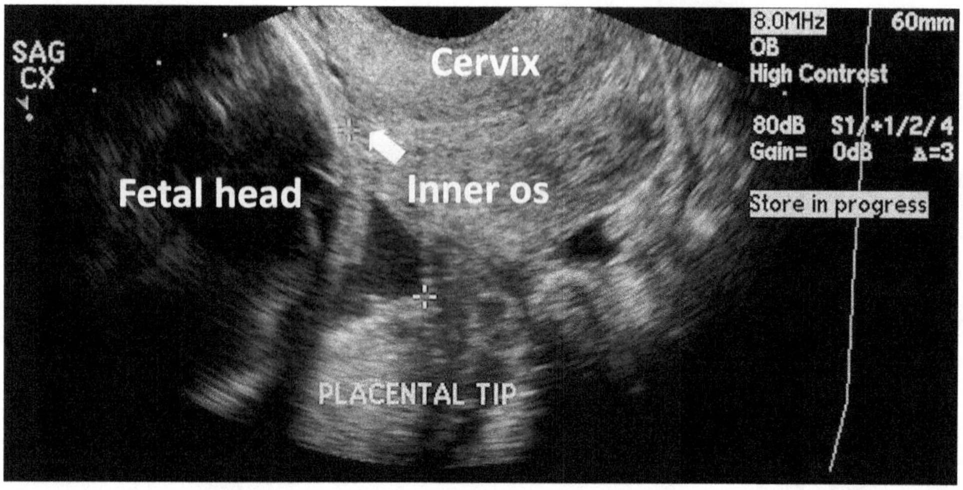

Figure 6-4. Resolved placenta previa. About 80% of cases of placenta previa or low-lying placenta diagnosed in the second trimester resolve by term. This third-trimester ultrasound shows a normal distance of 2.57 cm between the placental tip and the cervix and requires no further follow-up.

and 40% require more than *10 units* of packed RBCs (Mulla et al., 2019). Peripartum hysterectomy can be required to control or prevent intractable hemorrhage (Silver, 2022). Placenta accreta occurring in the absence of placenta previa is an uncommon cause of antepartum bleeding but is a strong risk factor for massive postpartum hemorrhage (Young & White, 2019).

The rate of PAS is higher for mothers who have both placenta previa and prior cesarean or other uterine surgery. In the United Kingdom, PAS has a prevalence of 1.7 cases per 10,000 births overall, but as high as 577 per 10,000 births in individuals with both a previous cesarean and current placenta previa (Jauniaux, Grønbeck, et al., 2019). Individuals with suspected PAS should give birth in a regional medical center with ready access to blood products and a highly experienced, multidisciplinary care team (Terlizzi, 2022). This team typically includes professionals such as experienced obstetricians and maternal–fetal medicine specialists; expert pelvic surgeons, urologists, interventional radiologists, anesthesiologists, and critical care specialists; skilled nurses; general surgeons, trauma surgeons, and neonatologists (American College of Obstetricians & Gynecologists [ACOG] & SMFM, 2018/2021).

Diagnosis of Placenta Previa

When the placenta clearly overlies the cervix or when it is positioned above the lower uterine segment, placenta previa can be diagnosed or excluded by transabdominal sonography (Cunningham et al., 2022, ch. 43). The false-positive rate for low-lying placenta on transabdominal sonography is as high as 26–60% (Heinrichs, 2020). The lower uterine segment can be difficult to visualize when the client is obese, and a false-positive result can occur when the bladder is full (Cunningham et al., 2022, ch. 43). When diagnosis is uncertain, transvaginal sonography allows safe and reliable visualization of the internal cervical os and affords accurate diagnosis.

Management

The antepartum management of placenta previa is dictated by whether the client is asymptomatic, actively bleeding, or stable after one or more episodes of active bleeding.

Bleeding Placenta Previa

Significant active bleeding from placenta previa is an obstetric emergency. Individuals with bright-red, painless vaginal bleeding in the second half of pregnancy should be presumed to have placenta previa until contradictory evidence appears. More than half of individuals with placenta previa persisting into the third trimester undergo emergency cesarean section for hemorrhage, and about one fourth of those undergoing cesarean for hemorrhage require a blood transfusion (Cunningham et al., 2022, ch. 43).

The gestational age at which a previa begins to bleed and the severity of the episode(s) are unpredictable (Kuribayashi et al., 2021). Although bleeding related to placenta previa can occur early in the second trimester, onset is usually in or near the third trimester (Cunningham et al., 2022, ch. 43; Francois & Foley, 2021). About one third begin bleeding before 30 weeks of gestation; these individuals tend to have worse outcomes than those who begin bleeding closer to term (Lockwood & Russo-Stieglitz, 2023a). Another one-third have an initial bleeding episode, known as the sentinel bleed, between 30 0/7 and 36 6/7 weeks of gestation. Most of the rest begin bleeding at or beyond 37 weeks of gestation (Lockwood & Russo-Stieglitz, 2023a). In about 10% of individuals with placenta previa, bleeding does not occur until the onset of term labor (Cunningham et al., 2022, ch. 43). Hemorrhage from placenta previa can occur unexpectedly in community settings when the individual has not had an antenatal ultrasound.

Up to 90% of individuals present with relatively painless vaginal bleeding, although some can have uterine contractions, pain, and bleeding similar in presentation to placental abruption (Lockwood & Russo-Stieglitz, 2023a). The sentinel bleed is rarely severe and usually resolves, only to reoccur (Cunningham et al., 2022, ch. 43). It is more likely to be serious when it occurs

For the client of a community midwifery practice who has declined antenatal ultrasound, the first sign of placenta previa can be massive hemorrhage in early labor.

Do not perform a digital examination of a client with antepartum bleeding until the diagnosis of placenta previa is excluded!

before 30 weeks of gestation (Francois & Foley, 2021; Kuribayashi et al., 2021). Severe bleeding is more strongly associated with anterior placenta previa than with posterior or lateral placental locations (Kuribayashi et al., 2021). A thick placental edge and short cervical length on ultrasound also carry higher risk of severe bleeding (Kuribayashi et al., 2021). Other risk factors for severe bleeding include repeated bleeding episodes, gravidity of 5 or greater, and history of intrauterine procedures such as cesarean section, myomectomy, intrauterine operations, elective abortion, or hysteroscopy (Huang et al., 2022).

Even the gentlest digital cervical examination can provoke torrential hemorrhage! Do *not* perform a digital examination until the diagnosis of placenta previa is excluded. Transvaginal ultrasound, however, can be performed safely in individuals with placenta previa because the vaginal probe is ideally positioned 20–30 mm away from the cervix and angled to prevent accidental slippage (Lockwood & Russo-Stieglitz, 2023a). In localities where sonography is not readily available, digital cervical examination should be performed in an operating room with preparations in place for immediate cesarean section (Cunningham et al., 2022, ch. 43).

The goals of managing an individual with an acutely bleeding placenta previa are to maintain maternal hemodynamic stability and determine whether emergency cesarean is required (Lockwood & Russo-Stieglitz, 2022). The obstetrician should move immediately to cesarean birth if the client is in active labor, is hemodynamically unstable, if there is a category III fetal heart rate (FHR) refractory to resuscitative measures, or if there is a large amount of bleeding after 34 weeks of gestation (Lockwood & Russo-Stieglitz, 2022). Upon removal of the placenta, there is a high risk (up to 29%) of major postpartum hemorrhage (Lockwood & Russo-Stieglitz, 2022) that can necessitate uterine balloon compression, compression sutures, uterine or internal iliac artery ligation, pelvic artery embolization, or hysterectomy (Cunningham et al., 2022, ch. 43).

Because most poor neonatal outcomes associated with placenta previa result from complications of prematurity, a main goal of management is to prolong pregnancy whenever possible. The mother should be evaluated in a hospital labor and delivery unit, and fetal monitoring should be used to determine wellbeing. Corticosteroid administration may be considered if gestational age is as early as 22 0/7 weeks or as late as 36 6/7 weeks to reduce the incidence and severity of neonatal respiratory distress syndrome, intraventricular hemorrhage, and necrotizing enterocolitis (ACOG, 2017/2024). See Chapter 14, "Pharmacological Treatment of PTL." Magnesium sulfate therapy for neuroprotection may be initiated for gestation at less than 32 0/7 weeks in which cesarean is planned within 24 hr but not emergently (Lockwood & Russo-Stieglitz, 2022).

There are no evidence-based recommendations to guide management of a small amount of third-trimester bleeding from placenta previa that has resolved by the time of presentation (Heinrichs, 2020). When fetal and maternal testing are reassuring, discharge can be considered after a period of observation (Heinrichs, 2020; Lockwood & Russo-Stieglitz, 2022). Candidates for outpatient management should be counseled on the risks and benefits, should be able to return to the hospital within 20 min, should maintain pelvic rest and avoid strenuous activity at home, and should have an adult companion present at all times who can call for an ambulance if hemorrhage occurs (Heinrichs, 2020; Lockwood & Russo-Stieglitz, 2022).

With more significant bleeding, inpatient observation for 24–48 hr is suggested (Heinrichs, 2020; Lockwood & Russo-Stieglitz, 2022). Individuals with three or more bleeding episodes are usually hospitalized until they give birth (Lockwood & Russo-Stieglitz, 2022). If the mother is significantly preterm, the obstetrician may opt for transfer to a perinatologist at a tertiary-care perinatal center, where staff is present around the clock to perform an emergency cesarean and the NICU can better meet the needs of the newborn should it become necessary (Cashion, 2016).

Asymptomatic Placenta Previa

Clients with persistent placenta previa in the third trimester should have serial ultrasounds to assess placental location and fetal growth. Refer the client to an obstetrician or a maternal-fetal medicine (MFM) specialist to determine whether comanagement or transfer of care is more appropriate. Discuss with the client that a cesarean birth is necessary and may be performed emergently if antepartum hemorrhage occurs. Counsel clients to call with *any* bleeding, leaking fluid, or signs of labor.

Although there is no hard evidence supporting the practice, individuals with placenta previa are customarily advised to observe pelvic rest—avoidance of vaginal or rectal penetration (Jain, Bos, & Bujold, 2020) and avoidance of orgasm by any means (Lockwood & Russo-Stieglitz, 2022). Orgasm is associated with uterine contractions which can provoke bleeding (Lockwood & Russo-Stieglitz, 2022). Insertion of a penis, sex toy, or other object deep into the vagina or rectum

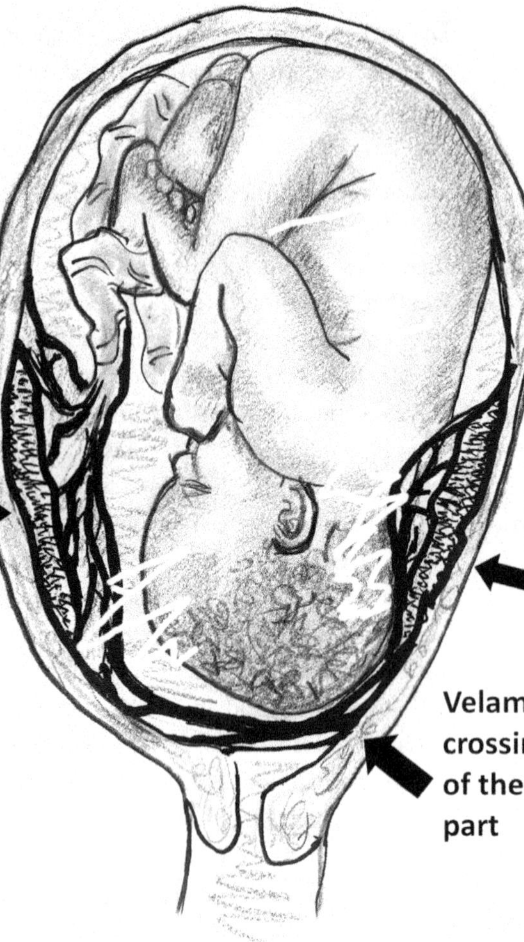

Figure 6-5. Vasa previa involves velamentous blood vessels crossing the cervix ahead of the fetal presenting part. These vessels often run from the placenta to a succenturiate lobe or arise from a bilobed placenta or velamentous cord insertion.

ACOG and SMFM recommend that individuals with uncomplicated placenta previa (without FGR, preeclampsia, or other issues that can indicate early intervention) undergo cesarean section at 36 0/7–37 6/7 weeks of gestation (ACOG & SMFM, 2021/2024; SMFM & Gyamfi-Bannerman, 2018). The risk of hemorrhage increases as the distance between the placental edge and internal os decreases (Lockwood & Russo-Stieglitz, 2022). ACOG (2017/2024) recommends a single course of betamethasone for planned cesarean at less than 37 0/7 weeks of gestation for those who have not previously received antenatal corticosteroids.

Vaginal birth in a hospital is appropriate for some clients with low-lying placenta if vasa previa is absent. In some cases, the descending fetal head compresses the placental bed and inhibits bleeding during labor. In others, the placental bed becomes disrupted and heavy bleeding occurs (Hull & Resnik, 2014). In one meta-analysis of individuals with a low-lying placenta undergoing a trial of labor, clients with a placental edge less than 10 mm from internal os had a 45% chance of emergency cesarean, whereas those with the placental edge 11–20 mm from internal os had a 14% chance of emergency cesarean (Jansen et al., 2019). Because of the high risk of intrapartum and postpartum hemorrhage, mothers with low-lying placentas should give birth in a hospital with the capacity for emergency cesarean.

could possibly cause direct trauma to the placenta previa. Clients with placenta previa can be advised to avoid moderate and strenuous exercise, lifting objects weighing 20 lb (9 kg) or greater, and standing for periods longer than 4 hr because these activities have been associated with a small but significant risk for PTL (Lockwood & Russo-Stieglitz, 2022). Bed rest or reduced activity, however, does not reduce the risk of bleeding and can cause physical deconditioning and psychosocial stress and may increase the risk for venous thromboembolism (Jain et al., 2020; SMFM, Lauder, Sciscione, Biggio, & Osmundson, 2020).

All clients, particularly those at risk for hemorrhage, should optimize nutrition to prevent anemia and increase iron intake when their hemoglobin level is low. Oral iron supplements are effective and best tolerated when lower doses (40–60 mg elemental iron) are taken every other day rather than daily (Auerbach & Landy, 2023). Intravenous (IV) iron infusion is advised when anemia is severe, when the client cannot tolerate oral iron, or when oral iron is ineffective in raising the hemoglobin level (Auerbach & Landy, 2023).

Vasa Previa

Vasa previa is a potentially catastrophic condition in which exposed, unsupported fetal vessels, unprotected by the placenta or umbilical cord, cross the membranes over the cervix. These vessels are vulnerable to spontaneous rupture and to tearing during rupture of membranes, digital examination, or labor. Furthermore, contractions can compress the presenting part against the unprotected vessels and result in fetal hypoxia and bradycardia (Lijoi & Brady, 2003). Velamentous vessels within 2 cm of the internal os are just as vulnerable to breakage and compression as those that cross the cervix. Whereas other etiologies of antepartum bleeding involve maternal blood loss, a ruptured vasa previa represents a fetal hemorrhage that can quickly become fatal.

Vasa previa occurs in about 1 in 1,300 to 1 in 2,500 births, but the use of assisted reproductive technologies increases the prevalence to as high as 1 in 202 (Lockwood & Russo-Stieglitz, 2023b). Around 85% of cases of vasa previa have identifiable risk factors including use of assisted reproductive technology; velamentous cord insertion; multiple gestation; and bilobed, succenturiate, or low-lying placenta (Jauniaux & Silver, 2020).

There are three types of vasa previa (Lockwood & Russo-Stieglitz, 2023b):

- Type 1: Membranous vessels with a velamentous or marginal cord insertion;
- Type 2: Membranous vessels connecting lobes of a bilobed placenta or a placenta and a succenturiate lobe; and
- Type 3: Membranous vessels on the margin of the placenta, more commonly during a resolving placenta previa.

Diagnosis

The diagnosis of vasa previa is made when velamentous vessels are visualized within 2 cm of the cervix (Catanzarite et al., 2016). This condition can be identified with 93–98% accuracy by routine sonography as early as the second trimester using a combination of transabdominal and transvaginal color Doppler imaging (Jauniaux, Alfirevic, et al., 2018; SMFM Pub. Cmte., Sinkey, Odibo, & Dashe, 2015). Antepartum recognition via ultrasound can be lifesaving for the fetus. When vasa previa is recognized prenatally, prelabor cesarean section should be planned to minimize the chance for vascular rupture. Prenatal diagnosis reduces perinatal mortality by approximately 95% and greatly reduces the risk of neurologic damage to survivors (Zhang et al., 2021). When vasa previa is discovered at the time of antepartum hemorrhage, perinatal death occurs in more than half of cases (Oyelese et al., 2004; Silver, 2015).

Although transvaginal ultrasound scanning is overall highly effective for diagnosing vasa previa, it can miss some cases even in the best circumstances (SMFM Pub. Cmte. et al., 2015). Routine ultrasound can sometimes reliably exclude vasa previa, which does not occur when the placenta is single-lobed and the cord is inserted into the center (Deng & Copel, 2016). Some cases of suspected second-trimester vasa previa (13–39%) resolve naturally as the lower segment elongates and shifts the velamentous vessels away from the cervix (Lockwood & Russo-Stieglitz, 2023b). Individuals with placenta previa or a low-lying placenta on second-trimester ultrasound examination should have a repeat transvaginal ultrasound with color and pulsed Doppler at 32 weeks of gestation to screen for vasa previa even if the low-lying placenta has resolved (Bronsteen et al., 2013; SMFM Pub. Cmte. et al., 2015).

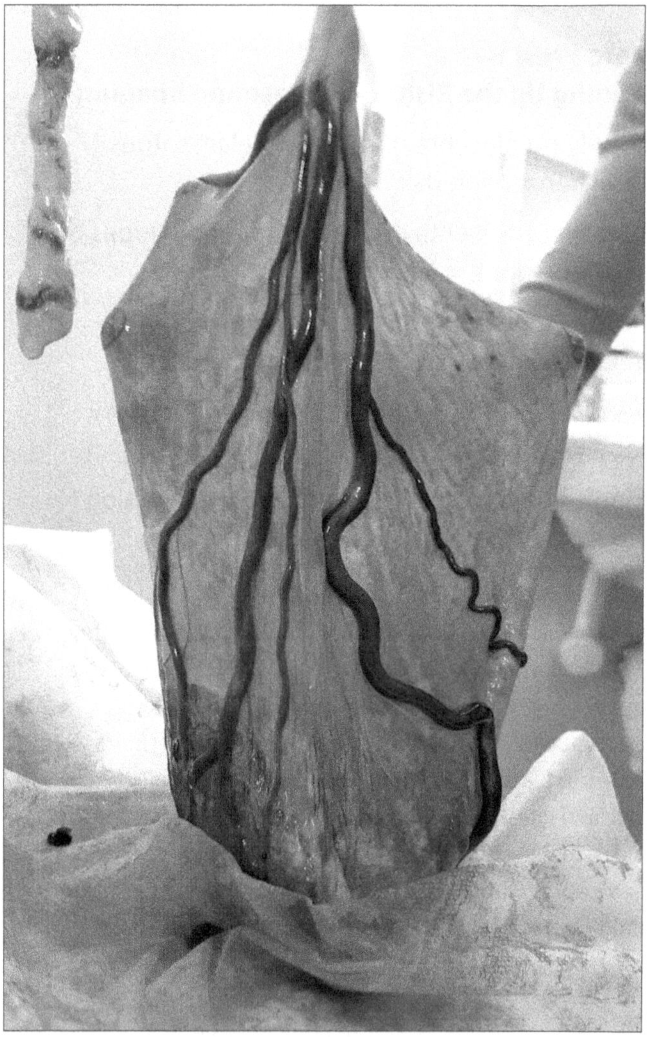

Figure 6-6. Velamentous cord insertion. The mother who delivered this placenta had declined prenatal ultrasound, so this remarkable case of velamentous cord insertion was a complete surprise to the birth center midwife who attended her labor. Note that rupture of membranes occurred disconcertingly close to the unprotected vessels. Velamentous vessels are also susceptible to compression in labor, which can lead to fetal compromise. If the midwife had used excessive cord traction during third stage labor, the cord could have avulsed from the placenta. Mother and baby were healthy, however, and birth was uneventful. Photograph by Kristen Harker.

Ruptured Vasa Previa

The vessels of a vasa previa are most likely to burst at the time of spontaneous or deliberate rupture of the membranes, but bleeding can occur with intact membranes. A hemorrhaging

Vasa Previa—
Adding Up the Risks on Ultrasound Imaging

Low-lying placenta or previa + velamentous insertion = High risk.

Low-lying placenta or previa + multiple lobes or accessory lobe = High risk.

Resolved placenta previa + marginal or velamentous cord insertion = Moderate risk.

Fundal placenta + multiple lobes or accessory lobe = Low risk.

Single-lobed placenta + central cord insertion = No risk.

vasa previa usually presents as profuse vaginal bleeding with FHR abnormalities. Because the entire fetal blood volume is usually less than 100 ml/kg (Silver, 2015), fetal death from exsanguination can occur in less than 10 min (Hull & Resnik, 2014). Typically, the fetus develops tachycardia followed by variable and late decelerations, bradycardia, or a preterminal sinusoidal rhythm (Hull & Resnik, 2014). A baby born severely anemic and hypovolemic can require emergent blood transfusion and fluid replacement (James, Steer, Weiner, & Gonik, 2011).

Management

SMFM recommends administration of antenatal steroids between 28 0/7 and 32 0/7 weeks of gestation in case of need for urgent preterm cesarean, consideration of hospital admission at 30 0/7–34 0/7 weeks of gestation, and scheduled cesarean at 34 0/7–37 0/7 weeks of gestation (SMFM Pub. Cmte. et al., 2015). In determining timing for planned cesarean, the risks of PTB should be weighed against the risks of emergency cesarean or stillbirth should rupture of membranes or labor occur. Emergency cesarean is also indicated for nonreassuring fetal testing, vaginal bleeding accompanied by fetal tachycardia, or a sinusoidal FHR pattern (Lockwood & Russo-Stieglitz, 2023b). About 28–42% of antenatally diagnosed cases of vasa previa require emergency cesarean (SMFM Pub. Cmte. et al., 2015). Although individuals at high risk for hemorrhage may be admitted to the hospital for close monitoring, those who live within about 15 min of the hospital and have a long, closed cervix; reassuring fetal testing; no contractions or vaginal bleeding; and no history of spontaneous PTB are sometimes offered outpatient management (Lockwood & Russo-Stieglitz, 2023b). Inpatient or outpatient, close antepartum surveillance should be used to monitor fetal growth and wellbeing, cervical length, and uterine activity (Hasegawa, Arakaki, Ichizuka, & Sekizawa, 2015).

When performing digital cervical examinations on clients in labor with intact membranes, consider the possibility of vasa previa, particularly when the client has not had an ultrasound examination. Before performing artificial rupture of membranes, very carefully use your fingertips to trace the membranes covering the presenting part and take note of any blood vessels. Sometimes these vessels pulsate. If you suspect vasa previa, transport the mother immediately to a hospital by ambulance. Consider a subcutaneous injection of 0.25 mg of terbutaline to weaken and space contractions during transport.

Consider ruptured vasa previa as a potential diagnosis when red bleeding and abnormal FHR patterns occur with rupture of membranes or with digital examination when membranes are intact. Ruptured vasa previa is a dire emergency. There are no temporizing measures that will improve outcomes in the community setting. The only chance for fetal survival is rapid transport to a facility with the capacity for immediate cesarean section and neonatal intensive care.

DIFFERENTIAL DIAGNOSES

Placental abruption, placenta previa, uterine rupture, bloody show, ruptured varicosity.

Placental Abruption

Placental abruption (*abruptio placentae*) refers to partial or complete separation of the placenta from the decidual-placental interface before birth of the fetus, generally after 20 weeks of gestation (Ananth & Kinzler, 2022). Because more than 600 ml/min of blood flows through the intervillous space at term, hemorrhage following antepartum separation of the placenta can be torrential (Cunningham et al., 2022, ch. 43). Placental abruption is a common cause of bleeding during pregnancy, responsible for about one third of all antepartum bleeding (Francois & Foley, 2021). If severe, it is one of the most serious obstetrical emergencies (Ghaheh et al., 2013). About 10% of all PTBs and 10%–20% of all perinatal deaths are associated with placental abruption (Odendaal, 2021).

Placental abruption can produce arterial or venous hemorrhage. A central abruption tends to involve acute high-pressure arterial hemorrhage, which can produce rapidly evolving symptoms such as severe pain, uterine tetany (unrelenting contraction) or tachysystole, and FHR abnormalities (Ananth & Kinzler, 2022). In a central abruption, vaginal bleeding can be profuse or entirely absent if the hemorrhage remains trapped behind the placenta. Marginal abruption tends to involve chronic low-pressure venous bleeding at the edge of the placenta (Ananth & Kinzler, 2022). Marginal abruption can spontaneously resolve or worsen over time.

Fifty-six percent of abruptions occur in the antepartum period; 44% occur during labor (Ananth & Kinzler, 2022). Two-thirds of abruptions are considered severe. A severe abruption is associated with maternal complications such as hypovolemic shock, disseminated intravascular coagulation (DIC), renal failure, need for hysterectomy, or death and with perinatal complications such as hypoxia, NICU admission, or death (Ananth & Kinzler, 2022).

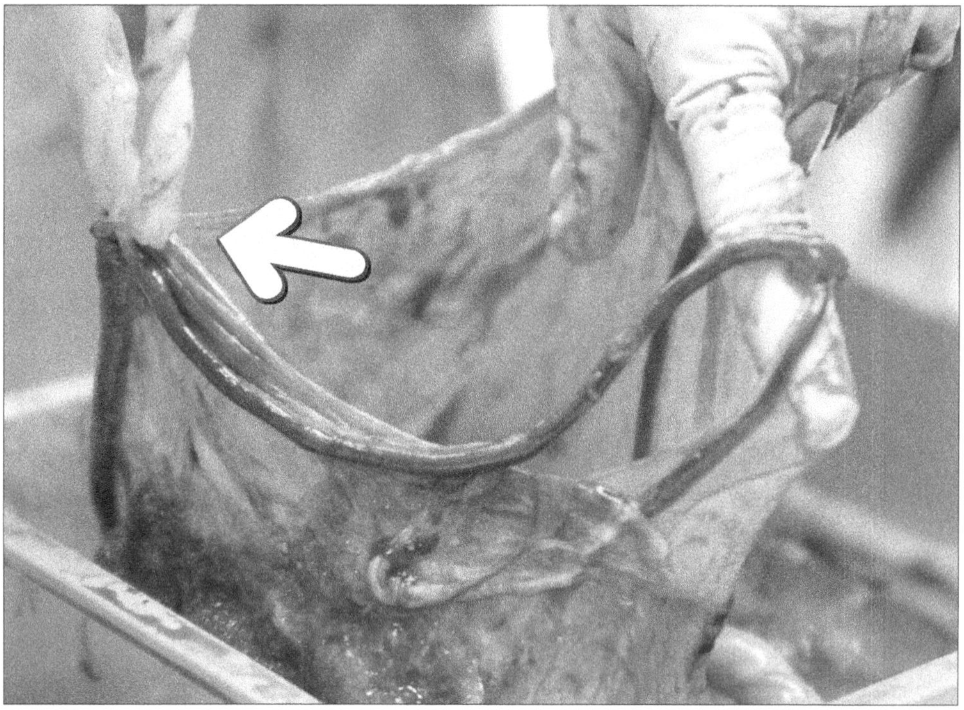

Figure 6-7. Vasa previa and large velamentous vessels on a dizygotic twin placenta. The arrow points to the site where an umbilical cord inserts into the membranes. Several large vessels crossed the lower uterine segment and cervix before connecting with the placenta. The amniotic membranes had ruptured spontaneously in the vicinity of the membranous vessels before presentation to the hospital, but fortunately the vessels remained intact. Cesarean section was performed before labor. Both babies were healthy, although the child with the velamentous vessels was 10 oz (283 g) lighter than her twin.

Pathophysiology

Abruption begins with the rupture of a maternal vessel in the decidua basalis at the interface with the placental villi (Cunningham et al., 2022, ch. 43). The collecting blood forms a retroplacental hematoma that acts as a wedge, splitting it from the decidual interface and lifting the placenta away from the uterus. This hematoma creates a barrier between the placental villi and the maternal blood supply that obstructs the exchange of gases. In the case of a severe abruption, the hematoma can expand until most of the placenta has detached. Decidual bleeding leads to the production of thrombin, which can result in inflammation and uterine contractions (Francois & Foley, 2021).

Abruption appears to occur as the result of either acute mechanical separation or chronically defective deep placentation (Visintine, 2022). Mechanical trauma (e.g., blunt trauma, deceleration injury from vehicular crash) or rapid decompression of a distended uterus (e.g., rupture of membranes with polyhydramnios, birth of a first twin) can generate shearing forces that cause the inflexible placenta to separate from the comparatively elastic uterine wall (Visintine, 2022). See Chapter 9 for a comprehensive discussion of trauma in pregnancy. Any placenta that implants over a uterine abnormality, cesarean scar, or fibroid is especially susceptible to abruption (Francois & Foley, 2021). A circumvallate placenta (chorionic plate is smaller than the basal plate, and the stiff, raised edges consist of folded membranes, degenerated decidua, and fibrin deposits) is relatively rigid and therefore is at higher risk for abruption (Celik et al., 2021).

Placental abruption, preeclampsia, and FGR can all arise from the same root cause: poor uteroplacental perfusion leading to chronic tissue hypoxia and ischemia (Ananth & Kinzler, 2022; Francois & Foley, 2021; Visintine, 2022). Abnormal trophoblastic invasion of uteroplacental arteries in the first trimester can lead to decidual necrosis and chronic placental inflammation, setting the stage for abruption, preeclampsia, or FGR (Ananth & Kinzler, 2022). Pregnant individuals with chronic hypertension or preeclampsia are five times more likely to experience abruption than normotensive people, but antihypertensive therapy does not appear to reduce the risk (Francois & Foley, 2021).

About 4–12% of individuals with preterm prelabor rupture of membranes (PPROM) develop placental abruption; those with greater latency between rupture of membranes and birth (24 hr or more) and those of lower gestational age are at increased risk (Tikkanen, 2011). Placental abruption can be both the cause and the result of PPROM (Tikkanen, 2011). Neutrophils, attracted to fibrin deposits at the site of decidual hemorrhage, release material that breaks down the amniotic membranes, predisposing them to prelabor rupture (Tikkanen, 2011). PPROM is frequently associated with ascending intrauterine infection, and uterine infection can lead to placental

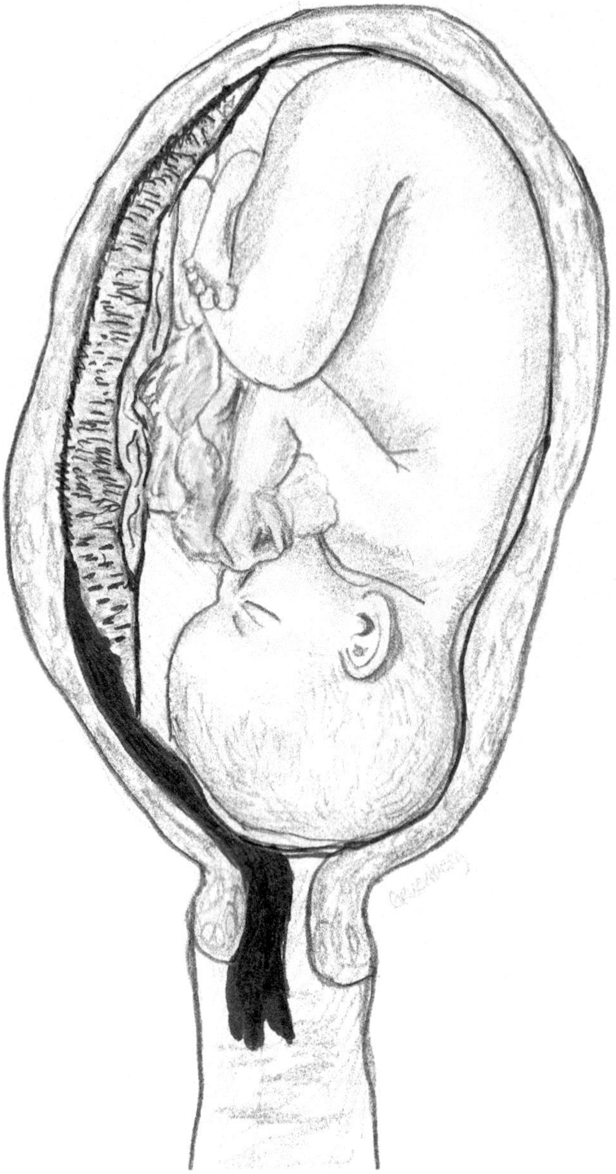

Figure 6-8. Marginal abruption occurs when the edge of the placenta separates from the uterine wall, causing bleeding.

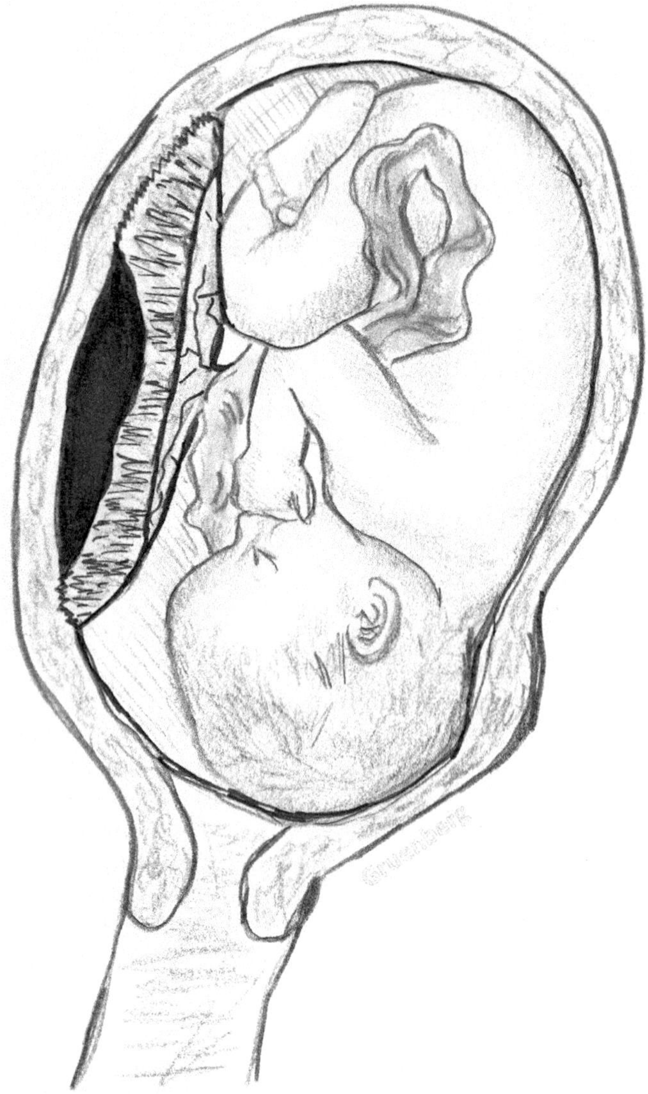

Figure 6-9. Central abruption involves bleeding behind the placenta while the margins remain intact, forming a hematoma that blocks perfusion without frank bleeding.

abruption. In some cases, the sudden reduction of uterine volume resulting from rupture of membranes can precipitate placental abruption.

Maternal and Perinatal Consequences

Sometimes a mild abruption at term has no adverse effect on mother or baby. Maternal risk depends largely on the severity of abruption (Ananth & Kinzler, 2022). Serious maternal outcomes include antepartum and/or postpartum hemorrhage, which can lead to acute blood-loss anemia; hypovolemic shock; DIC; acute kidney injury; acute respiratory distress syndrome; multiorgan failure; peripartum hysterectomy; and even death (ACOG Cmte. on Clinical Practice Guidelines—Obstetrics, Cahill, Raghuraman, Gandhi, & Kaimal, 2024; Ananth & Kinzler, 2022). Almost 30% of individuals with severe abruption develop DIC. Other serious maternal complications include pulmonary edema, acute myocardial infarction, cardiomyopathy, stroke, and amniotic fluid embolism (Visintine, 2022). Mothers who have had a placental abruption are at higher long-term risk of premature cardiovascular disease and death than those with no history of abruption (Ananth & Kinzler, 2022). When abruption necessitates cesarean birth, there is not only an immediate risk of intraoperative and postsurgical complications, but also an increased risk of complications in subsequent pregnancies related to uterine scarring.

The level of risk to the fetus is relative to the amount of placental separation and the gestational age when abruption occurs (Francois & Foley, 2021). The fetus can become deprived of oxygen if the remaining placenta is unable to meet its needs or if maternal hypovolemia and shock impair circulation. Fetal complications include hypoxemia, FGR, oligohydramnios,

PTB, asphyxia, and stillbirth. Up to 12% of recognized abruptions result in perinatal death; up to 50% of these deaths occur before birth (Ananth & Kinzler, 2022). The amount of vaginal bleeding does not indicate the extent of abruption, but fetal demise suggests that more than 45% of the placenta has detached (Ananth & Kinzler, 2022). Deaths in the first month of life are usually related to PTB (Ananth & Kinzler, 2022). Placental abruption also appears to increase the risk for adverse long-term neurobehavioral development, hypoxia-associated periventricular leukomalacia, and sudden infant death syndrome (Ananth & Kinzler, 2022; Francois & Foley, 2021).

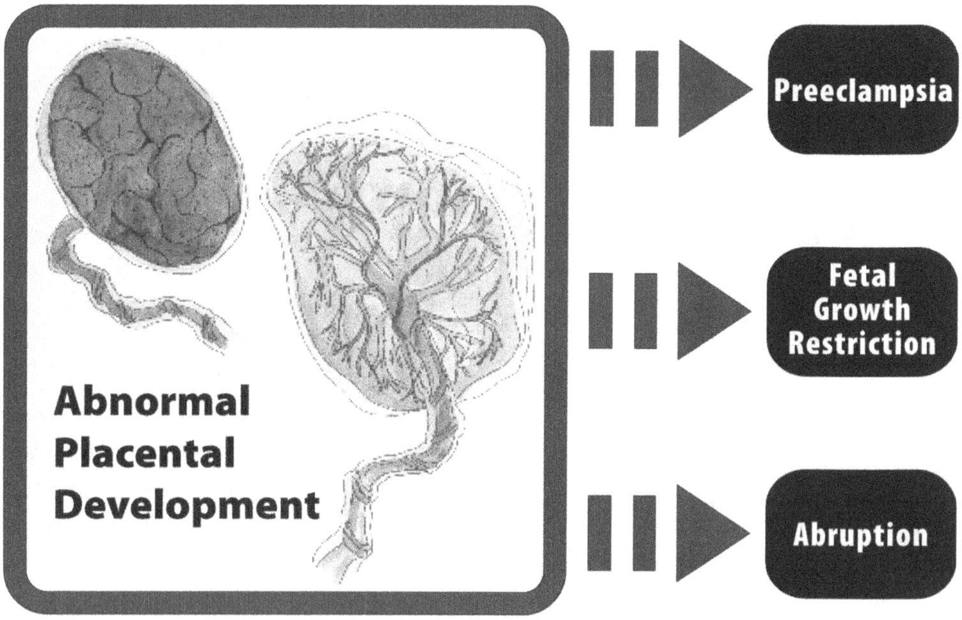

Figure 6-10. Abnormal placental development can lead to poor placental perfusion and can be the root cause for FGR, preeclampsia, and nontraumatic abruption.

Incidence and Risk Factors

Abruption is the most common cause of serious vaginal bleeding in pregnancy, occurring in 1% of pregnancies (Heinrichs, 2020). The rate of abruption is increasing in the United States and Canada and is dropping in the Netherlands, Spain, Finland, Sweden, Denmark, and Norway (Ananth & Kinzler, 2022). About 56% of abruptions develop antepartum, and about 44% develop intrapartum (Francois & Foley, 2021). About 60% develop at term, about 25% between 32 0/7 and 36 6/7 weeks of gestation, and about 14% before 32 0/7 weeks of gestation (Francois & Foley, 2021). Although nearly half of individuals with placental abruption have no identifiable risk factors, some conditions, such as the following, are associated with a higher risk.

History of abruption: The strongest risk factor for abruption is previous abruption. After one abruption, the risk of reoccurrence is 5%–17% (Visintine, 2022). After two, the risk of reoccurrence increases to 25% (Visintine, 2022). It also increases with the severity of the abruption. A mother who has an abruption that results in fetal demise has a 7% risk of abruption with fetal demise in a future pregnancy (Ananth & Kinzler, 2022; Oyelese & Ananth, 2022).

Maternal hypertensive disorders: Maternal hypertension (e.g., chronic hypertension, superimposed preeclampsia, preeclampsia with severe features, gestational hypertension, and eclampsia) increases the risk of abruption fivefold (Ananth & Kinzler, 2022). For individuals with chronic hypertension, antihypertensive therapy appears to reduce the risk of abruption. (Ananth & Kinzler, 2022).

Trauma: Blunt abdominal trauma (for example a kick to or fall on the abdomen) is associated with about 1% of cases of abruption (Visintine, 2022). Trauma such as a motor vehicle crash (MVC) can result in abruption through rapid deceleration and subsequent shearing injury, even without direct injury to the abdomen. Abruption can follow seemingly minor trauma (Cunningham et al., 2022, ch. 43), and it is usually evident within 24 hr after the incident (Ananth & Kinzler, 2022). Fetomaternal hemorrhage, uncommon with most spontaneous abruptions, can occur if traumatic injury tears the placenta (Cunningham et al., 2022). Abruption resulting from trauma is not likely to reoccur spontaneously (Ananth & Kinzler, 2022).

Tobacco smoking: Tobacco smoking is associated with a fivefold increase in risk for abruption (Ananth & Kinzler, 2022). Supplementation with vitamins C and E can reduce the risk of abruption associated with smoking (Abramovici et al., 2015; Rumbold, Ota, Hori, Miyazaki, & Crowther, 2015).

Physical exertion: Though it appears that fit, active mothers are at lower risk for abruption overall (Meah, Davies, & Davenport, 2020), strenuous activity has been associated with higher risk for abruption. In one study, individuals undertaking moderate or heavy physical exertion were 8 times more likely to have an abruption during the hour following the activity than individuals involved in light or no exertion (Chahal et al., 2018).

PPROM: As previously discussed, PPROM and associated intraamniotic infection can cause or result from placental abruption. Almost 40% of placentas from mothers with PPROM show evidence of old decidual hemorrhages (Visintine, 2022). For pregnancies between 20 0/7 and 36 6/7 weeks of gestation,

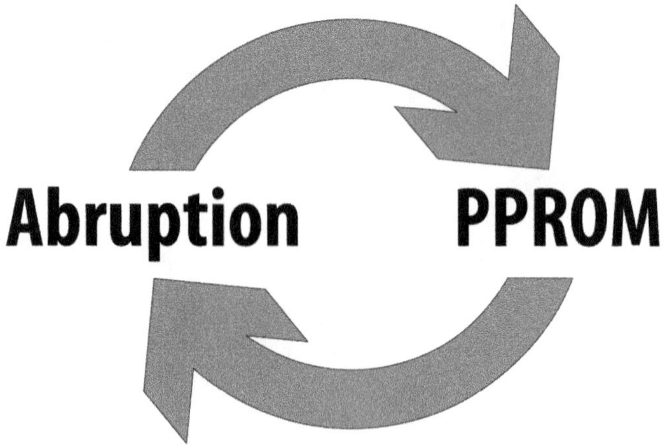

Figure 6-11. Preterm prelabor rupture of the membranes can be either the cause or the result of placental abruption.

the abruption rate is 5% overall and as high as 17% for the subset of individuals with previable prelabor ruptured membranes (Cunningham et al., 2022, ch. 43).

Rapid uterine decompression: Rapid decompression of a gravid uterus, especially one overdistended by multiple fetuses or polyhydramnios, can precipitate placental abruption (Francois & Foley, 2021). Amniotomy or spontaneous rupture of membranes can cause shearing of the inelastic placenta as the uterine cavity shrinks. Twin gestations have an almost threefold increase in the risk for placental abruption when compared to singletons.

Structural uterine abnormalities: Synechiae (intrauterine adhesions) and uterine fibroids provide mechanically and biologically unstable locations for the placenta to implant (Ananth & Kinzler, 2022). Müllerian duct anomalies increase the risk fivefold, and septate uterus carries the highest risk for abruption (Ananth & Kinzler, 2022).

Cocaine use: Up to 10% of pregnant individuals using cocaine in the third trimester have an abruption (Ananth & Kinzler, 2022).

More modest risk factors for abruption include asthma, subclinical hypothyroidism, major fetal congenital anomalies, prior cesarean birth, exposure to air pollution, conception through assisted reproductive technology, marginal placental cord insertion, grand multiparity, and short maternal stature (Ananth & Kinzler, 2022). Short umbilical cord and placenta previa are also risk factors for abruption. COVID-19 (SARS-CoV-2) infection has been demonstrated to increase the likelihood of abruption to as high as 2.2% (Litman et al., 2022). The risk is greatest when the diagnosis is within 30 days before admission for childbirth (Litman et al., 2022). Individuals who are underweight at conception can be at greater risk for abruption (Jenabi et al., 2022).

Presentation

Placental abruption is largely a clinical diagnosis that can be confirmed by radiographic, laboratory, or pathologic findings. Presentation is influenced by whether the abruption is acute or chronic, overt or concealed, severe or self-limiting (Francois & Foley, 2021). The four classic signs and symptoms of acute abruption are (Visintine, 2022)

- Vaginal bleeding (67–78%);
- Uterine tenderness or abdominal/back pain (52–66%);
- Category II or III electronic FHR tracing (60–78%); and
- Uterine hypertonus or tachysystole (more than 5 contractions in 10 min, averaged over 30 min; 17%).

Signs of abruption can be ambiguous, especially in less-severe cases. The individual with a small abruption can experience light to moderate bleeding (with or without pain and contractions), an inconclusive or negative sonogram report, and a reassuring FHR. Sometimes an abnormal fetal heart pattern is the only indication of abruption (Hall, 2009). About 10–20% of clients with abruptions experience uterine contractions/irritability and little else (Ananth & Kinzler, 2022; Cunningham et al., 2022). FHR abnormalities, abnormal maternal vital signs, and sudden onset of vaginal bleeding or abdominal pain suggest a large abruption that can result in severe maternal morbidity and fetal death (Ananth & Kinzler, 2022). Although the amount of bleeding does not correlate well with the amount of placental separation, degree of discomfort does: abdominal or back pain tends to become more intense with a severe abruption (Ananth & Kinzler, 2022).

Bleeding: Vaginal bleeding can be bright or dark red. Sometimes the mother passes formed clots that can be very large. Bleeding from the placental edge or beneath the membranes can enter the amniotic fluid and impart a distinctive "port wine" hue that is unique to abruption (Meserve, Sirois, Parast, & Boyd, 2018). In some cases of abruption, external bleeding is heavy, but placental separation is minimal, and the fetus is not compromised. In others, external bleeding is absent, but the concealed abruption is extensive enough to result in fetal demise and maternal compromise.

Mothers with a large abruption can sometimes lose more than half of their blood volume, leading to hemorrhagic shock, coagulopathy, and even death (Cunningham et al., 2022, ch. 43). Some degree of intravascular coagulation occurs with most large placental abruptions (Cunningham et al., 2022, ch. 43). DIC is more likely with a concealed abruption because the higher intrauterine pressure forces more thromboplastin into the large veins draining the implantation site (Cunningham et al., 2022, ch. 43).

Uterine tone and contractility: Although any contraction pattern is possible, the classic pattern seen in abruption is a low-amplitude tachysystole. The contractions usually have a sawtooth pattern with many low waves and minimal break between them. In a major abruption, blood can seep into the muscle fibers of the myometrium and extend to the serosal surface, causing the uterus to become enlarged and mottled with dark-purple blotches (Couvelaire uterus). This hemorrhagic infiltration of the myometrium can result in uterine irritability, hypertonicity (exaggerated uterine tone), or rapidly progressive labor (Sukumaran, Jia, & Chandraharan, 2021). A hypertonic uterus can feel as solid as a block of wood with no fetal parts palpable (Ananth & Kinzler, 2022; Stafford, Belfort, & Dildy, 2019).

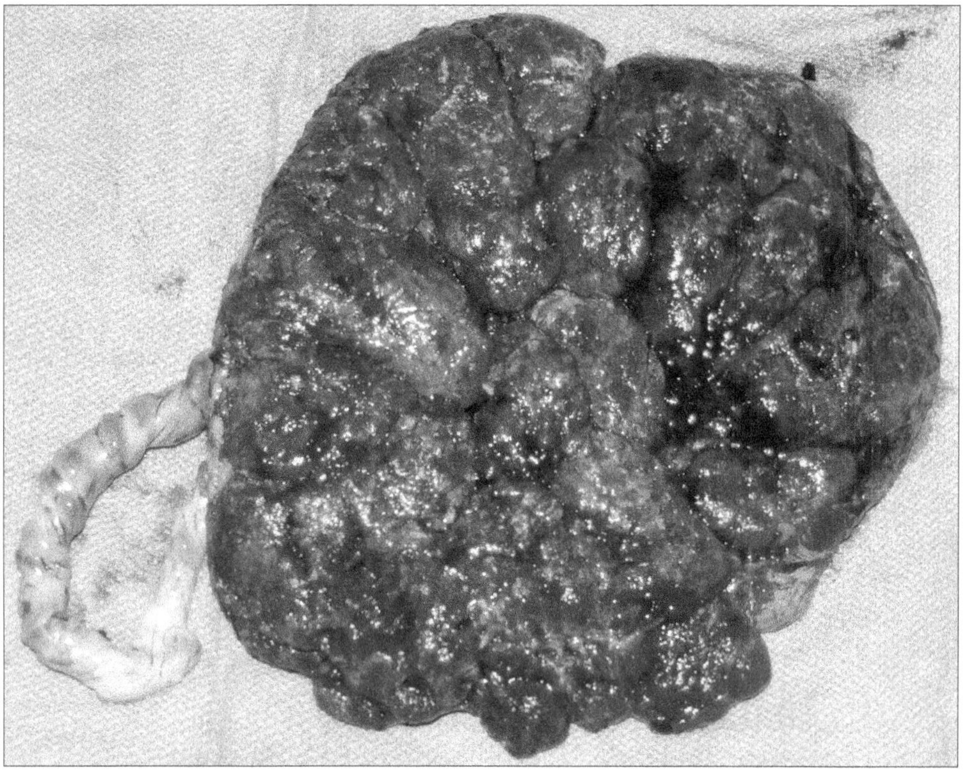

Figure 6-12. Extremely calcified placenta of a heavy smoker at 37 weeks of gestation. Tobacco use is associated with small, calcified placentas and high risk of abruption, preterm birth (PTB), and stillbirth.

Pain: The pain of abruption probably results from extravasation of blood into the myometrium and can be severe. Although this pain is usually located in the abdomen, back pain is common when the placenta is on the posterior wall of the uterus. It can be difficult to distinguish the pain caused by the abruption itself from that caused by uterine contractions stimulated by the abruption (Mei & Lin, 2018).

FHR pattern: Undetectable variability and bradycardia are the FHR patterns most strongly associated with low 5-min Apgar score, acidosis, and a large placental separation (Usui et al., 2008). When bradycardia related to abruption is sustained at a rate lower than 80 beats per min (bpm), 40% of fetuses have poor outcomes (Takano et al., 2013). Other concerning patterns associated with abruption include fetal tachycardia, late or variable decelerations, rising or decreasing baseline, or a sinusoidal pattern. The FHR pattern can be normal if placental circulation is largely intact and the mother is not hypovolemic. Early in the abruption process, maternal catecholamines can constrict blood vessels to maintain perfusion of the mother's heart and brain at the expense of uteroplacental blood flow (Hall, 2009). Consequently, abnormal FHR patterns can be an early sign of maternal hemodynamic compromise (Hull & Resnik, 2014).

Supportive Diagnostics

While there is no definitive test for placental abruption, certain assessments can support or refute the clinical impression. These assessments include the following:

Imaging: The sensitivity of ultrasound in recognizing placental abruption is only about 24%; more than 75% of abruptions are missed on sonography (Visintine, 2022). During the acute phase of the abruption, the blood appears similar in texture to the surrounding placental tissue on ultrasound, and intrauterine bleeding can be difficult to identify. The specificity, however, is 96%; if an abruption is seen on ultrasound, the provider can be confident that the diagnosis is accurate (Visintine, 2022). A retroplacental hematoma (located between the placenta and the myometrium) is the definitive ultrasound finding and can appear solid or complex with densities that vary with the timing of the bleed (Ananth & Kinzler, 2022). Other findings that suggest abruption include a subchorionic collection of fluid, echogenic (reflective on ultrasound) debris in the amniotic fluid, a thickened placenta, and a placenta that shimmers with maternal movement—"Jell-O®" sign (Ananth & Kinzler, 2022). Contrast-enhanced computerized tomography (CT) and magnetic-resonance imaging (MRI) can detect abruption and may be used in cases of abdominal trauma; but these tests are expensive, they are not always readily available, and positive findings are unlikely to change management (Ananth & Kinzler, 2022).

Laboratory findings: Laboratory findings associated with severe abruption can include a low hematocrit; a low platelet count; a high prothrombin time [PT] and partial thromboplastin time [PTT]; and low fibrinogen. Placental abruption is the

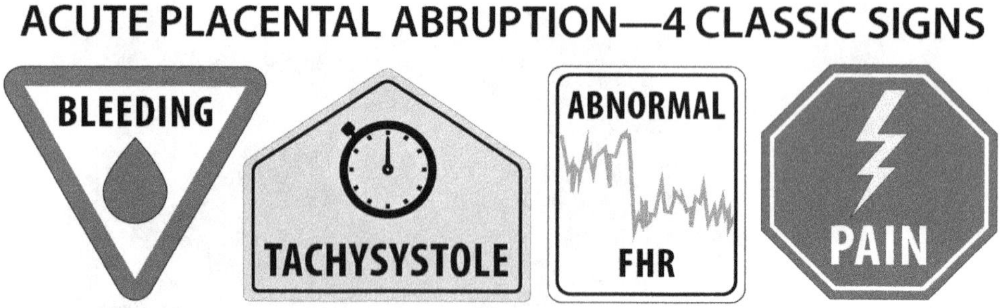

Figure 6-13. The four classic signs of acute placental abruption: bleeding, pain, tachysystole, and abnormal FHR. A client with a placental abruption may have any, all, or none of these signs, making clinical diagnosis difficult.

most common cause of DIC in obstetrics (Cunningham et al., 2022, ch. 43). By contrast, coagulopathy is rare with placenta previa, probably because placental thromboplastin (a substance that incites intravascular coagulation) tends to escape through the cervical canal rather than entering the maternal circulation when bleeding is caused by placenta previa (Cunningham et al., 2022, ch. 43).

Fibrinogen level is the best indicator of severe bleeding, DIC, and the need for transfusion of multiple blood products (Ananth & Kinzler, 2022). Fibrinogen levels are elevated in pregnancy, reaching mean values close to 5 g/L by term (Atallah et al., 2023). In pregnancy, fibrinogen levels that are within normal range for the nonpregnant individual can indicate a coagulation disorder (Atallah et al., 2023). An individual with placental abruption and a fibrinogen concentration of less than 3 g/L is at higher risk for intrauterine fetal demise (Atallah et al., 2023). The Kleihauer-Betke test for fetomaternal hemorrhage is not recommended for nontraumatic abruption because is positive in only 4% of individuals in this setting and is of questionable clinical benefit (Boller et al., 2020; Visintine, 2022).

Pathology findings: At delivery, the placenta often shows no evidence of recent abruption, although a fresh bleed can leave a loosely formed retroplacental clot on the maternal side that can easily be detached by the fingers. An abruption that is hours old can leave a firmer clot more solidly adherent to the placenta. A longstanding clot can indent the surface of the placenta and eventually solidify and turn pale (Mei & Lin, 2018). Placental pathological examination confirms the presence of acute abruption in only 25% of cases and chronic clinical abruption in about 60% (Visintine, 2022). The absence of pathologic findings does not exclude an abruption (Visintine, 2022).

Prognosis and Management

Any client with significant antepartum bleeding or suspected abruption should be evaluated in a hospital. The obstetric team usually performs an immediate cesarean if the mother or (viable) fetus is unstable and vaginal birth is not imminent. A category III tracing or a biophysical profile score of 0–4 of 10 indicates that the fetus is compromised and should be born quickly (Oyelese & Ananth, 2022). Although a category II fetal heart tracing is usually considered indeterminate, when associated with abruption it can presage sudden fetal deterioration and death (Oyelese & Ananth, 2022). The provider must weigh gestational age, cervical dilation, and whether maternal or fetal status seems to be worsening (Oyelese & Ananth, 2022).

When the mother is stable with no evidence of ongoing major blood loss or coagulopathy, the FHR pattern is reassuring (category I), and the fetus is less than 34 0/7 weeks of gestation, expectant management can be appropriate (Oyelese & Ananth, 2022). A course of corticosteroids should be given to promote fetal lung maturity in case further bleeding necessitates birth. Individuals who have had a placental abruption remain at risk for recurrent or progressive abruption (Oyelese & Ananth, 2022). Birth is recommended for clients presenting with acute bleeding from placental abruption at or beyond 36 0/7 weeks of gestation (Oyelese & Ananth, 2022).

When birth is required and mother and fetus are relatively stable, trial of labor is recommended if continuous fetal monitoring and provisions for emergency cesarean are available (Oyelese & Ananth, 2022). Labor usually progresses rapidly in the presence of placental abruption. Artificial rupture of the membranes and oxytocin augmentation can be used to hasten labor when necessary (Oyelese & Ananth, 2022).

Mothers with placental abruption often must surrender their birth plans to the bewildering need for emergency surgery or other interventions. Instead of the anticipated normal postpartum recovery, they frequently must cope with extended hospital stays, a compromised baby, obstacles to breastfeeding and bonding, and slower healing. Consequently, they can be at higher risk for postpartum depression and PTSD.

DIFFERENTIAL DIAGNOSES

Placenta previa, vasa previa, bloody show of labor, uterine rupture. Intrauterine bleeding can also originate from subchorionic (between the placenta and the membranes) and preplacental (between the placenta and the amniotic fluid) sites (Ananth & Kinzler, 2022).

Uterine Rupture

Although the rupture of any internal organ can be life-threatening, rupture of the large, well-perfused

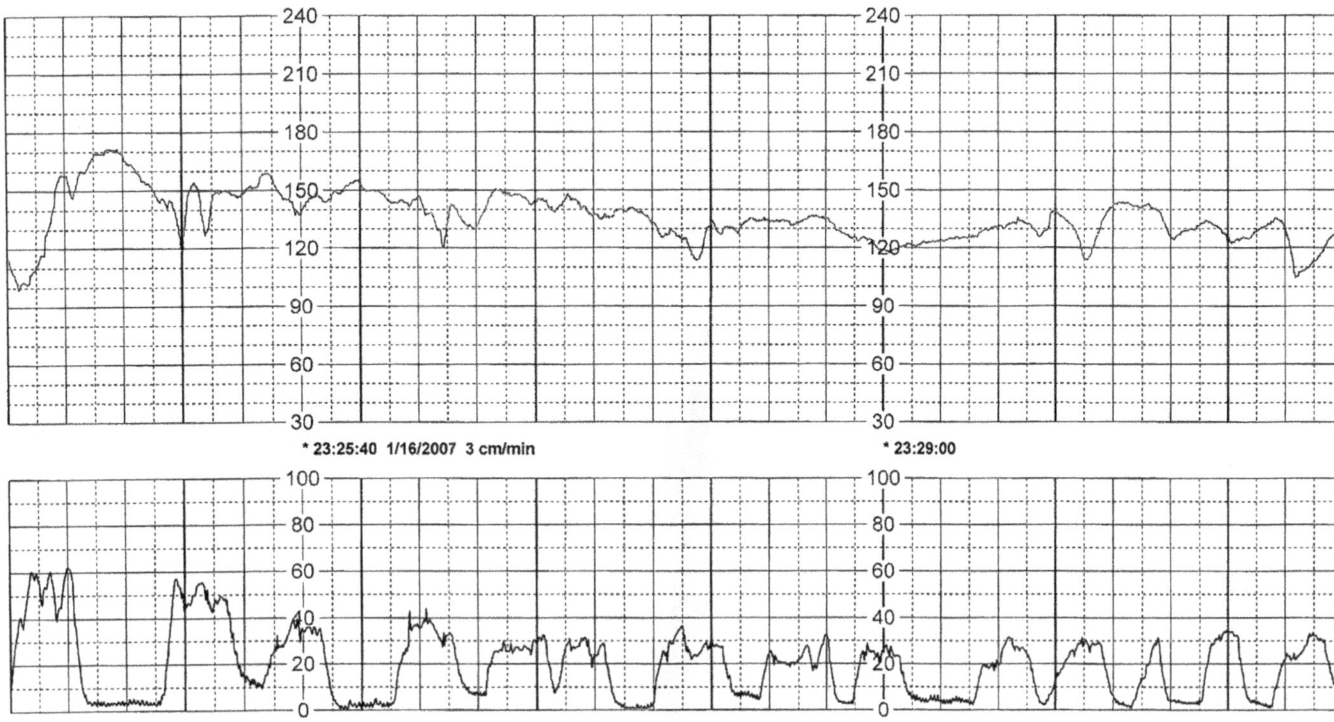

Figure 6-14. The low amplitude, high frequency contraction pattern often seen with significant abruption. This mother presented to the hospital with moderate bleeding, painful contractions, and a deep, severe backache. The fetal heart tracing was category II upon presentation and progressed quickly to category III. Emergency cesarean occurred soon after this tracing was obtained. Apgars were 2, 4, and 5, and the cord arterial pH was 6.9.

pregnant uterus is especially serious. A ruptured uterus can involve any part of the organ and can extend into the cervix, vagina, and bladder. Most uterine ruptures occur in individuals who have had surgical incisions through the myometrium to the uterine cavity, e.g., cesarean section, myomectomy, uterine resection (Smith & Wax, 2022). Rupture of the unscarred uterus is rare, but it is associated with greater risk to mother and fetus because it is more likely to occur outside the lower uterine segment and extend beyond the cervix (Al-Zirqi, Daltveit, & Vangen., 2019).

A ruptured uterus puts both mother and fetus at risk for serious morbidity and death. In one study of complete rupture of scarred and unscarred uteruses, 26.2% of newborns died, 6.1% of surviving infants had permanent brain damage from hypoxic ischemic encephalopathy, and 23.0% required NICU admission for severe hypoxia or other causes (Al-Zirqi et al., 2019). Another author found a 6% perinatal death rate for uterine rupture after cesarean (Guise et al., 2010). A study of the maternal consequences of uterine rupture found that 43.3% of mothers had severe postpartum hemorrhages without hysterectomies; 20.6% required peripartum hysterectomies; many developed serious cardiac, cerebral, renal, and respiratory complications; and 1.3% died (Al-Zirqi et al., 2019). A large Canadian study found a rate of 1 maternal death in 500 uterine ruptures (Wen et al., 2005).

Incidence

In developed countries, uterine rupture occurs in 1 of 1,428 pregnancies, but among mothers with prior cesarean, the rate jumps to 1 in 500 to 1 in 125—and the incidence is rising with the rate of cesarean section (Al-Zirqi, Stray-Pedersen, Forsén, Daltveit, & Vangen, 2016). Rupture of the unscarred pregnant uterus is extremely rare, occurring in 1 in 5,700–20,000 pregnancies and about 1 in 22,000 births in the United States (Smith & Wax, 2022). Risk is higher in resource-limited countries where higher parity, contracted pelvises due to nutritional deficiencies, and prolonged obstructed labor play a role (Smith & Wax, 2022).

Risk factors

Certain conditions put a mother at higher risk for uterine rupture. In combination, they seem to increase the risk. But no single factor or combination can consistently predict all instances (Francois & Foley, 2021). Risk factors include the following:

Myometrial Weakness or scarring. Congenital or acquired myometrial weakness can predispose an individual to uterine rupture. Acquired weaknesses include previous uterine surgery; prolonged labor or use of uterotonic drugs; previous uterine rupture; placenta accreta, increta, or percreta; prior cerclage; and uterine adenomyosis (Smith & Wax, 2022).

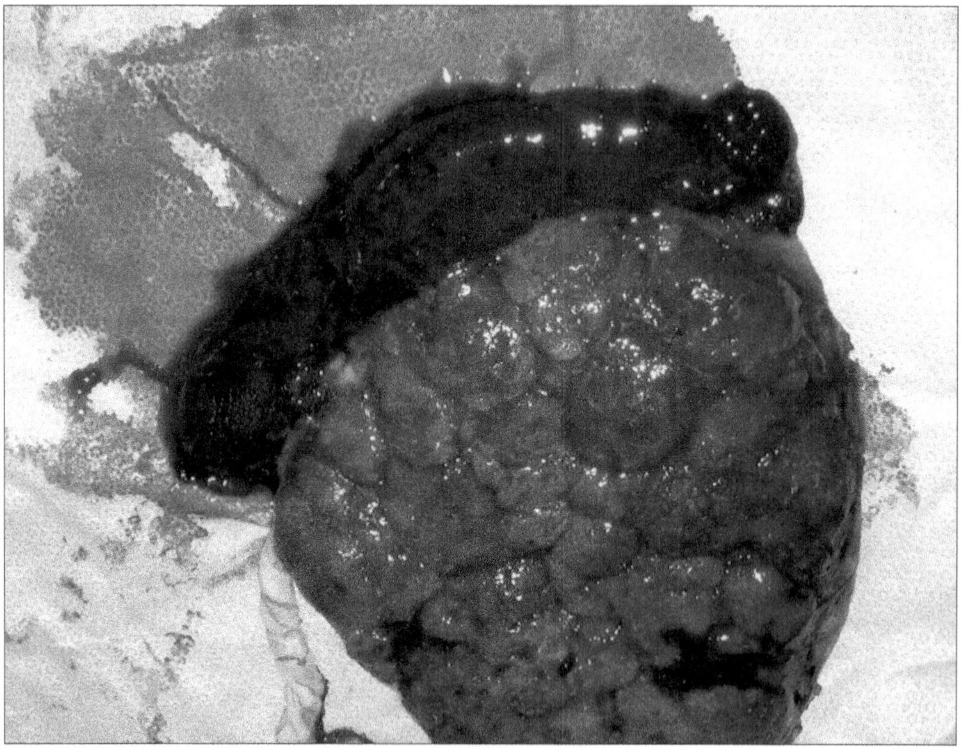

Figure 6-15. Placenta with acute abruption with a large adherent clot and smaller clots in other locations. Fortunately, emergency cesarean section was performed promptly, and mother and baby ultimately did well.

Prior uterine rupture carries risk of recurrent rupture or dehiscence from 6% if the rupture occurred in the lower uterine segment to 32% if it involved the upper segment (ACOG, 2019; Landon & Frey, 2022; Ness, 2022). Prelabor cesarean section about 36–37 weeks of gestation is recommended for mothers with prior uterine rupture (ACOG, 2019).

Other factors that can produce small increases in risk for uterine rupture include grand multiparity, cocaine use, uterine anomalies, adenomyosis, and invasive placenta (Smith & Wax, 2022).

Herbal preparations. Certain herbs have been associated with uterine rupture. A study conducted at a hospital in western Uganda noted that 35% of subjects with uterine rupture had used herbs given by traditional birth attendants to induce labor (Mukasa et al., 2013). In a large study at a hospital in Ghana, 58.5% of mothers with uterine rupture had consumed an herbal remedy known locally as *kalguteem* or *masuge*; 9.8% of those mothers and 82.9% of the affected babies died (Fofie & Baffoe, 2010).

Among individuals with a prior cesarean, the incidence of uterine rupture is approximately 1 in 100 to 1 in 200 cases (Francois & Foley, 2021). These ruptures usually occur during labor. Risk is highest for individuals with a classical (vertical) or T-shaped incision—4% and 9% risk of rupture, respectively (Francois & Foley, 2021). Other risk factors for rupture of a scarred uterus include maternal age over 30, birthweight greater than 8 lb 13 oz (4,000 g), less than 18 months between births (2.3%–4.8% risk), single-layer uterine closure, more than one cesarean birth (0.9% for one, 1.8% for two), and previous second-trimester cesarean birth (Ness, 2022). Prolonged second stage labor in the current pregnancy increases the risk from 0.7% for second stage less than1 hr to 3.1% for second stage of 3 hr or longer (Ness, 2022).

For the individual choosing a trial of labor after cesarean section (TOLAC), risk of uterine rupture is lower when the mother has had a prior vaginal birth and lower still after a successful vaginal birth after cesarean, or VBAC (Ness, 2022). TOLAC is most likely to be safe and successful when onset of labor is spontaneous. Augmentation with oxytocin can increase the risk of uterine rupture by about 1%, but this risk is largely associated with doses greater than 20 mU/min (Ness, 2022). The risk of uterine rupture after cesarean is as high as 2.5% when labor is induced with prostaglandins, and even higher with sequential use of prostaglandins and oxytocin (Ness, 2022).

Several researchers have developed calculators for predicting the likelihood of successful VBAC (Metz, 2023). The Maternal-Fetal Medicine Units Network (MFMU) offers two VBAC calculators free of charge online. One is designed to estimate the likelihood of successful vaginal birth at an early stage of pregnancy (MFMU, n.d.-a). The other (MFMU, n.d.-b) incorporates the individual's circumstances at the time of labor, including Bishop score and gestational age. Although algorithms and formulas cannot predict uterine rupture, they can clarify risk level to help provider and client plan for birth. VBAC calculator results are not intended to discourage strongly motivated individuals from attempting a vaginal birth, for many with low calculator scores succeed (Metz, 2023).

Mechanism

Uterine rupture can be a result of weakness of the myometrium, obstructed labor, or trauma (Smith & Wax, 2022). It is usually classified as complete if all uterine wall layers are separated or incomplete if uterine muscle is separated but the visceral peritoneum is intact; the latter is also known as uterine scar dehiscence or uterine window (Cunningham et al., 2022, ch. 42). Complete rupture of the uterus is an emergency involving complete disruption of all uterine layers that can lead to massive hemorrhage, expulsion of the fetus into the abdominal cavity, and perinatal hypoxemia or asphyxia (Landon & Grobman, 2021). Whereas complete uterine rupture is rare and catastrophic, uterine scar dehiscence is more common and seldom results in poor maternal or fetal outcome (Cunningham et al., 2022, ch. 42). More than 90% of uterine ruptures occur in the anterior lower uterine segment, but they can extend to the fundus, cervix, vagina, broad ligament, or through the posterior vaginal fornix (Evans & B-Lynch, 2012; Landon & Frey, 2022; Landon & Grobman, 2021).

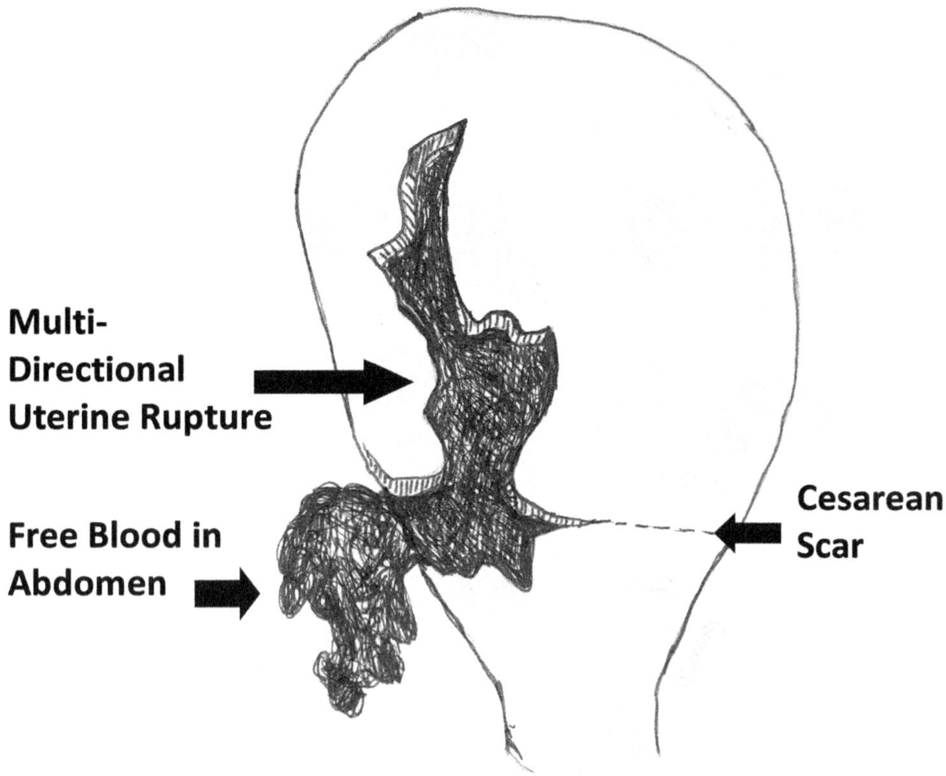

Figure 6-16. Whereas the separation of a cesarean scar can be a bloodless "window" into the uterus, uterine rupture involves full-thickness tearing of the uterine muscle and can expel the fetus into the mother's abdominal cavity. A simple window can rapidly turn into a uterine rupture, creating a complex, extensive laceration of the myometrium.

Obstructed Labor

During normal labor, the upper segment contracts, retracts, and expels the fetus while the lower segment remains softer, passive, and distensible. The muscle fibers of the upper segment shorten and shrink with each contraction, remaining relatively fixed at a shorter length and growing thicker as labor progresses. The lower segment forms a thin, stretchy tube through which the fetus can pass and is pulled upward and around the presenting part of the fetus (Cunningham et al., 2022, ch. 42).

If the fetal presenting part does not fit through the maternal pelvis, arrest of labor can occur. This disproportion is *absolute* when the fetus is too large for the bony birth canal or *relative* when the fetus is mispositioned and the presenting diameters are too large (Sinha, Talaulikar, & Arulkumaran, 2018). The multipara with obstructed labor tends to have frequent tetanic contractions until the obstruction is overcome or the uterus ruptures (Evans & B-Lynch, 2012; Saxena, 2014; Sinha et al., 2018). The contractions of a nullipara with obstructed labor, however, typically become weaker and less coordinated until labor ceases entirely (Evans & B-Lynch, 2012; Saxena, 2014; Sinha et al., 2018). Uterine rupture is both more common and more lethal in low-resource areas, largely because of neglected or obstructed labors. In remote areas, cesarean section can be delayed by hours or even days, leading to stillbirth. In these cases, prolonged pressure from impaction can cause the tissues of the birth canal to lose circulation and become necrotic, resulting in vesicovaginal, vesicocervical, or rectovaginal fistulas.

Other signs of obstructed labor include arrest of cervical dilation or descent, irregular contraction pattern, fetal head poorly applied to an edematous cervix, and pronounced caput

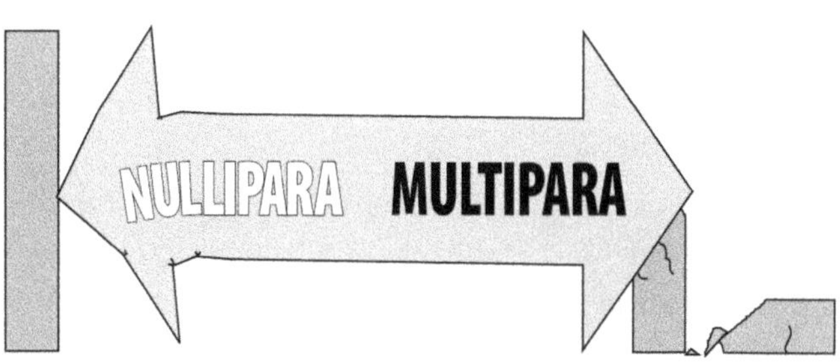

Figure 6-17. Nullipara with obstructed labor: contractions usually become weaker, less organized, and farther apart. Multipara with obstructed labor: contractions usually become abnormally strong to overcome the obstruction.

and exaggerated molding. Over time, the upper uterine segment can become thick and retracted, while the lower uterine segment becomes abnormally thin and overstretched. Bandl's ring, a rigid, pathologic constriction, can form at the junction of the uterine segments. It sometimes can be visualized and palpated at about the level of the umbilicus as a depression between the upper and lower halves of the uterus, like the two humps of a camel. Bandl's ring signifies impending rupture of the lower uterine segment due to extreme thinning and inability to move the fetus farther down the birth canal (Manoharan, Wuntakal, & Erskine, 2010; van den Broek, 2020). Diagnosis is typically made during cesarean section, when a thick transverse muscular band is observed dividing the upper and lower segments (Ehsanipoor & Satin, 2022).

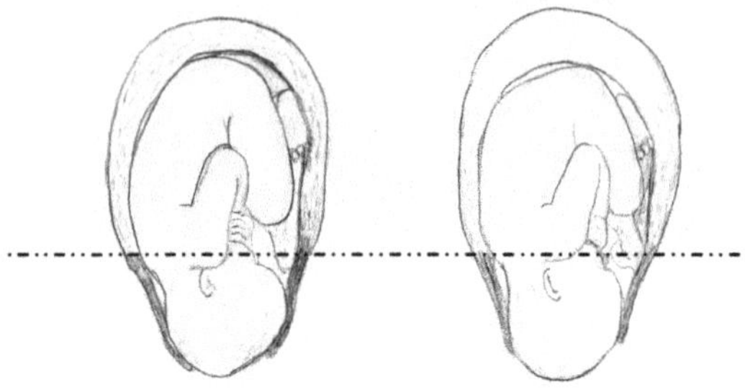

Figure 6-18. In normal labor, the upper uterine segment shortens and shrinks with each contraction, and the muscle fibers remain relatively fixed at a shorter length. The muscle of the lower uterine segment and cervix thins and stretches as it is pulled upward around the fetus.

Additionally, a pathologic uterine ring can trap the fetal neck, shoulder, thorax, or extremities and prevent birth. The fetus can be difficult to extract during cesarean section, and even a vertical incision through the ring might not readily allow birth (Berghella, 2022). Compression by the ring can result in fetal intracranial, intrathoracic, or intraabdominal injuries, though these are rare (Lauria, Barthold, Zimmerman, & Turrentine, 2007). A pathological ring can also present as an hourglass constriction of the uterus after the birth of a first twin, necessitating a prompt cesarean to rescue the second twin (Berghella, 2022).

Trauma

Trauma (from MVC, fall, assault, etc.) or an obstetric maneuver (e.g., internal or external cephalic version, fundal pressure) can result in traumatic uterine rupture (Smith & Wax, 2022). This topic is discussed in detail in Chapter 9, "Traumatic Uterine Rupture."

Presentation

Uterine dehiscence, occurring when a hysterotomy scar (healed wound from uterine surgery, commonly cesarean) opens partially or completely, can be asymptomatic and can be noted only as an incidental finding on ultrasound or during a repeat cesarean section (Landon & Frey, 2022). In contrast, complete uterine rupture is an emergency requiring rapid and decisive intervention. Classic signs of uterine rupture include the following abnormal findings:

1. **Abnormal fetal heart pattern.** Fetal wellbeing depends on how much of the placenta remains attached to the uterus and the mother's ability to perfuse it—both can change within minutes (Cunningham et al., 2022, ch. 42). The most common FHR pattern associated with uterine rupture, found in up to 70% of cases, is bradycardia (Ridgeway, Weyrich, & Benedetti, 2004). Late decelerations (19.0–87.5%) and variable decelerations (5.1–19.0%) have also been associated with uterine rupture (Ridgeway et al., 2004). Category III FHR tracings commonly occur in the hour before uterine rupture is diagnosed (Landon & Frey, 2022). Often, the attending physician proceeds to emergency cesarean because of an abnormal fetal heart tracing and discovers the uterine rupture upon opening the abdomen (Landon & Frey, 2022; Landon & Grobman, 2021).
2. **Abnormal bleeding**. Vaginal bleeding can be minimal despite catastrophic intraabdominal hemorrhage. Most of the blood lost during uterine rupture typically remains inside the abdomen (Togioka & Tonismae, 2022). Rupture extending through the cervix and upper vaginal wall usually involves much more vaginal bleeding than rupture involving the posterior uterus or parametrium. Rupture that results in injury to the bladder can present with acute gross hematuria (Landon & Grobman, 2021).
3. **Abnormal vital signs**. Heavy maternal blood loss can be associated with hypotension, tachycardia, and shock. Hypotension is often accompanied by lightheadedness, dizziness, nausea, vomiting, pallor, sweating, and anxiety. Often there is minimal external bleeding, and the source of shock is not readily apparent. Uterine rupture can produce symptoms and physical findings that mimic those of other disorders, such as referred pain to the chest and shoulder pain, when free blood in the abdomen irritates the diaphragm (Cunningham et al., 2022, ch. 42).

4. **Abnormal contractions.** Uterine rupture can present with a gradual decrease in the amplitude of consecutive contractions, known as the "staircase sign" (Heinrichs, 2020; Matsuo, Scanlon, Atlas, & Kopelman, 2008). After the fetus is expelled into the peritoneal cavity, contractions usually stop.
5. **Abnormal abdominal pain.** Abdominal pain is often severe and constant, unlike the intermittent pain of contractions, but the degree, character, and location of pain can vary (Smith & Wax, 2022). A ruptured uterus in a mother with epidural anesthesia can present with vital-sign changes and abnormal fetal heart pattern but minimal discomfort, or with severe pain unmitigated by anesthesia (Smith & Wax, 2022).

Obstructed Labor

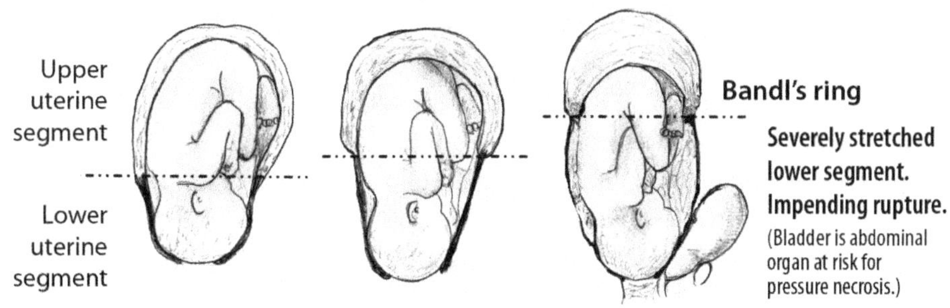

Figure 6-19. When labor is obstructed, the upper uterine segment becomes thick and retracted while the lower uterine segment becomes abnormally thin and overstretched. Bandl's ring, a rigid pathologic constriction ring, can form at the junction of the uterine segments. If a cesarean is not performed, the uterus is likely to rupture. Pressure on the bladder and/or rectum can result in tissue necrosis, increasing the likelihood of fistula formation.

6. **Abnormal change in fetal station.** A sudden change in the fetal position can occur if the fetus moves through a uterine laceration into the abdominal cavity. Sometimes the presenting part is no longer palpable in the pelvis or can assume a higher station.
7. **Abnormal change in abdominal contour.** If the fetus is expelled from the uterus, the shape of the abdomen can change, and fetal parts can be easily palpated through the abdominal wall. Intraabdominal hemorrhage can increase girth, abdominal rigidity, and rebound tenderness.

In rare cases, rupture is recognized only after vaginal birth. Uterine rupture should be suspected postpartum if the individual has heavy bleeding through the cervix despite a well-contracted uterus. The provider might be able to palpate the site of rupture on internal uterine examination after birth. Postpartum diagnosis appears to be more common with rupture of an unscarred uterus (Al-Zirqi, Daltveit, & Vangen, 2018).

Management

Early recognition of signs and symptoms and moving quickly to surgery improve outcomes of uterine rupture. Infants born by cesarean section within 18–20 min after uterine rupture have the best outcomes (Al-Zirqi et al., 2018; Holmgren, 2012); those with a decision-to-birth time of greater than 30 min are likely to have poor outcomes (Ness, 2022). The diagnosis is confirmed when the obstetrician opens the abdomen and visualizes complete disruption of all uterine layers, active bleeding, and free blood in the abdominal cavity (Smith & Wax, 2022). The fetus is born by emergency cesarean section, then the ruptured uterus must be removed or repaired. The decision to perform hysterectomy is influenced by the extent of uterine damage, the client's hemodynamic stability, the skill of the surgeon, and the client's desire for future pregnancy. Repair of an extensive laceration can be difficult and time-consuming. The surgeon must control hemorrhage and identify and repair damage to other organs such as the urinary tract. If the urinary tract is damaged, an experienced urologic surgeon is sometimes consulted intraoperatively (Sá, Arlindo, Raupp, Fortuna, & Cunha Filho, 2021).

VBAC in Community Settings

Although 13% of uterine ruptures occur outside a hospital (Heinrichs, 2020), only a small percentage of this number results from planned community birth. Because of the small but serious risk of uterine rupture, VBAC in community settings is a controversial topic. Mothers planning home VBAC are more likely to have successful vaginal births than their counterparts in the hospital (Bayrampour et al., 2021; Deline et al., 2012), but maternal transfer rates are high, risk to the newborn is greater, and risk of uterine rupture is significant (Cox, Bovbjerg, Cheyney, Leeman, 2015).

ACOG states that most mothers who have had one or two cesareans with a low-transverse incision are candidates for TOLAC (ACOG, 2019). Despite this recommendation, and an average success rate of 74%, only 13% of potential TOLAC candidates in the United States had a VBAC in 2018, and the rate has remained below 15% since 2002 (Basile Ibrahim et al., 2021). For many mothers, the most significant obstacle to having a VBAC is finding a supportive provider (Basile Ibrahim et al., 2021). By 2008, concerns about safety and liability led approximately half of U.S. physicians and one third of U.S. hospitals to stop offering TOLAC (MacDorman, Declercq, Mathews, & Stotland, 2012).

Mothers denied a hospital TOLAC are forced to choose between undergoing a repeat cesarean, traveling to a distant provider, or attempting a home VBAC (Basile Ibrahim et al., 2021). Because of the risks associated with TOLAC, however, and the unpredictable nature of uterine rupture, ACOG recommends that mothers attempt TOLAC in facilities able to provide continuous FHR monitoring during labor and perform emergency cesarean section (ACOG, 2019). Consequently, ACOG considers prior cesarean an absolute contraindication to planned home birth (ACOG, 2017/2024; ACOG, 2019).

TOLAC is permitted in some accredited birth centers if the facility uses an informed consent process with the client and documents it with a signed consent form. This discussion must include the birth center's resources for managing emergencies that can occur during TOLAC, resources at the client's preferred hospital, time considerations for emergency transport, and how delays can affect outcomes (Commission for the Accreditation of Birth Centers, 2023). Risk is lowest if only clients with a previous vaginal birth and an uncomplicated term, singleton, vertex pregnancy are accepted for TOLAC in a community setting, (Cox et al., 2015). Adverse outcomes are more likely when clients attempting TOLAC have additional risk factors such as multiple gestations and nonvertex presentations and when mothers have not had ultrasound imaging (Cox et al., 2015). In community settings, time delays between identification of early warning signs and accessing definitive care can affect outcomes and should be factored into the midwife's plan of care (N. Tharpe, personal communication, February 25, 2018). The best outcomes are seen with judicious client selection, collaborative relationships between community midwives and obstetricians, timely transfers, and access to ultrasound and laboratories for prenatal testing (Cox et al., 2015).

Vaginal or Cervical Sources of Bleeding

The bloody show of labor is usually mixed with mucus and can precede labor by more than 72 hr. Excluding bloody show, only about 5% of cases of third-trimester bleeding have a cervical or vaginal source (Pluym & Han, 2020). Lesions in these areas tend to cause spotting or pink discharge rather than frank hemorrhage.

Cervical ectropion. Cervical ectropion (eversion of the endocervix that exposes the lining of columnar epithelium to the vagina) is a common and normal finding in pregnancy. Exposed columnar epithelium can bleed during coitus or during a vaginal examination. Sometimes a bleeding ectropion is a sign of a vaginal infection, such as trichomonas, candida, or bacterial vaginosis (Sánchez, Rivera, Castillo, & Ortiz, 2012).

> When assessing antepartum bleeding outside a hospital, the goal is not to make a diagnosis, but to distinguish potentially serious hemorrhage from benign bleeding and transfer high-risk clients emergently.

Ruptured varicosity. Rupture of a vulvar, vaginal, or cervical varicose vein is a rare cause of antepartum hemorrhage. During pregnancy, varicose veins often develop in the legs, vulva, and hemorrhoidal plexus because of increased blood volume, compression of the inferior vena cava by the gravid uterus, and hormonal changes. About 2–4% of pregnancies are affected by vulvar varicosities, which typically develop after 12–26 weeks of gestation and resolve shortly after birth (Yaliwal, Kori, Mudanur, & Manne, 2021). Cervical varices occur more frequently in pregnancies complicated by placenta previa (Kumazawa et al., 2007; O'Brien & Smoleneic, 2013; Şükür, Yalçın, Kahraman, & Söylemez, 2011).

Vulvar varicose veins that rupture before or during labor can cause torrential hemorrhage (Furuta et al., 2013). A ruptured varicosity can also cause a significant hematoma if there is no outlet to the skin. In very rare cases, uterine varicosities can rupture and cause life-threatening intraabdominal bleeding.

When a ruptured varicosity is suspected, apply a pressure dressing, hemostatic gauze, or vaginal packing against the source of the bleeding and transport rapidly. Keep firm pressure on the wound and do not remove. If the dressing soaks through, add another dressing on top and resume applying pressure. In some cases, the wound must be sutured to achieve hemostasis. The McDonald cerclage has been used to control antepartum hemorrhage from a ruptured cervical varix (Fujibe, Mariya, Mizuuchi, Ishioka, & Saito, 2021; Polietkov & Kahn, 2022).

Management of Antepartum Bleeding

If you are unsure whether a problem exists, investigate to determine the source and severity of the bleeding. In community settings, the goal is to assess, stabilize if necessary, and transport the client with significant bleeding to a hospital maternity unit. Ideally the destination facility has laboratory and blood-transfusion resources, ability to perform emergency cesarean, and intensive-care support for mothers and babies (RCOG, 2011). It is not usually possible to determine the cause of antepartum hemorrhage in community settings. Even in a tertiary hospital with optimal staff and equipment, sometimes a diagnosis is obvious only in retrospect—or not at all.

Assess and Evaluate

GOLDCART History

When the client presents with third-trimester bleeding, take a GOLDCART history to determine the amount of bleeding, circumstances of onset, and associated symptoms. Because any delay in transport can worsen maternal or fetal outcomes, perform multiple tasks simultaneously and take the history while doing a physical examination and preparing to transfer the client to a hospital. Note the presence of risk factors and the nature of any abdominal pain as well as any history of recent intercourse, trauma, drug use, hypertension, or uterine surgery (Pluym & Han, 2020).

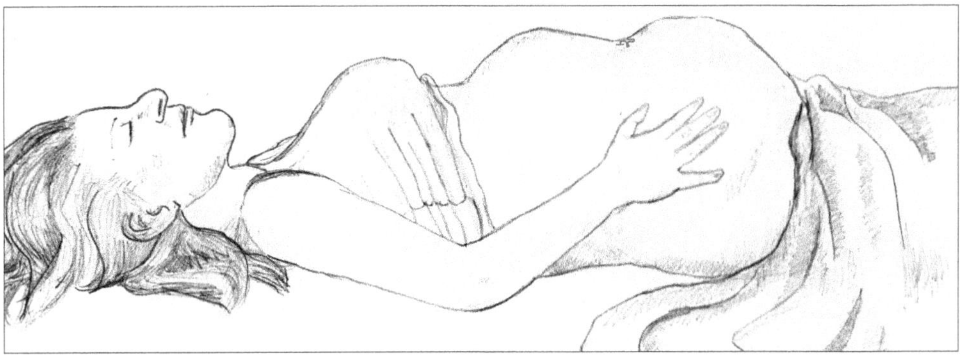

Figure 6-20. Bandl's ring causes the uterus to take on the shape off a two-humped camel with a depression near the umbilicus. An unengaged occiput posterior fetus and a distended maternal bladder can produce a similar contour.

Form a Clinical Impression

Certain characteristics of pain and bleeding can give clues to the nature of the problem. Although the classic presentations of complications fit into neat categories, symptoms experienced by real clients are much more variable. Keep in mind that more than one problem can coexist. Approach every situation with a truly open mind and be ready for anything. The following are hallmark characteristics of conditions that result in bleeding.

Placenta previa usually presents with bright-red, painless vaginal bleeding and sometimes with contractions. Often there is a mild or moderate sentinel bleed days or weeks before an intractable flow occurs (Cunningham et al., 2022, ch. 43). The uterus is soft and nontender between contractions. The fetus can be high in the abdomen and is commonly a nonvertex presentation. Heart tones are usually reassuring unless bleeding is severe. Coagulopathy seldom complicates placenta previa but can be a feature of placental abruption (Cunningham et al., 2022, ch. 43).

Placental abruption classically presents with acute onset of vaginal bleeding, uterine tenderness, uterine contractions, and abnormal FHR patterns, but any or all of these findings can be absent (Norwitz & Park, 2023). A marginal placental separation can present with light, intermittent bleeding like bloody show or with bloody amniotic fluid. The amount of vaginal bleeding does not always correlate with the severity of the abruption. In severe abruption, the uterus can become rigid and tender, and fetal parts can become difficult to palpate because of uterine tetany, especially when the hemorrhage is concealed behind the placenta. Shock and coagulopathy are sometimes present with severe abruption. Blood can be bright red, dark red, or purplish, like port wine. Sometimes a marginal abruption forms a clot, then leaks serum that can suggest rupture of the amniotic membranes (James et al., 2011).

Uterine rupture typically occurs during labor or after abdominal trauma but can occur (rarely) without an obvious antecedent. It is most likely in individuals who have had a previous cesarean section or other surgical incision through the uterine myometrium. Signs and symptoms can include vaginal bleeding (heavy or light), abnormal fetal heart pattern, maternal tachycardia, sudden change in the character of labor pain, abdominal tenderness (or unusual patterns of pain radiation), or severe shock. The mother sometimes feels the sensation of something tearing internally. The presenting part can become impalpable on vaginal examination, and fetal parts can suddenly become easy to palpate through the abdominal wall. Uterine contractions can cease.

Ruptured vasa previa typically presents as profuse vaginal bleeding—often starting when membranes rupture—with an abnormal fetal heart pattern.

Ruptured vaginal or cervical varicosity can result in a painless, copious hemorrhage of dark-red blood that can be difficult to control (Hurton, Morrill, Mascola, York, & Bromley, 1998).

Bloody show. The presence of only red, brown, or pink spotting suggests bloody show or other capillary bleeding from the cervix or vagina. Bloody show is usually mixed with mucus and is not usually enough to soak a sanitary pad or turn toilet water red. The individual with bloody show does not usually pass clots. In contrast to the rapid onset of symptoms that characterize the Big Four, labor usually develops more gradually, with contractions that become longer, stronger, and more frequent. The diagnosis of labor does not exclude a more serious source of bleeding; hemorrhage from placenta previa, vasa previa, abruption, or uterine rupture can have an intrapartum onset.

Antepartum hemorrhage is a true emergency that can result in severe blood loss within minutes. Rapid recognition of early signs and symptoms, accompanied by definitive action by the midwife can decrease rates of fetal and maternal injury

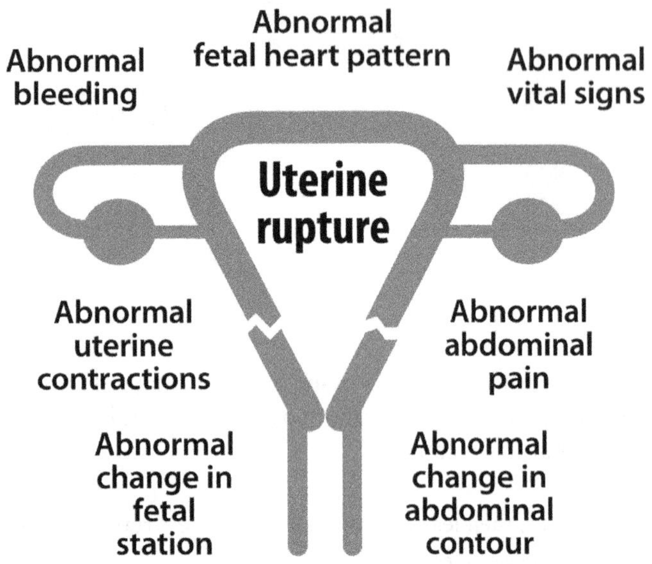

Figure 6-21. The "7 Abnormals" of uterine rupture. Classic warning signs of uterine rupture include abnormal fetal heart pattern, abnormal maternal vital signs, vaginal bleeding, sudden or worsening abdominal pain, and abnormal uterine contractions.

and death (N. Tharpe, personal communication, February 25, 2018). Timely cesarean is often the only path to a good outcome. Indecision and delay can result in the death of the fetus and the mother. Ideally, the client should be transferred to a hospital with the capacity for emergency cesarean section and a NICU. Your goal is to stabilize the mother without delaying transport, then tailor management to specific causes based on the clinical picture and the resources available (Winter, Crofts, Laxton, Barnfield, & Draycott, 2016). Immediate management includes ensuring a patent airway and effective respirations while maintaining circulation with IV fluids until blood products can be administered (Carillo & Chandraharan, 2021).

Stabilize and Transport

Teamwork yields optimal outcomes; ideally the midwife can work in partnership with emergency medical services (EMS) responders, nurses, physicians, and others along the chain. Move fast and accomplish multiple actions simultaneously. The order of these steps may vary with circumstances.

1. **Call for help** and mobilize all available providers. Expedite transfer of care! Transport by advanced life support ambulance or aircraft can be lifesaving for both the client with severe antepartum hemorrhage and the fetus. Provide support, information, and reassurance to the mother.
2. **Designate, recognize, or BE the team leader** to make decisions and reduce the confusion that results from many people trying to make decisions at once. The leader is usually the most qualified person and uses input from team members to streamline care. The team leader can change with circumstances—you in the client's home; you, the paramedic, or both working together *en route* to the hospital; a physician in the hospital.
3. **Take vital signs and do a primary survey.** Place the mother in whatever position yields the optimal maternal and fetal vital signs. Using the ABCDEF approach, assess and frequently monitor pulse, blood pressure (BP), respiratory rate and quality, FHR, and oxygen saturation. Bear in mind that vital signs can remain normal even with severe blood loss. Pregnant mothers can lose up 40% of their blood volume without going into shock (Cashion, 2016). The higher venous tone of an individual with hypertension can mask hypovolemia by keeping BP in the normal ranges despite large blood loss. Typically, pregnant individuals compensate for blood loss until unable to do so, then become tachycardic, hypotensive, and confused or agitated. When they cross this threshold, they can develop life-threatening pathologies such as DIC and acute kidney injury.
4. **Recognize and manage shock.** Assess for the signs of hypovolemic shock: tachycardia; tachypnea; cold, pale, sweaty, and/or bluish skin; restlessness and anxiety; confusion or unconsciousness; narrowed pulse pressure; and, as compensatory mechanisms fail, hypotension (see Chapter 9, "Shock"). If the mother is bleeding copiously, showing signs of shock, or has a low oxygen saturation, give high-flow oxygen at 15 L/min through a non-rebreathing mask (Aslih & Walfisch, 2011; RCOG, 2011; Taylor & Plaat, 2011). Encourage optimal perfusion by placing the client in a left lateral position. Provide warmth but do not overheat. Raise the foot of the bed or tuck something under the legs to raise them about 12 in. (30 cm) to encourage circulation to vital organs. Consider antishock garments for hemodynamically unstable hypovolemic clients in remote settings (see Chapter 7, "Other Temporizing Measures Involving Compression").
5. **Examine the abdomen.** Correlate gestational age with fundal height. Evaluate FHR and pattern and note any

First Thought, Worst Thought

What is the most likely cause of antepartum/intrapartum bleeding?

Bloody show, minor cervical trauma from coitus.

What is the worst it could be?

The Big Four: Placenta previa, placental abruption, vasa previa, uterine rupture.

abnormalities. Palpate fetal position. Note areas of discomfort and rebound tenderness. Note frequency and strength of contractions and baseline uterine tone. Continued intraabdominal hemorrhage may result in rebound tenderness and abdominal distension and rigidity. If you suspect a concealed abruption, mark the fundal height and time directly on the abdomen with marker or pen. If blood is collecting behind the placenta, in some cases you can observe a progressive rise in fundal height.

6. **Assess and monitor external blood loss.** In the case of abruption or uterine rupture, actual blood loss can be far greater than observed because of intraabdominal bleeding behind the placenta, into the abdomen, or into the amniotic sac. Quantify blood loss by weighing bloody pads and subtracting the weight of dry pads; the difference in grams equals the volume of blood in milliliters (see Chapter 7, "Quantify Blood Loss"). You can also collect blood in graduated measurement containers, including drapes with measuring pockets. Note the presence of amniotic fluid or urine, which can expand the volume and make blood loss appear greater. The use of visual aids and training sessions to memorize the capacity and appearance of certain soaked items can improve estimation of blood loss (Lockwood & Russo-Stieglitz, 2022; Zuckerwise, Pettker, Illuzzi, Raab, & Lipkind, 2014).
7. **Perform a digital and/or speculum cervical examination, as indicated.** *Do not perform a digital or sterile speculum examination until placenta previa has been excluded.* Although a digital examination is an important part of the evaluation of a laboring individual, it can trigger uncontrollable hemorrhage in the client with placenta previa or vasa previa. Although a few authorities recommend performing a gentle speculum examination to evaluate late-pregnancy bleeding with unknown placental location, most authors oppose a vaginal examination of any kind when there is a chance of placenta previa (Hacker, Gambone, & Hobel, 2016; Hull & Resnik, 2014; James et al., 2011; Tharpe, Farley, & Jordan, 2017; Tillett & Hanson, 1999; Wiedaseck & Monchek, 2014). A sonographer can safely perform transvaginal ultrasound because the probe does not normally touch the cervix (Lockwood & Russo-Stieglitz, 2023a).

   If the client had a previous ultrasound screening that excluded placenta previa, proceed with a sterile speculum examination. Blood coming through the cervix distinguishes a uterine source from a vaginal lesion or cervical ectropion. If the cervix has begun to open, the white bulge of membranes in the cervical os or a presenting fetal part is often visible. A large balloon of membranes filling the vagina can mean complete dilation or a partially dilated cervix with hour-glassing fetal membranes. Blood clots,

Table 6-3

Sample GOLDCART History for Antepartum/Intrapartum Bleeding

General situation and history—How many weeks pregnant are you? Do you have any health issues or pregnancy complications? How many pregnancies have you had and how many births? Is the baby moving? Have you had an ultrasound? Do you have any abnormalities with your placenta? Have you had any cesarean sections or other uterine surgeries?
Onset—When did you first start to bleed? What were you doing? Was the onset gradual or rapid? Did you hit your belly or have an accident? Did you have recent intercourse or put anything inside your vagina before the bleeding started?
Location—Are you sure the blood is coming from your vagina? Could it be from your bladder or rectum? Where do you feel pain? Does it start in one place and radiate to somewhere else? Where?
Duration—How long have you been bleeding? Has it been steady or does it come and go?
Characteristics—Is the blood brown, red, or pink? Is it watery, mixed with mucus, or free-flowing? How many pads have you soaked since the bleeding began? Large pads or small pads? How long does it take to soak a pad? Is blood on the tissue when you wipe? Is it soaking through your underwear? Is it turning the toilet water red? Are you passing clots?
Associated symptoms—Are you leaking fluid? Any nausea, vomiting, fever, dizziness, palpitations, or fainting? Is your uterus tight? Do you have pain? Is the pain sharp, dull, or crampy? Does it come and go like contractions? How would you rate the pain on a scale of 0–10, with 10 being the worst pain imaginable?
Relieving/aggravating factors—Do you get a gush of blood when you have a contraction? Does your abdomen hurt more when you press on it? Do you only bleed when you have a bowel movement?
Treatment—Have providers evaluated your bleeding previously? What did they recommend? Have you been following their recommendations? Have you been using any alternative remedies? Has your condition changed since these treatments?

Table 6-4
Possible Sources of Late-Pregnancy Bleeding

Possible Sources of Late-Pregnancy Bleeding
Placenta previa
Uterine rupture
Placental abruption
Vasa previa
Trauma
Cervical hemangioma
Infection
Cervicovaginal neoplasm
Bloody show
Cervicitis/polyps/ectropion
Vaginal or cervical varicosities

pools of free blood, or amniotic fluid can also make visualization of the cervix difficult. A gentle digital cervical examination can establish effacement, station, dilation, and presenting part if the client is in labor.

8. **Establish large-bore IV access at two sites.** Consider drawing a complete blood count (CBC), coagulation studies (PT/PTT/fibrinogen), blood type and crossmatch, blood urea nitrogen (BUN), and electrolytes if it will expedite treatment at the hospital. You may test for coagulopathy *en route* if doing so does not delay care. Draw 5 ml of blood into a red-top tube and put it aside. If a clot does not form within 6 min. or it forms and lyses within 30 min, a coagulation defect is most likely present (Johnson, Hallock, Bienstock, Fox, & Wallach, 2015).

   Rapidly infuse crystalloid solutions, e.g., normal saline (NS) or lactated Ringer's (LR), to refill the intravascular space and improve perfusion. In a critically ill individual, about 80% of these fluids will equilibrate into the extravascular space in an hour, so it is crucial to rapidly infuse a volume that is two to three times the estimated blood loss (Cunningham et al., 2022, ch. 44). Multiple infusions of crystalloid solutions, however, can result in a low hematocrit and depletion of platelets and clotting factors, potentially causing a dilutional coagulopathy that is clinically indistinguishable from DIC (Cunningham et al., 2022, ch. 44). Administration of blood products to restore red cells and clotting factors is an essential component of managing severe hemorrhage.

9. **Expedite birth when there is actual or impending maternal or fetal compromise.** Significant antepartum bleeding is a contraindication to planned birth in a community setting. Mode of birth is dependent on the gestational age, placental location, clinical circumstances, available resources, and the mother's hemodynamic stability. Anticipate the need for neonatal resuscitation if birth occurs.

Table 6-5
Targeted Physical Assessment for Late-Pregnancy Bleeding

Targeted Physical Assessment for Late-Pregnancy Bleeding
Vital signs and FHR—ABCDEF Tachycardia, hypotension, or orthostatic hypotension can indicate low blood volume due to hemorrhage. The heart rate of a compromised fetus can show decelerations, bradycardia, tachycardia, or a sinusoidal pattern.
Abdominal examination Correlate gestational age with fundal height. Palpate fetal position. Note areas of discomfort on palpation or rebound tenderness. Note frequency and strength of contractions and baseline uterine tone.
Visualize external genitalia; perform speculum examination after placenta previa has been excluded Quantify bleeding and determine origin. Clear away excess blood with swabs. Is blood or amniotic fluid coming through the cervix? Is the cervix open? Does it appear shortened? Look for cervical and vaginal lesions.
Digital examination after placenta previa has been excluded Is the cervix dilated or effaced? What is the presenting part? Is the client in labor, and if so, what stage? Is there blood on your fingers after the examination?

10. **Anticipate postpartum hemorrhage.** Antepartum hemorrhage increases the risk for postpartum hemorrhage (RCOG, 2011). Use active management of third stage labor if the mother gives birth before reaching the hospital.
11. **Ensure accurate documentation.** Record every assessment and action and fax or hand-carry prenatal records to the receiving hospital.

Definitive Care

Ideally antepartum bleeding with the potential for serious hemorrhage will be managed in a hospital with the ability to perform an immediate cesarean, facilities for blood transfusion, and intensive-care support for mother and infant. The most effective method of controlling severe antepartum hemorrhage, regardless of cause, is birth of the infant (Winter et al., 2016). The obstetrician should move to immediate cesarean for cases with heavy bleeding resulting in maternal or fetal compromise unless vaginal birth is imminent (Pluym & Han, 2020). When the mother is compromised, birth should not be delayed for fetal concerns, such as waiting a few days to allow a preterm fetus to benefit fully from steroids (Winter et al., 2016).

Ultrasound imaging can be crucial to diagnosis of antepartum bleeding. Transvaginal ultrasound can determine whether the placenta is across the cervical os and whether placenta accreta/increta/percreta is present. Ultrasound can

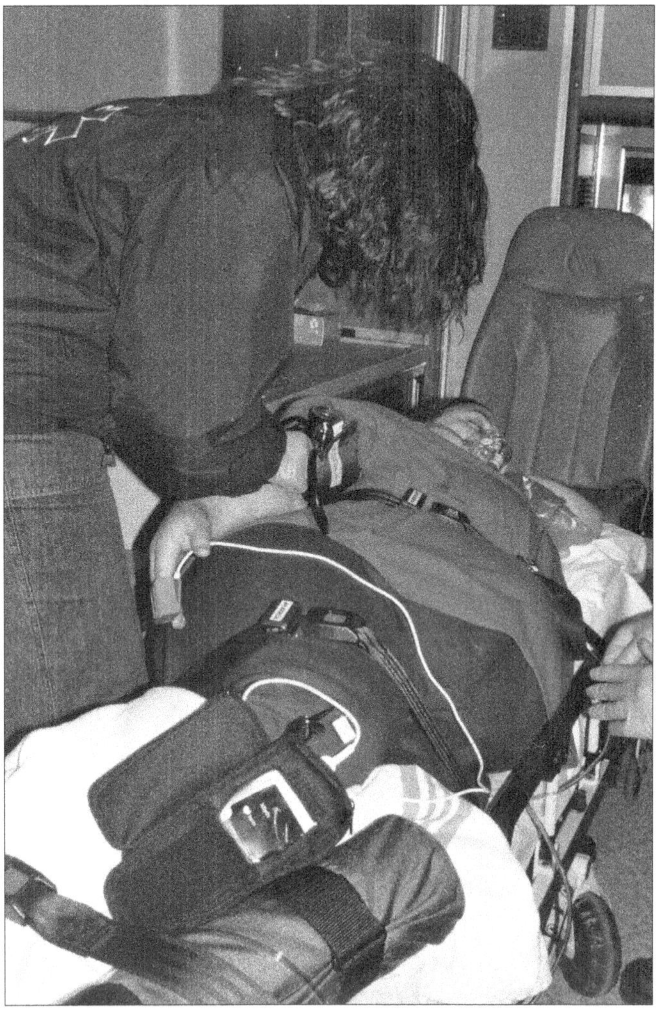

Figure 6-22. When a pregnant client is bleeding heavily, rapid transport to a hospital often provides the best chance for a good outcome.

Table 6-6 **The BLEEDERS Mnemonic**
BRING in help
Mobilize EMS.
Assemble people to assist.
LEAD
Take charge or designate a single team leader to direct management.
Encourage others on scene to coordinate with leader.
EVALUATE
Assess and frequently monitor vital signs, FHR, oxygen saturation, level of consciousness, pain, bleeding, signs, and symptoms.
EMPLOY stabilization measures
Perform appropriate procedures and interventions.
Give appropriate medications.
Establish intravenous (IV) access and give fluid bolus.
Give high-flow oxygen.
Position on side with feet elevated.
Provide warmth.
DIAGNOSE
Consider differential diagnoses, possible causes, and comorbidities and take steps to correct them.
EXPEDITE transport
Transfer to the closest hospital most able to manage maternal and neonatal issues.
RECORD and document
Complete the medical record.
SHARE
Share information with receiving providers.

identify a shortened or funneling cervix indicating PTL. Ultrasound can also verify fetal presentation. Abruption, however, is often not identifiable on ultrasound unless bleeding is severe (Oyelese & Ananth, 2006). The provider should not waste valuable time performing an ultrasound examination on an unstable mother or fetus when the placental site and presentation are already known.

Continuous fetal monitoring: When the fetus is viable, the FHR should be continuously monitored for abnormal patterns such as loss of reactivity, minimal variability, tachycardia, late decelerations, or a sinusoidal heart rate. The maternal rate and oxygen saturation should be tracked with a pulse oximeter.

Laboratory tests: Baseline tests can include CBC, crossmatch for units of blood, BUN, electrolytes, liver function tests, and coagulation studies (fibrinogen concentration, PT, activated PTT). Rh-negative individuals should undergo a Kleihauer-Betke test to determine the appropriate dose of anti-D immunoglobulin to prevent isoimmunization. A urine toxicology screen can be performed to rule out use of certain drugs, such as cocaine, that have been associated with antepartum bleeding.

Blood products: Most of the oxygen delivered to the tissues by the blood is bound to hemoglobin in red blood cells (RBCs). When large numbers of RBCs are lost to hemorrhage, oxygen delivery is reduced at the cellular level. Crystalloid fluids such as LR or NS can expand intravascular volume, stabilize vital signs, and improve urine output; transfusion of packed red cells can improve and maintain tissue oxygenation (Hess, 2023). When clotting factors are depleted, they must be replaced. If blood loss is excessive or the mother is unstable, the provider may initiate a massive transfusion protocol to maintain a hematocrit of at least 25–30%, a platelet count of at least 75,000/mcl, fibrinogen of at least 300 mg/dl, and a PT and PTT less than 150% of control (Oyelese & Ananth, 2022).

Considerations for Limited-Resource Settings

In low-resource settings, antepartum hemorrhage is more likely to result in maternal or perinatal death, especially in remote areas without accessible surgical care or anesthesia. Often death is related to delays in diagnosis, transportation, or management. Sometimes the midwife is the last point of referral, not the first (Christie et al., 2014). Many countries have not yet developed standards of care, and some have difficulty adapting international guidelines to local realities (Kongnyuy & van den Broek, 2009). The mother with antepartum hemorrhage will have the best outcomes when rapidly transported to a medical center with the capacity for emergency cesarean and neonatal intensive care capabilities.

Topics for Discussion

1. Ruby R. is recovering from an emergency cesarean undertaken when her placenta previa began to bleed copiously. She and the baby are stable and recovering, but Ruby feels physically and emotionally drained. She is grateful that she and her baby survived, but profoundly disappointed that she did not have the gentle waterbirth she had envisioned. How can you support Ruby as she processes these events? What comments or actions can be helpful?
2. Janetta W. is a 37-year-old G7 P6 who arrives at your birth center in labor at 37 weeks of gestation. She reports that her bloody show is heavier than usual with this labor. When she takes off her underwear, you see that her sanitary pad is thoroughly saturated with bright-red blood. How do you proceed?
3. Hawa is 25 weeks pregnant and had painless bright-red bleeding "like a period" during intercourse. What do you want to know? What are your differential diagnoses?
4. You arrive at the home of Molly M., a 28-year-old G3 P2002, to find her in active labor. After her membranes rupture spontaneously with a gush, she begins to bleed a steady stream of bright-red blood. What do you suspect? What should you do?
5. You are a volunteer midwife in a rural clinic in Uganda. A traditional birth attendant brings in Adaliya Z., a multigravida who has been laboring for days. Adaliya reports that she had been having strong, very frequent contractions, but now her uterus does not relax at all. You palpate her abdomen and notice that it is rounded at the fundus and above the pubis, but hollowed near the umbilicus. It is as firm as a brick and does not relax. The FHR is showing late decelerations. There is no vaginal bleeding. What problem do you suspect? What are your next steps? What is likely to happen if you do not act quickly?

References

Abramovici, A., Gandley, R. E., Clifton, R. G., Leveno, K. J., Myatt, L., Wapner, R. J., . . . Eunice Kennedy Shriver National Institute of Child Health Human Development Maternal-Fetal Medicine Units Network. (2015). Prenatal vitamin C and E supplementation in smokers is associated with reduced placental abruption and preterm birth: A secondary analysis. *BJOG, 122*(13), 1740–1747. https://doi.org/10.1111/1471-0528.13201

Al-Zirqi, I., Daltveit, A. K., & Vangen, S. (2019). Maternal outcome after complete uterine rupture. *Acta Obstetricia et Gynecologica Scandinavica, 98*(8), 1024–1031. https://doi.org/10.1111/aogs.13579

Al-Zirqi, I., Stray-Pedersen, B., Forsén, L., Daltveit, A. K., & Vangen, S. (2016). Uterine rupture: Trends over 40 years. *BJOG, 123*(5), 780-787. https://doi.org/10.1111/1471-0528.13394

American College of Obstetricians and Gynecologists. (2017, corrected and reaffirmed 2024). *Antenatal corticosteroid therapy for fetal maturation* (Committee Opinion 713). Retrieved from https://www.acog.org/clinical/clinical-guidance/committee-opinion/articles/2017/08/antenatal-corticosteroid-therapy-for-fetal-maturation

American College of Obstetricians and Gynecologists. (2019). *Vaginal birth after cesarean delivery* (Practice Bulletin 205). Retrieved from https://www.acog.org/clinical/clinical-guidance/practice-bulletin/articles/2019/02/vaginal-birth-after-cesarean-delivery

American College of Obstetricians and Gynecologists & Society for Maternal-Fetal Medicine. (2018, reaffirmed 2021). *Placenta accreta spectrum* (Obstetric Care Consensus 7). Retrieved from https://www.acog.org/clinical/clinical-guidance/obstetric-care-consensus/articles/2018/12/placenta-accreta-spectrum

American College of Obstetricians and Gynecologists & Society for Maternal-Fetal Medicine. (2021, reaffirmed 2024). *Medically indicated late-preterm and early-term deliveries* (Committee Opinion 831). Retrieved from https://www.acog.org/Clinical/Clinical-Guidance/Committee-Opinion/Articles/2021/07/Medically-Indicated-Late-Preterm-and-Early-Term-Deliveries

American College of Obstetricians and Gynecologists Committee on Obstetric Practice. (2017, reaffirmed 2023). *Planned home birth* (Committee Opinion 697, interim update). Retrieved from https://www.acog.org/clinical/clinical-guidance/committee-opinion/articles/2017/04/planned-home-birth

American College of Obstetricians and Gynecologists Committee on Clinical Practice Guidelines—Obstetrics, Cahill, A. G., Raghuraman, N., Gandhi, M., & Kaimal, A. J. (2024). *First and second stage labor management* (Clinical Practice Guideline 8). *Obstetrics & Gynecology, 143*(1), 144–162.

Ananth, C. V., & Kinzler, W. L. (2022). Acute placental abruption: Pathophysiology, clinical features, diagnosis, and consequences. In V. A. Barss (Ed.), *UpToDate*. Retrieved November 13, 2023, from https://www.uptodate.com/contents/acute-placental-abruption-pathophysiology-clinical-features-diagnosis-and-consequences

Aslih, N., & Walfisch, A. (2011). Clinical approach to pregnancy-related bleeding. In E. Sheiner (Ed.), *Bleeding during pregnancy: A comprehensive guide* (pp. 3–21). New York, NY: Springer.

Atallah, A., Piccin, G., Dubernard, G., Abdul-Hay, M. J., Cortet, M., & Huissoud, C. (2023). Fibrinogen for the prediction of severe maternal complications in placental abruption with fetal death after 24 weeks of gestation. *International Journal of Gynecology & Obstetrics, 160*(3), 900–905. https://doi.org/10.1002/ijgo.14417

Auerbach, M., & Landy, H. J. (2023). Anemia in pregnancy. In J. S Tirnauer & V. A Barss (Eds.), *UpToDate*. Retrieved November 13, 2023, from https://www.uptodate.com/contents/anemia-in-pregnancy

Baeseman, Z. J. (2022). Vaginal bleeding in pregnancy. In R. D. Kellerman & D. P. Rakel (Eds.), *Conn's current therapy 2022* (pp. 1251–1253). Philadelphia, PA: Elsevier.

Balayla, J., Desilets, J., & Shrem, G. (2019). Placenta previa and the risk of intrauterine growth restriction (IUGR): A systematic review and meta-analysis. *Journal of Perinatal Medicine, 47*(6), 577–584. https://doi.org/10.1515/jpm-2019-0116

Basile Ibrahim, B., Knobf, M. T., Shorten, A., Vedam, S., Cheyney, M., Illuzzi, J., & Kennedy, H. P. (2021). "I had to fight for my VBAC": A mixed methods exploration of women's experiences of pregnancy and vaginal birth after cesarean in the United States. *Birth, 48*(2), 164–177. https://doi.org/10.1111/birt.12513

Bayrampour, H., Lisonkova, S., Tamana, S., Wines, J., Vedam, S., & Janssen, P. (2021). Perinatal outcomes of planned home birth after cesarean and planned hospital vaginal birth after cesarean at term gestation in British Columbia, Canada: A retrospective population-based cohort study. *Birth, 48*(3), 301–308. https://doi.org/10.1111/birt.12539

Berghella, V. (2022). Cesarean birth: Surgical technique. In V. A. Barss (Ed.), *UpToDate*. Retrieved October 1, 2023, from https://www.uptodate.com/contents/cesarean-birth-surgical-technique

Boller, M., Navarrete, E., Hung, Y.-Y., Weintraub, M. R., Moore, G., & Schauer, G. (2020). Placental abruption is not associated with clinically significant fetomaternal hemorrhage. *Obstetrics & Gynecology, 135*,164S. https://doi.org/10.1097/01.AOG.0000664028.44953.c0

Bronsteen, R., Whitten, A., Balasubramanian, M., Lee, W., Lorenz, R., Redman, M., . . . Comstock C. (2013). Vasa previa: Clinical presentations, outcomes, and implications for management. *Obstetrics & Gynecology, 122*(2, Pt. 1), 352–357. https://doi.org/10.1097/AOG.0b013e31829cac58

Cameron, J. C., Davis, E. P., Dickinson, R. L., Earle, C. W., Etheridge, J. H., Garrigues, H. J., . . . Schwarz, H. (1897). *An American text-book of obstetrics for practitioners and students*. Philadelphia, PA: W. B. Saunders. Retrieved from https://archive.org/details/americantextbook00norr/

Carillo, A. P., & Chandraharan, E. (2021). Management of massive obstetric haemorrhage: Antepartum, intrapartum and postpartum. In E. Chandraharan & S. Arulkumaran (Eds.), *Obstetric and intrapartum emergencies: A practical guide to management* (2nd ed., Kindle version, ch. 5). Cambridge, United Kingdom: Cambridge University Press.

Cashion, K. (2016). Hemorrhagic disorders. In D. L. Lowdermilk, S. E. Perry, K. Cashion, K. Rhodes Alden, & E. F. Olshansky (Eds.), *Maternity and women's health care* (11th ed., pp. 669–686). St. Louis, MO: Elsevier.

Catanzarite, V., Cousins, L., Daneshmand, S., Schwendemann, W., Casele, H., Adamczak, J., . . . Patel, A. (2016). Prenatally diagnosed vasa previa: A single-institution series of 96 cases. *Obstetrics & Gynecology, 128*(5),1153–1161. https://doi.org/10.1097/AOG.0000000000001680

Celik, O. Y., Obut, M., Keles, A., Calık, M. G., Dagdeviren, G., Yucel, A., & Sahin, D. (2021). Outcomes of pregnancies diagnosed with circumvallate placenta, and use of uterine artery pulsatility index and maternal serum alpha-fetoprotein for prediction of adverse outcomes. *European Journal of Obstetrics & Gynecology and Reproductive Biology, 262*, 57–61. https://doi.org/0.1016/j.ejogrb.2021.05.008

Chahal, H. S., Gelaye, B., Mostofsky, E., Sanchez, S. E., Mittleman, M. A., Maclure, M., . . . Williams, M. A. (2018). Physical Exertion immediately prior to placental abruption: A case-crossover study. *American Journal of Epidemiology, 187*(10), 2073–2079. https://doi.org/10.1093/aje/kwy138

Christie, K., Clack, A., Creemers, J., Hayden, B., Kodindo, G., Sadia, S., . . . Wright, A. (2014). Pregnancy-related problems. In D. Southall (Ed.), *International maternal & child health care: A practical manual for hospitals worldwide* (pp. 135–338). London, United Kingdom: Radcliffe Publishing. Retrieved from https://www.mcai.org.uk/_files/ugd/dd2ba4_c5284b1b150f4d70a72fe1cd710d530d.pdf

Commission for the Accreditation of Birth Centers. (2023). *Indicators of compliance with standards for birth centers* (reference ed. 2.3). Hamburg, PA: Author. Retrieved from https://www.birthcenteraccreditation.org/wp-content/uploads/2023/09/CABC_IndicatorsRefEd-2.3_2023-0915.pdf

Cox, K. J., Bovbjerg, M. L., Cheyney, M., & Leeman, L. M. (2015). Planned home VBAC in the United States, 2004–2009: Outcomes, maternity care practices, and implications for shared decision making. *Birth, 42*(4), 299–308. https://doi.org/10.1111/birt.12188

Cunningham, F. G., Leveno, K. J., Dashe, J. S., Hoffman, B. L., Spong, C. Y., & Casey, B. M. (Eds.). (2022). *Williams obstetrics* (26th ed., Kindle version). New York, NY: McGraw-Hill.

Deline, J., Varnes-Epstein, L., Dresang, L. T., Gideonsen, M., Lynch, L., & Frey, J. J. (2012). Low primary cesarean rate and high VBAC rate with good outcomes in an Amish birthing center. *Annals of Family Medicine, 10*(6), 530–537. https://doi.org/10.1370/afm.1403

Deng, J., & Copel, J. (2016). Vasa previa. *Contemporary OB/GYN, 61*(2), 18. Retrieved from http://contemporaryobgyn.modernmedicine.com/contemporary-obgyn/news/vasa-previa

Ehsanipoor, R. M., & Satin, A. J. (2022). Labor: Overview of normal and abnormal progression. In V. A. Barss (Ed.), *UpToDate*. Retrieved October 1, 2023, from https://www.uptodate.com/contents/labor-overview-of-normal-and-abnormal-progression

Evans, D. G., & B-Lynch, C. (2012). Obstetric trauma. In S. Arulkumaran, M. Karoshi, L. G. Keith, A. B. Lalonde, & C. B-Lynch (Eds.), *A comprehensive textbook of postpartum hemorrhage: An essential clinical reference for effective management* (2nd ed., pp. 185–192). London, United Kingdom: Sapiens Publishing. Retrieved from https://www.glowm.com/pdf/PPH_2nd_edn_Chap-23.pdf

Fofie, C. O., & Baffoe, P. (2010). A two-year review of uterine rupture in a regional hospital. *Ghana Medical Journal, 44*(3), 98–102. Retrieved from https://www.ncbi.nlm.nih.gov/pmc/articles/PMC2996838/

Francois, K. E., & Foley, M. R. (2021). Antepartum and postpartum hemorrhage. In M. B. Landon, H. L. Galan, E. R. M. Jauniaux, D. A. Driscoll, V. Berghella, W. A. Grobman, . . . A. G. Cahill (Eds.), *Gabbe's obstetrics: Normal and problem pregnancies* (8th ed., Kindle version, ch. 18). Philadelphia, PA: Elsevier.

Fujibe, Y., Mariya, T., Mizuuchi, M., Ishioka, S., & Saito, T. (2021). Effectiveness of cross double McDonald cerclage for intractable bleeding from a cervical varix in pregnant women. *Gynecology and Minimally Invasive Therapy, 10*(3), 177–180. Retrieved from https://journals.lww.com/gmit/fulltext/2021/10030/effectiveness_of_cross_double_mcdonald_cerclage.10.aspx

Furuta, N., Kondoh, E., Yamada, S., Kawasaki, K., Ueda, A., Mogami, H., & Konishi, I. (2013). Vaginal delivery in the presence of huge vulvar varicosities: A case report with MRI evaluation. *European Journal of Obstetrics & Gynecology and Reproductive Biology, 167*(2), 127–131. https://doi.org/10.1016/j.ejogrb.2012.11.024

Ghaheh, H. S., Feizi, A., Mousavi, M., Sohrabi, D., Mesghari, L., & Hosseini, Z. (2013). Risk factors of placental abruption. *Journal of Research in Medical Sciences, 18*(5), 422–426. Retrieved from https://www.ncbi.nlm.nih.gov/pmc/articles/PMC3810579/

Guise, J.-M., Eden, K., Emeis, C., Denman, M. A., Marshall, N.; Fu, R., . . . McDonagh, M. (2010). *Vaginal birth after cesarean: New insights*. AHRQ Publication 10-E003. Retrieved from https://archive.ahrq.gov/research/findings/evidence-based-reports/vbacup-evidence-report.pdf

Hacker, N. F., Gambone, J. C., & Hobel, C. J. (2016). *Hacker and Moore's essentials of obstetrics and gynecology* (6th ed.). Philadelphia, PA: Saunders.

Hall, D. R. (2009). Abruptio placentae and disseminated intravascular coagulopathy. *Seminars in Perinatology, 33*(3), 189–195. Retrieved from https://www.researchgate.net/publication/26236131_Abruptio_Placentae_and_Disseminated_Intravascular_Coagulopathy

Hasegawa, J., Arakaki, T., Ichizuka, K., & Sekizawa, A. (2015). Management of vasa previa during pregnancy. *Journal of Perinatal Medicine, 43*(6), 783–784. https://doi.org/10.1515/jpm-2014-0047

Heinrichs, G. (2020). Late pregnancy bleeding. In L. Leeman, L. Dresang, J. S. Quinlan, & S. R. Magee (Eds.), *Advanced life support in obstetrics: Provider manual* (9th ed., pp. 95–109). Leawood, KS: American Academy of Family Physicians.

Hess, J. R. (2023). Massive blood transfusion. In J. S. Tirnauer (Ed.), *UpToDate*. Retrieved October 1, 2023, from http://www.uptodate.com/contents/massive-blood-transfusion

Holmgren, C. M. (2012). Uterine rupture associated with VBAC. *Clinical Obstetrics and Gynecology, 55*(4), 978–987. https://doi.org/10.1097/GRF.0b013e31826fd9b0

Huang, S., Zuo, Q., Wang, T., Tang, X., Ge, Z., Lu, H., . . . Jiang, Z. (2022). Maternal and neonatal outcomes of repeated antepartum bleeding in 493 placenta previa cases: A retrospective study. *Journal of Maternal-Fetal & Neonatal Medicine, 35*(25), 5318–5823. https://doi.org/10.1080/14767058.2021.1878495

Hull, A. D., & Resnik, R. (2014). Placenta previa, placenta accreta, abruptio placentae, and vasa previa. In R. Resnik, R. Creasy, J. Iams, C. Lockwood, T. Moore, & M. Greene (Eds.), *Creasy and Resnik's maternal-fetal medicine: Principles and practice* (7th ed., pp. 732–742). Philadelphia, PA: Elsevier Saunders.

Hurton, T., Morrill, H., Mascola, M., York, C., & Bromley, B. (1998). Cervical varices: An unusual etiology for third-trimester bleeding. *Journal of Clinical Ultrasound, 26*(6), 317–319. https://doi.org/10.1002/(SICI)1097-0096(199807/08)26:6<317::AID-JCU7>3.0.CO;2-L

Jain, V., Bos, H., & Bujold, E. (2020). Diagnosis and management of placenta previa (Guideline 402). *Journal of Obstetrics and Gynaecology Canada, 42*(7), 906–917.e1. https://doi.org/10.1016/j.jogc.2019.07.019

James, D., Steer, P., Weiner, C., & Gonik, B. (2011). *High risk pregnancy: Management options* (4th ed.). Philadelphia, PA: Elsevier Saunders.

Jansen, C. H. J. R., De Mooij, Y. M., Blomaard, C. M., Derks, J. B., Van Leeuwen, E., Limpens, J., . . . Pajkrt, E. (2019). Vaginal delivery in women with a low-lying placenta: A systematic review and meta-analysis. *BJOG, 126*(9), 1118–1126. https://doi.org/10.1111/1471-0528.15622

Jauniaux, E., Grønbeck, L., Bunce, C., Langhoff-Roos, J., & Collins, S. L. (2019). Epidemiology of placenta previa accreta: A systematic review and meta-analysis. *BMJ Open, 9*(11), e031193. Retrieved from https://www.ncbi.nlm.nih.gov/pmc/articles/PMC6858111/

Jauniaux, E., & Silver, R. (2020). Rethinking prenatal screening for anomalies of placental and umbilical cord implantation. *Obstetrics & Gynecology 136*(6), 1211–1216. https://doi.org/10.1097/AOG.0000000000004175

Jauniaux, E. R. M., Alfirevic, Z., Bhide, A., Burton, G., Collins, S., & Silver, R. (2018). Vasa praevia: Diagnosis and management (Green-top Guideline 27b). *BJOG, 126*(1), e49–e61. https://doi.org/0.1111/1471-0528.15307

Jenabi, E., Salimi, Z., Bashirian, S., Khazaei, S., & Ayubi, E. (2022). The risk factors associated with placenta previa: An umbrella review. *Placenta, 117*, 21–27. https://doi.org/10.1016/j.placenta.2021.10.009

Johnson, C. T., Hallock, J. L., Bienstock, J. L., Fox, H. E., & Wallach, E. E. (Eds.). (2015). *The Johns Hopkins manual of gynecology and obstetrics* (5th ed.). Philadelphia, PA: Wolters Kluwer/Lippincott Williams & Wilkins.

Kongnyuy, E. J., & van den Broek, N. (2009). Developing standards for postpartum hemorrhage in a resource-limited country. *Health Care for Women International, 30*(11), 989–1002. https://doi.org/10.1080/07399330902836126

Kumazawa, Y., Shimizu, D., Hosoya, N., Hirano, H., Ishiyama, K., & Tanaka, T. (2007). Cervical varix with placenta previa totalis. *Journal of Obstetrics and Gynaecology Research, 33*(4), 536–538. https://doi.org/10.1111/j.1447-0756.2007.00553.x

Kuribayashi, M., Tsuda, H., Ito, Y., Tezuka, A., Ando, T., Tamakoshi, K., & Mizuno, K. (2021). Evaluation of the risk factors for antepartum hemorrhage in cases of placenta previa: A retrospective cohort study. *Journal of International Medical Research, 49*(11). https://doi.org/10.1177/03000605211054706

Landon, M. B., & Frey, H. (2022). Uterine rupture: After previous cesarean birth. In V. A. Barss (Ed.), *UpToDate*. Retrieved October 1, 2023, from https://www.uptodate.com/contents/uterine-rupture-after-previous-cesarean-birth

Landon, M. B., & Grobman, W. A. (2021). Vaginal birth after cesarean delivery. In M. B. Landon, H. L. Galan, E. R. M. Jauniaux, D. A. Driscoll, V. Berghella, W. A. Grobman, . . . A. G. Cahill (Eds.), *Gabbe's obstetrics: Normal and problem pregnancies* (8th ed., Kindle version, ch. 20). Philadelphia, PA: Elsevier.

Lauria, M. R., Barthold, J. C., Zimmerman, R. A., & Turrentine, M. A. (2007). Pathologic uterine ring associated with fetal head trauma and subsequent cerebral palsy. *Obstetrics & Gynecology, 109*(2, Pt. 2), 495–497. https://doi.org/10.1097/01.AOG.0000231678.01757.73

Lijoi, A. F., & Brady, J. (2003). Vasa Previa Diagnosis and Management. *Journal of the American Board of Family Medicine, 16*(6), 543–548. https://doi.org/10.3122/jabfm.16.6.543

Litman, E. A., Yin, Y., Nelson, S. J., Capbarat, E., Kerchner, D., & Ahmadzia, H. K. (2022). Adverse perinatal outcomes in a large United States birth cohort during the COVID-19 pandemic. *American Journal of Obstetrics & Gynecology MFM, 4*(3),100577. https://doi.org/10.1016/j.ajogmf.2022.100577

Lockwood, C. J., & Russo-Stieglitz, K. (2022). Placenta previa: Management. In V. A. Barss (Ed.), *UpToDate*. Retrieved December 18, 2023, from https://www.uptodate.com/contents/placenta-previa-management

Lockwood, C. J., & Russo-Stieglitz, K. (2023a). Placenta previa: Epidemiology, clinical features, diagnosis, morbidity and mortality. In V. A. Barss (Ed.), *UpToDate*. Retrieved December 18, 2023, from https://www.uptodate.com/contents/placenta-previa-epidemiology-clinical-features-diagnosis-morbidity-and-mortality

Lockwood, C. J., & Russo-Stieglitz, K. (2023b). Velamentous umbilical cord insertion and vasa previa. In V. A. Barss (Ed.), *UpToDate*. Retrieved December 18, 2023, from http://www.uptodate.com/contents/velamentous-umbilical-cord-insertion-and-vasa-previa

MacDorman, M. F., Declercq, E., Mathews, T. J., & Stotland, N. (2012). Trends and characteristics of home vaginal birth after cesarean delivery in the United States and selected states. *Obstetrics & Gynecology, 119*(4), 737–744. https://doi.org/10.1097/AOG.0b013e31824bb050

Manoharan, M., Wuntakal, R., & Erskine, K. (2010). Uterine rupture: A revisit. *Obstetrician & Gynaecologist, 12*(4), 223–230. https://doi.org/10.1576/toag.12.4.223.27613

Maternal-Fetal Medicine Units Network (n.d.-a). *Vaginal birth after cesarean* [online calculator]. Retrieved June 1, 2017 from https://mfmunetwork.bsc.gwu.edu/PublicBSC/MFMU/VGBirthCalc/vagbirth.html

Maternal-Fetal Medicine Units Network (n.d.-b). *Vaginal birth after cesarean* [online calculator]. Retrieved June 1, 2017 from https://mfmunetwork.bsc.gwu.edu/PublicBSC/MFMU/VGBirthCalc/vagbrth2.html

Matsuo, K., Scanlon, J. T., Atlas, R. O., & Kopelman, J. N. (2008). Staircase sign: A newly described uterine contraction pattern seen in rupture of unscarred gravid uterus. *Journal of Obstetrics and Gynaecology Research, 34*(1), 100–104. https://doi.org/10.1111/j.1447-0756.2007.00709.x

Meah, V. L., Davies, G. A., & Davenport, M. H. (2020). Why can't I exercise during pregnancy? Time to revisit medical 'absolute' and 'relative' contraindications: Systematic review of evidence of harm and a call to action. *British Journal of Sports Medicine, 54*(23), 1395–1404. https://doi.org/10.1136/bjsports-2020-102042

Mei, Y., & Lin, Y. (2018). Clinical significance of primary symptoms in women with placental abruption. *Journal of Maternal-Fetal & Neonatal Medicine, 31*(18), 2446–2449. https://doi.org/10.1080/14767058.2017.1344830

Meserve, E. E., Sirois, K. F., Parast, M. M., & Boyd, T. K. (2018). Evaluation of the placenta. In C. P. Crum, M. R. Nucci, B. E. Howitt, S. R. Granter, M. M. Parast, T. K. Boyd, . . . W. A. Peters, III (Eds.), *Diagnostic gynecologic and obstetric pathology* (3rd ed., pp. 1137–1181). Philadelphia, PA: Elsevier.

Metz, T. D. (2023). Choosing the route of delivery after cesarean birth. In V. A. Barss (Ed.), *UpToDate*. Retrieved October 1, 2023, from https://www.uptodate.com/contents/choosing-the-route-of-delivery-after-cesarean-birth

Mhyre, J. M., & Khan, F. A. (2022). Anesthesia for the patient with peripartum hemorrhage. In M. Crowley (Ed.), *UpToDate*. Retrieved October 1, 2023, from https://www.uptodate.com/contents/anesthesia-for-the-patient-with-peripartum-hemorrhage

Mukasa, P. K., Kabakyenga, J., Senkungu, J. K., Ngonzi, J., Kyalimpa, M., & Roosmalen, V. J. (2013). Uterine rupture in a teaching hospital in Mbarara, western Uganda, unmatched case-control study. *Reproductive Health, 10*(1), 29–34. https://doi.org/10.1186/1742-4755-10-29

Mulla, B. M., Weatherford, R., Redhunt, A. M., Modest, A. M., Hacker, M. R., Hecht, J. L., . . . Shainker, S. A. (2019). Hemorrhagic morbidity in placenta accreta spectrum with and without placenta previa. *Archives of Gynecology and Obstetrics, 300*(6), 1601–1606. https://doi.org/10.1007/s00404-019-05338-y

Ness, A. (2022). Trial of labor after cesarean. In V. Berghella (Ed.), *Obstetric evidence based guidelines* (4th ed., pp. 180–194). Boca Raton, FL: CRC Press. https://www.taylorfrancis.com/chapters/edit/10.1201/9781003102342-15

Norwitz, E. R., & Park, J. S. (2023). Evaluation and differential diagnosis of vaginal bleeding after 20 weeks of gestation. In V. A. Barss (Ed.), *UpToDate*. Retrieved October 1, 2023, from https://sso.uptodate.com/contents/evaluation-and-differential-diagnosis-of-vaginal-bleeding-after-20-weeks-of-gestation

O'Brien, B., & Smoleneic, J. (2013). Cervical varicosities and placenta praevia. *Australian and New Zealand Journal of Obstetrics and Gynaecology, 53*(5), 451–454. https://doi.org/10.1111/ajo.12127

Odendaal, H. (2021). Association of concomitant drinking and smoking during pregnancy with placental abruption, fetal growth restriction and sudden infant death syndrome (SIDS). *Journal of Pulmonary Medicine, 5*(2), 1000111. Retrieved from https://pubmed.ncbi.nlm.nih.gov/34308437/

Oyelese, Y., & Ananth, C. V. (2006). Placental abruption. *Obstetrics & Gynecology, 108*(4), 1005–1016. https://doi.org/10.1097/01.AOG.0000239439.04364.9a

Oyelese, Y., & Ananth, C. V. (2022). Acute placental abruption: Management and long-term prognosis. In V. A. Barss (Ed.), *UpToDate*. Retrieved October 1, 2023, from https://www.uptodate.com/contents/acute-placental-abruption-management-and-long-term-prognosis

Oyelese, Y., & Canterino, J. C. (2011). Placenta previa and placenta accreta. In E. K. Sheiner (Ed.), *Bleeding during pregnancy: A comprehensive guide* (pp. 135–150). New York, NY: Springer.

Oyelese, Y., Catanzarite, V., Prefumo, F., Lashley, S., Schachter, M., Tovbin, Y., . . . Smulian, J. C. (2004). Vasa previa: The impact of prenatal diagnosis on outcomes. *Obstetrics & Gynecology, 103*(5, Pt. 1), 937–942. https://doi.org/10.1097/01.AOG.0000123245.48645.98

Oyelese, Y., & Smulian, J. C. (2006). Placenta previa, placenta accreta, and vasa previa. *Obstetrics & Gynecology, 107*(4), 927–941. https://doi.org/10.1097/01.AOG.0000207559.15715.98

Pluym, I. D., & Han, C. S. (2020). Third-trimester bleeding. In J. T. Queenan, C. Y. Spong, & C. J. Lockwood (Eds.), *Protocols for high-risk pregnancies: An evidence-based approach* (7th ed., pp. 493–505). Hoboken, NJ: Wiley. https://doi.org/10.1002/9781119635307.ch48

Ridgeway, J. J., Weyrich, Darin, L., & Benedetti, T. J. (2004). Fetal heart rate changes associated with uterine rupture. *Obstetrics & Gynecology 103*(3) 506–512. https://doi.org/10.1097/01.AOG.0000113619.67704.99

Royal College of Obstetricians & Gynaecologists. (2011). *Antepartum haemorrhage* (Green-top Guideline 63). Retrieved from https://www.rcog.org.uk/globalassets/documents/guidelines/gtg_63.pdf

Rumbold, A., Ota, E., Hori, H., Miyazaki, C., & Crowther, C. A. (2015). Vitamin E supplementation in pregnancy. *Cochrane Database of Systematic Reviews*. https://doi.org/10.1002/14651858.CD004069.pub3

Sá, C. P. N., Arlindo, E. M., Raupp, G. S., Fortuna, E. L., & Cunha Filho, E. V. (2021). Uterine rupture of the unscarred uterus: A case report. *Journal of Medical Case Reports and Case Series, 2*(13). https://doi.org/10.38207/JMCRCS/2021/0213179

Sánchez, A., Rivera, A., Castillo, F., & Ortiz, S. (2012). Cervical erosion as result of infectious vaginitis. *European Journal of Experimental Biology, 2*(5), 1659–1663. Retrieved from http://www.imedpub.com/articles/cervical-erosion-as-result-of-infectious-vaginitis.pdf

Saxena, R. (2014). *Bedside obstetrics and gynecology* (2nd ed.). New Delhi, India: Jaypee Brothers Medical Publishers.

Silver, R. (2022). Placenta accreta spectrum: Clinical features, diagnosis, and potential consequences. In V. A. Barss (Ed.), *UpToDate*. Retrieved October 1, 2023, from https://www.uptodate.com/contents/placenta-accreta-spectrum-clinical-features-diagnosis-and-potential-consequences

Silver, R. M. (2015). Abnormal placentation: Placenta previa, vasa previa, and placenta accreta. *Obstetrics & Gynecology, 126*(3), 654–668. https://doi.org/10.1097/AOG.0000000000001005

Sinclair, S., Masters, H. R., DeFranco, E., Rountree, S., & Warshak, C. R. (2021). Universal transvaginal cervical length screening during pregnancy increases the diagnostic incidence of low-lying placenta and placenta previa. *American Journal of Obstetrics & Gynecology MFM, 3*(1), 100255. https://doi.org/10.1016/j.ajogmf.2020.100255

Sinha, S., Talaulikar, V. S., & Arulkumaran, S. (2018). Malpositions and malpresentations of the fetal head. *Obstetrics, Gynaecology and Reproductive Medicine, 28*(3), 83–91. https://doi.org/10.1016/j.ogrm.2018.01.001

Smith, J. F., & Wax, J. R. (2022). Uterine rupture: Unscarred uterus. In V. A. Barss (Ed.), *UpToDate*. Retrieved October 1, 2023, from https://www.uptodate.com/contents/uterine-rupture-unscarred-uterus

Society for Maternal-Fetal Medicine & Gyamfi-Bannerman, C. (2018). Management of bleeding in the late preterm period (SMFM Consult Series 44). *American Journal of Obstetrics & Gynecology, 218*(1), B2–B8. https://doi.org/10.1016/j.ajog.2017.10.019

Society for Maternal-Fetal Medicine Publications Committee, Sinkey, R. G., Odibo, A. O., & Dashe, J. S. (2015). Diagnosis and management of vasa previa (SMFM Consult Series #37). *American Journal of Obstetrics & Gynecology, 213*(5), 615–619. https://doi.org/10.1016/j.ajog.2015.08.031

Society for Maternal-Fetal Medicine, Lauder, J., Sciscione, A., Biggio, J., & Osmundson, S. (2020). The role of activity restriction in obstetric management (SMFM Consult Series 50). *American Journal of Obstetrics & Gynecology, 223*(2), B2–B10. https://doi.org/10.1016/j.ajog.2020.04.031

Stafford, I. A., Belfort, M. A. & Dildy, G. A. (2019). Etiology and management of hemorrhage. In J. P. Phelan, L. D. Pacheco, M. R. Foley, G. R. Saade, G. A. Dildy,

& M. A. Belfort (Eds.), *Critical care obstetrics* (6th ed., Kindle version, ch. 37). Hoboken, NJ: Wiley Blackwell.

Sukumaran, S., Jia, Y. J., & Chandraharan, E. (2021). Uterine tachysystole, hypertonus and hyperstimulation: An urgent need to get the definitions right to avoid intrapartum hypoxic-ischaemic brain injury. *Global Journal of Reproductive Medicine, 8*(2), 5556735. Retrieved from https://juniperpublishers.com/gjorm/GJORM.MS.ID.555735.php

Şükür, Y. E., Yalçın, İ., Kahraman, K., & Söylemez, F. (2011). Cervical varix complicating marginal placenta previa: A unique coexistence. *Journal of Obstetrics and Gynaecology Research, 37*(10) 1515–1517. https://doi.org/10.1111/j.1447-0756.2011.01548.x

Takano, Y., Furukawa, S., Ohashi, M., Michikata, K., Sameshima, H., & Ikenoue, T. (2013). Fetal heart rate patterns related to neonatal brain damage and neonatal death in placental abruption. *Journal of Obstetrics and Gynaecology Research, 39*(1), 61–66. https://doi.org/10.1111/j.1447-0756.2012.01945.x

Taylor, J. A., & Plaat, F. (2011). Anesthesia and intensive care management of bleeding during pregnancy. In E. Sheiner (Ed.), *Bleeding during pregnancy: A comprehensive guide* (pp. 217–244). New York, NY: Springer.

Terlizzi, K. (2022). FAQ What do patients need to know? In D. Lagrew, J. McNulty, C. Sakowski, V. Cape, E. McCormick, & C. H. Morton (Eds.), *Improving health care response to obstetric hemorrhage, v. 3.0: A CMQCC quality improvement toolkit* (pp. 267–269). Palo Alto, CA: California Maternal Quality Care Collaborative. Retrieved from https://www.cmqcc.org/sites/default/files/HEMToolkit_03252022 Errata 7.2022 (2).pdf

Tharpe, N. L., Farley, C. L., & Jordan, R. G. (2022). *Clinical practice guidelines for midwifery & women's health* (6th ed., Kindle version). Burlington, MA: Jones & Bartlett Learning.

Tikkanen, M. (2011). Placental abruption: Epidemiology, risk factors and consequences. *Acta Obstetricia et Gynecologica Scandinavica, 90*(2), 140–149. https://doi.org/10.1111/j.1600-0412.2010.01030.x

Tillett, J., and Hanson, L. (1999). Midwifery triage and management of trauma and second/third trimester bleeding. *Journal of Nurse-Midwifery, 44*(5), 439–448. https://doi.org/10.1016/S0091-2182(99)00084-1

Togioka, B. M., & Tonismae, T. (2022). Uterine rupture. In *StatPearls*. Treasure Island, FL: StatPearls Publishing. Retrieved September 30, 2023, from https://www.ncbi.nlm.nih.gov/books/NBK559209/

Usui, R., Matsubara, S., Ohkuchi, A., Kuwata, T., Watanabe, T., Izumi, A., & Suzuki, M. (2008). Fetal heart rate pattern reflecting the severity of placental abruption. *Archives of Gynecology and Obstetrics, 277*(3), 249–253. https://doi.org/10.1007/s00404-007-0471-9

van den Broek, N. R. (2020). Maternal and newborn health. In E. T. Ryan, D. R. Hill, T. Solomon, N. E. Aronson, & T. P. Endy (Eds.), *Hunter's tropical medicine and emerging infectious diseases* (10th ed., pp. 133–140). Edinburgh, United Kingdom: Elsevier.

Varouxaki, N., Gnanasambanthan, S., Datta, S., & Amokrane, N. (2018). Antepartum haemorrhage. *Obstetrics, Gynaecology and Reproductive Medicine, 28*(8), 237–242. https://doi.org/10.1016/j.ogrm.2018.07.001.

Visintine, J. F. (2022). Placental abruption. In V. Berghella (Ed.), *Obstetric evidence based guidelines* (4th ed., pp. 345–353). Boca Raton, FL: CRC Press. https://www.taylorfrancis.com/chapters/edit/10.1201/9781003102342-30

Wen, S. W., Huang, L., Liston, R., Heaman, M., Baskett, T., Rusen, I. D., . . . Kramer, M. S. (2005). Severe maternal morbidity in Canada, 1991-2001. *CMAJ, 173*(7), 759–764. https://doi.org/10.1503/cmaj.045156

Wiedaseck, S., and Monchek, R. (2014), Placental and cord insertion pathologies: Screening, diagnosis, and management. *Journal of Midwifery & Women's Health, 59*(3), 328–335. https://doi.org/10.1111/jmwh.12189

Winter, C., Crofts, J., Laxton, C., Barnfield, S., & Draycott, T. (2016). *PROMPT (PRactical Obstetric Multi-Professional Training): Practical locally based training for obstetric emergencies, course manual* (North American ed.). C. P. Weiner (Ed.). Cambridge, United Kingdom: Cambridge University Press.

Yaliwal, R. G., Kori, S. S., Mudanur, S. R., & Manne, S. (2021). Spontaneous rupture of vaginal varicose veins mimicking placenta praevia. *International Journal of Reproduction, Contraception, Obstetrics and Gynecology, 10*(5), 2122–2124. https://doi.org//10.18203/2320-1770.ijrcog20211556

Young, J. S., & White, L. M. (2019). Vaginal bleeding in late pregnancy. *Emergency Medicine Clinics of North America, 37*(2), 251–264. https://doi.org/10.1016/j.emc.2019.01.006

Zhang, W., Geris, S., Al-Emara, N., Ramadan, G., Sotiriadis, A., & Akolekar, R. (2021). Perinatal outcome of pregnancies with prenatal diagnosis of vasa previa: Systematic review and meta-analysis. *Ultrasound in Obstetrics & Gynecology, 57*(5), 710–719. https://doi.org/10.1002/uog.22166

Zuckerwise, L. C., Pettker, C. M., Illuzzi, J., Raab, C. R., & Lipkind, H. S. (2014). Use of a novel visual aid to improve estimation of obstetric blood loss. *Obstetrics & Gynecology, 123*(5), 982–986. https://doi.org/10.1097/AOG.0000000000000233

7 Postpartum Hemorrhage

Objectives

- Compare and contrast expectant management and active management of the third stage of labor (AMTSL).
- Discuss how iron deficiency can precipitate or worsen postpartum hemorrhage.
- Formulate a plan of management for third stage hemorrhage, including pharmacological therapy.
- Compare the benefits and drawbacks of using an intrauterine balloon tamponade device, an intrauterine vacuum-induced hemorrhage-control device, a condom catheter, hemostatic-gauze packing, and untreated-gauze packing for controlling atonic postpartum hemorrhage.

Composite Case Study

It was a busy night at the birth center. At 11:45 p.m., Rosa W., a low-risk primigravida, pushed a robust baby boy into the hands of Amy Frasier, the CNM on duty. Rosa had lost 200 ml of blood while giving birth but was apparently stable as she sat nursing her newborn. About two hr postpartum, Lauren, the nurse, called Amy back into the room after she noticed a rising fundal height and fresh blood on Rosa's pad. Around 1:30 a.m., Amy used fundal massage to express 810 ml of soft, red clots from Rosa's uterus, bringing her quantitative blood loss (QBL) to 1,010 ml. Amy started an IV infusion of 500 ml normal saline containing oxytocin. Rosa resolutely declined transfer to the hospital. She was asymptomatic, and her vital signs were stable. Because Rosa's uterus was well-contracted and her lochia was minimal, Amy expected no further bleeding.

At 2:30 a.m., Rosa's uterus was again 2 cm above the umbilicus. Her fundus was firm. On the underpad, Amy found a 4 cm spot of bright-red blood with soft clots, surrounded by a serous pink halo. External uterine compression dislodged a few more small clots. Amy donned sterile gloves and inserted two fingers into the cervix. She felt a large gelatin-textured mass of clot in the lower uterine segment beyond the internal os. Amy made a beckoning gesture with her internal fingers while her opposite hand compressed the uterus externally. Bright-red clots and blood gushed from Rosa's uterus, whereupon the bleeding slowed, and her fundus contracted firmly at 2 cm below the umbilicus. The nurse weighed the pads and determined that they held 1,025 ml of blood, which brought the total blood loss to 2,035 ml.

At this point, Rosa felt nauseated and lightheaded, and she readily agreed to hospital transport. Lauren called emergency medical services (EMS) with her cell phone on speaker while starting a second intravenous (IV) line with an 18-gauge catheter. Lauren infused tranexamic acid (TXA) 1 g in 10 ml (100 mg/ml) IV at 1 ml/min while Amy administered 0.2 mg of methylergonovine (Methergine®), gave 400 mcg of buccal misoprostol (Cytotec®), and inserted a Foley catheter to keep Rosa's bladder empty. After the TXA treatment had finished, Amy infused lactated Ringer's with the clamp wide open.

Rosa's vital signs were normal when she lay flat, but she became tachycardic, nauseated, and dizzy when she moved to the ambulance stretcher. Amy accompanied Rosa in the ambulance for the 20-min transport. When Rosa's fundus became boggy again, Amy used fundal massage to control the bleeding. When atony persisted, she held external bimanual compression until the uterus was again firm.

En route, *Amy called in a report to the collaborating obstetrician and to the labor and delivery triage nurse. At the hospital, the receiving midwife and physician reviewed Rosa's records and strategized. The nurses prepared a room for managing a severe postpartum hemorrhage, with easy access to oxytocin, carboprost, TXA, methylergonovine, an intrauterine vacuum-induced hemorrhage-control device, and a balloon tamponade device. The team opened the operating room and notified the anesthesiologist in case surgical management was necessary. The hospital nurse-midwife alerted the blood bank that a massive transfusion protocol might be necessary.*

By the time Rosa was transferred to a bed, her uterus was again 2 cm (0.8 in.) above the umbilicus and deviated to the left. She was feeling crampy and complained of dizziness and nausea. Her pulse was 130, blood pressure 100/60, respirations 22. Anika Whitlock, the receiving midwife, placed both hands on Rosa's abdomen and expressed a large mass of dark, formed clots. The nurse put them on a scale and calculated the volume at 820 ml, bringing the total EBL loss to 2,855 ml. Anika calculated that Rosa, who weighed about 155 lb (70 kg), had lost about 40% of her circulating blood volume. Anika knew that such massive blood loss put Rosa at high risk for coagulopathy and organ damage.

The obstetrician ordered a complete blood count (CBC), complete metabolic panel (CMP), coagulation panel, and blood type and crossmatching, and ordered a transfusion of 1 unit of O-negative packed red blood cells. Anika ordered 250 mcg of carboprost and a second infusion of TXA while inserting an intrauterine vacuum-induced hemorrhage-control device. Soon Anika felt Rosa's uterus clench firmly at 3 cm below the umbilicus. As blood products and fluids infused, Rosa's bleeding stopped entirely, and her vital signs improved. Anika ordered repeat CBC tests at 12 hr and 24 hr after the bleeding stopped. Rosa's initial hemoglobin and hematocrit were 9.3 g/dl and 29.4%, respectively, and the values at her 12-hr assessment were 7.2 g/dl and 22 %. She agreed to daily IV iron infusions while she was in the hospital. Rosa was asymptomatic and was discharged at 3 days postpartum with instructions to take iron and prenatal vitamins and to consume a high-protein, nutrient-rich diet. At two weeks postpartum, her hemoglobin was 10.1 g/dl, and at 6 weeks, it was 12.2 g/dl. Her providers strongly recommended that future births take place in a hospital because of her risk of repeat postpartum hemorrhage.

Definition, Causes, and Risk Factors

Mughal Emperor Shah Jahan built the Taj Mahal (1632–1653 CE) as a monument to his beloved wife Mumtaz, who died of postpartum hemorrhage (PPH) after laboring 30 hr to give birth to their 14th child (A. Kumar, 2014). Despite many advances in treatment, PPH remains one of the leading causes of maternal mortality. Excessive bleeding after childbirth is associated with 25–35% of maternal deaths worldwide; in some countries, PPH is a factor in up to 55% of maternal deaths (Lalonde, Liljestrand, Rushwan, & Okong, 2012; Purwosunu, Sarkoen, Arulkumaran, & Segnitz, 2016). Globally, about 14 million women experience PPH every year, resulting in about 70,000 maternal deaths (World Health Organization [WHO], 2022).

In economically developed countries, about 8% of maternal deaths are attributable to PPH (Picetti et al., 2020). In the United States, PPH is a major cause of maternal mortality (Ende & Butwick, 2021) and the leading cause of severe maternal morbidity (American College of Obstetricians & Gynecologists [ACOG], 2017/2021). As many as 93% of hemorrhage-related maternal deaths may be preventable (ACOG, 2019/2022). Even so, the rate of postpartum hemorrhage in the United States increased 26% between 1994 and 2006, largely because of rising rates of uterine atony (ACOG, 2017/2021). Similar increases have occurred in Canada and the United Kingdom (Paterson-Brown & Bamber, 2014). This rise in PPH may be attributable to a greater proportion of mothers having risk factors for hemorrhage, such as placental abnormalities, preeclampsia, polyhydramnios, or macrosomia; those undergoing labor induction; and those with previous or current cesarean birth. Despite this increase, maternal mortality from postpartum hemorrhage has decreased since the late 1980s, largely due to increasing rates of transfusion and peripartum hysterectomy (ACOG, 2017/2021).

PPH can lead to shock, renal failure, acute respiratory distress syndrome, coagulopathy, pituitary necrosis (Sheehan syndrome), and acute renal failure (ACOG, 2017/2021). For some, surviving PPH involves the sacrificing of future childbearing. For each person who dies of PPH, another 15 require hysterectomy to stop the bleeding (Briley et al., 2014). Even moderately heavy blood loss can interfere with health by causing orthostatic hypotension, anemia, and exhaustion.

Defining PPH

When abnormal blood loss is identified quickly, the provider can intervene immediately to prevent major hemorrhage and its subsequent complications for the client (Main, Martin, Romine, & Thomas, 2022). Postpartum hemorrhage, however is defined in many ways across countries and guidelines (Hofer et al., 2023). This lack of consistency in these definitions has confounded the ability of researchers to determine prevalence and the ability of providers to determine severity (Escobar et al., 2022).

Classic Definition

Historically, PPH has been defined as blood loss greater than 500 ml for a vaginal birth or 1,000 ml for a cesarean birth (Mavrides et al., 2016). This definition first appeared more than a century ago in an influential textbook:

> In healthy gravidae a loss of blood up to one pint (500 gm.) is usually borne without any symptoms, and it is generally believed that the woman has gained about this amount during pregnancy. The average loss during labor is about 300 gm.—8 to 10 ounces. It is best to consider a loss above a pint as pathologic. (De Lee, 1914, p. 768)

Ever since, 500 ml has been the threshold of excessive blood loss, though the figure was evidently based on one physician's visual estimate and has been passed uncritically from one authority to the next. There are several problems with De Lee's definition. First is the arbitrary division between normal blood loss while giving birth and postpartum hemorrhage.

If a blood loss of 490 ml is normal, why is 510 ml abnormal if neither amount affects the hemodynamic status of a healthy individual? A nonpregnant adult can donate 500 ml to a blood bank without incident.

Another problem is that blood loss is difficult to quantify. Since the 1960s, it has been clear that visual assessment of postpartum blood loss, "a glance and a guess," is inaccurate (Main, Goffman, et al., 2015). Even experienced providers tend to overestimate small blood loss and underestimate hemorrhage (Kodkany, Dermain, & Sloan, 2012). Providers' inability to visually estimate blood loss invalidates most studies evaluating the frequency of postpartum hemorrhage.

Providers have attempted to diagnose PPH by measuring clients' hemoglobin and/or hematocrit before and after giving birth. The result, however, is retrospective diagnosis; usually the hemorrhage has been controlled by the time the laboratory values are assessed. Antepartum anemia, preeclampsia, dehydration, overhydration, or timing of the test can alter hemoglobin and hematocrit values irrespective of blood loss (Rath, 2011). Further, many clients in community settings do not have prelabor measurements for comparison. Some definitions consider the rate of blood loss (for example, greater than 150 ml/min), but the rate is difficult to quantify while it is occurring.

Revised Definitions

In 2014, ACOG's nomenclature-consensus conference (reVITALize) redefined early postpartum hemorrhage as "cumulative blood loss of ≥1,000 ml or blood loss accompanied by sign[s]/symptoms of hypovolemia within 24 hours following the birth process," including intrapartum loss (ACOG, 2014, p. 1). It added that "signs/symptoms of hypovolemia may include tachycardia, hypotension, tachypnea, oliguria, pallor, dizziness, or altered mental status" (ACOG, 2014, p. 1). For cumulative blood loss of 500–999 ml, ACOG recommends greater supervision and interventions as clinically indicated (ACOG, 2014, p. 1). Similarly, in the same year an international panel of experts in obstetrics, gynecology, hematology, transfusion, and anesthesiology redefined PPH as "active bleeding >1,000 ml within the 24 hours following birth that continues despite the use of initial measures including first-line uterotonic agents and uterine massage" (Abdul-Kadir et al., 2014, p. 1756).

The Royal College of Obstetricians and Gynaecologists classifies PPH as minor (500–1,000 ml) or major (more than 1,000 ml). The major hemorrhage category is further divided into moderate, 1,001–2,000 ml, and severe, more than 2,000 ml (Mavrides et al., 2016). Another definition of severe or massive PPH includes blood loss greater than 1,500–2,500 ml, a hemoglobin decrease of 4 g/dl or more, need for transfusion of least 4 units of packed red blood cells (PRBCs), and/or the need for embolization or operative intervention (Schorn & Phillippi, 2014).

American College of Obstetricians and Gynecologists (ACOG) "reVITALize" Definition of Early PPH

"Cumulative blood loss of ≥1,000 ml . . . within 24 hours following the birth process (includes intrapartum loss)."

OR

Blood loss within 24 hr "accompanied by sign[s]/symptoms of hypovolemia" such as "tachycardia, hypotension, tachypnea, oliguria, pallor, dizziness, or altered mental status."

"Cumulative blood loss of 500–999 ml alone is abnormal and should trigger increased supervision and potential interventions as clinically indicated."

From *"reVITALize Obstetric Data Definitions"* (version 1.0, p. 1), by American College of Obstetricians and Gynecologists, 2014 (https://www.acog.org/-/media/project/acog/acogorg/files/pdfs/publications/revitalize-ob.pdf?la=en&hash=D9ECE1577C2A0B535F42C1B8DC492070). Copyright by ACOG.

The California Maternal Quality Care Collaborative (CMQCC) obstetric hemorrhage toolkit describes stages of postpartum hemorrhage as follows (Main, Martin, Romine, et al., 2022):

Stage 0—Everyone in labor or giving birth.

Stage 1—Blood loss of 500 ml or more (vaginal birth) or 1,000 ml or more (cesarean birth) with

- Continued bleeding

  Or

- Signs of concealed hemorrhage: vital signs abnormal or trending toward abnormal: heart rate 110 or more beats per min (bpm), blood pressure (BP) 85/45 mm Hg or lower, O_2 saturation less than 95%, shock index 0.9 (see "Shock Index" in Chapter 9)

  Or

- Confusion.

Stage 2—Continued bleeding or vital sign instability, and less than 1,500 ml cumulative blood loss.

Stage 3—Continued bleeding with cumulative blood loss greater than 1,500 ml

Or

- Transfusion of more than 2 units of PRBCs

  Or

- Abnormal vital signs

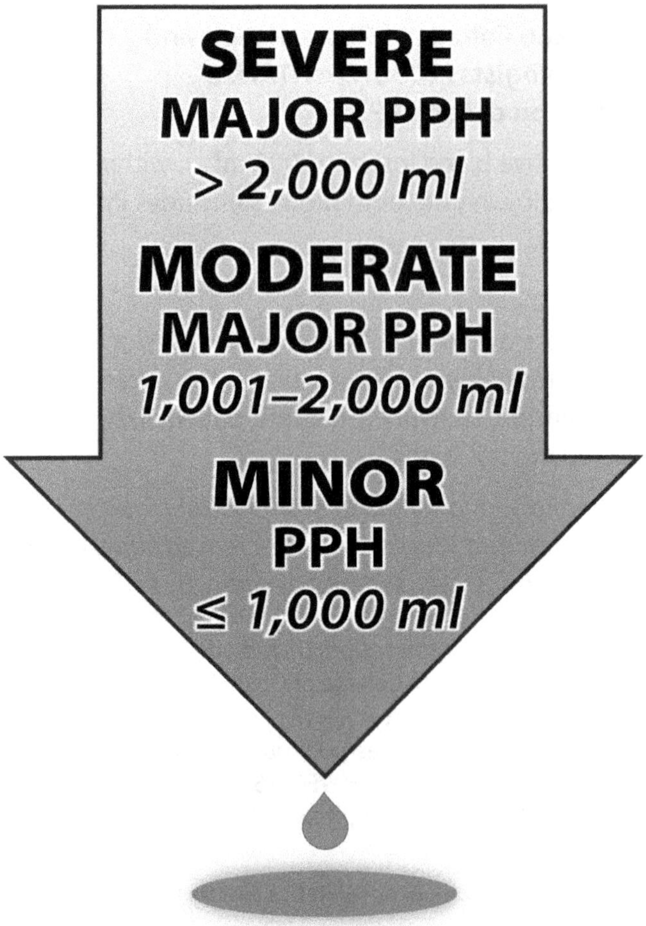

Figure 7-1. The Royal College of Obstetricians and Gynaecologists recognizes degrees of PPH based on blood loss. Adapted from "Prevention and Management of Postpartum Haemorrhage," by E. Mavrides et al., 2016, *BJOG*, 124, p. e113. Copyright by Royal College of Obstetricians and Gynaecologists.

Or

- Suspicion of disseminated intravascular coagulation (DIC).

Excessive Blood Loss

On average, blood volume increases by about 50% during a healthy pregnancy with a range of 30–60%, or 1,500–2,000 ml for an average-sized mother (F. G. Cunningham et al., 2022, ch. 42). The number of red blood cells (RBCs) in circulation increases by about 21% (Kodkany et al., 2012). Changes in coagulation factors during pregnancy allow blood to clot more readily. Healthy mothers with adequate intrapartum hemoglobin and hematocrit levels generally tolerate up to 1,000 ml of blood loss without hemodynamic compromise (Borovac-Pinheiro et al., 2018). Although these physiologic adaptations are a buffer against large blood loss while giving birth, they can also mask the signs of hypovolemia until blood loss is extreme (Main, Martin, Romine, et al., 2022).

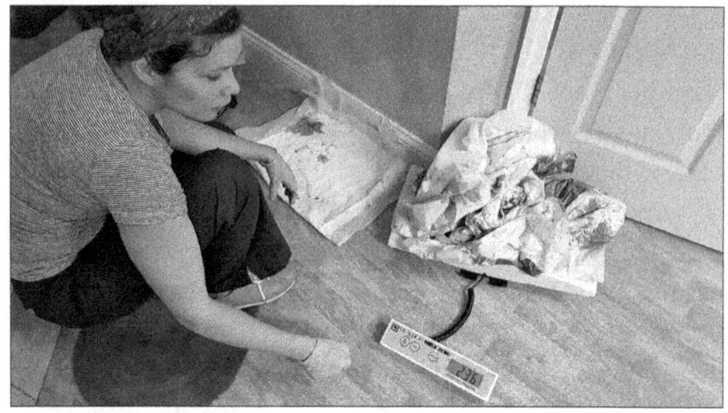

Figure 7-3. A birth center midwife weighs blood loss on an infant scale at intervals while managing a postpartum hemorrhage.

The risk of death from postpartum hemorrhage depends not only on the volume of blood lost, but also on overall health (Marwaha, Singh, & Naniwal, 2016). Any uncontrolled blood loss will eventually lead to shock and tissue damage, but every hemorrhage is unique. Response to blood loss involves the victim's size and weight, how much blood volume has expanded during pregnancy, hematocrit level at onset of labor, platelet count, hydration status, and quantity and rate of blood loss. Clients with preeclampsia can have little or no blood-volume increase over nonpregnant levels and can develop shock with relatively low blood loss (Kodkany et al., 2012; Schorn & Phillippi, 2014). Likewise, clients with anemia have fewer RBCs overall and are less able to tolerate a large blood loss (Main, Martin, Romine, et al., 2022).

Quantification of Blood Loss

Quantitative blood loss (QBL) assessment allows the midwife to recognize and respond to hemorrhage at an earlier stage, improves maternal outcomes, and speeds implementation of necessary interventions. Birth attendants estimate the amount of blood lost visually by how much is present on drapes, pads, sponges, the floor, etc., after a birth.

Handful Method

Rapid estimate of blood loss based on a glove size of 7/medium:

- One handful = about ½ cup = about 125 ml
- Two hands cupped together = about 1 cup = about 250 ml
- Blood clot the size of a fist = about 1 cup = about 250 ml

People with larger or smaller hands should adjust the estimate accordingly. Note: 1 cup (U.S. customary) = 236.5 ml; 1 cup (metric) = 250 ml.

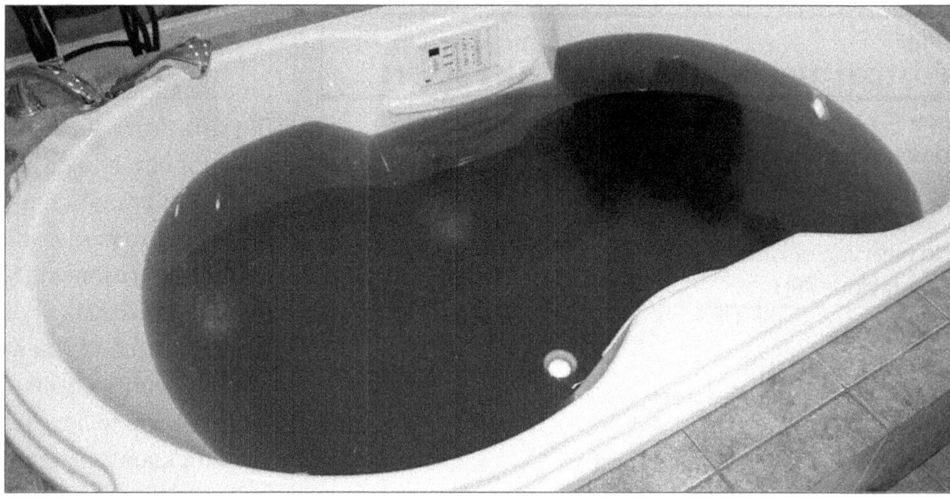

Figure 7-2. Quantifying blood loss is impossible in a waterbirth. Many midwives estimate blood loss in a tub or pool by assessing water clarity. For example, excessive blood loss is possible if one cannot easily visualize the mother's legs under the water. In this image, a maroon towel is visible in the spa tub, which suggests that blood loss was not excessive. Bear in mind that water clarity also depends on the size of the tub and the amount of water it contains. In practice drills, adding measured amounts of artificial blood mixture to a birth pool can improve the midwife's ability to estimate blood loss in a tub that size.

Visual estimation of blood loss—"a glance and a guess"—can result in providers underestimating large-volume blood loss by 33–50% when compared to direct measurement (Butwick, Romine, McNulty, Main, & Rosenstein, 2022). Simulation and visual-assessment training can improve accuracy, but it declines without regular practice (Butwick, Romine, et al., 2022).

Blood loss can be easily quantified with a scale. First, determine the dry weight of an absorbent item in grams, for example, a disposable underpad. Subtract the dry weight in grams from the weight of the soaked pad. The weight-to-volume ratio of blood is 1:1 (1 g = 1 ml), so the difference in grams is the amount of blood in ml. A pad with a dry weight of 100g (3.5 oz) that weighs 600 g (1 lb 5 oz) soaked with blood contains 500 ml of blood. Blood from the umbilical cord, amniotic fluid, and urine do not count toward the total.

In most physiologic births, QBL involves some degree of guesswork, but several techniques can improve your accuracy:

- Weigh or measure all blood clots and blood-soaked materials to determine volume.
- Quantify and *communicate* cumulative blood loss at short intervals when the client is actively bleeding. Slow-trickle bleeding and repeated uterine expression of clots and blood can add up to significant quantities.
- Before the placenta delivers, assess the amount of amniotic fluid, urine, and stool present to subtract from total weight.
- Consider using graduated-measurement containers such as calibrated drapes, emesis basins, or a plastic bag to collect blood.
- Replace soiled pads quickly.
- Regularly attend training that improves assessment skills.
- Learn how the appearance of blood on underpads, sheets, towels, and sanitary pads correlates with the amount of blood loss. Under research conditions, memorizing the appearance of measured volumes of artificial blood on common obstetric materials improves the accuracy of estimating blood loss (Zuckerwise, Pettker, Illuzzi, Raab, & Lipkind, 2014).
- Consider weighing the usual pads and linens used for birth and keeping a laminated list of dry weights in the birth bag or on the wall.
- When the membranes rupture at the time of birth and mix with the blood, you can estimate the amount of amniotic fluid as about 700 ml if the amniotic fluid volume is average, 300 ml if oligohydramnios is present, and 1,400 ml if polyhydramnios is present (Butwick, Romine, et al., 2022).

Risk Factors

Any mother can experience a postpartum hemorrhage regardless of health, risk factors, or management. PPH occurs in about about 0.4–4.4% of individuals deemed at low risk for PPH and about 5.1–23.0% of those considered at high risk (Butwick, Main, McCormick, & Sakowski, 2022). Because low-risk mothers far outnumber high-risk mothers, fully 40% of PPH occurs in the absence of risk factors—anyone who gives birth is potentially vulnerable (Butwick, Main, et al., 2022).

With low-risk clients, postpartum hemorrhage occurs infrequently, is often unexpected, and can catch a provider by surprise. An unprepared provider can be the biggest risk factor for life-threatening postpartum hemorrhage (Karoshi, Palacios-Jaraquemada, & Keith, 2012). In the United Kingdom, a 25-year analysis of maternal deaths revealed that substandard care played a role in the outcome of 60–70% of deaths from postpartum hemorrhage (Karoshi et al., 2012). Even a conscientious, capable provider can

Table 7-1
Postpartum Hemorrhage Risk Factors

Low
Unscarred uterus
Single gestation
Fewer than 4 previous vaginal births
No bleeding disorder
No previous PPH
Medium
Prior cesarean birth
Full-thickness uterine surgery
Multiple gestation
More than 4 previous vaginal births
Intrauterine infection
History of previous PPH
Large or multiple uterine fibroids
Platelets 50,000–100,000/mcl
Hematocrit less than 30%
Gestational age less than 37 0/7 or greater than 41 6/7 weeks
Preeclampsia
Prolonged labor/induction (longer than 24hr)
Estimated fetal weight greater than 8 lb 13 oz (4,000 g)
Morbid obesity (body mass index [BMI] greater than 40 kg/m^2)
Polyhydramnios
Operative vaginal birth
Genital tract trauma, including 2nd- and 3rd-degree lacerations
High
Multiple full-thickness uterine surgeries
Placenta previa or low-lying placenta
Suspected or known placenta accreta
Placental abruption or bleeding greater than show
Coagulopathy
History of more than 1 PPH
HELLP syndrome
Platelets less than 50,000/mcl
Hematocrit less than 24% (hemoglobin lower than 8)
Fetal demise
2 or more medium risk factors
Active postpartum bleeding, soaking more than 1 pad/hr or passing a 6 cm or larger clot
Retained placenta
Vertical incision with prior cesarean
Uterine rupture
Emergent or urgent cesarean section, especially when performed in labor

Adapted from "Obstetric Hemorrhage Risk Factor Assessment," by A. Butwick, E. Main, E. McCormick, and C. Sakowski, in D. Lagrew et al. (Eds.), *Improving Health Care Response to Obstetric Hemorrhage, V. 3.0: A CMQCC quality improvement toolkit* (pp. 30–40), 2022, Palo Alto, CA: California Maternal Quality Care Collaborative. Copyright by publisher.

neglect or fail to appreciate the magnitude of a postpartum hemorrhage, especially when fatigued, distracted, or ill (Karoshi et al., 2012). Overconfidence in the perceived safety of physiologic birth despite warning signs of hemorrhage—or hesitation to do a thorough examination for fear of causing maternal discomfort—can impede recognition and timely treatment (S. Adkins, personal communication, January 25, 2022).

Evaluation of risk factors can help the community midwife to identify clients who are unacceptably high risk and transfer them to hospital care. In some cases, such as the client with known placenta previa, community birth is contraindicated. In others, such as a healthy grand multipara, some risk exists, but the client and provider may find giving birth at home or in a birth center an acceptable option. Although neither race nor ethnicity puts anyone physiologically at higher risk for hemorrhage, in the United States black and Native American mothers have higher rates of morbidity due to hemorrhage, most likely caused by inequitable care (Butwick, Main, et al., 2022).

Ask clients if they would be willing to accept a blood transfusion if it became necessary; people who refuse blood products are at greater risk for complications from hemorrhage (Butwick, Main, et al., 2022). Counsel clients about the risks and benefits of giving birth in and out of the hospital. If they choose to give birth in a community setting, document the conversation thoroughly.

At intervals throughout the antepartum course, evaluate every pregnant client for risk factors associated with major obstetric hemorrhage (see Table 7-1). Reevaluate the risk status of clients when they start labor, when they enter the second stage of labor, after giving birth, and any time the client's condition changes (Butwick, Main, et al., 2022). Plan for intrapartum management and consider what uterotonics can be used and what supplies should be on hand. Create an action plan in case of emergency and explain it thoroughly to both the client and team members to reduce confusion or resistance in a life-and-death situation.

The Causes of PPH

To manage postpartum hemorrhage, the provider must first recognize that the mother's bleeding is excessive, next identify the site of bleeding, then direct corrective measures at the source (ACOG, 2017/2021). A client with PPH can have more than one source of bleeding that require recognition and treatment, for example a cervical laceration together with uterine atony. Primary PPH occurs within the first 24 hr of birth; secondary PPH occurs between 24 hr after giving birth and 12 weeks postpartum (ACOG, 2017/2021).

Consider Possible Causes of PPH

- Uterine atony
- Retained placenta
- Placenta accreta
- Trauma/laceration/uterine rupture
- Uterine inversion
- Amniotic fluid embolism syndrome (AFES)
- Coagulopathy

There are four major etiologies for postpartum hemorrhage, although any given mother can suffer from more than one of these. From most common to least common, they are

- **Uterine atony** (lack of effective contraction after giving birth) is by far the most common cause of PPH.
- **Retained placenta/membranes/clots** prevent effective uterine contraction.
- **Trauma** can include lacerations of the perineum, vulva, vagina, cervix, or uterine myometrium, uterine rupture, uterine inversion, or surgical incisions.
- **Coagulation abnormalities** occur in individuals with an inherited or acquired bleeding disorder or as a result of acute conditions such as hemorrhage or sepsis.

Management of Postpartum Hemorrhage

The key factors in preventing maternal death from PPH are early recognition of persistent bleeding; early involvement of a senior clinician; early determination of the source of bleeding; early assessment of severity of blood loss and presence of coagulopathy; and timely intervention to control bleeding including initiation of surgical interventions (Ramler et al., 2022). **Be ready to manage PPH at every birth.** Early recognition and timely intervention can limit overall blood loss and prevent hemorrhage complication (Main, Martin, Romine, et al., 2022). Act quickly when blood loss is 500 ml or more and increasing or when there is a rapid loss of lesser amounts. Clinical signs of excessive blood loss or hypovolemia include increased heart rate and respiratory rate, decrease in BP, reduction in urine output, dizziness, pallor, confusion, lethargy, anxiety, or change from baseline mental status (Main, Martin, Romine, et al., 2022). Even where absolute values are normal, trends in vital signs can be significant, for example, if the client who normally has a pulse of 64 develops a heart rate in the 90s (Main, Martin, Romine, et al., 2022).

A postpartum hemorrhage can be a stressful situation for all people involved. Anxiety and stress can increase distractibility and affect judgment, working memory, decision-making, and prioritization skills of team members (Gabr, 2019).

ALERT

Assess tone
Look for injury
Express clots
Remove retained products
Track coagulation

Figure 7-4. The mnemonic ALERT guides the provider through assessing and managing the causes of postpartum hemorrhage.

Your calm demeanor can emotionally stabilize everyone in the room. Panic is contagious, but so is calm. Slow the cadence of your speech, lower the pitch of your voice, stand tall, and slow your nonverbal gestures. Keep the conversation in the room about the mother and her situation and avoid extraneous chatter unless the mother finds it beneficially distracting (Kodkany et al., 2012). Maintain a caring and professional focus on the client.

Take Action

Failure to identify and manage excessive blood loss during childbirth is a major cause of maternal mortality and morbidity (Joint Commission, 2010). Use assessment thresholds to recognize and respond to excessive blood loss (Belfort, 2023d; Butwick, Romine, et al., 2022; Florida Perinatal Quality Collaborative, 2015). Remember the "Four As of Response":

- **Accept** less than 500 ml blood loss when bleeding is controlled. This is normal. Monitor and continue physiologic care.
- **Alert** when blood loss is 500–1,000 ml. Control bleeding and prepare for severe hemorrhage.
- **Action** required for blood loss of 1,000–1,500 ml, *or for bleeding of a lesser amount that is increasing*. The vital functions of the client are in danger. Treat for hemorrhage while transporting to the hospital.
- **Alarm** when blood loss is greater than 1,500 ml. Treat for severe hemorrhage.

Get Help

Any birth has the potential for PPH. Any PPH has the potential for maternal collapse. Although excessive bleeding at birth usually responds to uterine massage, uterotonics, and emptying the uterus, severe PPH can be difficult to resolve, especially in community settings far from potential help (Ward, 2012). The goal is to activate EMS *before* the mother's life is in danger. When emergency personnel arrive, there are usually enough hands to perform many tasks simultaneously.

Move It Along

Move quickly from one step to the next while keeping one eye on the clock (Karoshi et al., 2012). Unchecked postpartum hemorrhage can kill a healthy mother in less than 2 hr, and almost 90% of PPH deaths occur within 4 hr of giving birth (Belfort, 2023b). The Golden Hour is the first hour after the onset of hemorrhage; the Silver Hour is the second. Ideally, by the end of the Golden Hour, the client with significant PPH should be in a hospital, benefiting from interventions such as blood products and from therapies such as intrauterine tamponade or an intrauterine vacuum device. When the midwife waits until the Silver Hour to initiate treatment and transport, valuable time has been lost, and the likelihood of poor outcomes increases.

As discussed previously, treatment options for PPH are geared to etiology and include:

For atony: Uterine massage and manual compression, uterotonic medications, intrauterine vacuum device, intrauterine tamponade with a balloon catheter, uterine packing. Transport as indicated.

For retained placenta, membrane, or clots: Empty the uterus. Transport as indicated.

For trauma: Use direct pressure or suturing to control bleeding from lacerations. Replace inverted uterus and give uterotonics. Transport as indicated.

For coagulopathy: Transport for blood product transfusions.

TXA is useful for controlling hemorrhage of any etiology. When initial treatments fail, management options available at a hospital for the appropriate level can include uterine artery embolization, compression sutures, uterine or internal iliac artery ligation, or emergency hysterectomy.

A Stepwise Approach to Management of PPH

Postpartum hemorrhage usually begins abruptly and, with proper treatment, ends quickly. The operating room is the safest place to manage the unstable client with ongoing postpartum hemorrhage (Belfort, 2023d). Your job is to get your client to definitive care without unnecessary delay. Stop the bleeding and maintain perfusion to vital organs without delaying transport, tailoring management to specific causes as you identify them:

If your client is bleeding significantly after giving birth, move fast and accomplish multiple actions simultaneously. Decisively move from one intervention to the next while considering modifications that might apply to this client. With each intervention, reassess and note whether the treatment has been successful. If bleeding continues, move on to the next intervention. Delays and indecisiveness can increase total blood loss. As blood loss increases, the risk of major morbidity from hemorrhagic shock and death increases, and the hemorrhage becomes much more difficult to control (Belfort, 2023b). The steps of managing postpartum hemorrhage fit into the mnemonic "MULES BITE."

- **M**assage the uterus.
- **U**terotonics.
- **L**ocate and address source of bleeding.
- **E**mpty the uterus.
- **S**tart IV fluids, maintain life support.
- **B**ladder catheter.
- **I**ntrauterine **T**amponade (or vacuum device).
- **E**vacuate (Expedite transport).

Perform Interventions

An organized, stepwise response to bleeding forms a structure for optimal care and teamwork (Main, Goffman, et al., 2015). The order of these steps can vary with circumstances; many can be performed simultaneously. The midwife, as the first link in the chain of survival, provides the initial steps of care. Further interventions may be performed as needed by EMS responders, hospital personnel, or others.

1. *Call for help.* Mobilize all available providers. Call EMS and do not delay transport. Provide interventions *en route* whenever possible. Call the receiving hospital and give an SBAR report (see "The SBAR Tool" in Chapter 4).
2. *Provide support.* Give information and reassurance to the client.
3. *Assume leadership or designate a team leader.* Having a team leader reduces the confusion that results from many people trying to make decisions at once. The leader, usually the most qualified person, uses input from team members to streamline care. Ideally, the leader does not leave the client's side.
4. *Attend to the ABCs.* Attending to the client's Airway, Breathing, and Circulation is fundamental to any resuscitation. A client who stops breathing needs ventilation.
5. *Quantify blood loss.* Keep a running total.
6. *Massage and compress the uterus.* Because most PPH is due to atony, check the uterus for tone and use massage or compression if it is boggy.
7. *Give medications.* If the uterus is boggy or no other source of bleeding is apparent, give uterotonics. Oxytocin

Table 7-2

Stages of Postpartum Hemorrhage and Management in a Community Setting

	Quantitative Blood Loss (QBL)	**Typical Clinical Signs**	**Action**
Stage 0	Prepare for hemorrhage. Quantify postpartum blood loss.	Normal.	Evaluate risk factors. Treat multiple risk factors as high risk. Support physiologic birth. Use active management of third stage labor.
Stage 1	Blood loss: 500–999 ml with ongoing bleeding OR Abnormal bleeding during recovery or postpartum.	Slight change in BP. Heart rate normal and/or palpitations. Respiratory rate normal. Dizziness. Normal urine output.	**M**assage the uterus. **U**terotonics. **L**ocate source of bleeding. **E**mpty the uterus. **S**tart IV fluids, oxygen. **B**ladder catheter. **I**ntrauterine **T**amponade. **E**xpedite Transport.
Stage 2	Blood loss: 1,000–1,500 ml	Vital signs may remain as in Stage 1. OR Narrowed pulse pressure. Heart rate >100 bpm. Respiratory rate 20–30. Diaphoretic. Weak. Urine output 20–30 ml/hr.	Continue with MULES BITE. Start second large-bore IV line.
Stage 3	Blood loss: 1,500–2,499 ml	Hypotension. Narrowed pulse pressure. Heart rate >120 bpm. Respiratory rate 30–40. Pallor. Cool extremities. Restlessness. Urine output 5–15 ml/hr.	
	Blood loss: ≥2,500 ml	Profound hypotension. Heart rate >140 bpm. Pulse rate is higher than SBP. Respiratory rate >40. Little or no urine output.	Continue with MULES BITE. Keep client warm. Consider pneumatic antishock garment. Watch for coagulopathy. Call ahead to alert blood bank of situation and expedite access to blood products. At hospital, do not wait for laboratory results; transfuse 2 units packed red blood cells (PRBCs). When blood loss is severe and/or client is still hemorrhaging upon arrival at hospital, activate massive transfusion protocol upon arrival.
!	Weigh, calculate, announce, and record total blood loss every 5 min. Obtain, announce, and record vital signs, including O_2 saturation, every 5 min.		

Adapted from *Improving Health Care Response to Obstetric Hemorrhage, v. 3.0: A CMQCC Quality Improvement Toolkit* (pp. 189–192), by D. Lagrew et al. (Eds.), 2022, Palo Alto, CA: California Maternal Quality Care Collaborative. Copyright by publisher.

When the mother's heart rate is greater than the systolic blood pressure (SBP), hemodynamic compromise is likely. Monitor closely and treat proactively. See "Hypovolemic Shock" in Chapter 9.

is the recommended first-line uterotonic; other options include misoprostol, methylergonovine, and carboprost. TXA, ideally given early during treatment, is effective in controlling PPH due to trauma or atony.

8. *Check for trauma.* Examine the perineum, vulva, vagina, and cervix for lacerations.
9. *Keep the uterus and bladder empty.* Express clots. Remove any retained placenta or membrane. Insert an indwelling urinary catheter and monitor urinary output.
10. *Manually explore and empty the uterus.* Check for retained placenta, membranes, and blood clots. Check for uterine inversion or uterine rupture.
11. *"Pack or vac" the uterus.* When atony is unresponsive to uterotonics, pack the uterus or use a vacuum-induced hemorrhage control device. Consider intrauterine balloon tamponade, hemostatic-gauze packing, or sterile cotton-based gauze packing.

While measures listed above are in progress, accomplish the following:

12. *Monitor hemodynamic stability and assess for shock.* Assess and frequently monitor pulse, BP, respiratory rate, and oxygen saturation. Recognize the signs of hypovolemic shock: tachycardia; tachypnea; cold, pale, sweaty, or bluish skin; confusion or unconsciousness; narrowed pulse pressure; and, as compensatory mechanisms fail, hypotension. (See "Hypovolemic Shock" in Chapter 9.) Watch for coagulopathy and renal failure. Position the client flat on the side or back. Give oxygen to maintain oxygen saturation above 95%. Provide warmth, but do not overheat. Consider antishock garments for hemodynamically unstable hypovolemic clients far from definitive care. Watch for signs of coagulopathy, including petechiae or purpura and bleeding from the bladder, rectum, nose, or IV site.
13. *Establish large-bore (18-gauge or larger) IV access at two sites, ideally bilateral antecubital fossae.* Consider drawing a complete blood count; coagulation studies—prothrombin time (PT), partial thromboplastin time (PTT), and fibrinogen; blood type and crossmatch; blood urea nitrogen (BUN); and electrolytes if it will expedite treatment at the hospital.
14. *Give fluids.* Bolus at least 1,000–2,000 ml of LR or NS. A BP cuff inflated around the bag of IV fluid can increase the flow rate. Do not allow the client to eat or drink.

Blood Product Basics

Packed red blood cells (PRBCs)

- Best first-line product
- 1 unit = 200 ml
- When the antibody screen is positive, crossmatch can take 1–24 hr

Fresh frozen plasma (FFP)

- Approximately 35–45 min to thaw
- Highly beneficial if >2 units PRBCs given, or for prolonged prothrombin time (PT) or partial thromboplastin time (PTT)
- 1 unit = 18 ml

Platelets (PLTs)

- Priority for clients with platelets <50,000
- Single-donor apheresis unit (= 6 units of platelet concentrates) provides 40,000–50,000 transient increase in platelets

Cryoprecipitate (CRYO)

- Approximately 35–45 min to thaw
- Priority for clients with fibrinogen levels <80
- 10-unit pack raises fibrinogen 80–100 mg/dl
- Best for DIC with low fibrinogen that does not need volume replacement
- Caution: 10 units can come from 10 different donors, so infection risk is proportionate

Adapted from "Blood Product Replacement: Obstetric Hemorrhage," by A. Butwick, R. Lee, J. McNulty, and D. Redell, in D. Lagrew et al. (Eds.), *Improving Health Care Response to Obstetric Hemorrhage, v. 3.0: A CMQCC Quality Improvement Toolkit* (pp. 131–132), 2022, Palo Alto, CA: California Maternal Quality Care Collaborative. Copyright by publisher.

15. *Anticipate need for blood products.* Consider notifying the hospital blood bank of your client's ETA.
16. *Share records.* Fax or hand-carry your client's prenatal and intrapartum care records to the receiving hospital.
17. *Document.* Use a PPH charting document to record vital signs, bleeding amount and total QBL, fundal height and firmness, mental status, and any interventions.

Ongoing documentation during emergency treatment increases accuracy and can provide a timeline of events (Ward, 2012). Accurate records are also useful during debriefing sessions, to help providers understand what worked and what did not, and to find ways to do better next time. All team members should coordinate charting so that actions, events, and times are consistent across all documents related to the case.

Read the Bleeding

Bleeding resulting from PPH can have one source or several, e.g., atony plus a vaginal sulcus laceration or a retained placental fragment plus a cervical laceration plus intermittent atony. When bleeding primarily is from a single source, color, texture, and opacity of the bleeding give the provider clues to its origin. With practice, the provider who recognizes these distinctions can more quickly identify the source of the bleeding. Bleeding from postpartum hemorrhage tends to fall into one of three categories:

Rapid Red: fast-flowing "stop-sign red" blood. It is the texture of whole milk, and it can be a flood, a moderate flow, or a trickle. Clots are gelatinous and usually amorphous.

Rapid Red indicates active bleeding that can be arterial. Consider atony or trauma. Move fast to stop the hemorrhage.

Decreasing Dark: dark red to burgundy or maroon. The texture varies. Clots can be soft and formed or dark, solid, and textured. Fibrin strands within the clots can cause them to resemble placental fragments, but unlike placental tissue, they readily break apart under finger pressure. When placental fragments are placed in water, chorionic villi can be seen.

Decreasing Dark can suggest that bleeding is slowing. Sometimes this kind of bleeding appears a few minutes after giving a uterotonic, which causes a strong contraction that forces older clots from the uterus. Consider intermittent atony. If blood loss is much lower than in earlier assessments, watchful waiting may be appropriate; otherwise, move fast to stop the hemorrhage.

Sneaky Serous: serosanguineous, translucent, thin, the texture of skim milk or thinner. Firm, dark clots may emerge when the uterus is compressed. The blood spot can form a lighter-colored halo around the edges.

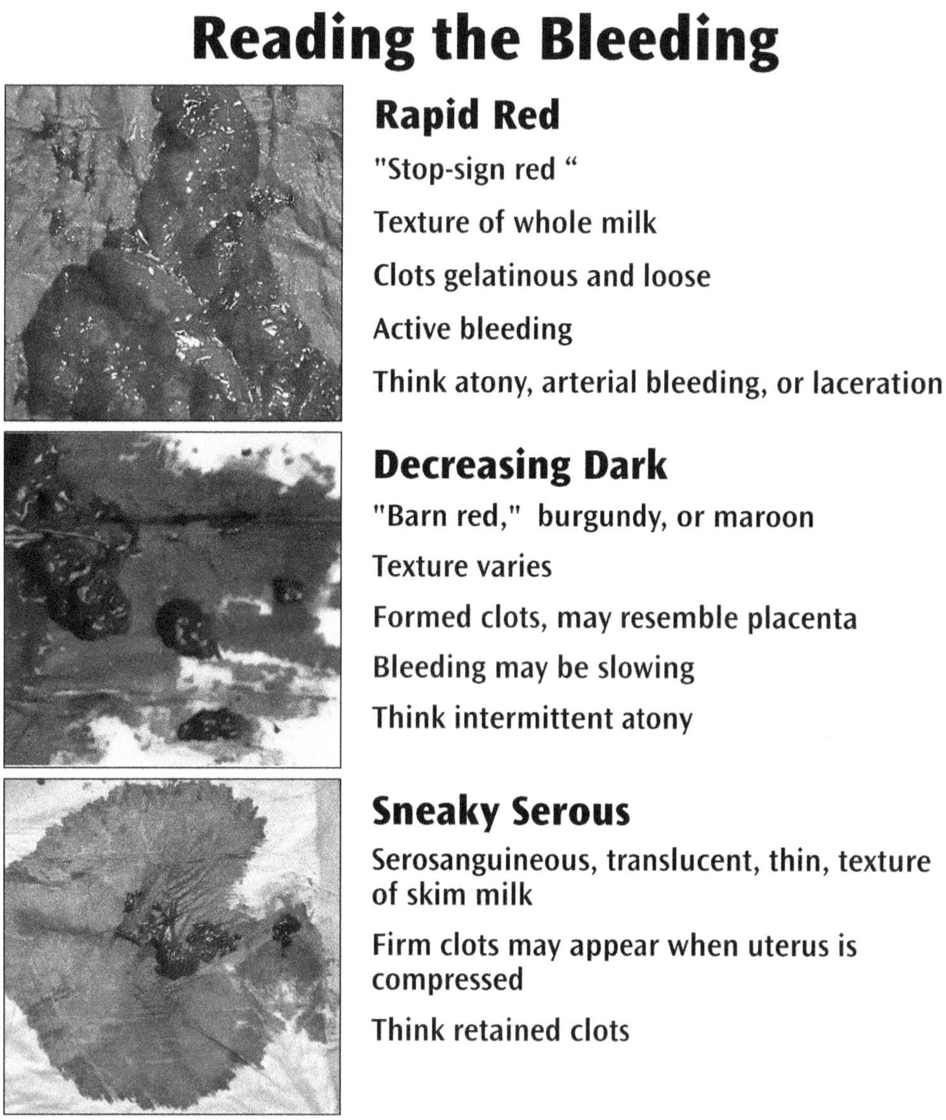

Figure 7-5. The texture and color of vaginal blood loss shortly after the baby is born can give important insight into the etiology of postpartum hemorrhage.

Sneaky Serous indicates retained clots. Assess fundus and express or extract clots. Ensure empty bladder. Consider uterotonics to prevent reoccurrence.

Addressing the Causes of PPH

Because PPH can result from any combination of the four etiologies of PPH, effective management involves recognizing that blood loss is excessive, identifying the source or sources of bleeding, and targeting management to controlling bleeding from that source. Often, bleeding originates from multiple sources, such as a hemorrhage that involves both uterine atony and several gushing lacerations. A severe hemorrhage from atony, retained products, or trauma can lead to coagulopathy that persists even after the instigating problem is managed. The following section addresses management targeted to the 4 causes of PPH As outlined in the AFFLICT mnemonic:

- Atony (poorly contracted uterus)
- Flesh & Fragments (uterus distended with clots, retained placenta, or tissue fragments)
- Laceration/Injury (tissue damage)
- Clotting Trouble

AFFLICT: Etiologies of PPH: Atony

During pregnancy, maternal vessels pass through a latticework of interwoven uterine muscle fibers to supply the placenta with a robust blood flow of 700–900 ml/min at term (Schorn & Phillippi, 2014). Separation of the placenta exposes large venous sinuses that can rapidly expel substantial quantities of blood. After the placenta separates, the uterine myometrium contracts strongly, and coils of muscle mechanically compress the vessels supplying the placental bed. These "living ligatures" squeeze the vessels closed, staunching the flow of blood (Begley et al., 2019). Local decidual hemostatic factors (such as tissue factor type-1 plasminogen activator inhibitor) and systemic coagulation components (such as platelets and circulating clotting factors) create a fibrin mesh over the placental site to further reduce bleeding.

Uterine atony is the absence of effective contraction after giving birth. In the United States, at least 80% of primary PPH cases are caused by uterine atony, a condition which complicates 1 in 40 U.S. births (Belfort, 2023b). The incidence of PPH due to atony is increasing in the United States, Canada, and Australia (Wetta et al., 2013). The cause of this increase is unclear but seems related to the upsurge in interventions such as induction of labor, cesarean birth, and operative vaginal birth (assisted by forceps or vacuum extraction).

With diffuse atony, the uterus dilates and fills with a large quantity of blood, often without significant external blood loss. With focal atony, the fundus can feel firm and well contracted while the lower segment is dilated with clots (Belfort, 2023b). A low-lying placental site can bleed persistently because the lower uterine segment is not as contractile and is less efficient at preventing bleeding.

Primiparity and high parity (especially 7 or more previous births) are both risk factors for PPH (F. G. Cunningham et al., 2022, ch. 42). Abnormal placentation or retained tissue can set the stage for postpartum atony. Hypotonic and hypertonic contractions and protracted labor are clearly associated with atony, although it is debatable whether this atony is related to uterine fatigue or if an underlying uterine dysfunction leads to both abnormal labor and postpartum atony (Baskett, 2012; Kodkany et al., 2012). The overdistended uterus (macrosomia, multiple gestation, polyhydramnios) is prone to hypotonia immediately after childbirth (F. G. Cunningham et al., 2022, ch. 42). Labor induction or augmentation increases the risk for postpartum atony, as do previous atonic PPH, therapeutic use of magnesium sulfate, and third stage labor lasting more than 20 min (F. G. Cunningham et al., 2022, ch. 42).

The AFFLICT Mnemonic for Etiologies of PPH

Atony (poorly contracted uterus)

Flesh & **F**ragments (uterus distended with clots, retained placenta, or tissue fragments)

Laceration/**I**njury (tissue damage)

Clotting **T**rouble (abnormal coagulation)

RECAPS: Steps of Intervention for Uterine Atony

The use of mnemonics can reduce the likelihood of error by providing a sequence of actions for the clinician to follow. When everyone on the team uses the same mnemonic, all members approach the situation similarly and can improve teamwork and client safety. The mnemonic RECAPS guides the provider through the steps of managing atonic PPH (see Table 7-3). Though the mnemonic is presented as a series of steps to enhance learning, multiple interventions should be accomplished simultaneously, for example uterotonics should be given as indicated while a clinician rubs, empties, or compresses the uterus.

RECAPS Step 1: Rub

Immediately postpartum, the uterus should contract into a solid mass palpable at or below the umbilicus. The fundus of a poorly contracted uterus is usually above the umbilicus and can be deviated from midline. Whereas a well-contracted uterus is firm and rounded like a coconut, the atonic uterus feels boggy and pliable, like bread dough, when palpated through the abdominal wall. To correct atony, support the lower uterine segment with one hand and rub the fundus gently but firmly in a circular motion. As you massage, the uterus should feel progressively firmer. The muscle of a well-contracted uterus cannot be indented with your fingers. Often, external uterine massage is all that is necessary to stop excessive bleeding. In some cases,

First Thought, Worst Thought:

What is the most likely cause of postpartum hemorrhage?

Atony

What is the worst it could be?

Shock, coagulopathy

Table 7-3

RECAPS: Steps of Intervention for Uterine Atony

Rub	Fundal massage
Empty	Remove clots and retained products Empty bladder
Compress	Bimanual compression Aortic compression
Administer	Oxytocin Prostaglandins (PGs) Methylergonovine/ergometrine Intravenous (IV) fluids Tranexamic acid (TXA) Blood products Clotting factors
Pack or Vac	Intrauterine balloon Vacuum-induced PPH control device Gauze packing Hemostatic-gauze packing
Surgery	Arterial embolization Compression sutures Artery ligation Hysterotomy Hysterectomy

The steps of intervention for managing uterine atony can be recalled easily by using the mnemonic RECAPS: Rub-Empty-Compress-Administer-Pack-Surgery. Multiple interventions can be tried simultaneously.

however, atony is intermittent, and the uterus becomes boggy again when the provider stops rubbing.

RECAPS Step 2: Empty the Uterus and Bladder

Remove any retained products of conception: Inspect the placenta and membranes. If there are pieces missing, perform a manual exploration of the uterus and remove them. Retained membranes can adhere to the uterine wall and prove tricky to identify and remove. They will feel smooth in contrast to the rough texture of the uterine lining.

Evacuate blood clots: Uterine spiral arteries that perfuse the placenta are uniquely devoid of musculature and cannot contract to limit bleeding (Gill, Patel, & Van Hook, 2023). After the placenta is expelled, hemostasis is achieved by uterine contraction that mechanically compresses the blood vessels supplying the placental bed. When the uterus is effectively contracted, the sidewalls compress the interior and eliminate dead space, and the vessels remain compressed.

When the uterus is relaxed, the sidewalls collapse outward, removing compression from the spiral arteries and forming a central cavity that can fill with blood. The blood then coagulates, filling the uterus with a mass of firm clots that prevents effective contraction. Bleeding and clotting continue, and the uterus can distend with what can be 1,000 ml or more of blood and clots. When the uterus is filled with clots, the fundus can rise well above the umbilicus, often deviated to the right or left. If only the lower uterine segment is atonic, the fundus will feel firm to palpation while the lower segment distends with blood and clots (Belfort, 2023b). External bleeding can be serosanguineous or appear watery if there are formed clots in the uterus.

Evacuation of clots from the uterine cavity controls bleeding by allowing the uterus to contract (ACOG, 2017/2021). Often clots spontaneously evacuate during uterine massage. To express clots from the uterus using external pressure, grasp the lower uterine segment above the pubic bone and place your other hand on the fundus. Curl your hand around the fundus until your fingertips point toward the posterior surface of the uterus. Gently and firmly, bring the fundus anterior and toward the pubis, as if bending it forward over the lower segment. This maneuver can also be performed one-handed. Do not push the fundus directly down toward the vagina, doing so can encourage uterine prolapse or inversion.

If clots do not expel, do a digital examination and insert two fingers through the cervix. Compress the uterus with a hand on the abdomen or have your assistant provide fundal pressure. If there are clots in the lower uterine segment, they will feel like gelatin and will usually slide out in chunks if you disrupt them with a beckoning movement of your fingers. In some cases, it is necessary to reach an entire hand into the uterus to evacuate. After clot evacuation the uterus should immediately become firm. Watch closely for reoccurrence. If atony persists, the uterus can refill with clots in 3–5 min. Consider following uterine exploration with antibiotic therapy to reduce the risk of infection.

Empty the bladder: A distended bladder can prevent normal uterine contraction (Mavrides et al., 2016). Suspect a full bladder when the fundus is palpable above the umbilicus and to the right of midline. Insert either a single use or indwelling bladder catheter to ensure complete emptying of the bladder. An indwelling urinary catheter often helps maintain uterine tone (Evensen & Anderson, 2020).

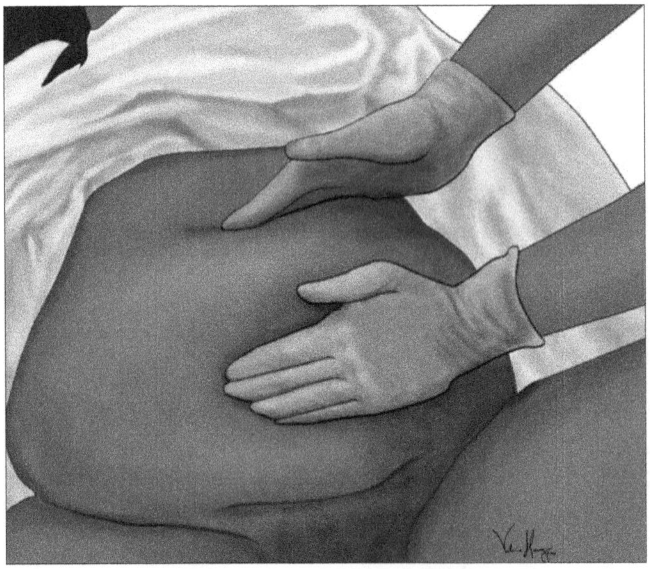

Figure 7-6. The initial action in the management of uterine atony is to stimulate uterine contraction by rubbing it between the hands. "Front View of Postpartum Uterine Massage," by V. Henry, 2016 (https://upload.wikimedia.org/wikipedia/commons/f/fe/Front_View_of_Postpartum_Uterine_Massage.png). CC BY-SA 4.0.

RECAPS Step 3: Compress the Uterus

Bimanual Compression

Bimanual uterine massage—manually compressing the uterus between the clinician's two hands—can reduce or resolve hemorrhage due to atony while other therapeutic measures are undertaken (Bailey et al., 2016). Bimanual compression stops bleeding by putting pressure on the open wound of the placental attachment site, staunching blood flow and encouraging clotting. It can be performed internally or externally.

External bimanual compression: To perform external bimanual compression, ensure an empty bladder by catheterizing when necessary. Using your nondominant hand, grasp the lower uterine segment between your thumb and fingers or position it against the flat of your hand. Cup your dominant hand lightly over the fundus with your fingertips directed toward the mother's spine. Grasp the fundus and bring it firmly forward toward your lower fist, as if trying to bend the uterus in half over the lower segment. You can also perform bimanual compression by squeezing the uterus between two fists or two palms, or between a fist and a palm. Use whatever method is most effective. This intervention is extremely uncomfortable for the client, but it can effectively stop the bleeding.

Maintain compression for at least 5–10 min. Hemostasis can require 20 min or more. If you let go too soon to check if bleeding has stopped, bleeding is likely to reoccur, and you will need to begin again. You will feel the uterus become harder and smaller beneath your hands if compression stimulates uterine contraction.

External Bimanual Compression

- Press the edge of one hand into the abdomen above the fundus. Cup the fundus in your hand or make a fist.
- Place the other hand on the abdomen just above the symphysis pubis.
- Press the hands toward each other as if trying to fold the fundus over the lower segment.

Internal Bimanual Compression

- Don sterile gloves.
- Place your nondominant hand on the fundus or have an assistant hold it for you.
- Place the dominant hand into the vagina and form it into a fist in the anterior vaginal fornix.
- Grasp the uterus through the abdominal wall and bend it onto lower uterine segment.
- Compress the uterus between your two hands until it is adequately contracted.
- If the uterus remains atonic and the hemorrhage continues, continue bimanual compression until a uterine balloon or packing is ready to insert or until surgical management is available.

Internal bimanual compression: Internal bimanual compression involves compressing the uterus between a fist in the vagina and a hand on the fundus through the abdominal wall. Locate the fundus through the abdominal wall with your nondominant hand. Insert your entire gloved dominant hand into the vagina. When you feel the soft, floppy lips of the open cervix, bring your hand to the front of it and make a fist in the anterior fornix, as far above the cervix as you can reach, pressing against the lower uterine wall. Press firmly toward the mother's umbilicus (Frye, 2013).

The external hand puts pressure on the uterus through the abdominal wall by firmly compressing it against the vaginal hand. Maintain compression and massage while other interventions are initiated and continue until the uterus remains firm and bleeding has abated or until the uterus is packed with gauze or a balloon compression device. About 10 min of bimanual compression tends to decrease or stop bleeding even in the absence of adequate contraction and can even control the bleeding from a ruptured uterus. In some cases, 30–60 min of compression is required (Andreatta, Perosky, & Johnson, 2012).

Two-person bimanual compression: It takes great strength and endurance to maintain bimanual compression for long periods. For comparison, try compressing a book between your fist and your hand at chest level: most people tire after only a minute or two (Andreatta et al., 2012; C. Cunningham et al., 2017). The two-person method of bimanual compression allows providers to sustain effective bimanual compression for a much longer time (Andreatta et al., 2012; Martins, de Souza, Khanum, Naz, & Souza, 2016). In this procedure, an assistant compresses the uterus with two hands on the abdomen while the provider applies pressure with a fist in the anterior fornix (Andreatta et al., 2012; C. Cunningham et al., 2017). The provider's other hand can then support the elbow of the compressing arm.

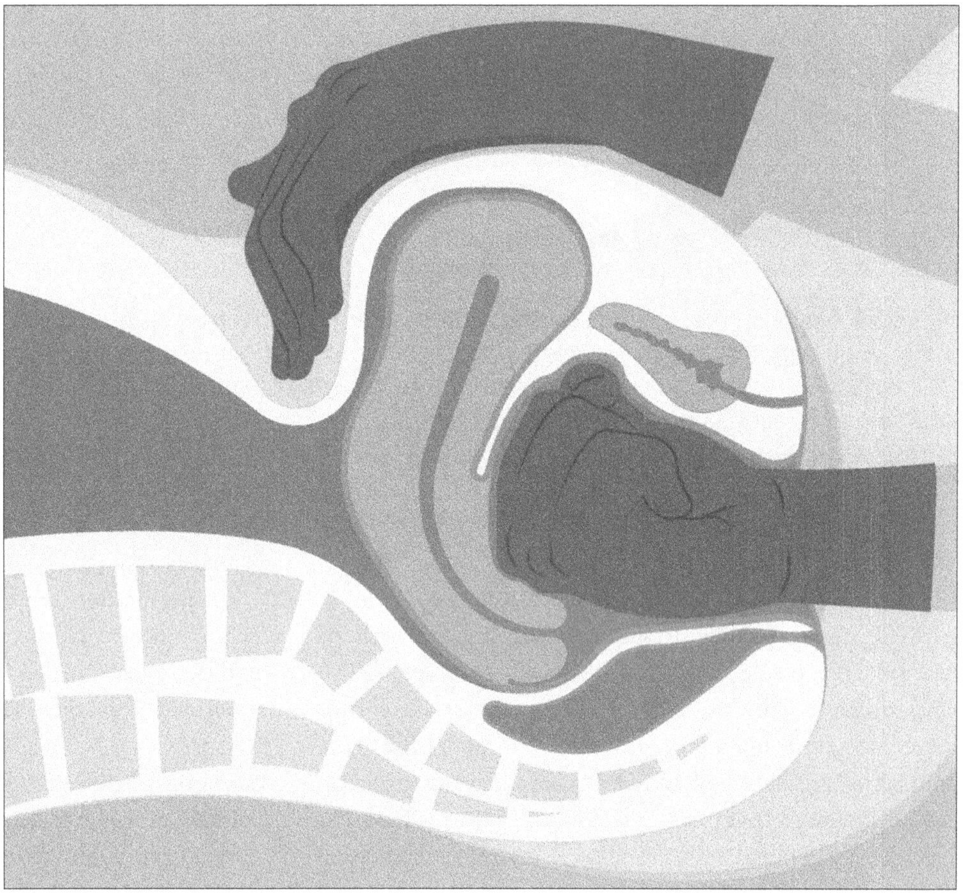

Figure 7-7. Internal bimanual compression involves folding the uterus toward the symphysis and compressing it between the external and internal hands (©rumruay/Adobe Stock).

During prolonged transport to hospitals in remote regions, such as in economically developing countries, it is often necessary for teams to switch off when fatigue limits their effectiveness.

Researchers are currently testing a slim, insertable device called the PPH Butterfly which would help the provider to sustain effective bimanual compression over time (C. Cunningham et al., 2017; Weeks et al., 2021). Instead of inserting a fist into the vagina, the provider inserts the speculum-sized device and wedges the handle against the bed, putting pressure on the uterus.

Other Compression Techniques

Lower uterine segment compression: Compression of the lower uterine segment through the abdominal wall can effectively control a hemorrhage due to focal atony (Chantrapitak, Srijuntuek, & Wattanaluangarun, 2011). Make a fist and position it just above the symphysis. Straighten your elbows and bring your shoulders directly over your fist, as if preparing to do cardiopulmonary resuscitation (CPR). Press down by using your body weight to sink your fist into the soft tissue proximal to the symphysis. Deep pressure compresses the uterus against the sacral promontory and decreases blood loss. If you rely only on the strength of your arms, you will tire more quickly, and the force of compression will be oblique rather than perpendicular. This technique has also been used to prevent postpartum hemorrhage (Anansakunwat, Iamurairat, & Boonyoung, 2018; Chantrapitak, Anansakalwat, Suwikrom, Wattanaluangarun, & Puangsa-art, 2018; Chantrapitak, Srijanteok, & Puangsa-art, 2009).

Cervical traction: Light traction on the cervix seems to compress and distort the blood vessels supplying the lower uterine segment and induces uterine contraction (Yüksel, 2015). This technique can stop postpartum hemorrhage without harm to the mother or adverse effects in future pregnancies (Hamdy et al., 2019; Matsubara, Kuwata, Usui, & Ohkuchi, 2013; Yüksel, 2015). It appears especially useful for bleeding from a boggy lower uterine segment (Yüksel, 2015).

There are several methods of cervical traction described in the literature, mostly as case studies. These include

- *Using one instrument:* Apply a ring forceps to the anterior and posterior surfaces of the open cervix, as if grasping a sandwich between your thumb and forefinger (see Figure 7-8).

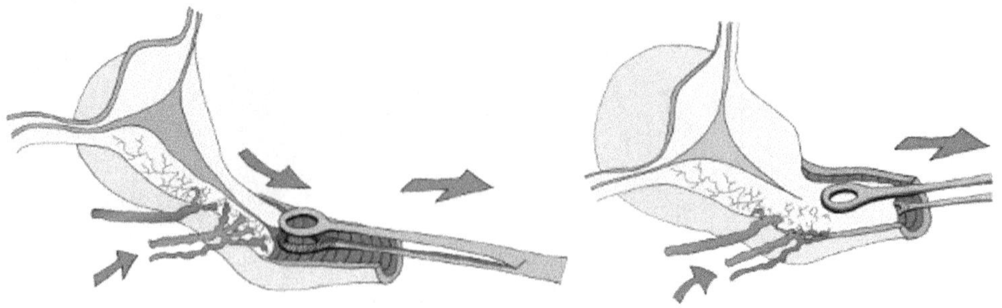

Figure 7-8. Gentle cervical traction can stretch the uterine muscle, stopping postpartum hemorrhage by obstructing the vessels that supply blood to the lower uterine segment. This procedure is especially useful after expulsion of a low-lying placenta. From "A Novel Approach to Primary Lower Uterine Segment Atony," by H. Yüksel, 2015, *Taiwanese Journal of Obstetrics & Gynecology, 54*(4), 453. CC BY-NC-ND 4.0.

- *Using two instruments:* Visualizing the cervix as a clock face, apply one ring forceps from 6 o'clock to 2 and the other from 6 to 10 (Brown & Fletcher, 2013).

The cervix-holding technique can be used with or without an intrauterine balloon (Matsubara et al., 2013). To perform the procedure, insert a speculum. Gently draw the cervix down toward the introitus with about the same amount of pressure you would use to pull your lower lip away from your teeth. When traction is applied, bleeding should slow dramatically or stop. If traction is released, bleeding can restart. Apply light traction—just enough to stop bleeding—for at least 10 min. In a hospital, the forceps are sometimes allowed to maintain tension by dangling off the edge of the bed. Holding the cervix carries a small risk of cervical laceration or uterine rupture, particularly if traction is excessive.

Other Temporizing Measures Involving Compression

External aortic compression, the nonpneumatic antishock garment (NASG), and bimanual uterine compression can be used as temporizing measures (El Ayadi, Robinson, Geller, & Miller, 2013). Bear in mind that temporizing measures buy time for other treatments to take effect but do not in themselves control hemorrhage.

External aortic compression: When bleeding is significant and there is a delay in definitive treatment, aortic compression can temporarily control bleeding and encourage clotting of the placental site (Belfort, 2023d; Lalonde & the International Federation of Gynecology and Obstetrics [FIGO] Safe Motherhood & Newborn Health Cmte., 2012). It is used along with other steps of PPH management and is not a standalone treatment. Compression of the aorta can improve BP, minimize blood loss, and increase perfusion of the vital organs (Lalonde & FIGO, 2012).

To compress the aorta, stand on the side of the client. If standing on the left side, make a fist with your right hand and place it on the abdomen just above and to the left of the umbilicus (the abdominal aorta passes just to the left of the midline). Your index finger should be at the umbilicus and your knuckles should be in line with the spine. Palpate for a femoral pulse with your right hand.

Lean over the mother and let your body weight compress the aorta against the spine. Do not use your arm muscles; they will quickly tire. You will feel a strong pulse under your fist. Compress until the femoral pulse disappears.

This procedure can be very painful to the client and tiring for the provider, but it can prevent exsanguination while the mother is transported to the hospital or while interventions are performed. If the client's legs become numb and tingly, release pressure somewhat to allow for some circulation, then resume. Whenever possible, this procedure should be maintained by an assistant or teams of helpers, freeing the midwife to perform other interventions (Lalonde & FIGO, 2012). Compression belts have been devised to achieve aortic compression without provider fatigue during postpartum hemorrhage (Dias et al., 2017).

Nonpneumatic antishock garment (NASG), a lightweight neoprene garment that secures with hook-and-loop (Velcro®-type) fasteners in horizontal segments. It helps to stabilize a client in hypovolemic shock by compressing the abdomen and lower extremities. By increasing vascular resistance within the compressed region of the body, the NASG effectively decreases the size of the container through which the blood must circulate, increasing perfusion to vital organs and tamponading bleeding sites below the level of the diaphragm (Lalonde & FIGO, 2012; S. Miller, Lester, & Hensleigh, 2004). The NASG can mitigate shock, decrease blood loss, reduce the need for emergency hysterectomy, and save lives (Lalonde & FIGO, 2012).

Secure the garment from the bottom up, starting with the ankle segments and working upward quickly until the abdominal segment is closed. A foam ball compresses the uterus. Leave the perineal area open, maintaining access for monitoring bleeding, managing lacerations, or inserting a urinary catheter. The NASG can remain in place during surgery or any vaginal procedure. The abdominal part can be opened for laparotomy.

The NASG is recommended as a temporizing measure for PPH by WHO and FIGO, and it is endorsed by the British Royal College of Obstetricians and Gynaecologists for use during transfer of community births (El Ayadi et al., 2013). It is especially useful in low-resource settings where mothers with severe postpartum hemorrhage must be stabilized for many hours awaiting blood transfusion or surgical intervention (S. Miller et al., 2004).

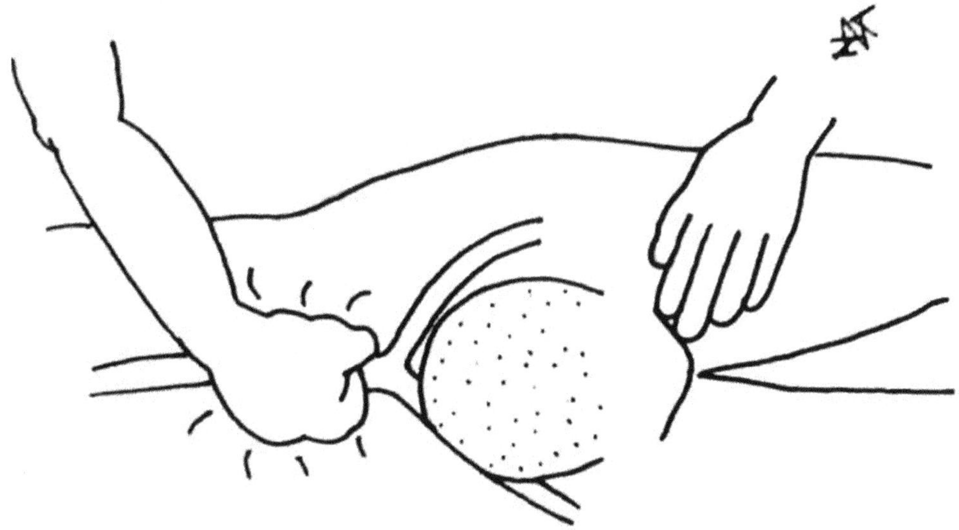

Figure 7-9. Aortic compression can reduce blood loss when severe hemorrhage occurs and there is a delay in definitive care. From "Uterine Atony: Management Strategies," by P. S. Lim et al., in P. Kochhar (Ed.), Blood Transfusion in Clinical Practice (p. 105), 2012, Rijeka, Croatia: InTech. CC BY 3.0.

RECAPS Step 4: Administer Uterotonic Medications

Uterotonic Medications

Uterotonic medications cause uterine contraction that can correct both focal and generalized uterine atony. Because uterine atony is the most common cause of PPH, *give uterotonic medications immediately* if the mother is bleeding excessively while implementing other interventions such as uterine massage, bimanual compression, and emptying the uterus. Timeliness is more important than the sequence of medications given. ACOG recommends oxytocin as the first-line medication (ACOG, 2017/2021). If uterotonics are not effective within 30 min, or if three different uterotonics are given, the provider should move on to the next level of intervention (Belfort, 2023d; Karoshi et al., 2012).

Oxytocin (Pitocin®)

Oxytocin, a hormone produced by both mother and fetus, is the first-line agent for preventing and treating PPH because it is optimally effective and has few side effects. It stimulates rhythmic contractions of the upper uterine segment which constrict spiral arteries and reduce blood flow through the uterus (Anderson & Etches, 2007). For clinical use, oxytocin is synthesized from mammal pituitary extracts to reduce contamination (U.S. Food and Drug Administration [FDA], 2014) and sold as Pitocin® (U.S.) and Syntocinon®. One regimen (Belfort, 2023d) is 40 units in 1 L of normal saline (NS) or lactated Ringer's (LR) infused intravenously (IV) at a rate sufficient to control uterine atony (usually 10–15 ml/min), or 10 units intramuscularly (IM). CMQCC recommends 10–30 units in 500 ml NS (see Table 7-4). The uterus responds to IV infusion almost immediately, and effects last up to 1 hr. IM injection causes uterine contraction within 3–5 min and effects persist 2–3 hr (FDA, 2014). Oxytocin administered with birth of the anterior shoulder has about the same efficacy of oxytocin given with the expulsion of the placenta (Main, Goffman, et al., 2015). Administration of oxytocin before expulsion of the placenta does not increase the likelihood of retained placenta. Rapid infusion of high-dose oxytocin (for example, 40 units in 100 ml of NS) can cause severe hypotension and cardiovascular collapse (Belfort, 2023d).

Methylergonovine (Methergine®) and Ergometrine

Methylergonovine maleate (Methergine®) is a semisynthetic ergot alkaloid that is FDA-approved for routine management of the third stage of labor and postpartum atony. Ergometrine (not available in the United States) is a similar drug. The CMQCC recommends either IM methylergonovine 0.2 mg or carboprost 250 mcg as the second-line agent after oxytocin for uterine atony (Adams, Butwick, & McNulty, 2022). Ergot alkaloids cause generalized tetanic contraction of the smooth muscle of the upper and lower uterine segments (Anderson & Etches, 2007). Ergot, a fungus that grows on rye and other grasses, was used as an abortifacient and labor stimulant as early as the 12th century BCE in China (Schiff, 2006). It remained in wide use to augment labor until an investigation in 1824 linked it to a high rate of stillbirth (Schiff, 2006).

Methylergonovine is a fast-acting compound that stimulates uterine contractions, usually without significant vasoconstriction (Giger & Engel, 2006). It is supplied in ampules containing 0.2 mg in a volume of 1 ml and as a 0.2 mg tablet. When administered orally, the onset of action occurs within 5–10 min; as an IM injection, it begins to work within 2–5 min (Adams, Butwick, et al., 2022). IM methylergonovine can

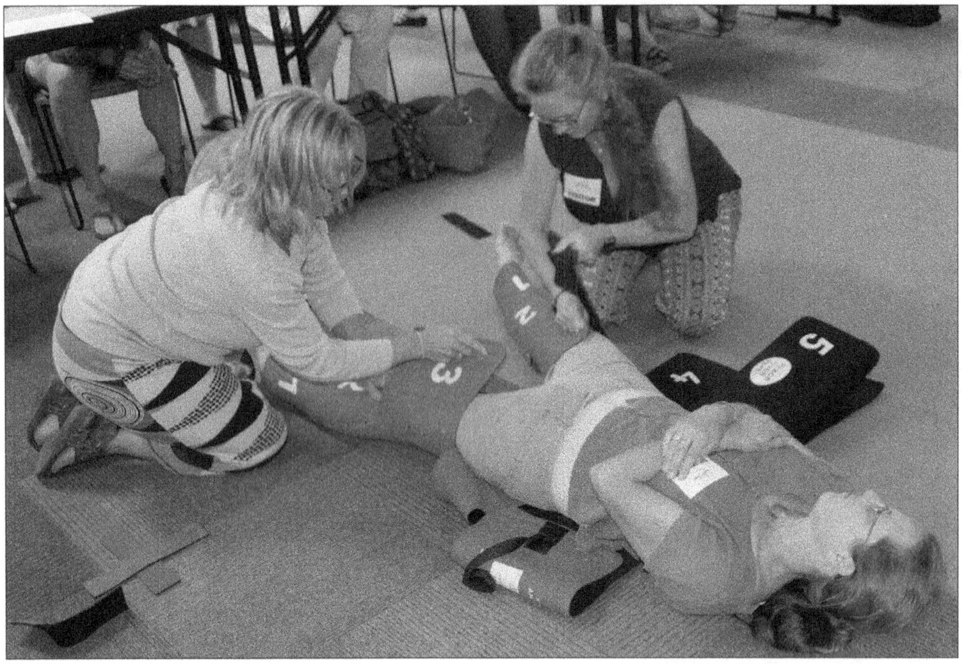

Figure 7-10. An instructor and two participants practice securing the NASG garment at a Birth Emergency Skills Training workshop. When properly applied, the garment can stabilize the client in hemorrhagic shock.

be repeated at 2–4 hr intervals, if necessary, and the oral dose can be repeated every 6–8 hr. The IM preparation requires refrigeration. Do not use methylergonovine if the client has hypertension, Raynaud's phenomenon, or coronary artery disease. Although methylergonovine is generally safe, severe side-effects, including tachycardia, hypertension, vomiting, bradycardia, hypotension, diffuse coronary spasm, and myocardial infarction have been reported (Ibrahim, Mustafa, & Louon, 2008). There have also been numerous reports of serious medication errors occurring when a vial of methylergonovine was mistaken for a vial of vitamin K and inadvertently administered to an infant (Wilson, Santiago, Preziosi, Fisher, & Hall, 2021).

Prostaglandin (PG) Analogs

PG analogs are drugs that bind to a PG receptor to enhance uterine contractility and cause vasoconstriction (Anderson & Etches, 2007).

Carboprost (Hemabate®)

Carboprost, or 15-methyl-PGF2alpha, is FDA-approved for the treatment of postpartum hemorrhage secondary to uterine atony unresponsive to massage and oxytocin. CMQCC considers carboprost a second-line drug for administration after oxytocin (Adams, Butwick, et al., 2022). The dose is one 250-mcg ampule given as an IM injection. Plasma level peaks about 30 min after administration. About 75% of clients require only one dose (Adams, Butwick, et al., 2022). Additional doses can be given every 15–90 min to a maximum of 8 doses, but if the mother continues to bleed after one or two doses, additional carboprost will probably be ineffective (Belfort, 2023d). Carboprost must be refrigerated. Side effects often include nausea, vomiting, and explosive diarrhea; consider giving antidiarrheal and antiemetic medications when administering carboprost. Fever, bronchospasm, and hypertension are other potential adverse effects. Asthma is a strong contraindication to the use of carboprost because it can cause bronchoconstriction (Francois & Foley, 2021). Do not use with clients with liver disease, cardiovascular disease, or asthma.

Misoprostol (Cytotec®)

Misoprostol is a synthetic prostaglandin E1 analog that is available in 100 or 200 mcg tablets. The drug is water-soluble and can be administered by the sublingual, buccal, oral, vaginal, and rectal routes. The optimal dose is unclear. CMQCC no longer recommends misoprostol as a second line uterotonic because research indicates that misoprostol given with oxytocin is no more effective than oxytocin alone and because misoprostol is associated with high rates of shivering and fever in 22–58% of recipients (Adams, Butwick, et al., 2022). It is often used for clients with contraindications to methylergonovine or carboprost, such as those with asthma or hypertension.

Sublingual or buccal misoprostol avoids first-pass hepatic metabolism and is absorbed quickly, reaching a peak concentration within 30 min that persists for about 3 hr whereas rectal administration requires about an hour to reach peak concentration, even with higher doses of 800 and 1,000 mg (Belfort, 2023d). Oral misoprostol is also absorbed rapidly and reaches a peak concentration within 30 min, but the peak is lower and declines more quickly (Belfort, 2023d). Whereas misoprostol administered by the sublingual or buccal routes is effective for about 3 hr, rectally administered misoprostol is therapeutic for about 4 hr (Belfort, 2023d). A 400-mcg dose appears to be as effective as 600 mcg, but with

> Uterotonics and other medications can lose potency when subjected to temperature extremes and can become less effective when birth bags are kept in a very hot or cold vehicle

Table 7-4

Recommended Medications for Atony Treatment

Recommended Medications for Atony Treatment
Administer first-line agent Oxytocin 10–30 units in 500 ml or 20–60 units in 1,000 ml normal saline (NS) or lactated Ringer's (LR) solution, time-limited bolus infusion over 10–15 min, followed by maintenance infusion at a lower rate. Alternatively, 10 units given intramuscularly (IM). *Avoid high doses of oxytocin infusion greater than 30–40 units/hr.* *Closely monitor maternal heart rate (using pulse oximeter) and blood pressure (BP) when delivering higher-rate oxytocin infusions or boluses for active hemorrhage.*
Choose a standard second-line agent Methylergonovine 0.2 mg IM or Carboprost 250 mcg IM or Misoprostol 600 mcg orally or 800 mcg sublingually. (Rectal administration is no longer recommended due to the late onset of action.) *Consider misoprostol only for clients with asthma and hypertension. Misoprostol is no longer recommended otherwise due to high rates of side effects and inconsistent efficacy.*
Unresponsive to uterotonics Move quickly to nonpharmacologic methods of treatment based on etiology, e.g., uterine balloon tamponade, B-Lynch suture, interventional radiology, trauma repair, dilation and curettage. Consider TXA 1 g intravenously (IV) within 3 hr of recognizing PPH. You may give a second dose of 1 g if bleeding continues after 30 min or if bleeding stops and then restarts within 24 hr of completing the first dose.
Adapted from "Medications for Prevention and Treatment of Postpartum Hemorrhage," by S. M. Adams, A. Butwick, and J. McNulty, in D. Lagrew et al. (Eds.), *Improving Health Care Response to Obstetric Hemorrhage, v. 3.0: A CMQCC Quality Improvement Toolkit* (p. 114), 2022, Palo Alto, CA: California Maternal Quality Care Collaborative. Copyright by publisher.

fewer side effects such as fever and chills (Belfort, 2023d). Other acceptable approaches combine giving 200 mcg orally plus 400 mcg sublingually, or giving 400, 600, or 800 mcg sublingually (Belfort, 2023d). CMQCC recommends Misoprostol dosage of 600 mcg orally or 800 mcg sublingually, and no longer recommends rectal administration due to the late onset of action (Adams, Butwick, et al., 2022). WHO suggests 800 mcg sublingually in a single dose (WHO, 2012). Vaginal administration is not recommended because the flow of blood can wash the tablet away and limit absorption.

Side effects are dose-related and include fever, which can reach 104°F (40°C), accompanied by shaking chills. Treat fever promptly with acetaminophen. Because it can be difficult to determine whether the fever is related to misoprostol administration or infection (such as endometritis or urinary tract infection), consult your collaborating physician and initiate hospital transfer for any mother with postpartum fever. Diarrhea and headaches are also possible. Unlike carboprost (below), misoprostol can be used in clients with asthma. It does not require refrigeration and is inexpensive.

Tranexamic Acid (TXA)

TXA is an antifibrinolytic medication that is used to arrest or prevent bleeding. TXA inhibits fibrinolysis and the destruction of clots, thus stabilizing the fibrin meshwork produced by the coagulation cascade and reducing excess bleeding (Franchini & Mannucci, 2020). At the onset of severe postpartum hemorrhage, fibrin can break down at an accelerated rate and deplete the mother's fibrinogen (Belfort, 2023d). TXA, a synthetic derivative of the amino acid lysine, competitively blocks the lysine binding sites on plasminogen which prevents lysine from interacting with formed plasmin and fibrin. TXA is effective in controlling postpartum hemorrhage regardless of whether the bleeding is due to genital tract trauma or uterine atony and is quickly becoming the standard of care (Della Corte et al., 2020; Kroener & Toman, 2020; Tang & Stetz, 2020).

The World Maternal Antifibrinolytic (WOMAN) Trial found that TXA decreased death due to postpartum hemorrhage by 31% without adverse effects (Shakur, Roberts, et al., 2017). WHO and other key reproductive health organizations consider TXA effective, safe, and cost-effective, and recommend IV TXA in addition to standard care for mothers with PPH after vaginal birth or cesarean section (ACOG, 2017/2021; Adams, Butwick, et al., 2022; Della Corte et al., 2020; Evensen, Anderson, & Fontaine, 2017; Queensland Clinical Guidelines, 2021; Shakur, Beaumont, et al., 2018; Sudhof, Shainker, & Einerson, 2019; WHO, 2017). There is also evidence that TXA is effective in preventing PPH when used within 10 min after vaginal birth together with oxytocin, controlled cord traction, and uterine massage (Saccone et al., 2020).

TXA administration can be helpful in many PPH situations, including when

Methylergonovine and Human Milk

The manufacturer of Methergine® and the U.S. Food and Drug Administration (FDA) recommend that mothers avoid nursing and discard breastmilk for at least 12 hr after receiving methylergonovine. There is **no** evidence however, that a single dose of IM methylergonovine is harmful to the infant or to the mother's milk supply. Given the small volume of colostrum ingested by an infant in the first 12 hr of life, a single maternal 0.2 mg IM injection probably exposes the infant minimally, if at all. Documented harm to infants is limited to accidental oral poisonings and 40 cases in which providers inadvertently injected newborns with a full maternal dose packaged very similarly to the newborn dose of vitamin K. A few case reports correlate short-term decrease in milk volume with use of methylergonovine to treat postpartum hemorrhage. Methylergonovine and ergotamine are contraindicated once milk supply is established because of potential adverse effects on the infant.

Ashwal et al., 2022; Bangh, Hughes, Roberts, & Kovarik, 2005; Gilad, Merlob, Stahl, Averbuch, & Klinger, 2017; Lupin Pharmaceuticals, 2017; National Institute of Child Health and Human Development, 2018.

- The postpartum client continues to bleed after uterotonics (oxytocin, prostaglandins, methylergonovine) have been given.
- Balloon tamponade or uterine packing is necessary.
- The client is hemorrhaging from a deep or complex laceration and the midwife cannot achieve hemostasis.
- There is an expanding genital-tract hematoma.
- The client is actively bleeding and facing a long transport.
- The client has a small habitus or is known to be anemic and is bleeding excessively.
- There is excessive bleeding of any etiology.

TXA is available as a 1 g/10 ml vial as well as a 1,000 mg/100 ml IV piggyback medication (Adams, Butwick, et al., 2022; Belfort, 2023d). Infuse the 1 g/10 ml vial over 10 min as undiluted drug or infuse the piggyback at a rate of 1 g (10 ml of a 100 mg/ml solution) over 10–20 min. *The mother can develop hypotension when the infusion rate exceeds 100 mg/min* (Belfort, 2023d). When PPH is caused by atony, use TXA alongside other standard treatments including oxytocin, PGs, ergot alkaloids, bimanual compression, or uterine tamponade.

A second 1-g dose can be given after 30 min if bleeding persists. TXA is most effective when started immediately after birth of the infant and must be initiated within 3 hr postpartum. Potential treatment benefits decrease by about 10% for every 15-min delay and become negligible after 3 hr. Onset of action for IV TXA is 5–15 min, the half-life is about 2 hr, and therapeutic effect is sustained for 7–8 hr (Belfort, 2023d). TXA appears in human milk at about .01 of the maternal serum peak concentration; it is unlikely to affect the nursing infant (Belfort, 2023d).

TXA can be mixed with NS or lactated Ringer's and can be infused through the same IV cannula used for hydration. Its compatibility with oxytocin is unclear. One study found that oxytocin can lose potency when mixed with TXA in the same solution (Pacheco et al., 2017). Until compatibility is determined, either infuse TXA through a second IV site *or* give oxytocin IM while giving TXA IV. Do not mix TXA with solutions containing penicillin. Do not administer to clients with history of a thromboembolic event or known hypersensitivity to TXA (Mielke & Obermeyer, 2020). TXA is contraindicated for clients with significant renal disease.

Oral administration of TXA tablets is of no benefit in an emergency PPH situation because it requires about 1 hr to reach a therapeutic plasma concentration (Shakur-Still et al., 2022). Moreover, in treating PPH, misoprostol with oral TXA is no more effective than misoprostol alone (Diop et al., 2020). In a hospital, however, oral TXA can be used to reduce bleeding in the clinically stable postpartum client with a congenital bleeding disorder such as von Willebrand disease or hemophilia (Pacheco et al., 2017).

RECAPS Step 5: Pack or "Vac" the Uterus

Intrauterine Tamponade

Uterine atony usually responds well to massage, compression, and medications. Occasionally, these therapies fail to sustain effective contraction when labor has been prolonged or when uterine infection has taken hold (Baskett, 2012; Kodkany et al., 2012). In these cases, intrauterine tamponade with a balloon device, hemostatic gauze, or sterile gauze can save lives by controlling bleeding until the client can receive care in a facility with surgical facilities and the capacity for blood transfusion (Bagga, Jain, Chopra, Kalra, & Gopalan, 2004; Fox, 2023). The efficacy of intrauterine tamponade as a stand-alone treatment is unclear because it can increase blood loss if a cervical laceration or uterine perforation occurs during insertion (Fox, 2023).

Uterine Balloon Tamponade

Uterine balloon tamponade (UBT) is an effective second-line treatment for PPH that is much less invasive than surgical management but has comparable efficacy (Tindell et al., 2013). UBT involves inserting an inflatable object into the uterus and distending it with NS. The hydrostatic pressure applied to the uterine wall reduces uterine artery perfusion, compresses blood vessels in the placental bed, and encourages clotting and contraction (Tindell et al., 2013). A meta-analysis by Suarez et al. (2020), showed that UBT devices were 85.9% effective in stopping PPH overall, 87.1% in cases of uterine atony, and 88.6% in cases of placenta previa, but much less effective against hemorrhage due to invasive placenta (placenta accreta spectrum [PAS], 66.7%) or retained products of conception (76.8%). UBT can be used by itself or in conjunction with a B-Lynch uterine compression suture, a technique that squeezes the myometrium between the internal balloon and the external suture to make a "uterine sandwich" (Fox, 2023).

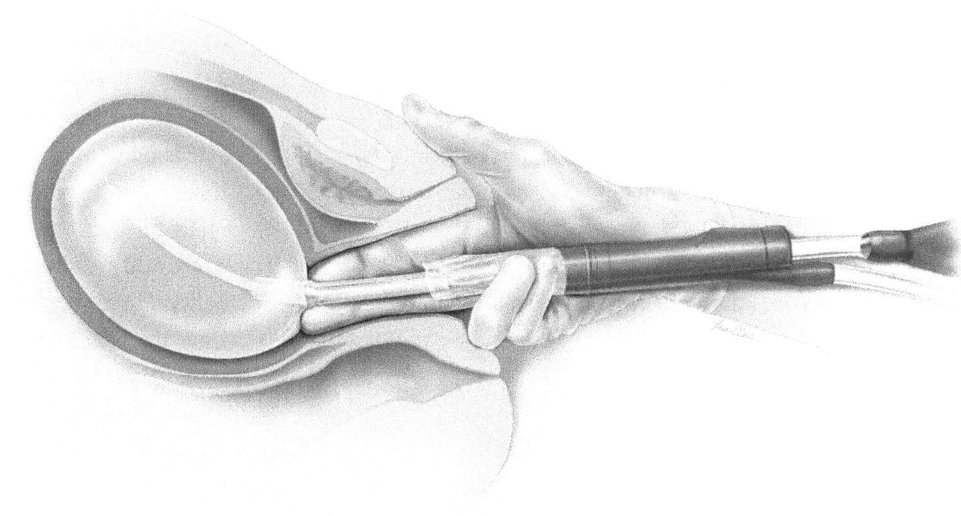

Figure 7-11. The Ebb® Complete Tamponade System is a dual-balloon tamponade designed to treat postpartum hemorrhage quickly and effectively. Image courtesy of Clinical Innovations, LLC; used with permission.

Uterine balloon tamponade should not be used

- When the client is allergic to the materials that make up the device.
- With known bicornuate uterus.
- When uterine rupture is suspected.
- When the client has cervical cancer.
- When a purulent infection of the vagina, cervix, or uterus is present.

Monitor vital signs closely after placing a balloon, even if bleeding seems to stop. It is possible to have concealed intra-abdominal bleeding with a balloon in place (Main, Martin, McNulty, & Vincent, 2022). If pain medication is available, offer it to the mother before inserting the device. Carefully check for bleeding lacerations before placing a balloon. Balloons should be inflated with only fluid; inflation with air or carbon dioxide can lead to air embolism (Fox, 2023).

Balloons Designed for Use With PPH

Several balloon catheters were designed specifically for one-time use in postpartum hemorrhage (Fox, 2023).

- **The Bakri® postpartum balloon** was the first product on the market for the purpose of controlling PPH. It is also best studied and the most expensive of these products. It can be inserted quickly, allows assessment of continued bleeding, and is optimally effective (Belfort, 2023d). The Bakri® tamponade kit includes a silicone catheter and a 500-ml silicone balloon that can accept as much as 1,300 ml of NS (Fox, 2023). The provider inserts the deflated balloon into the uterus and fills it with NS. The balloon conforms to the uterine interior and tamponades the bleeding. Because the central lumen of the catheter allows drainage, the provider can easily monitor ongoing bleeding.
- **The BT-Cath® balloon tamponade** is a pear-shaped silicone balloon that conforms to the shape of the uterine cavity when filled with 500 ml of fluid. One lumen of the catheter serves as a conduit for infusing NS while the other drains blood from the fundus.
- **The Ebb® Complete Tamponade System** is a single-use double balloon system with a drainage catheter. The upper balloon is positioned in the fundus with a maximum volume of 750 ml while the lower balloon is inflated in the vagina with a maximum volume of 300 ml. The provider fills each balloon by attaching an IV fluid bag of isotonic solution to the infusion port and squeezing it.

Insertion of UBT Device

Although UBT devices differ, their insertion processes are very similar. Refer to manufacturer's instructions for specific information on the device you are using. It is helpful to have someone read you the instructions as you perform the steps. General instructions are as follows:

Assemble Equipment

- Balloon device and at least 500–1,000 ml of warmed sterile crystalloid (sterile NS, water, or LR) to instill into the balloon device. Warming fluids to 90–100°F (32–38°C) enhances the coagulation cascade and can be more effective than using room-temperature solution (Fox, 2023). A sealed bag of IV fluid can be quickly heated by placing it in a bowl of warm tap water or under warm running water.

- Two or more Luer lock syringes (60 ml or larger).
- 1,000 ml basin. Empty the crystalloid solution into the basin for faster filling of the syringes.
- The largest speculum available.
- Ring forceps.
- Antiseptic solution (e.g., povidone-iodine).
- Gauze or vaginal packing to stabilize balloon if necessary.
- Bladder catheter.
- Collection bag to measure ongoing blood loss, such as a urinary catheter bag.

Insert Balloon

Though balloons differ, the insertion process is similar for most (Fox, 2023; Main, Martin, McNulty, et al., 2022). Refer to the package insert for instructions specific to your device. The placement process is most efficient if the provider inserts the catheter and assesses uterine filling and tone while an assistant manages the saline infusion and turns the stopcocks (Main, Martin, McNulty, et al., 2022).

- Place the client in a dorsal lithotomy position.
- Cleanse the cervix and vagina with antiseptic solution.
- Guide the deflated balloon through the dilated cervix and as high as possible into the uterine cavity.
- Some providers use ring forceps to facilitate placement. If so,
    - Insert a speculum into the vagina.
    - Grasp the anterior cervical lip with ring forceps.
    - Apply gentle traction so the cervical canal and uterine cavity are aligned. Sometimes cervical traction slows or stops the bleeding by itself.
    - Use a second ring forceps to insert the balloon as high in the cavity as possible. Use caution; using excessive force can perforate the uterus.
- If you encounter resistance before the entire balloon is in the uterus, shift the angle of insertion or have your assistant press into the abdomen to straighten the axis of the uterus. If the obstruction persists, discontinue the procedure. Do not try to push through resistance.
- While you hold the device in place, ask your assistant to fill the balloon(s) with warm sterile fluid by aspirating crystalloid solution from the basin with a syringe and instilling it into the port. You will feel slight resistance when the balloon is full, and you should notice a decrease in bleeding.
- Hold the balloon within the uterine cavity to prevent extrusion while it is filling. Do not kink the tubing.
- If bleeding stops when the balloon is partially or maximally filled, the tamponade is effective. After the bleeding stops, add an additional 50–100 ml of fluid to keep the balloon in place.
- Once the balloon is optimally filled, tug gently on the stem to seat the balloon within the lower uterine segment. Do not pull it out of the uterus.
- If a double balloon device is used, fill the vaginal balloon to maintain positioning. If the balloon does not stay in position, place vaginal packing to aid retention.
- Mark the fundal height on the maternal abdomen with a pen or marker. If the fundal height rises, consider the presence of a concealed intrauterine hemorrhage.
- Monitor for hemodynamic instability: pallor, dizziness, hypotension, tachycardia, confusion, uterine enlargement, abdominal pain, abdominal distension, or oliguria.
- Attach a collection bag to the drainage port. Flush the port with sterile NS occasionally to keep it patent.
- If hemorrhage continues with the balloon filled, the balloon is ineffective, and another method should be tried.

Other Balloon Tamponade Devices

Inflatable latex, silicone, or polyurethane devices meant for other purposes can be used for tamponading the uterus to control postpartum hemorrhage (Fox, 2023). They tend to be almost as effective as products designed for intrauterine use and often cost much less.

Condom Balloon Intrauterine Catheter

The condom catheter is a device that can be constructed from a condom, a Foley-type catheter, and a bag of NS or LR. The concept of using a condom for balloon tamponade was developed by Sayeba Akhter in Bangladesh as an alternative to the expensive devices marketed for the purpose (Akhter et al., 2003). In her initial 23 subjects, bleeding stopped within 15 min and did not reoccur, and there was no postpartum infection (Akhter et al., 2003). Condoms are usually available in low-resource areas, and condom balloon catheters are easy to use, effective, inexpensive, and safe (Ahmad, Seth, Agarwal, & Choudhary, 2017; Akhter et al., 2003; Hasabe, Gupta, & Rathode, 2016; Maya, Buntugu, Aki, & Srofenyoh, 2015). The provider can position a condom balloon catheter in the uterus using a speculum and ring forceps, or by introducing it through a digital cervical examination.

Assembling and Inserting the Condom Catheter Using Ring Forceps

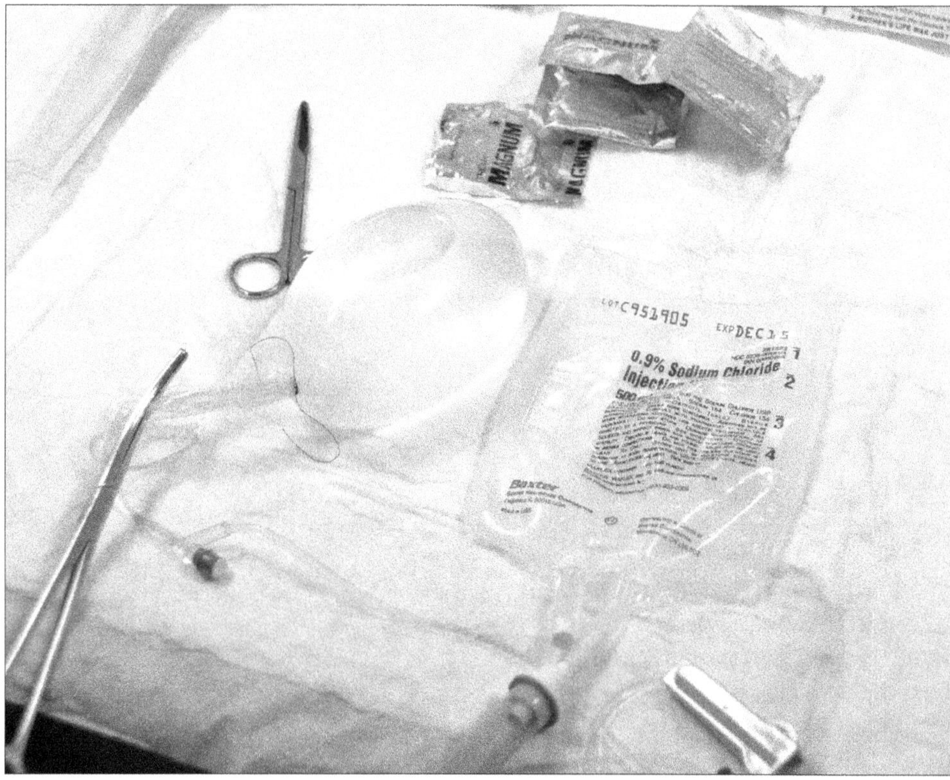

Figure 7-12. The condom catheter can easily hold 500 ml of fluid and can be quickly constructed from readily available materials. This version was created by inserting IV tubing directly into the condom. More commonly, a Foley-type catheter is inserted into the condom, and IV tubing is attached to the catheter.

1. Insert a size 18–22 Fr (6–7.3 mm) Foley-type catheter (the largest available) or IV catheter tubing aseptically into an unrolled male condom to about two thirds of its length (Maya et al., 2015).
2. Tie the proximal end of the unrolled condom with sterile string or with the thickest, heaviest suture material available to prevent leakage after inflation. Some providers use two ties 1 cm apart. The tie should be tight enough to secure the catheter, but not tight enough to occlude the lumen.
3. Test for leaks by attaching an IV infusion set and filling it with warm NS. Empty the condom and prepare for insertion.
4. Insert a speculum and visualize the cervix.
5. Grasp the cervix with two ring forceps (one anterior and one posterior) and gently coax the cervix toward the introitus. The act of grasping, pulling, and holding the cervix with ring forceps can decrease or stop postpartum hemorrhage without further intervention.
6. Use a third ring forceps to grasp the catheter just distal to the tie and introduce it into the uterus. Take care not to accidentally puncture the condom or perforate the uterus.
7. The provider can also insert the condom catheter digitally. Guide the condom catheter between the first two fingers of the dominant hand, as you would when inserting an intrauterine pressure catheter (Hasabe et al., 2016). Hold the catheter with your fingers as the catheter fills, and release when you can feel the balloon bulging against the cervix.
8. One at a time, reposition the ring forceps that are clamped to the cervix so that the cervical opening narrows and keeps the catheter in place. One forceps grips the cervix at the 10 and 2 o'clock positions, and the other at 4 and 8 (see Figure 7-13). Alternatively, you can pack the vagina with gauze to keep the balloon in place.
9. Remove the introducer forceps and connect the end of the catheter to an infusion set attached to a 500 ml bag of NS warmed to 90–100°F (32–38°C) and fill the condom with 250–500 ml of the solution (350 ml is average). Raise the infusion bag at least 4–6 ft (1.2–1.9 m) above the uterus to increase the flow. Fill until bleeding stops. As the pressure increases in the balloon, the infusion rate slows. To prevent uterine overdistension, lower the bag until flow stops or reverse flow begins. The provider can digitally hold the balloon in place as the assistant infuses fluids.
10. Attach an umbilical cord clamp to the distal end of the Foley catheter about 5–6 in. (13–15 cm) below the introitus to retain fluid in the balloon.
11. Watch for continued external or internal bleeding. Mark the fundal height on the maternal abdomen with a pen or marker. A rising fundal height indicates concealed hemorrhage.
12. Infuse oxytocin IV diluted in 500 or 1,000 ml of NS or LR.
13. Insert an indwelling catheter into the client's bladder to keep it empty and monitor output.

The Every Second Matters for Mothers-Uterine Balloon Tamponade Device® (ESM-UBT) is an inexpensive condom-balloon kit designed for global use. In

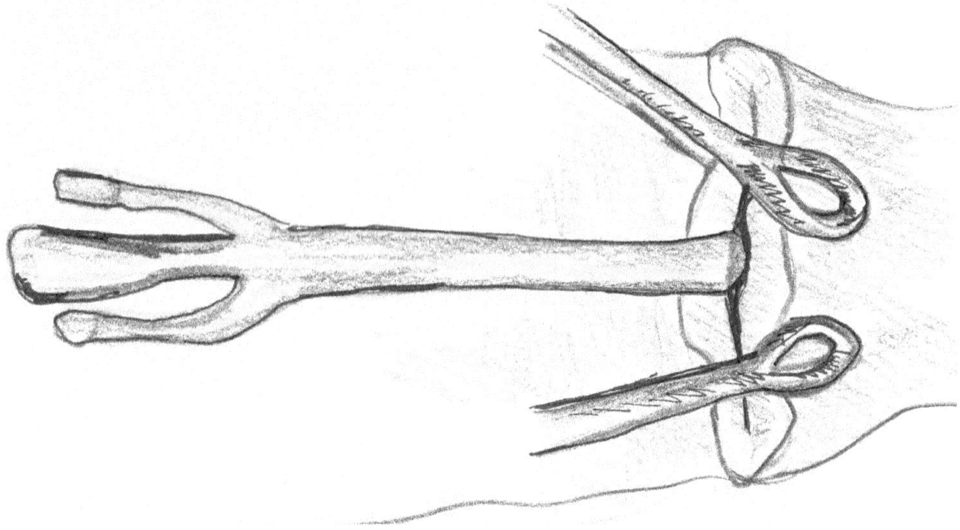

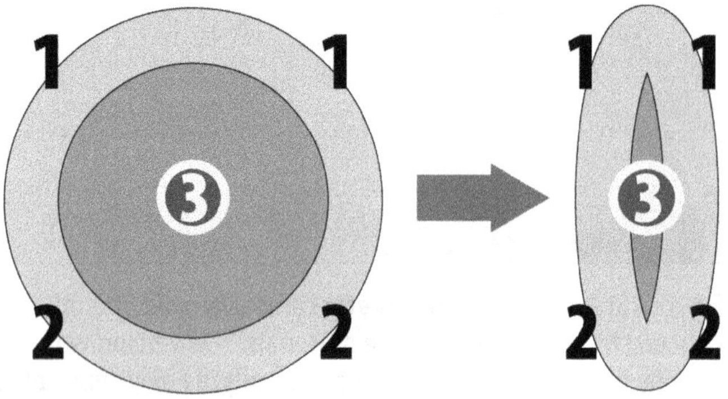

Figure 7-13. Above: Using ring forceps to close the cervix around the catheter to aid retention of the intra-uterine balloon. Right: 1. Forceps #1. 2. Forceps #2. 3 Catheter.

resource-limited settings, skilled birth attendants often find commercial UBT devices unaffordable and find improvised balloon tamponade devices time-consuming and intimidating. The ESM-UBT kit, introduced in 2010 by the Massachusetts General Hospital Division of Global Health Innovation (Mollazadeh-Moghaddam et al., 2019), bridges the gap. It includes a condom and a catheter (neither of which may be readily available in some settings), an O-ring to secure the condom to the catheter without a suture tie, a syringe, and instructions for assembly and insertion.

Condom Catheter Hints

A condom catheter lacks a drainage channel. Consider inserting a Foley-type catheter alongside it to prevent blood from accumulating in the uterine cavity. If a catheter without a collection bag is used to drain the uterus, a plastic bag or glove can be attached to the distal end to collect drainage for quantification of ongoing blood loss.

A condom becomes wobbly when filled with fluid. One team describes a "trio" condom catheter, which involves fitting 3 condoms over the Foley catheter, one inside another. The suture tie is placed over all three layers to secure them to the catheter (Simaika, 2010). When inflated, these condoms can hold more fluid and provide firmer tamponade. This device also maintains pressure if one layer should leak.

Surgical Glove Intrauterine Balloon Catheter

A sterile surgical glove tied to a Foley catheter, nasogastric tube, or IV infusion tubing is assembled in much the same way as the condom catheter. When expanded with sterile fluid, glove balloon catheters are about as effective as condom catheters in controlling atonic hemorrhage (Fox, 2023; Lalonde & FIGO, 2012). Compared to the condom catheter, a latex glove is more durable, less likely to slip, easier to handle, and shaped more like a uterus when inflated (Nalini, Singh, Bijeta, & Singh, 2017).

Fingers-Up Method: To use the fingers-up method, thread the catheter through the sleeve of the glove and tie it to the catheter in the same fashion as the condom catheter. Insert the device fingers-first into the uterus (Lalonde & FIGO, 2012). Clamp the catheter with an umbilical cord clamp.

Sleeve-up method: Knot the sleeve with the fingers pointing downward. This knot will be in the fundus. Cut a small hole or slit in the middle finger of the glove and insert the tip of a 16 Fr (5.3 mm) nasogastric tube through the hole to about 8 cm (Theron, 2010). Tie the glove to the tubing. Tie the ring and index fingers of the glove around the catheter, which is now within the middle finger of the glove. After they are knotted, give them a stretch and tie several more knots in them to reduce the risk of leakage. Remove air from the balloon, prime the IV tubing, and insert it into the NG catheter. Insert the device into the cervix with one hand and open the saline administration set. Remove your fingers from the uterus once the glove has filled with saline. Clamp the catheter with an umbilical cord clamp.

JH Glove Balloon

The JH glove balloon optimally fits the contours of the uterine cavity. First, mark the fundal height with a pen mark on the mother's abdomen. Tie off the fingers of a #7 sterile glove, then turn it inside out to create a uterus-shaped balloon (Nalini et al., 2017). Insert the proximal end of a Foley-type catheter about 2–3 cm into the sleeve of the glove and tie it

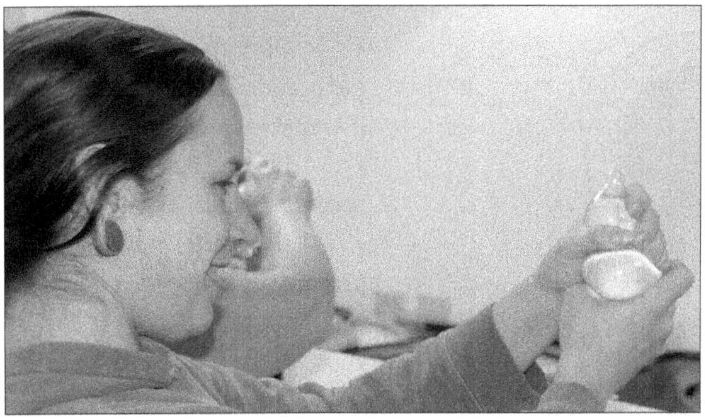

Figure 7-14. Condoms are designed to be durable, even under pressure. This condom, filled with 500 ml of NS and tied to IV tubing, withstood the determined squeezing of a Birth Emergency Skills Training workshop participant.

firmly. Cut the distal end of the catheter and connect it to a suction catheter. Fill a 50-ml syringe with warm NS and attach it to the suction catheter. Insert and fill the balloon. Add fluid 50 ml at a time to a maximum of 500 ml. Stop adding saline to the balloon if the fundal height rises more than 1.5 cm above the pen mark or if significant resistance is encountered when injecting saline (Nalini et al., 2017). Clamp the catheter with an umbilical cord clamp.

Single or Multiple Hyperfilled Foley-Type Bladder Catheters

The balloons of Foley-type bladder catheters can effectively provide intrauterine tamponade when hyperdistended and used singly or in bunches (Fox, 2023). In one case study, providers inserted 5 Foley catheters simultaneously into the uterus of a hemorrhaging mother, filled each one with 80 ml of saline, and successfully stopped a hemorrhage that was refractory to uterine curettage and gauze packing (Georgiou, 2009). Other case studies involving single Foley catheters filled with 30–50, 80, and 110 ml of NS also resolved PPH that failed to respond to uterotonics and uterine curette (Georgiou, 2009).

Sengstaken-Blakemore Tube

The Sengstaken-Blakemore tube, designed to control bleeding from esophageal varices, can effectively stop postpartum hemorrhage (Jan, Beenish, & Hamid, 2015). The upper tip of the drainage channel, however, is too long for the uterine cavity (Grönvall, Tikkanen, Tallberg, Paavonen, & Stefanovic, 2013). To improve the fit between the balloon and the uterine fundus, the provider must either cut off the tip of the drainage tube or fold the drainage tube and distal gastric balloon back and fill only the proximal esophageal balloon (Georgiou, 2009). Although the Bakri® intrauterine balloon and the Sengstaken-Blakemore esophageal tube appear equally effective for controlling uterine bleeding, balloons designed for obstetric use are recommended because they are made of hypoallergenic silicone or polyurethane rather than latex, their shapes conform better to the uterine cavity, they are easier to manage, and they come ready to use (Fox, 2023).

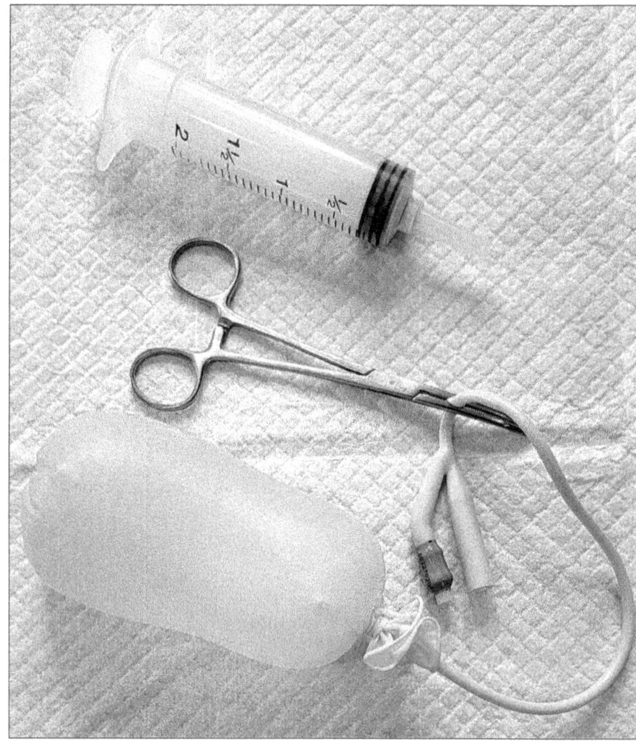

Figure 7-15. A surgical glove can be tied to a Foley-type urinary catheter or IV tubing and filled with NS to provide uterine tamponade. Photograph by Avril Bowens.

Rusch Urologic Balloon

The Rusch balloon is a durable, large-capacity balloon normally used for distending the bladder (Johanson, Kumar, Obhrai, & Young, 2001). It can hold up to 1,500 ml when filled but should be filled with only 300–500 ml when positioned in the uterus. It is made of latex and is unsuitable for clients with latex allergy (Keriakos & Mukhopadhyay, 2006).

Uterine Packing

Like uterine balloon tamponade, packing with plain or hemostatic gauze can stop the bleeding of an atonic uterus or allow time to coordinate a definitive procedure or transportation to another facility where embolization is available (Bagga et al., 2004; Kobayashi et al., 2020). Intrauterine balloon tamponade, however, is safer and more effective than gauze packing (Abul, Al-Naseem, Althuwaini, Al-Muhanna, & Clement, 2023).

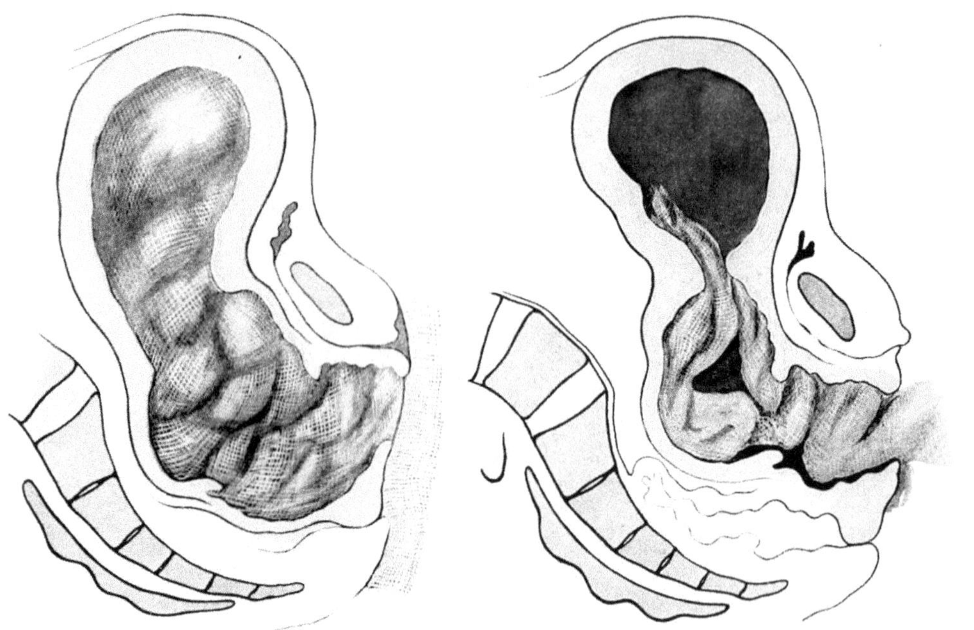

Figure 7-16. Gauze uterine packing should fill all dead space in the uterus. If it is too loose, a concealed hemorrhage can result. From *The Principles and Practice of Obstetrics* (pp. 785–786), by J. B. De Lee, 1914, Philadelphia, PA: W. B. Saunders. In the public domain.

Cotton-Gauze Uterine Packing

Packing the uterus with rolled gauze ribbons controls postpartum hemorrhage mechanically by compressing uterine vascular sinuses (Ali, Ghazi, & Siddiq, 2008; Nizam & Haider, 2010). Gauze packing was a popular method of controlling PPH before the 1960s, after which concern for infection caused the medical community to abandon its routine use (Bagga et al., 2004). Providers were also uncomfortable with the tendency of gauze to hide ongoing bleeding which must soak many yards of packing material before becoming visible at the vagina (Bagga et al., 2004). In 2012, WHO discouraged its use, instead strongly recommending the use of intrauterine balloon tamponade (Main, Martin, McNulty, et al., 2022; WHO, 2012).

When no intrauterine balloon device is available, uterine packing with gauze is safe, simple, and effective for controlling otherwise intractable postpartum hemorrhage (Bagga et al., 2004; Francois & Foley, 2021; Kobayashi et al., 2020). Even providers with limited training and few supplies can learn the technique (Ali et al., 2008). Uterine packing can limit blood loss during transport and arrangements for surgery. Sometimes packing is so effective that surgery is no longer needed (Bagga et al., 2004). Of more than 1,000 cases of uterine gauze packing reported in the literature, the majority had successful outcomes and did not require hysterectomy (Maier, 1993).

Packing the uterus with gauze:

The provider needs three to six long rolls of continuous gauze such as Kerlix™, ideally in a 6-ply, 4.5 in. x 4.1 yards (11.4 cm x 3.75 m) roll (Bagga et al., 2004).

- Offer the mother pain medication or anesthesia if available.
- Insert a Foley catheter to keep the bladder empty.
- Use sterile gloves and prepare the gauze on a sterile surface, if possible.
- Unroll the gauze and tie the strips tightly together until they form one long continuous length. Roll them into a sphere like a ball of yarn.
- Soak the ball of gauze in NS, or NS with Povidone-iodine (contraindicated in shellfish or iodine allergy).
- If the cervix is sufficiently dilated, you can pack the uterus manually. Pack the moist gauze tightly deep within the uterine cavity, beginning at the fundus and moving from side to side, layering the gauze without forming gaps or holes where blood can pool. If the cervix is partially closed and will not admit a hand, some providers use a speculum and ring forceps to introduce the packing. *Take care not to perforate the uterus!*
- When the uterus is full, pack the vagina firmly in the same fashion, leaving a tail of bandage protruding from the vagina.
- Document the procedure, including the number of gauze rolls inserted and their effect on the bleeding.
- If the tip of the gauze begins to trickle blood over the next 5–10 min, the client is still bleeding. If the tip remains dry, the procedure is presumed successful (Jan et al., 2015).
- If bleeding continues, do not repack the uterine cavity with gauze. Choose another intervention.
- Administer broad-spectrum antibiotics.
- The pack should be removed within 24–36 hr. If the gauze is removed in this timeframe, serious infection is unlikely (Bagga et al., 2004).

Chitosan-Coated Gauze Uterine Packing

New hemostatic agents containing chitosan, a hypoallergenic substance derived from shrimp and crab shells, shows great promise for treating postpartum hemorrhage or severe lacerations, particularly when far from definitive care (Dueckelmann et al., 2019; Maul et al., 2015; Patton-Molitors, Gubin,

Gross, & Bartlett, 2015; Schmid, Rezniczek, Rolf, & Maul, 2012; Schmid, Rezniczek, Rolf, Saade, et al., 2013). When chitosan gauze is applied to a laceration or to the placental bed in an atonic uterus, it swells and becomes gelatinous. The electrostatic attraction between the positively charged chitosan and the negatively charged red-blood-cell membranes produces stable blood clots that seal open vessels within lacerations or on the placental bed (Schmid, Rezniczek, Rolf, Saade et al., 2013). Chitosan does not contract the atonic uterus, but immediately stops the time-critical bleeding from the placental bed that can lead to shock, coagulopathy, and death (Carles et al., 2016; Maul et al., 2015; Schmid, Rezniczek, Rolf, Saade, et al., 2013). Because this mechanism of action is independent of the clotting cascade, chitosan can stop bleeding even in the presence of DIC or another coagulopathy. When used on the battlefield with gravely wounded soldiers, chitosan agents were 97% successful in controlling hemorrhage without adverse effects (Cox, Schreiber, McManus, Wade, & Holcomb, 2009; Schmid, Rezniczek, Rolf, & Maul, 2012; Wedmore, McManus, Pusateri, & Holcomb, 2006; Zhang, Gao, & Liu, 2015).

Chitosan, a hydrophilic polysaccharide (long chain of sugars that dissolves in water), has natural antibacterial and antifungal properties (Carles et al., 2016; Jayakumar, Prabaharan, Sudheesh Kumar, Nair, & Tamura, 2011). It reduces the risk of wound infection by damaging the cytoplasmic membranes of both gram-positive and gram-negative bacteria in a way that does not produce resistant pathogens (Jayakumar et al., 2011). It is broken down by lysozyme, which is naturally present in tears, saliva, and mucus (D. T. Miller, Roque, & Santin, 2015).

Chitosan-covered gauze packing can gain control of an atonic uterine hemorrhage when medical and surgical interventions fail (Bennett et al., 2014; Dueckelmann et al., 2019; Maul et al., 2015; Schmid, Rezniczek, Rolf, & Maul, 2012). Suitable for use also in low-resource countries (Maul et al., 2015), it is available for purchase by unlicensed providers, relatively low in cost, easy to use, and effective. Large randomized trials are needed to confirm the safety of using chitosan gauze to manage postpartum hemorrhage (Maul et al., 2015; Schmid, Rezniczek, Rolf, Saade, et al., 2013)

Minisponge Uterine Tamponade

Still in clinical trials, the minisponge uterine tamponade device allows the provider to deploy a strong and flexible pouch containing small sponges into the atonic uterus using a preloaded applicator (Phillips, Eppes, Rodriguez, & Sakamoto, 2022; Rodriguez et al., 2017). It was adapted for use in PPH from the XStat® minisponge tamponade device, a wound dressing approved by the FDA for treatment of traumatic, noncompressible bleeding on battlefields and elsewhere

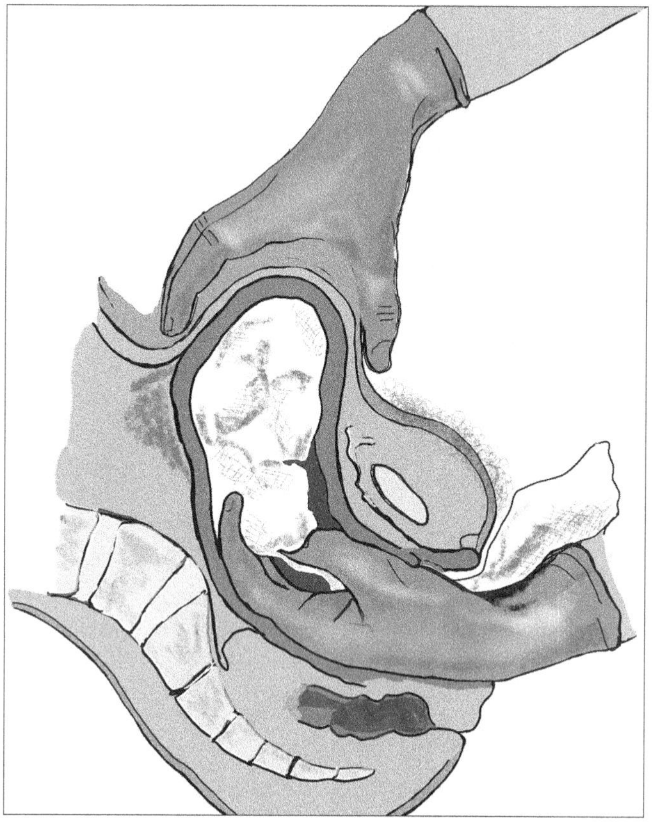

Figure 7-17. Uterine packing can be introduced by hand or with ring forceps. Methodically layer the gauze from side to side, being sure to eliminate dead spaces. Illustration after *The Principles and Practice of Obstetrics* (p. 782), by J. B. De Lee, 1914, Philadelphia, PA: W. B. Saunders. In the public domain.

(Rodriguez et al., 2017). Each minisponge is compressed to 4–5 mm but expands to 40–50 mm within 20 sec of contact with blood, conforming to the natural shape of the uterine cavity (Phillips et al., 2022). The expanded sponges exert an outward force to facilitate tamponade. The device remains in place until hemostasis is achieved and the mother is clinically stable, usually about an hour. It is easily removed with gentle traction.

Postplacement Care for Balloons or Packing

- Anyone requiring uterine packing to control a postpartum hemorrhage should be transported to a hospital for further management.
- Monitor for signs and symptoms of ongoing hemorrhage, including air hunger or shortness of breath, palpitations, dizziness, decreased level of consciousness, bleeding from IV access sites, fainting, pallor, hypotension, tachycardia, confusion, uterine enlargement, abdominal pain/distension, and decreased urine output.
- Consider infusing broad-spectrum antibiotic prophylaxis while the balloon/pack is in place to reduce the risk of endometritis.

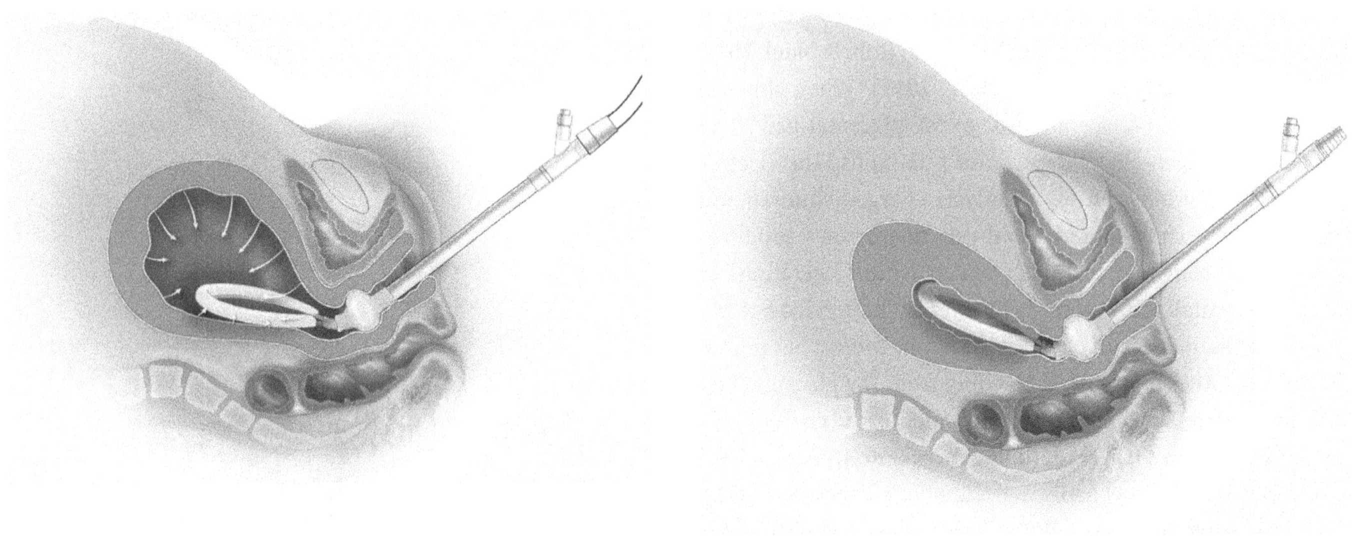

Figure 7-18. Vacuum-induced uterine tamponade. The Jada System with low-level vacuum connected creates a vacuum within the uterus, causing the uterus to collapse onto itself and the inner uterine walls to compress the bleeding vessels. In a clinical study, collapse of the uterus occurred within minutes, and control of bleeding and uterine contraction followed soon thereafter. Images courtesy of Alydia Health.

- Oxytocin infusion can be continued for 6–12 hr to prevent uterine atony (Fox, 2023). Additional uterotonics can be used if necessary.
- Blood products are administered as indicated.
- If the drain port becomes occluded with clots, periodically flush it with sterile NS.
- The balloon should be removed only in a hospital by an obstetrician capable of surgical intervention if bleeding continues. Balloons and gauze packs typically stay in place 2–12 hr if bleeding has decreased or for up to 24 hr if the client remains unstable (Fox, 2023). Vaginal gauze packing is sometimes easier to remove if it is first moistened with NS.

Vacuum-Induced Uterine Tamponade

The intrauterine vacuum-induced hemorrhage control device (Jada® System) is a silicone loop that connects to a vacuum source. When the loop is placed inside a hemorrhaging atonic uterus after birth and attached to suction, 20 vacuum pores facilitate creation of vacuum within the uterine cavity (D'Alton, Rood, Smid, et al., 2020). Pooled blood is sucked from the uterus and the uterine cavity collapses, simulating a contraction that tamponades the placental site and controls the hemorrhage, usually within 3–5 min (D'Alton, Rood, Smid, et al., 2020). Continued application of low-level vacuum maintains hemostasis while physiologic or medication-induced uterine contractions occlude vessels and facilitate sustained control of bleeding (Segnitz & Arulkumaran, 2017). In contrast with methods that expand the uterine cavity and use outward pressure to control bleeding, the intrauterine vacuum-induced hemorrhage control device works to facilitate the normal contraction of the uterus. This novel device is 94% effective in controlling postpartum hemorrhage due to atony (D'Alton, Rood, Smid, et al., 2020), superior to the 87% effectiveness reported for balloon tamponade devices (Suarez et al., 2020).

The Jada® System should not be used with uterine rupture, unresolved uterine inversion, current cervical cancer, known uterine anomaly, or current infection of the vagina, cervix, or uterus (D'Alton, Rood, Simhan, & Goffman, 2021). The cervix must be dilated at least 3 cm for safe placement (D'Alton, Rood, Simhan, et al., 2021). It has not been evaluated for use in mothers who give birth before 34 gestational weeks (D'Alton, Rood, Simhan, et al., 2021).

Using the Intrauterine Vacuum-Induced Hemorrhage Control Device

1. Perform a manual sweep of the uterine cavity to remove retained products and clots and to rule out uterine rupture.
2. Introduce the device through the cervix into the uterine cavity manually or with ring forceps. Place the uterine loop inside the uterine cavity so that the donut-shaped cervical seal lies just outside the external os in the proximal vagina.
3. Fill the cervical seal with sterile fluid (60–120 ml) to limit vacuum application to the uterus only.
4. Apply low-level vacuum (70–90 mm Hg) using an appropriate vacuum system (not a portable unit). The uterus will collapse in 1–2 min from the time of vacuum connection, and bleeding should stop within 3–5 min (D'Alton, Rood, Smid, et al., 2020).
5. The intrauterine vacuum-induced hemorrhage control device remains in the uterus with the vacuum applied for at least 1 hr after control of hemorrhage to give uterine

contractions time to further collapse the uterine cavity and occlude vessels.

6. Evaluate effectiveness by watching for blood flow through the system and palpating for a firm uterine fundus. The device should be left in place for no more than 24 hr.
7. After the hemorrhage has been controlled for at least an hour, disconnect the vacuum and deflate the cervical seal. Leave the device in place for at least 30 min more and watch for atony or continued bleeding.
8. Support the fundus with one hand on the abdomen and gently withdraw the device from the uterus through the vagina.

The vacuum device has a reassuring safety profile, can be placed quickly and easily, and can stop bleeding in minutes while encouraging the uterus to regain tone. A major drawback of the device is the necessity of access to a suction unit with a constant, regulated vacuum. Alydia® is currently exploring alternatives to a regulated vacuum source to facilitate use in community settings and in places with limited resources (R. Lange, personal communication, January 4, 2021).

RECAPS Step 6: Surgical Treatment

Surgical Management and Embolization

Rarely, surgical intervention is needed to stop PPH. The surgeon enters the abdomen with either a subumbilical vertical incision or a Pfannenstiel incision; removes any free blood; and examines the pelvic organs for laceration, rupture, or hematoma. In the case of uterine rupture, the surgeon must quickly decide whether to repair the defect or perform a hysterectomy. If atony is the cause of the hemorrhage, a tourniquet can be used to mechanically occlude the uterine blood supply as a temporizing measure. The surgeon can wrap a Penrose drain or urinary catheter around the lower uterine segment, cross the ends, and pull them in opposite directions to restrict blood loss while blood products are infused (Belfort, 2023c).

Uterine compression sutures control atonic hemorrhage by squeezing the uterus between ligatures preventing it from relaxing and filling with blood. The B-Lynch technique compresses the uterine walls with single large suture to create an effect like that of bimanual compression (Gilmandyar & Thornburg, 2019). The technique involves opening the lower uterine segment, suturing through the posterior wall and over the fundus with absorbable suture, and then tying the suture anteriorly. The B-Lynch suture can effectively control bleeding from atony when other methods are unsuccessful. Other methods of surgical uterine compression have also been described. Uterine compression sutures are safe and preserve the potential for future reproduction (Belfort, 2023c). Compression sutures can also be used in conjunction with a uterine balloon tamponade in a technique known as the "uterine sandwich."

Ligation of uterine and utero-ovarian arteries can slow or stop uterine bleeding. It is less effective if bleeding results from uterine atony or PAS. It does not harm the uterus or seem to affect future fertility (Belfort, 2023c).

Arterial embolization is an option at some facilities for hemodynamically stable clients. A catheter is inserted into a femoral artery, and internal iliac arteriography is performed. An occlusive thrombotic agent administered through the catheter occludes the arteries responsible for the hemorrhage. Arterial embolization can be useful when the client wishes to have more children and surgical options have been exhausted. Arterial embolization is also used to manage large postpartum hematomas.

Hysterectomy should be performed without delay when postpartum hemorrhage fails to respond to any other therapy. Clients who hemorrhage from complications of placenta previa or placenta accreta syndrome are more likely to require hysterectomy to control the bleeding (Huque et al., 2018). Other risk factors for hysterectomy are advanced maternal age and prior cesarean section.

AFFLICT: Etiologies of PPH: Flesh & Fragments

Retained Clots and Tissue

An empty uterus can usually control its own bleeding by remaining contracted. Retained blood clots, placenta, membranes, and other detritus can disrupt the uterine contractions necessary to constrict placental-bed vessels (Baskett, 2012; Kodkany et al., 2012; Koh, Di Filippo, Bisits, & Welsh, 2020). Likewise, uterine fibroids can contribute to postpartum hemorrhage by preventing uterine involution, therefore prolonging bleeding from the placental bed (Groom & Jacobson, 2012). Bimanual clot evacuation involves holding the fundus of the uterus with one hand on the abdomen while performing a vaginal examination to digitally break down and expel any blood clots (Koh et al., 2020). This procedure can improve the contraction of the uterus and reduce need for surgical intervention in the management of severe postpartum hemorrhage (Koh et al., 2020).

As a standard part of initial postpartum assessment, carefully examine the placenta for completeness of tissue and membranes. Cup the placenta in your hands and view the maternal side to ensure the presence of all cotyledons. Piece together any torn fragments. Rough areas of the placenta or discontinuous vessels can indicate that part of the placenta is retained. Assess the membranes carefully to ensure that

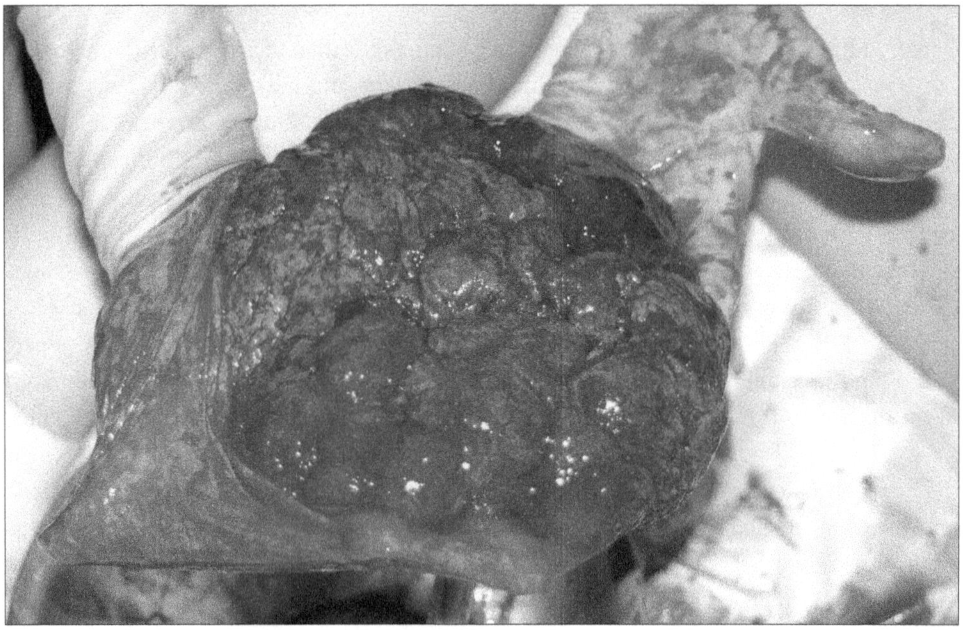

Figure 7-19. Intact placenta. When an intact placenta is slightly cupped in the midwife's hands, the spaces between the cotyledons close and the surface appears smooth.

both layers (amnion and chorion) are complete. The chorion (tougher outer membrane) is somewhat hazy and opaque, containing the fragments of old blood vessels. The amnion is thin and translucent. Place a hand into the opening of the membrane, then spread your fingers to assess the size of the cavity within and whether the membranes are intact or shredded.

If a client continues to hemorrhage after bimanual compression, massage, and uterotonics, give analgesia and manually explore the uterus to remove clots, membrane, and placental fragments. Consider wrapping moist gauze around one hand, then carefully inserting it into the uterus to remove retained placental tissue by gently sweeping the inner wall of the uterus. Persistently adherent placental fragments can require curettage by a physician in the operating room.

Retained Placenta

Retained placenta is generally defined as failure of the placenta to deliver within 30 min (Evensen et al., 2017; Weeks, 2023). The average length of third stage labor appears to be 5–6 min, and 90% of placentas are delivered within 15 min (Funai & Norwitz, 2023b). When active management of third stage labor (AMTSL) is used, 98% of placentas are expelled within 30 min (Weeks, 2023). Preterm births (PTBs) tend to have a longer third stage than term births (Funai & Norwitz, 2023b). Retained placenta is associated with about 10% of maternal deaths worldwide, most of them in low-resource countries (Nayak, 2020). When a mother has had a retained placenta, the risk of reoccurrence in a future pregnancy is about 6–12% (Weeks, 2023).

Mechanism of Third Stage Labor

During the third stage of labor, the body must detach and expel the placenta while staunching the flow of blood to the placental bed (Weeks & Fawcus, 2020). Detachment occurs in a four-step sequence (Weeks & Fawcus, 2020):

First (latent) phase: The myometrium contracts and thickens after the birth of the baby, but the area beneath the placenta remains thin and uncontracted. The length of this stage generally determines the length of third stage labor.

Second (contraction) phase: A sustained contraction causes the muscle fibers behind the placenta to become shorter and thicker, encouraging the relatively inflexible placenta to shear along the cleavage plane where it meets the uterus. A hematoma forms behind the placenta, accelerating the process of release.

Third (detachment) phase: The placenta releases in a wave of separation that progresses from the lower uterine segment to the fundus (Funai & Norwitz, 2023b).

Fourth (expulsion) phase: Spontaneous uterine contractions, downward pressure from the developing retroplacental hematoma, and an increase in maternal intraabdominal pressure expel the placenta (Funai & Norwitz, 2023b).

Placental retention occurs when one or more of these steps are abnormal or fail to occur. There are three mechanisms for retained placenta:

- *Placenta adherens:* The placenta remains attached due to inadequate uterine contraction and lack of shearing force. It easily separates on manual removal.
- *Trapped or incarcerated placenta:* The placenta separates but is held in the uterus by abnormal uterine contraction. The signs of placental separation might be present (cord lengthens, uterus rises and hardens, and there is a gush of blood), and the edge of the placenta might be palpable through a constricted cervix (Weeks, 2023).
- *Placenta accreta spectrum (PAS):* A decidual defect has allowed the placenta to pathologically invade the myometrium. It cannot cleanly separate.

Encouraging Placental Delivery

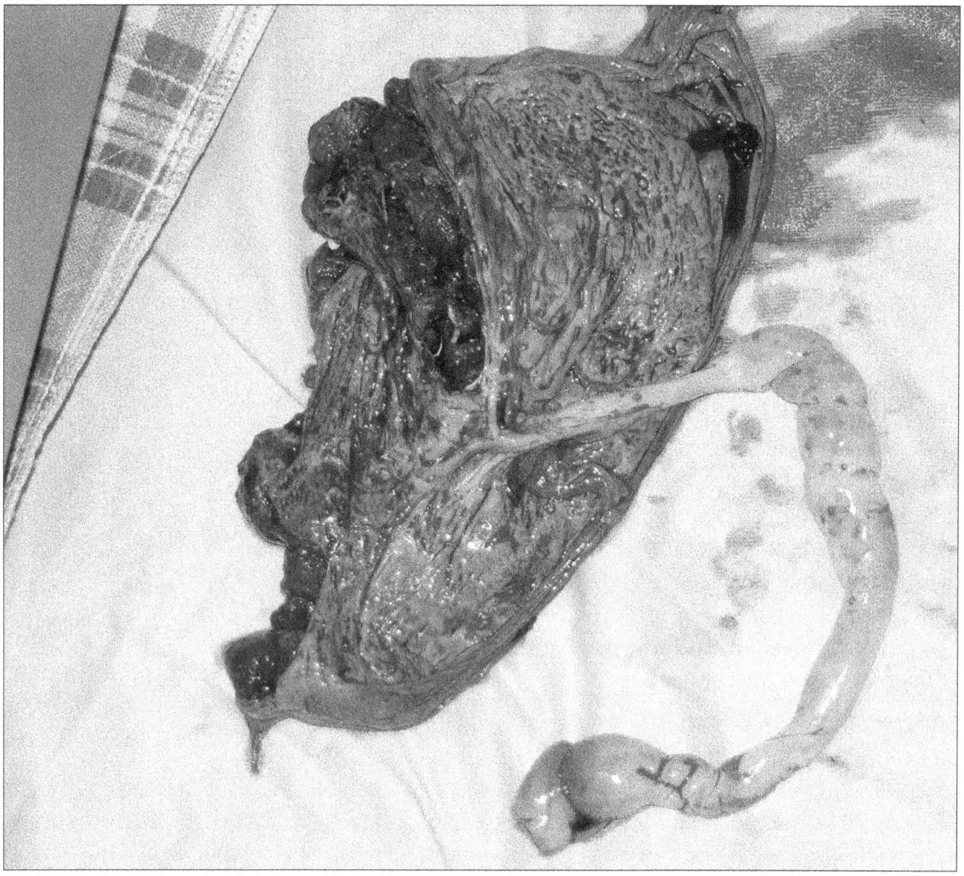

Figure 7-20. Nonintact placenta. Rough edges and obvious disruptions indicate that this placenta is not intact. The midwife undertook manual removal and was unable to extract the placenta in one piece. When pieces of the placenta remain in the uterus, the mother is at high risk for severe hemorrhage.

It is not always possible to identify the mechanism of retained placenta by clinical assessment, even in a hospital. The treatment that would be appropriate for placenta adherens (uterotonics) can worsen an incarcerated placenta by constricting the cervix (Akol & Weeks, 2016; Weeks, 2023). The appropriate treatment for a trapped placenta (uterine relaxants) could result in hemorrhage with placenta adherens (Akol & Weeks, 2016). Generally, retained placentas must be removed manually or surgically.

Controlled Cord Traction

Controlled cord traction is a technique that involves applying steady traction on the cord together with stabilization or counter-traction of the contracted uterus (Hofmeyr, Mshweshwe, & Gülmezoglu, 2015). Controlled cord traction can encourage the expulsion of a trapped placenta and promote the separation of placenta adherens (Du, Ye, & Zheng, 2014; Weeks, 2023). The benefits of routine controlled cord traction are small but significant; it slightly decreases the need for manual removal of the placenta, reduces mean blood loss (by only about 10 ml), shortens third stage (by 3 min), and decreases the risk of mild PPH—from 12.7% to 11.8% (Du et al., 2014; Funai & Norwitz, 2023b; Gülmezoglu et al., 2012; Hofmeyr et al., 2015; Rouse, 2013; Weeks & Fawcus, 2020). Controlled cord traction does not appear to reduce the risk of moderate or severe PPH (Weeks & Fawcus, 2020).

The provider can weigh these benefits against the potential for discomfort or disruption of physiologic third stage and bonding and decide on the most appropriate course. Traction on a weak cord insertion can cause the cord to avulse, particularly in the case of velamentous insertion. When the cord avulses while the placenta is in the uterus, the placenta often comes out spontaneously if the mother assumes an upright position and pushes.

To perform controlled cord traction using the Brandt Andrews method:

- Watch for signs of detachment.
- Grasp the cord in one hand (hold the clamp, hold the cord with a gauze square, or wrap the cord around your fingers).
- Place your opposite hand on the lower abdomen just above the client's pubic bone.
- Keep gentle tension on the cord and wait for a uterine contraction.
- Ask the client to push with the contraction.
- Maintain tension on the cord or apply *careful* traction at a downward angle in line with the pelvic curve. At the same time, press the edge of your hand into the abdomen and angle it toward the umbilicus with moderate pressure. Your two hands will move away from each other as you execute this maneuver. Traction should be as gentle as possible but as firm as necessary. Caution! Excessive traction will avulse the cord, possibly necessitating manual removal.
- The mother's pushing is the primary force that expels the placenta. Cord traction assists her efforts.

Table 7-5
Risk Factors for Retained Placenta

Risk factors due to poor uterine contraction
High parity
Prolonged use of oxytocin
Intrauterine infection
Risk factors due to abnormal placentation
Prior uterine surgery (cesarean section, myomectomy, dilation and curettage)
In vitro fertilization
Previous PAS
Uterine fibroids
Adenomyosis
Other risk factors
Preterm birth (PTB)
Congenital uterine abnormality
History of retained placenta
Stillbirth
Use of ergot alkaloids with the placenta *in utero*
Small for gestational age infant

Adapted from (1) "Underlying Mechanisms of Retained Placenta: Evidence from a Population Based Cohort Study," by S. Greenbaum, T. Wainstock, D. Dukler, E. Leron, and E. Erez, 2017, *European Journal of Obstetrics & Gynecology and Reproductive Biology, 216*, 12–17. Copyright by Elsevier B.V. (2) "Retained Placenta After Vaginal Delivery: Risk Factors and Management," by N. C. Perlman and D. A. Carusi, 2019, *International Journal of Women's Health*, 527–534. CC BY-NC 3.0.

- When the placenta descends, you will see the cord lengthen and the placenta appear at the introitus. If it is not yet ready, you will feel resistance. In that case, wait until the uterus contacts again and repeat the maneuver.

Windmill Technique

The windmill technique is a variation of controlled cord traction in which traction is applied laterally in a circular fashion, moving slowly like the hands of a clock. The provider gently applies tension to the cord laterally, perpendicular to the birth canal, and slowly moves the cord in a circle with the vagina at its center (Nayak, 2020). At some point in the circle, traction aligns with the unreleased part of the placenta and helps detach it from the uterus. Use of the windmill technique encourages spontaneous placental expulsion and lessens the need for manual removal, surgical curettage, anesthesia, or antibiotics (Nayak, 2020).

One study tested the windmill technique when placentas were retained for more than 30 min after term vaginal birth (Hinkson, Suermann, Hinkson, & Henrich, 2017).

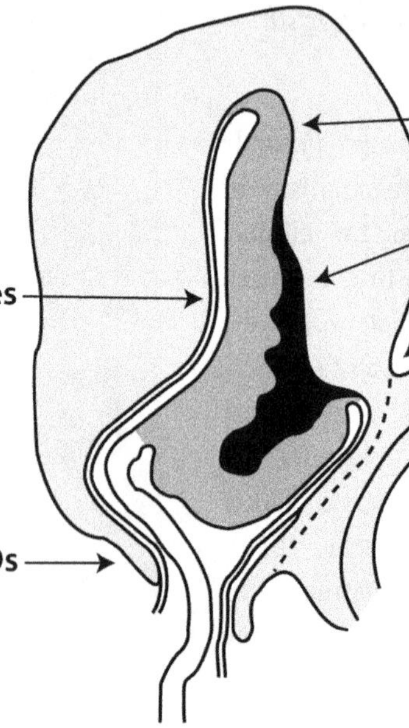

Figure 7-21. The uppermost part of the placenta is usually the last to release. Adapted from *A Handbook of Midwifery* (p. 123), by W. R. Dakin, 1897, London, United Kingdom: Longmans, Green, & Co. In the public domain.

After traditional interventions had failed (oxytocin infusion, bladder emptying, controlled cord traction, acupuncture, homeopathy, breastfeeding), clients were offered the windmill technique as an alternative to manual removal of the placenta. It was successful 86% of the time (Hinkson et al., 2017).

To perform the windmill technique, grasp the cord and *slowly* rotate the cord through 360°, mimicking the blade of a windmill. With your other hand, provide counter-traction on the uterus through the abdomen. If the cord lengthens, the placenta has released. On average, it takes about 7 min (range 4–15 min) for the windmill technique to release the placenta. Stop the procedure if the cord does not lengthen, if there is abnormal bleeding, or if the cord begins to tear.

Umbilical Cord Drainage

When cord clamping is delayed, placental drainage has no clinical benefit and does not decrease the incidence of postpartum hemorrhage or retained placenta (Funai & Norwitz, 2023b). When cord clamping is immediate, there is some evidence that allowing the umbilical cord to drain shortens the third stage of labor by about 2.28 min (Wu, Chen, Wang, & Wang, 2017). To use this technique, remove the clamp from the maternal end of the cord after the infant's cord clamp has been placed and the umbilical cord has been severed. Drain the blood remaining in the placenta. The blood obtained from the placenta is fetal in origin and is not part of maternal blood loss calculations.

Umbilical Vein Injection (UVI)

There has been much debate about the effectiveness of NS and uterotonic medications injected or infused into the umbilical vein to treat retained placenta due to placenta adherens. The concept is to administer a uterotonic drug directly to the retroplacental myometrium to stimulate effective contractions that can release the placenta (N. Kumar, Shayesteh, Haas, & Weeks, 2021). Whereas some research has suggested that intraumbilical oxytocin is modestly effective in reducing blood loss at birth (Baig, Shahzad, Khurshid, & Malik, 2015) and in managing retained placenta (Shompa, Akhter, Nazneen, & Begum, 2014), other studies have concluded that oxytocin or saline administered via umbilical vein injection is probably ineffective (Weeks, 2023).

A Cochrane review (N. Kumar et al., 2021) evaluated 24 random controlled trials involving 2,348 mothers receiving UVI and concluded that there may be a small benefit to UVI of oxytocin, but as many as 18 mothers would need to be treated to prevent one retained placenta (N. Kumar et al., 2021). The authors noted, however, that no harmful effects are associated with its administration, it is inexpensive, and it can be given while awaiting placental delivery (N. Kumar et al., 2021). They also suggest that it may slightly reduce the incidence of retained placenta if undertaken within 15–30 min after the birth of the infant. This benefit, albeit small, could be important outside a hospital or in resource-limited areas. The use of oxytocin via UVI solution does not affect the length of third stage labor, postpartum blood loss, or incidence of infection (N. Kumar et al., 2021). Carbetocin is similarly effective (Elfayomy, 2015; Salem, Saraya, Badr, & Soliman, 2019). UVI is unlikely to have any effect in clients with retained placenta due to PAS, but it may cause cervical contraction in the client with a trapped placenta, worsening the problem and making spontaneous birth less likely (N. Kumar et al., 2021).

Prostaglandin solutions appear more effective than oxytocin in releasing placenta adherens (N. Kumar et al., 2021). Misoprostol infused into the umbilical vein appears to reduce the duration of the third stage of labor and total blood loss (Najafian, Ghasemi, & Hajiha-Esfahani, 2018; Nazeer, Rehman, Tahir, Saeed, & Gul, 2016; Patra et al., 2017; Rajab & Alalaf, 2014). More research is needed.

A variety of solutions have been used (N. Kumar et al., 2021), including

- Oxytocin 10–30 IU (or more) in 10–30 ml NS;
- Misoprostol 800 mcg in 20–30 ml NS; and
- Carbetocin 100 mcg in 20–40 ml NS.

The umbilical vein is the preferred route because it is wider and more distensible than either artery and because injection into the artery can induce vasoconstriction (Lashin, 2020).

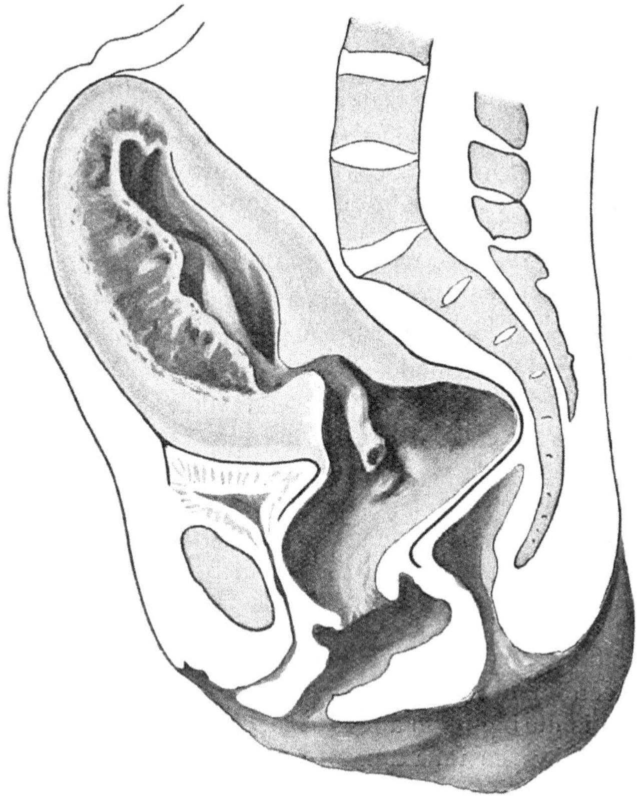

Figure 7-22. An incarcerated placenta is trapped by abnormal uterine contraction that prevents expulsion. In this illustration the contraction occurred well above the cervical os. From *The Practice of Midwifery* (7th ed., p. 976), by A. L. Galabin and G. Blacker, 1910, New York, NY: Macmillan. In the public domain.

Insert the needle of a sterile 20-ml syringe into the vein and inject a solution of diluted medication (N. Kumar et al., 2021). After injection, milk the cord upward to push the solution into the placenta (Lashin, 2020).

The Pipingas technique involves threading a catheter into the umbilical vein, then injecting the medication in at least 30 ml of saline (N. Kumar et al., 2021). A size 10 pediatric nasogastric tube can be used (Alalaf et al., 2020). After the cord is double-clamped and cut, access the part hanging out of the vagina. Recut between the clamp and the vagina and advance the catheter into the umbilical vein. When you feel resistance, retract the catheter slightly to ensure that the injected fluid is distributed equally to all the vascular branches, then inject the solution (Alalaf et al., 2020).

Indications for Intervention

Retained Placenta Without Hemorrhage

In a community setting, when the client is not bleeding and the placenta shows no signs of detachment, at some point it becomes necessary to transport the client to a higher level of

Table 7-6

Manual Removal of Placenta and Uterine Exploration

- Prepare for hemorrhage. Start IV access and prepare an infusion of NS or LR with Pitocin® simultaneously with other steps.
- Offer pain medication, if available, before uterine exploration. Removal of retained tissue can be difficult and painful.
- Don a gown and sterile gloves. For this procedure, you can have your arm inserted into the mother's body nearly up to the elbow.
- Press your fingertips together (as if donning a bracelet) and insert your entire dominant hand into the vagina. Your nondominant hand or the hand of an assistant holds the fundus through the abdominal wall.
- Pass your hand through the cervix and explore the wall of the uterus with your fingertips. It will feel rough, like corrugated cardboard. On the fetal surface of the placenta, you will feel membranes, vessels, and the umbilical cord attachment. Following the cord will lead you to the placenta.
- Find the cleavage plane where the placenta joins the uterine wall and work your fingers into the space, using them like a spatula, with the same pressure you would use to separate the edible part of a tangerine from the rind.
- Your goal is to quickly detach the entire placenta and bring it out in one piece. After the placenta is detached, collect it into the palm of your hand and gently ease it out. Ideally, placenta, cord, and membranes will come out in one mass, and it will be obvious that it is intact. When the uterus is empty, it should contract firmly, and bleeding should stop. Give oxytocin to encourage hemostasis.
- If the placenta fragments and comes out in pieces, wrap moistened gauze around your fingertips, enter the uterus again, and gently scrape the uterus to retrieve stray bits of tissue.
- If you cannot find the cleavage plane or if the placenta does not come away neatly, it is possible that the placenta is invasive (attached to muscle instead of the uterine lining). STOP IMMEDIATELY and perform bimanual compression instead. Further attempts at removal can result in intractable hemorrhage (McCall et al., 2022).

care. When the placenta is undelivered after 20–30 min, a hemorrhage is more likely, and this risk increases with the passing of time (Weeks, 2023). Manual removal of the placenta may resolve the problem but carries the risk of severe hemorrhage that may be difficult to manage in a community setting. The timing of transport is determined by considerations such as local guidelines, maternal risk factors, distance to the hospital, the availability of first responders, the providers and equipment on hand, and shared decision-making with the family. Many providers will initiate a transfer if the placenta is undelivered at 30 min, particularly when the hospital is distant or when the midwife does not have IV access or medications.

Retained Placenta With Hemorrhage (Third Stage Hemorrhage)

Third stage hemorrhage is excessive bleeding after the birth of the infant with the placenta *in utero*. If you notice abnormal bleeding while the cord is still attached to the baby, first check for cord rupture. Sometimes the blood from a torn cord will spray and splatter in a manner unlike the steady flow of maternal bleeding. When the cord is torn or broken, the blood you see is coming directly from the infant's circulation, and quick recognition is key to a good neonatal outcome. Immediately clamp the cord between the damaged area and the infant, cut the cord between the clamp and the damaged area, then evaluate the newborn for signs of hypovolemia.

Next, check for placental detachment by performing controlled cord traction using the Brandt-Andrews maneuver. Take care not to cause uterine inversion by using excessive traction. If the placenta does not come easily and the client is bleeding significantly, move to manual removal (see Table 7-6). The Commission for the Accreditation of Birth Centers (CABC) permits manual removal of the placenta or uterine exploration in the birth center *only* in cases of uncontrollable postpartum hemorrhage when the mother cannot be stabilized for transport (CABC, 2023).

After exploration and evacuation of the uterus, continue massage and uterotonics. Often bleeding can be controlled by removal of clots and placental fragments, but in some cases surgical management is necessary. After manual uterine exploration, IV broad-spectrum antibiotics are commonly administered to reduce the risk of endometritis (Weeks, 2023).

Placenta Accreta Spectrum (PAS, Invasive Placenta)

PAS is a rare condition in which the placenta invades beyond the normal cleavage plane and grows into or through the uterine myometrium. It is most likely to develop when the placenta grows over decidua that is thin, poorly formed, or absent. PAS carries a significant risk of intractable hemorrhage, hysterectomy, coagulopathy, multisystem organ failure, and even death. The potential for hemorrhage correlates with the amount of placental invasion into the myometrium, the size of the area affected, and whether the placenta has invaded into extrauterine tissues such as the bladder (Silver & Branch, 2018). Surgery that disturbs the decidua or abnormal uterine anatomy seems to predispose to placental invasion. About 80% of cases of adherent placenta are associated with a history of cesarean birth, curettage, or myomectomy (Silver, 2023).

Types of PAS include (Silver, 2023)

- Placenta accreta (63%): chorionic villi of the placenta attach to myometrium in the absence of the decidual layer.
- Placenta increta (15%): chorionic villi penetrate deeply into the myometrium reaching the external layer.
- Placenta percreta (22%): chorionic villi penetrate through the uterine serosa, sometimes growing into adjacent organs, such as the bladder or bowel.

Of clients with retained placenta, only one in 440 has complete placenta accreta (Weeks, 2023); it is more common to have small invasive areas on an otherwise normal placenta. Previous cesarean is the strongest risk factor for PAS; more than 90% of clients with PAS have a history of cesarean birth (Pandey, Neogi, Gautam, & Raushan, 2023). Though it is still a relatively rare condition, the incidence of PAS has increased with the rising rate of cesarean section. In 1950, the rate of PAS was 1 in 30,000 (Silver, 2023). Between 2008 and 2011, the rate increased to 1 in 731 births in the United States; in a similar period, it rose to 1 in 695 births in Canada (Silver, 2023). Up to 80% of accretas are associated with placenta previa (ACOG et al., 2018/2021). Clients with placenta previa who have had two or more cesarean births have up to 11% risk of developing PAS; with five or more cesareans, risk increases to 61% (Silver et al., 2006). In the absence of placenta previa, the rate of PAS is 0.2% for mothers having a second cesarean birth and a rate of nearly 5% for mothers having six or more cesarean births (Perlman & Carusi, 2019). The risk for PAS is also higher when a client has had a procedure that causes damage to the endometrium, such as curettage, manual removal of the placenta, hysteroscopic removal of intrauterine adhesions, uterine-artery embolization, endometrial ablation, or myomectomy entering the uterine cavity (Silver, 2023). Additional risk factors are advanced maternal age, high parity, *in vitro* fertilization, a diagnosis of PAS in a previous pregnancy, and, possibly, multiple gestations (Silver, 2023).

Placenta accreta can be discovered on ultrasound examination when the normal hypoechoic area behind the placenta is irregular or absent, the myometrium behind the placenta is abnormally thin, or the bladder wall appears abnormal (Rac et al., 2015). Although placental lakes (enlarged intervillous spaces filled with turbulent venous blood) are usually a normal finding on ultrasound, the presence of multiple venous lakes close to an abnormal myometrium is suspicious for PAS (Bowman & Kennedy, 2014). The absence of ultrasound findings does not rule out PAS (ACOG et al., 2018/2021). Magnetic-resonance imaging (MRI) is unable to reliably predict the depth of invasion or type of PAS (ACOG et al., 2018/2021)

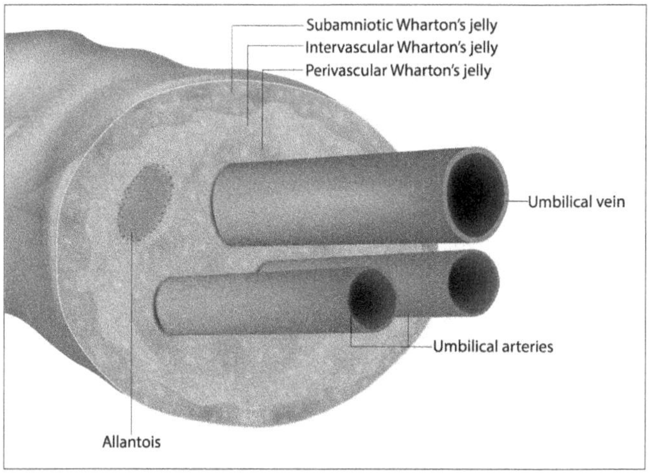

Figure 7-23. Cross-section of a human umbilical cord (©sakurra/Adobe Stock).

Always consider the possibility of undiagnosed PAS when attempting manual removal of a placenta. An invasive placenta is firmly attached to the uterine wall, and you will be unable to develop a line of separation if you try to remove it. *Stop immediately* if all or part of the placenta does not readily detach, if you are unable to find a cleavage plane, or if something feels abnormal about the placental attachment. The first clinical manifestation of PAS can be massive, life-threatening hemorrhage that occurs when the provider attempts manual removal of the placenta (ACOG et al., 2018/2021). Withdraw your hand from the uterus and arrange for emergency transport. This client is at high risk for uncontrollable bleeding and can require a hysterectomy (ACOG et al., 2018/2021).

In general, if a client is known to have PAS, cesarean birth or cesarean hysterectomy is recommended at 34 0/7–35 6/7 weeks of gestation if the client is stable (ACOG et al., 2018/2021). Roughly 50% of clients with PAS beyond 36 weeks of gestation require emergent cesarean for hemorrhage (ACOG et al., 2018/2021). For the client with antepartally diagnosed PAS, ACOG recommends planned birth at a tertiary-care center with continuously available, experienced medical staff including critical care subspecialists, hematologists, and cardiologists, and neonatologists (ACOG et al., 2018/2021). Access to a blood bank with protocols in place for massive transfusion is crucial to management.

When only a small part of the placenta is adherent, conservative or expectant management may be considered. Uterine preservation management involves removal of placenta or uteroplacental tissue without removal of the uterus (ACOG et al., 2018/2021). In some cases, mothers with a small area of invasive placenta can be treated by removing a small wedge of

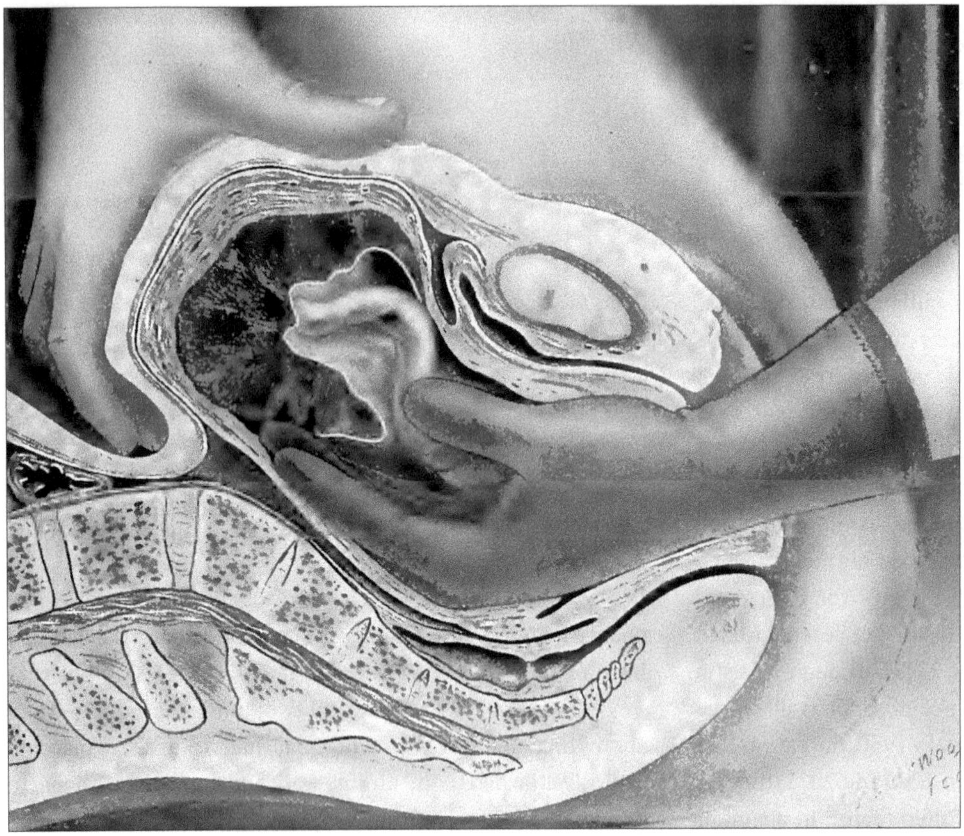

Figure 7-24. Manual removal of the placenta should be attempted in a community setting only if the client is bleeding excessively with the placenta undelivered and there is no suspicion of placenta accreta. From *Obstetrics: A Text-Book for the Use of Students and Practitioners* (3rd ed., p. 487), by J. W. Williams, 1912, New York, NY: D. Appleton. In the public domain.

uterine tissue containing the region of adherent placenta during cesarean birth (ACOG et al., 2018/2021; Silver, 2023). Expectant management involves leaving the placenta either partially or totally *in situ* (ACOG et al., 2018/2021). Over time, the placenta is resorbed by the body, but the risk of hemorrhage and sepsis remain high. Expectant management is only likely to be successful if the region of placental invasion is small and shallow.

AFFLICT: Etiologies of PPH: Laceration/Injury

Trauma

When bleeding persists despite a well-contracted uterus, consider perineal, vaginal, or cervical trauma. Common sites for lacerations include the perineum, the vaginal floor behind the perineum (where the fetal chin was situated during crowning), the labia (particularly at the level where the fetal ears emerged), vaginal sidewalls, the vaginal sulcus (groove between the vaginal sidewall and the vaginal floor), the periurethral region, and the periclitoral region. Less common sites include 3rd- and 4th-degree perineal lacerations (involving the anal sphincter and rectal mucosa, respectively) and cervical lacerations. Some clients sustain several of these lacerations simultaneously, potentially causing a multiple-site traumatic hemorrhage. A large vulvar, vaginal, or pelvic hematoma is a concealed hemorrhage that can produce severe pain and signs of shock without any visible bleeding. Uterine inversion is a rare but life-threatening traumatic event in which the uterus turns itself inside out and presents its inner surface through the cervix or even out of the vagina.

Half of a vaginal speculum, held by an assistant, is a serviceable retractor for visualizing vaginal lacerations.

Lacerations

Most lacerations sustained in childbirth involve the perineum, labia, periurethral or periclitoral regions, vaginal sulcus, or vaginal sidewalls. A first-degree laceration involves only the mucosa or skin; a second-degree laceration affects the underlying muscle. Bleeding from lacerations is bright red in color and continues despite a well-contracted uterus. It may be apparent immediately after the baby is born. Bleeding from a vaginal sidewall or sulcus laceration may be evident as red bleeding while the baby is descending in second stage or after the birth when the fetus is no longer tamponading the wound. If a laceration is bleeding, immediately press gauze against it and hold pressure until you are ready to repair it. Do not peek to see whether the bleeding has stopped. If the gauze becomes saturated, add more gauze on top. Sprinkling chitosan granules on the wound before applying gauze or applying chitosan-coated gauze can expedite hemostasis (Carles et al., 2017). Complex vaginal lacerations sometimes stop bleeding entirely when dusted with chitosan hemostatic powder and compressed with gauze for 5 min (Carles et al., 2016).

Assemble everything you will require for wound repair (lighting, local anesthetic, sutures, instruments, gauze, etc.) and then remove the pressure dressing to inspect the wound.

When blood is flowing briskly, it can be difficult to localize the injury. To perform a complete examination for obstetrical injury in a community setting, position the client at the edge of the bed with the legs supported for maximal visualization. Ensure adequate lighting and offer analgesia if available. Inspect the genital tract from cervix to perineum and, if necessary, palpate the uterine cavity for defects indicating uterine rupture. Inspect the labial, clitoral and periurethral areas carefully—a laceration in these places can temporarily close when the client's posture changes, then reopen and bleed persistently. Use a retractor to visualize the cervix and anterior and posterior fornix. When a retractor is unavailable, insert half of a vaginal speculum and have an assistant provide gentle traction to expose the tissues.

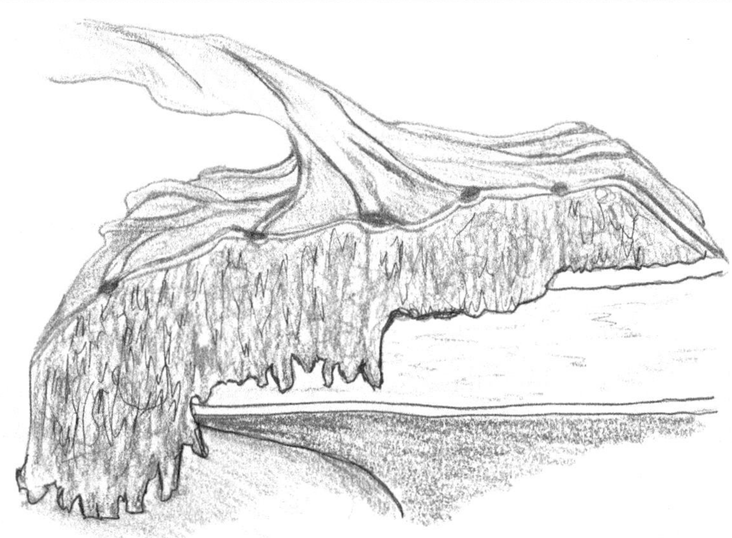

Figure 7-25. An invasive placenta grows beyond the physiologic endometrial cleavage plane into the uterine muscle (accreta, increta) or through the myometrium and uterine serosa and sometimes into adjacent organs such as the bladder (percreta). Illustration after "Placenta Accreta Spectrum," by R. M. Silver and D. W. Branch, 2018, *New England Journal of Medicine, 378*(16), p.1530. Copyright 2020 by Massachusetts Medical Society.

After inspecting the vagina, perform a rectal examination to identify any laceration to the rectal mucosa and anal sphincter. Palpate the sphincter between thumb and forefinger. Shearing forces produced by descent of the fetal head can separate the sphincter of a mother with an otherwise intact perineum (Toglia, 2022). Look carefully for deep lacerations that create a fourth-degree "buttonhole" by extending into the rectum. Rarely, buttonhole lacerations can occur in the presence of an intact perineum and rectal sphincter when a laceration of the vaginal floor extends into the rectum (Roper, Thakar, & Sultan, 2021).

Bleeding from lacerated tissues can usually be controlled by suturing using a running locked stitch or figure-eight sutures placed just proximal to the apex. Large or deep lacerations often require more than one layer for closure. TXA infusion can slow the flow of blood from obstetrical wounds as effectively as it controls hemorrhage in cases of uterine atony (Mielke & Obermeyer, 2020). Active bleeding from a long vaginal sidewall laceration usually involves an artery that has retracted under the vaginal wall (Karoshi et al., 2012). Place a figure-eight suture proximal and lateral to the apex of the laceration and apply light traction to the suture. This technique can reduce bleeding by compressing the vessels while bringing the laceration into easier reach. Repair each layer of tissue and close any dead space. When the surface of the wound is closed but bleeding continues within the tissues, a hematoma can form. When placing deep sutures to gain control of a bleeding vaginal laceration, guard against accidental stitching of adjacent structures, such as the bladder anteriorly, small bowel and rectum posteriorly, and the ureters and uterine vessels deep in the lateral fornices of the vagina. Although sutures can usually control the bleeding of typical childbirth-related lacerations, a surgical suite with optimal anesthesia, lighting, and assistants to obtain adequate exposure may be necessary for the repair of deep, complicated, or nonhemostatic vaginal lacerations (Laufer & Makai, 2023).

If you are unable to stop bleeding by suturing, insert a Foley-type catheter into the bladder and pack gauze into the wound. Consider applying chitosan powder before applying gauze and/or using chitosan-coated gauze. Hold firm pressure on the wound. If the dressing soaks through, add more gauze on top of it, do not replace it. If suturing is not an option or is ineffective and the client is hemorrhaging from a laceration, balloon tamponade can be used to apply pressure to a wound during transport until surgical hemostasis can be achieved (Ghirardini, Alboni, & Mabrouk, 2012). With the mother's permission, a Rusch balloon (Srivastava, Bartlett, & Thakur, 2012), Bakri® uterine tamponade balloon (Yoong, Sivashanmugarajan, et al., 2014), Sengstaken-Blakemore tube (Yoong, Sivashanmugarajan, et al., 2014) or condom catheter (Georgiou, 2014; Makin, Suarez-Rebling, Varma Shivkumar, Tarimo,

Table 7-7
Classification of Perineal Lacerations

First degree: Injury to skin of perineum only
Second degree: Injury to perineal muscles but not to anal sphincter
Third degree: Injury to anal sphincter complex

- *3a*: Less than 50% of external anal sphincter thickness torn
- *3b*: More than 50% external anal sphincter thickness torn
- *3c*. Both external and internal anal sphincter torn

Fourth degree: Injury to anal sphincter complex (external and internal) and anal epithelium

Adapted from "Prevention and Management of Obstetric Lacerations at Vaginal Delivery" (Practice Bulletin 198), by American College of Obstetricians and Gynecologists, 2018/2022, *Obstetrics & Gynecology, 132*(3), e97–e102. Copyright by ACOG.

& Burke, 2018; Yoong, Ray, & Phillip, 2009) can be placed in the vagina to control postpartum hemorrhage due to vaginal lacerations. If a balloon device is unavailable and the client is still hemorrhaging, the provider can wrap a small BP cuff around a bag of 250 ml NS, place it in a sterile bag and insert it into the vagina (Cameron & Menticoglou, 2011). The cuff is then inflated to as much as 220 mm Hg (Cameron & Menticoglou, 2011). The tubes leading to the cuff are then sealed with umbilical cord clamps to maintain the pressure in the cuff. Another approach is to place the BP cuff in a sterile glove (Pinborg, Bødker, & Høgdall, 2000).

Third- and Fourth-Degree Perineal Lacerations

Perineal lacerations involving the anal sphincter complex are considered severe, because they increase the risk of pelvic floor injury, fecal and urinary incontinence, pain, and sexual dysfunction that can persist for many years after giving birth (Toglia, 2022). Third-degree lacerations extend through the fascia and musculature of the perineal body and external anal sphincter and can involve the internal anal sphincter. Fourth-degree lacerations involve both the anal sphincter complex and anal mucosa. Five years after giving birth, 17% of mothers with obstetric anal sphincter lacerations report some liquid stool incontinence compared with 8% of mothers without such injuries (Arnold, Sadler, & Leli, 2021). Risk factors include higher maternal age, nulliparity, higher birthweight, precipitous delivery, instrumented vaginal birth, occiput posterior fetal position, and midline (median) episiotomy (Landy et al., 2011). Unless you have expertise with repair of 3rd- and 4th-degree lacerations, refer clients with anal sphincter injury to an experienced gynecologic or general surgeon to minimize the risk of infection, wound breakdown, rectovaginal fistula formation, and fecal incontinence (Laufer & Makai, 2023).

PPH with Bradycardia

Think uterine inversion—uterine ligaments tug on the peritoneum and can trigger a parasympathetic response or neurogenic shock. (See "Neurogenic Shock" in Chapter 9.)

Cervical Lacerations

Clinically significant cervical lacerations occur in 0.2–1.7% of vaginal births (Jashnani & Wani, 2022). Risk factors include instrumental births (especially with use of forceps), manual dilation of the cervix, induction with oxytocin, and precipitate labor (Jashnani & Wani, 2022). Predisposing factors include cervical edema from prolonged labor (Jashnani & Wani, 2022) and use of cerclage. A deep cervical laceration can extend into the lower segment of the uterus (ruptured uterus) or through the ureters, necessitating open abdominal surgery for repair (Jashnani & Wani, 2022). A poorly healed deep cervical laceration can weaken the cervix and predispose to preterm birth in future pregnancies (Arulkumaran, Karoshi, Keith, Lalonde, & B-Lynch, 2012; Hamou, Sheiner, Coreanu, Walfisch, & Silberstein, 2020).

Suspect a cervical laceration when the uterus is well-contracted, the bleeding is bright red, uterine rupture has been ruled out, and there is an absence of bleeding lacerations in the lower genital tract. The injury may be felt upon digital exploration as a discontinuity of the cervical tissue. Cervical lacerations (Jashnani & Wani, 2022) can be unilateral (more common on the left side due to dextrorotation of the uterus) or stellate (star-shaped); they can also involve detachment of an anterior or posterior cervical lip or annular detachment (complete or partial separation of the cervix from the uterus).

Large cervical lacerations or those with intractable bleeding require repair by a physician or other skilled provider following hospital transport. In many cases, the repair is undertaken in the operating room under regional or general anesthesia for optimal visualization and client comfort. It can be extremely difficult to locate the site of bleeding when hemorrhage involves a laceration of the cervix or proximal vagina. Do not waste time. Vaginal packing with gauze or chitosan-coated gauze ribbons can be used as a temporizing strategy to limit blood loss during transport.

To examine the cervix, insert a speculum and grasp the anterior cervix with a ring forceps. Place a second ring forceps at the 2 o'clock position and systematically inspect the entire

Signs of Uterine Inversion

- Vaginal bleeding—mild or severe
- Lower abdominal pain—mild or severe
- A mass of tissue protruding through cervix or vagina
- Urinary retention
- Bradycardia
- Fundus nonpalpable
- Severe postpartum hemorrhage
- Shock out of proportion to blood loss

From "Puerperal Uterine Inversion," by G. Macones, 2023, in V. A. Barss (Ed.), *UpToDate*. Copyright by UpToDate.

cervix by placing one forceps ahead of the next, proceeding around the circumference. A retractor is sometimes necessary to expose the area in need of suturing. Suture small cervical lacerations only when they are actively bleeding.

Hematomas

Postpartum hematomas can develop in the vulva, vaginal/paravaginal area, and retroperitoneum, usually within 24 hr after birth (Roman, 2023). They are most common when episiotomy, vacuum extraction, or forceps have been used, but they can sometimes occur in a mother without a laceration, especially with first births, large babies, preeclampsia, prolonged second stage of labor, multiple gestation, vulvar varicosities, or clotting disorders (Roman, 2023). A vulvar hematoma is usually formed by venous bleeding from multiple sites. Sometimes the source is a vaginal hematoma that has protruded through soft tissue to distend the vulva (Roman, 2023). Broad-ligament hematomas can be palpated as masses adjacent to the uterus. Small vaginal and vulvar hematomas are usually managed conservatively with ice packs and analgesics until the body reabsorbs the contents.

The client with a large vaginal or vulvar hematoma usually complains of intense vulvar or rectal pain and pressure. A firm, painful purple mass may be observable, or the collection of blood may be undetectable deep within the tissues. Vital sign abnormalities can include tachycardia and hypotension out of proportion to visible blood loss. Clients are frequently pale and sweaty and can appear restless or anxious.

If the hematoma greatly expands or if the client shows signs of hypovolemia, surgical intervention may be necessary to achieve hemostasis. A hematoma that is expanding often requires drainage, packing, or embolization at a hospital (Belfort, 2023d). Ultrasound, computerized tomography (CT) scanning, and MRI can be used to assess for broad-ligament and retroperitoneal hematoma.

Four Degrees of Uterine Inversion

- **First degree (incomplete):** The inverted fundus reaches the cervical os but does not protrude through.
- **Second degree (incomplete):** The inverted fundus extends through the cervix but is contained by the vagina.
- **Third degree (complete):** The inverted fundus reaches the introitus and may protrude out of the body.
- **Fourth degree (total):** The vagina is also inverted, and the entire uterus is out of the body.

Ruptured Varicosity

Varicose veins affect about 15% of pregnancies and can involve the uterus, perineum, or vagina (Kikuchi et al., 2016). Although varicosities seldom break during birth, rupture of a large vaginal varix can result in a life-threatening hemorrhage which can be difficult to control. If you are unable to stop the hemorrhage by suturing the injury, apply moist gauze or hemostatic gauze, apply firm pressure, and transport immediately. In some cases, hemorrhage can reoccur if the gauze is removed even days later (V. Choudhary & Bellad, 2017).

Uterine Rupture

After vaginal birth, suspect that the uterus has ruptured if the client has pain and persistent uterine bleeding despite use of uterotonic agents (Belfort, 2023d). See Chapter 6 for a full discussion of uterine rupture. Blood can exit through the vagina or collect in great volumes within the abdominal cavity. The client sometimes shows abdominal distension and signs of shock out of proportion to observed blood loss. Hematuria can occur if the laceration involves the bladder. During digital uterine exploration, the provider can sometimes palpate the site of rupture with the fingertips (J. F. Smith & Wax, 2022). The client with uterine rupture requires immediate transport for surgical repair and life support measures.

Puerperal Uterine Inversion

Uterine inversion occurs when the uterus turns inside-out and protrudes through the cervical os, into the vagina, or beyond the vulva. The result is usually life-threatening hemorrhage and shock. Even in hospitals, one in six victims of uterine inversion dies if the problem is not corrected quickly (Karoshi et al., 2012). In community settings, mortality can be even higher.

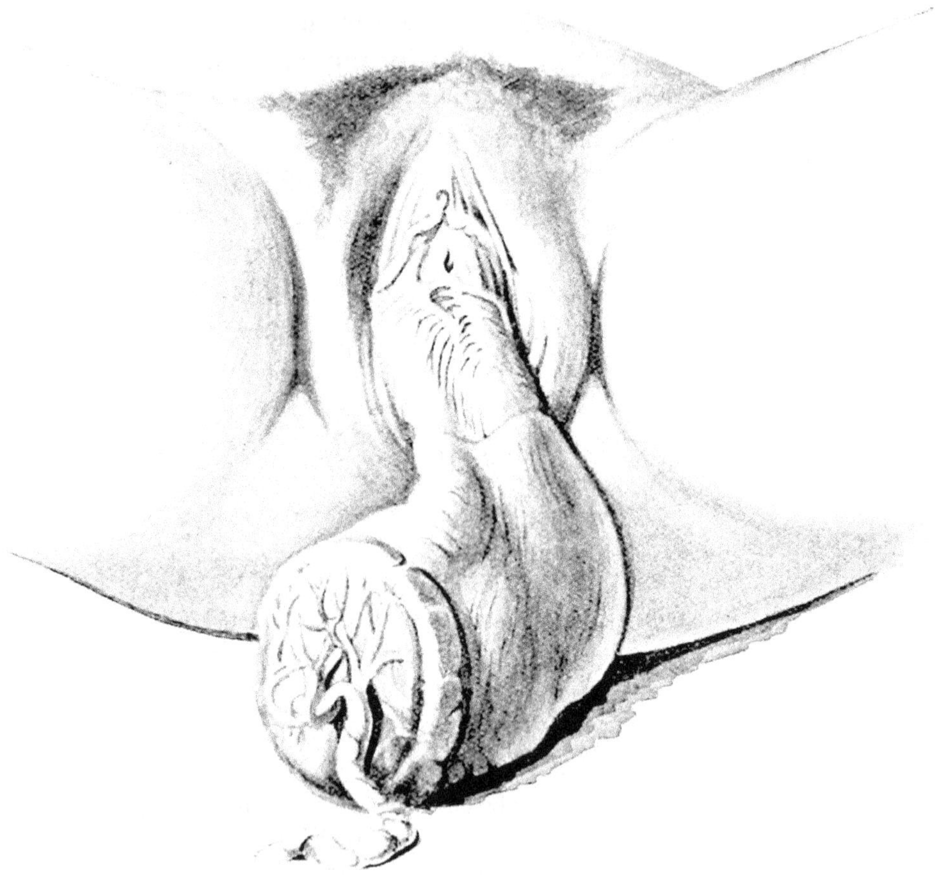

Figure 7-26. A total, 4th-degree uterine inversion involves inversion of the vagina and the uterus. The placenta is usually attached to the uterus. Expect hemorrhage and severe shock. From *The Practice of Midwifery* (7th ed., p. 966), by A. L. Galabin and G. Blacker, 1910, New York, NY: Macmillan. In the public domain.

Uterine inversion is a rare complication with an incidence of 1 in 3,500–20,000 births (Macones, 2023). It has been attributed to the use of excessive cord traction with fundal pressure, but evidence for a causal relationship is inconsistent (Macones, 2023). Risk factors for inversion, present in fewer than 50% of cases, include macrosomia, rapid or prolonged labor and birth, short umbilical cord, preeclampsia with severe features, use of uterine relaxants, nulliparity, uterine anomalies or leiomyoma, retained placenta, and placenta accreta (Macones, 2023). Maternal connective tissue disorders such as Marfan syndrome and Ehlers-Danlos syndrome can predispose to uterine inversion (Gadappa, Yelikar, & Wanjare, 2015). Uterine inversion can even occur spontaneously during a cesarean birth when the uterus turns itself inside-out through the incision (Macones, 2023).

Uterine inversion can present with severe and sudden shock, which can be caused by massive blood loss (hypovolemic shock) or by bradycardia (neurogenic shock). The uterine ligaments placing traction on the peritoneum are thought to trigger a parasympathetic response that can result in profound bradycardia or even cardiac arrest (Nag, Datta, Samaddar, & Panigrahi, 2015). Severe abdominal pain and urinary retention can be present. Uterine inversion is usually accompanied by severe hemorrhage. In the case of complete inversion, the uterus, a dark gray-purple mass, hangs out of the vulva, typically with the placenta and cord attached. You will be unable to feel the uterine fundus on abdominal palpation.

If you suspect an incomplete uterine inversion, perform a digital vaginal examination. An inverted uterus has a rough, corrugated texture. Attached placenta palpates as spongy and veiny, and the membranes feel slick and smooth. Upon digital exploration, the inverted fundus can feel like a mass in the vagina, and upon abdominal palpation a cuplike indentation is sometimes appreciated at the fundus (Macones, 2023).

When your client suffers a uterine inversion, *immediately* attempt to replace the uterus. Over time the lower uterine segment and cervix will contract, creating a constriction ring that makes manual replacement more difficult. Manual replacement outside the operating room is effective in only about two thirds of cases (Macones, 2023). Act fast and perform multiple actions simultaneously.

1. Call emergency medical services (EMS). The mother's chances for survival are much higher if you rapidly transport to a facility with experienced in-house obstetricians, anesthesiology staff, and operating-room personnel to minimize delays in treatment.
2. If you are running oxytocin for third stage management, turn it off (Evensen & Anderson, 2020). You cannot replace a contracted uterus.
3. Do not remove the placenta. Doing so will cause intractable hemorrhage.
4. Take the inverted uterus into the palm of your hand and forcefully push the fundus into the abdominal cavity along the long axis of the vagina, restoring it to its proper location. This action is like placing your hand at the toe of

RAMP: Goals in Managing Uterine Inversion

Rapid transport

Attempt immediate replacement of uterus

Manage Hemorrhage and Shock

Prevent Reoccurrence

an inverted sock and pushing to turn the sock right side out. Aim your force toward the umbilicus. Take care not to perforate the uterus with your fingertips. As the uterus moves back into place make a fist and continue pushing the uterus toward the umbilicus.

5. When a constriction ring is present, apply pressure to the part of the fundus nearest the ring and coax it through, bottom to top, squeezing a smaller part of the mass through the ring first. This action is like stuffing a down pillow into a narrow drawstring bag.
6. Hold the uterus in place for 3–5 min with your hands placed internally, externally, or both (Macones, 2023). The uterine ligaments should eventually retract and hold it in place.
7. Give uterotonic agents after the uterus is replaced to promote uterine tone, prevent reoccurrence, and control bleeding (Evensen & Anderson, 2020).
8. Monitor the position of the uterus, maternal vital signs, and signs of hemorrhage *en route* to the hospital.

Definitive Care for Uterine Inversion

At a hospital, the obstetrician may employ the following treatments if the uterus remains inverted.

- Administer medications (nitroglycerin, terbutaline, magnesium sulfate, or inhalational anesthetics) to relax pelvic tone, then try again to manually replace the uterus in the operating room.
- Perform surgical correction of the inversion by opening the abdomen. The surgeon can apply traction to the inverted fundus or incise the posterior uterine wall to transect the constriction ring (Macones, 2023).
- Perform hydrostatic reduction using a flow of 2–5 L of NS to push the uterus back into its usual position (Karoshi et al., 2012).
- Employ measures to prevent reoccurrence include cerclage, intrauterine balloons, and uterine compression sutures (Macones, 2023).
- Administer broad-spectrum IV antibiotics reduce the risk of severe infection.

DIFFERENTIAL DIAGNOSES

A prolapsed uterine fibroid appears very much like a uterine inversion. With a prolapsed fibroid, the fundus is palpable in its normal position; with uterine inversion, it is absent. Uterine inversion is not to be confused with a prolapsed cervix due to poor pelvic tone. In the latter case, the cervix is often visible at the introitus after birth, but the uterus does not protrude through it.

AFFLICT: Etiologies of PPH: Clotting Trouble

Coagulopathies

A coagulopathy is a disorder of impaired blood clotting that can lead to prolonged or excessive bleeding. Some coagulopathies are primary medical conditions. Others develop as complications of primary health disorders, including PPH. Whereas coagulopathy complicates about 1 in 500 births in the United States, it is an uncommon *primary* cause of PPH, occurring in 7% of cases (Belfort, 2022). In high-resource settings, most clients with bleeding disorders (such as idiopathic thrombocytopenic purpura, thrombotic thrombocytopenic purpura, von Willebrand disease, and hemophilia) are identified before pregnancy, and hospital birth is planned. Clients who have had limited medical care all their lives, however, do not always realize they have a bleeding disorder.

Normal hemostasis requires a delicate balance between the opposing mechanisms of coagulation (clot-forming) and fibrinolytic (clot-dissolving) factors in the blood (Hall, 2009). When injured vessels spill blood from the intravascular space, the hemostatic system stops the flow first with a platelet plug, then by the formation of a fibrin clot (Cashion, 2016). Coagulation factors that circulate in the bloodstream interact like a progression of falling dominoes, each factor sequentially activating the next in line. The fibrinolytic system breaks up clots to restore circulation.

Disseminated intravascular coagulation (DIC), also known as consumptive coagulopathy, is a life-threatening derangement of the clotting cascade and fibrinolytic system that results in simultaneous bleeding and clotting. Abnormal coagulation compromises perfusion and can ultimately result in multiple organ dysfunction. DIC begins when an event triggers the formation of innumerable microscopic clots, either by the release of large quantities of tissue thromboplastin or by widespread vascular injury (Cashion, 2016). The body responds by attempting to dissolve the unneeded clots, causing bleeding. The response to bleeding is more clotting, which consumes clotting factors at an accelerated rate. The byproducts of widespread

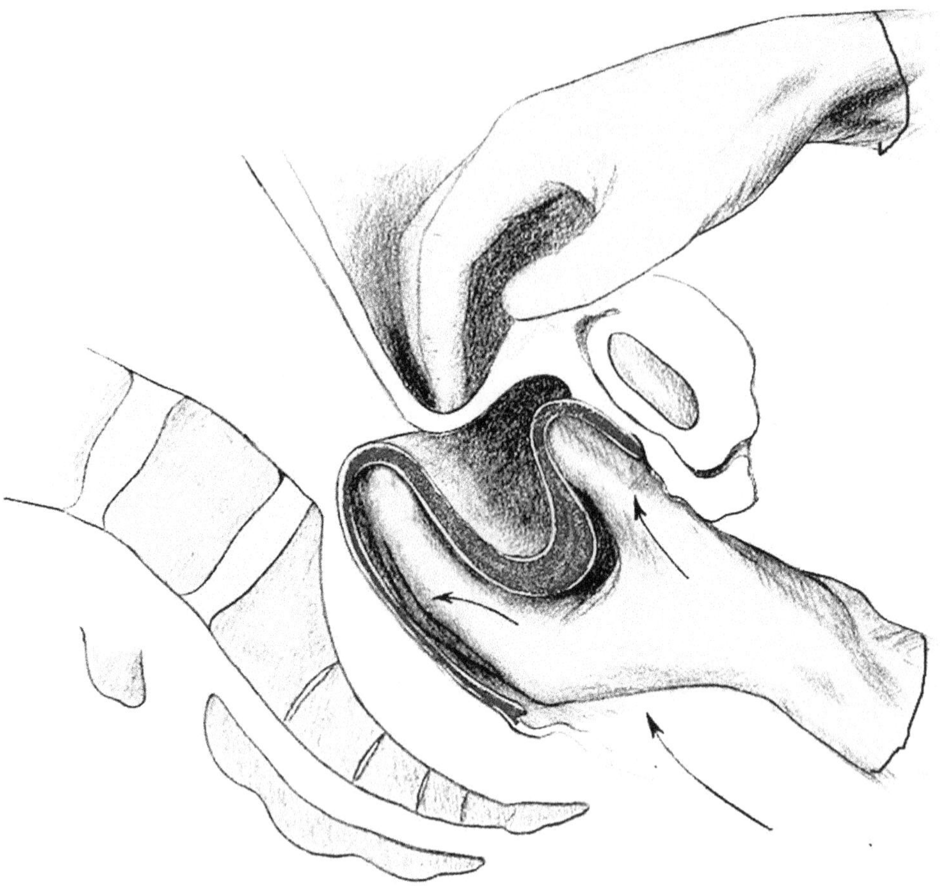

Figure 7-27. Reduction of a uterine inversion is most likely to be successful when you replace the uterus immediately after it inverts. From *The Principles and Practice of Obstetrics* (p. 762), by J. B. De Lee, 1914, Philadelphia, PA: W. B. Saunders. In the public domain.

clot formation and dissolution interfere with the ability of the blood to coagulate and cause excessive bleeding. Fibrin-narrowed vessels obstruct blood flow, causing ischemia and tissue death, and damage or destroy blood cells, causing anemia.

Coagulopathy can lead to PPH, and PPH can lead to coagulopathy (Belfort, 2022, 2023d). DIC can also occur with HELLP syndrome (**H**emolysis, **E**levated **L**iver enzymes, **L**ow **P**latelets), placental abruption, sepsis, fetal demise, major trauma, or amniotic fluid embolism. The client with DIC can develop severe vaginal, intrauterine, or intraabdominal bleeding or diffuse oozing of blood from IV or bladder catheter sites (Belfort, 2023a). Bruising, purpura, and petechiae are commonly noted on the skin. Abnormal clotting can manifest as deep-vein thrombosis (DVT) or with signs of microvascular thrombosis, such as renal failure. Some people develop difficulty breathing, coughing, and spitting blood (Levi, 2022). Signs of shock usually include tachycardia, hypotension, thready pulses, altered mental status, cool extremities, narrow pulse pressure, and organ involvement such as hepatic dysfunction or acute lung injury (Belfort, 2023a). Low fibrinogen level (less than 300 mg/dl), thrombocytopenia (less than 100,000/mcl), prolonged prothrombin time (PT), high international normalized ratio (INR, greater than 1.5), and/or prolonged activated partial thromboplastin time (aPTT) are laboratory abnormalities seen with DIC (Belfort, 2022).

Because *all* unabated bleeding eventually leads to shock and coagulopathy, the passage of time can make a straightforward PPH more complex. At the onset of postpartum hemorrhage, massage and uterotonics are usually enough to control the bleeding. When coagulopathy develops, however, even high-level interventions such as compression sutures, embolization, the use of blood products, or even hysterectomy sometimes fail to stop the bleeding (Karoshi et al., 2012). Blood-product replacement is necessary to achieve hemostasis, so rapid transport is crucial. Treatment consists of managing the underlying condition while providing hemodynamic support with PRBCs, platelets, fresh frozen plasma, and cryoprecipitate.

Care Following PPH

Physical Recovery

Few clients experiencing PPH require invasive procedures such as a hysterectomy or central arterial or venous line. Those who do are generally managed in the intensive-care unit. During and after significant hemorrhage, hospital providers monitor the client's level of consciousness, vital signs, and urine output, as well as blood count, electrolytes, and coagulation-panel values. Pulse oximetry monitors heart rate, oxygen saturation, and perfusion status. In the days after postpartum hemorrhage, clients can become edematous from crystalloid overload coupled with the fluid-retaining effects of oxytocin. Frequent lung auscultation monitors for the onset of pulmonary edema or acute respiratory distress syndrome. Within a few days, the client with healthy kidneys will eliminate the excess fluid. The pulse should remain less than 90 and the systolic blood pressure (SBP) should be over 100. Urinary output and hemoglobin should be adequate, and the client should be able to walk to the bathroom without dizziness or a significant change in vital signs. The fundus should be firm, and bleeding should be minimal. When the client meets these goals, the provider can consider discharge.

Emotional Care

Hemorrhage can be terrifying and disruptive for anyone, especially when it includes transport and admission to a hospital. At first, the midwife must focus on the hemorrhaging client's physical condition. As the client stabilizes or is managed by other providers, the midwife can begin to focus on the emotional needs of the client and family (Ward, 2012). Empower the client by providing choices and soliciting input when decisions are made. Incorporate as many of the client's preferences as are safe to include. Skin-to-skin contact is important to bonding and can be initiated while other procedures are in progress.

A mother's satisfaction with the birth experience is influenced by expectations, the amount of support received, the quality of the provider-client relationship, and ability to participate in decision-making (Funai & Norwitz, 2023a). Acknowledge the intense, conflicting emotions that often follow a health crisis and express warmth, empathy, and patience. Assess for signs of trauma, depression, and anxiety in the days and weeks after the event. A mother recovering from postpartum hemorrhage is often physically weak and requires help at home, particularly if there are other children. Family members can live too far away to be helpful, and partners may need to return to work.

Everyone processes emotional trauma uniquely. Some mothers or their family members develop traumatic stress reactions after a severe hemorrhage (Carrasco et al., 2022). Inform clients and their families of the signs and symptoms of PTSD and provide referrals for counseling as needed. The emotional distress associated with trauma may be more about the client's sense of threat, loss of control, or loss of trust in caregivers than about actual complications or events (Carrasco et al., 2022). Sensitive care can support resiliency and healing.

Sheehan Syndrome

Sheehan syndrome is a rare condition in which severe postpartum hemorrhage impairs blood flow to the anterior lobe of the pituitary, causing infarction and necrosis (Schorn & Phillippi, 2014). It affects about 1–2% of mothers who suffer postpartum hemorrhage severe enough to cause shock and to require the transfusion of multiple units of blood (Hale & Habib, 2014). Rarely, infarction can occur shortly after giving birth in the absence of overt hemorrhage. Postpartum pituitary infarction is a common cause of hypopituitarism in resource-limited countries but occurs infrequently in high-resource countries due to improvements in obstetrical care (Snyder, 2022).

Table 7-8

Enhancements and Disruptions to Physiologic Childbirth

Enhancements
- Spontaneous onset and progression of labor
- Physical and emotional support
- Freedom to eat, drink, and choose activities
- Intermittent auscultation
- Nonintervention in normal birth process of infant and placenta
- Skin-to-skin continuous contact between mother and infant
- Early and frequent breastfeeding

Disruptions
- Induction or augmentation of labor
- Intrusions, bright lights, uncomfortable room, lack of privacy, multiple providers, lack of supportive companions
- Time constraints
- Lack of access to food or drink
- Restriction of movement
- Continuous fetal monitoring
- Opiates, regional or general analgesia, episiotomy, operative vaginal or cesarean birth
- Immediate cord clamping
- Separation of mother and infant

Signs and symptoms of severe Sheehan syndrome include lethargy and fatigue, anorexia, weight loss, and inability to lactate. Less-severe symptoms can include poor milk production, failure to resume menses, and loss of pubic and axillary hair. Some clients experience nonspecific symptoms that can elude diagnosis for decades after the inciting event (Snyder, 2022). Some mothers with Sheehan's syndrome require lifelong hormone-replacement therapy (G. Choudhary, Soni, & Mohammed, 2020).

Secondary PPH

Secondary or late PPH is excessive bleeding occurring between 24 hr and 12 weeks postpartum. It is most likely to occur 1–2 weeks postpartum, and it follows 0.2–2.5% of births in high-resource countries (Belfort & Huisman, 2022). About 10% of cases present with massive bleeding (Groom & Jacobson, 2012). Secondary PPH most commonly results from subinvolution related to retained products of conception (including focal placenta accreta), subinvolution of the placental bed, and infection (Belfort & Huisman, 2022). Less commonly, late postpartum hemorrhage is related to a previously undiagnosed bleeding disorder or to the use of medications that predispose to bleeding, such as anticoagulants. Missed vaginal lacerations or hematomas or wound breakdown from infected suture lines can also lead to hemorrhage (Groom & Jacobson, 2012). A poorly healing cesarean incision can open, causing internal or external bleeding and occasionally evisceration of the bowel. Abnormal blood vessels such as arteriovenous malformations and false aneurysms and neoplasms such as choriocarcinomas are rare causes of secondary PPH.

On sonographic examination, findings can include an intrauterine mass, endometrial fluid, thickened endometrium, or abnormal vascularity, which can be difficult to distinguish from normal postpartum findings (Sellmyer, Desser, Maturen, Jeffrey, & Kamaya, 2013). Treatment is aimed at resolving the root cause. Give uterotonic agents if the uterus is poorly contracted. Surgical procedures (dilation and curettage, suction curettage) may be indicated for the removal of retained products. Broad-spectrum antibiotic therapy is indicated when endometritis is suspected, as indicated by fever, uterine tenderness, or foul-smelling discharge. Uncomplicated endometritis is usually managed outpatient with oral antibiotics, but clients with systemic symptoms can require admission for IV antibiotic therapy. Untreated endometritis can progress to sepsis.

Prevention of PPH

Antepartum Prevention

Minimize a client's risk of excess bleeding by encouraging good nutrition. A mother with a low hemoglobin value is often less able to tolerate blood loss after childbirth. Severe antepartum prenatal anemia carries a higher risk of placental abruption, maternal shock, and maternal intensive-care unit admission, and it appears to increase the risk that PPH will occur (Auerbach & Landy, 2024). For the client with preeclampsia, even mild anemia is associated with higher risk of PPH and blood transfusion (Burwick, Newman, & Rincon, 2022). Infants of mothers with antepartum anemia are more likely to experience fetal growth restriction and preterm birth and are at higher risk for autism spectrum disorder, attention deficit hyperactivity disorder, cognitive deficits, and intellectual disabilities (Auerbach & Landy, 2024).

Iron deficiency, the most common pathologic cause of anemia in pregnancy, can result from insufficient intake of dietary iron or from conditions that decrease iron absorption such as inflammatory bowel disease or a history of bariatric surgery. Individuals with heavy blood losses from menstruation or a short interval between pregnancies can enter the pregnancy with anemia or low iron stores (Auerbach & Landy, 2023). Low-dose iron supplementation at the level found in prenatal vitamin supplements is recommended from the first trimester to decrease the incidence of maternal anemia at term (ACOG, 2021). It is unclear, however, whether iron supplementation in well-nourished pregnant clients without anemia affects perinatal outcomes (ACOG, 2021). IV iron is an option for improving iron-deficiency anemia when oral iron is poorly tolerated or when rapid iron repletion is required (Adams, McNulty, & Rosenstein, 2022). Modern IV iron infusions with low-molecular-weight dextran carry a 1 in 200,000 risk of anaphylaxis and a 2–6% rate of mild, transient, and self-resolving reactions, in contrast to the high rate of adverse reactions associated with high-molecular-weight dextran (Adams, McNulty, et al., 2022).

Folate deficiency can cause megaloblastic anemia during pregnancy when the maternal diet is deficient in animal proteins, fresh leafy vegetables, and legumes (Auerbach & Landy, 2023). Daily folate at a dose of 400–800 mcg should be taken daily from one month before conception and continued throughout pregnancy. Vitamin B_{12} deficiency can cause macrocytic anemia in pregnancy, especially in individuals with Crohn's disease or who have had bariatric surgery. Other nutrient deficiencies such as inadequate vitamin A or chronic infections such as parasitic worm infestation can also cause anemia, often in low-resource settings (Auerbach & Landy, 2023).

Intrapartum Prevention

More mothers die during third stage labor than at any other time in pregnancy, birth, or the postpartum period (Weeks & Fawcus, 2020). When healthy individuals labor without disruptions, normal hemostatic processes unfold optimally and reduce the likelihood of excessive bleeding (Weeks & Fawcus, 2020). Reduce the risk of PPH by encouraging mothers to remain mobile and suggesting methods of pain management that are less likely to disrupt natural labor (Ward, 2012). Encourage hydration to compensate for insensible fluid loss (unmeasurable losses through lungs, skin, and respiratory tract) and to maximize circulating volume. Protect the sanctity of the birth area by fostering a private environment where the mother feels safe and protected. Throughout labor, reassess for risk PPH risk factors that can develop, including prolonged labor (longer than 12 hr), prolonged third stage (longer than 30 min), retained placenta, fever, hypertension, or abruption.

Active Versus Physiologic Management of Third Stage

Physiologic Management

The terms *physiological management*, *conservative management*, and *expectant management* are often used interchangeably to indicate a "hands-off" policy. The provider awaits signs of placenta separation and allows the placenta to deliver spontaneously or with the aid of gravity, maternal pushing, or

When the client has not had an ultrasound, consider the possibility of an undiagnosed twin before giving postpartum uterotonics or applying cord traction.

nipple stimulation (Begley et al., 2019). The attendant does not clamp or cut the cord until pulsations have ceased or the placenta is delivered, and prophylactic uterotonic medications are not used.

True psychophysiological care, however, is a complete package that supports the client's body, mind, heart, and soul to engage in the work of birth (Fahy et al., 2010; "Supporting Healthy and Normal Physiologic Childbirth," 2013). It is difficult to pry this package apart into components and attempt to determine which parts are most beneficial. To give birth normally, a mother needs privacy; confidence and trust in the provider; and to feel safe, secure, cared about, and respected. Many interrelated maternal and fetal factors such as corticotropin-releasing hormone, cortisol, and prostaglandins affect oxytocin release, as does the mother's emotional state. Because adrenaline competes with oxytocin on the myometrial binding sites, fear, anxiety, pain, and tension can put the brakes on a normally progressing labor and contribute to PPH (Saxton, Fahy, & Hastie, 2014).

When a client's pregnancy, labor, and birth have been normal, a psychophysiological approach optimizes the delicate balance of reproductive hormones and minimizes the risk of PPH (Hastie & Fahy, 2009). True physiologic labor and birth require a setting where the client feels safe and providers support immediate and sustained skin-to-skin contact between mother and infant, early breastfeeding, unobtrusive monitoring that does not interfere with bonding, and placenta expulsion by gravity and maternal effort (Fahy et al., 2010). Mother-infant skin contact alone has been shown to decrease the duration of the third stage of labor, decrease postpartum blood loss, and improve uterine contractility and involution (Erickson, Bovbjerg, & Cheyney, 2020; Karimi, Miri, Salehian, Khadivzadeh, & Bakhshi, 2019). Expectant management is most appropriate when the mother is well supported by the midwife and honors the body's cues regarding movement, positioning, hydration, and nutrition (Begley et al., 2019). When any component is missing or discordant, risk for hemorrhage can increase (Fahy et al., 2010).

For healthy mothers having a physiologic birth, less is more. Prophylactic oxytocin in the third stage does not appear to reduce total blood loss or the rate of PPH for a low-risk client having a completely natural birth (Davis et al., 2012; Dixon et al., 2013; Erickson, Bovbjerg, et al., 2020; Erickson, Lee, Grose, & Emeis, 2019; Fahy et al., 2010). In fact, for clients laboring physiologically, AMTSL appears to be associated with a *higher* risk for PPH (Davis et al., 2012; Dixon et al., 2013; Erickson, Lee, et al., 2019; Fahy et al., 2010).

Table 7-9

Oxytocin Dosages for AMTSL

Oxytocin infusion
Oxytocin 10–30 units in 500 ml or 20–60 units in 1,000 ml NS or LR controlled infusion with a standardized rate.
An example for a typical oxytocin regimen for atony prophylaxis is as follows: In 500 ml NS containing 30 units oxytocin—start with 334 ml/hr (10 units oxytocin given over 30 min). After 30 min, change to a maintenance rate 125 ml/hour (7.5 units oxytocin over 60 min).
OR
Oxytocin bolus
Oxytocin IV bolus of 1–3 units to initiate adequate uterine tone followed by an infusion to maintain adequate tone—30 units in 500 ml running at 125 ml/hr (7.5 units/hr).
OR
Oxytocin IM
Oxytocin 10 units IM when no IV access is possible.

Adapted from "Medications for Prevention and Treatment of Postpartum Hemorrhage," by S. M. Adams, A. Butwick, and J. McNulty, in D. Lagrew et al. (Eds.), *Improving Health Care Response to Obstetric Hemorrhage, v. 3.0: A CMQCC Quality Improvement Toolkit* (p. 115), 2022, Palo Alto, CA: California Maternal Quality Care Collaborative. Copyright by publisher.

Active Management of Third Stage Labor (AMTSL)

For many years, experts recommended a three-step regimen for AMTSL: giving a uterotonic agent before placental separation, early cord clamping, and controlled cord traction, sometimes with uterine massage (Berghella, 2023). Research has suggested that oxytocin administration alone may be the only effective component of AMTSL (Lagrew, Libova, & Lyndon, 2022). In hospital-based studies, active management with oxytocin has been shown to reduce total blood loss and the rate of postpartum hemorrhage (Berghella, 2023). The hospital-based client, however, is more likely to undergo interventions that raise the risk of postpartum hemorrhage, including oxytocin induction or augmentation and instrumental vaginal birth.

It has been hypothesized that if uterotonic drugs such as oxytocin were administered in the third stage of labor at every birth, the rate of PPH would decrease by 50% (Belfort, 2023b). WHO, ACOG, the American Academy of Family Physicians, the International Federation of Gynecologists and Obstetricians, the Association of Women's Health, Obstetric and Neonatal Nurses, and the International Confederation of Midwives recommend that *every* provider administer

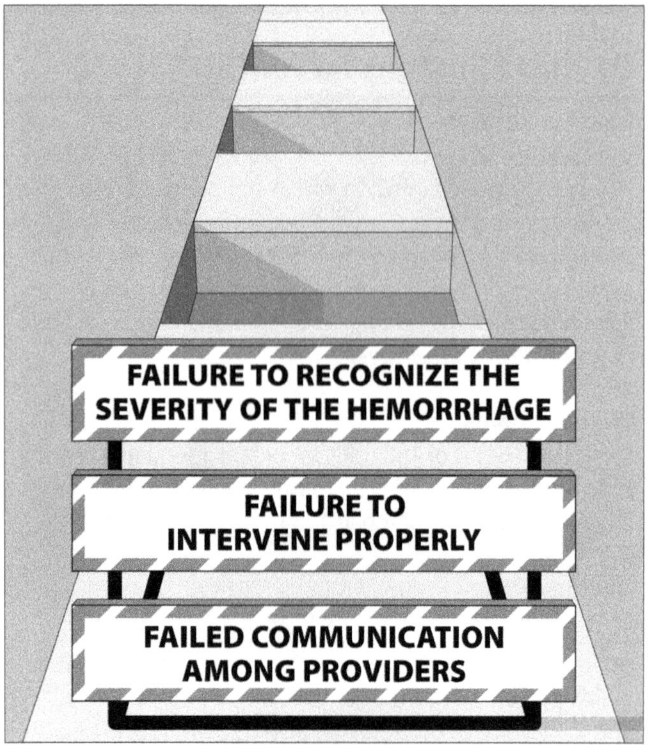
FAILURE TO RECOGNIZE THE SEVERITY OF THE HEMORRHAGE
FAILURE TO INTERVENE PROPERLY
FAILED COMMUNICATION AMONG PROVIDERS

Figure 7-28. Provider pitfalls are hazardous but avoidable.

oxytocin after *every* birth, but also note that low-risk mothers choosing physiologic birth should be supported when they decide to forgo prophylactic oxytocin (Main, Goffman, et al., 2015). A Cochrane Review considers conservative management of the third stage of labor appropriate *only* if the natural flow of oxytocin has not been disrupted by labor augmentation, induction, epidural, or narcotic analgesia (Begley et al., 2019).

For high-risk mothers, AMTSL reduces blood loss and can prevent hemorrhage. Conditions such as grand multiparity, rapid or slow labor, fetal macrosomia, shoulder dystocia, polyhydramnios, preeclampsia, or intraamniotic infection (IAI, chorioamnionitis) can put a client at higher risk for PPH. For these clients, prophylactic oxytocin minimizes blood loss and can be lifesaving. Ideally, active management should be integrated with the physiologic approach as much as possible, including immediate and ongoing skin-to-skin contact, early breastfeeding, and minimal disruption to the mother and infant.

Uterotonics for Third Stage Management

Oxytocin administration in the third stage of labor is the only intervention consistently proven to reduce the incidence of PPH, and it carries the lowest risk of side effects (ACOG, 2017/2021). Opinions differ over agents to be given in addition or instead—for example, oxytocin and TXA, oxytocin and misoprostol, oxytocin and methylergonovine (methylergometrine, Methergine®), carbetocin—in active third stage management for the prevention of postpartum hemorrhage after vaginal birth (ACOG, 2017/2021; Angarita & Berghella, 2023; Ottun et al., 2022). Some researchers have found no benefit from the use of multiple agents (Somanathan, Balu, Jacob, & Illickal, 2021).

Oxytocin

In the United States, oxytocin alone is the standard of care for AMTSL (Berghella, 2023). The usual dose is 10–40 units per 500 ml of NS, titrated to uterine response (Berghella, 2023). CMQCC recommends 10–30 units per 500 ml NS (Adams, Butwick, et al., 2022). When IV access is not available, give 10 units of IM oxytocin after the baby is born. IM oxytocin has a slower onset of action, 3–5 min compared with less than 1 min with the IV route (Berghella, 2023). For clients at high risk of PPH, some authors consider uterotonic therapy most effective when oxytocin is given along with methylergonovine or misoprostol (Berghella, 2023).

There is no difference in efficacy if oxytocin is given upon birth of the anterior shoulder or after expulsion of the placenta (Jackson et al., 2001). When the client has not had an ultrasound, consider the presence of an undiagnosed twin before giving postpartum uterotonics or applying controlled cord traction (Berghella, 2023). Potential adverse effects of prophylactic oxytocin are associated with rapid infusions of highly concentrated bags of oxytocin or large IV bolus doses and include hypotension, tachycardia, flushing, nausea, and vomiting (Adams, Butwick, et al., 2022).

Prostaglandins

Authorities disagree on the effectiveness of misoprostol for the prevention of PPH, used as a single agent or together with oxytocin. Recent studies, including a Cochrane review, have found that misoprostol is ineffective at preventing PPH due to its long onset of action (ACOG, 2017; Adams, Butwick, et al., 2022; W. R. P. Smith et al., 2020). Moreover, misoprostol use increases the likelihood of significant fever, diarrhea, and vomiting. CMQCC no longer recommends misoprostol for prevention or treatment of PPH unless it is the only agent available (Adams, Butwick, et al., 2022). Some authors, however, recommend using misoprostol (typical dose 200–400 mcg buccally) together with oxytocin for active third stage management (Angarita & Berghella, 2023; Berghella, 2023; Mishra, Nekkanti, Barma, & Mishra, 2021; Powell & Slaughter, 2021).

Ergot Alkaloids

Methylergonovine (Methergine®) can be given 0.2 mg IM to clients without hypertension, Raynaud's phenomenon, or history of migraine (Berghella, 2023). Ergot medications produce uterine contractions that are stronger and longer lasting than oxytocin. Whereas oxytocin acts specifically on uterine smooth muscle, ergot preparations act on smooth muscle throughout the body (Berghella, 2023). Methylergonovine is associated with higher incidence of retained placenta (Weeks, 2023). Potential adverse effects include nausea and vomiting (18%), blood-pressure elevation (1.7%), and severe afterpains (Weeks & Fawcus, 2020). This medication must be refrigerated and protected from light, so its usefulness is limited in remote regions lacking electricity.

Oxytocin Agonists

Carbetocin, a long-acting synthetic oxytocin agonist, works much like natural oxytocin, but has a longer duration of action. It is not available in the United States, but it is used in many other countries for prevention of uterine atony and hemorrhage (Berghella, 2023). Carbetocin is administered by giving 100 mcg as a single slow IV injection; lower doses can also be effective.

Tranexamic Acid (TXA)

TXA is highly effective when used relatively early in the hemorrhage protocol and appears beneficial when used prophylactically (Saccone et al., 2020). Some authorities recommend prophylactic use for clients at high risk for hemorrhage (Robinson, Basso, Chan, Duckitt, & Lett, 2022). TXA 1 g is administered IV over 10 min. The most common effects reported with TXA administration include nausea, vomiting, and diarrhea (Adams, Butwick, et al., 2022). Hypotension is possible if TXA is given more rapidly than recommended.

Complementary Treatment

Nipple Stimulation

Nipple stimulation through breastfeeding or digital rolling can sometimes decrease the incidence of postpartum hemorrhage by promoting the natural release of oxytocin. When uterotonics are not available or are declined by the client, nipple stimulation is a safe, inexpensive, and convenient intervention (Berghella, 2023), although there is insufficient evidence to recommend the practice (Abedi, Jahanfar, Namvar, & Lee, 2016).

Table 7-10

Preventing Postpartum Hemorrhage in Low-Resource Settings

In low-resource settings, up to two-thirds of significant PPH could be prevented through

- Programs to improve nutrition and increase iron stores.
- Providing or training skilled health care providers able to recognize risk factors at their earliest presentation.
- Access to uterotonic medications.
- Accurate QBL.
- Availability of telephone consultation with a more experienced health care provider.

Adapted from (1) *Oxytocin in the Uniject® Prefilled Injection Device*, by G. Batres, B. Aragón, M. Guy, and E. Jacoby, 2021, n.p.: Ministerio de Salud Publica y Asistencia Social, U.S. Agency for International Development, & PATH. (2) "Management of Postpartum Hemorrhage in Low Resource Settings," by V. Walvekar, A. Virkud, and R. Majumder, in S. Arulkumaran, M. Karoshi, L. G. Keith, A. B. Lalonde, and C. B-Lynch (Eds.), *A Comprehensive Textbook of Postpartum Hemorrhage* (2nd ed., pp. 539–544), 2012, London, United Kingdom: Sapiens Publishing. Copyright by publisher.

Improving Outcomes

Most deaths and morbidity from obstetric hemorrhage in the United States are thought to be preventable. Because PPH usually responds to treatment long before it becomes a life-threatening situation, experienced providers who have seen many good outcomes sometimes regard it as a benign issue that can be easily resolved (Lalonde et al., 2012; Marwaha et al., 2016). Because obstetric providers tend to underestimate large blood loss, overconfidence can prevent them from recognizing the volume and significance of PPH until the client has lost a dangerous amount of blood.

Poor outcomes are more likely to occur with

- Inexperienced providers or providers new to the practice.
- Fatigued providers on night shift.
- Incompetent or inexperienced assistants.
- Providers distracted by other issues, such as telephone calls or other clients in labor.
- Denial: providers do not acknowledge bleeding and fail to respond.
- Disregarding signs of worsening bleeding (dizziness, rising fundus, increasing tachycardia, falling BP, increasing respiratory rate, increasing abdominal girth, unusual pain).
- Delayed treatment because of underestimation of blood loss.
- Delayed availability of blood products.
- Lack of treatment algorithms/guidelines.
- Lack of knowledge and training.
- Insufficient communication between midwives, assistants, nurses, EMS, physicians, and other involved professionals.
- Poor organization (Kodkany et al., 2012).

Emergency Management Plan

Postpartum hemorrhage is often unexpected and cannot be reliably predicted or prevented. An early, aggressive response to bleeding minimizes blood loss (Main, Goffman, et al., 2015). Every birth provider should develop a plan for managing obstetric hemorrhage (Main, Goffman, et al., 2015). Preparedness is that much more important to the community midwife, whose clients are usually farther away from definitive care in time and distance.

To ready your practice for optimal response to PPH:

1. Identify your chain of support (see Chapter 4) and have telephone numbers for receiving providers and facilities easily accessible.
2. Keep hemorrhage supplies (medications, balloons, gauze) in one easily accessible location.
3. Conduct emergency drills and postdrill debriefings that include EMS responders and hospital providers if possible.
4. Assess hemorrhage risk at intake into practice, at 36 weeks of gestation, at onset of labor, every few hours through the laboring process, and periodically through the postpartum recovery.
5. Measure blood loss directly.
6. Offer uterotonics to manage the third stage of labor.
7. Debrief and review with other providers after the event to applaud successes, identify shortcomings, and improve flaws in the system.

Practice Considerations

Waterbirth

Individuals who give birth in the water have a lower incidence of major PPH, a higher risk of 1st- and 2nd-degree tears, and no difference in third- and 4th-degree perineal lacerations, retained placenta, and minor PPH when compared to those who deliver out of the water (Bovbjerg, Cheyney, & Caughey, 2022; Taliento et al., 2022). The provider should manage the third stage of labor as in any other birth. Active management can be safely conducted with clients in the tub, but they should be prepared to leave the tub if there is any evidence of excessive bleeding ("Model Practice Template," 2017). Mothers at greater risk for PPH should get out of the water to deliver the placenta so that the provider can better quantify and manage bleeding ("Model Practice Template," 2017).

Umbilical cord avulsion or rupture can occur during waterbirth. Some cases involve infants with short cords; others occur when the mother stresses the cord by lifting the infant rapidly from the water (Bovbjerg et al., 2022). Blood loss from umbilical cord avulsion comes directly from the baby's circulation. When recognition is delayed, the neonate can develop anemia requiring blood transfusion and intensive care, or even shock or death. One review found a cord avulsion rate of 2.4 per 1,000 waterbirths, but, lacking matched controls, it is unclear whether this rate is higher or lower than would be seen with a comparable group of healthy individuals having nonwaterbirths (Nutter, Meyer, Shaw-Battista, & Marowitz, 2014). Providers should avoid undue cord traction. When umbilical cord rupture is the suspected source of excess bleeding, immediately clamp and cut the cord between the site of bleeding and the infant's umbilicus, then quickly remove the newborn from the tub for assessment (Nutter et al., 2014). If possible, clamp the cord at least 4 in. (10 cm) from the infant's body as a potential route for vascular access if neonatal resuscitation is required.

Low-Resource Settings

Worldwide, severe postpartum hemorrhage is the leading cause of maternal mortality and severe maternal morbidities, responsible for 27.1% of maternal deaths, from 8% in high-resource regions to 32% in Northern Africa (Liu et al., 2021). In resource-poor countries, many hospitals that offer maternity care lack basic services such as a blood storage center, emergency facilities, emergency transport, and continuous in-house surgical capability, and they are often significant time and distance away from clients in need (Bhate-Deosthali, Khatri, & Wagle, 2011; Tindell et al., 2013). In the absence of local health facilities or trained birth professionals, many births in low-resource areas occur in the home or rudimentary health centers, attended by minimally skilled or untrained birth attendants (Batres, Aragón, Guy, & Jacoby, 2010; S. Miller et al., 2004). Moreover, even in locations where there are modern hospitals, many mothers cannot afford to access that care.

Many individuals in economically developing countries have little knowledge of obstetric danger signs. They often do not seek help until very ill or may decline treatment. Many view bleeding after childbirth as necessary, healthy, and cleansing and think that it should not be treated (Thaddeus & Nangalia, 2004). One survey in Bangladesh showed that most mothers did not consider complications such as placental abruption, obstructed labor, or excessive bleeding potentially life-threatening (Thaddeus & Nangalia, 2004).

Universal Precautions

Universal precautions protect the provider from bloodborne pathogens. In postpartum hemorrhage, blood can be difficult to contain. Manual removal of the placenta exposes the provider to blood nearly to the elbow. Standard gloves barely extend above the wrist. The provider who manages PPH in a setting with high rates of bloodborne disease and limited supplies of gloves and gowns faces many challenges in maintaining universal precautions. HIV/AIDS is always a concern and is prevalent in some economically developing countries.

Topics for Discussion

1. Carina K. gave birth to a healthy baby about 30 min ago in the master bedroom, and her midwife Alisha G. was sitting at the kitchen table finishing paperwork. The birth assistant called Alisha back to the bedroom to assess Carina's bleeding. Alisha found that her fundus was palpable 2 cm above the umbilicus and expelled 300 ml of clots from Carina's uterus. After the intervention, the fundus became firm and was palpable 2 cm below the umbilicus. Carina declined oxytocin and put the baby to the breast. When Alisha assessed Carina 20 min later, her uterus was again high and boggy, and Alisha expelled another 200 ml of clots. What could be causing Carina's bleeding? What should Alisha do next?
2. What kinds of uterine tamponade would you consider using if you were working in a low-resource setting, such as an isolated clinic in Cambodia or Papua New Guinea?
3. A term infant with a very short, thick cord was born precipitously to a grand multipara. The mother immediately tried to lift the baby to her abdomen, but suddenly grew faint, pale, nauseated, and confused. Her pulse dropped to 30, and her fundus was nonpalpable. What do you suspect? What are your next steps?
4. Ura C. is 2 weeks postpartum. After bleeding lightly to moderately every day since giving birth, today she has been soaking a pad an hour with bright-red blood. What problem do you suspect? What is your management plan?
5. Yelka R. gave birth to a healthy infant 15 min ago over an intact perineum after a rapid, intense labor. Throughout third stage labor, there was a steady trickle of red blood, which has continued since the birth of the placenta 5 min ago. The fundus is firm and 2 fingerbreadths below the umbilicus, and Yelka's bladder is empty. What do you suspect? How do you respond?

References

Abdul-Kadir, R., McLintock, C., Ducloy, A. S., El-Refaey, H., England, A., Federici, A. B., . . . Winikoff, R. (2014). Evaluation and management of postpartum hemorrhage: Consensus from an international expert panel. *Transfusion, 54*(7), 1756–1768. https://doi.org/10.1111/trf.12550

Abedi, P., Jahanfar, S., Namvar, F., & Lee, J. (2016). Breastfeeding or nipple stimulation for reducing postpartum haemorrhage in the third stage of labour. *Cochrane Database of Systematic Reviews, 2016*(1). https://doi.org/10.1002/14651858.CD010845.pub2

Abul, A., Al-Naseem, A., Althuwaini, A., Al-Muhanna, A., & Clement, N. S. (2022). Safety and efficacy of intrauterine balloon tamponade vs uterine gauze packing in managing postpartum hemorrhage: A systematic review and meta-analysis. *AJOG Global Reports, 3*(1), 100135. https://doi.org/10.1016/j.xagr.2022.100135

Adams, S. M., Butwick, A., & McNulty, J. (2022). Medications for prevention and treatment of postpartum hemorrhage. In D. Lagrew, J. McNulty, C. Sakowski, V. Cape, E. McCormick, & C. H. Morton (Eds.), *Improving health care response to obstetric hemorrhage, v. 3.0: A CMQCC quality improvement toolkit* (pp. 114–123). Palo Alto, CA: California Maternal Quality Care Collaborative. Retrieved from https://www.cmqcc.org/sites/default/files/HEMToolkit_03252022 Errata 7.2022 (2).pdf

Adams, S. M., McNulty, J., & Rosenstein, M. G. (2022). Management of iron deficiency anemia. In D. Lagrew, J. McNulty, C. Sakowski, V. Cape, E. McCormick, & C. H. Morton (Eds.), *Improving health care response to obstetric hemorrhage, v. 3.0: A CMQCC quality improvement toolkit* (pp. 41–50). Palo Alto, CA: California Maternal Quality Care Collaborative. Retrieved from https://www.cmqcc.org/sites/default/files/HEMToolkit_03252022 Errata 7.2022 (2).pdf

Ahmad, S. N., Seth, S., Agarwal, S., & Choudhary, S. (2017). Evaluating condom catheter balloon tamponade in non-traumatic postpartum haemorrhage resistant to medical management. *International Journal of Reproduction, Contraception, Obstetrics and Gynecology, 5*(6), 1874–1878. https://doi.org/10.18203/2320-1770.ijrcog20161681

Akhter, S., Begum, M. R., Kabir, Z., Rashid, M., Laila, T. R., & Zabeen, F. (2003). Use of a condom to control massive postpartum hemorrhage. *Medscape General Medicine, 5*(3), 38. Retrieved from https://www.medscape.com/viewarticle/459894

Akol, A. D., & Weeks, A. D. (2016). Retained placenta: Will medical treatment ever be possible? *Acta Obstetricia et Gynecologica Scandinavica, 95*(5), 501–504. https://doi.org/10.1111/aogs.12848

Alalaf, S. K., Al Tawil, N. G., Jawad, A. K., Mahmoud, M. B., Muhamad, B. Q., Abdul Rahman, K. H., . . . Bawadikji, A. A. (2020). Umbilical vein injection of 400 versus 800 µg misoprostol for the treatment of retained placenta: A multicenter, randomized double-blind controlled trial. *Journal of Obstetrics and Gynaecology Research, 46*(5), 727–735. https://doi.org/10.1111/jog.14232

Ali, T., Ghazi, A., & Siddiq, N. M. (2008). Uterovaginal packing in massive postpartum hemorrhage—A reappraisal. *Pakistan Journal of Surgery, 24*(1), 57–9. Retrieved from http://www.pjs.com.pk/journal_pdfs/jan_march08/15.pdf

American College of Obstetricians and Gynecologists. (2014). *reVITALize obstetric data definitions* (version 1.0). Retrieved from https://www.acog.org/-/media/project/acog/acogorg/files/pdfs/publications/revitalize-ob.pdf?la=en&hash=-D9ECE1577C2A0B535F42C1B8DC492070

American College of Obstetricians and Gynecologists. (2017, reaffirmed 2021). *Postpartum hemorrhage* (Practice Bulletin 183). Retrieved from https://www.acog.org/clinical/clinical-guidance/practice-bulletin/articles/2017/10/postpartum-hemorrhage

American College of Obstetricians and Gynecologists. (2018, reaffirmed 2022). *Prevention and management of obstetric lacerations at vaginal delivery* (Practice Bulletin 198). Retrieved from https://www.acog.org/clinical/clinical-guidance/practice-bulletin/articles/2018/09/prevention-and-management-of-obstetric-lacerations-at-vaginal-delivery

American College of Obstetricians and Gynecologists. (2019, reaffirmed 2022). *Quantitative blood loss in obstetric hemorrhage* (Committee Opinion 794). Retrieved from https://www.acog.org/clinical/clinical-guidance/committee-opinion/articles/2019/12/quantitative-blood-loss-in-obstetric-hemorrhage

American College of Obstetricians and Gynecologists. (2021). *Anemia in pregnancy* (Practice Bulletin 233). Retrieved from https://www.acog.org/clinical/clinical-guidance/practice-bulletin/articles/2021/08/anemia-in-pregnancy

American College of Obstetricians and Gynecologists, Society for Maternal-Fetal Medicine, Cahill, A. G., Beigi, R., Heine, R. P., Silver, R. M., & Wax, J. R. (2018, reaffirmed 2021). *Placenta accreta spectrum* (Obstetric Care Consensus 7). Retrieved from https://www.acog.org/clinical/clinical-guidance/obstetric-care-consensus/articles/2018/12/placenta-accreta-spectrum

Anansakunwat, W., Iamurairat, W., & Boonyoung, P. (2018). Lower uterine segment compression for 20 minutes to prevent early postpartum hemorrhage. *Journal of the Medical Association of Thailand, 101*(9), 1151–1156. Retrieved from http://www.thaiscience.info/Journals/Article/JMAT/10989499.pdf

Anderson, J. M., & Etches, D. (2007). Prevention and management of postpartum hemorrhage. *American Family Physician, 75*(6), 875–882. Retrieved from https://www.aafp.org/pubs/afp/issues/2007/0315/p875.html

Andreatta, P., Perosky, J., & Johnson, T. R. B. (2012). Two-provider technique for bimanual uterine compression to control postpartum hemorrhage. *Journal of Midwifery & Women's Health, 57*(4), 371–375. https://doi.org/10.1111/j.1542-2011.2011.00152.x

Angarita, A. M., & Berghella, V. (2023). Evidence-based labor management: Third stage of labor (part 5). *American Journal of Obstetrics & Gynecology MFM, 4*(5). https://doi.org/10.1016/j.ajogmf.2022.100661

Arnold, M. J., Sadler, K., & Leli, K. (2021). Obstetric lacerations: Prevention and repair. *American Family Physician, 103*(12), 745–752. Retrieved from https://www.aafp.org/pubs/afp/issues/2021/0615/p745.html

Arulkumaran, S., Karoshi, M., Keith, L. G., Lalonde, A. B., & B-Lynch, C. (Eds.). (2012). *A comprehensive textbook of postpartum hemorrhage: An essential clinical reference for effective management* (2nd ed.). London, United Kingdom: Sapiens Publishing. Retrieved from http://www.glowm.com/resource_type/resource/textbook/title/a-comprehensive-textbook-of-postpartum-hemorrhage-2<sup>nd<-sup >-edition/resource_doc/1275

Ashwal, E., Bergel Bson, R., Aviram, A., Hadar, E., Yogev, Y., & Hiersch, L. (2022). Risk factors for postpartum hemorrhage following cesarean delivery. *Journal of Maternal-Fetal & Neonatal Medicine, 35*(18), 3626-3630. https://doi.org/10.1080/14767058.2020.1834533

Auerbach, M., & Landy, H. J. (2023). Anemia in pregnancy. In J. S. Timauer & V. A, Barss (Eds.), *UpToDate*. Retrieved November 13, 2023, from https://www.uptodate.com/contents/anemia-in-pregnancy

Bagga, R., Jain, V., Chopra, S., Kalra, J., & Gopalan, S. (2004). Uterovaginal packing with rolled gauze in postpartum hemorrhage: Case report. *Medscape General Medicine, 6*(1), 50. Retrieved from https://www.ncbi.nlm.nih.gov/pmc/articles/PMC1140727/

Baig, F. S., Shahzad, N., Khurshid, H. N., & Malik, A. (2015). Postpartum haemorrhage: Comparison of intra umbilical and intra venous injection of oxytocin on blood loss in third stage of labour. *Professional Medical Journal, 22*(6), 793–797. Retrieved from http://theprofesional.com/article/vol. 22 no. 06/prof-2797.pdf

Bailey, R., Foley, M. R., Hall, N., Fleischer, A., D'Alton, M., Dildy, G. A., . . . Clark, S. L. (2016). The active management of postpartum uterine atony—A checklist based approach. *Open Journal of Obstetrics and Gynecology, 6*(11), 646. https://doi.org/10.4236/ojog.2016.611081

Bangh, S. A., Hughes, K. A., Roberts, D. J., & Kovarik, S. M. (2005). Neonatal ergot poisoning: A persistent iatrogenic illness. *American Journal of Perinatology, 22*(5), 239–243. https://doi.org/10.1055/s-2005-866604

Baskett, T. F. (2012). Preparedness for postpartum hemorrhage: An obstetric hemorrhage equipment tray. In S. Arulkumaran, M. Karoshi, L. G. Keith, A. B. Lalonde, & C. B-Lynch (Eds.), *A comprehensive textbook of postpartum hemorrhage: An essential clinical reference for effective management* (2nd ed., pp. 64–70). London, United Kingdom: Sapiens Publishing. Retrieved from http://www.glowm.com/pdf/PPH_2nd_edn_Chap-37.pdf

Batres, G., Aragón, B., Guy, M., & Jacoby, E. (2010). *Oxytocin in the Uniject® prefilled injection device: Guatemala pilot introduction: cost analysis of replacing oxytocin in ampoules with oxytocin in the Uniject® prefilled injection device for active management of the third stage of labor at the institutional level in Guatemala*. n.p.: Ministerio de Salud Publica y Asistencia Social, U.S. Agency for International Development, & PATH. Retrieved from https://www.path.org/publications/files/TS_oiu_cost_guatemala.pdf

Begley, C. M., Gyte, G. M. L., Devane, D., McGuire, W., Weeks, A., & Biesty, L. M. (2019). Active versus expectant management for women in the third stage of labour. *Cochrane Database of Systematic Reviews*. https://doi.org/10.1002/14651858.CD007412.pub5

Belfort, M. A. (2022). Disseminated intravascular coagulation (DIC) during pregnancy: Management and prognosis. In V. A. Barss (Ed.), *UpToDate*. Retrieved November 13, 2023, from https://www.uptodate.com/contents/disseminated-intravascular-coagulation-dic-during-pregnancy-management-and-prognosis

Belfort, M. A. (2023a). Disseminated intravascular coagulation (DIC) during pregnancy: Clinical findings, etiology, and diagnosis. In V. A. Barss (Ed.), *UpToDate*. Retrieved November 13, 2023, from https://www.uptodate.com/contents/disseminated-intravascular-coagulation-dic-during-pregnancy-clinical-indings-etiology-and-diagnosis

Belfort, M. A. (2023b). Overview of postpartum hemorrhage. In V. A. Barss (Ed.), *UpToDate*. Retrieved November 13, 2023, from https://www.uptodate.com/contents/overview-of-postpartum-hemorrhage

Belfort, M. A. (2023c). Postpartum hemorrhage: Management approaches requiring laparotomy. In V. A. Barss (Ed.), *UpToDate*. Retrieved November 13, 2023, from https://www.uptodate.com/contents/postpartum-hemorrhage-management-approaches-requiring-laparotomy#!

Belfort, M. A. (2023d). Postpartum hemorrhage: Medical and minimally invasive management. In V. A. Barss (Ed.), *UpToDate*. Retrieved November 13, 2023, from https://www.uptodate.com/contents/postpartum-hemorrhage-medical-and-minimally-invasive-management

Belfort, M. A., & Huisman, T. A. G. M. (2022). Secondary (late) postpartum hemorrhage. In V. A. Barss (Ed.), *UpToDate*. Retrieved November 13, 2023, from https://www.uptodate.com/contents/secondary-late-postpartum-hemorrhage

Bennett, B. L., Littlejohn, L. F., Kheirabadi, B. S., Butler, F. K., Kotwal R. S., Dubick, M. A., & Bailey J. A. (2014). Management of external hemorrhage in tactical combat casualty care: Chitosan-based hemostatic gauze dressings. *Journal of Special Operations Medicine, 14*(3), 40–57. Retrieved from https://www.jsomonline.org/Subscriber/articles/1403/2014340Bennett.pdf

Berghella, V. (2023). Management of the third stage of labor: Prophylactic pharmacotherapy to minimize hemorrhage. In V. A. Barss (Ed.), *UpToDate*. Retrieved November 13, 2023, from https://www.uptodate.com/contents/management-of-the-third-stage-of-labor-prophylactic-pharmacotherapy-to-minimize-hemorrhage

Bhate-Deosthali, P., Khatri, R., & Wagle, S. (2011). Poor standards of care in small, private hospitals in Maharashtra, India: Implications for public–private partnerships for maternity care. *Reproductive Health Matters, 19*(37), 32–41. https://doi.org/10.1016/S0968-8080(11)37560-X

Borovac-Pinheiro, A., Pacagnella, R. C., Cecatti, J. G., Miller, S., El Ayadi, A. M., Souza, J. P., . . . Winikoff, B. (2018). Postpartum hemorrhage: New insights for definition and diagnosis. *American Journal of Obstetrics & Gynecology, 219*(2), 162-168. https://doi.org/10.1016/j.ajog.2018.04.013

Bovbjerg, M. L., Cheyney, M., & Caughey, A. B. (2022). Maternal and neonatal outcomes following waterbirth: A cohort study of 17 530 waterbirths and 17 530 propensity score-matched land births. *BJOG, 129*(6), 950–958. https://doi.org/10.1111/1471-0528.17009

Bowman, Z. S., & Kennedy, A. M. (2014). Sonographic appearance of the placenta. *Current Problems in Diagnostic Radiology, 43*(6), 356–373. https://doi.org/10.1067/j.cpradiol.2014.05.006

Briley, A., Seed, P. T., Tydeman, G., Ballard, H., Waterstone, M., Sandall, J., . . . Bewley, S. (2014). Reporting errors, incidence and risk factors for postpartum haemorrhage (PPH) and progression to severe PPH: A prospective observational study. *BJOG, 121*(7), 876–888. https://doi.org/10.1111/1471-0528.12588

Brown, D. A., & Fletcher, H. (2013). Use of mediolateral cervical clamping to control postpartum hemorrhage. *International Journal of Gynecology & Obstetrics, 123*(2), 164–165. https://doi.org/10.1016/j.ijgo.2013.06.014

Burwick, R. M., Newman, R. A., & Rincon, M. (2022). Mild anemia and risk of postpartum hemorrhage or blood transfusion in preeclampsia. *American Journal of Obstetrics & Gynecology, 226*(1, Suppl.), S281–S282. https://doi.org/10.1016/j.ajog.2021.11.478

Butwick, A., Lee, R., McNulty, J., & Redell, D. (2022). Blood product replacement: Obstetric Hemorrhage. In D. Lagrew, J. McNulty, C. Sakowski, V. Cape, E. McCormick, & C. H. Morton (Eds.), *Improving health care response to obstetric hemorrhage, v. 3.0: A CMQCC quality improvement toolkit* (pp. 124–133). Palo Alto, CA: California Maternal Quality Care Collaborative. Retrieved from https://www.cmqcc.org/sites/default/files/HEMToolkit_03252022 Errata 7.2022 (2).pdf

Butwick, A., Main, E., McCormick, E., & Sakowski, C. (2022). Obstetric hemorrhage risk factor assessment. In D. Lagrew, J. McNulty, C. Sakowski, V. Cape, E. McCormick, & C. H. Morton (Eds.), *Improving health care response to obstetric hemorrhage, v. 3.0: A CMQCC quality improvement toolkit* (pp. 30–40). Palo Alto, CA: California Maternal Quality Care Collaborative. Retrieved from https://www.cmqcc.org/sites/default/files/HEMToolkit_03252022 Errata 7.2022 (2).pdf

Butwick, A., Romine, L., McNulty, J., Main, E., & Rosenstein, M. G. (2022). Best practice techniques to assess quantitative cumulative blood loss. In D. Lagrew, J. McNulty, C. Sakowski, V. Cape, E. McCormick, & C. H. Morton (Eds.), *Improving health care response to obstetric hemorrhage, v. 3.0: A CMQCC quality improvement toolkit* (pp. 104–112). Palo Alto, CA: California Maternal Quality Care Collaborative. Retrieved from https://www.cmqcc.org/sites/default/files/HEMToolkit_03252022 Errata 7.2022 (2).pdf

Cameron, A., & Menticoglou, S. (2011). Blood pressure cuff tamponade of vaginal lacerations causing significant postpartum hemorrhage. *Journal of Obstetrics and Gynaecology Canada, 33*(12), 1207–1207. https://doi.org/10.1016/S1701-2163(16)35103-9

Carles, G., Dabiri, C., Mchirgui, A., Saoudi, E. O., Hcini, N., Pouget, K., . . . de Matteis, B. (2017). Uses of chitosan for treating different forms of serious obstetrics hemorrhages. *Journal of Gynecology Obstetrics and Human Reproduction, 46*(9), 693–695. https://doi.org/10.1016/j.jogoh.2017.08.003

Carles, G., Dabiri, C., Mchirgui, A., Saoudi, E. O., Hcini, N., Seve, B., & de Matteis, B. (2016). Different uses of chitosan for treating serious obstetric hemorrhages. *Gynecology and Obstetrics Research Open Journal, 3*(1), 13–15. https://doi.org/10.17140/GOROJ-3-129

Carrasco, N., Combs, A., Klein, V. R., Terlizzi, K., Turner, T., & Morton, C. (2022). Communicating with and supporting women, birthing people, and families after an obstetric hemorrhage. In D. Lagrew, J. McNulty, C. Sakowski, V. Cape, E. McCormick, & C. H. Morton (Eds.), *Improving health care response to obstetric hemorrhage, v. 3.0: A CMQCC quality improvement toolkit* (pp. 146–162). Palo Alto, CA: California Maternal Quality Care Collaborative. Retrieved from https://www.cmqcc.org/sites/default/files/HEMToolkit_03252022 Errata 7.2022 (2).pdf

Chantrapitak, W., Anansakalwat, W., Suwikrom, S., Wattanaluangarun, R., & Puangsa-art, S. (2018). Postpartum hemorrhage outcome in lower uterine segment compression maneuver: A 20-year experience in Charoenkrung Pracharak Hospital. *Journal of the Medical Association of Thailand, 101*(4), 495–500. Retrieved from http://www.thaiscience.info/Journals/Article/JMAT/10989499.pdf

Chantrapitak, W., Srijanteok, K., & Puangsa-art, S. (2009). Lower uterine segment compression for management of early postpartum hemorrhage after vaginal delivery at Charoenkrung Pracharak Hospital. *Journal of the Medical Association of Thailand, 92*(5), 600–605. Retrieved from https://pdfs.semanticscholar.org/a51c/ca693b83bebaedf873a17ee5e9ed36bf599e.pdf

Chantrapitak, W., Srijuntuek, K., & Wattanaluangarun, R. (2011). The efficacy of lower uterine segment compression for prevention of early postpartum hemorrhage after vaginal delivery. *Journal of the Medical Association of Thailand, 94*(6), 649–656. Retrieved from https://pdfs.semanticscholar.org/1f63/5241cd1392c3f326b974ed8de12ec3ac573b.pdf

Choudhary, G., Soni, S., & Mohammed, S. (2020). Sheehan's syndrome: A rare cause of delayed recovery after anesthesia. *Journal of Obstetric Anaesthesia and Critical Care, 10*(1), 58. https://doi.org/10.4103/joacc.JOACC_9_19

Choudhary, V., & Bellad, M. B. (2017). Varicosities of vulva during pregnancy—A rare case report. *IOSR Journal of Dental and Medical Sciences, 16*(1), 75–76. Retrieved from https://iosrjournals.org/iosr-jdms/papers/Vol16-issue1/Version-9/P1601097576.pdf

Commission for the Accreditation of Birth Centers. (2023). *CABC indicators of compliance with standards for birth centers* (reference ed. 2.3). Hamburg, PA: Author. Retrieved from https://www.birthcenteraccreditation.org/wp-content/uploads/2023/09/CABC_IndicatorsRefEd-2.3_2023-0915.pdf

Cox, E. D., Schreiber, M. A., McManus, J., Wade, C. E., & Holcomb, J. B. (2009). New hemostatic agents in the combat setting. *Transfusion, 49*(Suppl. 5), 248S-255S. https://doi.org/10.1111/j.1537-2995.2008.01988.x

Cunningham, C., Watt, P., Aflaifel, N., Collins, S., Lambert, D., Porter, J., . . . Weeks, A. (2017). PPH Butterfly: A novel device to treat postpartum haemorrhage through uterine compression. *BMJ Innovations, 3*(1), 45–54. https://doi.org/10.1136/bmjinnov-2016-000144

Cunningham, F. G., Leveno, K. J., Dashe, J. S., Hoffman, B. L., Spong, C. Y., & Casey, B. M. (Eds.). (2022). *Williams obstetrics* (26th ed., Kindle version). New York, NY: McGraw-Hill.

D'Alton, M. E., Rood, K. M., Smid, M. C., Simhan, H. N., Skupski, D. W., Subramaniam, A., . . . Goffman, D. (2020). Intrauterine vacuum-induced hemorrhage-control device for rapid treatment of postpartum hemorrhage. *Obstetrics & Gynecology, 136*(5), 882–891. https://doi.org/10.1097/AOG.0000000000004138

D'Alton, M., Rood, K., Simhan, H., & Goffman, D. (2021). Profile of the Jada® System: the vacuum-induced hemorrhage control device for treating abnormal postpartum uterine bleeding and postpartum hemorrhage. *Expert Review of Medical Devices, 18*(9), 849–853. https://doi.org/10.1080/17434440.2021.1962288

Dakin, W. R. (1897). *A handbook of midwifery*. London, United Kingdom: Longmans, Green, & Co. Retrieved from https://archive.org/details/handbookofmidwif00daki

Davis, D., Baddock, S., Pairman, S., Hunter, M., Benn, C., Anderson, J., . . . Herbison, P. (2012). Risk of severe postpartum hemorrhage in low-risk childbearing women in New Zealand: Exploring the effect of place of birth and comparing third stage management of labor. *Birth, 39*(2), 98–105. https://doi.org/10.1111/j.1523-536X.2012.00531.x

De Lee, J. B. (1914). *The principles and practice of obstetrics*. Philadelphia, PA: W. B. Saunders. Retrieved from https://archive.org/details/principlespracti00dele

Della Corte, L., Saccone, G., Locci, M., Carbone, L., Raffone, A., Giampaolino, P., . . . Zullo, F. (2020). Tranexamic acid for treatment of primary postpartum hemorrhage after vaginal delivery: A systematic review and meta-analysis of randomized controlled trials. *Journal of Maternal-Fetal & Neonatal Medicine, 33*(5), 869–874. https://doi.org/10.1080/14767058.2018.1500544

Dias, T., Patabendige, M., Herath, R. P., Garvik, T. I., Liland, F., & Arulkumaran, S. (2017). Blood flow changes in pelvic vessels associated with the application of an abdominal compression belt in healthy postpartum women. *Ceylon Medical Journal, 62*(4), 228–232. https://doi.org/10.4038/cmj.v62i4.8572

Diop, A., Abbas, D., Martin, R., Razafi, A., Tuyet, H. T. D., & Winikoff, B. (2020). A double-blind, randomized controlled trial to explore oral tranexamic acid as adjunct for the treatment for postpartum hemorrhage. *Reproductive Health, 17*(1), 34. https://doi.org/10.1186/s12978-020-0887-2

Dixon, L., Tracy, S. K., Guilliland, K., Fletcher, L., Hendry, C., & Pairman, S. (2013). Outcomes of physiological and active third stage labour care amongst women in New Zealand. *Midwifery, 29*(1), 67–74. https://doi.org/10.1016/j.midw.2011.11.003

Du, Y., Ye, M., & Zheng, F. (2014). Active management of the third stage of labor with and without controlled cord traction: A systematic review and meta-analysis of randomized controlled trials. *Acta Obstetricia et Gynecologica Scandinavica, 93*(7), 626–633. https://doi.org/10.1111/aogs.12424

Dueckelmann, A. M., Hinkson, L., Nonnenmacher, A., Siedentopf, J. P., Schoenborn, I., Weizsaecker, K., . . . Braun, T. (2019). Uterine packing with chitosan-covered gauze compared to balloon tamponade for managing postpartum hemorrhage. *European Journal of Obstetrics & Gynecology and Reproductive Biology, 240*, 151–155. https://doi.org/10.1016/j.ejogrb.2019.06.003

El Ayadi, A. M., Robinson, N., Geller, S., & Miller, S. (2013). Advances in the treatment of postpartum hemorrhage. *Expert Review of Obstetrics & Gynecology, 8*(6), 525–537. Retrieved from https://www.researchgate.net/publication/262794851_Advances_in_the_treatment_of_postpartum_hemorrhage

Elfayomy, A. K. (2015). Carbetocin versus intra-umbilical oxytocin in the management of retained placenta: A randomized clinical study. *Journal of Obstetrics and Gynaecology Research, 41*(8), 1207–1213. https://doi.org/10.1111/jog.12702

Ende, H. B., & Butwick, A. J. (2021). Current state and future direction of postpartum hemorrhage risk assessment. *Obstetrics & Gynecology, 138*(6). 924–930. https://doi.org/10.1097/AOG.0000000000004579

Erickson, E. N., Bovbjerg, M. L., & Cheyney, M. J. (2020). Factors affecting third-stage management and postpartum hemorrhage in planned midwife-led home and birth center births in the United States. *Birth, 47*(4), 397–408. https://doi.org/10.1111/birt.12497

Erickson, E. N., Lee, C. S., Grose, E., & Emeis, C. (2019). Physiologic childbirth and active management of the third stage of labor: A latent class model of risk for postpartum hemorrhage. *Birth, 46*(1), 69–79. https://doi.org/10.1111/birt.12384

Escobar, M. F., Nassar, A. H., Theron, G., Barnea, E. R., Nicholson, W., Ramasauskaite, D., . . . Wright, A. (2022). FIGO recommendations on the management of postpartum hemorrhage 2022. *International Journal of Gynecology & Obstetrics, 157*(S1), 3–50. https://doi.org/10.1002/ijgo.14116

Evensen, A., Anderson, J. M., & Fontaine, P. (2017). Postpartum hemorrhage: Prevention and treatment [Updated version of printed article]. *American Family Physician, 95*(7), 442–449. Retrieved from http://www.aafp.org/afp/2017/0401/p442.html

Evensen, A. E., & Anderson, J. M. (2020). Postpartum hemorrhage. In L. Leeman, L. Dresang, J. S. Quinlan, & S. R. Magee (Eds.), *Advanced life support in obstetrics: Provider manual* (9th ed., pp. 187–204). Leawood, KS: American Academy of Family Physicians.

Fahy, K., Hastie, C., Bisits, A., Marsh, C., Smith, L., & Saxton, A. (2010). Holistic physiological care compared with active management of the third stage of labour for women at low risk of postpartum haemorrhage: A cohort study. *Women and Birth, 23*(4), 146–152. https://doi.org/10.1016/j.wombi.2010.02.003

Florida Perinatal Quality Collaborative. (2015). *Florida Obstetric Hemorrhage Initiative (OHI) tool kit: A quality improvement initiative for obstetric hemorrhage management* (version 10). Retrieved from http://health.usf.edu/publichealth/chiles/fpqc/~/media/5EB396812B504B2ABC336812AE82D412.ashx

Fox, K. A. (2023). Postpartum hemorrhage: Use of intrauterine tamponade to control bleeding. In A. Chakrabarti (Ed.), *UpToDate*. Retrieved November 13, 2023, from https://www.uptodate.com/contents/postpartum-hemorrhage-use-of-intrauterine-tamponade-to-control-bleeding

Franchini, M., & Mannucci, P. M. (2020). The never ending success story of tranexamic acid in acquired bleeding. *Haematologica, 105*(5), 1201–1205. https://doi.org/10.3324/haematol.2020.250720

Francois, K. E., & Foley, M. R. (2021). Antepartum and postpartum hemorrhage. In M. B. Landon, H. L. Galan, E. R. M. Jauniaux, D. A. Driscoll, V. Berghella, W. A. Grobman, . . . A. G. Cahill (Eds.), *Gabbe's obstetrics: Normal and problem pregnancies* (8th ed., Kindle version, ch. 18). Philadelphia, PA: Elsevier.

Frye, A. (2013). *Holistic midwifery: A comprehensive textbook for midwives in homebirth practice, vol. II: Care of the mother and baby from the onset of labor through the first hours after birth* (2nd ed.). Portland, OR: Labrys Press.

Funai, E. F., & Norwitz, E. R. (2023a). Labor and delivery: Management of the normal first stage. In V. A. Barss (Ed.), *UpToDate*. Retrieved November 13, 2023, from https://www.uptodate.com/contents/labor-and-delivery-management-of-the-normal-first-stage

Funai, E. F., & Norwitz, E. R. (2023b). Labor and delivery: Management of the normal third stage after vaginal birth. In V. A. Barss (Ed.), *UpToDate*. Retrieved November 13, 2023, from https://www.uptodate.com/contents/labor-and-delivery-management-of-the-normal-third-stage-after-vaginal-birth

Gabr, A. K. (2019). The importance of nontechnical skills in leading cardiopulmonary resuscitation teams. *Journal of the Royal College of Physicians of Edinburgh, 49*(2), 112–116. https://doi.org/10.4997/jrcpe.2019.205

Gadappa, S., Yelikar, K., & Wanjare, N. (2015). Study of inversion of uterus in tertiary care hospital. *Journal of Evolution of Medical and Dental Sciences, 4*(98), 16305–16308. https://doi.org/10.14260/jemds/2015/2406

Galabin, A. L., & Blacker, G. (1910). *The practice of midwifery* (7th ed.). New York, NY: Macmillan. Retrieved from https://babel.hathitrust.org/cgi/pt?id=nnc2.ark:/13960/t5r79382m&view=1up&seq=7

Georgiou, C. (2009). Balloon tamponade in the management of postpartum haemorrhage: A review. *BJOG, 116* (6), 748–757. https://doi.org/10.1111/j.1471-0528.2009.02113.x

Georgiou, C. (2014). A review of current practice in using balloon tamponade technology in the management of postpartum haemorrhage. *Hypertension Research in Pregnancy, 2*(1), 1–10. https://doi.org/10.14390/jsshp.2.1

Ghirardini, G., Alboni, C., & Mabrouk, M. (2012). Use of balloon tamponade in management of severe vaginal postpartum hemorrhage and vaginal hematoma: A case series. *Gynecologic and Obstetric Investigation, 74*(4), 320–323. https://doi.org/10.1159/000339931

Giger, R. K. A., & Engel, G. (2006). Albert Hofmann's pioneering work on ergot alkaloids and its impact on the search of novel drugs at Sandoz, a predecessor company of Novartis: Dedicated to Dr. Albert Hofmann on the occasion of his 100th birthday. *CHIMIA International Journal for Chemistry, 60*(1–2), 83–87. https://doi.org/10.2533/000942906777675164

Gilad, O., Merlob, P., Stahl, B., Averbuch, N., & Klinger, G. (2017). Outcome of breastfed infants following post-partum methylergonovine treatment. *Journal of Maternal-Fetal & Neonatal Medicine, 30*(13), 1569–1573. https://doi.org/10.1080/14767058.2016.1212831

Gill, P., Patel, A., & Van Hook, J. W. (2023). Uterine atony. In *StatPearls*. Treasure Island, FL: StatPearls Publishing. Retrieved November 13, 2023, from https://www.ncbi.nlm.nih.gov/books/NBK493238/

Gilmandyar, D., & Thornburg, L. L. (2019). Surgical management of postpartum hemorrhage. *Seminars in Perinatology, 43*(1), 27–34. https://doi.org/10.1053/j.semperi.2018.11.006

Greenbaum, S., Wainstock, T., Dukler, D., Leron, E., & Erez, E. (2017). Underlying mechanisms of retained placenta: Evidence from a population based cohort study. *European Journal of Obstetrics & Gynecology and Reproductive Biology 216*, 12–17. https://doi.org/10.1016/j.ejogrb.2017.06.035

Grönvall, M., Tikkanen, M., Tallberg, E., Paavonen, J., & Stefanovic, V. (2013). Use of Bakri balloon tamponade in the treatment of postpartum hemorrhage: A series of 50 cases from a tertiary teaching hospital. *Acta Obstetricia et Gynecologica Scandinavica, 92*(4), 433–43. https://doi.org/10.1111/j.1600-0412.2012.01531.x

Groom, K. M., & Jacobson, T. Z. (2012). The management of secondary postpartum hemorrhage. In S. Arulkumaran, M. Karoshi, L. G. Keith, A. B. Lalonde, & C. B-Lynch (Eds.), *A comprehensive textbook of postpartum hemorrhage: An essential clinical reference for effective management* (2nd ed.), pp. 466–473. London, United Kingdom: Sapiens Publishing. Retrieved from http://www.glowm.com/pdf/PPH_2nd_edn_Chap-56.pdf

Gülmezoglu, A. M., Lumbiganon, P., Landoulsi, S., Widmer, M., Abdel-Aleem, H., Festin, M., . . . Elbourne, D. (2012). Active management of the third stage of labour with and without controlled cord traction: A randomised, controlled, non-inferiority trial. *Lancet, 379*(9827), 1721–1727. https://doi.org/10.1016/S0140-6736(12)60206-2

Hale, B., & Habib, A. S. (2014). Sheehan syndrome: Acute presentation with severe headache. *International Journal of Obstetric Anesthesia, 23*(4), 383–386. https://doi.org/10.1016/j.ijoa.2014.04.011

Hamou, B., Sheiner, E., Coreanu, T., Walfisch, A., & Silberstein, T. (2020). Intrapartum cervical lacerations and their impact on future pregnancy outcome. *Journal of Maternal-Fetal & Neonatal Medicine, 33*(5), 883–887. https://doi.org/10.1080/14767058.2018.1505852

Hasabe, R., Gupta, K., & Rathode, P. (2016). Use of condom tamponade to manage massive obstetric hemorrhage at a tertiary center in Rajasthan. *Journal of Obstetrics and Gynecology of India, 66*(Suppl. 1), 88–93. https://doi.org/10.1007/s13224-015-0790-x

Hastie, C., & Fahy, K. M. (2009). Optimising psychophysiology in the third stage of labour: Theory applied to practice. *Women and Birth, 22*(3), 89–96. https://doi.org/10.1016/j.wombi.2009.02.004

Henry, V. (2016). *Front view of postpartum uterine massage* [Illustration]. Retrieved from https://en.m.wikipedia.org/wiki/File:Front_View_of_Postpartum_Uterine_Massage.png

Hinkson, L., Suermann, M. A., Hinkson, S., & Henrich, W. (2017). The windmill technique avoids manual removal of the retained placenta—A new solution for an old problem. *European Journal of Obstetrics & Gynecology and Reproductive Biology, 215*, 6–11. https://doi.org/10.1016/j.ejogrb.2017.05.028

Hofer, S., Blaha, J., Collins, P. W., Ducloy-Bouthors, A. S., Guasch, E., Labate, F., . . . Van de Velde, M. (2023). Haemostatic support in postpartum haemorrhage: A review of the literature and expert opinion. *European Journal of Anaesthesiology, 40*(1), 29–8. https://doi.org/10.1097/EJA.0000000000001744

Hofmeyr, G. J., Mshweshwe, N. T., & Gülmezoglu, A. M. (2015). Controlled cord traction for the third stage of labour. *Cochrane Database of Systematic Reviews, 2015*(1). https://doi.org/10.1002/14651858.CD008020.pub2

Huque, S., Roberts, I., Fawole, B., Chaudhri, R., Arulkumaran, S., & Shakur-Still, H. (2018). Risk factors for peripartum hysterectomy among women with postpartum haemorrhage: Analysis of data from the WOMAN trial. *BMC Pregnancy and Childbirth, 18*(1), 186. https://doi.org/10.1186/s12884-018-1829-7

Ibrahim, S. M., Mustafa, E., & Louon, A. (2008). Postpartum severe sinus bradycardia following methylergonovine administration. *Journal of International Medical Research, 36*(5), 1129–1133. https://doi.org/10.1177/147323000803600534

Jackson, K. W., Jr., Allbert, J. R., Schemmer, G. K., Elliot, M., Humphrey, A., & Taylor, J. (2001). A randomized controlled trial comparing oxytocin administration before and after placental delivery in the prevention of postpartum hemorrhage. *American Journal of Obstetrics & Gynecology, 185*(4), 873–877. https://doi.org/10.1067/mob.2001.117363

Jan, A., Beenish, Mr. [*sic*], & Hamid, A. (2015). Comparative study of uterine gauze packaging [*sic*] and Sangestaken Blackmore [*sic*] esophageal catheter for the management of PPH. *International Journal of Advanced Research, 3*(9), 398–401. Retrieved from http://www.journalijar.com/uploads/722_IJAR-6990.pdf

Jashnani, K. D., & Wani, R. J. (2022). Cervical trauma: Clinical conundrum and correlation. In K. D. Jashnani (Ed.), *Maternal mortality—Lessons learnt from autopsy* (pp. 25–30). Singapore: Springer. https://doi.org/10.1007/978-981-19-3420-9_6

Jauniaux, E. R. M., Alfirevic, Z., Bhide, A. G., Belfort, M. A., Burton, G. J., Collins, S. L., . . . Sentilhes, L. (2018). Placenta praevia and placenta accreta: Diagnosis and Management (Green-top Guideline 27a). *BJOG, 126*(1), e1–e48. https://doi.org/10.1111/1471-0528.15306

Jayakumar, R., Prabaharan, M., Sudheesh Kumar, P. T., Nair, S. V., & Tamura, H. (2011). Biomaterials based on chitin and chitosan in wound dressing applications. *Biotechnology Advances, 29*(3), 322–337. https://doi.org/10.1016/j.biotechadv.2011.01.005

Johanson, R., Kumar, M., Obhrai, M., & Young, P. (2001). Management of massive postpartum haemorrhage: Use of a hydrostatic balloon catheter to avoid laparotomy. *BJOG, 108*(4), 420–422. https://doi.org/10.1111/j.1471-0528.2001.00102.x

Joint Commission. (2010). *Preventing maternal death* (Sentinel Event Alert 44). Retrieved from https://web.archive.org/web/20151015002935/https://www.jointcommission.org/assets/1/18/SEA_44.PDF

Karimi, F. Z., Miri, H. H., Salehian, M., Khadivzadeh, T., & Bakhshi, M. (2019). The effect of mother-infant skin to skin contact after birth on third stage of labor: A systematic review and meta-analysis. *Iranian Journal of Public Health, 48*(4), 612–620. Retrieved from https://www.ncbi.nlm.nih.gov/pmc/articles/PMC6500522/

Karoshi, M., Palacios-Jaraquemada, J. M., & Keith, L. G. (2012). Managing the ten most common life-threatening scenarios associated with postpartum hemorrhage. In S. Arulkumaran, M. Karoshi, L. G. Keith, A. B. Lalonde, & C. B. Lynch (Eds.), *A comprehensive textbook of postpartum hemorrhage: An essential clinical reference for effective management* (2nd ed., pp. 3–18). London, United Kingdom: Sapiens Publishing. Retrieved from https://www.glowm.com/pdf/PPH_2nd_edn_Chap-01.pdf

Keriakos, R., & Mukhopadhyay, A. (2006). The use of the Rusch balloon for management of severe postpartum haemorrhage. *Journal of Obstetrics and Gynaecology, 26*(4), 335–338. https://doi.org/10.1080/01443610600595077

Kikuchi, N., Ohira, S., Asaka, R., Takatsu, A., Kobara, H., Ando, H., . . . Shiozawa, T. (2016). A case of vaginal varices that caused massive bleeding after vaginal delivery. *Shinshu Medical Journal, 64*(1), 35–39. https://doi.org/10.11441/shinshumedj.64.35

Kobayashi, T., Tanaka, T., Kawata, M., Oguma, K., Ito, S., Matsuzawa, N., . . . Kaneda, H. (2020). Intrauterine gauze or balloon tamponade for the management of postpartum hemorrhage due to uterine atony during maternal transportation. *Hypertension Research in Pregnancy, 8*(2), 57–60. https://doi.org/10.14390/jsshp.HRP2020-003

Kodkany, B. S., Derman, R. J., & Sloan, N. L. (2012). Pitfalls in assessing blood loss and decision to transfer. In S. Arulkumaran, M. Karoshi, L. G. Keith, A. B. Lalonde, & C. B-Lynch (Eds.), *A comprehensive textbook of postpartum hemorrhage: An essential clinical reference for effective management* (2nd ed., pp. 81–88). London, United Kingdom: Sapiens Publishing. Retrieved from http://www.glowm.com/pdf/PPH_2nd_edn_Chap-11.pdf

Koh, P. R., Di Filippo, D., Bisits, A., & Welsh, A. W. (2020). Bimanual examination for clot evacuation: A retrospective cohort study of women with postpartum haemorrhage after vaginal delivery. *BMC Pregnancy and Childbirth, 20*, 245. https://doi.org/10.1186/s12884-020-02916-w

Kroener, B., & Toman, R. (2020). In patients with PPH, does IV infusion of tranexamic acid reduce morbidity and mortality? *Evidence-Based Practice, 23*(1), 13–14. https://doi.org/10.1097/EBP.0000000000000479

Kumar, A. (2014). Monument of love or symbol of maternal death: The story behind the Taj Mahal. *Case Reports in Women's Health, 1*(2),4–7. https://doi.org/10.1016/j.crwh.2014.07.001

Kumar, N., Shayesteh, J., Haas, D. M., & Weeks, A. D. (2021). Umbilical vein injection for management of retained placenta. *Cochrane Database of Systematic Reviews, 2021*(3). https://doi.org/10.1002/14651858.CD001337.pub3

Lagrew, D., Libova, O., & Lyndon, A. (2022). Active management of third stage labor. In D. Lagrew, J. McNulty, C. Sakowski, V. Cape, E. McCormick, & C. H. Morton (Eds.), *Improving health care response to obstetric hemorrhage, v. 3.0: A CMQCC quality improvement toolkit* (pp. 89–92). Palo Alto, CA: California Maternal Quality Care Collaborative. Retrieved from https://www.cmqcc.org/sites/default/files/HEMToolkit_03252022 Errata 7.2022 (2).pdf

Lalonde, A., & FIGO Safe Motherhood Committee. (2012). Prevention and treatment of postpartum hemorrhage in low-resource settings. *International Journal of Gynecology & Obstetrics, 117*(2), 108–118. https://doi.org/10.1016/j.ijgo.2012.03.001

Lalonde, A. B., Liljestrand, J., Rushwan, H., & Okong, P. (2012). Postpartum hemorrhage today: Living in the shadow of the Taj Mahal. In S. Arulkumaran, M. Karoshi, L. G. Keith, A. B. Lalonde, & C. B-Lynch (Eds.), *A comprehensive textbook of postpartum hemorrhage: An essential clinical reference for effective management* (2nd ed., pp. 64–70). London, United Kingdom: Sapiens Publishing. Retrieved from http://www.glowm.com/pdf/PPH_2nd_edn_Chap-08.pdf

Landy, H. J., Laughon, S. K., Bailit, J. L., Kominiarek, M. A., Gonzalez-Quintero, V. H., Ramirez, M., . . . Consortium on Safe Labor. (2011). Characteristics associated with severe perineal and cervical lacerations during vaginal delivery. *Obstetrics & Gynecology, 117*(3), 627–635. https://doi.org/10.1097/aog.0b013e31820afaf2

Lashin, M. E.-B. (2020). Umbilical vein oxytocin injection versus umbilical cord drainage in management of third stage of normal vaginal delivery: A randomized controlled trial. *Open Journal of Obstetrics and Gynecology, 10*(5), 634–643. https://doi.org/10.4236/ojog.2020.1050057

Laufer, M. R., & Makai, G. (2023). Evaluation and management of female lower genital tract trauma. In A. Chakrabarti (Ed.*), UpToDate*. Retrieved November 13, 2023, from https://www.uptodate.com/contents/evaluation-and-management-of-female-lower-genital-tract-trauma

Levi, M. M. (2022, Aug. 23). Disseminated intravascular coagulation (DIC) clinical presentation. *Medscape*. Retrieved from https://emedicine.medscape.com/article/199627-clinical?0=reg=1

Lim, P. S., Shafiee, M. N., Kampan, N. C., Sulaiman, A. S., Ghani, N. A. A., Ismail, N. M., . . . Yassin, M. A. J. M. (2012). Uterine atony: Management strategies. In P. Kochhar (Ed.), *Blood transfusion in clinical practice* (pp. 97–128). Rijeka, Croatia: InTech. https://doi.org/10.5772/33272

Liu, C.-N., Yu, F.-B., Xu, Y.-Z., Li, J.-S., Guan, Z.-H., Sun, M.-N., . . . Chen, D.-J. (2021). Prevalence and risk factors of severe postpartum hemorrhage: A retrospective cohort study. *BMC Pregnancy and Childbirth, 21*(1), 1–8. https://doi.org/10.1186/s12884-021-03818-1

Lupin Pharmaceuticals. (2017). *About Methergine*. Retrieved from https://www.methergine.com/about-methergine

Macones, G. (2023). Puerperal uterine inversion. In V. A. Barss (Ed.), *UpToDate*. Retrieved November 13, 2023, from https://www.uptodate.com/contents/puerperal-uterine-inversion

Maier, R. C. (1993). Control of postpartum hemorrhage with uterine packing. *American Journal of Obstetrics & Gynecology, 169*(2, Pt. 1), 317–323. https://doi.org/10.1016/0002-9378(93)90082-T

Main, E., Martin, C., McNulty, J., & Vincent, J. (2022). Uterine tamponade for postpartum hemorrhage: Internal balloons and external compression stitches. In D. Lagrew, J. McNulty, C. Sakowski, V. Cape, E. McCormick, & C. H. Morton (Eds.), *Improving health care response to obstetric hemorrhage, v. 3.0: A CMQCC quality improvement toolkit* (pp. 134–142). Palo Alto, CA: California Maternal Quality Care Collaborative. Retrieved from https://www.cmqcc.org/sites/default/files/HEMToolkit_03252022 Errata 7.2022 (2).pdf

Main, E., Martin, C., Romine, L., & Thomas, A. (2022). Definition, early recognition and rapid response to obstetric hemorrhage using triggers. In D. Lagrew, J. McNulty, C. Sakowski, V. Cape, E. McCormick, & C. H. Morton (Eds.), *Improving health care response to obstetric hemorrhage, v. 3.0: A CMQCC quality improvement toolkit* (pp. 93–103). Palo Alto, CA: California Maternal Quality Care Collaborative. Retrieved from https://www.cmqcc.org/sites/default/files/HEMToolkit_03252022 Errata 7.2022 (2).pdf

Main, E. K., Goffman, D., Scavone, B. M., Low, L. K., Bingham, D., Fontaine, P. L., . . . Levy, B. S. (2015). National partnership for maternal safety: Consensus bundle on obstetric hemorrhage. *Journal of Obstetric, Gynecologic, & Neonatal Nursing, 44*(4), 462–470. https://doi.org/10.1111/1552-6909.12723

Makin, J., Suarez-Rebling, D. I., Varma Shivkumar, P., Tarimo, V., & Burke, T. F. (2018). Innovative uses of condom uterine balloon tamponade for postpartum hemorrhage in India and Tanzania. *Case Reports in Obstetrics and Gynecology, 2018*. https://doi.org/10.1155%2F2018%2F4952048

Martins, H. E. L., de Souza, M. L., Khanum, S., Naz, N., & Souza, A. C. R. H. (2016). The practice of nursing in the prevention and control of postpartum hemorrhage: An integrative review. *American Journal of Nursing Science, 5*(1), 8–15. https://doi.org/10.11648/j.ajns.20160501.12

Marwaha, A., Singh, P., & Naniwal, A. (2016). Role of intrauterine packing in primary post partum haemorrhage. *International Journal of Scientific Research, 5*(7). https://www.worldwidejournals.com/international-journal-of-scientific-research-(IJSR)/article/role-of-intrauterine-packing-in-primary-post-partum-haemorrhage/ODQxNw==/

Matsubara, S., Kuwata, T., Usui, R., & Ohkuchi, A. (2013). 'Holding the cervix' technique for post-partum hemorrhage for achieving hemostasis as well as preventing prolapse of an intrauterine balloon. *Journal of Obstetrics and Gynaecology Research, 39*(5), 1116–1117. https://doi.org/10.1111/jog.12019

Maul, H., Steinmacher, S., Saade, G., Gebauer, G., Rolf, N., & Schmid, B. (2015). Uterine packing with chitosan-covered gauze (Celox) for control of postpartum hemorrhage (PPH). *American Journal of Obstetrics & Gynecology, 212*(1, Suppl.), S358–S359. https://doi.org/10.1016/j.ajog.2014.10.940

Mavrides, E., Allard, S., Chandraharan, E., Collins, P., Green, L., Hunt, B. J., . . . Thomson, A. J. (2016). Prevention and management of postpartum haemorrhage (Green-top Guideline 52). *BJOG, 124*, e106–e149. Retrieved from https://www.rcog.org.uk/en/guidelines-research-services/guidelines/gtg52/

Maya, E. T., Buntugu, K. A., Aki, L., & Srofenyoh, E. K. (2015). Condom tamponade in the management of primary postpartum haemorrhage: A report of three cases in Ghana. *African Journal of Reproductive Health, 19*(3), 151–157. Retrieved from https://www.ajrh.info/index.php/ajrh/article/view/862

McCall, S. J., Deneux-Tharaux, C., Sentilhes, L., Ramakrishnan, R., Collins, S. L., Seco, A., . . . Kayem, G. (2022). Placenta accreta spectrum—variations in clinical practice and maternal morbidity between the UK and France: A population-based comparative study. *BJOG, 129*(10), 1676–1685. https://doi.org/10.1111/1471-0528.17169

Mielke, R. T., & Obermeyer, S. (2020). The use of tranexamic acid to prevent postpartum hemorrhage. *Journal of Midwifery & Women's Health, 65*(3), 410–416. https://doi.org/10.1111/jmwh.13101

Miller, D. T., Roque, D. M., & Santin, A. D. (2015). Use of Monsel's solution to treat obstetrical hemorrhage: A review and comparison to other topical hemostatic agents. *American Journal of Obstetrics & Gynecology, 212*(6), 725–735. https://doi.org/10.1016/j.ajog.2014.12.029

Miller, S., Lester, F., & Hensleigh, P. (2004). CEU: prevention and treatment of postpartum hemorrhage: New advances for low-resource settings. *Journal of Midwifery & Women's Health, 49*(4), 283–292. https://doi.org/10.1016/j.jmwh.2004.04.001

Mishra, N., Nekkanti, L. P., Barma, P., & Mishra, I. (2021). Adjunctive misoprostol for prevention of post-partum haemorrhage: A pragmatic strategy of selective sequential administration. *International Journal of Reproduction, Contraception, Obstetrics and Gynecology, 10*(2), 669–676. https://doi.org/10.18203/2320-1770.ijrcog20210325

A model practice template for hydrotherapy in labor and birth. (2017). *Journal of Midwifery & Women's Health, 62*(1), 120–126. https://doi.org/10.1111/jmwh.12587

Mollazadeh-Moghaddam, K., Dundek, M., Bellare, A., Borovac-Pinheiro, A., Won, A., & Burke, T. F. (2019). Mechanical properties of the Every Second Matters for Mothers-Uterine Balloon Tamponade (ESM-UBT) device: In vitro tests. *AJP Reports, 9*(4), e376–e383. https://doi.org/10.1055/s-0039-1697653

Nag, D. S., Datta, M. R., Samaddar, D. P., & Panigrahi, B. (2015). Cardiac arrest following acute puerperal uterine inversion. *Case Reports, 2015*. https://doi.org/10.1136/bcr-2014-207175

Najafian, A., Ghasemi, M., & Hajiha-Esfahani, N. (2018). Umbilical vein injection of misoprostol versus oxytocin for managing retained placenta after parturition: A randomized clinical trial. *International Journal of Women's Health and Reproduction Sciences, 6*(3), 297–301. Retrieved from https://ijwhr.net/pdf/pdf_IJWHR_297.pdf

Nalini, N., Singh, A. V., Bijeta, S. S., & Singh, J. K. (2017). Uterine balloon tamponade by JH balloon: A simple, efficient and cost effective method. *Journal of Contemporary Medical Research, 4*(3), 645–649. Retrieved from https://www.ijcmr.com/uploads/7/7/4/6/77464738/ijcmr_1335_march_32.pdf

National Institute of Child Health and Human Development. (2018, Oct 31). *Methylergonovine*. Retrieved from https://www.ncbi.nlm.nih.gov/books/NBK501342/

Nayak, M. (2020). Retained placenta delivery using Windmill technique: A novel step towards solution with self-developed conceptual model. *European Journal of Molecular & Clinical Medicine, 7*(8), 1470–1476. Retrieved from https://ejmcm.com/article_4318_2eb619833f287d186c7e7fda673faf3a.pdf

Nazeer, S., Rehman, M., Tahir, S., Saeed, K., & Gul, A. (2016). Umbilical vein injection of misoprostol vs Syntocinon in normal saline for the treatment of retained placenta: Randomized control trial. *Pakistan journal of Medical and Health Sciences, 10*(4), 1374–1377. Retrieved from https://pjmhsonline.com/2016/oct_dec/pdf/1374.pdf

Nizam, K., & Haider, G. (2010). Role of uterovaginal packing in postpartum hemorrhage. *Journal of the Liaquat University of Medical and Health Sciences, 9*(1), 27–29. Retrieved from http://lumhs.edu.pk/jlumhs/Vol09No01/pdfs/v9n1oa06.pdf

Nutter, E., Meyer, S., Shaw-Battista, J., & Marowitz, A. (2014). Waterbirth: An integrative analysis of peer-reviewed literature. *Journal of Midwifery & Women's Health, 59*(3), 286–319. https://doi.org/10.1111/jmwh.12194

Ottun, T. A., Adewunmi, A. A., Rabiu, A. K., Olumodeji, A. M., Oladipo, O. M., & Olalere, H. F. (2022). Misoprostol and oxytocin versus oxytocin alone in the active management of the third stage of labour: A randomized, double-blind, placebo-controlled trial. *Journal of Obstetrics and Gynaecology, 42*(5), 1048–1053. https://doi.org/10.1080/01443615.2021.1995342

Pacheco, L. D., Hankins, G. D. V., Saad, A. F., Costantine, M. M., Chiossi, G., & Saade, G. R. (2017). Tranexamic acid for the management of obstetric hemorrhage. *Obstetrics & Gynecology, 130*(4), 765–769. https://doi.org/10.1097/aog.0000000000002253

Pandey, A. K., Neogi, S. B., Gautam, D., & Raushan, M. R. (2023). New realm of placenta accreta spectrum disorder: Are we doing enough? *Lancet Regional Health—Southeast Asia, 14*. https://doi.org/10.1016/j.lansea.2023.100173

Paterson-Brown, S. & Bamber, J. (2014). Prevention and treatment of haemorrhage. In M. Knight, S. Kenyon, P. Brocklehurst, J. Neilson, J. Shakespeare, & J. J. Kurinczuk (Eds.), *Saving lives, improving mothers' care—Lessons learned to inform future maternity care from the UK and Ireland confidential enquiries into maternal deaths and morbidity 2009–2012* (pp. 45–55). Oxford, United Kingdom: National Perinatal Epidemiology Unit.

Patra, K. K., Chattopadhyay, S., Dey, A., Sarkar, C., Chakraborty, A., & Bhattacharyya, S. (2017). Umbilical vein injection of misoprostol versus normal saline for the treatment of retained placenta in a tertiary care centre—A non-randomised controlled trial. *Journal of Evolution of Medical and Dental Sciences, 6*(60), 4384–4387. http://dx.doi.org/10.14260/Jemds/2017/948

Patton-Molitors, R., Gubin, R., Gross, M., & Bartlett, L. (2015). *Literature Review: Improving management of postpartum hemorrhage with blood innovations*. Baltimore, MD: Jhpiego. Retrieved from http://reprolineplus.org/system/files/resources/PPH-blood-lit-review-2015Decrev.pdf

Perlman, N. C., & Carusi, D. A. (2019). Retained placenta after vaginal delivery: Risk factors and management. *International Journal of Women's Health, 2019*(11), 527–534. https://doi.org/10.2147/IJWH.S218933

Phillips, J. M., Eppes, C., Rodriguez, M., & Sakamoto, S. (2022). Traditional uterine tamponade and vacuum-induced uterine tamponade devices in obstetric hemorrhage management. *American Journal of Obstetrics & Gynecology MFM, 5*(25), 100739. https://doi.org/10.1016/j.ajogmf.2022.100739

Picetti, R., Miller, L., Shakur-Still, H., Pepple, T., Beaumont, D., Balogun, E., . . . WOMAN Trial Collaborators. (2020). The WOMAN trial: Clinical and contextual factors surrounding the deaths of 483 women following post-partum haemorrhage in developing countries. *BMC Pregnancy and Childbirth, 20*, 409. https://doi.org/10.1186/s12884-020-03091-8

Pinborg, A., Bødker, B., & Høgdall, C. (2000). Postpartum hematoma and vaginal packing with a blood pressure cuff. *Acta Obstetricia et Gynecologica Scandinavica, 79*(10), 887–889. https://doi.org/10.1034/j.1600-0412.2000.079010887.x

Powell, C., & Slaughter, J. (2021). Does the addition of misoprostol to the active management of the third stage of labor result in fewer postpartum hemorrhages? *Evidence-Based Practice, 24*(8), 12–13. https://doi.org/10.1097/EBP.0000000000001081

Purwosunu, Y., Sarkoen, W., Arulkumaran, S., & Segnitz, J. (2016). Control of postpartum hemorrhage using vacuum-induced uterine tamponade. *Obstetrics & Gynecology, 128*(1), 33–36. https://doi.org/10.1097/AOG.0000000000001473

Queensland Clinical Guidelines. (2021). *Primary postpartum haemorrhage*. Brisbane, Australia: Queensland Health. Retrieved from https://www.health.qld.gov.au/__data/assets/pdf_file/0015/140136/g-pph.pdf

Rac, M. W. F., Dashe, J. S., Wells, C. E., Moschos, E., McIntire, D. D., & Twickler, D. M. (2015). Ultrasound predictors of placental invasion: The placenta accreta index. *American Journal of Obstetrics & Gynecology, 212*(3), 343.e1–343.e7. https://doi.org/10.1016/j.ajog.2014.10.022

Rajab, S. S., & Alalaf, S. K. (2014). Umbilical vein injection of misoprostol versus normal saline for the treatment of retained placenta: Intrapartum placebo-controlled trial. *BMC Pregnancy and Childbirth, 14*, 37. https://doi.org/10.1186/1471-2393-14–37

Ramler, P. I., Beenakkers, I. C. M., Bloemenkamp, K. W. M., Van der Bom, J. G., Braams-Lisman, B. A. M., Cornette, J. M. J., . . . Van den Akker, T. (2022). Nationwide confidential enquiries into maternal deaths because of obstetric hemorrhage in the Netherlands between 2006 and 2019. *Acta Obstetricia et Gynecologica Scandinavica, 101*(4), 450–460. https://doi.org/10.1111/aogs.14321

Rath, W. H. (2011), Postpartum hemorrhage—Update on problems of definitions and diagnosis. *Acta Obstetricia et Gynecologica Scandinavica, 90*(5), 421–428. https://doi.org/10.1111/j.1600-0412.2011.01107.x

Robinson, D., Basso, M., Chan, C., Duckitt, K., & Lett, R. (2022). Postpartum Hemorrhage and Hemorrhagic Shock (Guideline 431). *Journal of Obstetrics and Gynaecology Canada, 44*(12), 1293–1310.e1. https://doi.org/10.1016/j.jogc.2022.10.002

Rodriguez, M. I., Jensen, J. T., Gregory, K., Bullard, M., Longo, P., Heidel, J., & Edelman, A. (2017). A novel tamponade agent for management of post partum hemorrhage: adaptation of the Xstat mini-sponge applicator for obstetric use. *BMC Pregnancy and Childbirth 17*, 187. https://doi.org/10.1186/s12884-017-1373-x

Roman, A. S. (2023). Management of hematomas incurred as a result of obstetric delivery. In K. Eckler (Ed.*), UpToDate*. Retrieved November 13, 2023, from https://www.uptodate.com/contents/management-of-hematomas-incurred-as-a-result-of-obstetric-delivery

Roper, J. C., Thakar, R. & Sultan, A. H. (2021). Isolated rectal buttonhole tears in obstetrics: Case series and review of the literature. *International Urogynecology Journal, 32*(7), 1761–1769. https://doi.org/10.1007/s00192-020-04502-2

Rouse, D. J. (2013). What is new in postpartum hemorrhage? Best articles from the past year. *Obstetrics & Gynecology, 122*(3), 693–4. https://doi.org/10.1097/AOG.0b013e3182a2c357

Saccone, G., Della Corte, L., D'Alessandro, P., Ardino, B., Carbone, L., Raffone, A., . . . Berghella, V. (2020). Prophylactic use of tranexamic acid after vaginal delivery reduces the risk of primary postpartum hemorrhage. *Journal of Maternal-Fetal & Neonatal Medicine, 33*(19), 3368–3376. https://doi.org/10.1080/14767058.2019.1571576

Salem, M. A. A., Saraya, Y. S., Badr, M. S., & Soliman, A.-Z. M. (2019). Intra-umbilical vein injection of carbetocin versus oxytocin in the management of retained placenta. *Sexual & Reproductive Healthcare, 21*, 21–25. https://doi.org/10.1016/j.srhc.2019.05.002

Saxton, A., Fahy, K., & Hastie, C. (2014). Effects of skin-to-skin contact and breastfeeding at birth on the incidence of PPH: A physiologically based theory. *Women and Birth, 27*(4), 250–253. https://doi.org/10.1016/j.wombi.2014.06.004

Schiff, P. L., Jr. (2006). Ergot and its alkaloids. *American Journal of Pharmaceutical Education, 70*(5), 98.

Schmid, B. C., Rezniczek, G. A., Rolf, N., & Maul, H. (2012). Postpartum hemorrhage: Use of hemostatic combat gauze. *American Journal of Obstetrics & Gynecology, 209*(1), e12–13. https://doi.org/10.1016/j.ajog.2011.09.018

Schmid, B. C., Rezniczek, G. A., Rolf, N., Saade, G., Gebauer, G., & Maul, H. (2013). Uterine packing with chitosan-covered gauze for control of postpartum hemorrhage. *American Journal of Obstetrics & Gynecology, 209*(3), 225.e1–5. https://doi.org/10.1016/j.ajog.2013.05.055

Schorn, M. N., & Phillippi, J. C. (2014). Volume replacement following severe postpartum hemorrhage. *Journal of Midwifery & Women's Health, 59*(3), 336–343. https://doi.org/10.1111/jmwh.12186

Segnitz, J., & Arulkumaran, S. (2017). Control of postpartum hemorrhage using vacuum-induced uterine tamponade [31M]. *Obstetrics & Gynecology, 129*(5), S140–S141. https://doi.org/10.1097/01.AOG.0000514702.64479.d1

Sellmyer, M. A., Desser, T. S., Maturen, K. E., Jeffrey, Jr., R. B., & Kamaya, A. (2013). Physiologic, histologic, and imaging features of retained products of conception. *RadioGraphics, 33*(3), 781–796. https://doi.org/10.1148/rg.333125177

Shakur, H., Beaumont, D., Pavord, S., Gayet-Ageron, A., Ker, K., & Mousa, H. A. (2018). Antifibrinolytic drugs for treating primary postpartum haemorrhage. *Cochrane Database of Systematic Reviews, 2018*(2). https://doi.org/10.1002/14651858.CD012964

Shakur, H., Roberts, I., Fawole, B., Chaudhri, R., El-Sheikh, M., Akintan, A., . . . Arakulmaran, S. (2017). Effect of early tranexamic acid administration on mortality, hysterectomy, and other morbidities in women with post-partum haemorrhage (WOMAN): An international, randomised, double-blind, placebo-controlled trial. *Lancet, 389*(10084), 2105–2116. https://doi.org/10.1016/S0140-6736(17)30638-4

Shakur-Still, H., Grassin-Delyle, S., Muhunthan, K., Ahmadzia, H. K., Faraoni, D., Arribas, M., & Roberts, I. (2022). Alternative routes to intravenous tranexamic acid for postpartum hemorrhage: A systematic search and narrative review. *International Journal of Gynecology & Obstetrics, 158*(Suppl. 1), 40–45. https://doi.org/10.1002/ijgo.14201

Shompa, L., Akhter, S., Nazneen, K., & Begum, M. (2014). Effect of oxytocin injection into umbilical vein for management of retained placenta. *Journal of Enam Medical College, 4*(2), 102–105. https://doi.org/10.3329/jemc.v4i2.19678

Silver, R. (2023). Placenta accreta spectrum: Clinical features, diagnosis, and potential consequences. In V. A. Barss (Ed.), *UpToDate*. Retrieved November 13, 2023, from https://www.uptodate.com/contents/placenta-accreta-spectrum-clinical-features-diagnosis-and-potential-consequences

Silver, R. M., & Branch, D. W. (2018). Placenta accreta spectrum. *New England Journal of Medicine, 378*(16), 1529–1536. https://doi.org/10.1056/NEJMcp1709324

Silver, R. M., Landon, M. B., Rouse, D. J., Leveno, K., Spong, C. Y., Thom, E. A., . . . Mercer, B. M. (2006). Maternal morbidity associated with multiple repeat cesarean deliveries. *Obstetrics & Gynecology, 107*(6),1226–1232. https://doi.org/10.1097/01.AOG.0000219750.79480.84

Simaika, Y. S. (2010). The 'trio' condom catheter: A modification of the condom catheter in the management of postpartum haemorrhage. *BJOG, 117*(3), 372. https://doi.org/10.1111/j.1471-0528.2009.02443.x

Smith, J. F., & Wax, J. R. (2022). Uterine rupture: Unscarred uterus. In V. A. Barss (Ed.), *UpToDate*. Retrieved November 13, 2023, from https://www.uptodate.com/contents/uterine-rupture-unscarred-uterus

Smith, W. R. P., Papadopoulou, A., Thomas, E., Tobias, A., Price, M. J., Meher, S., . . . Gallos, I. D. (2020). Uterotonic agents for first-line treatment of postpartum haemorrhage: A network meta-analysis. *Cochrane Database of Systematic Reviews*. https://doi.org/10.1002/14651858.cd012754.pub2

Snyder, P. J. (2022). Causes of hypopituitarism. In K. A. Martin (Ed.), *UpToDate*. Retrieved November 13, 2023, from https://www.uptodate.com/contents/causes-of-hypopituitarism

Somanathan, R., Balu, M., Jacob, E., & Illickal, S. M. (2021). A randomised controlled study for the prevention of post-partum haemorrhage with oxytocin plus methyl ergometrine versus oxytocin alone in the third stage of labour. *International Journal of Reproduction, Contraception, Obstetrics and Gynecology, 10*(5), 1906–1913. https://doi.org/10.18203/2320-1770.ijrcog20211509

Srivastava, G., Bartlett, C., & Thakur, Y. (2012). Successful use of Rusch balloon to control postpartum haemorrhage due to vaginal lacerations. *Journal of Obstetrics and Gynaecology, 32*(1), 36. https://doi.org/10.3109/01443615.2011.615416

Suarez, S., Conde-Agudelo, A., Borovac-Pinheiro, A., Suarez-Rebling, D., Eckardt, M., Theron, G., & Burke, T. F. (2020). Uterine balloon tamponade for the treatment of postpartum hemorrhage: A systematic review and meta-analysis. *American Journal of Obstetrics & Gynecology, 222*(4), 293.e1–293.e52. https://doi.org/10.1016/j.ajog.2019.11.1287

Sudhof, L. S., Shainker, S. A., & Einerson, B. D. (2019). Tranexamic acid in the routine treatment of postpartum hemorrhage in the United States: A cost-effectiveness analysis. *American Journal of Obstetrics & Gynecology, 221*(3), 275-e1–275.e12. https://doi.org/10.1016/j.ajog.2019.06.030

Supporting healthy and normal physiologic childbirth: A consensus statement by ACNM, MANA, and NACPM. (2013). *Journal of Perinatal Education, 22*(1), 14–18. https://doi.org/10.1891/1058-1243.22.1.14

Taliento, C., Tormen, M., Sabattini, A., Scutiero, G., Cappadona, R., & Greco, P. (2022). Impact of waterbirth on post-partum hemorrhage, genital trauma, retained placenta and shoulder dystocia: A systematic review and meta-analysis. *European Journal of Obstetrics, Gynecology, and Reproductive Biology, 276*, 26–37. https://doi.org/10.1016/j.ejogrb.2022.06.016

Tang, E., & Stetz, J. (2020). Tranexamic acid for postpartum hemorrhage. *American Family Physician, 101*(9). Retrieved from https://www.aafp.org/afp/2020/0501/od2.html

Thaddeus, S., & Nangalia, R. (2004). Perceptions matter: Barriers to treatment of postpartum hemorrhage. *Journal of Midwifery & Women's Health, 49*(4), 293–297. https://doi.org/10.1016/j.jmwh.2004.04.010

Theron, G. B. (2010). Surgical management of postpartum haemorrhage. In S. Fawcus & J. Moodley (Eds.), *A monograph of the management of postpartum haemorrhage* (pp. 45–63). (n.p.): National Department of Health, South Africa. Retrieved from http://www.hst.org.za/publications/NonHST Publications/Monograph Postpartum Haemorrhage.pdf

Tindell, K., Garfinkel, R., Abu-Haydar, E., Ahn, R., Burke, T. F., Conn, K., & Eckardt, M. (2013). Uterine balloon tamponade for the treatment of postpartum haemorrhage in resource-poor settings: A systematic review. *BJOG, 120*(1), 5–14. https://doi.org/10.1111/j.1471-0528.2012.03454.x

Toglia, M. R. (2022). Repair of episiotomy and perineal lacerations associated with childbirth. In K. Eckler (Ed.), *UpToDate*. Retrieved November 13, from https://www.uptodate.com/contents/repair-of-perineal-and-other-lacerations-associated-with-childbirth

U.S. Food and Drug Administration. (2014). *Pitocin®* [Package insert/label]. Retrieved from https://www.accessdata.fda.gov/drugsatfda_docs/label/2014/018261s031lbl.pdf

Walvekar, V., Virkud, A., & Majumder, R. (2012). Management of postpartum hemorrhage in low resource settings. In S. Arulkumaran, M. Karoshi, L. G. Keith, A. B. Lalonde, & C. B-Lynch (Eds.), *A comprehensive textbook of postpartum hemorrhage: An essential clinical reference for effective management* (2nd ed., pp. 539–544). London, United Kingdom: Sapiens Publishing. Retrieved from https://www.glowm.com/pdf/PPH_2nd_edn_Chap-64.pdf

Ward, A. M. (2012). The midwife confronts postpartum hemorrhage. In S. Arulkumaran, M. Karoshi, L. G. Keith, A. B. Lalonde, & C. B-Lynch (Eds.), *A comprehensive textbook of postpartum hemorrhage: An essential clinical reference for effective management* (2nd ed., pp. 549–554). London, United Kingdom: Sapiens Publishing. Retrieved from http://www.glowm.com/pdf/PPH_2nd_edn_Chap-66.pdf

Wedmore, I., McManus, J. G., Pusateri, A. E., & Holcomb, J. B. (2006). A special report on the chitosan-based hemostatic dressing: Experience in current combat operations. *Journal of Trauma: Injury, Infection, and Critical Care, 60*(3), 655–658. https://doi.org/10.1097/01.ta.0000199392.91772.44

Weeks, A. (2023). Retained placenta after vaginal birth. In V. A. Barss (Ed.), *UpToDate*. Retrieved November 13, 2023, from https://www.uptodate.com/contents/retained-placenta-after-vaginal-birth

Weeks, A., Cunningham, C., Taylor, W., Rosala-Hallas, A., Watt, P., Bryning, L., . . . Lavender, T. (2021). A phase 2 clinical trial of the PPH Butterfly, a new device to 'turn off the tap' of post-partum hemorrhage. *Authorea*. https://doi.org/10.22541/au.162015824.47500455/v1

Weeks, A. D., & Fawcus, S. (2020). Management of the third stage of labour. *Best Practice & Research Clinical Obstetrics & Gynaecology, 67*, 65–79. https://doi.org/10.1016/j.bpobgyn.2020.03.003

Wetta, L. A., Szychowski, J. M., Seals, M. S., Mancuso, M. S., Biggio, J. R., & Tita, A. T. N. (2013). Risk factors for uterine atony/postpartum hemorrhage requiring treatment after vaginal delivery. *American Journal of Obstetrics & Gynecology, 209*(1), 51.e1–51.e6. https://doi.org/10.1016/j.ajog.2013.03.011

Williams, J. W. (1912). *Obstetrics: A text-book for the use of students and practitioners* (3rd ed.). New York, NY: Appleton. Retrieved from https://archive.org/details/obstetricstextbo1912will/

Wilson, K., Santiago, R., Preziosi, M., Fisher, R., & Hall, A. B. (2021). Inadvertent methylergonovine administration to a newborn. *American Journal of Emergency Medicine, 44*, 479-e1.–479.e2. https://doi.org/10.1016/j.ajem.2020.10.079

World Health Organization. (2012). *WHO recommendations for the prevention and treatment of postpartum haemorrhage*. Geneva, Switzerland: WHO Press. Retrieved from http://apps.who.int/iris/bitstream/10665/75411/1/9789241548502_eng.pdf

World Health Organization. (2017). *Updated WHO recommendation on tranexamic acid for the treatment of postpartum haemorrhage: Highlights and key messages from the World Health Organization's 2017 global recommendation*. Geneva, Switzerland: WHO. Retrieved from https://apps.who.int/iris/bitstream/handle/10665/259379/WHO-RHR-17.21-eng.pdf

World Health Organization. (2022). *WHO postpartum haemorrhage (PPH) summit*. Retrieved from https://www.who.int/publications/m/item/who-postpartum-haemorrhage-(pph)-summit

Wu, H.-L., Chen, X.-W., Wang, P. & Wang, Q-M. (2017). Effects of placental cord drainage in the third stage of labour: A meta-analysis. *Scientific Reports, 7*, 7067. https://doi.org/10.1038/s41598-017-07722-7

Yoong, W., Ray, A., & Phillip, S. A. (2009). Balloon tamponade for postpartum vaginal lacerations in a woman refusing blood transfusion. *International Journal of Gynaecology & Obstetrics, 106*(3), 261. https://doi.org/10.1016/j.ijgo.2009.03.052

Yoong, W., Sivashanmugarajan, V., McMonagle, M., Hamilton, J., Karoshi, M., & Lodhi, W. (2014). Pelvic and vaginal packing for intractable venous obstetric haemorrhage: Practical tips for the obstetrician. *Obstetrician & Gynecologist, 16*(4), 276–280. https://doi.org/10.1111/tog.12129

Zhang, Y. J., Gao, B., & Liu, X. W. (2015). Topical and effective hemostatic medicines in the battlefield. *International Journal of Clinical and Experimental Medicine, 8*(1), 10–19. Retrieved from https://www.ncbi.nlm.nih.gov/pmc/articles/PMC4358424/

Zuckerwise, L. C., Pettker, C. M., Illuzzi, J., Raab, C. R., & Lipkind, H. S. (2014). Use of a novel visual aid to improve estimation of obstetric blood loss. *Obstetrics & Gynecology, 123*(5), 982–986. https://doi.org/10.1097/AOG.0000000000000233

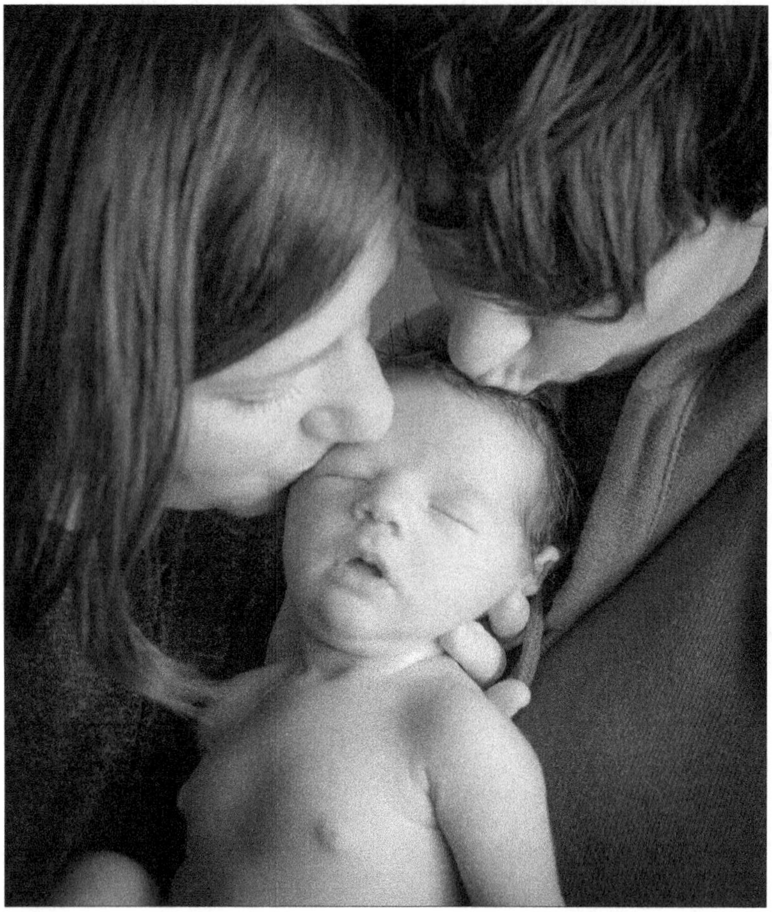

Abdominal Pain and Difficulty Breathing 8

Objectives

- Identify the signs and symptoms of deep-vein thrombosis (DVT) and pulmonary embolism (PE); discuss treatment modalities.
- Discuss the clinical signs of pulmonary edema and list three possible etiologies.
- Distinguish between the clinical signs and symptoms of appendicitis, renal calculi, and round-ligament pain.
- List two risk factors for ovarian torsion.

Composite Case Study

Kay W. called the birth center office to say she was unable to urinate. She had awakened at 6 a.m. with lower abdominal cramping that had been getting worse over the last few hours. Julia Sparks, CNM, was concerned, and asked Kay a series of questions using the GOLDCART framework. Kay was 16 weeks pregnant with her eighth baby. She had coitus with her husband at about 9 p.m. Since then, she had been leaking small amounts of urine, but she was unable to completely empty her bladder. In previous pregnancies she had occasional difficulty voiding during the second trimester, but she never before had a complete inability to urinate.

Julia asked Kay to come to the birth center for evaluation. On examination, the cause of the problem became clear to Julia. The uterine fundus was not palpable through Kay's abdomen, but the swell of a distended bladder was present above her pubic symphysis. On examination, the cervix was displaced so far forward that she had to angle her speculum sharply to visualize it tucked behind the pubic arch. On digital examination, the firm bulge of a retroflexed uterus was palpable in the posterior cul-de-sac.

Julia explained to Kay that her uterus was retroflexed, with her fundus sharply angled backwards in her pelvis towards her tail bone. During intercourse in the missionary position the night before, her uterus had become wedged in the pelvis between the sacral promontory and the pubic symphysis. The trapped cervix became elongated and shifted forward, compressing the lower bladder and obstructing drainage.

Julia inserted a urinary catheter and drained 1,000 ml of clear urine, to Kay's grateful relief. Julia then placed Kay in knee-chest position and performed a digital examination, gently applying pressure to the uterus through the vaginal wall to encourage it to move forward. Julia felt a slight forward shift in uterine position.

Julia told Kay that lax muscle tone and a retroverted uterus can predispose to uterine retention in the early second trimester. This condition can often be corrected by bladder drainage and uterine repositioning. In some cases, however, uterine abnormalities or large fibroids can cause persistent incarceration that requires expert management. If Kay developed pelvic pain, was unable to void within 6 hours after catheterization, or had recurring episodes of urinary retention, she would require evaluation by an obstetrician or maternal-fetal medicine specialist. If Kay was persistently unable to void, she might need an indwelling catheter to drain her bladder or a pessary to support the uterus in its correct position. Even if the urinary symptoms resolved, Julia said that Kay should have a pelvic exam in the office in the next week or two to ensure that the uterus was not pathologically incarcerated. Julia discussed the risk of urinary tract infection and urged Kay to call with the first signs and symptoms.

Julia told Kay to perform pelvic rocking exercises on hands and knees several times a day to encourage the uterus to move anteriorly. She recommended that Kay lie prone for a few minutes to bring her uterus forward before getting up at night to void. She suggested that Kay try coitus in a hands-and-knees position for the next few weeks to move the uterus forward in the abdomen rather than impacting it into the pelvis. Julia also said that Kay should limit fluids before bedtime, refrain from using the Valsalva maneuver while voiding or defecating, and lean forward at the start of urination. If urination becomes difficult again, Kay could try urinating while seated backwards on the toilet or on hands and knees in the tub. She added that Kay might help her bladder empty by applying suprapubic pressure while voiding.

Julia explained that usually by 20 weeks of gestation, the uterus has outgrown the pelvis and usually is no longer in danger of getting trapped. In rare cases, the uterus becomes incarcerated below the sacral promontory and is unable to escape. Because the uterus is unable to grow properly, abnormal pressure on the uterus and surrounding organs can lead to irreversible uterine ischemia, hydronephrosis, kidney injury, bladder or uterine rupture, rectal gangrene, stillbirth, or miscarriage.

Kay had no further reoccurrence of urinary retention. By 19 weeks of gestation, her uterus was in a normal position. She had an uneventful pregnancy and gave birth to an 8 lb 11 oz (3,950 g) boy at 39 weeks of gestation.

Abdominal and Pelvic Pain

Abdominal pain and shortness of breath are discomforts experienced at some point in nearly every pregnancy. Some of these complaints result from normal physiologic changes of pregnancy while others can indicate the presence of serious pathology. It can be challenging for the midwife to unravel the clues and form an accurate clinical impression.

Abdominal pain in pregnancy presents many diagnostic challenges to the midwife. Normal pregnancy discomfort can mimic serious abdominal pathology, and vice versa. Nausea, vomiting, abdominal pain, indigestion, and bowel irregularity are common symptoms of both abdominal pathology and of normal pregnancy. When the pregnant uterus becomes an abdominal organ at about 12 weeks of gestation, it begins to compress and displace the adjacent viscera. This reorganization of organs can change the character and quality of abdominal pain. Moreover, pain from elsewhere in the body can refer to the abdomen, confounding the clinical picture. It can be difficult for the provider to know when to reassure and when to respond.

Most pregnant individuals experience abdominal discomfort at times, frequently in the lower quadrants. Stretching of the round ligaments, Braxton Hicks contractions, fetal movement, gastric reflux, constipation, flatulence, or the pressure of uterine enlargement can cause a client to seek medical attention, fearing that something is wrong. In some instances, however, abdominal pain can indicate the presence of a gastrointestinal, gynecologic, urologic, or obstetric problem that necessitates intervention. Pregnancy creates conditions that can cause abdominal pain. The gravid uterus puts pressure on the urinary tract, encouraging hydroureter and hydronephrosis. Elevated progesterone levels decrease intestinal motility and gallbladder emptying, increasing the likelihood of gastroesophageal reflux, constipation, cholelithiasis, and kidney stones. The midwife's challenge is to distinguish a client with the normal discomforts of pregnancy from one with an abnormal condition.

Obstetrical Causes of Abdominal Pain

In early pregnancy, abdominal pain can be the initial symptom of an abnormal condition such as ectopic pregnancy, spontaneous abortion, or septic abortion. Later in pregnancy, pain can be a sign of placental abruption, placenta percreta, HELLP syndrome (**H**emolysis, **E**levated **L**iver enzymes, **L**ow **P**latelets), or uterine rupture. These conditions are discussed at length elsewhere in this book.

Round-Ligament Pain

Round ligaments attach near the uterine cornua, run through the inguinal ring and along the inguinal canal, and attach in the labia majora. Ligament pain appears related to stretching or spasm of the ligament or irritation of nearby nerve fibers (Bastian & Brown, 2023). The discomfort is usually felt on the right side of the lower abdomen but can be on the left or bilateral. Round-ligament pain can be triggered or exacerbated by walking, rolling over in bed, fetal movements, Braxton Hicks contractions, sneezing, vigorous activity, or prolonged standing. The pain is physiologically harmless but is often sharp and severe enough to interfere with daily activities. Splinting the painful area with the hand, flexing the hip on the affected side, applying heat, and wearing a maternity abdominal support belt can improve symptoms. Round ligament pain is a diagnosis of exclusion; consider alternative sources of pain before attributing symptoms to this condition (Bastian & Brown, 2023).

Placental Abruption

Placental abruption is the separation of the placenta from the uterine lining at or beyond 20 weeks of gestation while the fetus is *in utero*. Classic signs of placental abruption include vaginal bleeding, abdominal pain, uterine tachysystole (more than 5 contractions in a 10-min interval); a tense, boardlike abdomen; uterine tenderness; and a nonreassuring fetal heart rate (FHR) pattern (Ananth & Kinzler, 2022). Some cases, however, are subtle and have few or none of these signs. Antepartum and intrapartum abruption are discussed at length in detail in Chapter 6, and traumatic abruption is discussed fully in Chapter 9.

Acute Urinary Retention / Uterine Incarceration

Up to 20% of pregnant individuals have a retroverted or retroflexed uterus in the first trimester (Vidaeff & Schneider, 2022). By the early second trimester, the fundus normally rises from the hollow of the sacrum to an anterior ventral position within the abdominal cavity. Occasionally, the enlarging uterus becomes intermittently or persistently entrapped in the pelvis between the sacral promontory and the pubic symphysis (Vidaeff & Schneider, 2022). This condition, generally known as *uterine incarceration* when persistent, is sometimes termed *uterine impaction* when mild or intermittent. Risk factors include postsurgical adhesions, pelvic inflammatory disease, endometriosis, large uterine fibroids, multifetal gestation,

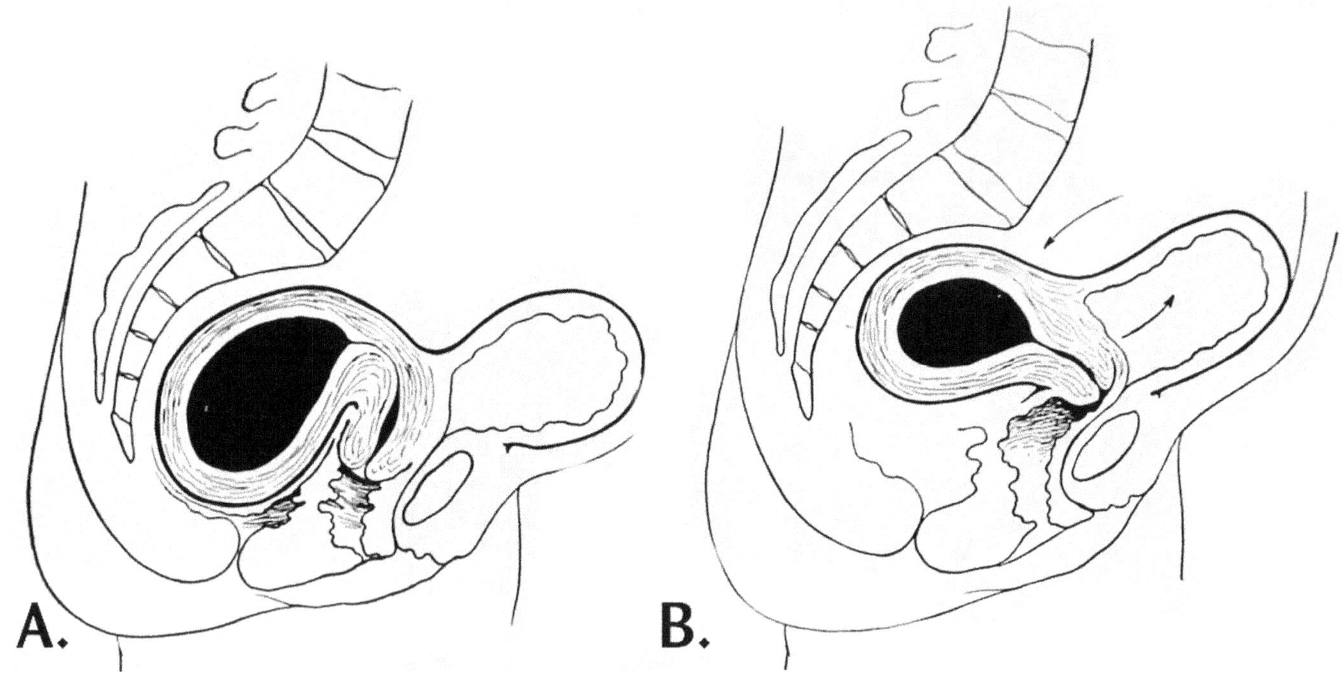

Figure 8-1. Urinary retention can occur when a retroflexed (A) or retroverted (B) gravid uterus presses on the neck of the bladder. The elongated cervix is adjacent to the pubic bone. If the uterus remains entrapped in the posterior pelvis, miscarriage, preterm birth (PTB), fetal demise, uterine wall necrosis, uterine rupture, cervicovaginal fistula, or rectal gangrene can occur. From *The Principles and Practice of Obstetrics* (p. 405), by J. B. De Lee, 1914, Philadelphia, PA: W. B. Saunders. In the public domain.

ovarian cysts, abnormal uterine structure, prior uterine incarceration, and weak supporting tissues.

Acute urinary retention can develop when the impacted uterus wedges against the neck of the bladder and urethra, obstructing the flow of urine (Vidaeff & Schneider, 2022). This obstruction usually develops between 9 and 16 weeks of gestation (Brahmantara et al., 2022). Symptoms usually begin overnight. As the individual sleeps, recumbent position and infrequent urination cause the lower bladder to flatten. The upper bladder fills and can press the uterus deeper into the pelvis (Yang & Huang, 2004). Having vaginal intercourse while in a supine position can also push the uterus backwards into the pelvis. Upon awakening, the client has difficulty starting a stream of urine and strains to overcome the obstruction. The Valsalva maneuver (increasing the pressure in the abdomen by pushing with a closed glottis) puts pressure on the uterus and can worsen the impaction. The client can also experience rectal pressure; constipation; pain in the pelvis, lower abdomen, and back; and urinary overflow, dribbling, urgency, and frequency (Vidaeff & Schneider, 2022).

On physical examination, the uterine fundus may be much lower than expected for gestational age or non-palpable. On speculum examination, the cervix is displaced to behind the pubic symphysis and sometimes can be visualized only by holding the speculum almost vertically. The retroflexed uterus is palpable in the posterior fornix as a firm bulge. The provider can also palpate the uterus by performing a rectal examination.

Urinary retention caused by uterine impaction is an emergency. Failure to empty the bladder and free the uterus can lead to hydronephrosis, urinary tract infection (UTI), rupture of the bladder, sepsis, peritonitis, miscarriage, or fetal demise (Slama, Barry, McManus, Latham, & Berniard, 2015). Urinary catheterization can relieve the obstruction and empty the bladder. If the catheter does not pass easily into the bladder, try lifting the cervix, which is usually palpable behind the symphysis.

If the client is less than 16 weeks of gestation, consider gently repositioning the retroflexed uterus. After the bladder has been drained with a urinary catheter, perform a digital examination and apply firm but gentle pressure to the uterus through the posterior fornix to shift the uterus anteriorly. If you are successful, you will feel the uterus move slightly forward, or the client will notice an improvement in symptoms. This maneuver can be more effective if the client assumes a knee-chest position or side-lying with pillows under the hips. Do not attempt to reposition the uterus after 19–20 weeks of gestation (Zhuang, Wang, Sang, Xu, & He, 2021). Past this stage, the risk of preterm labor (PTL) seems to increase with manual reduction (Zhuang et al., 2021).

If attempts at repositioning the uterus are unsuccessful or the client experiences significant discomfort during the intervention, refer semi-urgently to an obstetrician or

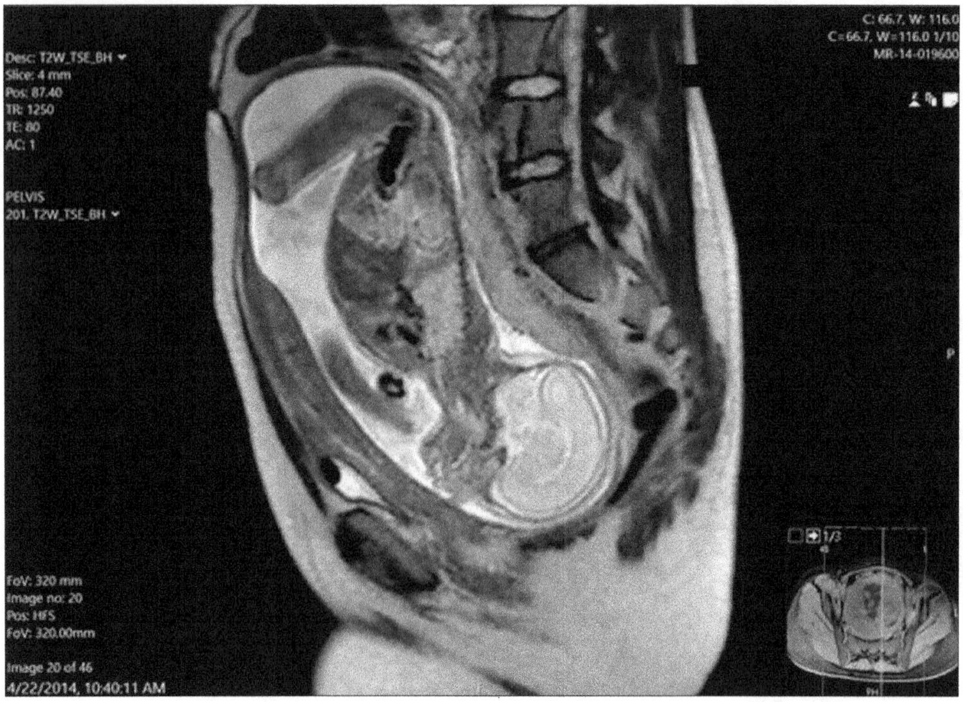

Figure 8-2. People with connective tissue disorders are at greater risk for incarceration of the uterus due to abnormal laxity of tissues. In this case, a woman with Ehlers-Danlos syndrome (EDS) was found to have an incarcerated uterus at 24 0/7 weeks of gestation. Because the uterus is inverted into the posterior pelvis, anatomical landmarks are distorted. The placenta implanted along the inverted *anterior* uterine wall, which is positioned by the maternal spine. The cervix is elongated to more than 13 cm in length and located just under the umbilicus. The fetal head is near the maternal coccyx and is compressing the rectum. The fundus overlying the fetal head is extremely thin and at risk for uterine rupture. From "A Case of Incarceration of the Gravid Uterus & the Ehlers-Danlos Syndromes with Literature Review," by M. H. Campbell, A. T. Sandlin, P. L. Wendel, and M. L. Racher, 2021, *Obstetrics and Gynaecology Cases—Reviews, 8*(2), p. 197, fig. 1. CC BY 4.0.

emergency department for assessment. Ultrasound or magnetic-resonance imaging (MRI) can exclude obstruction caused by cysts, bladder or pelvic tumors, or ectopic pregnancy (Lam & Suen, 2015). If urinary retention persists, an indwelling catheter or intermittent catheterization is sometimes necessary; both increase the risk of UTI, however (Vidaeff & Schneider, 2022).

To prevent reoccurrence of urinary retention due to uterine entrapment, the client can try exercises and postures that can shift the uterus into the abdomen. After voiding, the client can try holding a knee-chest position at least three times daily for 10 min per session for a minimum of one week (Vidaeff & Schneider, 2022). If voiding is difficult, the client can try applying suprapubic pressure while voiding (Zhuang et al., 2021), leaning forward at the start of urination, or urinating while seated backwards on the toilet or on hands and knees in a bathtub. Vaginal intercourse in a hands-and-knees or knee-chest position may shift the uterus anteriorly. Voiding after intercourse helps reduce the likelihood of uterine impaction and bladder infection. Before getting out of bed to void, the client should lie prone for a few minutes to bring the uterus forward (Zhuang et al., 2021). The client should limit fluids before bedtime and avoid using the Valsalva maneuver while voiding or defecating (Yang & Huang, 2004).

A retroflexed uterus usually moves into the abdominal cavity by 16–18 weeks of gestation (78.5% of cases) and the urinary symptoms typically resolve by that time (Tachibana et al., 2021). If the uterus remains retroverted in weeks 17–19 or if the client requires repeated catheterization, refer to a physician for evaluation. If the impaction is persistent, an obstetrician may attempt reduction using a cervical tenaculum for leverage (Zhuang et al., 2021). If manual reduction fails, invasive surgery such as colonoscopy-assisted repositioning, laparoscopy, or laparotomy may be considered (Zhuang et al., 2021). If fibroid tumors are the cause of the incarceration, myomectomy may be required.

Persistent Uterine Incarceration

Persistent uterine incarceration beyond 20 weeks of gestation is a rare (1 in 3,000 pregnancies) but serious complication (Pina Moreno et al., 2023). Whereas an impacted retroverted uterus is mobile and usually resolves spontaneously or with minimally invasive measures, a true incarcerated uterus can be serious or even life-threatening for mother and fetus. With gravid uterine incarceration, the growing uterus remains trapped in the pelvis between the sacral promontory and pubic symphysis until it becomes too large to fit (Vidaeff & Schneider, 2022). As the uterus enlarges, the anterior uterine wall thins and pouches out into the abdomen while the fundus remains wedged in the pelvis (Vidaeff & Schneider, 2022). The cervix can stretch to more than 10 cm in length, and the bladder and cervix can displace into the abdominal cavity (Vidaeff & Schneider, 2022). This abnormal positioning of the uterus can reduce uterine arterial blood flow, which can lead to miscarriage, oligohydramnios, fetal growth restriction, prelabor rupture of membranes (PROM), preterm birth (PTB), or fetal demise (Vidaeff & Schneider, 2022). Other case reports describe uterine wall necrosis, uterine rupture, cervicovaginal fistula, pulmonary embolism (PE), severe hydronephrosis, and rectal gangrene as complications (Vidaeff & Schneider, 2022).

Like the client with intermittent impaction from a retroverted uterus, a client with persistent uterine incarceration can present with pain in the back, abdomen, or suprapubic region; pelvic or rectal pressure; or urinary retention. Severe pain or PTL are likely to develop. About 9% of cases are asymptomatic (Pina Moreno et al., 2023).

The client with uterine incarceration should be under the care of an obstetrician. In one review of persistent uterine incarceration, only about 20% of cases reached term (Lacoste, Seffert, & Chauleur, 2013). If the client is asymptomatic or has only mild symptoms, uterine reduction is not usually attempted after 20 weeks of gestation because it is not likely to succeed and may result in pregnancy loss (Vidaeff & Schneider, 2022). Any urinary retention is treated by intermittent self-catheterization or an indwelling urinary catheter (Vidaeff & Schneider, 2022). Case reports have described spontaneous resolution of uterine incarceration in the second and third trimesters (Vidaeff & Schneider, 2022).

In the unlikely case of incarcerated uterus persisting into the third trimester, cesarean birth is recommended at 36 weeks of gestation to avoid subjecting the uterus to labor. Vaginal birth is contraindicated because displacement of the cervix prevents the normal progress of labor and increases the risk for uterine rupture. The distortion of anatomical relationships with this condition makes cesarean section complex. Upon entering the abdomen, the physician may find the posterior uterine wall, bladder, vagina, and elongated cervix where the lower uterine segment is normally located; a misplaced uterine incision can transect the bladder, cervix, or vagina (Vidaeff & Schneider, 2022). A preoperative MRI may be necessary to determine the location of key structures.

DIFFERENTIAL DIAGNOSES

UTI, uterine fibroid, ovarian mass, ectopic pregnancy.

Intrauterine Infection

Intraamniotic Infection (IAI) / Chorioamnionitis

Intraamniotic infection (IAI), also termed chorioamnionitis, is a condition in which the membranes and fetal part of the placenta (chorion) become inflamed, usually because of polymicrobial infection following rupture of membranes (Tita, 2023). It is associated with severe adverse maternal, fetal, and neonatal outcomes, including higher long-term risks for cerebral palsy and other neurodevelopmental disabilities for the infant (Tita, 2023). Although the term *chorioamnionitis* is widely used to indicate infection of the fetal membranes, *intraamniotic infection* is more precise because infection often involves the amniotic fluid, fetus, umbilical cord, or placenta as well as the chorion and amnion (Tita, 2023). Another term for the condition is "Triple I," which refers to "intrauterine inflammation or infection or both" (Higgins et al., 2016, p. 426).

Presumed Intraamniotic Infection (IAI) Criteria

ONE reading of fever ≥102.2°F (39.0°C)

OR

TWO readings of fever 100.4–102.1°F (38.0–38.9°C) 30 min apart

PLUS

- Fetal Tachycardia
- Elevated maternal white blood cells (WBCs)
- Cloudy, yellow, or foul-smelling fluid

Tita, (2023).

PTL with intact membranes or preterm prelabor rupture of membranes (PPROM) can be a sign of subclinical infection. It is thought that about 25% of mothers who give birth preterm have subclinical chorioamnionitis (Duff, 2021). At term, IAI affects 1–3% of pregnancies with intact membranes and 6–10% of those with PROM (Tita, 2023). The risk for IAI appears to increase after 40 completed weeks of gestation (American College of Obstetricians & Gynecologists [ACOG] Cmte. on Obstetric Practice, 2017/2022). IAI affects 7% of clients who spontaneously rupture membranes before labor at term (PROM) and 40% of those with PROM more than 24 hr before giving birth (Tita, 2023).

The contents of the amniotic sac ideally remain sterile because the cervix remains corked with a sticky mucus plug through most of pregnancy. Moreover, the amniotic membranes themselves seem to have antimicrobial properties (Tita, 2023). Lactobacilli in the vaginal flora also appear to weaken pathogenic microorganisms.

IAI occurs when disease-causing microorganisms invade the sterile environment within the pregnant uterus. Most cases of IAI develop when microorganisms that colonize the intestines or vagina ascend through the cervix. Bacterial colonization can cause inflammation, which can lead to prelabor rupture of membranes. Most infections are polymicrobial and involve anaerobic and aerobic microorganisms, typically

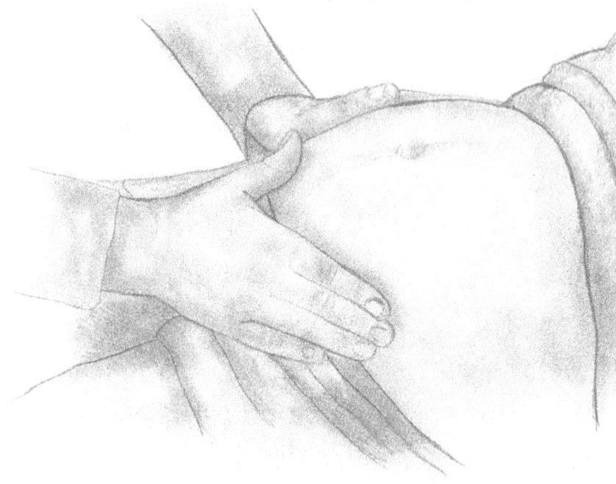

Figure 8-3. Clinical signs of IAI can include uterine tenderness, maternal malaise, fever, maternal leukocytosis, maternal or fetal tachycardia, fetal tachycardia, bacteremia, and foul-smelling amniotic fluid.

Group B *Streptococcus* (GBS), *Ureaplasma* and *Mycoplasma* species, *Gardnerella vaginalis*, and *Escherichia coli*, (ACOG Cmte. on Obstetric Practice, 2017/2022; Tita, 2023).

Occasionally, IAI results from amniocentesis or other procedures that penetrate the amniotic cavity or when pathogens such as *Listeria monocytogenes* cross into the uterus from the mother's bloodstream. Viruses such as cytomegalovirus, adenovirus, enterovirus, respiratory syncytial virus, and Epstein-Barr virus have been found in amniotic fluid, but there is no proof these that organisms cause IAI (Czikk, McCarthy, & Murphy, 2011). Very rarely, vaginal *Candida* infections can ascend into the uterus to cause acute IAI, putting the newborn at risk for congenital systemic candidiasis (Czikk et al., 2011; Tita, 2023). IAI can cause uteroplacental bleeding, placental abruption, or a precipitous birth. Intrauterine infection is associated with many if not most PTBs and appears to be an independent risk factor for cerebral palsy.

Primary risk factors include young maternal age, nulliparity, extended duration of labor and ruptured membranes, multiple vaginal examinations, and preexisting vaginal infections such as bacterial vaginosis and GBS colonization (Duff, 2021). Other risk factors include the use of an intracervical balloon catheter for cervical ripening, internal fetal or uterine contraction monitoring, digital rather than speculum examination in clients with PPROM, meconium-stained amniotic fluid, alcohol or tobacco use, and previous IAI (Tita, 2023).

IAI can be the cause or the result of dysfunctional labor (Duff, 2021). Longer labors usually involve more digital cervical examinations than shorter labors, and each cervical examination can increase the risk for IAI, especially after membranes have ruptured (Tita, 2023). Inflammation associated with IAI appears to cause abnormal contractions that result in nonprogressive labor. About 75% of mothers with IAI require oxytocin for augmentation of labor, and up to 40% require cesarean section, generally for failure to progress in labor (Duff, 2021). This impaired myometrial contractility can also lead to postpartum hemorrhage due to uterine atony (Tita, 2023).

Classic signs of IAI include (Tita, 2023)

- Fever above 100.4°F (38°C), 100%.
- Maternal leukocytosis (white blood cell [WBC] count greater than 12,000/mm–15,000/mm), 70–90%.
- Maternal tachycardia above 100 beats per min (bpm), 50–80%.
- Uterine tenderness, 4–25%.
- Bacteremia, 5–10%. GBS and *E. coli* are the most common pathogens that cause bacteremia.
- Purulent or malodorous amniotic fluid.
- FHR abnormalities—usually tachycardia and decreased variability, greater than 75% (Duff, 2021).

A presumptive diagnosis of IAI can be made in pregnant people with **one** episode of fever at or above 102.2°F (39.0°C) OR **two** readings of 100.4–102.1°F (38.0–38.9°C) 30 min apart, without another clear source of infection PLUS one or more of the following:

- Baseline FHR greater than 160 bpm for 10 min or longer, excluding accelerations, decelerations, and periods of marked variability.
- Maternal WBC count greater than 15,000/mm^3 in the absence of corticosteroid administration.
- Purulent (cloudy or yellowish) or foul-smelling fluid seen to be draining through the cervical os upon speculum examination.

Maternal complications from IAI include endometritis, peritonitis, sepsis, coagulopathy, and occasionally death (ACOG Cmte. on Obstetric Practice, 2017/2022). About 15–20% of cases of maternal sepsis result from IAI (Tita, 2023). Postpartum uterine atony with severe hemorrhage is a significant risk (ACOG Cmte. on Obstetric Practice, 2017/2022). Antibiotic therapy greatly reduces the risk of poor maternal outcome.

When the mother has IAI, the fetus is literally floating in a pool of infection. Bacteria can infiltrate the lungs, the digestive tract, all skin surfaces, the eyes, and the nasal passages. Consequently, the fetus exposed to intrauterine infection is at high risk for adverse outcomes. Serious fetal/neonatal complications of IAI include septic shock, pulmonary hypertension, respiratory failure, pneumonia, brain damage, meningitis, and death (ACOG Cmte. on Obstetric Practice, 2017/2022). Systemic fetal inflammatory syndrome involves the fetal response to intrauterine infection and can lead to PTL, growth restriction, severe newborn illness, brain injury, and chronic lung disease (Tita, 2023). Up to 40% of cases of early-onset neonatal sepsis appear to begin with intrauterine infection (Tita, 2023).

Tita (2023) notes that preterm infants fare worse than full-term infants and have a higher rate of perinatal death (25% versus 6% in preterm and term infants), newborn sepsis (28% versus 6%), pneumonia (20% versus 3%), severe intraventricular brain hemorrhage (24% versus 8%), and respiratory distress (62% versus 35%). Preterm infants also must contend with morbidity associated with immaturity while fighting infection. The infant is at higher risk for long-term complications including bronchopulmonary dysplasia and cerebral palsy, presumably due to inflammation, but the overall likelihood of these outcomes is low (ACOG Cmte. on Obstetric Practice, 2017/2022).

IAI is always an emergency and is potentially life-threatening to both mother and fetus. Because there is a high likelihood that the infant will require antibiotic therapy and close surveillance, transport the mother with IAI to a hospital with the capacity for neonatal intensive care. Management of IAI includes initiating continuous fetal monitoring, administering broad-spectrum intravenous (IV) antibiotics, giving antipyretics to reduce fever, and expediting birth. IAI can be resolved only by delivery of the infected products of conception and treatment with antibiotics. Vaginal birth is preferred but cesarean section might become necessary if labor does not progress, if the fetus does not tolerate labor, or if the mother's vital signs become unstable (Tita, 2023). IAI increases the risk of wound infection, endometritis, and venous thrombosis with cesarean birth.

The recommended antibiotic regimen is ampicillin 2 g IV every 6 hr PLUS gentamicin 5 mg/kg once daily (Tita, 2023). Alternative IV antibiotic therapies include ampicillin-sulbactam 3 g every 6 hr, ticarcillin-clavulanate 3.1 g every 4 hr, cefoxitin 2 g every 8 hr, cefotetan 2 g every 12 hr, piperacillin-tazobactam 3.375 g every 6 hr, or ertapenem 1 g every 24 hr (Tita, 2023).

DIFFERENTIAL DIAGNOSES

Pyelonephritis, influenza, appendicitis, and pneumonia among others. The laboring client with epidural anesthesia can become febrile in the absence of sepsis. Epidural anesthesia can also lead to fetal tachycardia and neonatal temperature above 100.4°F (38°C).

Postpartum Endometritis

Postpartum endometritis should be suspected if the client has an oral temperature 100.4°F (38.0°C) or higher on any two of the first 10 days postpartum, exclusive of the first 24 hr (Chen, 2023). Endometritis typically invades the decidual lining first, then attacks the uterine muscle as the infection progresses.

Risk factors for postpartum endometritis include

- Cesarean birth
- IAI/chorioamnionitis
- Prolonged labor
- Prolonged rupture of membranes
- Multiple cervical examinations with ruptured membranes
- Internal fetal or uterine monitoring
- Large amount of meconium in amniotic fluid
- Manual removal of the placenta
- Maternal diabetes mellitus or severe anemia
- PTB
- Vacuum or forceps assisted vaginal birth
- Postterm pregnancy
- HIV infection
- Colonization by GBS
- Heavy vaginal colonization by *E. coli*

The diagnosis of postpartum endometriosis is made when the client has two of the three hallmark signs: fever 100.4°F (38.0°C) or higher, pain or tenderness (uterine or abdominal) with no other known cause, and purulent drainage from uterus (Chen, 2023). Other signs and symptoms include malaise, tachycardia, body aches, chills, and foul-smelling lochia. The uterus is commonly larger than normal and soft on palpation. Lochia can be abnormally heavy or persistent.

Postpartum endometritis is typically a polymicrobial infection caused by microorganisms that ascend from the lower genital tract (Chen, 2023). Enterobacteriaceae (50%), gram-negative cocci (45%), and/or anaerobes (23%) are involved in most cases of postpartum endometritis (Rojas-Suarez & Suarez Rueda, 2020). Endometritis caused by *Streptococcus pyogenes* (group A) or *S. agalactiae* (group B) carries a significant risk of serious illness. Endometritis caused by *Clostridium sordellii* or *C. perfringens* or that involves streptococcal or staphylococcal toxic shock syndrome is rare but deadly (Chen, 2023).

Consult your collaborative physician when you suspect your client has endometritis. Treatment of postpartum endometritis includes IV broad-spectrum antibiotics, usually clindamycin 900 mg every 8 hr plus gentamicin 5 mg/kg every 24 hr if the client is not a carrier of GBS (Chen, 2023). If the client is colonized with GBS, ampicillin 2 g IV every 6 hr or ampicillin-sulbactam 3 g IV every 6 hr is added to the above regimen of clindamycin and gentamicin (Chen, 2023). IV antibiotics are continued until the client is afebrile for 24–48 hr and no longer has uterine tenderness (Chen, 2023). After successful treatment, it is not necessary to continue treatment with oral antibiotics.

PRURITUS + ELEVATED BILE ACIDS *or* TRANSAMINASES = ICP

Figure 8-4. ICP is diagnosed when the client experiences itching and has elevated bile acids or transaminases if there are no other conditions present that would explain the findings.

Preeclampsia / HELLP Syndrome

Preeclampsia is a multisystem progressive disorder which involves both abnormal placentation and maternal systemic vascular dysfunction (August & Sibai, 2023b). See "Preeclampsia" in Chapter 10. It develops in the second half of pregnancy or postpartum and is characterized either by the new onset of hypertension with proteinuria or by hypertension with end-organ dysfunction, with or without proteinuria (August & Sibai, 2023b). HELLP Syndrome, a disorder characterized by **H**emolysis, **E**levated **L**iver enzymes, and a **L**ow **P**latelet count, may be a severe form of preeclampsia or a variant of preeclampsia.

Pain in the right upper quadrant (RUQ), in the epigastrium, or below the sternum can be associated with severe preeclampsia or HELLP syndrome. The pain suggests liver damage and is thought to be caused by the stretching of the fibrous capsule covering the liver (Glisson's capsule) due to bleeding within the liver or, rarely, hepatic rupture (Kilpatrick & Shamshirsaz, 2022). When HELLP syndrome presents with nausea, vomiting, and malaise, it can be difficult to distinguish from nonspecific viral illness or viral hepatitis. Blood pressure (BP) of 140/90 mm Hg or higher and proteinuria are usually present, but either or both markers are sometimes absent in people with severe HELLP syndrome (Kilpatrick & Shamshirsaz, 2022).

Acute Fatty Liver of Pregnancy

Acute fatty liver of pregnancy (AFLP) is a rare but potentially fatal complication in which bubbles of fat replace the cytoplasm within the cells of the liver (Ko & Yoshida, 2006). Although the cause is unknown, genetic disorders leading to abnormal maternal or fetal fatty acid metabolism appear to predispose the pregnant person to this disease (R. H. Lee & Reau, 2023). Normally, maternal free fatty acids increase to meet the needs of a growing fetus, especially late in gestation. Defective maternal-fetal fatty acid metabolism can cause intermediate products of metabolism to accumulate in maternal blood and hepatocytes, damaging them. Fat accumulates in liver cells and perhaps in the kidney, placenta, and other sites. Untreated, the disease will progress to liver failure, encephalopathy, disseminated intravascular coagulation (DIC), and fetal demise. The victim of AFLP requires intensive care that can include blood transfusions, dialysis, or even liver transplantation (Liu, Ghaziani, & Wolf, 2017).

AFLP usually presents in the third trimester but can occur as early as 22 weeks of gestation and as late as 4 days postpartum (R. H. Lee & Reau, 2023). Signs and symptoms include nausea and vomiting, abdominal pain (primarily epigastric), jaundice, hypertension, and malaise. Preeclampsia with severe features or HELLP syndrome (hemolysis, elevated liver enzymes, low platelet count) is diagnosed in up to 40% of clients with AFLP (R. H. Lee & Reau, 2023). Clients with liver failure can rapidly develop ascites, encephalopathy, DIC, hypoglycemia, acute kidney injury, and multiorgan failure (R. H. Lee & Reau, 2023).

Clients with acute fatty liver of pregnancy (AFLP) have elevations in aspartate aminotransferase (AST) or alanine aminotransferase (ALT) typically reaching 5–10 times the upper limit of normal (R. H. Lee & Reau, 2023). Other laboratory findings can include elevated serum bilirubin levels, Low serum glucose, elevated serum creatinine, elevated white blood cell count, elevated ammonia level, elevated urate level, prolonged prothrombin time, international normalized ratio, activated partial thromboplastin time, low platelets, low fibrinogen, proteinuria, fragmented red blood cells, and burr cells (R. H. Lee & Reau, 2023). Liver biopsy will show microvesicular fat.

DIFFERENTIAL DIAGNOSES

Severe preeclampsia, HELLP syndrome, hepatitis.

Intrahepatic Cholestasis of Pregnancy

Intrahepatic cholestasis of pregnancy (ICP) is a condition of maternal elevated total serum bile acids, pruritus (itching), and abnormal liver function tests. This disorder impairs the release of bile from liver cells, causing it to accumulate until it impairs liver function (Williamson & Geenes, 2014). Bile levels increase in the maternal blood and cross the placenta, accumulating in the amniotic fluid and fetal blood, putting the fetus at risk for PTB, meconium-stained fluid, and stillbirth. ICP usually develops in the second and third trimesters and resolves quickly in the postpartum period (Lindor & Lee, 2023).

ICP is the most common liver disease unique to pregnancy, affecting 0.2–5.6% of pregnant people worldwide (Mitchell et al., 2021). There are wide geographic and ethnic variations in incidence of this disease, however, ranging from less than1% in parts of the United States to 27.6% among the indigenous Mapuche in Chile (Lindor & Lee, 2023). The etiology remains unidentified, but appears to involve genetic, hormonal, and environmental factors (Diken, Usta, & Nassar, 2014). Cholestasis reoccurs in about two-thirds of subsequent pregnancies (Durnwald, 2021). Pregnancy-related increases in estrogen and alterations in progesterone metabolism appear to trigger ICP, and in nonpregnant people, hormonal contraceptives can cause a similar condition. It is more common in people with underlying liver disease. Preeclampsia and gestational diabetes are more likely to occur in pregnancies complicated by ICP than in pregnancies without ICP (Ovadia et al., 2019).

Diagnosis

ICP is characterized by severe pruritus (itching), an elevation in serum bile acid concentrations, or abnormal liver function. Pruritus is usually worse at night and can be intolerable. It is especially intense on the palms and soles and can appear before laboratory tests become abnormal. In severe cases, itching affects ears, eyelids, and the inside of the mouth. RUQ pain, nausea, poor appetite, sleeplessness, steatorrhea (fatty stools), or jaundice can occur. There is no rash, but there may be skin excoriations caused by scratching. Some people have dark urine and pale stools (Williamson & Geenes, 2014); others develop gallstones (Diken et al., 2014).

More than 90% of clients with ICP have a significant increase in serum bile acids; sometimes this finding is the only laboratory abnormality (Lindor & Lee, 2023). Because itching can develop several weeks before bile acid elevation, if blood test results appear normal, consider repeating total bile acid and aminotransferase levels weekly if symptoms persist. Even in major laboratories, bile acid results can take several days.

Severe ICP, defined as bile acids greater than 40 mcmol/L affects about 20% of pregnant people with ICP. High concentrations of bile acids in amniotic fluid can damage fetal lungs and precipitate neonatal respiratory distress syndrome. The risk of stillbirth is low (0.4% mortality) when serum bile acids are less than 40 mcmol/L and highest (6.8% mortality) when they exceed 100 mcmol/L (Di Mascio et al., 2021). Most people with ICP remain well below this threshold. Possible explanations for sudden fetal death include sudden fetal arrhythmia or vasospasm of the placental surface vessels (Lindor & Lee, 2023). Coexisting pregnancy complications, such as preeclampsia or gestational diabetes, might increase the risk of stillbirth (Chappell et al., 2019). People who develop ICP are at higher risk for liver disease in later life.

Approximately 60% of people with ICP develop elevated serum liver enzymes, typically less than double the upper limit of normal (Lindor & Lee, 2023). Although alkaline phosphatase can be 4 times higher nonpregnant values, placental production of this enzyme sometimes raises values in healthy pregnant people (Lindor & Lee, 2023). Total and direct bilirubin may also rise.

Management

Treatment goals for ICP focus on managing maternal symptoms and preventing maternal and fetal complications. Oral dosing of ursodeoxycholic acid (ursodiol) increases bile flow, reduces itching, and improves liver biochemical tests for most mothers, but does not improve fetal/neonatal outcomes (Chappell et al., 2019; Lindor & Lee, 2023). The usual dose is 300 mg three times a day (or 15 mg/kg per day) until the baby is born. It can take one to two weeks for pruritus to improve, and three to four weeks to see improvement in liver function tests. If ursodeoxycholic acid is started empirically in the presence of normal laboratory test results, bile acid and transaminase levels may remain normal in the presence of ICP (Lindor & Lee, 2023).

Antepartum fetal surveillance tests (biophysical profile score, nonstress tests, daily fetal kick count) can fail to identify fetuses at risk of demise because fetal death seems to be a sudden event rather than the result of a chronic process (Lindor & Lee, 2023). About 90% of perinatal deaths occur after 37 weeks of gestation (median 38 weeks) and can occur shortly after surveillance testing that indicates a healthy fetus (Sheibani, Uhrinak, Lee, Fong, & Pathak, 2014). Nonetheless, ACOG and the Society for Maternal-Fetal Medicine (SMFM) suggest that it is appropriate to monitor pregnancies with ICP with antenatal fetal surveillance once or twice weekly beginning at diagnosis or at the gestational age when birth would be considered because of abnormal test results (ACOG Cmte. on Obstetric Practice & SMFM, 2021/2024).

With regard to timing of birth, ACOG recommends

- Total bile acid levels less than 100 mcmol/L: birth at 36–39 weeks of gestation or at diagnosis if 39 weeks or greater when diagnosed.
- Total bile acid levels equaling or exceeding 100 mcmol/L: birth at 36 weeks of gestation or at diagnosis if beyond 36 weeks.

Because of the risk of sudden fetal death and asphyxia, continuous fetal monitoring during labor is indicated (Lindor & Lee, 2023).

Pruritus usually subsides within days postpartum, and liver function tests spontaneously normalize soon after. Ursodiol does not pose a risk to breastfeeding babies but should be discontinued when labor begins. Bile acid concentration and liver function tests should be rechecked 6–8 weeks postpartum. About 60–70% of people experience reoccurrence of ICP in subsequent pregnancies (Lindor & Lee, 2023).

DIFFERENTIAL DIAGNOSES

Conditions characterized by elevated transaminase levels include HELLP syndrome, preeclampsia with severe features, hepatitis, biliary obstruction, or acute fatty liver of pregnancy—but pruritus is not a clinical feature in any of these disorders. Differential diagnoses for pruritus include skin diseases, dermatoses of pregnancy, skin irritants, or allergic reactions.

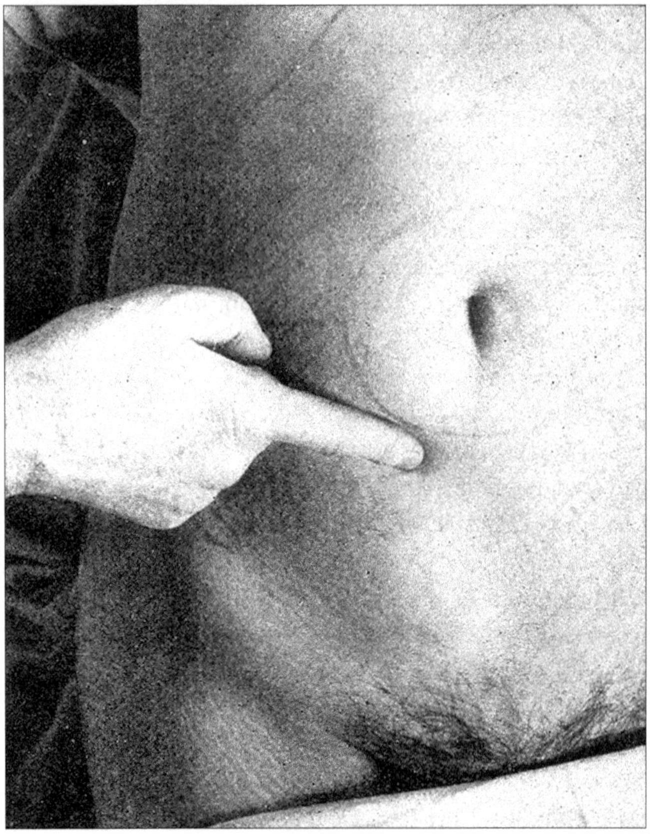

Figure 8-5. McBurney's point. In most people, the appendix attaches to the cecum beneath McBurney's point, a location on the right side of the abdomen one third of the distance from the anterior superior iliac spine to the umbilicus. In most pregnant people, the right-lower-quadrant (RLQ) pain associated with appendicitis occurs close to McBurney's point. In the third trimester, the expanding uterus pushes the appendix up, and the person may experience pain in the mid- or upper-right abdomen. From *The Diagnosis and Treatment of Diseases of Women* (p. 140), by H. S. Crossen, 1907, St. Louis, MO: C. V. Mosby. In the public domain.

Nonobstetrical Causes of Abdominal Pain

Gastroesophageal Reflux

Reflux, heartburn (pyrosis), water brash, and gastroesophageal reflux disease (GERD) affect 40–85% of pregnant individuals, commonly toward the end of gestation (Bianco, 2023). In pregnancy, high levels of estrogen and progesterone soften the lower esophageal sphincter and the enlarging uterus exerts pressure on the stomach as pregnancy progresses. Interestingly, one study showed that mothers with severe heartburn really do have babies with more hair, giving credibility to the folklore (Costigan, Sipsma, & DiPietro, 2006).

Symptoms of gastroesophageal reflux include chest or epigastric pain, regurgitation, painful or difficult swallowing, and nausea. Retrosternal burning discomfort can occur when the lower esophageal sphincter relaxes and gastric reflux inflames the esophagus (Cunningham et al., 2022, ch. 4). Water brash (regurgitation of saliva, sometimes laced with acid, from the lower part of the esophagus) may also occur (Kilpatrick & Shamshirsaz, 2022).

Reflux symptoms can improve if the client avoids tobacco, alcohol, and "trigger" foods and eats small, frequent meals. Heartburn is less likely to affect sleep if the head of the bed is elevated and the client avoids lying down for 2–3 hr after a meal. Oral antacids—including calcium, magnesium, or aluminum compounds—are considered safe and provide adequate relief in about half of gravidas with GERD (Bonthala & Wong, 2021). If severe symptoms persist, sucralfate, famotidine, or ranitidine may be prescribed (Bonthala & Wong, 2021). If these are not helpful, the next line of therapy is a proton-pump inhibitor such as omeprazole or pantoprazole. Endoscopy is for intractable cases.

Pelvic Congestion Syndrome (PCS) and Vulvovaginal Varicosities

During pregnancy, greater blood volume, altered hormonal balance, and the weight of the gravid uterus can cause varicose veins to develop, not only in the legs, labia, and anal canal, but also in the ovarian and internal iliac veins (Bałabuszek, Toborek, & Pietura, 2022). Pelvic congestion syndrome (PCS) is a painful condition caused by engorgement of these varicosities (N. R. Johnson, 2023). It most commonly affects multiparous people of reproductive age, can worsen during pregnancy, and subsides with menopause.

Some clients with pelvic varicosities experience dull, heavy, aching pain in the lower abdomen or pelvis. Others experience hip pain or persistent genital arousal (Phillips, Deipolyi, Hesketh, Midia, & Oklu, 2014). If varicose veins affect the bladder, the client can experience bladder irritability, urinary urgency, or dysuria (Bałabuszek et al., 2022). Occasionally, PCS presents with acute pain in the abdomen, lower back, hips, or legs (Bałabuszek et al., 2022).

Pain and discomfort tend to increase with lifting and with long periods of standing, walking, or sitting (Bałabuszek et al., 2022). Coitus tends to exacerbate symptoms of PCS, and the client can have a persistent throbbing ache for hours afterward. The initial onset can occur during pregnancy, and symptoms can worsen with each pregnancy thereafter. Rest in a lateral recumbent posture empties the veins and decreases symptoms. In nonpregnant people, symptoms are worst just before menstruation.

Ultrasound imaging can detect pelvic varicosities. Bimanual examination might reveal tender ovaries, cervical motion tenderness, and uterine tenderness and is particularly useful in nonpregnant clients. Vulvovaginal varicosities are identified visually and can appear as purple-blue distensible folds in the vaginal mucosa or as a grapelike cluster of veins in the labia (N. R. Johnson, 2023). Because upright positions enhance venous distension, examine the client in both the supine and upright positions when checking for vulvar and vaginal varicosities.

Table 8-1
Urinalysis Basics for Urinary Tract Infection (UTI)

Urinary specific gravity (USG)
Reflects hydration status and the concentrating ability of the kidneys. USG ≤1.010 = relative hydration, ≥1.020 = relative dehydration.
Urinary pH
Varies with serum pH, diet, medications, and pathology. Alkaline urine (pH 8.5–9.0) can indicate infection with urea-splitting organisms such as Proteus, Klebsiella, or Ureaplasma.
Blood
Bacterial infection of the bladder lining is the most common cause of hematuria. Other causes include kidney stones, renal disease, medications, trauma, and tumors. Vaginitis and urethritis do not cause hematuria.
Leukocyte esterase
Leukocyte esterase indicates WBCs in the urine with a specificity of only 55% for UTI. Leukocyte esterase can also indicate an inflammatory disorder or contamination by vaginal discharge.
Nitrites
A positive nitrites test identifies urinary infection, indicating the presence of bacteria that reduce urinary nitrates to nitrites. Some bacteria, including *Enterococcus*, *Pseudomonas*, and *Acinetobacter*, do not perform this conversion; therefore, infection can be present with a negative nitrite test. (Nitrite dipsticks left open to the air will yield a false positive.)
Casts
Casts are formed in the kidneys. If there are symptoms of infection and white cell casts are present, suspect pyelonephritis.
WBCs
WBC count greater than 5 per high-powered field is suggestive of UTI in symptomatic clients. Elevated WBCs can also indicate an inflammatory disorder or contamination by vaginal discharge.
Bacteria
Bacteria present in the urine is an abnormal finding, representing either a UTI or contamination of the sample with microorganisms from the skin or the vagina.
Adapted from (1) "Understanding Urinalysis: Clues for the Obstetrician–Gynecologist," by S. Coad, B. Friedman, and R. Geoffrion, 2012, *Expert Review of Obstetrics & Gynecology, 7*(3), pp. 269–279. Copyright by Expert Reviews Ltd. (2) "Urinalysis: A Comprehensive Review," by J. A. Simerville, W. C. Maxted, and J. J. Pahira, 2005, *American Family Physician, 71*(6), pp. 1153–1162. Copyright by American Academy of Family Physicians.

Comfort measures include vulvar support and compression (elastic pelvic support device), elevation of the legs, sleeping on the left side, exercise, and avoidance of long intervals of standing or sitting (N. R. Johnson, 2023). Most mothers with vulvovaginal varicosities can give birth vaginally (Giannella, Montanari, Delli Carpini, Di Giuseppe, & Ciavattini, 2022). Vulvar varicosities are unlikely to rupture or become lacerated during vaginal birth, but those that do can cause severe hemorrhage that is difficult to control. For this reason, a client with extremely large vulvovaginal varicosities may choose to give birth in a hospital that offers interventional radiology procedures and has readily available vascular surgeons (Giannella et al., 2022). Thrombosis of vulvar varicosities can also (rarely) occur.

Vulvovaginal varicosities usually disappear within approximately 30–40 days postpartum (N. R. Johnson, 2023), and pelvic varicosities tend to improve within this same timeframe. If the condition persists after pregnancy, treatment may include nonsteroidal antiinflammatory drugs (NSAIDs), acupuncture, physical therapy, or suppression of ovulation. In severe cases, embolization surgery can be used to stop blood flow to the affected veins.

Appendicitis

Appendicitis is inflammation of the vermiform appendix, a hollow structure located at the base of the cecum. The lumen of the appendix can become blocked by hard fecal masses, calculi, or other obstructions. Initial inflammation of the wall of the appendix can lead to localized ischemia, infection, and the development of an intraabdominal abscess or generalized peritonitis (Martin, 2022). The lifetime risk for appendicitis is about 7–10% (Cunningham et al., 2022, ch. 57).

Although appendicitis is more likely to occur in people who are not pregnant, appendicitis is the most common nonobstetrical surgical emergency during pregnancy, affecting about 1 pregnancy per 800–1,500 (Rebarber & Jacob, 2023). The physiologic changes and common discomforts of pregnancy can mask acute appendicitis. Appendiceal rupture occurs more frequently in pregnant clients, especially in the third trimester,

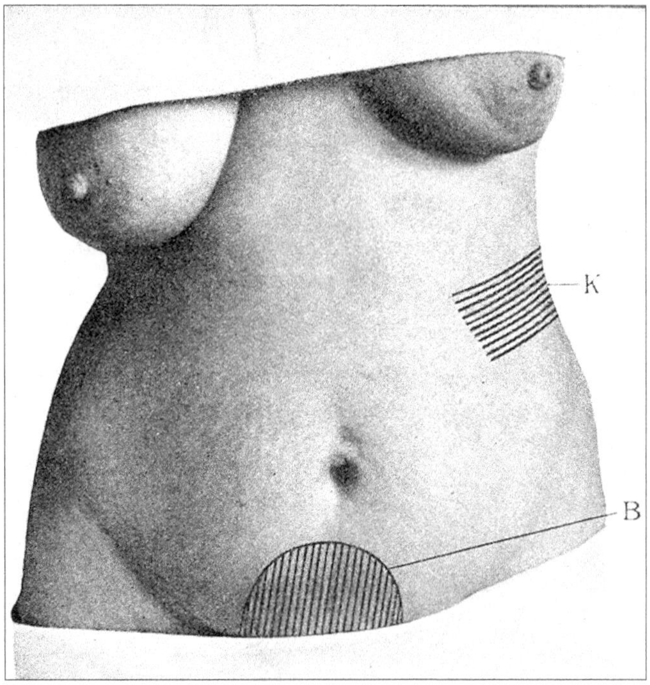

Figure 8-6. Kidney and bladder pain. The shaded areas in the photograph indicate the usual pain distribution for kidney (K) and bladder (B) disorders. From *A Treatise on the Diseases of Women for Students and Practitioners* (p. 853), by P. Findley, 1913, Philadelphia, PA: Lea & Febiger. In the public domain.

perhaps because of delay in diagnosis and the reluctance of some surgeons to operate (Rebarber & Jacob, 2023).

Appendicitis usually presents as dull, poorly localized periumbilical pain in both the pregnant and nonpregnant, but later localizes to sharp focal pain in the right lower quadrant (RLQ). Like their nonpregnant counterparts, most pregnant people with appendicitis experience maximal tenderness at McBurney's point, which is 3.8–5.1 cm (1.5–2 in.) below a line drawn from the right anterior superior iliac spine to the umbilicus (see Figure 8-5). In the third trimester, the appendix migrates a few centimeters cephalad as the uterus grows, and the pain of appendicitis can localize to the mid or upper right of the abdomen. Rebarber and Jacob (2023) note that pregnant clients with appendicitis often have vague or nonspecific signs and symptoms including nausea (85%), RLQ tenderness (85%), rebound tenderness (80%), RLQ pain (75%), vomiting (70%), anorexia (65%), abdominal guarding (50%), rectal tenderness (45%), RUQ pain or tenderness (20%), fever above 100.0°F (37.8°C, 20%), and dysuria (8%).

Graded-compression ultrasound (a technique of applying gradual transducer pressure to displace the bowel over the site of maximal pain) is the first-line imaging modality, offering excellent specificity but limited sensitivity (Mostbeck et al., 2016). Gestational age, maternal body mass index (BMI), and the training and experience of the sonographer can influence the accuracy of sonography for diagnosis. When ultrasound examination is inconclusive, MRI has a high sensitivity and specificity for diagnosing appendicitis during pregnancy. Computerized tomography (CT) can be performed if MRI is not readily available.

The treatment for suspected appendicitis is appendectomy with antibiotic therapy. The surgeon may choose a laparoscopic or open procedure. When there is a delay greater than 24 hr from onset of symptoms to surgery, 14–43% of clients suffer ruptured appendix (Rebarber & Jacob, 2023). Whereas appendectomy with an unruptured appendicitis carries a fetal loss rate of 1.5%, a ruptured appendix carries a 36% rate of fetal loss (Rebarber & Jacob, 2023). Peritoneal abscess and peritonitis also elevate the rate of fetal loss.

DIFFERENTIAL DIAGNOSES

Ectopic pregnancy, ruptured ovarian cyst, adnexal torsion, pelvic inflammatory disease (PID), ovarian cancer, placental abruption, IAI, uterine fibroid degeneration, labor, ectopic pregnancy, Crohn's disease, diverticulitis, ureteral stone, and HELLP syndrome.

Urinary Tract Infection (UTI)

Pregnancy predisposes individuals to UTI, the severity of which can range from mild and asymptomatic to critical. Pregnancy hormones relax smooth muscle in the ureters, which can kink and allow urine to pool, supporting bacterial growth. Pregnant people with a history of UTI, or those with urinary tract abnormalities, diabetes mellitus (but not gestational diabetes), sickle cell anemia, or PTL are at higher risk for infection.

Asymptomatic Bacteriuria

Asymptomatic bacteriuria occurs in 2–7% of pregnant people and is most common during early pregnancy (Cunningham et al., 2022, ch. 56; Gupta, 2023). Asymptomatic bacteriuria is defined as isolation of the same bacterial strain in the urine in counts of 100,000 or more colony-forming units (cfu)/ml (ACOG, 2023). Risk factors include prior UTI, diabetes mellitus, multiparity, and low socioeconomic status. Without treatment, up to 30–40% of these individuals develop symptomatic infection of the bladder or kidneys; with treatment, this risk falls by 70–80% (Gupta, 2023). Many studies associate untreated bacteriuria with greater risk of PTB, low birthweight, and higher perinatal mortality (Gupta, 2023).

Cystitis

Cystitis, a symptomatic infection of the bladder, occurs in approximately 7% of pregnancies in the United States (Cunningham et al., 2022, ch. 56; Gupta, 2023). It can present with

Consider treating UTI in pregnancy with a 10–14-day course of any of the following medications:

Cephalexin 500 mg 4 times daily

Ampicillin 500 mg 4 times daily

Nitrofurantoin 100 mg twice daily (second and third trimesters)

Sulfisoxazole 1 g 4 times daily (second and third trimesters)

About 20–40% of *Escherichia coli* infections are resistant to ampicillin and amoxicillin.

A test-of-cure urine culture should be negative 1–2 weeks after treatment begins.

Adapted from "Urinary Tract Infections in Pregnancy," by E. K. Johnson and E. D. Kim, 2017, *Medscape*, article 452604.

UTI Prevention for Client Education

Avoid adding scented agents to tub baths.

Wash hands before using the toilet.

Wash front to back.

Wipe front to back.

Never wipe twice with same tissue.

Use unscented soap, lotion, lubricants, and toilet paper.

Empty the bladder at least every 4 hr while awake.

Urinate when you need to; avoid suppressing the urge.

Avoid tight-fitting synthetic underpants; wear cotton.

Increase fluid intake until urine is pale or clear.

Empty the bladder before and after coitus.

Launder washcloths in hot water.

Disinfect sex toys.

frequent urination, urgency, lower pelvic cramping (especially while voiding), a burning sensation with urination, and sometimes a low-grade fever. Sometimes urinary-tract infection mimics or triggers PTL. Urine can be cloudy, bloody, or bad-smelling. Hematuria and pyuria (WBCs in the urine) are also frequently seen on urinalysis.

Urinalysis and urine culture are recommended for any client with dysuria. While a urine culture showing 100,000 cfu/ml or more is considered positive, in the presence of symptoms it may be appropriate to treat the client with antibiotics if the culture grows 1,000 cfu/ml or more of pathogenic bacteria (ACOG, 2023). *E. coli* causes the majority of UTIs in female individuals, pregnant or not (Gupta, 2023). Other pathogenic microorganisms include *Klebsiella* and *Enterobacter*, and gram-positive organisms such as GBS. If a culture has no growth in 24–48 hr, there is no infection present. False negatives can occur if the urine is very dilute. If the pregnant client's urine culture contains mixed gram-positive bacteria, lactobacilli, or *Staphylococcus* species (other than *S. saprophyticus*), these microorganisms are presumed to be contaminants rather than a true infection and do not constitute a UTI unless counts are 100,000 cfu/ml or higher (ACOG, 2023).

Urinalysis uses chemical, microscopic, and visual inspections of the urine to detect cells, cell fragments, and substances such as crystals or casts associated with UTI or other conditions. Some bacteria (such as *E. coli*) convert the nitrates that are present in healthy urine into a different kind of nitrite that can be tested for on urinalysis. Therefore, the presence of nitrites in urine is an indicator of UTI. Leukocyte esterase is an enzyme that is released by WBCs. Its presence indicates pyuria and is suspicious for UTI (Appenheimer & Ford, 2020). A voided sample contaminated with vaginal discharge might test positive for leukocyte esterase, however, especially during pregnancy (O'Leary, Armstrong, Byrne, Talento, & O'Coigligh, 2020) or when sexually transmitted infections or bacterial vaginosis is present (Appenheimer & Ford, 2020). Clients with positive leukocyte esterase do not require a urine culture unless they also have positive nitrates or symptoms of UTI (Coad, Friedman, & Geoffrion, 2012).

Treatment

If your client has signs and symptoms consistent with UTI, send clean-catch or catheter urine sample for culture. Empiric therapy can be started for the symptomatic client before culture results are available to alleviate discomfort and to decrease the likelihood of progression to pyelonephritis. The culture and sensitivity report issued by the laboratory will identify the causative microorganism and which antibiotics are the most effective treatments. A test of cure is necessary after antibiotic therapy because up to 30% of clients have persistent bacteriuria after treatment (Gupta, 2023).

There is some evidence that nutritional supplements such as cranberries, lactobacilli, and vitamin C taken separately can prevent recurrent UTIs in susceptible people, but work much better when taken together (Montorsi, Gandaglia, Salonia, Briganti, & Mirone, 2016). Although cranberry products alone can reduce the occurrence of

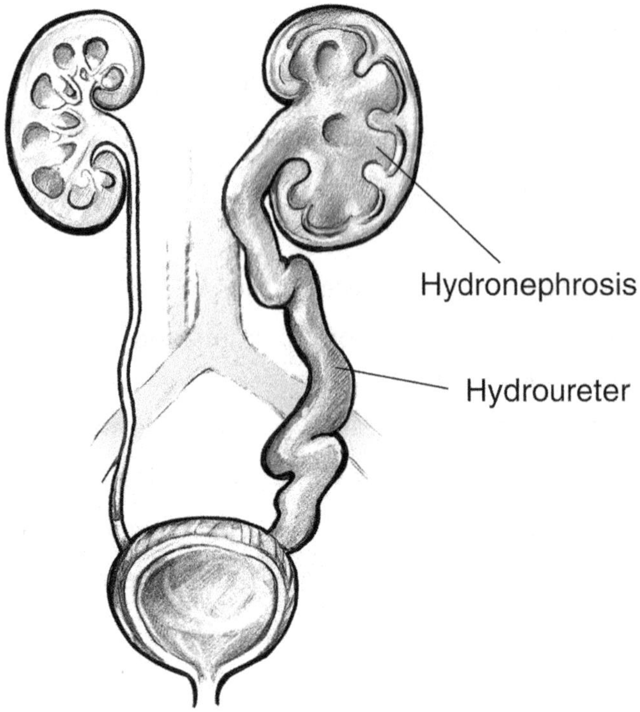

Figure 8-7. Hydronephrosis and hydroureter. "Drawing of Swollen Kidney and Ureter," by National Institute of Diabetes and Digestive and Kidney Diseases, n.d. (https://www.niddk.nih.gov/news/media-library/17590). In the public domain.

symptomatic UTI in some people, it does not seem to be effective in pregnancy (Dante, Pedrielli, Annessi, & Facchinetti, 2013). D-mannose, a simple sugar extracted from the larch tree, appears to prevent UTI by preventing bacteria from adhering to the bladder wall (Domenici et al., 2016). It has not, however, been studied in pregnancy.

Pyelonephritis

Pyelonephritis (infection of the upper urinary tract and kidneys) occurs in 0.5–2% of pregnant people, usually during the second and third trimesters (Gupta, 2023). Cystitis precedes pyelonephritis in almost 40% of cases (Cunningham et al., 2022, ch. 56). Symptoms include sudden onset of high fever, shaking chills, nausea, vomiting, urinary pain and urgency, flank or low-back pain, costovertebral angle tenderness, and malaise. Signs of cystitis are not always evident, but pyuria and hematuria are common. Untreated pyelonephritis can cause PTL or septic shock.

Pyelonephritis is a serious condition that can become life-threatening. Potential complications include anemia (from hemolysis due to endotoxins), bacteremia, respiratory insufficiency, pulmonary edema, preterm contractions, and renal injury or failure (Cunningham et al., 2022, ch. 56). As many as 20% of pregnant individuals with severe pyelonephritis develop complications including acute respiratory distress syndrome (ARDS) and septic shock syndrome (Gupta, 2023).

Management generally requires hospital admission and administration of parenteral broad-spectrum beta-lactams, along with IV hydration, antipyretics, and pain management. After the client has been afebrile for 24–48 hr and symptoms have improved, the provider may transition the client to oral antibiotics in accordance with susceptibility results and discharge to complete 10–14 days of treatment. Pyelonephritis in pregnancy reoccurs in 6–8% of clients (Gupta, 2023). Some providers give low-dose antibiotics for the remainder of the pregnancy to prevent reinfection.

Hydroureter and Hydronephrosis

Dilation of the ureters and renal pelvis (hydroureter and hydronephrosis) occurs when an obstructed urinary tract causes urine buildup in the upper urinary tract. Pregnancy hormones relax the smooth muscle of the ureter and allow it to become compressed by the enlarging uterus at the pelvic brim, obstructing urine flow (Farr et al., 2017). This dilated collecting system can contain 200–300 ml of urine, which favors the growth of bacteria and increases the risk of pyelonephritis (Thadhani & Maynard, 2022). Up to 80% of pregnant individuals have some degree of hydronephrosis or hydroureter, which typically begins in the second trimester and resolves by 6–12 weeks postpartum (Thadhani & Maynard, 2022).

While most cases of hydronephrosis remain asymptomatic, some clients experience acute or chronic flank pain. The right kidney is more likely to be affected. There appears to be no association between the volume of maternal hydronephrosis and the degree of flank pain experienced (Farr et al., 2017). Many clients are managed on analgesics and taught techniques to reduce pressure on the kidneys and ureters, such as urinating while on hands and knees in a bathtub. Pain from hydronephrosis can increase if the condition worsens or if urinary-tract infection develops. If hydronephrosis threatens kidney function, the client can require percutaneous or stent drainage. Rarely, hydronephrosis can exacerbate hypertension or cause renal failure.

DIFFERENTIAL DIAGNOSES

Renal stones, pyelonephrosis.

Kidney/Ureter Stones

Calculi in the kidney (nephrolithiasis) or ureter (ureterolithiasis) complicate 0.03–0.4-% of pregnancies, and are among the most common nonobstetric causes of hospital admission during pregnancy (Burwick, 2021). Certain physiologic changes during pregnancy encourage the formation of renal calculi. Higher calcium demand can increase the mobilization of calcium from the bones and suppress parathyroid function. Kidneys grow larger and filter blood at an increased rate. Calcium excretion doubles, and uric acid secretion increases out of proportion to urine citrate and magnesium excretion, creating favorable conditions for the formation of calcium oxalate or phosphate stones (Mandal, Saha, & Pal, 2017).

The client with renal or ureteral stones typically experiences severe pain in the flank, abdomen or groin. There is often blood or pus in the urine (Preminger & Curhan, 2021). Pain from upper-ureteral stones tends to radiate to the flank, and pain from lower ureteral obstruction typically radiates to the labia. The location and character of the pain can change as the stone migrates. Pain comes in waves as the stone moves in the ureter and causes ureteral spasm. Kidney infection can accompany nephrolithiasis, causing fever and malaise. Uncommonly, renal calculi can lead to premature labor or preeclampsia. Urinary obstruction with concurrent infection is unusual, but when present, it carries a high risk of spontaneous abortion and premature labor.

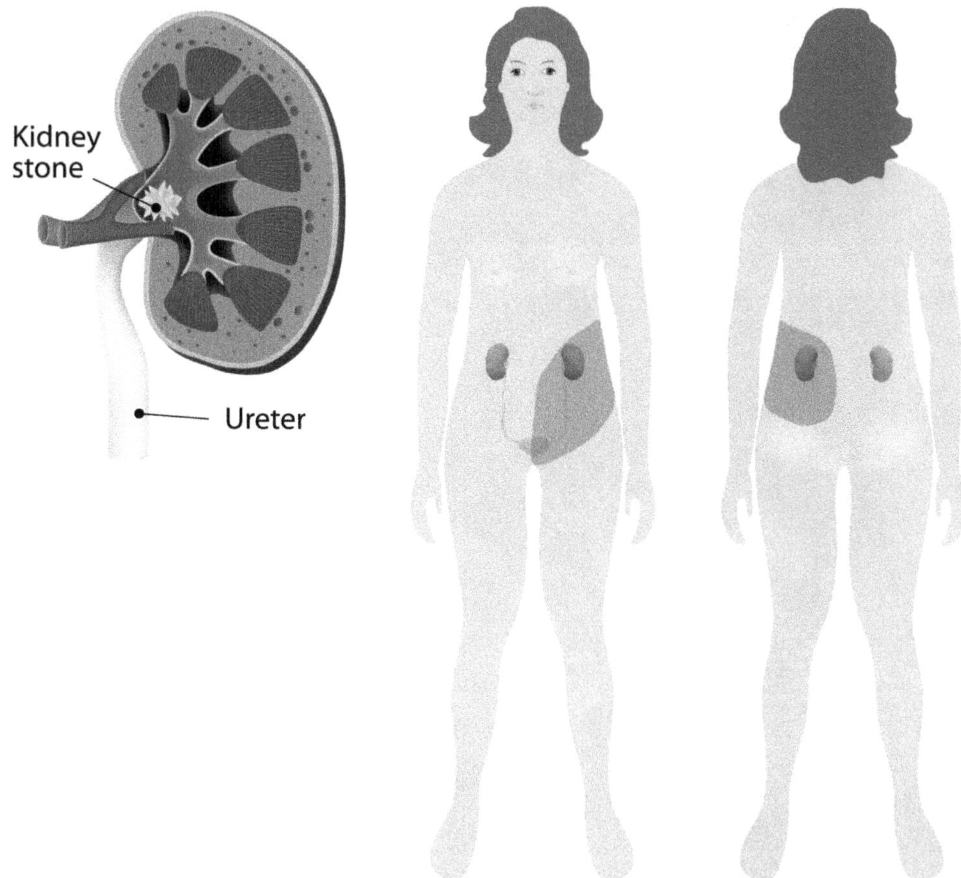

Figure 8-8. Typical pain distribution for renal calculi. The pain of kidney stones tends to occur in a flank—abdomen-groin distribution (©designua/Adobe Stock).

Renal and pelvic ultrasound detects kidney and ureteral stones in about 60% of cases (Preminger & Curhan, 2021). If transabdominal ultrasound is negative, transvaginal and Doppler sonography can detect distal ureteral stones. MRI may be considered in any trimester, and low-dose CT scans may be used in the second and third trimesters (Preminger & Curhan, 2021).

Most cases of renal colic present in the second or third trimester of pregnancy and can affect either side. Urolithiasis in pregnancy is usually managed with hydration and analgesia while laying the client on the asymptomatic side (Preminger & Curhan, 2021). About 70–80% of stones pass through the urinary tract spontaneously (Preminger & Curhan, 2021). Occasionally, emergent surgical management of renal stones is necessary in the case of obstructing stones with evidence of UTI, sepsis, or acute kidney injury. If there are no indications for emergency surgery, stone removal is often delayed until after birth.

DIFFERENTIAL DIAGNOSES

Appendicitis, bowel obstruction, cholecystitis.

Ovarian Cyst

Ovarian cysts are a common finding in pregnancy, and seldom cause complications or pain. Generally, ovarian cysts identified in pregnant clients are benign simple cysts less than 5 cm in diameter (Runowicz & Brewer, 2023). Most of these are either follicular or corpus luteum cysts that occur as part of the normal function of the ovary, and most spontaneously resolve by the early second trimester. Some ovarian cysts become symptomatic due to their size or location, or cause pain when they compress adjacent structures. Persistent ovarian cysts, particularly those larger than 5 cm, can cause torsion or labor obstruction, or they can rupture and cause intraabdominal hemorrhage (D'Ambrosio et al., 2021).

Rupture of an ovarian cyst into the peritoneal cavity or bleeding into an ovarian cyst is a rare occurrence in pregnancy but is most likely to happen in the first or early second trimester. Rupture can occur spontaneously, but typically

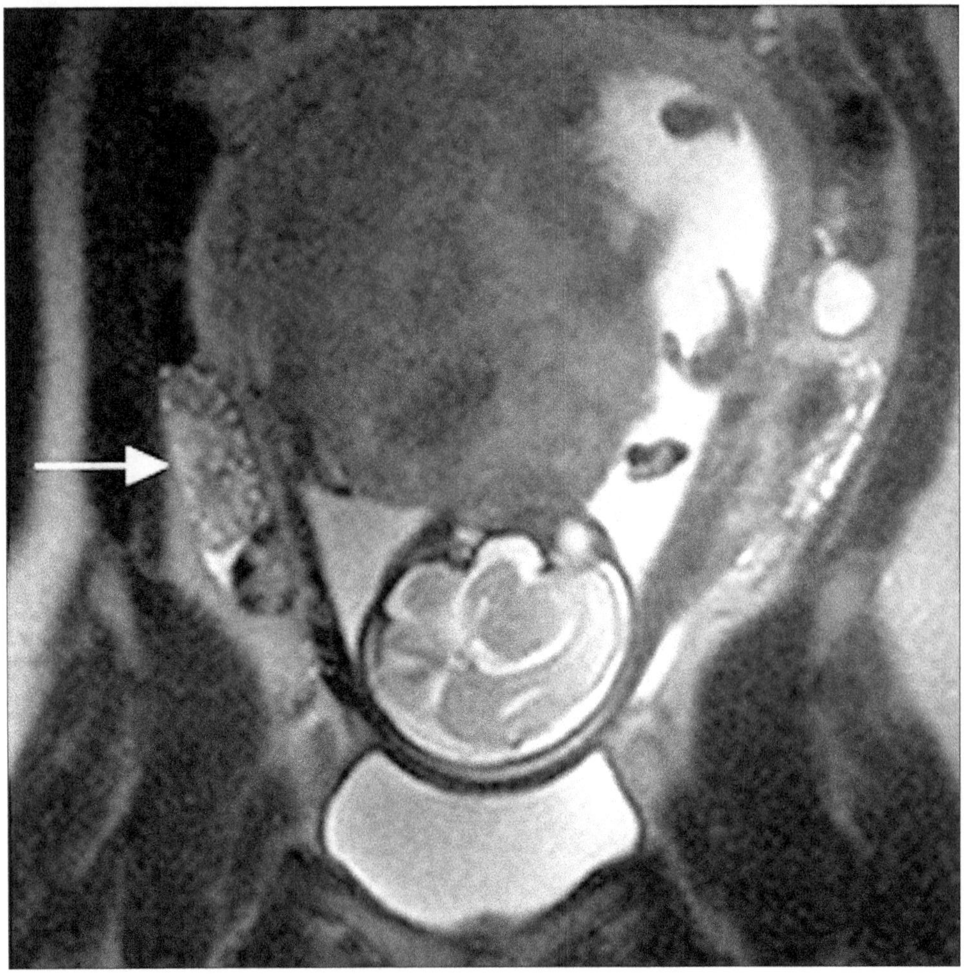

Figure 8-9. A 30-year-old woman presented with RLQ pain at 28 weeks gestational age. Magnetic-resonance imaging (MRI) demonstrated an enlarged right ovary (arrow) and a normal appearing left ovary. The right ovary, torsed repeatedly to 720°, was surgically removed. From "Magnetic Resonance Imaging Performance for Diagnosis of Ovarian Torsion in Pregnant Women with Stimulated Ovaries," by E. Asch et al., 2017, *Fertility Research and Practice, 3*, p. 13. CC BY 4.0.

follows strenuous physical activity, such as exercise or sexual intercourse. Pain is usually sudden and is moderate to severe on one side of the lower abdomen, probably caused by the irritating effects of blood flowing into the abdomen or stretching the ovarian cortex (Sharp, 2023). One side of the lower abdomen may be tender to palpation. A ruptured dermoid cyst can release sebaceous material or blood into the abdomen and cause peritonitis with rigidity of the abdominal wall and rebound tenderness (Sharp, 2023).

Rarely, bleeding from a ruptured cyst can cause hemodynamic instability. Intraabdominal hemorrhage can be associated with Cullen's sign (bluish discoloration around the umbilicus). Ultrasound examination can show an adnexal mass and fluid in the pelvis or just free fluid. Most people with a ruptured ovarian cyst are discharged home after diagnosis, but surgery (usually via laparoscopy) may be indicated in cases complicated by extreme pain or hemorrhage.

DIFFERENTIAL DIAGNOSES

Ectopic pregnancy, appendicitis, degenerating fibroid.

Adnexal Torsion

Adnexal torsion occurs when the ovary or fallopian tube twists with the vascular pedicle, crimping off blood vessels and compromising perfusion. Tissues beyond the obstruction become hypoxic and eventually necrotic and inflamed. Adnexal torsion is a surgical emergency, and delay in diagnosis can result in loss of an ovary, peritonitis, and even death.

Torsion occurs in female individuals of all ages—even female fetuses—but is especially common during pregnancy, particularly between 10 and 17 weeks of gestation. Risk is greatest for people with ovarian masses or with large, hyperstimulated ovaries due to infertility therapies (Bras, Braga, Tomé, & Ferreira, 2017). Pregnant individuals with a persistent adnexal mass (4 cm or larger) have about a 15% chance of ovarian or adnexal torsion (Laufer, 2023). Torsion can also occur in the postpartum period because of a sudden increase in adnexal mobility (Laufer, 2023).

The classic presentation is severe, colicky, unilateral lower abdominal and pelvic pain. The pain is often constant but can be intermittent if the ovary twists and untwists with change in posture or activity (Sasaki & Miller, 2014). Signs and symptoms can include severe pain in the lower abdomen and flank, nausea, vomiting, and possibly low-grade fever. Physical examination does not always yield concrete information about the source of the problem. Though rebound tenderness can occur, up to 30% of clients with confirmed torsion had no pain upon abdominal palpation or release of pressure (Sasaki & Miller, 2014). The clinician sometimes elicits cervical motion tenderness or palpates a tender adnexal mass.

Sonographic imaging can reveal an ovarian mass, enlargement, displacement, free fluid in the cul-de-sac, or uniform peripheral cystic structures formed by edema of the follicles (Sasaki & Miller, 2014). A torsed fallopian tube may be enlarged and filled with fluid. Doppler studies can document lack of blood flow to the ovarian tissue. If adnexal torsion is suspected, emergency laparoscopy or laparotomy is performed either to restore circulation or to remove the tube and ovary. Adnexal torsion is very difficult to diagnose preoperatively. Laparoscopy confirms the diagnosis in only about 10%–44% of clients suspected of torsion (Sasaki & Miller, 2014).

DIFFERENTIAL DIAGNOSES

Ectopic pregnancy, degenerating uterine fibroid, ruptured ovarian cyst, appendicitis, renal stones, placental abruption.

Uterine Fibroids

Uterine fibroids (leiomyomas), benign smooth muscle cell tumors of the uterus, are common among individuals of childbearing age. Fibroids can grow or shrink during pregnancy but usually do not (Ouyang & Norwitz, 2022). Larger fibroids (more than 5 cm in diameter) are more likely to grow, typically increasing during the first trimester and remaining stable thereafter.

Uterine fibroids are usually asymptomatic in pregnancy, but can cause localized or generalized discomfort, especially if more than 5 cm in diameter. Degeneration, torsion, or impaction of a uterine fibroid can cause severe abdominal pain during pregnancy. Submucosal and retroplacental fibroids increase the risk of placental abruption, especially when they are large.

Large submucosal fibroids that distort the uterine cavity can cause fetal malpresentation. Fibroids have been associated with dysfunctional labor and higher rates of tachysystole. Large fibroids in the lower uterine segment can obstruct labor.

Red or carneous degeneration occurs when a fibroid outgrows its blood supply, usually in the second trimester (Bhave, Shah, & Chaudhari, 2016). Lack of perfusion leads to tissue necrosis and infarction, which is typically accompanied by significant localized abdominal pain, nausea, vomiting, low-grade fever, and leukocytosis. Fibroid degeneration is a self-limited process. Treatment often involves pain management with acetaminophen or short-term opioid administration. For pregnancies less than 32 weeks of gestation, a 48-hr course of NSAIDs may be used (Ouyang & Norwitz, 2022). Using NSAIDs after 32 0/7 weeks of gestation or for longer than 48 hr can cause the fetus to develop premature closure of the ductus arteriosus, neonatal pulmonary hypertension, oligohydramnios, or platelet dysfunction (Ouyang & Norwitz, 2022).

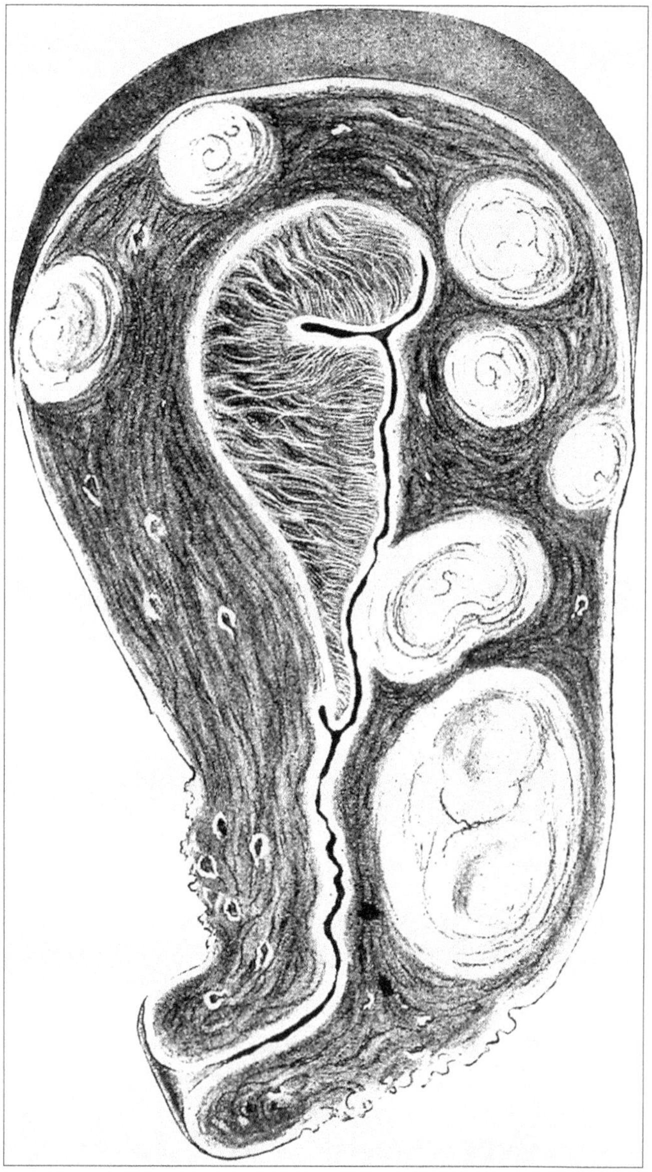

Figure 8-10. Multiple intramural fibroids in a uterus immediately postpartum. The uterus was removed immediately after cesarean section following a long, dysfunctional labor. The placenta is retained in the uterine cavity. From *A Treatise on the Diseases of Women for Students and Practitioners* (p. 95), by P. Findley, 1913, Philadelphia, PA: Lea & Febiger. In the public domain.

DIFFERENTIAL DIAGNOSES

Appendicitis, pyelonephritis, cholecystitis, placental abruption.

Cholecystitis and Cholelithiasis

The term *cholecystitis* refers to inflammation of the gallbladder, usually in association with cholelithiasis (gallstones). When there is an imbalance or change in the composition of bile, cholesterol crystals and calcium salts can form rocklike gallstones and biliary sludge that can interfere with drainage of the gallbladder and cause inflammation. Cholelithiasis is more

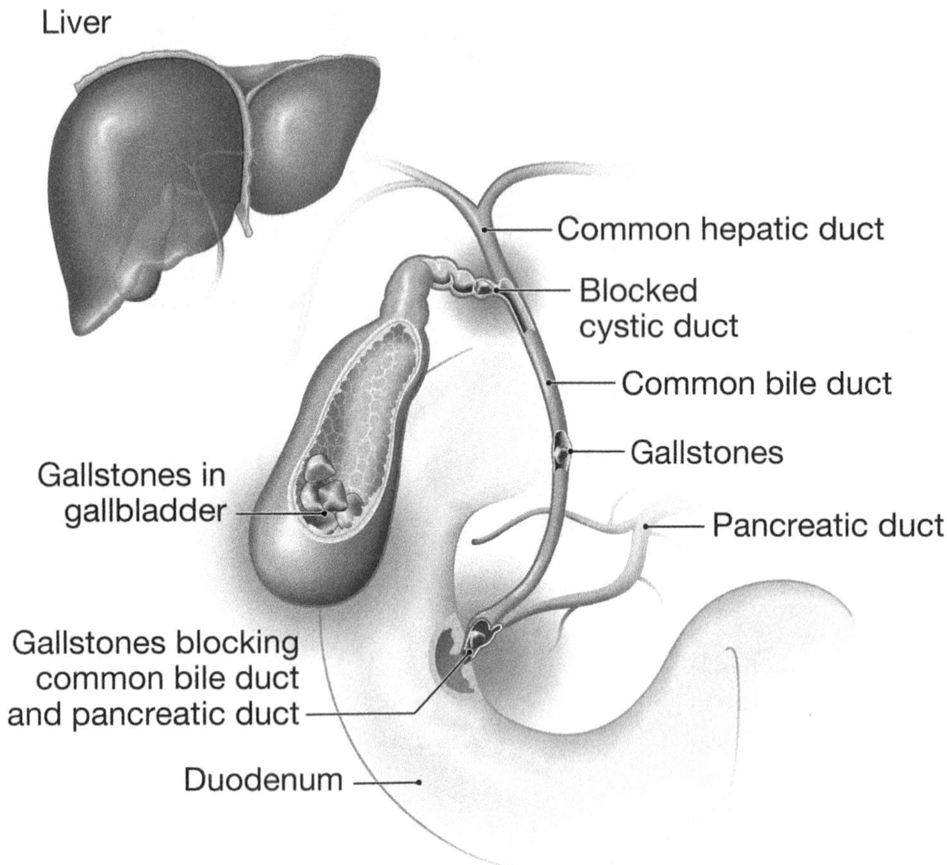

Figure 8-11. Common sites of pain and obstruction with cholelithiasis. Physiologic changes of pregnancy such as slowed gallbladder emptying and increased cholesterol saturation of bile encourage the formation of gallstones (©Axel Kock/Adobe Stock)

common during pregnancy because of slowed gallbladder emptying and increased cholesterol saturation of bile (Brooks, 2022). About 30% of pregnant individuals have biliary sludge, and 1–3% develop gallstones (Durnwald, 2021).

Biliary colic occurs when the gallbladder contracts, usually after a fatty meal, and pushes a stone or sludge against its outlet. Rising pressure within the gallbladder causes pain, which typically persists for 4–6 hr. Then, as the gallbladder relaxes, the stones shift, and pain subsides (Brooks, 2022).

The classic presentation of acute cholecystitis is deep, gnawing RUQ or epigastric pain, sometimes radiating to the shoulder, back, or chest; anorexia; nausea; vomiting; and fever. This pain, known as biliary colic, tends to develop an hour or more after a meal containing fatty food. The client with gallbladder pain often has tenderness to palpation in the RUQ (Murphy's sign). Press your fingers at the costal margin in the RUQ on the right midclavicular line. Ask the client to inhale. As air fills the lungs, press deeply into the subcostal region. If the client experiences pain or suddenly stops inhaling, Murphy's sign is positive, suggesting an inflamed gallbladder. A sonographic Murphy's sign occurs when the client experiences pain when the ultrasound transducer scans the area over the gallbladder.

Pale or gray stools can occur if the bile duct is completely obstructed. Laboratory studies can show leukocytosis (elevated WBC count), elevated band count, and elevated liver enzymes. Ultrasound studies can identify gallstones and biliary sludge, inflammation of the gallbladder, and dilation of the common bile duct.

Expectant management of cholecystitis is the safest approach in the pregnant client, but surgery is often indicated if pancreatitis, common bile-duct obstruction, or cholangitis (infection of the bile duct) occurs. Severe cholecystitis can lead to abscess and gangrene. Uncommonly, severe cholecystitis with or without cholelithiasis can lead to perforation of the gallbladder and peritonitis caused by bile spilling into the abdominal cavity. After appendicitis, acute cholecystitis is the most common nonobstetrical indication for surgery in pregnant people (Athwal, Bhogal, Hodson, & Ramcharan, 2016). Laparoscopic removal of the gallbladder (cholecystectomy) is the most common laparoscopic procedure performed in pregnancy. It is safest when undertaken in the second trimester (Durnwald, 2021). PTB and fetal loss are rare complications of cholecystectomy during pregnancy (Athwal et al., 2016). Most cases of biliary colic and some cases of mild acute cholecystitis can be managed with supportive care and expectant management until cholecystectomy can be performed shortly after giving birth (Durnwald, 2021). Cholecystectomy is indicated during pregnancy when the client has recurrent biliary colic or severe acute cholecystitis (Durnwald, 2021).

Gallstone Pancreatitis

Acute pancreatitis during pregnancy, a rare but serious disease, is almost always associated with gallstones (Cunningham et al., 2022, ch. 58). If a gallstone lodges within the ampule of Vater, blocking drainage of the pancreatic duct, digestive enzymes back up and become activated. The pancreas begins to digest itself, causing massive inflammation and tissue damage. High estrogen levels and a genetic predisposition toward high triglyceride levels can also precipitate pancreatitis. One in 5 pregnant clients with acute pancreatitis will develop severe disease; mortality for severe pancreatitis can reach 25% (Cunningham et al., 2022, ch. 58; Ducarme, Maire, Chatel, Luton, & Hammel, 2014). Fetal risks include PTL and intrauterine fetal death.

Pancreatitis is most likely to develop during the third trimester or the early postpartum period (Ducarme et al., 2014). The pain of acute pancreatitis is typically sudden and severe, starting in the upper abdomen and radiating to the back. Leaning forward lessens its severity. Nausea, vomiting, abdominal distension, low-grade fever, tachycardia, hypotension, and abdominal tenderness may be present. About 10% develop sepsis, which causes widespread inflammation throughout the body and can lead to ARDS (Cunningham et al., 2022, ch. 58).

Serum amylase levels 300% of upper normal values or higher and elevated serum lipase support the diagnosis of acute pancreatitis. The degree of enzyme elevation, however, does not reliably correlate with the severity of disease (Cunningham et al., 2022, ch. 58). Symptoms usually resolve in about 5 days with conservative treatment, including bowel rest, pain medication, IV hydration, and sometimes nasogastric suction. Although nonsurgical management of gallstone pancreatitis is recommended in the first trimester, laparoscopic cholecystectomy is preferred in the second (Ducarme et al., 2014). Third-trimester management ranges from conservative treatment to surgery.

DIFFERENTIAL DIAGNOSES

Gastric or duodenal ulcer, bowel obstruction, ectopic pregnancy, biliary colic, diverticulitis. intraabdominal abscess, acute fatty liver of pregnancy.

Bowel Obstruction

Bowel obstruction is a very rare but serious cause of abdominal pain in pregnancy. The risk of bowel obstruction during pregnancy increases with advancing gestation and is most frequently caused by the pressure of the growing uterus on adhesions from previous abdominal surgeries, including appendectomy or gastric bypass (Cunningham et al., 2022, ch. 57). It can also occur immediately postpartum when the uterus rapidly becomes smaller (Cunningham et al., 2022, ch. 57). Other causes of bowel obstruction in pregnancy include colorectal cancer, volvulus (twisting of a loop of intestine around its mesenteric attachment), intussusception (one segment of intestine telescopes inside another), or hernia (Kilpatrick & Shamshirsaz, 2022). Fetal mortality secondary to maternal bowel obstruction is 17%,

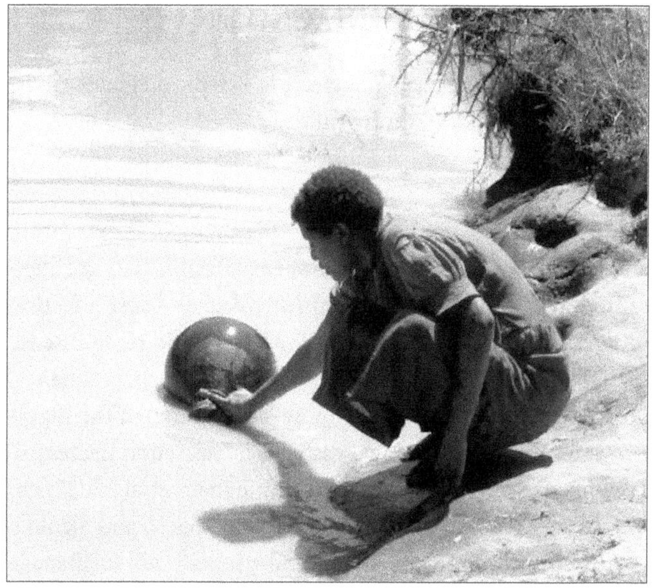

Figure 8-12. Giardiasis, an intestinal infection caused by the protozoan parasite *Giardia lamblia*, can cause abdominal cramps, flatulence, vomiting, or watery diarrhea. Giardiasis usually spreads through drinking water contaminated with feces from infected people or animals. "Unsafe Drinking Water, Ethiopia," by D. Lantagne, 2006, Centers for Disease Control and Prevention Public Health Image Library image 22472 (https://phil.cdc.gov/Details.aspx?pid=2247). In the public domain.

and the maternal mortality rate is 2% (Webster, Bailey, Wilson, & Burke, 2015).

Typical signs of acute bowel obstruction in pregnancy include (Cunningham et al., 2022, ch. 57)

- Abdominal pain (98%)
- Nausea and vomiting (82%)
- Abdominal tenderness (70%)
- Abnormal bowel sounds (55%)

Often the victim is unable to pass any stool or gas (Kilpatrick & Shamshirsaz, 2022). Pain is usually diffuse and poorly localized. Small-bowel obstruction is more painful than colonic obstruction. Pain typically comes in waves—every 4–5 min for upper-bowel obstruction (Bordeianou & Yeh, 2021), or every 20–30 min for lower-bowel (Yeh & Bordeianou, 2023).

Diagnosis is confirmed by examination and imaging. Abdominal ultrasound scans, radiographs, or MRI usually reveal the site and degree of obstruction. Bowel obstruction is managed similarly in pregnant and nonpregnant clients. If there are no signs of peritonitis, the provider may opt for a conservative approach, which includes nasogastric aspiration and IV fluids. Bowel obstruction is potentially life-threatening. Immediate surgery is indicated when bowel ischemia, necrosis, or perforation is suspected (Bordeianou & Yeh, 2022).

DIFFERENTIAL DIAGNOSES

Gastric or duodenal ulcer, pancreatitis, ectopic pregnancy, biliary colic, appendicitis, diverticulitis.

Perforated Ulcer

Peptic ulcers are open sores in the lining of the stomach, duodenum, or occasionally the lower esophagus. They are often caused by chronic gastritis from *Helicobacter pylori* infection or overuse of aspirin or other NSAIDs. Peptic ulcer disease (PUD) is an uncommon cause of abdominal pain in pregnancy, probably because food moves more slowly through the digestive tract during pregnancy, gastric acid secretion decreases, and mucus secretion increases (Cunningham et al., 2022, ch. 57). A pregnant individual should avoid tobacco and alcohol, improve nutrition, avoid stress, and use antacids to manage heartburn—practices that encourage peptic ulcers to heal (Goel, Rani, Huria, Gupta, & Dalal, 2014).

PUD is characterized by epigastric pain, which can be worse at night or after eating, and is often accompanied by nausea and vomiting. When PUD is diagnosed in pregnancy, treatment includes acid suppression with a proton pump inhibitor and testing for *Helicobacter pylori* infection. If *H. pylori* is present, antimicrobial treatment is usually initiated during the postpartum period (Vakil, 2022).

A perforated peptic ulcer is a medical emergency in which acid, digestive enzymes, and partially digested food leak into the abdominal cavity, causing sudden, agonizing pain. The pain of a perforated ulcer is severe and diffuse, and it may be felt in the abdomen, epigastrium, neck, or chest. Deep breathing or movement can worsen the pain. The client sometimes has grossly bloody or "coffee-ground" emesis containing partially digested blood. As shock sets in, the client becomes pale, sweaty, tachycardic, and hypotensive with a boardlike abdomen (Kilpatrick & Shamshirsaz, 2022). The client usually does well if the condition is diagnosed within 6 hr after perforation but deteriorates with more than a 12-hr delay (Kilpatrick & Shamshirsaz, 2022). Most perforations of the stomach and duodenum are surgical emergencies (Søreide et al., 2015).

DIFFERENTIAL DIAGNOSES

Ruptured abdominal aortic aneurysm, biliary colic, pancreatitis.

Other Abdominal Pain

In addition to the conditions mentioned above, abdominal pain in a pregnant person can indicate placental abruption, uterine rupture, labor, miscarriage, ectopic pregnancy, or trauma. These conditions are discussed elsewhere in the book. Musculoskeletal issues are a common cause of pain during pregnancy. A highly active or malpositioned fetus can cause discomfort that a client or provider can mistake for a more serious issue. For example, the unyielding head of a breech fetus wedged against the rib cage can cause pain.

Table 8-2
Etiologies to Consider for Abdominal Pain

Epigastric
Consider gastric or duodenal ulcer, early appendicitis, hiatal hernia, HELLP syndrome, heartburn, gallbladder disease, pancreatitis, or (rarely) myocardial infarction.

Right-upper-quadrant (RUQ)
Consider abruption, uterine rupture, cholecystitis, hepatitis, HELLP syndrome, constipation, pneumonia, diverticulitis, diarrhea, intestinal gas, pressure from fetus, appendicitis. Right flank pain from renal calculi or hydronephrosis can radiate to the RUQ.

Left-upper-quadrant (LUQ)
Consider abruption, uterine rupture, heartburn, ulcers, constipation, diarrhea, diverticulitis, or enlarged spleen (such as with infectious mononucleosis).

Right-lower-quadrant (RLQ)
Consider abruption, uterine rupture, round-ligament pain, intestinal gas, appendicitis, ectopic pregnancy, postsurgical adhesions, ureteral stones, diverticulitis, inguinal hernia, endometriosis lesions, ovarian cysts and tumors, ovarian torsion, fibroids, cystitis.

Left-lower-quadrant (LLQ)
Consider abruption, uterine rupture, round-ligament pain, colon pain, intestinal gas, ectopic pregnancy, postsurgical adhesions, ureteral stones, diverticulitis, inguinal hernia, endometriosis lesions, ovarian cysts and tumors, ovarian torsion, fibroids, cystitis.

Intestinal gas and diarrhea cramps are just as common as in the nonpregnant population. Acute diarrhea is usually caused by viruses, bacteria, or parasites. Foodborne diseases can present with nausea, vomiting, fever, abdominal pain, and diarrhea developing anywhere from 1 hr to several days after the contaminated food is consumed (Kendall & Moreira, 2023). Constipation can cause persistent abdominal pain. Abdominal pain can also result when pain is referred from another site.

About half of individuals with sickle cell disease have acutely painful vasoocclusive episodes while pregnant (Kilpatrick & Shamshirsaz, 2022). RUQ pain is often associated with liver involvement. About half of vasoocclusive episodes are accompanied by fever, swelling, tenderness, tachypnea, hypertension, nausea, or vomiting (Kilpatrick & Shamshirsaz, 2022).

Somatization Syndrome

Somatization disorder belongs to a category of psychiatric disorders in which the client experiences various physical

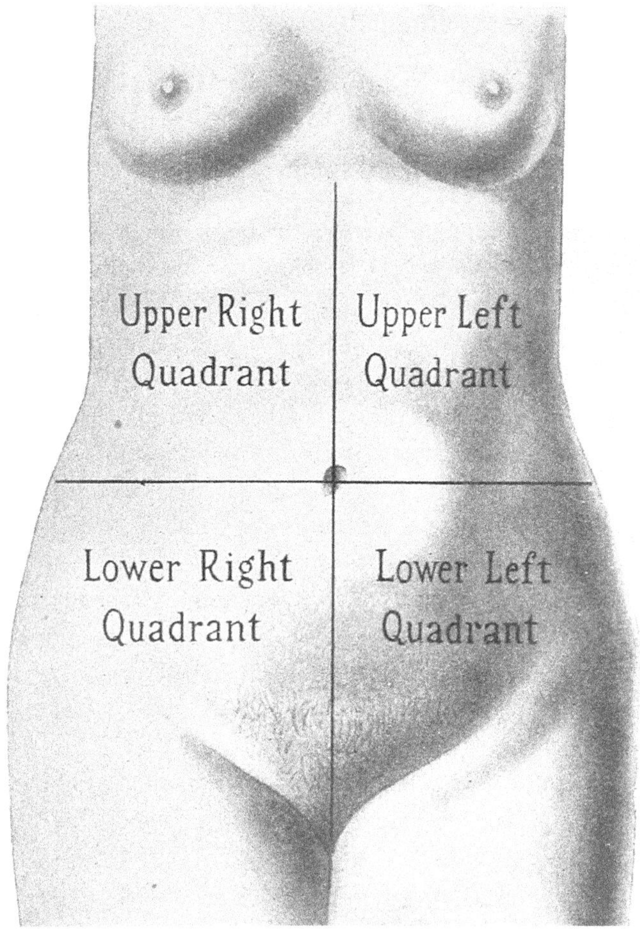

Figure 8-13. Where is the pain? Location can be an important clue to diagnosis. From *A Treatise on the Diseases of Women for Students and Practitioners* (p. 95), by P. Findley, 1913, Philadelphia, PA: Lea & Febiger. In the public domain.

symptoms, attributes them to physical illness, and seeks medical help for them (Iloson, Möller, Sundfeldt, & Bernhardsson, 2021). Clients with somatization can present with multiple unexplained symptoms, vague and inconsistent history, lack of factors that exacerbate or alleviate symptoms, and lack of positive findings on physical examination (Levenson, 2022).

Common complaints include headache; pain in the pelvis, abdomen, back or joints; gastrointestinal symptoms such as nausea, vomiting, bloating, gas, and diarrhea; cardiopulmonary symptoms such as chest pain, dizziness, shortness of breath, and palpitations; neurologic symptoms such as fainting, pseudoseizures, amnesia, muscle weakness, dysphagia, visual disturbances, and difficulty walking; and gynecological complaints such as dyspareunia, chronic dysmenorrhea, and vulvodynia (Levenson, 2022). Adult somatization often follows childhood or adult trauma, especially sexual trauma (Iloson et al., 2021). Symptoms are frequently triggered by present-day anxiety, depression, or interpersonal conflicts (Levenson, 2022). They are real to the client and can be disabling.

Table 8-3
Risk Factors for Venous Thromboembolism (VTE)

Antepartum

- Multiple gestation
- Varicose veins
- Inflammatory bowel disease
- UTI
- Diabetes
- Hospitalization for >3 days for condition unrelated to giving birth
- Body mass index (BMI) ≥30 kg/m^2
- Maternal age ≥35 years

Postpartum

- Cesarean, especially emergent
- Medical comorbidities
- BMI ≥25 kg/m^2
- PTB before 36 0/7 weeks of gestation
- Antepartum or postpartum hemorrhage
- Stillbirth
- Maternal age ≥35 years
- Hypertension
- Smoking
- Eclampsia or preeclampsia
- Postpartum infection

Adapted from "Deep Vein Thrombosis in Pregnancy: Epidemiology, Pathogenesis, and Diagnosis," by A. Malhotra and S. E. Weinberger, 2023a, in G. Finlay (Ed.), *UpToDate*. Copyright by UpToDate.

DIFFERENTIAL DIAGNOSES

Diseases such as Lyme disease, lupus, Ehlers-Danlos syndrome, and Marfan syndrome are examples of diseases with diverse physical manifestations that can cause pain and dysfunction in many different body systems.

Assessment and Management of Acute Abdomen in Pregnancy

The term *acute abdomen* can describe any spontaneous, nontraumatic disorder with rapid onset of symptoms that can indicate serious intraabdominal pathology (Leath & Phippen, 2022). Pathologic abdominal pain can be especially difficult to diagnose during pregnancy. Some conditions that cause abdominal pain, such as acute bowel obstruction, appendicitis, ectopic pregnancy, or placental abruption, can be immediately life-threatening and require immediate referral to an emergency department (Kendall & Moreira, 2023).

In contrast with symptoms from benign issues, pain associated with acute abdomen is typically moderate or severe and can be accompanied by vomiting, diarrhea, vaginal bleeding, headache, fever, or fainting (Kilpatrick & Shamshirsaz, 2022). Hemodynamic instability is always serious, and it necessitates rapid transport by ambulance to a hospital. Peritoneal signs (rebound tenderness, abdominal guarding) or pain confined to one part of the abdomen suggest significant abdominal pathology. A client with peritonitis avoids movement and keeps the knees flexed. Any bump, cough, or palpation of the abdomen causes severe pain. Rebound tenderness and abdominal-wall rigidity (involuntary guarding) are also signs of peritonitis.

Management priorities for acute abdomen include

- Obtain GOLDCART history.
- Assess airway, breathing, and circulation; monitor vital signs; and perform targeted physical examination.
- If vital signs are unstable, start an intravenous (IV) infusion of normal saline or lactated Ringer's, consider administering oxygen, position for comfort and optimal vital signs, and transport rapidly to a facility with the capacity for immediate surgery.
- If client is stable, consult or transfer care as indicated, and arrange for transport as recommended by a physician.
- Chart essential data and history for the receiving facility and send records.

Difficulty Breathing in Pregnancy

It can be a challenge to distinguish the normal physiologic dyspnea of pregnancy from the signs and symptoms of pulmonary or cardiac pathology. Sixty to 70% of healthy pregnant people complain of shortness of breath at some point in the pregnancy (Weinberger, 2023). Many clients report a sensation of air hunger that begins in the first or second trimester, increases during the second trimester, and then usually improves in the third trimester (Weinberger, 2023). One explanation is that high levels of progesterone cause hyperventilation and mild respiratory alkalosis, causing the feeling of breathlessness. When a client reports shortness of breath, perform a thorough assessment and refer to a higher level of care if there is any possibility that the symptoms are abnormal.

Abnormal breathing can be caused by (Schwartzstein, 2023)

- Lack of fitness
- Anemia
- Neuromuscular, airway, chest wall, or lung conditions reducing ability to move air
- Alterations in the ability of the lung to exchange gases
- Alterations in cardiovascular system function
- Alterations of the respiratory center in the brain
- Ketoacidosis

Venous Thromboembolism (VTE)

Thrombosis is the partial or complete blockage of a vessel by a blood clot. Pulmonary embolus (PE) is the partial or complete blockage of the pulmonary artery or one of its branches. About 90% of blood clots in the lung arise from a deep-vein thrombosis (DVT) elsewhere in the body, usually in the leg (Merriam & Pettker, 2021). Venous thromboembolism (VTE) is the term to describe disorders which involve DVT and/or pulmonary embolism (PE). VTE complicates approximately 1 in 1,500 pregnancies (Merriam & Pettker, 2021). It is the seventh leading cause of maternal mortality in the United States, accounting for 9% of maternal deaths (Malhotra & Weinberger, 2023a). About half of these cases develop antepartum, and the other half develop postpartum, most often in the first weeks (ACOG Cmte. on Clinical Practice, 2018/2022).

Pregnancy induces profound changes to the hemostatic system. To support the growth of a fetus, the pregnant individual must develop high-volume, high-flow, low-resistance uteroplacental circulation. To avoid potentially lethal postpartum hemorrhage, the mother's blood must clot more readily. Because of this hypercoagulability, the incidence of VTE is 4 times higher during pregnancy than it is in the nonpregnant state (Malhotra & Weinberger, 2023a). VTE is most likely to develop under conditions of vascular disruption, venous stasis, and a hypercoagulable state (Virchow's triad), all of which can be present in pregnancy. Risk increases when the enlarging uterus compresses the inferior vena cava and pelvic veins (ACOG Cmte. on Clinical Practice, 2018/2022). Up to 25% of all cases of VTE in pregnancy occur in mothers who have had a previous event (ACOG Cmte. on Clinical Practice, 2018/2022). The presence of inherited thrombophilias such as Factor V Leiden or antiphospholipid antibody syndrome is another major risk factor. Cesarean birth increases the risk of VTE fourfold as compared with vaginal birth (ACOG Cmte. on Clinical Practice, 2018/2022). Other conditions that increase risk include the presence of varicosities, postpartum hemorrhage, infection, hypertension, autoimmune disease, heart disease, sickle cell disease, multiple gestation, and preeclampsia.

Deep-vein Thrombosis (DVT)

DVT occurs when a blood clot forms in one or more deep veins. Most DVTs in pregnancy form in the femoral vein; relatively few arise in the calf. DVT can also occur in the iliac veins of the pelvis, causing pain in the lower abdomen. In pregnancy, DVT is most likely to involve the left leg (70–90%) because of compression of the left iliac vein by the right iliac artery and from pressure of the pregnant uterus on the inferior vena cava (Malhotra & Weinberger, 2023a).

Diffuse pain and swelling, redness, warmth, and tenderness may develop. Sometimes a thrombosed vein feels like a palpable cord of tissue. A positive test for Homans' sign (pain elicited by while dorsiflexing the foot) suggests DVT; but Homans' sign may be present with many other conditions, such as cellulitis, muscle or tendon injury, trauma, or lymphedema (Merriam & Pettker, 2021). If circulation is intact, the client may have no signs or symptoms. Iliac-vein thrombosis may present with swelling of the entire leg, which can be accompanied by flank, lower-abdomen, buttock, or back pain. Many clients with superficial venous thrombosis also have or develop DVT that is not apparent (Cannegieter et al., 2015). Diagnosis of DVT is made using venous ultrasonography with or without color Doppler (Merriam & Pettker, 2021).

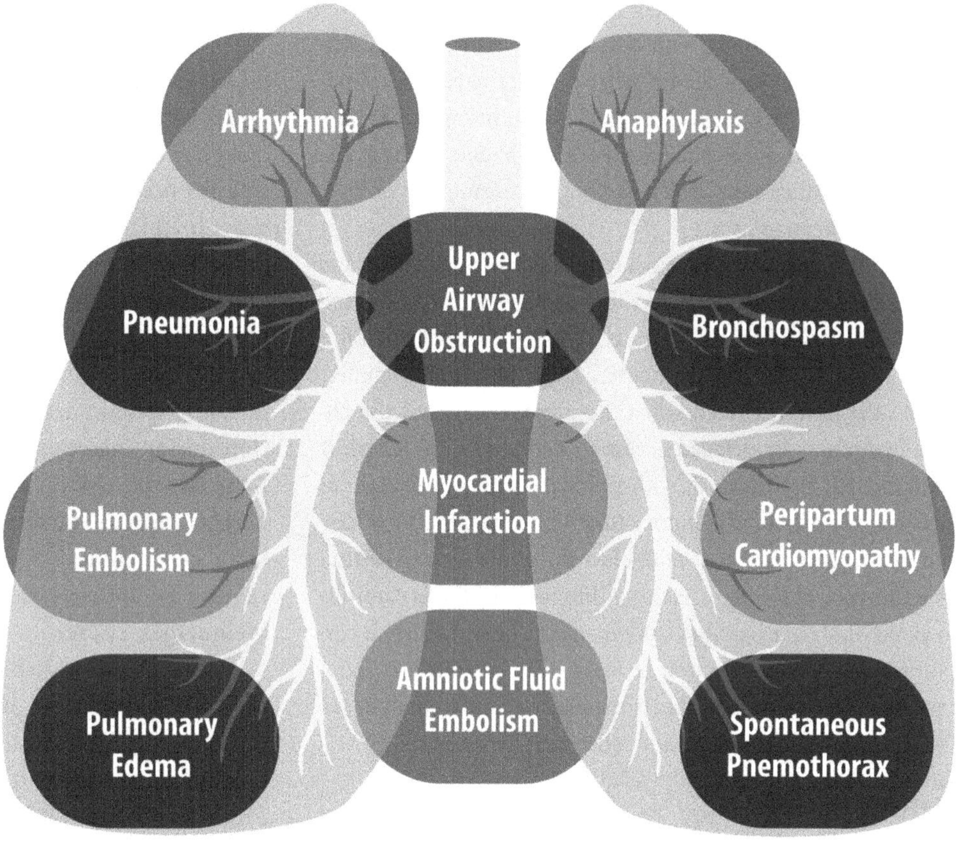

Figure 8-14. Causes of sudden-onset dyspnea in pregnancy.

Varicose Veins

Varicose veins, which affect about 40% of pregnant and postpartum people, are a risk factor for phlebitis and thrombosis (Smyth, Aflaifel, & Bamigboye, 2015). A varicosity develops when valves within a vein weaken and allow blood to pool. As the vein distends, its walls stretch and lose elasticity. Veins in the legs, vulva, rectum, and pelvis are most commonly affected. Increased blood volume, compression from uterine enlargement, and the vasodilatory effects of progesterone during pregnancy increase pressure in the leg veins, encouraging the development of varicosities. A pregnant client with varicose veins can experience pain, swelling, or leg cramps, any of which can be mistaken for DVT.

Pulmonary Embolism (PE)

PE, the blockage of an artery in the lungs by a migrant clot or substance, produces hypoxemia by obstructing the arteries carrying deoxygenated blood to the lungs, causing affected lung tissue to be ventilated but not perfused (Parker & Wilson, 2016). Blood oxygen levels fall, and the client experiences respiratory distress. The poorly perfused lung tissue can become ischemic or die, causing chest pain. PE is always serious and can lead to severe hypoxemia, respiratory failure requiring intubation and mechanical ventilation, or death.

Additionally, the blockage can restrict the flow of blood as it circulates through the lungs and into the left ventricle, thereby decreasing cardiac preload. The body attempts to compensate for this volume deficit with tachycardia. If the body is unable to maintain cardiac output by increasing the heart rate, BP will fall. PE also triggers an inflammatory response that can cause pain, fever, malaise, hemoptysis, and pleural effusions. Large emboli produce sudden occlusion of a significant area of lung tissue, causing sudden respiratory and circulatory compromise (Parker & Wilson, 2016). Smaller emboli can lodge deeper within the lung and cause tissue death over hours or days, often producing gradual and subtle signs and symptoms.

The clinical presentations of PE are ambiguous and easy to mistake (Malhotra & Weinberger, 2023a). Most commonly, the client presents with dyspnea (62%), pleuritic chest pain (55%), cough (24%), sweating (18%), and sometimes hemoptysis—expectorating blood (Malhotra & Weinberger, 2023b). Other manifestations, such as hypoxia, tachycardia, tachypnea, fever, apprehension, hypotension, syncope, and shock, are nonspecific for any single disorder. Of the people who fit the clinical picture of PE, a diagnosis of pneumonia is more likely than PE (Bajc, Olsson, Gottsäter, Hindorf, & Jögi, 2015). Sudden chest pain and dyspnea along with a hot, red, swollen leg reliably indicate PE, but 30% of clients with PE do not have clinical evidence of DVT (Clark & Hankins, 2012). If symptoms are subtle, providers sometimes mistake a client's complaints of chest discomfort, breathlessness, or leg swelling for normal physiologic changes of pregnancy.

If you suspect PE, act quickly to stabilize your client and transport emergently to a facility capable of diagnosis and treatment. Death from PE is most likely to occur within a few hours of onset, so minutes matter. Many preventable maternal deaths have occurred when the provider ignored the client's symptoms or delayed access to definitive care (Clark & Hankins, 2012). Transport with the client sitting as upright as possible to improve respiratory function. Give high-flow oxygen if the pulse oximeter shows less than 95% oxygen saturation (Murphy & Cullinan, 2020). Administer IV fluids carefully to avoid fluid overload that can precipitate heart failure. If cardiovascular collapse occurs, resuscitate as appropriate. Paramedics (and their counterparts outside the United States) can initiate cardiac monitoring and intubate if necessary.

Definitive Care

In a hospital, the pregnant client with acute chest pain or symptoms consistent with PE usually undergoes the following tests:

- Chest x-ray.
- A ventilation/perfusion (V/Q) scan if the chest x-ray is normal. A V/Q scan is a nuclear medicine procedure that uses radioactive material to evaluate airflow and blood flow in the lungs. V/Q scanning is both sensitive and specific for the diagnosis of PE. The benefits of determining the presence of a PE generally outweigh any risks to mother and fetus associated with the small dose of radiation.
- Computerized tomography pulmonary angiography (CTPA) if the chest x-ray is abnormal or if the V/Q scan is indeterminate. The procedure involves IV injection of radioactive material followed by a CT scan of the chest. CTPA testing accurately identifies the presence of a PE but exposes mother and fetus to higher levels of radiation than a V/Q scan and higher risk of breast cancer or neonatal thyroid function depression (van Mens et al., 2017).
- Proximal vein compression sonography (CUS) if the client has clinical signs of DVT, such as leg pain, swelling, or erythema.
- In emergencies, the physician may consider thrombolysis, surgical embolectomy, or transvenous catheter embolectomy despite possible risks to the fetus.

Anticoagulation

In most VTE cases, the mainstay of management is therapeutic anticoagulation, which helps to prevent reoccurrence of clots. Low-molecular-weight (LMW) heparin is safe for pregnant and lactating people because it does not cross the placenta and is not secreted in breast milk (Malhotra & Weinberger, 2023c). Because anticoagulant therapy can increase the risk of postpartum hemorrhage, anticoagulants are typically discontinued before induction of labor or cesarean section. This is particularly important if epidural or spinal anesthesia is desired because anticoagulation during insertion (or removal) of an epidural catheter increases the risk for spinal hematoma (Malhotra & Weinberger, 2023c). The client at high risk for acute PE during labor can require a temporary inferior vena cava filter or require IV anticoagulants while giving birth (Malhotra & Weinberger, 2023c).

Most clients at risk for VTE are maintained antenatally on LMW heparin. At 36–37 weeks of gestation, the pharmacological regimen should be changed to an SC adjusted dose of unfractionated heparin (ACOG Cmte. on Clinical Practice, 2018/2022). The goal is to achieve birth of the infant at least 24 hr after the last dose of LMW heparin, or at least 12 hr after the last dose of unfractionated heparin. Because most postpartum bleeding is controlled by uterine contraction rather than by clotting, anticoagulation does not usually increase postpartum blood loss unless there is a complex laceration. The concern is for the extremely small risk of a potentially devastating epidural or spinal hematoma with regional anesthesia (ACOG Cmte. on Clinical Practice, 2018/2022). Protamine sulfate can effectively reverse unfractionated heparin (and less reliably, LMW heparin) but is rarely required and is not indicated with a prophylactic dose of heparin.

In the absence of postpartum hemorrhage, a heparin regimen is typically restarted 12 hr after a cesarean birth or 6 hr after a vaginal birth. Anticoagulant medication should be continued for at least 6 weeks postpartum (Malhotra & Weinberger, 2023c). The total duration of anticoagulant therapy (including both pregnancy and postpartum) should be at least 3–6 months for people with transient risk factors such as pregnancy and longer for people with persistent risk factors such as inherited thrombophilia. *People with DVT or PE in pregnancy and those on anticoagulant therapy are not suitable candidates for birth in community settings.*

DIFFERENTIAL DIAGNOSES

Pneumonia, peripartum cardiomyopathy, pulmonary edema, amniotic fluid embolism.

Pulmonary Edema

Pulmonary edema is an abnormal accumulation of fluid in the alveoli and interstitial spaces of the lungs which compromises gas exchange. Pulmonary edema can result from heart dysfunction, chronic hypertension, dysrhythmias, cardiac diseases, inhaled toxins, or near drowning (American Academy of Orthopedic Surgeons [AAOS], 2018). In pregnancy, pulmonary edema can develop antepartum, intrapartum, or postpartum, and is usually associated with use of tocolytic medications (especially terbutaline), preeclampsia, IV fluid overload, or underlying cardiac disease (Reardon & Chen, 2023). Tocolytics are more likely to cause pulmonary edema in combination, especially when IV magnesium sulfate is used with SC terbutaline.

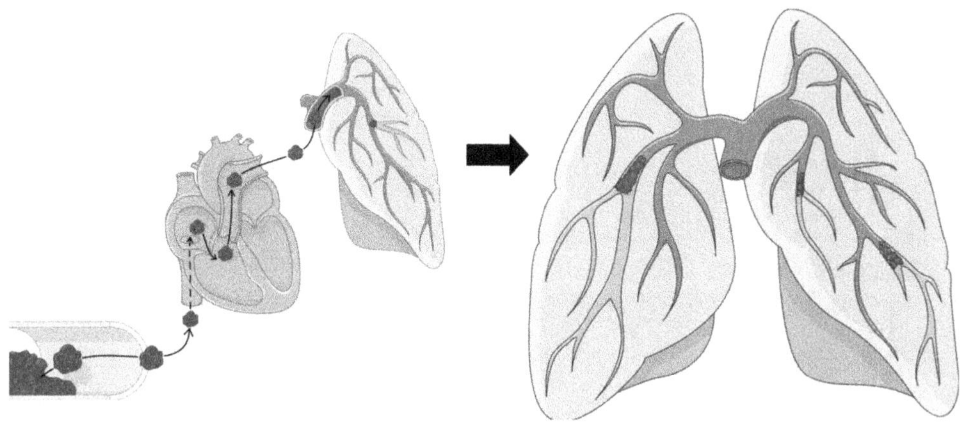

Figure 8-15. Process by which a deep-vein thrombosis (DVT) becomes a pulmonary embolism (PE). A thrombus forms in a deep vein, usually in the leg or pelvis. It dislodges and travels up the vena cava to the heart. The clot enters the heart via the right atrium, and the next heartbeat moves it to the right ventricle. From the right ventricle, the thrombus travels into the pulmonary artery. It lodges in a lung artery and blocks perfusion of the tissue beyond, leading to hypoxia and tissue damage. Adapted from "Pulmonary Embolism [1]" and "Pulmonary Embolism [7]," by Servier Medical Art, 2016b, 2016c (https://smart.servier.com/wp-content/uploads/2016/10/Embolie_pulmonaire_01-680x574.png). CC BY 3.0.

Signs and symptoms include difficulty breathing, cough, orthopnea, chest pain, diaphoresis, restlessness, and anxiety with a sense of suffocation. In early pulmonary edema, signs of compromise can be subtle or undetectable. In severe cases of pulmonary edema related to heart failure, the victim sometimes expectorates pink foam.

Upon auscultating the lungs, fine crackles audible in the bases of the lungs at the end of inspiration indicate that the alveolar walls are swollen and the alveoli are filling with fluid. The crackling sound is caused by wet alveoli popping open as the lungs reach maximal inflation (AAOS, 2018). Providers inexperienced with auscultating abnormal lung sounds can miss subtle crackles and assume the lungs are clear (Clark & Hankins, 2012). They can also miss crackles when evaluating clients in noisy settings or when listening through clothing.

Untreated pulmonary edema can be fatal, more often if there are delays to accessing definitive care. Call emergency medical services (EMS) and request a paramedic (U.S.) or equivalent response because the client requires cardiac monitoring and medications *en route*. Address the cause of the pulmonary edema if possible. Sit the client upright to reduce pressure on the diaphragm from the uterus and other abdominal organs. Position the client with the legs dependent over the side of the bed to encourage blood to pool in the legs, which lowers central venous pressure and reduces cardiac preload (Parker & Wilson, 2016). Apply a pulse oximeter and give oxygen if the oxygen saturation is less than 95% (Murphy & Cullinan, 2020).

At the hospital, the priorities will be to establish effective ventilation, to treat the pulmonary edema, and to address the underlying condition that led to the presenting issue. If the preeclamptic client has critical hypertension that precipitated pulmonary edema, a priority may be to rapidly reduce the BP. If the problem is hypervolemia or heart failure, the diuretic furosemide (Lasix®) can reduce intravascular volume. Furosemide acts initially as a vasodilator, opening peripheral vessels and moving fluid from the lungs to the extremities. Then it blocks the absorption of sodium, chloride, and water from the filtered fluid in the kidney tubules, increasing urine output.

DIFFERENTIAL DIAGNOSES

Pneumonia, asthma, bronchitis, congestive heart failure (CHF) related to peripartum cardiomyopathy, PE.

Asthma

Asthma is a chronic inflammatory disorder of the small airways with episodes of acute exacerbation. Asthma restricts airflow to alveoli by constricting the bronchioles and obstructing the lower airways. In some cases of severe asthma, air becomes trapped in the lungs by extreme narrowing and closure of airways.

Deep within the small airways of the lungs, immune cells such as mast cells, eosinophils, and neutrophils stand ready to launch an immune response if challenged. In a healthy person, these cells launch an inflammatory response to invading

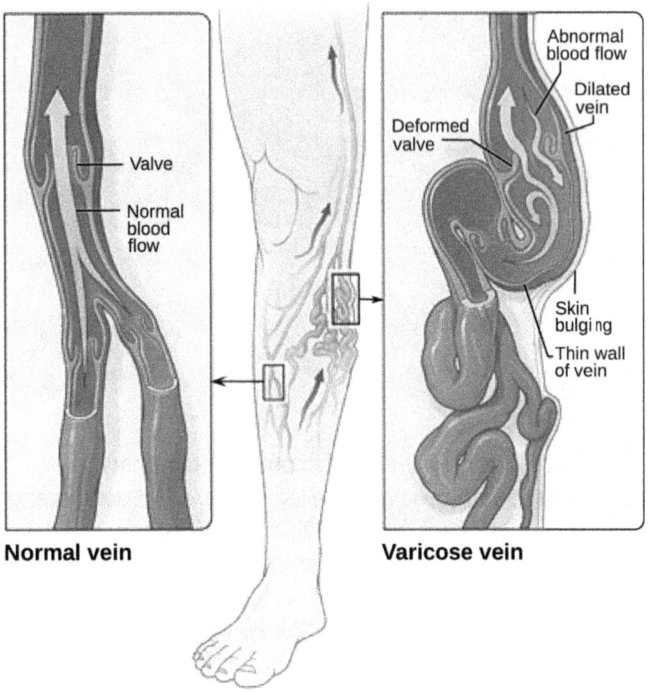

Figure 8-16. Varicose veins are a risk factor for DVT. Pregnancy predisposes people to varicose veins in the pelvis, vulva, rectum, and lower extremities. "Varicose Veins," by Jmarchn, 2017 (https://commons.wikimedia.org/wiki/File:-Varicose_veins-en.svg). CC BY-SA-3.0.

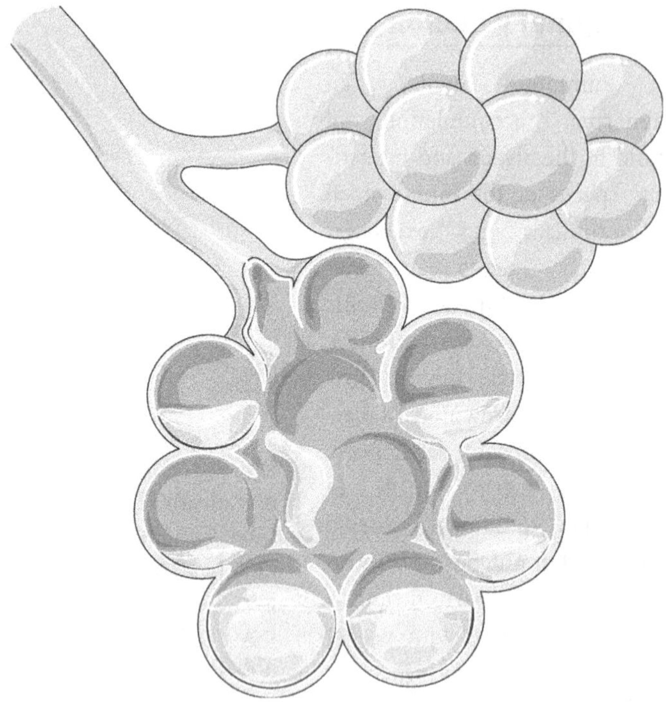

Figure 8-17. Pulmonary edema refers to a collection of fluid in the tissue and alveoli of the lungs. This condition causes hypoxia by blocking gas exchange and can lead to respiratory failure. "Pulmonary Edema," by Servier Medical Art, 2016a (https://smart.servier.com/wp-content/uploads/2016/10/Oedeme_poumons-637x680.png). CC BY 3.0.

pathogens (Parker & Wilson, 2016). Goblet cells secrete mucus to snare invaders and block their advance, and the muscular walls of the lower airways contract and become edematous (Parker & Wilson, 2016).

In the asthmatic person, the inflammatory mediators overreact, creating abnormal swelling, bronchoconstriction, and mucus plugging in large areas of the lungs (Parker & Wilson, 2016). Asthma attacks can be triggered by upper-respiratory-tract infection, gastroesophageal reflux, sinusitis, exercise, aspirin, NSAIDs, tobacco smoke, chemical fumes, humidity, cold, emotional upset, and allergens such as house mites, animal hair, and pollen. As the asthma exacerbation worsens, the narrowed passages can collapse and trap air between the alveoli and the small airways. This trapped air hyperinflates the lungs but is not available for gas exchange. If the process continues, the lungs will eventually be unable to draw in any more air. Severe hypoxia may develop, and intrathoracic pressure increases. If this pressure compresses the vena cava, cardiac output and BP may decrease.

Asthma is one of the most common medical conditions, affecting 8% of pregnancies (Cunningham et al., 2022, ch. 54). In some clients, it is diagnosed for the first time during pregnancy (Cunningham et al., 2022, ch. 54; Lao & Hui, 2022). Maternal asthma increases the risk for gestational diabetes, PTB, placental abruption, and adverse obstetric outcomes, including congenital malformations especially when it is poorly controlled (Lao & Hui, 2022).

In pregnancy, asthma remains stable in about one third of people, worsens in about one third, and improves in about one third. Clients who improve tend to do so gradually over the course of the pregnancy and see the most improvement in the last 4 weeks. Exacerbations, usually triggered by viral infection or nonadherence to inhaled corticosteroid medications, are most likely early in the third trimester. Intrapartum and postpartum exacerbations are less common (Lao & Hui, 2022). Carboprost tromethamine (Hemabate®) is contraindicated for the asthmatic client with postpartum hemorrhage.

Pregnant clients with asthma are usually managed on bronchodilators and inhaled glucocorticoids, as are most asthma sufferers. In the United States, albuterol (salbutamol, Proventil® et al.) is the recommended short-acting beta-agonist, budesonide (Pulmicort®) the preferred inhaled glucocorticoid, and Salmeterol (Serevent®) the inhaled long-acting beta-agonist of choice (Schatz & Weinberger, 2023). Acute asthma exacerbations are managed similarly to those in nonpregnant clients and may include treatment with inhaled short-acting beta-agonist albuterol, inhaled ipratropium, oral or IV glucocorticoids, or IV magnesium sulfate (Schatz & Weinberger, 2023).

Consider asthma when evaluating any pregnant client complaining of wheezing, cough, or dyspnea. If your client is having an asthma attack, rapidly address the ABCs and POP. Mild-to-moderate asthma can present with slightly increased breathing effort, tachycardia, tachypnea, cough, chest tightness, or wheezes (Parker & Wilson, 2016). The expiratory phase of respiration is often longer than the inspiratory phase. Wheezing related to asthma usually involves multiple high-pitched lung sounds, audible most prominently during expiration (Fanta & Lange-Vaidya, 2022). If bronchospasm is severe, wheeze is sometimes absent because of decreased airflow.

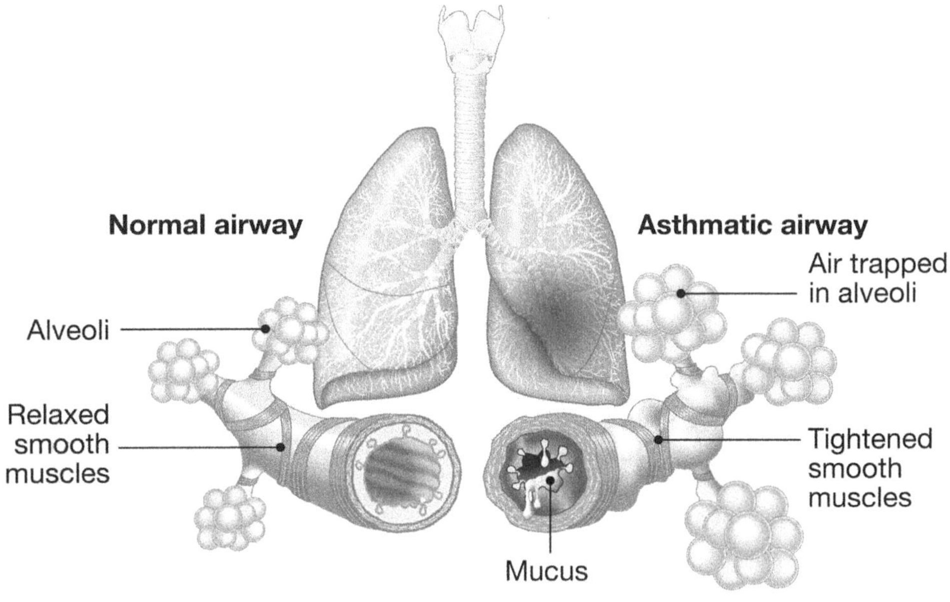

Figure 8-18. During an asthma episode, airways become inflamed and constricted in reaction to environmental triggers such as smoke, dust, or pollen (©Axel Kock/Adobe Stock).

Severe dyspnea can present with tachypnea greater than 30 breaths/min, tachycardia greater than 120 bpm, sweating, inability to speak in full sentences or phrases, restless anxiety, or inability to lie supine (Fanta & Lange-Vaidya, 2022). Up to 50% of clients with severe compromise do not show any of these signs (Fanta & Lange-Vaidya, 2022). Status asthmaticus is a severe, prolonged asthmatic attack that continues despite conventional treatment.

Many clients choose to self-treat mild asthma exacerbation with a rescue inhaler as advised by their physicians. The goals of treatment are to improve gas exchange, reduce bronchospasm, and reduce mucus production and airway edema (Parker & Wilson, 2016). Provide oxygen if needed, whatever is necessary to keep oxygen saturation at least 95% (Schatz & Weinberger, 2023). Consider EMS for transport if respiratory distress becomes significant. Establish IV access without delaying transport. Frequently assess the client, the severity of the attack, and the client's response to treatment.

In the ambulance, EMS personnel sometimes initiate cardiac monitoring and may give an albuterol nebulizer treatment. At the hospital, providers will typically continue treatments of short-acting beta-agonists and consider the use of other medications such as systemic glucocorticoids. Fetal monitoring should be initiated if the fetus is near or above the threshold of viability. If the client does not respond well to treatment after 4–6 hr of attentive care, hospital admission is often required for vigilant ongoing management (Schatz & Weinberger, 2023). Very few pregnant people require intubation or mechanical ventilation. The pulmonologist may consider alternative pharmacological regimens to reduce the likelihood of future attacks and educate the client about triggers to avoid.

DIFFERENTIAL DIAGNOSES

Anaphylaxis, drug reaction, airway obstruction, anxiety, arrhythmia, PE, amniotic fluid embolism, congestive heart failure (CHF) related to peripartum cardiomyopathy, physiologic dyspnea of pregnancy.

Respiratory Infection

Bronchitis

Acute bronchitis involves inflammation of the bronchi, which usually presents as a cough with sputum production. At onset, acute bronchitis can be indistinguishable from the common cold, but the cough of bronchitis lingers after cold symptoms resolve. Suspect bronchitis in clients who have an acute onset of a persistent cough which can last 1–3 weeks who do not have signs of pneumonia (see below). About half of individuals with bronchitis expectorate purulent sputum when coughing but usually do not have a fever. More than 90% of cases of bronchitis are viral (Larson & File, 2023). Because antibiotics are not indicated for a viral infection, bronchitis is managed with supportive care (Larson & File, 2023).

Pneumonia

Pneumonia, an inflammatory condition of the lung primarily affecting the alveoli, is a leading cause of death in the United

States (Cunningham et al., 2022, ch. 54). Alterations in immune status make the pregnant person especially vulnerable to pneumonia and increase the severity of viral, fungal, and tuberculous infections. The elevated intragastric pressure of pregnancy increases risk of aspiration pneumonia as well. The pregnant client with pneumonia is at risk for complications such as respiratory failure sepsis, pneumothorax, pericardial effusion, and pericardial tamponade (Pacheco, Saad, A., La Rosa De Los Rios, & Webb, 2021). Maternal pneumonia is also associated with adverse perinatal outcomes such as low birthweight, PTB, low Apgar scores, cesarean birth, and preeclampsia/eclampsia (Pacheco et al., 2021).

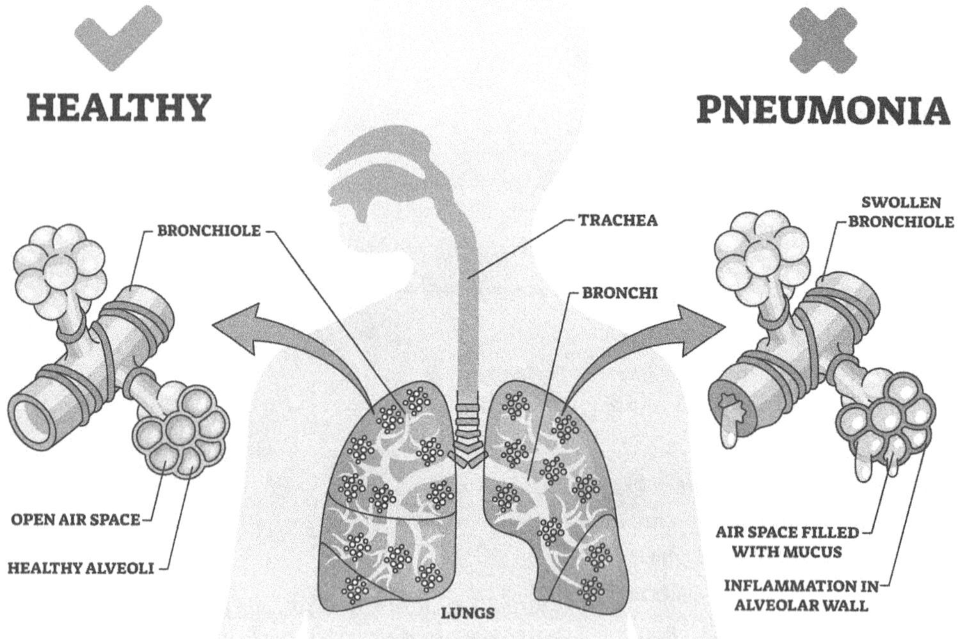

Figure 8-19. Pneumonia causes hypoxia by blocking gas exchange (©VectorMine/Adobe Stock).

Pneumonia can occur at any stage of gestation but is most likely to occur midway through the third trimester (Pacheco et al., 2021). Community-acquired pneumonia is frequently caused by bacteria (usually *Haemophilus influenzae* or *Streptococcus pneumoniae*); atypical bacteria such as *Mycoplasma pneumoniae, Chlamydophila pneumoniae,* or *Legionella pneumophila* (Pacheco et al., 2021), or viruses, including influenza A and B, COVID-19 (SARS-CoV-2), metapneumovirus, adenovirus, and respiratory syncytial virus (Cunningham et al., 2022, ch. 54). Rarely, the infection is caused by fungi or protozoa (Cunningham et al., 2022, ch. 54).

Although the classic presentation of pneumonia includes rigors, fever, pleuritic chest pain, dyspnea, and cough, symptoms vary and overlap those of bronchitis, influenza, and other respiratory infections. Clients with pneumonia usually appear quite ill. Signs and symptoms of pneumonia during pregnancy are similar to those experienced by the nonpregnant and typically include (Pacheco et al., 2021)

- Cough (90%)
- Productive sputum (66%)
- Dyspnea (66%)
- Pleuritic chest pain when breathing or coughing (50%)

The cough can sometimes be triggered by turning from one side to the other (AAOS, 2018). Sputum can be purulent and very thick if the client is dehydrated. There can be fever, tachypnea, tachycardia, decreased oxygen saturation, headaches, sweats, and malaise (Larson & File, 2023).

Lung assessment findings can include dullness on percussion, crackles, and diminished breath sounds over the affected lobe(s). Bronchial or bronchovesicular breath sounds or a pleural friction rub are sometimes noted over areas of consolidation. Consolidation occurs when the normally air-filled alveoli contain fluid or other material like blood, pus, or cellular exudate. Besides infectious pneumonia, lung consolidation can occur with conditions such as atelectasis, pulmonary edema, pulmonary hemorrhage, aspiration pneumonia, or pulmonary neoplasm. In severe disease, breath sounds can be decreased or absent.

Delay in diagnosis can result in severe complications such as sepsis. Chest x-rays (posteroanterior and lateral views) are recommended for any client with a history and physical examination suggestive of pneumonia (Pacheco et al., 2021). Typical labs include complete blood count (CBC) with differential, chemistry panel, blood cultures at two sites, and sputum Gram stain and culture. The pregnant client with severe pneumonia or with comorbidities such as asthma, diabetes, compromised immune system, or cardiac or renal disease requires hospitalization and aggressive management (Pacheco et al., 2021). The plan of care typically includes IV antibiotics and hydration, supplemental oxygen if the maternal oxygen saturation is less than 95%, and close maternal-fetal monitoring until there is clinical improvement (Larson & File, 2023). Pregnant clients with nonsevere pneumonia who are otherwise healthy can sometimes opt for outpatient management with close follow-up (Pacheco et al., 2021). Antibiotic therapy for bacterial pneumonia is determined by the drug's safety profile and its effectiveness against typical and atypical pathogens.

DIFFERENTIAL DIAGNOSES

PE, pulmonary edema, asthma.

COVID-19

The 2019 novel coronavirus disease COVID-19 is a recently discovered zoonotic virus that is pathogenic to humans. In early 2020, COVID-19 achieved community spread and become a pandemic. The virus enters the body through the upper airway and lungs, infecting the ACE2 receptors on the cells that line the respiratory tract (Smith, 2020; Varga et al., 2020). By damaging the lungs, the virus gains access to the pulmonary vessels, which also have abundant ACE2 receptors. The infection spreads throughout the vasculature of the body in a tempest of hyperinflammation, affecting the endothelium and stimulating an immune response that can become a dangerous cytokine storm (Smith, 2020; Varga et al., 2020). This damage to endothelial cells appears to be the cause of many COVID-related complications such as myocardial infarction, VTE, PE, DIC, and stroke (Becker, 2020; Di Renzo & Giardina, 2020).

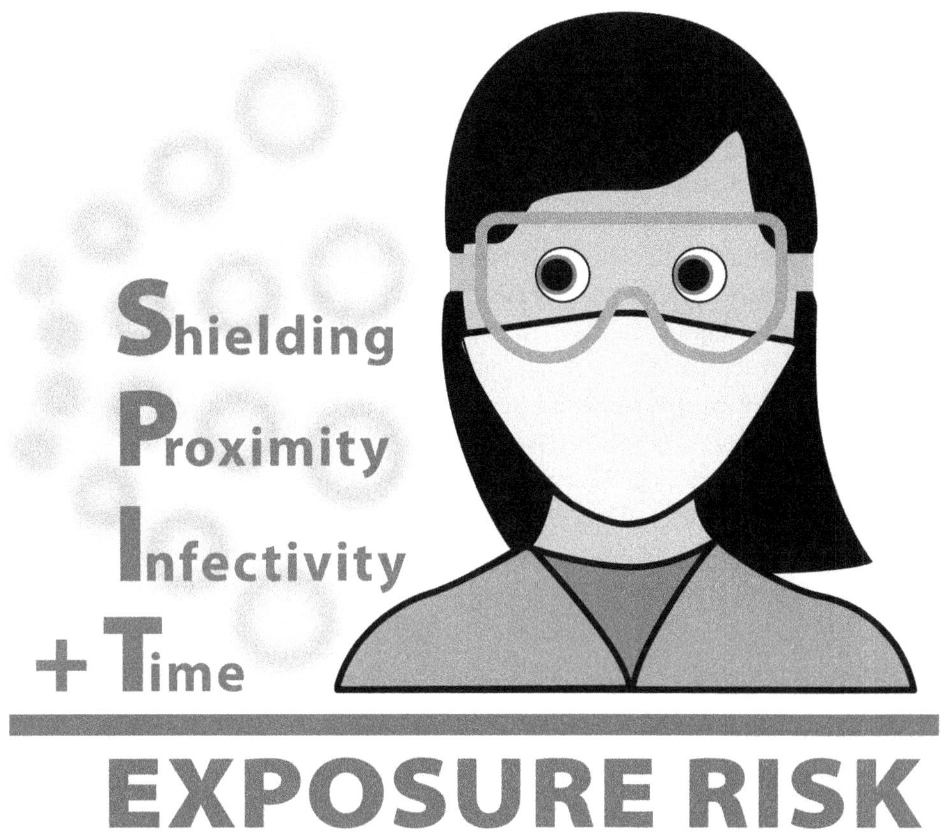

Figure 8-20. Consider SPIT when assessing COVID-19 risk: Shielding, Proximity, Infectivity, and Time. COVID-19 exposure risk appears to increase when the health care worker has unprotected physical contact with infectious droplets or fluids or prolonged proximity to clients with active COVID-19 infections (beginning 48 hr before onset of symptoms). This risk can be mitigated by using personal protective equipment (PPE) and negative-pressure rooms, minimizing close contact, testing for the virus, requiring infected clients to wear a mask to contain secretions, and decreasing exposure times.

COVID-19 can cause widespread complications throughout the body including (Berghella & Hughes, 2023; McIntosh, 2023)

- *Respiratory disorders*: Pneumonia, respiratory failure, ARDS.
- *Cardiac disorders*: Arrhythmias, myocardial injury, heart failure, and shock.
- *Thromboembolic complications*: VTE including extensive DVT and PE, stroke, limb ischemia.
- *Kidney disorders*: Acute kidney injury, glomerular disease.
- *Neurologic disorders*: Encephalopathy, strokes, seizures, weakness headache, dizziness, altered mental status, disorders of smell and taste.
- *Gastrointestinal issues*: anorexia, diarrhea, nausea.
- *Psychiatric illness*: anxiety disorders, depressive disorders, insomnia disorder, posttraumatic stress disorder.

COVID-19 is transmitted through respiratory droplets and infected body fluids that reach another person's eyes, nose, or mouth or an open cut, wound, or abrasion (Poon et al., 2020). The virus also spreads via fomites and can remain viable on plastic and stainless-steel objects for up to 72 hr and on copper and cardboard for up to 24 hr (Poon et al., 2020). Respiratory emissions contain clusters of minuscule droplets that can remain suspended in a cloud for long periods. Alterations in temperature, humidity, turbulence, and speed can affect the rate and distance that these droplets travel and how quickly they evaporate. A cough or sneeze containing pathogen-bearing droplets can travel up to 8 m, and the respiratory emissions of active labor can travel even further (Mok et al., 2021). Mok et al. (2021, p. 618) demonstrated that during active labor and with pushing efforts, "a warm and vigorous cloud" of respiratory droplet emissions can travel approximately 30% faster than with voluntary breathing in early labor and at least 6% faster than with coughing (Mok et al., 2021).

Although most pregnant individuals with COVID-19 do not develop severe disease, they are at higher risk for ICU admission, a 3-fold higher risk of mechanical ventilation and ventilatory support, and 70% higher risk of death than non-pregnant people with COVID-19 (SMFM, 2021). This elevated risk for severe disease and death is higher for black individuals, presumably because of inequitable care (SMFM, 2021). Vertical transmission is extremely rare: most cases of neonatal infection with COVID-19 appear to result from postnatal transmission from their mothers or other caregivers with COVID-19.

Berghella and Hughes (2023) concluded that COVID-19 infection during pregnancy

- Does not increase risk for miscarriage or congenital anomalies.
- Appears to increase risk for PTB, cesarean birth, and stillbirth, especially if the mother is critically ill with COVID-19 in the third trimester.
- Strongly increases the risk for preeclampsia, especially among nulliparas—even if the infection is asymptomatic (Papageorghiou et al., 2021).
- Minimally increases risk of infection of the newborn.

Like their nonpregnant counterparts, pregnant clients with COVID-19 pneumonia often present with fever or cough (Berghella & Hughes, 2023). Less commonly, they present with myalgia, malaise, sore throat, diarrhea, loss of taste or smell, or shortness of breath. Clinical presentation varies widely from client to client, however. Many COVID-19 infections are asymptomatic or involve only minor nasal congestion. After resolution of the infection, many experience persistent symptoms, including fatigue, dyspnea, chest pain, and cough, for months or years. Many experience persistent psychological symptoms following COVID-19, including anxiety, depression, posttraumatic stress disorder (PTSD), and deficits in memory and concentration (Mikkelsen & Abramoff, 2023). These persistent symptoms are termed *long COVID*, *post-COVID conditions*, or *postacute sequelae of COVID-19 infection*.

Laboratory tests sometimes show an abnormally low WBC or lymphocyte count or high concentrations of AST, ALT, or C-reactive protein. Initial chest imaging with high-resolution CT may show small, patchy shadows and interstitial changes. As the disease worsens, the lesions increase in size and number, evolving into ground-glass opacities (hazy areas caused by inflammation) and infiltrating consolidation (Li et al., 2020).

Any pregnant individual, like anyone else seeking health care, should be screened for signs and symptoms of respiratory infection. Ask about the presence of fever, cough, chills, muscle aches, new loss of taste or smell, sore throat, or shortness of breath. If the screen is positive, direct the client to a testing site to be swabbed for likely pathogens, including COVID-19 and influenza.

Providers managing clients with potential or confirmed COVID-19 should use personal protective equipment (PPE) including N95 respirators, gowns, gloves, shoe coverings, hair coverings, and eye protection (ACOG, 2021). Use continuous pulse oximetry; oxygen therapy is indicated if maternal oxygen saturation falls below 95% (Rasmussen, Smulian, Lednicky, Wen, & Jamieson, 2020). Continuous fetal monitoring is indicated, not only to evaluate fetal wellbeing, but also because an abnormal fetal heart rate (FHR) tracing can be an early sign of maternal respiratory compromise. Mechanical ventilation should be initiated if respiratory failure is imminent. Superimposed bacterial and viral infections are common with COVID-19, and antimicrobial therapy is sometimes indicated (Rasmussen et al., 2020).

At this writing, an oral COVID-19 protease inhibitor, Paxlovid (which includes nirmatrelvir, a COVID-19 main protease inhibitor, and ritonavir, an HIV-1 protease inhibitor and CYP3A inhibitor) is available for emergency use for the treatment of outpatients with mild to moderate COVID-19 infection who are at high risk of clinical progression (ACOG, 2021). Pregnant clients are eligible to receive outpatient oral COVID-19 protease inhibitor therapy even if pregnancy is their only risk factor but stand to gain greater benefit if they have additional risk factors such as BMI greater than 25, chronic kidney disease, diabetes mellitus, or cardiovascular disease. Clinicians should weigh the available data against the individual risks of COVID-19 in pregnancy in each situation. There are no human data on the use of nirmatrelvir during pregnancy, and the risks of short-term exposure to these medications must be balanced against the risks associated with untreated COVID-19 during pregnancy (ACOG, 2021).

During the COVID-19 pandemic, many pregnant individuals became concerned about contracting the virus in hospitals or during prenatal visits (Davis-Floyd, Gutschow, & Schwartz, 2020). Innumerable mothers who had previously favored hospital birth—many of them late in gestation—scrambled to find community midwives who would accept them as clients (Davis-Floyd et al., 2020). The Society of Obstetricians and Gynaecologists of Canada recommended hospital birth for those who tested positive for COVID-19 to address the increased likelihood of fetal distress, the need for full PPE, and the challenges involved in sanitizing surfaces at home (Elwood et al., 2020). The Association of Ontario Midwives in Canada advises hospital birth for clients with confirmed or suspected COVID-19 who are febrile or who have comorbidities; afebrile clients with mild illness and no comorbidities can make an informed choice of birthplace after a comprehensive discussion of risks and benefits with a provider (Bourgeois et al., 2021). The Royal College of Obstetricians & Gynaecologists of the United Kingdom recommends fetal monitoring for symptomatic people with COVID-19 in the active phase of labor, but not for asymptomatic people (RCOG, 2020). In the United States, the American Academy of Pediatrics does not recommend home births in any circumstances, and ACOG maintains its long-standing position that the safest place for birth is a hospital, hospital-based birth center, or accredited freestanding birth center (ACOG, 2022).

In August 2021, 22 professional health care organizations, including ACOG, the American College of Nurse-Midwives (ACNM), and the American Academy of Pediatrics, issued a joint statement strongly urging all who are pregnant, recently pregnant, planning to become pregnant, or lactating to become fully vaccinated against COVID-19 (ACOG, 2020/2023; ACOG et al., 2021). Elsewhere, one of the signatories, ACOG, declared that health care professionals have an ethical obligation to be vaccinated themselves and to encourage clients to do likewise (ACOG Cmte. on Obstetric Practice, 2021). ACOG maintains that vaccination of health care providers not only gives them evidence-based protection against the virus, but also helps them prevent its spread among those they serve and inspires public confidence in the vaccines (ACOG, 2020/2023).

Spontaneous Pneumothorax

Pneumothorax is a collection of air in the pleural space between the visceral and parietal pleura that can impair lung expansion or cause the lung to collapse. When a healthy individual draws a breath, the chest wall expands outward and the diaphragm descends, increasing the volume of the chest cavity and lowering the pressure within the chest so that room air rushes in to fill the void (Parker & Wilson, 2016). The lungs are bound to the chest wall and diaphragm by an airtight seal between the internal lining of the chest wall and the external layer of the lungs (Parker & Wilson, 2016). Any air, blood, or fluid that accumulates between the lungs and chest wall disrupts this seal and increases intrapleural pressure, causing part or all of the lung to collapse.

Air can enter the pleural space through a breach of the chest wall (penetrating trauma) or the lung wall (rupture of an air sac). From the pleural space, trapped air can migrate from lung and vascular connective tissue into subcutaneous tissue, forming crunchy pockets of air under the skin—subcutaneous emphysema (Kandiah, Iswariah, & Elgey, 2013). Pneumothorax can be the consequence of a traumatic injury such as a penetrating chest wound or a rib fracture (Y. C. G. Lee, 2023).

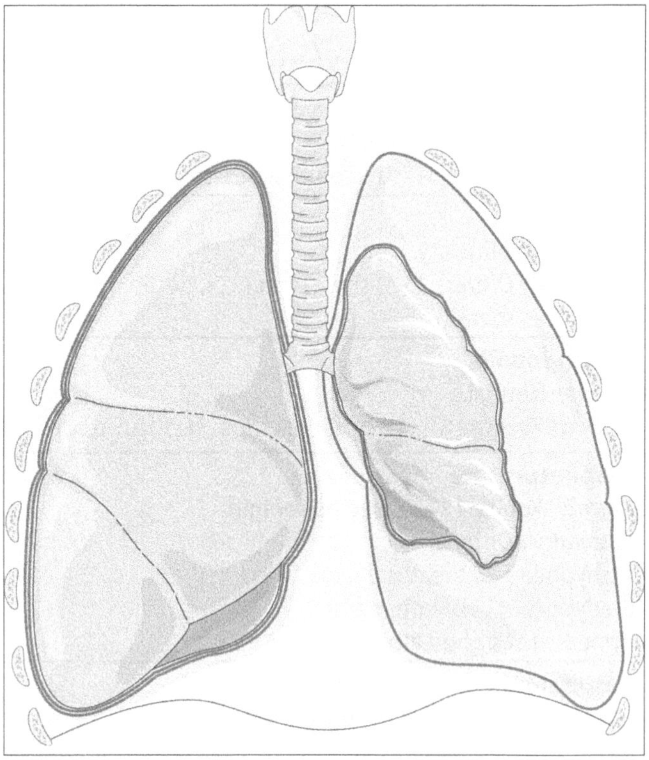

Figure 8-21. A pneumothorax is a collection of air within the pleural space that can result in the partial or complete collapse of a lung (©rumruay/Adobe Stock).

Spontaneous pneumothorax and pneumomediastinum occur when weakened areas of lung tissue (blebs or bullae) blow out like bulges on a weak inner tube (Scala et al., 2016). An undiagnosed bleb can develop into a pneumothorax when a client bears down forcefully or screams loudly during labor; retches while vomiting; coughs forcefully, especially with asthma or pertussis (Khurram, Patel, & Farra, 2015); or even sneezes (Parker & Wilson, 2016). Spontaneous pneumothorax is more common in smokers and those with a connective-tissue disease such as Marfan syndrome or Ehlers-Danlos syndrome. Pneumomediastinum can result from esophageal rupture caused by severe vomiting (Liang, Ooka, Santo, & Kaibara, 2002). Spontaneous pneumomediastinum (air in the mediastinum) with subcutaneous emphysema is termed *Hamman's syndrome* (Khurram et al., 2015). Rarely, Hamman's syndrome can progress to life-threatening cardiac tamponade.

The classic presentation of spontaneous pneumothorax is dyspnea and sudden onset of pleuritic retrosternal chest pain radiating to the back or neck, but some cases present with only tachypnea or no symptoms at all. Subcutaneous emphysema can cause swelling, notably of the shoulders, neck, face, or breast. This swelling has a distinctive crackly texture when palpated and is a clear indication that a pneumothorax is present. Some people also feel a pop or a sharp chest pain when the lung tissue ruptures.

Table 8-4
Targeted Physical Examination for Dyspnea in Pregnancy

General appearance *Normal:* Calm, not anxious. *Respiratory Distress:* Distressed, anxious, struggling, or somnolent.
Speech *Normal:* No difficulty. *Respiratory Distress:* Uses short sentences, declining to phrases, single words, and inability to speak.
Breath sounds *Normal:* Normal. *Respiratory distress:* wheeze, crackles, stridor, decreased breath sounds.
Respiratory rate *Normal:* Adults: 12–20 breaths per min. *Respiratory Distress:* Tachypnea >20 breaths per min. Bradypnea <12 breaths per min. Apnea—Lack of breathing.
Respiratory effort *Normal:* Easy respirations, small chest and abdominal movement. *Respiratory Distress:* Pronounced chest and abdominal movement. Use of accessory muscles (sternocleidomastoid, abdominal, pectoral). Tripod posture (leans forward to support the upper body on hands). Orthopnea (difficulty breathing when lying flat on side).
Heart rate *Normal:* 60–100, regular rhythm. *Respiratory Distress:* Tachycardia >100 bpm. Bradycardia <60 bpm. Irregular rhythm.
Skin *Normal:* Warm dry, well-perfused. *Respiratory Distress:* Diaphoretic, pale, dusky, cyanotic, clammy.
Mental status *Normal:* Alert. *Respiratory Distress:* Anxious, combative, somnolent.
Oximetry *Normal:* Oximetry ≥95% on room air. *Respiratory Distress:* Oximetry <95% (<90% = serious hypoxia).

In rare cases, tension pneumothorax develops when trapped air within the pleural space increases with each inspiration. Intrathoracic pressure progressively rises until the affected lung collapses and the mediastinum is pushed toward the opposite side of the chest. Compression of the vena cava reduces cardiac preload and output, and compression of the unaffected lung further reduces gas exchange. Early signs of tension pneumothorax include chest pain, anxiety, dyspnea, "air hunger," use of accessory muscles, rapid shallow breathing, pallor, and tachycardia. Late-stage signs include distended neck veins, hypotension, tracheal deviation, decreased breath sounds, chest hyperresonance, hypoxia, cyanosis, apnea, shock, and cardiac arrest (Parker & Wilson, 2016).

Surprisingly, spontaneous pneumothorax and Hamman's syndrome in pregnancy are usually benign conditions that resolve spontaneously and do not reoccur (Fernando & Edmonds, 2015). In most cases, the volume of air that moves from the lung to the pleural space is usually small, and the amount does not usually increase after the initial event (Parker & Wilson, 2016). The condition is usually diagnosed with a standard inspiratory chest x-ray, followed by CT scan if more information is needed (Khurram et al., 2015). In most cases, the affected client should be managed with reassurance, oxygen, sedatives, and analgesics (Lou, 2017). Routine follow-up is not necessary (Khurram et al., 2015). Resuscitate hemodynamically unstable clients by attending to the ABCs—airway, breathing, and circulation. Clinically unstable clients require immediate chest tube thoracostomy. If chest-tube insertion is delayed, a paramedic (U.S.) or equivalent may perform needle decompression in the field.

DIFFERENTIAL DIAGNOSES

PE, pneumonia, myocardial infarction, musculoskeletal pain, esophageal rupture.

Cardiac Disease

Although significant maternal cardiac disease is a contraindication for birth in community settings, a client with undiagnosed heart problems can become symptomatic while in the care of a midwife. Consider cardiac disease in any pregnant client who develops dyspnea, chest pain, pulmonary edema, palpitations, unexplained tachycardia, bradycardia, irregular pulse, orthopnea, or fainting (Van der Merwe, Hall, Herbst, & Doubell, 2014; Wenstrom, 2015). Fatigue and exercise intolerance can be normal parts of pregnancy; when symptoms are extreme, however, consider a cardiac issue.

Table 8-5

Sample GOLDCART History for Difficulty Breathing

Sample GOLDCART History for Difficulty Breathing
General situation and history—Has this ever happened to you before? Do you have a medical condition that causes difficulty breathing? Are you taking any medications? Have you been ill? Are other family members ill? How many weeks pregnant are you? Do you have any health issues or pregnancy complications? How many pregnancies have you had? How many babies? Is the baby moving?
Onset—What were you doing when this problem began? Was the onset gradual or rapid? Was there a cause or trigger?
Location—Where do you feel discomfort? Does it start in one place and radiate to somewhere else? Where?
Duration—When did you first have trouble breathing? Is the problem constant or recurrent? How often does this occur? How long has this been occurring?
Characteristics—Is what you are experiencing today what you usually feel when you are short of breath? Do you have chest pressure or tightness? Do you have pain? Is the pain sharp, dull, or crampy? How would you rate the pain on a scale of 0–10, 10 being the worst pain imaginable? Does the pain change when you take a deep breath?
Associated symptoms—Do you have a cough? What does the cough sound like and when does it occur? Do you bring up sputum when you cough? What does the sputum look like? Do you have a fever? Any nausea, vomiting, dizziness, palpitations, or fainting? Are you spitting up blood?
Relieving/aggravating factors—Does anything you do make your breathing better or worse? Is it worse if you change position?
Treatment—Have you done or taken anything to treat your shortness of breath? Have providers evaluated your difficulty breathing previously? What did they recommend? Have you been following the recommendations? Did they work? Have you taken your medication? Have you been using any alternative remedies? Has your condition changed since these treatments?

Airway Obstruction

Difficulty breathing can be caused by acute upper-airway obstruction. Choking on food is one of the most common causes of airway obstruction in a healthy adult. Angioedema of the tongue or larynx related to anaphylaxis or peritonsillar abscess can also cause airway obstruction.

Hyperventilation Syndrome

Hyperventilation syndrome involves a transient increase in respiratory rate out of proportion to metabolic needs. The episode can last several minutes to an hour and usually resolves spontaneously. Hyperventilation syndrome usually begins with the sensation of being unable to get enough air while at rest. Respirations are often irregular with periods of fast breathing that can include frequent sighs. Episodes of acute hyperventilation are associated with anxiety and fear and a sense of impending doom. Associated complaints can include dizziness or lightheadedness; chest pain or tightness; numbness in hands, feet, and lips; palpitations; and involuntary muscle contractions in the hands and feet (Schwartzstein, Richards, Edlow, & Roy-Byrne, 2021). Most people who are hyperventilating are usually unaware that they are breathing rapidly.

Contrary to popular wisdom, people who are hyperventilating should NOT breathe into a paper bag. This therapy can cause hypoxemia if the client has underlying acidosis, respiratory compromise, or cardiovascular disease. Coaching the breath can quickly resolve the episode as follows (Schwartzstein et al., 2021):

- Ask the client to place one hand on the abdomen and one hand on the chest.
- Ask the client to notice which hand moves the farthest while inhaling. In hyperventilating clients, the hand on the chest will almost always move much more than the hand on the abdomen.
- Ask the client to breathe in such a manner that the hand on the abdomen makes large outward movements and the hand on the chest is nearly still. Reassure the client that this breathing technique will take some practice to learn.
- Ask the client to inhale slowly over 4 sec, pause for a few seconds, and then exhale over 8 sec. After 5–10 such breathing cycles, the client should feel calmer and notice an improvement in hyperventilation. Continuation of this breathing exercise usually resolves hyperventilation.

Although hyperventilation syndrome generally resolves without complications, many serious disorders present with

Table 8-6

Causes of Chest Pain in Pregnancy

Myocardial ischemia or infarction (angina, heart attack)
Rare. Classic presentation of cardiac pain includes pressure, heaviness, tightness, or constriction in the center or left of the chest with referred pain to the neck, jaw, or shoulder. Worse with exertion, cold, or emotional stress; relieved by rest. Can be accompanied by dyspnea, nausea and vomiting, diaphoresis, presyncope, or palpitations. More common in people with preexisting cardiac issues, hypertensive crisis, or intoxication with cocaine or methamphetamine.

Aortic dissection
Rare. Classic presentation includes acute radiating chest and back pain that is severe and sharp with ripping and tearing sensation. More common in people with connective tissue disorders.

Heart failure
Rare. Chest discomfort, usually with progressive dyspnea, cough, fatigue, and peripheral edema.

Pericarditis
Rare. Pleuritic chest pain that improves with sitting up and leaning forward.

Pulmonary embolism (PE)
Uncommon, but a leading cause of maternal mortality. Dyspnea followed by pleuritic chest pain, cough, and symptoms of deep venous thrombosis.

Pneumothorax
Rare. Sudden onset of sharp, localized pleuritic chest pain and dyspnea. More common in people with connective tissue disorders.

Pneumonia
Relatively uncommon. Pleuritic chest pain, fever, and productive cough.

Lung cancer
Rare. Chest pain on the side of the primary tumor, cough, hemoptysis, and dyspnea.

Pleuritis (inflammation of the lung pleura)
Uncommon. Chest pain that is worse with deep breathing. Provider sometimes auscultates a pleural friction rub.

Gastroesophageal reflux disease (GERD)
Common. Squeezing or burning substernal chest pain radiating to the back, neck, jaw, or arms. Can mimic cardiac pain.

Hiatus hernias
Fairly common. Can present with dysphagia, epigastric or chest pain, heartburn, or regurgitation.

Esophageal rupture
Very rare. Spontaneous perforation of the esophagus, often preceded by forceful vomiting. Can present with excruciating chest pain, subcutaneous emphysema, abdominal pain, vomiting blood, hypotension, and fever. More common in people with connective tissue disorders.

Referred pain
Somewhat common. Ulcers, gallbladder disease, pancreatitis, bowel disorders and other problems can present with chest pain. Chest pain can develop when nerves that supply tissues near the lungs, the diaphragm, or the lining of the abdomen also supply the chest wall. When one part of the nerve is irritated, the pain is perceived elsewhere.

Musculoskeletal chest pain
Common. Local or regional chest tenderness without other symptoms. Pain often increases with palpation or with certain movements.

- Costochondritis: Multiple areas of tenderness, usually involving the cartilages at the costochondral or costosternal junctions. There is no heat, erythema, cough, fever, or localized swelling.
- Trauma: Localized tenderness, and reproduction of the pain by pressing on the spot. There may be redness or bruising. Spasm of intercostal muscles can cause pain.
- Rib subluxation: Sharp pain at rib attachment sites at the sternum and the corresponding vertebrae; rib subluxation is more common in people with connective tissue disorders or those who have severe coughing episodes.

Psychiatric

- Panic attack/disorder: *Common*. Panic attacks involve spontaneous episodes of intense fear that begin abruptly and last for several minutes to an hour. Panic disorder may be present in 30% or more of clients with chest pain in the absence of significant heart disease.
- Other psychiatric etiologies: *Common*. People with depression, somatization, or factitious disorder may present with chest pain.

Cocaine or methamphetamine intoxication
Fairly common in some populations. Can cause myocardial ischemia, aortic dissection, coronary artery aneurysm, cardiomyopathy, acute pulmonary toxicity ("crack lung"), and arrhythmias.

Herpes zoster (shingles)
Uncommon. Chest pain can be the presenting symptom of shingles, developing before the rash.

Adapted from "Outpatient Evaluation of the Adult with Chest Pain," by J. R. McConaghy, 2023, in J. Givens (Ed.), *UpToDate*. Copyright by UpToDate.

similar signs and symptoms. When your client is breathing rapidly, attempt to find the cause. Attend to ABCs with POP, monitor lung sounds, and reassure the client. If there are signs of compromise (see Table 8-4), if the client's oxygen saturation is less than 95%, or if hyperventilation persists, consult a physician or transfer to the hospital as indicated.

DIFFERENTIAL DIAGNOSES

Ketoacidosis, toxic ingestion or exposure, lactic acidosis, myocardial infarction, heart failure, PE, pneumothorax, asthma exacerbation, respiratory infection.

Assessment and Management

A pregnant (or recently pregnant) client who complains of shortness of breath may be experiencing normal pregnancy discomfort, the exacerbation of underlying disease such as asthma, or the onset of a new disorder such as acute PE (Weinberger, 2023). Careful assessment will usually determine whether the client is genuinely having trouble breathing. Do not waste time interviewing and examining the client who is experiencing significant dyspnea. Activate EMS immediately, then assess and treat while waiting for the ambulance. Clients who are not breathing adequately require bag-mask ventilation with supplemental oxygen or advanced airway management (AAOS, 2018).

History and Assessment

Start by ensuring that the client has an open airway, then assess breathing. Form a visual impression as you enter the room. Is the client gasping for air or working hard to breathe? Use of accessory muscles to breathe (sternocleidomastoid, abdominal, pectoral), confusion, lethargy, cyanosis, and inability to maintain respiratory effort herald impending respiratory arrest (Ahmed & Graber, 2022). The client may display a frantic apprehension that can be difficult to distinguish from a panic attack. Other signs of severe respiratory distress include (Ahmed & Graber, 2022)

- Inability to speak more than a few words at a time. Assess for fragmented speech by asking the client to count to 10 in one breath.
- Tachypnea greater than 25 breaths per min.
- Inability to lie flat. A client with significant dyspnea sometimes instinctively assumes a tripod position to reduce the work of breathing. In tripod position, the client holds an upright posture with the torso inclined slightly forward to minimize airway resistance, the neck extended to the "sniffing" position, and the hands thrust forward.
- Diaphoresis (extreme sweating).
- Stridor or wheezing audible without a stethoscope can indicate upper airway obstruction or severe bronchospasm.
- Dusky skin or cyanosis indicates poor perfusion and/or hypoxemia.

GOLDCART History

Obtaining an accurate history is the first important step in determining the source of the problem. The client, bystanders, and the client's surroundings can usually supply important clues. Often, if you elicit relevant information and put it into context, you can form a clinical impression based on the history alone.

Physiologic breathlessness during pregnancy has a gradual onset. Onset during exercise can be related to physical deconditioning or normal changes of pregnancy. Dyspnea related to more serious issues such as PE, cardiac disease, airway obstruction, pneumothorax, or bronchospasm tend to have a more abrupt onset independent of activity.

Dyspnea after exposure to cold or allergens can indicate asthma exacerbation (Ahmed & Graber, 2022). Acute dyspnea immediately after eating or taking a medicine or supplement suggests an allergic reaction. Dyspnea after an interval of bed rest, immobility, or surgery suggests PE, as does dyspnea with a painful leg. Difficulty breathing after a fall or automobile accident suggests pneumothorax, rib fracture, or pulmonary contusion.

Physiological breathlessness of pregnancy is not associated with a cough. Acute respiratory infection is the most common cause of coughing, and it can be accompanied by fever, mucus production, or sore throat. Acute bronchitis can present with coughing or wheezing. Asthma exacerbation can present with a new or worsening cough, sometimes with wheezing, chest tightness, or shortness of breath. Pulmonary edema can also present with a wheeze. Pulmonary tuberculosis (TB) presents with fever, cough, weight loss, night sweats, and malaise (Weinberger, 2023). A cough that has been present for three or more weeks is either chronic or subacute. Chronic sinusitis or gastroesophageal reflux can cause a chronic cough or hoarseness.

Expectoration of yellow or green mucus suggests bronchitis or pneumonia. Coughing clear, white, or pink foam suggests pulmonary edema. Grossly bloody sputum is associated with PE, tuberculosis, and lung cancer. Asthma, heart failure, respiratory infection, or PE may present with a nonproductive cough.

Pulmonary Assessment

A targeted physical examination identifies issues requiring intervention and establishes a baseline from which to measure improvement or deterioration. A healthy adult, including one who is pregnant, breathes 12–20 times per min with adequate tidal volume and a regular pattern of inhalation and exhalation. At rest, breathing should appear effortless with subtle changes in rate and regularity. On auscultation, lung sounds should be clear. People with dyspnea can have a fast, normal, or slow respiratory rate. A client can be hypoxic without significant dyspnea.

Chest pain (see Table 8-6) is present with many disorders that cause dyspnea. The characteristics of the pain can give clues to the etiology of dyspnea. The pain of a myocardial infarction is usually a heavy substernal pressure that can radiate to the arms or jaw and is unchanged by taking a deep breath. Pleuritic pain increases with deep inspiration and indicates inflammation of the pleural membranes surrounding the lungs. A pneumothorax is usually accompanied by sharp pain in a specific area of the chest.

Hypoxemia (low oxygen in the blood) can cause restlessness, confusion, or even combative behavior (AAOS, 2018). In pregnancy, oxygen saturation should be 95% or higher. Standard pulse oximeters often display inaccurate readings when used on people with hypothermia, shock, or carbon monoxide poisoning.

Hypercapnia (high carbon dioxide) manifests as lethargy and sleepiness.

Crackles (rales) suggest the presence of fluid in the alveoli. Crackles suggest a problem deep within the lung, such as pulmonary edema. When fluid or mucus collects in the lung bases, alveoli collapse and the walls of the alveoli stick together. When the client takes a breath, the alveolar walls are forced open with a popping sound. Fine crackles are usually late-inspiratory, soft, high-pitched, and very brief. The sound is like that of a lock of hair rolled between the fingers near the ears. Coarse crackles are early inspiratory, louder, and lower-pitched, and they last longer than fine crackles. The sound is like the snap of opening hook and loop closures (Velcro®). Crackles confined to a small area suggest pneumonia, especially when associated with cough, fever, pleuritic chest pain, dyspnea, or sputum production (Weinberger, 2023).

Wheezing is a high-pitched whistling sound that can occur during inspiration or expiration. Wheezing can be caused by partial blockage to air flow below the trachea. Asthma, anaphylaxis, bronchitis, a foreign body in a main-stem bronchus, or congestive heart failure can present with wheezing.

Stridor is a harsh, high-pitched sound that indicates partial airway obstruction. Stridor is usually audible without a stethoscope and less musical than the whistle of a wheeze. Inspiratory stridor suggests blockage above the vocal cords, such as epiglottitis or aspirated foreign body. Expiratory stridor and stridor on both inspiration and expiration suggest obstruction below the vocal cords, such as croup or a foreign body (Parker & Wilson, 2016).

Diminished breath sounds indicate that there is less air movement in the lungs. Conditions that present diminished breath sounds include severe asthma, pneumonia, pneumothorax, and tension pneumothorax.

Cardiovascular Assessment

An abnormal heart rhythm can be the cause of dyspnea or indicate underlying disease. Heart murmurs or extra heart sounds can be audible with congestive heart failure, abnormal heart valves, severe hypertension, or other heart disease. Any disease process that reduces right-heart filling can cause jugular venous distension. (See "Cardiogenic Shock" in Chapter 9.)

Pulsus paradoxus is an abnormal decrease in stroke volume, systolic blood pressure (SBP), and pulse wave during inspiration that can develop when right-heart function is compromised by severe asthma, PE, or cardiac tamponade (Ahmed & Graber, 2022). To assess for pulsus paradoxus, measure the client's SBP after a normal exhalation, then retake the BP when the lungs expand after normal inspiration. A difference between SBPs greater than 10 mm Hg indicates pulsus paradoxus. The pulse may feel weaker during inhalation and stronger during exhalation.

Management of Dyspnea

Call EMS if your client is having difficulty breathing. As a community midwife, you can do little to alter a client's respiratory condition. Your role is to recognize that there is a problem, provide supportive care, give supplementary oxygen if oxygen saturation is less than 95%, and transport emergently to the nearest facility. If the client is stable, consult or transfer care as indicated, and arrange for transport as recommended by the receiving provider. Chart essential data and history and fax records to the receiving facility.

At the hospital, the primary goals for the emergency clinician managing a client with acute dyspnea include optimizing oxygenation, determining the need for emergency airway management and ventilatory support, and determining whether a life-threatening condition exists (Ahmed & Graber, 2022). Most clients will require chest x-rays, an electrocardiogram (ECG), a CBC, serum chemistries, and, if the fetus is viable, continuous fetal monitoring. After a diagnosis is determined, care is tailored to address the underlying issue while optimizing vital signs.

Topics for Discussion

1. Maribeth H. 26-year-old gravida 2, para 1 (G2 P1) at 18 weeks of gestation, calls at 1 a.m. with chest pain and

"stomach cramps" that spread from her RUQ into her back. She states that she experienced this pain once previously, but now the pain has returned and is worse. The pain woke her from sleep an hour ago. She had fettuccine alfredo for dinner and cheesecake for dessert a few hours before bed. What do you suspect? What would you recommend?

2. Your client Madison Z., G1 P0 at 37 0/7 weeks of gestation, has intrahepatic cholestasis of pregnancy (ICP) with significantly elevated serum bile acids (more than 100 mcmol/L) and severe itchiness. The maternal-fetal medicine specialist recommends that she undergo induction of labor tonight in a hospital with continuous fetal monitoring. Madison wants a home birth with a naturally occurring labor. How would you counsel this client?
3. Puja B., 28-year-old G3 P2 at 28 weeks of gestation, called to report pain in her RLQ. What questions would you ask her? What disorders can present with this symptom?
4. Dennie F., age 42, is in labor with her third child at your birth center when she suddenly feels extremely short of breath. How do you respond?
5. Robert S., a 35-year-old G1P0 transgender man at 18 weeks of gestation, arrives at his scheduled prenatal appointment short of breath and coughing. He has been sick for about 4 days and thinks he has a fever. Assess his symptoms using the GOLDCART framework.

References

Ahmed, A., & Graber, M. A. (2022). Approach to the adult with dyspnea in the emergency department. In M. Ganetsky (Ed.), *UpToDate*. Retrieved November 13, 2023, from https://www.uptodate.com/contents/approach-to-the-adult-with-dyspnea-in-the-emergency-department

American Academy of Orthopedic Surgeons. (2018). *Nancy Caroline's emergency care in the streets* (8th ed.). Burlington, MA: Jones & Bartlett Learning.

American College of Obstetricians and Gynecologists. (2020, revised 2023). *COVID-19 Vaccination considerations for obstetric–gynecologic care* (Practice Advisory). Retrieved from https://www.acog.org/clinical/clinical-guidance/practice-advisory/articles/2020/12/covid-19-vaccination-considerations-for-obstetric-gynecologic-care

American College of Obstetricians and Gynecologists. (2021). *COVID-19 FAQs for obstetricians-gynecologists, obstetrics*. Retrieved from https://www.acog.org/clinical-information/physician-faqs/covid-19-faqs-for-ob-gyns-obstetrics

American College of Obstetricians and Gynecologists. (2022). *COVID-19, pregnancy, childbirth, and breastfeeding: Answers from ob-gyns*. Retrieved from https://www.acog.org/womens-health/faqs/coronavirus-covid-19-pregnancy-and-breastfeeding

American College of Obstetricians and Gynecologists. (2023). *Urinary tract infections in pregnant individuals* (Clinical Consensus 4). Retrieved from https://www.acog.org/clinical/clinical-guidance/clinical-consensus/articles/2023/08/urinary-tract-infections-in-pregnant-individuals

American College of Obstetricians and Gynecologists, American Academy of Family Physicians, American Academy of PAs, American Academy of Pediatrics, American Association of Nurse Practitioners, American College of Nurse-Midwives . . . Vaccinate Your Family. (2021, August 9). *Statement of strong medical consensus for vaccination of pregnant individuals against COVID-19*. Retrieved from https://www.acog.org/news/news-releases/2021/08/statement-of-strong-medical-consensus-for-vaccination-of-pregnant-individuals-against-covid-19

American College of Obstetricians and Gynecologists Committee on Clinical Practice. (2018, reaffirmed 2022). *Thromboembolism in pregnancy* (Practice Bulletin 196). Retrieved from https://www.acog.org/clinical/clinical-guidance/practice-bulletin/articles/2018/07/thromboembolism-in-pregnancy

American College of Obstetricians and Gynecologists Committee on Obstetric Practice. (2017, reaffirmed 2022). *Intrapartum management of intraamniotic infection* (Committee Opinion 712). Retrieved from https://www.acog.org/clinical/clinical-guidance/committee-opinion/articles/2017/08/intrapartum-management-of-intraamniotic-infection

American College of Obstetricians and Gynecologists Committee on Obstetric Practice. (2021). *Ethical issues with vaccination in obstetrics and gynecology* (Committee Opinion 829). Retrieved from https://www.acog.org/clinical/clinical-guidance/committee-opinion/articles/2021/07/ethical-issues-with-vaccination-in-obstetrics-and-gynecology

American College of Obstetricians and Gynecologists Committee on Obstetric Practice & Society for Maternal-Fetal Medicine. (2021, reaffirmed 2024). *Indications for outpatient antenatal fetal surveillance* (Committee Opinion 828). Retrieved from https://www.acog.org/clinical/clinical-guidance/committee-opinion/articles/2021/06/indications-for-outpatient-antenatal-fetal-surveillance

Ananth, C. V., & Kinzler, W. L. (2022). Acute placental abruption: Pathophysiology, clinical features, diagnosis, and consequences. In V. A. Barss (Ed.), *UpToDate*. Retrieved November 13, 2023, from https://www.uptodate.com/contents/acute-placental-abruption-pathophysiology-clinical-features-diagnosis-and-consequences

Appenheimer, A. B., & Ford, B. (2020). Urine dipstick: Urinary nitrites and leukocyte esterase—Dipping into murky waters. In V. Sharp, L. Antes, M. Sanders, & G. Lockwood (Eds.), *Urine tests* (pp. 97–115). Cham, Switzerland: Springer https://doi.org/10.1007/978-3-030-29138-9_6

Asch, E., Wei, J., Mortele, K. J., Humm, K., Thornton, K., & Levine, D. (2017). Magnetic resonance imaging performance for diagnosis of ovarian torsion in pregnant women with stimulated ovaries. *Fertility Research and Practice, 3*, 13. https://doi.org/10.1186/s40738-017-0040-2

Athwal, R., Bhogal, R. H., Hodson, J., & Ramcharan, S. (2016). Surgery for gallstone disease during pregnancy does not increase fetal or maternal mortality: a meta-analysis. *HepatoBiliary Surgery and Nutrition, 5*(1), 53–57. https://doi.org/10.3978/j.issn.2304-3881.2015.11.02

August, P., & Sibai, B. M. (2023). Preeclampsia: Clinical features and diagnosis. In V. A. Barss (Ed.), *UpToDate*. Retrieved November 13, 2023, from https://www.uptodate.com/contents/preeclampsia-clinical-features-and-diagnosis

Bajc, M., Olsson, B., Gottsäter, A., Hindorf, C., & Jögi, J. (2015). V/P SPECT as a diagnostic tool for pregnant women with suspected pulmonary embolism. *European Journal of Nuclear Medicine and Molecular Imaging, 42*(8), 1325–1330. https://doi.org/10.1007/s00259-015-3056-z

Bałabuszek, K., Toborek, M., & Pietura, R. (2022). Comprehensive overview of the venous disorder known as pelvic congestion syndrome. *Annals of Medicine, 54*(1), 22–36. https://doi.org/10.1080/07853890.2021.2014556

Bastian, L. A. & Brown, H. L. (2023). Clinical manifestations and diagnosis of early pregnancy. In V. A. Barss (Ed.), *UpToDate*. Retrieved November 13, 2023, from https://www.uptodate.com/contents/clinical-manifestations-and-diagnosis-of-early-pregnancy

Becker, R. C. (2020). COVID-19 update: Covid-19-associated coagulopathy. *Journal of Thrombosis and Thrombolysis, 50*(1), 54–67. https://doi.org/10.1007/s11239-020-02134-3

Berghella, V., & Hughes, B. L. (2023). COVID-19: Overview of pregnancy issues. In V. A. Barss (Ed.), *UpToDate*. Retrieved November 13, 2023, from https://www.uptodate.com/contents/covid-19-overview-of-pregnancy-issues

Bhave, N. V., Shah, P. K., & Chaudhari, H. (2016). An unusual presentation of degenerating fibroid. *International Journal of Reproduction, Contraception, Obstetrics and Gynecology, 5*(2), 582–584. https://doi.org/10.18203/2320-1770.ijrcog20160420

Bianco, A. (2023). Maternal adaptations to pregnancy: Gastrointestinal tract. In V. A. Barss (Ed.), *UpToDate*. Retrieved November 13, 2023, from https://www.uptodate.com/contents/maternal-adaptations-to-pregnancy-gastrointestinal-tract

Bonthala, N., & Wong, M. S. (2021). Gastrointestinal diseases in pregnancy. In M. B. Landon, H. L. Galan, E. R. M. Jauniaux, D. A. Driscoll, V. Berghella, W. A. Grobman, . . . A. G. Cahill (Eds.), *Gabbe's obstetrics: Normal and problem pregnancies* (8th ed., Kindle version, ch. 53). Philadelphia, PA: Elsevier.

Bordeianou, L., & Yeh, D. D. (2021). Etiologies, clinical manifestations, and diagnosis of mechanical small bowel obstruction in adults. In W. Chen (Ed.), *UpToDate*. Retrieved November 13, 2023, from https://www.uptodate.com/contents/etiologies-clinical-manifestations-and-diagnosis-of-mechanical-small-bowel-obstruction-in-adults

Bordeianou, L., & Yeh, D. D. (2022). Management of small bowel obstruction in adults. In W. Chen (Ed.), *UpToDate*. Retrieved November 13, 2023, from https://www.uptodate.com/contents/management-of-small-bowel-obstruction-in-adults

Bourgeois, C., Ejiwunmi, R., Erdman, J., Hope, N., MacDonald, T., Meuser, A., . . . Wolfe, S. (2021). *Home birth during the COVID-19 pandemic: A viable option for all clients at low risk of complications*. Retrieved from https://www.ontariomidwives.ca/sites/default/files/AOM - Choice of Birthplace during the COVID-19 Pandemic - APRIL 2021.pdf

Brahmantara, B. N., Harjoto, B. S., Setiawan, W. A., Wanaditya, G. K., Santoso, M. I., Suarlin, I. K. Y. A., & Bay, G. P. (2022). Acute urinary retention in early pregnancy: A case report. *European Journal of Medical and Health Sciences, 4*(5), 35–37. https://dx.doi.org/10.24018/ejmed.2022.4.5.1494

Bras, R., Braga, J., Tomé, A., & Ferreira, H. (2017). Adnexal torsion in the first trimester of pregnancy: Diagnosis, laparoscopic management, and review of the literature. *Surgical Technology International, 30*, 210–214. Retrieved from https://europepmc.org/article/MED/28537347

Brooks, D. C. (2022). Gallstone diseases in pregnancy. In W. Chen & A. Chakrabarti (Eds.), *UpToDate*. Retrieved November 13, 2023, from https://www.uptodate.com/contents/gallstone-diseases-in-pregnancy

Burwick, R. M. (2021). Renal disease in pregnancy. In M. B. Landon, H. L. Galan, E. R. M. Jauniaux, D. A. Driscoll, V. Berghella, W. A. Grobman, . . . A. G. Cahill (Eds.), *Gabbe's obstetrics: Normal and problem pregnancies* (8th ed., Kindle version, ch. 44). Philadelphia, PA: Elsevier.

Campbell, M. H., Sandlin, A. T., Wendel, P. L., & Racher, M. L. (2021). A case of incarceration of the gravid uterus & the Ehlers-Danlos Syndromes with literature review. *Obstetrics and Gynaecology Cases—Reviews, 8*(2), 197. https://doi.org/10.23937/2377-9004/1410197

Cannegieter, S. C., Horváth-Puhó, E., Schmidt, M., Dekkers, O. M., Pedersen, L., Vandenbroucke, J. P., & Sørensen, H. T. (2015). Risk of venous and arterial thrombotic events in patients diagnosed with superficial vein thrombosis: A nationwide cohort study. *Blood, 125*(2), 229–235. https://doi.org/10.1182/blood-2014-06-577783

Chappell, L. C., Bell, J. L., Smith, A., Linsell, L., Juszczak, E., Dixon, P. H., . . . Thornton, J. G. (2019). Ursodeoxycholic acid versus placebo in women with intrahepatic cholestasis of pregnancy (PITCHES): A randomised controlled trial. *Lancet, 394*(10201), 849–860. https://doi.org/10.1016/S0140-6736(19)31270-X

Chen, K. T. (2023). Postpartum endometritis. In V. A. Barss (Ed.), *UpToDate*. Retrieved November 13, 2023, from https://www.uptodate.com/contents/postpartum-endometritis

Clark, S. L., & Hankins, G. D. V. (2012). Preventing maternal death: 10 clinical diamonds. *Obstetrics & Gynecology, 119*(2, Pt. 1), 360–364. https://doi.org/10.1097/AOG.0b013e3182411907

Coad, S., Friedman, B., & Geoffrion, R. (2012). Understanding urinalysis: Clues for the obstetrician-gynecologist. *Expert Review of Obstetrics & Gynecology, 7*(3), 269–279. https://doi.org/10.1586/eog.12.21

Costigan, K. A., Sipsma, H. L., & DiPietro, J. A. (2006). Pregnancy folklore revisited: The case of heartburn and hair. *Birth, 33*(4), 311–314. https://doi.org/10.1111/j.1523-536X.2006.00128.x

Crossen, H. S. (1907). The diagnosis and treatment of diseases of women. St. Louis, MO: C. V. Mosby. Retrieved from https://commons.wikimedia.org/wiki/File:The_diagnosis_and_treatment_of_diseases_of_women_(1907)_(14597924687).jpg

Cunningham, F. G., Leveno, K. J., Dashe, J. S., Hoffman, B. L., Spong, C. Y., & Casey, B. M. (Eds.). (2022). *Williams obstetrics* (26th ed., Kindle version). New York, NY: McGraw-Hill.

Czikk, M. J., McCarthy, F. P., & Murphy, K. E. (2011). Chorioamnionitis: From pathogenesis to treatment. *Clinical Microbiology and Infection, 17*(9), 1304–1311. https://doi.org/10.1111/j.1469-0691.2011.03574.x

D'Ambrosio, V., Brunelli, R., Musacchio, L., Del Negro, V., Vena, F., Boccuzzi, G., . . . Giancotti, A. (2021). Adnexal masses in pregnancy: An updated review on diagnosis and treatment. *Tumori Journal, 107*(1), 12–16. https://doi.org/10.1177/0300891620909144

Dante, G., Pedrielli, G., Annessi, E., & Facchinetti, F. (2013). Herb remedies during pregnancy: A systematic review of controlled clinical trials. *Journal of Maternal-Fetal & Neonatal Medicine, 26*(3), 306–312. https://doi.org/10.3109/14767058.2012.722732

Davis-Floyd, R., Gutschow, K., & Schwartz, D. A. (2020). Pregnancy, birth and the COVID-19 pandemic in the United States. *Medical Anthropology, 39*(5), 413–427. https://doi.org/10.1080/01459740.2020.1761804

De Lee, J. B. (1914). *The principles and practice of obstetrics*. Philadelphia, PA: W. B. Saunders. Retrieved from https://archive.org/details/principlespracti00dele

Di Mascio, D., Quist-Nelson, J., Riegel, M., George, B., Saccone, G., Brun, R., . . . Berghella, V. (2021). Perinatal death by bile acid levels in intrahepatic cholestasis of pregnancy: A systematic review. *Journal of Maternal-Fetal & Neonatal Medicine, 34*(21), 3614–3622. https://doi.org/10.1080/14767058.2019.1685965

Di Renzo, G. C., & Giardina, I. (2020). Coronavirus disease 2019 in pregnancy: Consider thromboembolic disorders and thromboprophylaxis. *American Journal of Obstetrics & Gynecology, 223*(1), 135. https://doi.org/10.1016/j.ajog.2020.04.017

Diken, Z., Usta, I. M., & Nassar, A. H. (2014). A clinical approach to intrahepatic cholestasis of pregnancy. *American Journal of Perinatology, 31*(01), 001–008. https://doi.org/10.1055/s-0033-1333673

Domenici, L., Monti, M., Bracchi, C., Giorgini, M., Colagiovanni, V., Muzii, L., & Benedetti Panici, P. (2016). D-mannose: A promising support for acute urinary tract infections in women. A pilot study. *European Review for Medical and Pharmacological Sciences, 20*(13), 2920–2925. Retrieved from https://www.europeanreview.org/article/11121

Ducarme, G., Maire, F., Chatel, P., Luton, D., & Hammel, P. (2014). Acute pancreatitis during pregnancy: A review. *Journal of Perinatology, 34*(2), 87–94. https://doi.org/10.1038/jp.2013.161

Duff, W. P. (2021). Maternal and perinatal infection in pregnancy: Bacterial. In M. B. Landon, H. L. Galan, E. R. M. Jauniaux, D. A. Driscoll, V. Berghella, W. A. Grobman, . . . A. G. Cahill (Eds.), *Gabbe's obstetrics: Normal and problem pregnancies* (8th ed., Kindle version, ch. 58). Philadelphia, PA: Elsevier.

Durnwald, C. P. (2021). Hepatic disorders during pregnancy. In M. B. Landon, H. L. Galan, E. R. M. Jauniaux, D. A. Driscoll, V. Berghella, W. A. Grobman, . . . A. G. Cahill (Eds.), *Gabbe's obstetrics: Normal and problem pregnancies* (8th ed., Kindle version, ch. 52). Philadelphia, PA: Elsevier.

Elwood, C., Raeside, A., Boucoiran, I., Van Schalkwyk, J., Money, D., Yudin, M., . . . Poliquin, V. (2020, July 27). *COVID-19 and pregnancy*. Retrieved from https://sogc.org/common/Uploaded%20files/Media%20Updates/EN_Statement-COVID_Pregnancy.pdf

Fanta, C. H., & Lange-Vaidya, N. (2022). Asthma in adolescents and adults: Evaluation and diagnosis. In P. Dieffenbach (Ed.), *UpToDate*. Retrieved November 13, 2023, from https://www.uptodate.com/contents/diagnosis-of-asthma-in-adolescents-and-adults

Farr, A., Ott, J., Kueronya, V., Margreiter, M., Javadli, E., Einig, S., . . . Bancher-Todesca, D. (2017). The association between maternal hydronephrosis and acute flank pain during pregnancy: A prospective pilot-study. *Journal of Maternal-Fetal & Neonatal Medicine, 30*(20), 2417–2421. https://doi.org/10.1080/14767058.2016.1252328

Fernando, M., & Edmonds, H. (2015). Spontaneous pneumomediastinum and subcutaneous emphysema during labour in an uncomplicated pregnancy (EP10.38). *BJOG, 122*(S1), 173.

Findley, P. (1913). *A treatise on the diseases of women for students and practitioners*. Philadelphia, PA: Lea & Febiger. Retrieved from https://books.google.com/books?id=eBQ1AQAAMAAJ&printsec=frontcover&source=gbs_ViewAPI#v=onepage&q&f=false

Giannella, L., Montanari, M., Delli Carpini, G., Di Giuseppe, J., & Ciavattini, A. (2022). Huge vulvar varicosities in pregnancy: Case report and systematic review. *Journal of International Medical Research, 50*(5). https://doi.org/10.1177/03000605221097764

Goel, B., Rani, J., Huria, A., Gupta, P., & Dalal, U. (2014). Perforated duodenal ulcer—A rare cause of acute abdomen in pregnancy. *Journal of Clinical and Diagnostic Research, 8*(9), OD03–OD04. https://doi.org/10.7860/JCDR/2014/9130.4846

Gupta, K. (2023). Urinary tract infections and asymptomatic bacteriuria in pregnancy. In A. Bloom (Ed.), *UpToDate*. Retrieved November 13, 2023, from https://www.uptodate.com/contents/urinary-tract-infections-and-asymptomatic-bacteriuria-in-pregnancy

Higgins, R. D., Saade, G., Polin, R. A., Grobman, W. A., Buhimschi, I. A., Watterberg, K., . . . Raju, T. N. K. (2016). Evaluation and management of women and newborns with a maternal diagnosis of chorioamnionitis: Summary of a workshop. *Obstetrics & Gynecology, 127*(3), 426–436. https://doi.org/10.1097/AOG.0000000000001246

Iloson, C., Möller, A., Sundfeldt, K., & Bernhardsson, S. (2021). Symptoms within somatization after sexual abuse among women: A scoping review. *Acta Obstetricia et Gynecologica Scandinavica, 100*(4), 758–767. https://doi.org/10.1111/aogs.14084

Jmarchn [Screen name]. (2017). *Varicose veins*. Retrieved from https://commons.wikimedia.org/wiki/File:Varicose_veins-en.svg

Johnson, E. K., & Kim, E. D. (2017). Urinary tract infections in pregnancy. *Medscape*. Retrieved from https://emedicine.medscape.com/article/452604-overview

Johnson, N. R. (2023). Vulvovaginal varicosities and pelvic congestion syndrome. In K. Eckler (Ed.), *UpToDate*. Retrieved November 13, 2023, from https://www.uptodate.com/contents/vulvovaginal-varicosities-and-pelvic-congestion-syndrome

Kandiah, S., Iswariah, H., & Elgey, S. (2013). Postpartum pneumomediastinum and subcutaneous emphysema: Two case reports. *Case Reports in Obstetrics and Gynecology, 2013*. https://doi.org/10.1155/2013/735154

Kendall, J. L>, & Moreira, M. E. (2023). Evaluation of the adult with abdominal or flank pain in the emergency department. In M. Ganetsky, (Ed.), *UpToDate*. Retrieved November 13, 2023, from https://www.uptodate.com/contents/evaluation-of-the-adult-with-nontraumatic-abdominal-or-flank-pain-in-the-emergency-department

Khurram, D., Patel, B. & Farra, M. W. (2015). Hamman's syndrome: A rare cause of chest pain in a postpartum patient. *Case Reports in Pulmonology, 2015*. https://doi.org/10.1155/2015/201051

Kilpatrick, C. C., & Shamshirsaz, A. A. (2022). Approach to acute abdominal/pelvic pain in pregnant and postpartum patients. In V. A. Barss (Ed.), *UpToDate*. Retrieved November 13, 2023, from https://www.uptodate.com/contents/approach-to-acute-abdominal-pelvic-pain-in-pregnant-and-postpartum-patients

Ko, H. H., & Yoshida, E. M. (2006). Acute fatty liver of pregnancy. *Canadian Journal of Gastroenterology, 20*(1), 25–30. https://doi.org/10.1155/2006/638131

Lacoste, C. R., Seffert, P., & Chauleur, C. (2013). Acute urinary retention and retroverted uterus during pregnancy. *Gynécologie Obstétrique & Fertilité, 41*(4), 265–268. https://doi.org/10.1016/j.gyobfe.2013.02.004

Lam, K., & Suen, C. F. D. L. W. (2015). Stranded under the Prom: Impacted gravid uterus presenting as acute urinary retention. *BMJ Case Reports, 2015*, bcr2015211064. https://doi.org/10.1136/bcr-2015-211064

Lantagne, D. (2006). *Unsafe drinking water, Ethiopia* [Photograph]. Centers for Disease Control and Prevention Public Health Image Library image 22472. Retrieved from https://phil.cdc.gov/Details.aspx?pid=2247

Lao, T. T., & Hui, S.-Y. A. (2022). The obstetric aspects of maternal asthma. *Best Practice & Research Clinical Obstetrics & Gynaecology, 85*(Pt. A), 57–69. https://doi.org/10.1016/j.bpobgyn.2022.08.005

Larson, L. E., & File, T. M., Jr. (2023). Approach to the pregnant patient with a respiratory infection. In V. A. Barss & S. Bond (Eds.), *UpToDate*. Retrieved November 13, 2023, from https://www.uptodate.com/contents/approach-to-the-pregnant-patient-with-a-respiratory-infection

Laufer, M. R. (2023). Ovarian and fallopian tube torsion. In A. Chakrabarti (Ed.), *UpToDate*. Retrieved November 13, 2023, from https://www.uptodate.com/contents/ovarian-and-fallopian-tube-torsion

Leath, C. A., & Phippen, N. T. (2022). Evaluation of acute abdomen. *BMJ Best Practice*. Retrieved 21 April 2023, from https://bestpractice.bmj.com/topics/en-us/503

Lee, R. H., & Reau, N. (2023). Acute fatty liver of pregnancy. In K. M. Robson & V. A. Barss (Eds.), *UpToDate*. Retrieved November 13, from https://www.uptodate.com/contents/acute-fatty-liver-of-pregnancy

Lee, Y. C. G. (2023). Pneumothorax in adults: Epidemiology and etiology. In G. Finlay (Ed.), *UpToDate*. Retrieved November 13, 2023, from https://www.uptodate.com/contents/pneumothorax-in-adults-epidemiology-and-etiology

Levenson, J. L. (2022). Somatic symptom disorder: Assessment and diagnosis. In D. Solomon (Ed.), *UpToDate*. Retrieved November 13, 2023, from https://www.uptodate.com/contents/somatic-symptom-disorder-assessment-and-diagnosis

Li, M., Lei, P., Zeng, B., Li, Z., Yu, P., Fan, B., . . . Liu, H. (2020). Coronavirus disease (COVID-19): Spectrum of CT findings and temporal progression of the disease. *Academic Radiology, 27*(5), 603–608. https://doi.org/0.1016/j.acra.2020.03.003

Liang, S.-G., Ooka, F., Santo, A., & Kaibara, M. (2002). Pneumomediastinum following esophageal rupture associated with hyperemesis gravidarum.

Journal of Obstetrics and Gynaecology Research, 28(3), 172–175. https://doi.org/10.1046/j.1341-8076.2002.00033.x

Lindor, K. D., & Lee, R. H. (2023). Intrahepatic cholestasis of pregnancy. In K. M. Robson & V. A. Barss (Eds.), *UpToDate*. Retrieved November 13, 2023, from https://www.uptodate.com/contents/intrahepatic-cholestasis-of-pregnancy

Liu, J., Ghaziani, T. T., & Wolf, J. L. (2017). Acute fatty liver disease of pregnancy: Updates in pathogenesis, diagnosis, and management. *American Journal of Gastroenterology, 112*(6), 838–846. https://doi.org/10.1038/ajg.2017.54

Lou, Y. Y. (2017). Hamman's syndrome: Spontaneous pneumomediastinum and subcutaneous emphysema during second stage of labour. *International Journal of Reproduction, Contraception, Obstetrics and Gynecology, 6*(6), 2622–2624. https://doi.org/10.18203/2320-1770.ijrcog20172365

Malhotra, A., & Weinberger, S. E. (2023a). Deep vein thrombosis in pregnancy: Epidemiology, pathogenesis, and diagnosis. In G. Finlay (Ed.), *UpToDate*. Retrieved November 13, 2023, from https://www.uptodate.com/contents/deep-vein-thrombosis-in-pregnancy-epidemiology-pathogenesis-and-diagnosis

Malhotra, A., & Weinberger, S. E. (2023b). Pulmonary embolism in pregnancy: Clinical presentation and diagnosis. In G. Finlay (Ed.), *UpToDate*. Retrieved November 13, 2023, from https://www.uptodate.com/contents/pulmonary-embolism-in-pregnancy-clinical-presentation-and-diagnosis

Malhotra, A., & Weinberger, S. E. (2023c). Venous thromboembolism in pregnancy and postpartum: Treatment. In G. Finlay (Ed.), *UpToDate*. Retrieved November 13, 2023, from https://www.uptodate.com/contents/venous-thromboembolism-in-pregnancy-and-postpartum-treatment

Mandal, D., Saha, M. M., & Pal, D. K. (2017). Urological disorders and pregnancy: An overall experience. *Urology Annals, 9*(1), 32–36. https://doi.org/10.4103/0974-7796.198901

Martin, R. F. (2022). Acute appendicitis in adults: Clinical manifestations and differential diagnosis. In W. Chen (Ed.), *UpToDate*. Retrieved November 13, 2023, from https://www.uptodate.com/contents/1386#!

McConaghy, J. R. (2023). Outpatient evaluation of the adult with chest pain. In S. Swenson (Ed.), *UpToDate*. Retrieved November 13, 2023, from https://www.uptodate.com/contents/outpatient-evaluation-of-the-adult-with-chest-pain

McIntosh, K. (2023). COVID-19: Clinical features. In M. Bogorodskaya (Ed.), *UpToDate*. Retrieved November 13, 2023, from https://www.uptodate.com/contents/covid-19-clinical-features

Merriam, A. A., & Pettker, C. M. (2021). Thromboembolic disorders in pregnancy. In M. B. Landon, H. L. Galan, E. R. M. Jauniaux, D. A. Driscoll, V. Berghella, W. A. Grobman, . . . A. G. Cahill (Eds.), *Gabbe's obstetrics: Normal and problem pregnancies* (8th ed., Kindle version, ch. 50). Philadelphia, PA: Elsevier.

Mikkelsen, M. E., & Abramoff, B. (2023). COVID-19: Evaluation and management of adults with persistent symptoms following acute illness ("Long COVID"). In G. Finlay (Ed.), *UpToDate*. Retrieved November 13, 2023, from https://www.uptodate.com/contents/covid-19-evaluation-and-management-of-adults-with-persistent-symptoms-following-acute-illness-long-covid

Mitchell, A. L., Ovadia, C., Syngelaki, A., Souretis, K., Martineau, M., Girling, J., . . . Williamson, C. (2021). Re-evaluating diagnostic thresholds for intrahepatic cholestasis of pregnancy: case-control and cohort study. *BJOG: An International Journal of Obstetrics & Gynaecology.*

Mok, T., Harris, E., Vargas, A., Afshar, Y., Han, C. S., Karagozian, A., & Rao, R. (2021). Evaluation of respiratory emissions during labor and delivery: Potential implications for transmission of severe acute respiratory syndrome coronavirus 2 (SARS-CoV-2). *Obstetrics & Gynecology, 138*(4), 616–621. https://doi.org/10.1097/AOG.0000000000004533

Montorsi, F., Gandaglia, G., Salonia, A., Briganti, A., & Mirone, V. (2016). Effectiveness of a combination of cranberries, *Lactobacillus rhamnosus*, and vitamin C for the management of recurrent urinary tract infections in women: Results of a pilot study. *European Urology, 70*(6), 912–915. https://doi.org/10.1016/j.eururo.2016.05.042

Mostbeck, G., Adam, E. J., Nielsen, M. B., Claudon, M., Clevert, D., Nicolau, C., . . . Owens, C. M. (2016). How to diagnose acute appendicitis: Ultrasound first. *Insights into Imaging, 7*(2), 255–263. https://doi.org/10.1007/s13244-016-0469-6

Murphy, N., & Cullinan, B. (2020). Maternal resuscitation and trauma. In L. Leeman, L. Dresang, J. S. Quinlan, & S. R. Magee (Eds.), *Advanced life support in obstetrics: Provider manual* (9th ed., pp. 205–226). Leawood, KS: American Academy of Family Physicians.

National Institute of Diabetes and Digestive and Kidney Diseases. (n.d.). Drawing of swollen kidney and ureter. Retrieved from https://www.niddk.nih.gov/news/media-library/17590

O'Leary, B. D., Armstrong, F. M., Byrne, S., Talento, A. F., & O'Coigligh, S. (2020). The prevalence of positive urine dipstick testing and urine culture in the asymptomatic pregnant woman: A cross-sectional study. *European Journal of Obstetrics & Gynecology and Reproductive Biology, 253*, 103–107. https://doi.org/10.1016/j.ejogrb.2020.08.004

Ouyang, D. W., & Norwitz, E. R. (2022). Uterine fibroids (leiomyomas): Issues in pregnancy. In V. A. Barss (Ed.), *UpToDate*. Retrieved November 13, 2023, from https://www.uptodate.com/contents/uterine-fibroids-leiomyomas-issues-in-pregnancy

Ovadia, C., Seed, P. T., Sklavounos, A., Geenes, V., Di Ilio, C., Chambers, J., . . . Bull, L. (2019). Association of adverse perinatal outcomes of intrahepatic cholestasis of pregnancy with biochemical markers: Results of aggregate and individual patient data meta-analyses. *Lancet, 393*(10174), 899–909. https://doi.org/10.1016/S0140-6736(18)31877-4

Pacheco, L. D., Saad, A., La Rosa De Los Rios, M., & Webb, C. M. (2021). Respiratory disease in pregnancy. In M. B. Landon, H. L. Galan, E. R. M. Jauniaux, D. A. Driscoll, V. Berghella, W. A. Grobman, . . . A. G. Cahill (Eds.), *Gabbe's obstetrics: Normal and problem pregnancies* (8th ed., Kindle version, ch. 43). Philadelphia, PA: Elsevier.

Papageorghiou, A. T., Deruelle, P., Gunier, R. B., Rauch, S., García-May, P. K., Mhatre, M., . . . Villar, J. (2021). Preeclampsia and COVID-19: Results from the INTERCOVID prospective longitudinal study. *American Journal of Obstetrics & Gynecology, 225*(3), 289.e1–289.e17. https://doi.org/10.1016/j.ajog.2021.05.014

Parker, L., & Wilson, A. (2016). *Paramedic principles and practice ANZ SLS*. Chatswood, NSW: Elsevier Australia.

Phillips, D., Deipolyi, A. R., Hesketh, R. L., Midia, M., & Oklu, R. (2014). Pelvic congestion syndrome: Etiology of pain, diagnosis, and clinical management. *Journal of Vascular and Interventional Radiology, 25*(5), 725–733. https://doi.org/10.1016/j.jvir.2014.01.030

Pina Moreno, J. M., Ruiz Minaya, M., Fraile López, A., Feltrer Hidalgo, M., Ortega Abad, V., & García-Tizón Larroca, S. (2023). Importance of the early diagnosis of incarcerated gravid uterus: Case report and systematic review. *International Journal of Gynecology & Obstetrics, 162*(1), 193–201. https://doi.org/10.1002/ijgo.14615

Poon, L. C., Yang, H., Kapur, A., Melamed, N., Dao, B., Divakar, H., . . . Hod, M. (2020). Global interim guidance on coronavirus disease 2019 (COVID-19) during pregnancy and puerperium from FIGO and allied partners: Information for healthcare professionals. *International Journal of Gynecology & Obstetrics, 149*(3), 273–286. https://doi.org/10.1002/ijgo.13156

Preminger, G. M., & Curhan, G. C. (2021). Kidney stones in adults: Kidney stones during pregnancy. In A. Q. Lam (Ed.), *UpToDate*. Retrieved November 13, 2023, from https://www.uptodate.com/contents/kidney-stones-in-adults-kidney-stones-during-pregnancy

Rasmussen, S. A., Smulian, J. C., Lednicky, J. A., Wen, T. S., & Jamieson, D. J. (2020). Coronavirus Disease 2019 (COVID-19) and pregnancy: What obstetricians need to know. *American Journal of Obstetrics & Gynecology, 222*(5), 415–426. https://doi.org/10.1016/j.ajog.2020.02.017

Reardon, C. C., & Chen, F. (2023). Acute respiratory failure during pregnancy and the peripartum period. In G. Finlay (Ed.), *UpToDate*. Retrieved November 13, 2023, from https://www.uptodate.com/contents/acute-respiratory-failure-during-pregnancy-and-the-peripartum-period

Rebarber, A., & Jacob, B. P. (2023). Acute appendicitis in pregnancy. In K. Eckler (Ed.), *UpToDate*. Retrieved November 13, 2023, from https://www.uptodate.com/contents/acute-appendicitis-in-pregnancy

Rojas-Suarez, J. A., & Suarez Rueda, N. (2020). Maternal sepsis. In L. Leeman, L. Dresang, J. S. Quinlan, & S. R. Magee (Eds.), *Advanced life support in obstetrics: Provider manual* (9th ed., pp. 275–295). Leawood, KS: American Academy of Family Physicians.

Royal College of Obstetricians & Gynaecologists. (2020, July 24). *Coronavirus (COVID-19) infection in pregnancy* (version 11). Retrieved from https://www.rcog.org.uk/globalassets/documents/guidelines/2020-07-24-coronavirus-covid-19-infection-in-pregnancy.pdf

Runowicz, C. D., & Brewer, M. (2023). Adnexal mass: Evaluation and management in pregnancy. In A. Chakrabarti (Ed.), *UpToDate*. Retrieved November 13, 2023, from https://www.uptodate.com/contents/adnexal-mass-evaluation-and-management-in-pregnancy

Sasaki, K. J., & Miller, C. E. (2014). Adnexal torsion: Review of the literature. *Journal of Minimally Invasive Gynecology, 21*(2), 196–202. https://doi.org/10.1016/j.jmig.2013.09.010

Scala, R., Madioni, C., Manta, C., Maggiorelli, C., Maccari, U., & Ciarleglio, G. (2016). Spontaneous pneumomediastinum in pregnancy: A case report. *Revista Portuguesa de Pneumologia, 22*(2), 129–131. https://doi.org/10.1016/j.rppnen.2015.09.004

Schatz, M. & Weinberger, S. E. (2023). Management of asthma during pregnancy. In P. Dieffenbach (Ed.), *UpToDate*. Retrieved November 13, 2023, from https://www.uptodate.com/contents/management-of-asthma-during-pregnancy

Schwartzstein, R. M. (2023). Approach to the patient with dyspnea. In P. Dieffenbach (Ed.), *UpToDate*. Retrieved November 13, 2023, from https://www.uptodate.com/contents/approach-to-the-patient-with-dyspnea

Schwartzstein, R. M., Richards, J., Edlow, J. A., & Roy-Byrne, P. P. (2021). Hyperventilation syndrome in adults. In J. Givens (Ed.), *UpToDate*. Retrieved November 13, 2023, from https://www.uptodate.com/contents/hyperventilation-syndrome-in-adults

Servier Medical Art. (2016a). *Pulmonary edema* [Graphic]. Retrieved from https://smart.servier.com/wp-content/uploads/2016/10/Oedeme_poumons-637x680.png

Servier Medical Art. (2016b). *Pulmonary embolism* [1] [Graphic]. Retrieved from https://smart.servier.com/wp-content/uploads/2016/10/Embolie_pulmonaire_01-680x574.png

Servier Medical Art. (2016c). *Pulmonary embolism* [7] [Graphic]. Retrieved from https://smart.servier.com/wp-content/uploads/2016/10/Embolie_pulmonaire_07-680x645.png

Sharp, H. T. (2023). Evaluation and management of ruptured ovarian cyst. In A. Chakrabarti (Ed.), *UpToDate*. Retrieved November 13, 2023, from https://www.uptodate.com/contents/evaluation-and-management-of-ruptured-ovarian-cyst

Sheibani, L., Uhrinak, A., Lee, R. H., Fong, A., & Pathak, B. (2014). Intrahepatic cholestasis of pregnancy: The effect of bile acids on fetal heart rate tracings. *Obstetrics & Gynecology, 123*(Suppl. 1), 78S–79S. https://doi.org/10.1097/01.AOG.0000447401.84270.a7

Simerville, J. A., Maxted, W. C., & Pahira, J. J. (2005). Urinalysis: A comprehensive review. *American Family Physician, 71*(6), 1153–1162. Retrieved from https://www.aafp.org/afp/2005/0315/p1153.pdf

Slama, R., Barry, M., McManus, K., Latham, D., & Berniard, M. (2015). Uterine incarceration: Rare cause of urinary retention in healthy pregnant patients. *Western Journal of Emergency Medicine, 16*(5), 790–792. https://doi.org/10.5811/westjem.2015.7.27185

Smith, D. B. (2020). Coronavirus may be a blood vessel disease, which explains everything. *Elemental*. Retrieved from https://elemental.medium.com/coronavirus-may-be-a-blood-vessel-disease-which-explains-everything-2c4032481ab2

Smyth, R. M. D., Aflaifel, N., & Bamigboye, A. A. (2015). Interventions for varicose veins and leg oedema in pregnancy. *Cochrane Database of Systematic Reviews 2015*(10). https://doi.org/10.1002/14651858.CD001066.pub3

Society for Maternal-Fetal Medicine. (2021). *COVID-19 and pregnancy: What maternal-fetal medicine subspecialists need to know*. Washington, DC: SMFM. Retrieved from https://s3.amazonaws.com/cdn.smfm.org/media/3238/PDF.pdf

Søreide, K., Thorsen, K., Harrison, E. M., Bingener, J., Møller, M. H., Ohene-Yeboah, M., & Søreide, J. A. (2015). Perforated peptic ulcer. *Lancet, 386*(10000), 1288–1298. https://doi.org/10.1016/S0140-6736(15)00276-7

Tachibana, D., Misugi, T., Kitada, K., Kurihara, Y., Tahara, M., Hamuro, A., . . . Koyama, M. (2021). Incarcerated gravid uterus: Spontaneous resolution is not rare. *Diagnostics, 11*(9), 1544. https://doi.org/10.3390/diagnostics11091544

Thadhani, R. I., & Maynard, S. E. (2022). Maternal adaptations to pregnancy: Renal and urinary tract physiology. In A. Chakrabarti (Ed.), *UpToDate*. Retrieved November 13, 2023, from https://www.uptodate.com/contents/maternal-adaptations-to-pregnancy-renal-and-urinary-tract-physiology

Tita, A. T. N. (2023). Clinical chorioamnionitis. In V. A. Barss (Ed.), *UpToDate*. Retrieved November 13, 2023, from https://www.uptodate.com/contents/clinical-chorioamnionitis

Vakil, N. B. (2022). Peptic ulcer disease: Treatment and secondary prevention. In S. Grover (Ed.), *UpToDate*. Retrieved November 13, 2023, from https://www.uptodate.com/contents/peptic-ulcer-disease-treatment-and-secondary-prevention

Van der Merwe, J. L., Hall, D. R., Herbst, P., & Doubell, A. (2014). Patient profile of a tertiary obstetric-cardiac clinic: Management of cardiac disease in pregnancy. *SA Heart, 11*(2), 80–85. Retrieved from https://journals.co.za/content/saheart/11/2/EJC157342

van Mens, T. E., Scheres, L. J. J., de Jong, P. G., Leeflang, M. M. G., Nijkeuter, M, Middeldorp, S., & Cochrane Vascular Group. (2017). Imaging for the exclusion of pulmonary embolism in pregnancy. *Cochrane Database of Systematic Reviews*. https://doi.org/10.1002/14651858.CD011053.pub2

Varga, Z., Flammer, A. J., Steiger, P., Haberdecker, M., Andermatt, R., Zinkernagel, A. S., . . . Moch, H. (2020). Endothelial cell infection and endotheliitis in COVID-19. *Lancet, 395*(10234), 1417–1418. https://doi.org/10.1016/S0140-6736(20)30937-5

Vidaeff, A. C., & Schneider, K. M. (2022). Incarcerated gravid uterus. In V. A. Barss (Ed.), *UpToDate*. Retrieved November 13, 2023, from https://www.uptodate.com/contents/incarcerated-gravid-uterus

Webster, P. J., Bailey, M. A., Wilson, J., & Burke, D. A. (2015). Small bowel obstruction in pregnancy is a complex surgical problem with a high risk of fetal loss. *Annals of the Royal College of Surgeons of England, 97*(5), 339–344. https://doi.org/10.1308/003588415X14181254789844

Weinberger, S. E. (2023). Maternal adaptations to pregnancy: Dyspnea and other physiologic respiratory changes. In V. A. Barss (Ed.), *UpToDate*. Retrieved November 13, 2023, from https://www.uptodate.com/contents/maternal-adaptations-to-pregnancy-dyspnea-and-other-physiologic-respiratory-changes

Wenstrom, K. D. (2015). Cardiac disease. In J. T. Queenan, C. Y. Spong, & C. J. Lockwood (Eds.), *Protocols for high-risk pregnancies: An evidence-based approach* (pp. 128–138). Chichester, United Kingdom: John Wiley & Sons. https://doi.org/10.1002/9781119001256.ch15

Williamson, C., & Geenes, V. (2014). Intrahepatic cholestasis of pregnancy. *Obstetrics & Gynecology, 124*(1), 120–133. https://doi.org/10.1097/AOG.0000000000000346

Yang, J. M., & Huang, W.-C. (2004). Sonographic findings in acute urinary retention secondary to retroverted gravid uterus: Pathophysiology and preventive measures. *Ultrasound in Obstetrics & Gynecology, 23*(5), 490–495. https://doi.org/10.1002/uog.1039

Yeh, D. D., & Bordeianou, L. (2023). Large bowel obstruction. In W. Chen (Ed.), *UpToDate*. Retrieved November 13, 2023, from https://www.uptodate.com/contents/large-bowel-obstruction

Zhuang, L., Wang, X.-Y., Sang, Y., Xu, J., & He, X.-L. (2021). Acute urinary retention in the first and second-trimester of pregnancy: Three case reports. *World Journal of Clinical Cases, 9*(13), 3130–3139. https://doi.org/10.12998/wjcc.v9.i13.3130

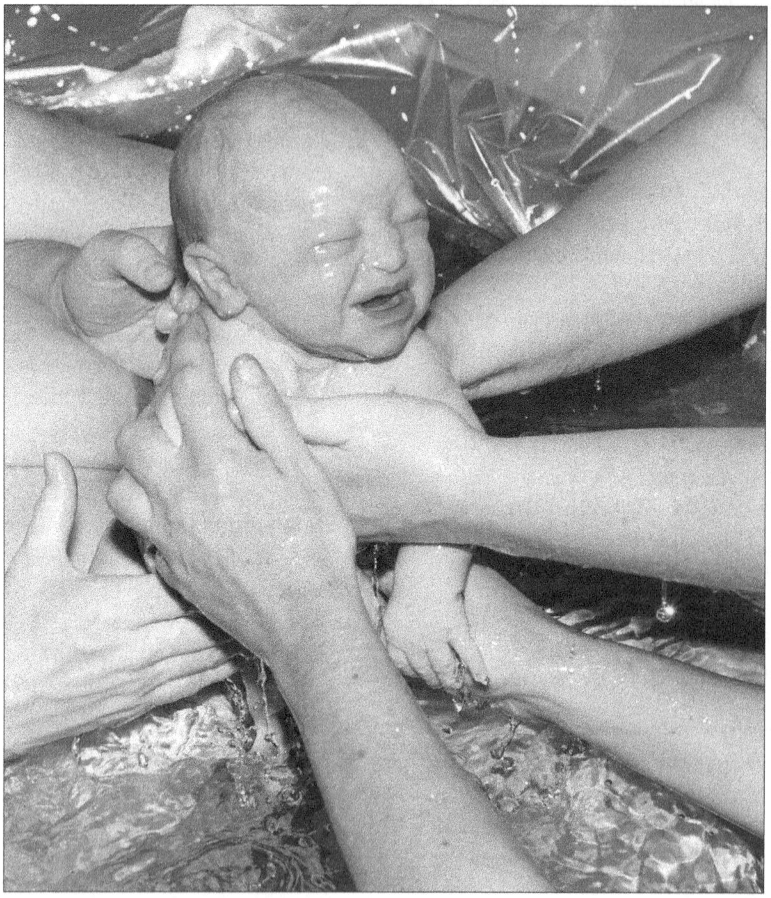

Trauma, Shock, Altered Level of Consciousness, and Cardiac Arrest

9

Objectives

- Identify the presenting symptoms and signs of shock and describe immediate and specific management.
- Give three examples of how the normal physiologic changes of pregnancy can affect responses to traumatic injury.
- Identify cardiopulmonary resuscitation (CPR) modifications that improve blood flow when giving chest compressions to a pregnant client in cardiac arrest.
- Identify three etiologies of shock that can develop intrapartum.
- List three conditions that can cause fainting in a healthy pregnant person.

Composite Case Study

As Mingi Nam, CPM, left her office one evening, she noticed an unmoving human form on the ground at the shopping center across the street. She rushed to assist, and found Margaret M., her 36-week-pregnant client, lying on the concrete near the foot of a staircase. Margaret was on her left side, and blood was pooling under her head. Mingi flung open the door of the nearest shop and yelled, "I need help out here! Someone call an ambulance! There's a bleeding pregnant woman on the ground!"

As the storekeeper activated emergency medical services (EMS), Mingi and two helpful shoppers rushed to Margaret's side. "Margaret! Margaret! Can you hear me?" Mingi said, quickly checking for breathing and consciousness. Margaret moaned but did not answer or make eye contact. Mingi saw that she was breathing adequately and began checking for injuries, starting at the head.

A laceration on the side of Margaret's head was bleeding copiously but appeared superficial. Mingi pulled a clean scarf out of her handbag and instructed another bystander to apply pressure to the wound to stop the bleeding. No blood was coming from Margaret's ears, nose, or mouth, and there was none inside her unbuttoned coat. There was no blood on her tights that might indicate vaginal bleeding. Mingi ran her hands over Margaret's body as far as she could reach, and Margaret showed no sign of pain. Mingi did notice that Margaret's right wrist was bent at an abnormal angle, like a dinner fork.

Margaret's eyes fluttered open and she began to struggle and argue as Mingi and the bystanders discouraged her from rising. Mingi spoke words of reassurance and proceeded through the GOLDCART line of questioning. Margaret, fully lucid now, explained that she had slipped on the stairs and fallen to the ground. She remembers reaching out a hand to break her fall, but everything went black when she hit her head on the pavement. She was not dizzy before she fell. Her wrist, head, right hip, and neck hurt. She was not contracting. The baby was not moving.

EMS personnel arrived within 8 min of the call and worked quickly to immobilize Margaret's spine with a backboard and cervical collar. They placed a wedge under her right hip to displace her pregnant abdomen from the midline. The crew applied a splint on Margaret's wrist and loaded her into the ambulance. Mingi slid onto the bench seat beside her. As the ambulance began to move, EMS personnel obtained intravenous access, infused IV fluids, and initiated cardiac monitoring. Mingi provided reassurance and monitored the fetal heart rate with her Doppler device. The scalp laceration was no longer bleeding. En route *Margaret was alert and oriented but distracted by significant pain in her head and wrist. She was also feeling nauseated.*

Upon arrival at the hospital, Margaret received morphine sulfate for pain management. She underwent 4 hr of continuous fetal monitoring and had an ultrasound evaluation of the fetus and placenta. The tracing was category I and the biophysical profile was 10 of 10; there was no sign of abruption. The Kleihauer-Betke test did not detect fetal red blood cells in her circulation, but because she was Rh negative, she received 300 mcg Rh immune globulin IM prophylactically.

The CT scan of Margaret's head showed no intracranial bleeding. She was diagnosed with acute mild traumatic brain injury (concussion), and her head laceration was repaired. Her wrist was splinted, and after discharge she began active range-of-motion exercises of the shoulder and fingers. Four weeks later her wrist splint was removed. Soon after, she gave birth to a healthy baby. It was at least 5 months before her wrist felt fully healed.

Trauma in Pregnancy

Many of us feel an overpowering urge to help when someone is injured. In the United States and other high-resource countries, life-threatening trauma and critical emergencies are fortunately rare among healthy people who give birth in community settings. Traumatic injury, however, can happen when we least expect it. A client can suffer a fall, or the midwife can happen upon a motor vehicle crash (MVC) or a victim of assault. A shooter in a mall or sporting event can injure dozens of people in a matter of seconds. Midwives can improve outcomes for pregnant victims of trauma by acting quickly, summoning help, and providing supportive care until they are stabilized or transferred to a higher level of care. When obstetrical providers volunteer in remote areas or assist pregnant people at disaster sites, a basic knowledge of trauma management can be lifesaving.

Traumatic injury occurs when tissues are exposed to energy levels beyond their tolerance (American Academy of Orthopedic Surgeons [AAOS], 2018). Trauma in pregnancy is both common and potentially deadly. In the United States, trauma complicates 1 in 12 pregnancies and is a leading nonobstetric cause of maternal death (Morris & Hueppchen, 2021). Most maternal traumatic injuries in pregnancy (Neuman & Promes, 2021) follow MVCs, (48%), falls (25%), and domestic violence (17%). Other mechanisms of trauma in pregnancy include penetrating trauma, toxic exposure, burns, drowning, and electrocution, as well as suicide and homicide (Kilpatrick, 2023).

Although severe maternal injuries are much more likely than nonsevere injuries to result in fetal death, minor injuries are more common and are responsible for 60–70% of trauma-related fetal deaths (Brown & Small, 2021; Murphy & Cullinan, 2020; Neuman & Promes, 2021). Lack of seatbelt use is a major risk factor for fetal morbidity and death. The mechanisms of injury most likely to lead to fetal death include MVCs, gunshot wounds, and falls (Brown & Small, 2021). Penetrating trauma carries an especially high risk of fetal death, up to 40% after stabbings and 71% after gunshot wounds (Brown & Small, 2021).

In the United States between 2000 and 2008, the number of active-shooter incidents averaged five per year (Jacobs, Warshaw, & Burns, 2016). Between 2009 and 2016, this number tripled, and the number shot and killed in such events increased by almost 150% (Jacobs et al., 2016). The incidence continues to climb. In 2023, mass shootings in the United States occurred at a record pace, averaging one per week—17 such incidents in 111 days (January to late April) with 88 deaths ("One Mass Killing Every 6.53 Days," 2023). About 31% of public mass shootings in the world occur in the United States (K. A. Fowler, Leavitt, Betz, Yuan, & Dahlberg, 2021).

Bombings are mostly likely to occur in densely populated areas during military or social conflict, but explosions can also result anytime from unintended events involving gas lines, fuel storage, and even grain elevators (Deitchman, Ashkenazi, & Falk, 2020). Blast incidents tend to affect large numbers of people who sustain many different types of injuries ranging from minor to catastrophic, potentially overwhelming the resources available at receiving hospitals. For example, the 2013 Boston Marathon bombing killed three people and injured 264.

In war zones, health facilities are often destroyed or inaccessible, raising the risk of maternal/child morbidity and death (Valand, Miles, & Pandya, 2020). Rape, often involving torture and multiple attackers, occurs in areas of conflict and in refugee camps. People can be emotionally traumatized by losing their homes or by witnessing the murder, rape, or injury of loved ones.

Pregnancy and Vulnerability to Trauma

Traumatic injury affects the pregnant, the nonpregnant, and the fetus differently. Anatomically and physiologically, pregnancy alters nearly every organ system in the body. Pregnancy-related changes can also affect the victim's response to trauma and to resuscitation (American College of Surgeons, Cmte. on Trauma [ACS], 2018). These modifications can mask and mimic signs and symptoms, increase the risk of accidents, and alter the pattern and severity of injury (D'Argent, Verelst, & Sabbe, 2020). For example, because the pregnant uterus can elevate the diaphragm as much as 4 cm at term, an injury to the chest can potentially damage intraabdominal organs (Narvaez & Vrees, 2021).

Higher blood volume, lower vascular resistance, and rising maternal heart rate increase maternal cardiac output by 40% by the end of the first trimester (Neuman & Promes, 2021). By the third trimester, uterine blood flow is as high as 600 ml/min (Kilpatrick, 2023). Cardiac output increases further during labor. With each contraction, vessels within the uterine muscle compress and return 300–500 ml of maternal blood to the circulating volume, like water from a squeezed sponge (Soma-Pillay, Catherine, Tolppanen, & Mebazaa, 2016). The vessels refill when the contraction subsides. The body's sympathetic response to pain and anxiety also increases cardiac output by raising blood pressure (BP) and heart rate. Immediately postpartum, cardiac output surges by 60–80% as the uterus shrinks and pushes blood into the systemic circulation (Soma-Pillay et al., 2016). Within the first hour postpartum, cardiac output returns to prelabor values.

These cardiovascular changes affect reactions to trauma. Injury to uterine or pelvic vessels can result in rapid exsanguination (Kilpatrick, 2023). Blood vessels in the pregnant uterus remain maximally dilated throughout pregnancy and have no mechanism for increasing perfusion to the fetus when maternal cardiac output is low. A drop in cardiac output can quickly result in decreased placental blood flow, and as a result the fetus can become severely compromised even when the mother's condition is stable. Beyond 20 weeks of gestation, simply lying supine can reduce cardiac output by as much as 30% (Kilpatrick, 2023).

Plasma volume increases by 50% before 32 weeks of gestation, but the total red-cell mass increases only by 20–30% (Narvaez & Vrees, 2021). This state of relative dilutional anemia can affect oxygen delivery to the tissues and change responses to acute blood loss. The pregnant trauma victim can lose 30–35% of circulating blood volume before showing signs of shock (Petrone & Marini, 2015).

During pregnancy, there is a 15% increase in the metabolic rate and a 20% increase in oxygen consumption associated with the fetus, placenta, and uterus (Soma-Pillay et al., 2016). A pregnant person has a reduced oxygen reserve and develops anoxia more quickly than others (Kilpatrick, 2023). The respiratory rate does not increase, but the pregnant person moves nearly 50% more air per breath (Weinberger, 2023). The pregnant individual is at greater risk for aspiration (because of lower esophageal tone) and is more difficult to intubate because of edema and friability of the airway (Sakamoto, Michels, Eisfelder, & Joshi, 2019).

Mechanism of Injury

The type and severity of trauma depend on the strength, direction, and nature of traumatic forces and what body parts they affect (AAOS, 2018). Each form of energy—mechanical, chemical, thermal, electrical, and barometric—is likely to produce certain characteristic types of injury. By considering the mechanism of injury, the provider can identify victims at risk of significant hemorrhage, disability, or death. For example, a person who falls three stories has a 50% likelihood of dying, and no one is likely to survive a free fall greater than five stories (Warner, Grabo, & Schwab, 2020). Additionally, certain mechanisms are associated with specific patterns of injury. A fall victim who lands on both feet from a height greater than 10–15 ft (3.0–4.6 m) can suffer calcaneal (heel), leg, pelvis, and spine fractures; injury to the thoracic aorta; or renal injuries (Warner et al., 2020).

Interpersonal Violence

Violence affects all cultures and socioeconomic groups. More than one in three women worldwide have experienced physical and/or sexual partner violence or sexual violence by a nonpartner (Wu, Chen, Fang, & Wan, 2020).

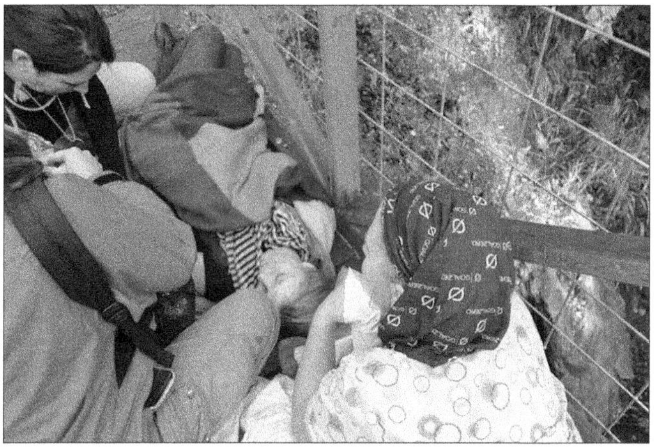

Figure 9-1. Midwives who volunteer to help at a disaster scene are often tasked with providing care to the nonpregnant. In this training exercise, midwives help a simulated shock victim who collapsed on a bridge.

Most commonly, the aggressor is the victim's intimate male partner (Ludermir, Lewis, Valongueiro, de Araújo, & Araya, 2010). Intimate partner violence (IPV) can involve physical or sexual assault, psychological abuse, progressive isolation, stalking, deprivation, intimidation, and reproductive coercion (Lévesque et al., 2021).

In the United States, some minorities are disproportionately affected by violent crime. The reported rate of IPV is highest in American Indian/Alaska Native women (Heck et al., 2021). Within this demographic, homicide is the third leading cause of death among women and girls between 10 and 24 years of age and the fifth leading cause of death among women between 25 and 34 (Joseph, 2021). On some U.S. reservations, indigenous women are murdered at a rate more than 10 times the national average, and many others go missing and are never found (Joseph, 2021). Although rates of intimate partner homicide among the nonpregnant are similar in white and black populations, pregnant black individuals are victims at more than three times the rate of pregnant white individuals and more than eight times higher than that of nonpregnant black females (Wallace, Gillispie-Bell, Cruz, Davis, & Vilda, 2021).

Intimate partner homicide is the leading nonobstetric cause of maternal death in the United States (Morrison et al., 2020; Narvaez & Vrees, 2021). Pregnant individuals are more likely to experience interpersonal violence than their nonpregnant counterparts and are also more likely to sustain lethal injuries from the attack (Wallace et al., 2021). Conflict with present or former partners is a factor in more than half of suicides by pregnant individuals (Morrison et al., 2020). IPV during pregnancy is associated with low birthweight, preterm labor (PTL) or preterm birth (PTB), poor weight gain, obstetric complications, pelvic fracture, placental abruption, fetal

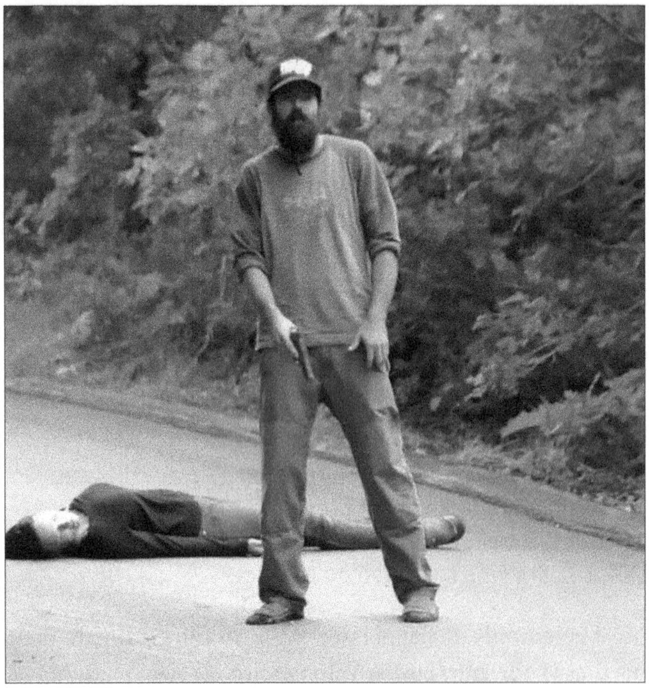

Figure 9-2. More than 38% of all murdered women are killed by an intimate partner (WHO, 2011). During pregnancy that number goes up to more than 45% (Palladino, Singh, Campbell, Flynn, & Gold., 2011). Photograph taken by the author during a crisis-response drill.

injury, sexually transmitted infections, pregnancy loss, delayed prenatal care, depression, and poor parenting (Román-Gálvez, Martín-Peláez, Martínez-Galiano, Khan, & Bueno-Cavanillas, 2021; World Health Organization [WHO], 2011).

Injuries resulting from IPV during pregnancy can include broken bones, cuts, burns, hemorrhages, broken teeth, stab wounds, gunshot wounds, and head injuries. Abusers attacking pregnant individuals often target the abdomen, buttocks, breasts, genitals, head, neck, and extremities. Posttraumatic stress disorder caused by abuse is commonly associated with depression, anxiety, and substance abuse (American College of Obstetricians & Gynecologists, 2012/2022). An abused pregnant client sometimes somatizes psychological distress and presents with vague complaints, headaches, sleep and appetite disturbances, palpitations, chronic pelvic pain, urinary frequency or urgency, irritable bowel syndrome, sexual dysfunction, abdominal symptoms, or recurrent vaginal infections (ACOG, 2012/2022).

Suspect intimate partner abuse when a client's injuries are inconsistent with the stated history or if a client frequently presents with injuries or health issues. Isolated injuries to the gravid abdomen should raise concern. Other red flags include the partner answering for the client and insisting on being present throughout the office visit, including trips to the restroom. If you suspect intimate partner violence, document your findings carefully and objectively and report any suspicion of abuse to the relevant authorities.

Falls

About 25–27% of pregnant people experience a fall during pregnancy (Hrvatin & Rugelj, 2021). Pregnancy-related risk factors include joint laxity, weight gain, low back pain, and an altered sense of balance. People are more likely to fall when negotiating slippery floors, stairways, cluttered areas, or uneven ground; when wearing inappropriate shoes, hurrying, or carrying additional loads; or when lighting is poor (Hrvatin & Rugelj, 2021). Greater joint laxity increases the risk of musculoskeletal injury, including pelvic fracture, from a fall (Narvaez & Vrees, 2021). Maternal pelvic fractures can lead to retroperitoneal hemorrhage and organ injury, as well as fetal skull fracture and penetrating brain injury with advancing gestation (Narvaez & Vrees, 2021).

Distance from the ground, position at impact, the landing surface, and the age and health of the victim influence the severity of injuries sustained in a fall. Whereas children usually fall head first, adults often land on their feet, buttocks, or outstretched hands. Other common fall-related injuries include wrist, foot, leg, pelvic, hip, and vertebral fractures.

Vehicular Accidents

MVCs are a leading cause of trauma-associated fetal deaths in the United States (Brown & Small, 2021). Fifty percent of pregnant individuals involved in an MVC sustain injuries, most of them minor (Amezcua-Prieto et al., 2020).

Newton's first law of motion states that an object in motion will remain in motion until acted on by another force. A vehicle in motion will remain in motion unless something—the brakes, a tree, another vehicle—causes it to stop. People in the vehicle will continue to move at their original speed until something—a seat belt, a seat, the steering wheel, the dashboard, or an airbag—causes them to stop. The organs within the body will move at their original speed until stopped by other parts of the body (AAOS, 2018). For example, the brain continues to move forward until it is stopped by the inside of the skull, causing compression injury to the front part of the brain and stretching of the back part (AAOS, 2018). The damage caused by organs striking the inside of the body can be severe while displaying few external signs.

Unbelted drivers tend to bounce around the vehicle's interior and sustain injury with each impact, especially in a rollover accident (AAOS, 2018). If forward motion is not stopped by the seat belt, airbag, or car interior, occupants often go through the windshield, sustaining injuries when their bodies strike the ground or other objects. The risk of fetal mortality is great when the mother is ejected from a motor vehicle or is struck by one (Hanahara, Hitosugi, & Tateoka, 2020).

An abrupt stop—as when a car strikes a tree—causes more injury than a slow stop—as when a car runs off the road into a sandlot. Side impacts (T-bone collisions) are especially dangerous because forces are transferred directly to the occupant. Debris along the path of the vehicle can indicate multiple collisions and different force vectors in play (AAOS, 2018). If two vehicles hit head on, the forces contributed by each vehicle add up; two vehicles traveling 97 kph/60 mph generate forces equivalent to one vehicle hitting a stationary object at twice that speed (AAOS, 2018).

The angle of impact, the kind of vehicle, and the person's position at the time of impact influence the severity and pattern of injuries. Because the person inside the car experiences the same forces that cause damage to the vehicle, the provider can gain insight into potential injuries by considering where the vehicle is deformed, inside and out. A cracked windshield, bent steering wheel, or crushed dashboard indicate the potential for spinal injury. If the steering wheel is bent beneath the airbag, chest and abdominal injuries are probable. Significant injury is likely when another vehicle intrudes into the passenger compartment. Whiplash injuries can occur if the vehicle is struck from behind.

Traumatic contact with the steering wheel, a mechanism of severe injury in both front and rear collisions, can be prevented by proper use of a seatbelt (Hanahara et al., 2020). Use of a properly adjusted 3-point seatbelt restraint system dissipates deceleration forces, reducing MVC fatalities 65–70% and decreasing serious injury 10-fold (ACS, 2018). The shoulder restraint should cross the collar bone and lay between the breasts and the lap belt should cross the hips under the abdomen. A belt worn incorrectly across the upper abdomen can transmit enough direct force to the uterus to rupture it. With a lap belt only, on impact a pregnant person can flex forward and compress the uterus, increasing the risk for uterine rupture or abruption (ACS, 2018).

Seat belts reduce the risk of serious injury for everyone in the vehicle, pregnant or not. An unrestrained passenger is not only in danger, but likely to become a large projectile that can smash into other occupants at high speed. For occupants ejected from a vehicle, the likelihood of serious injury increases by more than 300% (ACS, 2018). Airbags reduce deaths by about 30% in direct frontal MVCs but are designed to be used with seatbelts for maximum benefit (Wallis & Greaves, 2002).

Vehicle v. Pedestrian

When an adult pedestrian is struck by a vehicle, the impact usually throws the body onto the hood of the car, causing injuries to the head, pelvis, and chest. A child is more likely to be knocked to the ground and run over. Anyone pinned under a tire or wreckage is likely to experience severe hypovolemic shock when the weight is removed.

Blunt and Penetrating Trauma

Blunt trauma involves injury from forceful impact with a dull object, for example a fist, a bat, or contact with the ground. Skin can appear almost undamaged despite serious internal injury. Vehicular accidents are the most common cause of blunt abdominal trauma in pregnancy (Brown & Small, 2021). Blunt abdominal trauma can result in hemorrhage and hypovolemia due to placental abruption or severe maternal splenic, hepatic, and retroperitoneal injuries (Brown & Small, 2021).

Penetrating trauma (for example a stabbing or cutting injury, dog bite, or bullet wound) involves a sharp object or projectile breaking the skin, causing both an external wound and internal damage. Gunshot wound severity depends on the type of gun used, range, and whether there is an exit wound. In stab wounds, the duller the weapon, the more force it takes to penetrate. A longer, thicker blade can do more damage than a short, narrow blade.

Obstetric Complications of Trauma

Trauma can cause any number of obstetric complications, including previable pregnancy loss, PTL and PTB, rupture of membranes, uterine rupture, fetal injury, and fetal demise (Morris & Hueppchen, 2021). Any decrease in maternal systolic blood pressure (SBP) can decrease blood flow to the uterus and decrease fetal oxygenation (Kilpatrick, 2023). Placental abruption or tearing often occurs with multisystem trauma or severe abdominal injury, but it can also occur after minor injuries (Warner et al., 2020). Fetomaternal hemorrhage—fetal blood loss into the maternal circulation—occurs in up to 30% of cases of maternal traumatic injury (Kilpatrick, 2023). The fetus can sustain skull fractures and intracerebral hemorrhage from maternal pelvic trauma or direct injuries from a penetrating wound.

Traumatic injury in pregnancy is classified as major or minor. A minor injury is one that does not involve rapid compression, deceleration, shearing forces, or direct injury to the abdomen and does not cause maternal pain, bleeding, or contractions. The likelihood of adverse fetal outcome, however, is unpredictable and does not necessarily correlate with the degree of trauma (D'Argent et al., 2020). Severe trauma carries a higher risk of fetal loss, but most fetal deaths (60–70%) follow minor trauma, which is more prevalent (D'Argent et al., 2020). The presence of contractions, vaginal bleeding, and abdominal

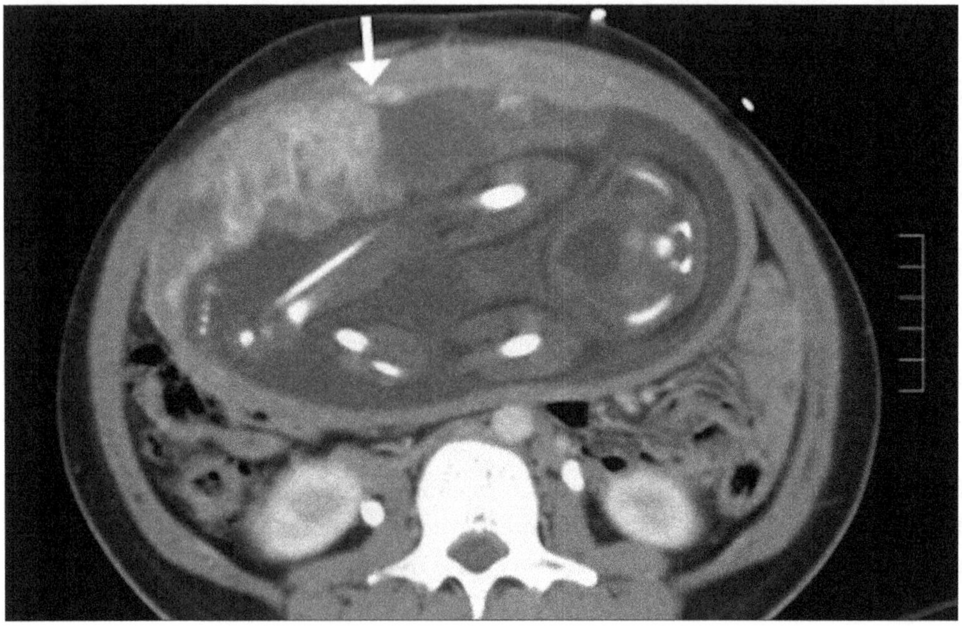

Figure 9-3. Computerized tomography (CT) scan of a trauma victim at 29 weeks gestational age shows a large placental abruption. The white arrow marks the border between perfused and nonperfused regions of the placenta; the darker half is not functional. From "CT Evaluation of Placental Abruption in Pregnant Trauma Patients," by S. H. Wei, M. Helmy, and A. J. Cohen, 2009, *Emergency Radiology, 16*(5), p. 371. Copyright by authors.

pain after the incident indicates a higher likelihood of preterm labor or abruption.

Placental Abruption

Placental abruption complicates 1–2% of cases of minor maternal trauma and up to 40% of severe maternal abdominal trauma (Brown & Small, 2021). Abruption occurs when maternal vessels that supply the placenta rupture, allowing blood to pool in the decidua (Schmidt, Skelly, & Raines, 2022). This collection of blood acts as an expanding wedge that forces the decidual-placental interface to separate (Page, Roloff, Modi, Dong, & Neeki, 2020). The disconnected part of the placenta is unavailable for gas exchange and other critical functions, putting the fetus at increasing risk as the defect expands. If more than half of the placenta is affected, the fetus usually dies (Page et al., 2020), and the mother is at high risk of shock and disseminated intravascular coagulation (DIC). Blunt abdominal trauma can cause direct injury to the uterus and placenta and lead to abruption, especially when the placenta is anterior, fundal, or lateral (Acar & Meric, 2017). Shearing forces created at the interface of placenta and uterine wall can also separate the placenta from its attachment even in the absence of blunt trauma (Brown & Small, 2021). When a mother is in a high-speed vehicular collision, the uterus continues to travel forward until it is stopped by an immovable object such as the steering wheel or seat belt, which then directs forces backward (Cunningham et al., 2022, ch. 50). The flexible uterine muscle can change shape when subjected to these forces of acceleration and deceleration, but the inelastic placenta cannot. Shearing forces are created which can cause placental abruption or tearing. A fetomaternal hemorrhage can occur if fetal blood is forced into placental bed venules and enters the maternal circulation (Cunningham et al., 2022, ch. 50). Even a minor MVC without significant maternal injury can cause abruption due to shearing acceleration-deceleration forces (Brown & Small, 2021).

Traumatic abruption is the most common cause of fetal death due to trauma and carries a 50–80% risk of fetal mortality (Brown & Small, 2021). In an MVC, the correct use of seatbelts greatly reduces the risk of abruption (Acar & Meric, 2017). Abruption can develop immediately after abdominal trauma occurs or hours after the impact (Brown & Small, 2021).

Signs of placental abruption include abdominal pain, vaginal bleeding, leakage of amniotic fluid, back pain, uterine tenderness, uterine rigidity, abnormal fetal heart rate (FHR), regular uterine contractions, intensity of contractions greater than expected for stage of labor, increasing fundal height, or maternal shock (D'Argent et al., 2020). The amount of vaginal bleeding does not indicate the severity of abruption; the uterine cavity can accommodate the entire blood volume of the placenta without any external evidence (D'Argent et al., 2020). The fetal heart tracing may be reassuring until 30% of the placenta is separated from the uterus (D'Argent et al., 2020). Abruption of more than 50% usually causes fetal death (D'Argent et al., 2020). Tachysystole, typically in a low-amplitude, high-frequency pattern, is strongly associated with abruption (Ananth & Kinzler, 2022).

Abruptions can be difficult to diagnose. They can be asymptomatic, produce classic or atypical signs, or cause catastrophic deterioration. Abruption is primarily a clinical diagnosis, but findings from imaging, laboratory, and postpartum pathologic studies can support the clinical impression (Kilpatrick, 2023). Laboratory assessments can be unremarkable despite significant pathology, however. Ultrasound imaging yields false negative results in about half of cases, though positive results are highly reliable indicators of abruption (Ananth & Kinzler, 2022).

Fetomaternal Hemorrhage

Fetomaternal hemorrhage (FMH) is the entry of significant amounts of fetal blood into the maternal circulation. Significant FMH is rare, occurring in about 1 in 1,000 to 1 in 5,000 births, but can result in tragic outcomes such as severe anemia, hypoxia, anoxia, or exsanguination of the fetus (D'Argent et al., 2020). FMH is much more common in trauma victims and can affect 10–30% of cases of significant maternal trauma (D'Argent et al., 2020), especially when there is an anterior placenta (Kilpatrick, 2023). Although uterine tenderness, contractions, vaginal bleeding, or an abnormal fetal heart tracing can be present, some FMH occurs with subtle or absent clinical signs (Moise, 2022).

When FMH occurs between an Rh-positive fetus and an Rh-negative mother, the maternal immune response becomes activated, and formation of RhD antibodies can occur (isoimmunization). Because these maternal antibodies easily cross the placenta and enter the fetus, they can attack the red blood cells (RBCs) of any Rh-positive fetus, potentially causing fetal hemolysis, anemia, hydrops, and death. As little as 0.01 ml of Rh-positive fetal blood can cause maternal isoimmunization (Neuman & Promes, 2021).

RhD immune globulin (RhIg) is administered to Rh-negative mother within 72 hr of any incidence of vaginal bleeding or suspected/potential abruption to block the maternal immune response to fetal hemoglobin. A standard 300 mcg dose of RhIg is given to treat an exchange of up to 30 ml of fetal whole blood or 15 ml of fetal RBCs as estimated by the Kleihauer-Betke (KB) test (Narvaez & Vrees, 2021). If a larger amount of blood is exchanged, multiple doses may be required. The KB test or flow cytometry can be used to quantify the amount of fetal hemoglobin in the maternal circulation to determine the dose of RhIg. It is not necessary to perform a KB test in Rh positive clients—in this situation antibodies will not form against fetal blood, and life-threatening fetal blood loss will reveal itself with an abnormal fetal heart tracing (Narvaez & Vrees, 2021).

Traumatic Uterine Rupture

Traumatic uterine rupture is a rare but devastating injury occurring in less than 1% of trauma cases, usually as a result of direct high-energy abdominal impact (D'Argent et al., 2020). During the first trimester, the thick-walled uterus is well protected within the bony pelvis. Toward the end of pregnancy, the uterus becomes larger and thinner-walled, characteristics that make it increasingly vulnerable to blunt trauma, penetration,

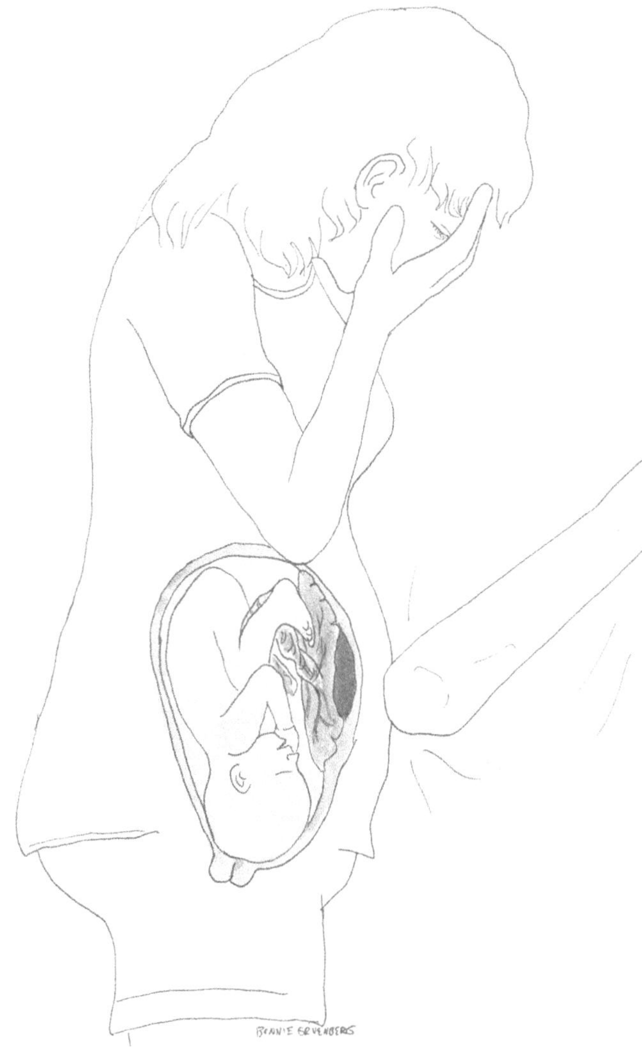

Figure 9-4. An anterior placenta is more vulnerable to abruption caused by blunt trauma.

or rupture. Maternal consequences of traumatic uterine rupture include severe hemorrhage, bladder laceration, hysterectomy, and death. Perinatal consequences include serious morbidity or mortality from prolonged intrauterine hypoxia (J. F. Smith & Wax, 2022).

Traumatic rupture of an unscarred uterus most commonly follows direct high-energy blunt or penetrating injury to the abdomen or pelvis such as that seen with assault, pelvic fracture, or a fall from a height onto the perineum (D'Argent et al., 2020). The well-perfused uterus bleeds copiously when injured and can be a major source of blood loss in trauma. Clinical signs of uterine rupture include maternal shock, uterine tenderness, guarding, rigidity, vaginal bleeding, peritonitis, irregular uterine contours, discrepancy between uterine size and gestational age, abnormal fetal heart pattern, and fetal death (D'Argent et al., 2020). If the fetus is expelled into the abdominal cavity after uterine rupture, it might be easily palpable through the abdominal wall, usually in oblique or transverse lie (ACS, 2018). The presenting part may be out of the pelvis on vaginal examination. The uterine fundus may be nonpalpable if there is fundal rupture. Emergency cesarean section is undertaken when uterine rupture is suspected; hysterectomy is often necessary to save the mother if the uterus is badly damaged (J. F. Smith & Wax, 2022).

Table 9-1
Sample GOLDCART History for Trauma

Always act quickly and treat life-threatening issues before taking a detailed history.
General situation and history—What happened? How many weeks pregnant are you? Do you have any health issues or pregnancy complications? Is the baby moving? How old are you? How many pregnancies and births have you had?
Onset—What were you doing when you had your accident? Were you dizzy before you fell? Did someone hurt you?
Location—Where is your pain? Does it start in one place and radiate to somewhere else? Where? What did you hit when you fell? Did you hit your head?
Duration—When did this happen? What have you been doing since then? How have your symptoms changed? Were you unconscious? Do you know how long?
Characteristics—Is the pain stabbing, shooting, or dull? Is there weakness in any of your limbs? Is the abnormal sensation tingly, prickly, itchy, or numb?
Associated symptoms—Any other pain, weakness, headache, sweating, visual changes, numbness, shortness of breath, nausea, vomiting, fever, diarrhea, dizziness, or fainting? Are you leaking fluid or having vaginal bleeding? Are you having contractions?
Relieving/aggravating factors—What makes it better or worse? Did your symptoms improve when you changed position?
Treatment—What have you done to manage your problem since your accident? Has it helped?

Fetal Injury

The fetus is protected from direct fetal injury by layers of tissue—abdominal wall, uterine myometrium, placenta, and amniotic fluid—that serve as buffers in most traumatic incidents. Most traumatic fetal deaths occur secondary to placental abruption or maternal shock and death (ACS, 2018). Rarely, however, blunt, or penetrating trauma can cause direct injury to the fetus, resulting in fetal spleen rupture, fracture of the fetal skull, fetal intracranial hemorrhage, and cerebral edema (Brown & Small, 2021). A displaced maternal pelvic fracture in late pregnancy can cause fetal skull fractures or brain injury (Kilpatrick, 2023). The fetus can occasionally suffer direct trauma when the abdominal wall strikes an object such as the dashboard or steering wheel (ACS, 2018). Most cases of fetal injury due to penetrating trauma (stab wound, gunshot) are fatal to the fetus, whereas the fetus injured by blunt maternal trauma has a better chance of survival (Hajduk, Nakamura, Ryan, & Puri, 2021).

Preterm Birth (PTB)

Preterm prelabor rupture of the amniotic membranes (PPROM), preterm contractions, and PTL commonly follow major trauma (Kilpatrick, 2023). Sometimes, planned PTB, usually by cesarean section, is undertaken to benefit survival of mother and infant (Kilpatrick, 2023). If the mother is stable, fetal death is not an indication for cesarean birth (Kilpatrick, 2023).

The Pregnant Victim of Trauma

The focus of trauma care in pregnancy is to provide optimal treatment of the mother, which in turn gives the fetus the best chance for survival (ACS, 2018). Initial treatment priorities remain the same regardless of whether the client is pregnant. The midwife's role is to call for help, address life-threatening issues as appropriate, and transfer to a higher level of care. Pregnant victims of significant trauma require treatment at a regional trauma center with obstetric services (MacArthur, Foley, Gray, & Sisley, 2019), but initial stabilization at a local hospital may be necessary. To gain competency in managing trauma, consider becoming certified in Prehospital Trauma Life Support® (PHTLS), Advanced Trauma Life Support® (ATLS), or the equivalent.

Priorities in Initial Trauma Care

A systematic approach to trauma assessment improves outcomes, but methods differ. WHO, the International Committee of the Red Cross [ICRC], and the ATLS program advocate the ABCDE approach to assessment (**A**irway, **B**reathing, **C**irculation, **D**isability, **E**xposure). This method considers airway management the first priority (WHO & ICRC, 2018). Other authorities (Ferrada et al., 2018; Petrosoniak & Hicks, 2018) maintain that the goal in trauma care is to maintain perfusion and that massive hemorrhage must be controlled immediately, giving the **C** of circulation priority over airway and breathing (**CAB**). The **CAB** model maintains that if blood is not circulating, gas exchange cannot occur within the body's tissues, even if the lungs are pumped with air. Prehospital Trauma Life Support now recommends using **XABCDE**, which gives **X** (*eXsanguinating hemorrhage*) priority in management (National Assn. of Emergency Medical Technicians [NAEMT] & ACS, 2020). Further research is necessary to clarify which approach yields better outcomes. Because ATLS® has set the standard for international trauma care since 1978, this book follows its guidelines.

The concept of a "golden hour" following injury that chiefly determines a critically injured client's likelihood of survival is attributed to a 1975 article by R. Adams Cowley, founder of Baltimore's renowned Shock Trauma Institute. He wrote the article in support of a shock trauma center at the University of Maryland with helicopter service that could fly any trauma victim in the state to Baltimore within a "golden hour" (Rogers, Rittenhouse, & Gross, 2015). In truth, although rapid intervention can improve outcome in some critical cases, the relationship between timing and mortality appears complex, and no field-based study has shown a significant association between response interval and survival (Raja & Zane, 2023). Most deaths from trauma occur either at the scene or within the first 4 hr of care at a trauma center (Raja & Zane, 2023). If the victim is alive after 24 hr, survival is likely (Raja & Zane, 2023).

Primary Survey

First, assess the scene for potential threats or hazards, for example downed power lines, an active shooter, or a snarling dog. Assure your own safety before helping anyone else (Klein & Tadi, 2023). *Do not attempt to help a victim if the scene is not safe.*

Activate emergency medical services (EMS) and stay on the telephone or radio to provide information to the dispatcher. In an accident, mass casually incident, or other event that obstructs access, such as a flood or riot, the dispatcher will use your report to determine the number and kind(s) of emergency service to send (medical, fire, police). When an ambulance arrives, provide a concise report in SBAR (**S**ituation, **B**ackground, **A**ssessment, and **R**ecommendation) format (see "The SBAR Tool" in Chapter 4).

Assess an unstable trauma victim quickly and efficiently by performing a rapid primary survey with simultaneous correction of critical issues, then a more thorough secondary survey and transport to provide definitive care. The ABCDEF approach allows the clinician to quickly identify and address any life-threatening conditions. See Chapter 4 for a full discussion on the steps of assessment. A client beyond 20 weeks of gestation without suspicion of spinal injury should be placed on the left side (Krywko, Toy, Mahan, & Kiel, 2022). Do not move the victim when there is any possibility of spinal injury. If injuries necessitate supine positioning, tilt the victim 15° to the left by placing a wedge under the right hip or under the right side of the spine board to avoid compression of the vena cava and aorta (Galvagno, Nahmias, & Young, 2019).

ABCs with POP

Airway (with c-spine stabilization if necessary)

Breathing

Circulation (with attention to bleeding)

Disability (level of consciousness)

Exposure (to identify other issues)

Fetal status

with

Placenta

Optimally

Perfused

Maintain warmth by covering the client with warm blankets as appropriate. Trauma victims with even mild hypothermia are more likely to die (AAOS, 2018). The lethal triad of trauma is a vicious cycle of three interlinked factors—hypothermia, coagulopathy, and acidosis—that decrease survival in trauma (van Veelen & Brodmann Maeder, 2021). Because the coagulation mechanism functions within a narrow range of temperature and pH, a hypothermic trauma victim develops abnormal platelet function, inhibition of clotting, and inappropriate clot dissolution. Increased bleeding leads to shock. The poor perfusion of shock decreases oxygen delivery to the tissues, which triggers anaerobic metabolism, lactate production, and metabolic acidosis. Anaerobic metabolism reduces heat production and worsens hypothermia (Chatrath, Khetarpal, & Ahuja, 2015). Acidosis decreases cardiac contractility. Without intervention, the process continues in a downward spiral until the victim dies.

Secondary Survey

The secondary survey is a head-to-toe assessment of the trauma victim, including a GOLDCART history, evaluation of mechanism of injury, physical examination, and reassessment of vital signs. If the victim cannot provide the information, ask witnesses and bystanders. Begin the secondary survey after the primary survey is completed, resuscitative efforts have been started, and the victim's vital functions have begun to improve (ACS, 2018). If there is more than one rescuer, one can perform the secondary survey while other team members manage the primary survey and begin resuscitation (ACS, 2018). If

Trauma Tactics

- Act quickly.
- Treat the greatest threat to life first.
- Apply indicated treatment even if you do not know the diagnosis.
- Evaluate the victim *without* taking a detailed history.

Adapted from *Advanced Trauma Life Support® Student Course Manual* (10th ed., p. xxxvi), by American College of Surgeons Committee on Trauma, 2018, Chicago, IL: American College of Surgeons. Copyright by publisher.

the victim's condition worsens during the secondary survey, go back and reassess the primary survey.

Physical Examination

Physical examination of a trauma victim involves visualizing and palpating as much of the body as is accessible or is appropriate given the mechanism of injury. Begin at the head and systematically examine the entire body, including the spine and neck, chest, abdomen and pelvis, limbs, and neurological function. Protect the spinal cord from unnecessary movement until a spinal injury is excluded (NAEMT & ACS, 2020).

Head: Evaluate for lacerations, punctures, bruising, evidence of fractures, and neurologic injuries. Evaluate eyes for injury and assess pupil size, equality, and reactiveness. Evaluate the bony structures of the face, look inside the mouth, and consider potential risks to the airway such as swelling or loose teeth.

Cervical Spine and Neck: Evaluate for cervical spine tenderness, subcutaneous emphysema, punctures, lacerations, or bruising.

Chest: Evaluate for lacerations, punctures, bruising, and evidence of fractures on the thorax. A client with a significant chest injury may have pain, difficulty breathing, or hypoxia. Auscultate the lungs, assessing for symmetrical breath sounds and adequate air movement. Auscultate the heart and look for signs of cardiac issues such as scars from open heart surgery or a pacemaker.

Abdomen and Pelvis: Evaluate for lacerations, punctures, and bruising. Intraabdominal bleeding can enlarge the abdomen over time. Pain on palpation of the pelvic ring and deep bruising over the iliac crests, pubis, or labia can indicate pelvic fracture.

Extremities: Evaluate for lacerations, punctures, bruising, fractures and abnormal motor and sensory function.

Buttocks, perineum, genitalia: Evaluate for bruising or lacerations. Assess for vaginal bleeding, leaking, and hematoma. If the client is contracting and appears to be in labor, perform a digital examination for cervical dilation. If a pregnant client has vaginal bleeding, do not perform a vaginal examination until placenta previa has been ruled out.

Neurological System: Evaluate for paralysis, weakness, and loss of sensation, which would suggest significant injury to the spinal column or peripheral nervous system.

Intravenous (IV) Fluids

When managing a trauma victim, support intravascular volume by inserting two large-bore peripheral venous catheters or by intraosseous infusion. Bolus 1–3 L of an isotonic solution to increase intravascular volume and support circulation. Additionally, tranexamic acid (TXA) administered promptly can improve survival for hemorrhaging clients (Almuwallad, Cole, Ross, Perkins, & Davenport, 2021). When possible, warm IV solutions to body temperature to decrease the risk of hypothermia. IV fluids supply intravascular volume, but do not contain essential blood components such as oxygen-carrying red cells or clotting factors. If the victim has lost a significant amount of blood, transfusion of blood products is often required to support circulation. Aggressively infusing crystalloid solutions while the victim is actively bleeding can dilute the blood and increase the risk of coagulopathy. Trauma victims receiving more than 3 L of crystalloids are more likely to die (ACS, 2018). When a victim of trauma is hemorrhaging, expedite transport to a trauma center for definitive care.

Forensic Evidence

If you suspect that the injury is the result of a criminal act, be mindful of preserving the evidence as you attend to the victim's needs (Ozsaker, Kaya, Alcan, van Giersbergen, & Aktas, 2020). Disturb the scene as little as possible. If you disrobe the victim to expose an injury, save the victim's clothing for law enforcement personnel. In cases of sexual violence, do not undress or touch the victim unless it is medically necessary. To preserve evidence, the victim should refrain from washing, changing clothes, urinating, defecating, smoking, drinking, eating, grooming hair, brushing teeth, or rinsing the mouth until a medical forensic specialist can conduct an examination.

Reassess

Reevaluate the victim repeatedly for new signs and symptoms or changes in condition. Frequently assess and document findings and vital signs.

Transport

A team of EMS professionals is well equipped to immobilize and stabilize a trauma victim. If spinal trauma is suspected, encourage the client to remain still until EMS immobilizes the spine with a rigid cervical collar and backboard, as indicated. In the United States, an emergency medical technician (EMT) is trained in life support to the basic or intermediate level. A paramedic (U.S.) or equivalent is certified in advanced life support and uses many of the same lifesaving medications, devices, and procedures as the emergency-room physician. EMTs and paramedics may be certified in Prehospital Trauma Life Support (PHTLS). Pregnant clients with major injuries or a significant mechanism of injury should be transported to a facility that can provide comprehensive trauma and obstetrical care even if the client appears stable (ACS, 2018).

Definitive Care for Trauma in Pregnancy

Major trauma in pregnancy is optimally managed by a multidisciplinary team of experts at a regional trauma center. The primary goals are to evaluate and stabilize maternal injuries, ventilate the lungs, arrest hemorrhage, and treat hypovolemia. Maternal oxygen saturation (SaO_2) should be maintained at 95% or higher with the use of supplemental oxygen as necessary (Kilpatrick, 2023). Initial assessment can include portable x-rays at the bedside (MacArthur et al., 2019). Focused assessment with sonography for trauma (FAST) and diagnostic peritoneal lavage can be used to detect intraabdominal blood suggesting a surgical emergency in the unstable victim (MacArthur et al., 2019). The stable victim of trauma may require computerized tomography (CT) scans or detailed x-rays (MacArthur et al., 2019). All trauma victims should be frequently reevaluated to identify signs of deterioration. If immediate surgery is not necessary, the client is frequently admitted to the hospital for stabilization or observation. Treatment should be directed toward maintaining hemodynamic stability and addressing specific injuries. Clients with minor injuries may be discharged shortly after evaluation (MacArthur et al., 2019).

Fetal Heart Monitoring

Mothers beyond the age of fetal viability who have experienced abdominal trauma should have continuous fetal and uterine monitoring with an external FHR monitor and tocodynamometer for at least 4 hr (Kilpatrick, 2023). If gestational age is unknown, if the fundus is at or above the level of the umbilicus, initiate monitoring until specific gestational age information is obtained (Greco, Day, & Pearlman, 2019). In the first 4 hr of tocodynamic monitoring after trauma, 4 contractions in an hour should raise suspicion, and more than 8 contractions suggest abruption (D'Argent et al., 2020). Although abruption can occur up to 6 days after trauma, the risk of a delayed abruption is very low (Kilpatrick, 2023). Continuous monitoring may be discontinued after 4 hr if the following criteria are met (Kilpatrick, 2023):

- Uterine contractions fewer than 6/hr
- Absence of vaginal bleeding
- Absence of abdominal/uterine pain
- Category I FHR tracing
- Maternal vital signs normal

Clients with the following findings should be continuously monitored for at least 24 hr (Kilpatrick, 2023):

- Abdominal bruising or other obvious abdominal injury
- Regular contractions (1 or more in 10 min or 6/hr)
- Vaginal bleeding
- Abnormal FHR tracing
- Abdominal/uterine pain
- Coagulopathy, e.g., low platelets or low fibrinogen (less than 200 mg/dl)

Ultrasound Imaging

Ultrasound is used to determine fetal age, position, and amniotic fluid volume. When there is a possibility of direct fetal injury, a fetal anatomic survey is indicated. A biophysical profile is often used to evaluate the fetus for signs of compromise at any gestational age when birth is likely to benefit the fetus (Kilpatrick, 2023). Placental abruption, however, is frequently undetectable on ultrasound and yields false-negative rates of about 50% (Neuman & Promes, 2021).

Shock

Shock is a condition of cellular and tissue hypoxia (Gaieski & Mikkelsen, 2023a). Without oxygen, people die quickly. The average nonpregnant person carries enough fat stores to sustain life for 30 days and enough glucose for one day, but only enough oxygen reserves to survive for 5 min (NAEMT & ACS, 2020). If oxygen supply to the tissues stops, organ damage begins within minutes. If not corrected, it will decline to end-organ damage, failure of multiple organ systems, and death.

In pregnancy, blood volume expands by 1,500–1,600 ml, plasma volume by 1,200–1,300 ml, and RBCs by 300–400 ml (Antony, Racusin, Aagard, & Dildy, 2021). This increase in blood volume allows most individuals to remain hemodynamically stable despite large blood loss. In a healthy pregnant client, clinical signs of shock—SBP below 80 mm Hg, tachycardia, tachypnea, and altered level of consciousness—may not be evident until blood loss is 1,500 ml or more (Royal College of Obstetricians & Gynaecologists, 2016). In all cases of shock, early recognition, prompt treatment, and correcting the underlying problem are essential to good outcomes.

Signs of shock

- Tachycardia
- Bradycardia in neurogenic shock
- Hypotension
- Cool extremities (neurogenic shock can present with warm extremities)
- Weak peripheral pulses
- Prolonged capillary refill (>2 sec)
- Narrowing of the pulse pressure (<20 mm Hg)
- Increase in respiratory rate
- Change in skin color (e.g., pale, cyanotic)
- Altered mental status not due to head injury (from agitation to coma)

From "Approach to Shock in the Adult Trauma Patient," by C. Colwell, 2023, in M. Ganetsky (Ed.), *UpToDate*. Copyright by UpToDate.

Pathophysiology of Shock

To reach the tissues of the body, oxygen must first bind to the hemoglobin in RBCs (NAEMT & ACS, 2020). The delivery of oxygen to the tissues involves four life-sustaining mechanisms (R. Fowler, Pepe, Stevens, Ramirez, & Mell, 2018):

- Adequate air exchange in the lungs to allow oxygenation of the blood.
- Intact system of blood vessels to carry oxygenated blood to the tissues.
- Adequate heart function to drive circulation.
- Adequate volume of RBCs and plasma within the blood vessels.

Shock involves a progressive decline through three phases: compensated shock, decompensated shock, and irreversible shock (Gaieski & Mikkelsen, 2023a). The early stages of shock begin when acute injury or infection causes reduction in circulating blood volume, ineffective heart function, greatly increased peripheral vasodilation, or a combination of these (Collins, 2000). Because perfusion is impaired, the cells of the body become hypoxic and ion pumps within the cell membranes begin to fail (Gaieski & Mikkelsen, 2023a). This dysfunction leads to edema within cells. Deprived of oxygen, cells must generate energy with anaerobic metabolism, which is inefficient and produces harmful byproducts such as lactic acid. Changes in the microcirculation decrease regional blood flow and lead to tissue injury. Systemically, these changes can lead to acidosis, endothelial dysfunction, and widespread inflammation. Reduced cardiac output and decreased BP reduce perfusion of the vital organs, and they begin to malfunction in a downward spiral that can lead to death.

Tissue perfusion throughout the body depends on systemic vascular resistance (SVR) and adequate cardiac output.

- SVR, the amount of resistance the heart must push against, is determined by vessel diameter, vessel length, and blood viscosity.
- Cardiac output, the amount of blood the heart can pump, is determined by heart rate and stroke volume.
- Stroke volume (the amount of blood pumped per beat) is determined by preload (the stretch of a filled left ventricle before the heart contracts), amount of blood, heart contractility, and afterload (impedance to blood flow).

Compensated Shock (Preshock)

When the body detects low circulating blood volume and poor perfusion, it activates compensatory mechanisms to maintain perfusion to the brain and vital organs (Gaieski & Mikkelsen, 2023a). The signs and symptoms of compensated shock are as follows (R. Fowler et al., 2018; Gaieski & Mikkelsen, 2023b):

Mental status changes: Usually due to poor perfusion of the brain, shock-related mental status changes usually begin as agitation and decline to confusion, delirium, or coma.

Rapid heart rate: Tachycardia makes the most of inadequate oxygen delivery to the tissues by moving blood through the circuit faster. Tachycardia follows activation of the sympathetic nervous system, which causes the release of catecholamines (e.g., epinephrine, norepinephrine) from the adrenal glands

Narrowed pulse pressure: Pulse pressure is systolic blood pressure (SBP) minus diastolic blood pressure (DBP). A narrowed pulse pressure (less than 20 mm Hg difference between the systolic and diastolic pressures, for example, 100/85) can indicate that catecholamine release is causing vessels in the extremities to constrict, redirecting blood flow to the vital organs and increasing the DBP.

Pale, cool skin: Caused by peripheral vasoconstriction or by loss of circulating RBCs.

Warm, red skin: Can be present in early distributive shock because of peripheral vasodilation (see below).

Higher respiratory rate: When perfusion is poor, tachypnea increases the amount of oxygen available to the body and helps to compensate for metabolic acidosis.

Increasing heart rate and tachypnea in a pregnant client with stable systolic blood pressure (SBP) are signs of compensated shock until proven otherwise, even if bleeding is not apparent.

Sweating: Diaphoresis is caused by the effects of catecholamines on sweat glands.

Lower urinary output: Oliguria in shock can be due to shunting of renal blood flow to other vital organs, direct injury to the kidney, or intravascular volume depletion.

Thirst: Can be triggered by hypovolemia.

Hypotension: May be due to poor cardiac output.

Decompensated Shock (Shock)

Decompensated or uncompensated shock occurs when compensatory mechanisms are exhausted and the client shows signs of cellular hypoxia (Gaieski & Mikkelsen, 2023a). The body is no longer able to perfuse all of its tissues (AAOS, 2018). Cells in nonperfused tissues become starved for oxygen, leading to anaerobic metabolism (AAOS, 2018). Signs and symptoms of decompensated shock include tachycardia, dyspnea, diaphoresis, hypotension, low urine output, and cool, clammy skin. Extremities can become cool, cyanotic, mottled, or pulseless. Confusion, restlessness, and agitation are signs of imminent circulatory collapse in cardiogenic or hypovolemic shock (Bonanno, 2011).

End-Organ Dysfunction

End-organ dysfunction occurs when the heart, liver, kidneys, brain, and other vital organs are damaged, malfunction, or die. The victim stops producing urine, acidemia reduces the cardiac output and deranges cellular metabolism, and level of consciousness changes from alert restlessness to confusion, then coma. The client with end-organ dysfunction requires aggressive medical intervention to avoid death and can sustain permanent organ damage.

Classifications of Shock

There are four recognized classifications of shock (Gaieski & Mikkelsen, 2023a):

- *Distributive*: Involves vasodilation and abnormal distribution of blood flow leading to inadequate blood supply to tissues and organs. Some examples of distributive shock are septic shock, neurogenic shock, anaphylactic shock, and toxic shock.
- *Cardiogenic*: Involves cardiac dysfunction leading to inadequate tissue perfusion. Some examples of cardiogenic shock are myocardial infarction, atrial and ventricular arrhythmias, and valve or ventricle septal rupture.

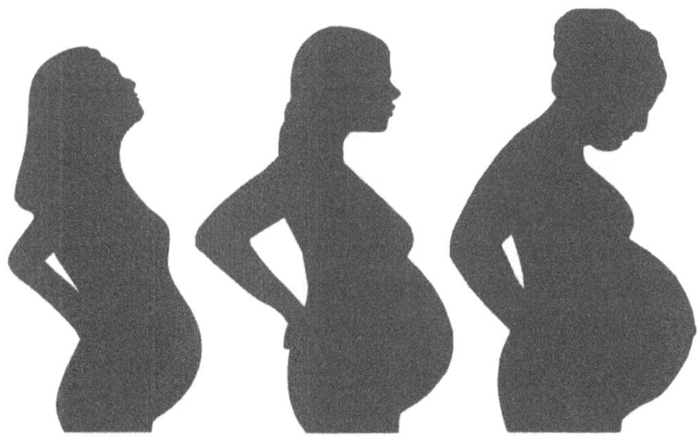

Figure 9-5. Relationship between estimated blood loss and blood volume in pregnant individuals of different weights. A small, slender mother has considerably less blood than a taller, heavier one, and a given loss is a higher percentage of total volume. Adapted from "Prevention and Treatment of Haemorrhage," by S. Paterson-Brown and J. Bamber, in M. Knight et al. (Eds.), *Saving Lives, Improving Mothers' Care* . . . (p. 49), 2014, Oxford, United Kingdom: National Perinatal Epidemiology Unit. Copyright by publisher.

- *Hypovolemic*: Involves low effective circulating blood volume. Some causes of hypovolemic shock are hemorrhage, dehydration, and fluid shifts from ascites or burns.
- *Obstructive*: Involves blockage to flow into or out of the heart, leading to inadequate oxygen and nutrient delivery to the organs and tissues. Some causes of obstructive shock are tension pneumothorax, pulmonary embolism (PE), cardiac tamponade, and restrictive cardiomyopathy.

An affected client can have more than one type of shock sequentially or simultaneously. Shock of unknown etiology is termed *undifferentiated shock*.

Hypovolemic Shock

In pregnancy, hypovolemic shock can follow antepartum or postpartum hemorrhage, miscarriage or ectopic pregnancy, trauma, or hemorrhage from other pathology such as gastrointestinal bleeding. Postpartum hemorrhage is the most common cause of pregnancy-related shock (Belfort, 2023a). Hypovolemic shock can also result from fluid loss related to diarrhea, vomiting, heatstroke, insensible losses, burns, or third-spacing of fluids into the interstitial space. Insufficient fluid in the intravascular space reduces blood return to the heart, causing decreased cardiac output and shock.

Maternal blood volume varies with body dimensions and other characteristics (Burtch, Scott, Zimmerman, &

Patel, 2016; Hernandez, Alexander, Sarode, McIntire, & Leveno, 2012). Those with more body surface area have greater blood volume than those with less and can lose more blood before reaching a critical physiologic threshold (Burtch et al., 2016). People with anemia or preeclampsia have lower intravascular volume and can decompensate with less blood loss (Main, Martin, Romine, & Thomas, 2022). Although high blood volume protects against hemorrhage, obese people are more likely to experience severe PPH and are less able to tolerate large blood loss, probably because obesity increases intraabdominal pressure and decreases venous return (Hernandez et al., 2012; Lisonkova et al., 2017; Sterling, Jones, Coleman, & Summers, 2015).

The ATLS program (ACS, 2018) describes four classes of hemorrhage with specific clinical signs that can indicate the progression of hypovolemic shock. This model was developed from studies involving nonpregnant adults. The values can differ during pregnancy; for instance, healthy pregnant or postpartum individuals can lose more than 30% of their blood volume before SBP begins to fall (Nathan et al., 2015).

Class I hemorrhage is the hemodynamic equivalent of donating a unit of blood: blood loss of up to 15% of total volume (ACS, 2018). The heart rate may be normal or minimally elevated, and there is no change in BP, pulse pressure, or respiratory rate.

Class II hemorrhage occurs when there is a 15–30% blood volume loss (ACS, 2018). Tachycardia (heart rate of 100–120) and tachypnea (respiratory rate of 20–24) in a pregnant client with stable SBP are signs of compensated shock until proven otherwise, even if bleeding is not apparent (Belfort, 2023a). Pulse pressure (the difference between SBP and DBP) narrows in hypovolemia, reflecting a rise in DBP related to vasoconstriction. Cool extremities, diaphoresis, pallor, and capillary refill longer than 2 sec can also indicate peripheral vasoconstriction. Decreased urine output can indicate reduced blood flow to the kidneys.

Class III hemorrhage occurs with a 30–40% blood volume loss (ACS, 2018). The client can display signs of inadequate perfusion such as decreased BP, tachypnea, pronounced mental status changes, and rapid, thready pulse. Urine output is decreased. Most people with class III hemorrhage require a crystalloid infusion and transfusion of packed red blood cells (PRBCs) and blood products to restore adequate perfusion (ACS, 2018).

Table 9-2

Clinical Signs and Symptoms of Hypovolemic Shock and Their Immediate Causes

Sign/Symptom	Immediate Cause
Rapid heart rate	Catecholamine response increases cardiac output.
Hypotension	Blood pressure (BP) decreases because of low intravascular volume.
Tachypnea	Respirations increase to raise the amount of oxygen in the blood and to compensate for metabolic acidosis by exhaling carbon dioxide and water.
Hypothermia	Peripheral vasoconstriction reduces blood flow to the extremities, so they get cold and lower the temperature of the rest of the body. Rapid intravascular infusion of room-temperature intravenous (IV) fluids can contribute to hypothermia.
Anxiety, restlessness, confusion, decreased level of consciousness	Decreased oxygen to the brain due to low blood flow or inadequate oxygenation.
Cool, clammy, pale skin	Catecholamine response constricts the blood vessels in the extremities and in the skin to improve central circulation.
Thirst and dry mucous membranes	Fluid depletion and dehydration.
Low urine output	Decreased kidney perfusion.

Adapted from "Volume Replacement Following Severe Postpartum Hemorrhage," by M. N. Schorn and J. C. Phillippi, 2014, *Journal of Midwifery & Women's Health, 59*(3), pp. 336–343. Copyright by John Wiley and Sons.

Class IV hemorrhage involves the urgently life-threatening loss of more than 40% of blood volume. Without aggressive resuscitation, the client can die (ACS, 2018). Blood transfusion is required. SBP is less than 80 mm Hg, tachycardia is greater than 140 beats per min (bpm), respiratory rate is greater than 40, skin is cold and pale, urine output is minimal or absent, and mental status is significantly depressed. The client either has a very narrow pulse pressure or an undetectable DBP. Bradycardia is a sign of impending death. Rapid transfusion and immediate surgical intervention are usually necessary to save the client's life.

Laboratory Values

Hemoglobin and hematocrit assessments are not helpful during acute hemorrhage (Belfort, 2023a) because values can remain normal or minimally decreased until interstitial fluid redistributes into the blood plasma (Hernandez et al., 2012). Hemoglobin levels fall by about 1 g/dl with every 500 ml of blood loss, *but it can take 8–12 hr for the complete blood count (CBC) to accurately reflect this decrease* (Belfort, 2023b). Hematocrit and hemoglobin begin to fall 4 hr after acute blood loss, but the peak change may not occur until as late as 48–72 hr after birth (Main et al., 2022).

At term, a healthy pregnant individual has a fibrinogen level of 350–650 mg/dl, nearly twice the nonpregnant range of 200–400 mg/dl (Belfort, 2023b). With hemorrhage, fibrinogen usually drops to critically low levels, so the fibrinogen level is a more sensitive indicator of ongoing major blood loss than the prothrombin time (PT), activated partial thromboplastin time (aPTT), or platelet count before other coagulation factors become abnormal. A hemorrhaging pregnant or postpartum client with a fibrinogen level less than 200 mg/dl is at high risk of death and usually requires multiple units of blood and blood products to correct the coagulopathy (Belfort, 2023b).

Blood Products

During or after severe hemorrhage, the client often requires PRBCs, fresh frozen plasma, platelets, and recombinant Factor VIIa to restore blood volume, enhance tissue oxygenation, and promote clot formation (Belfort, 2023b; Schorn & Phillippi, 2014). These products can be used together as part of a massive transfusion protocol (Schorn & Phillippi, 2014). Blood typing and Rh and antibody screening should be evaluated in the antenatal period. PRBCs are usually transfused to enhance the oxygen-carrying ability of the circulating volume and to improve intravascular volume by increasing osmolality. One unit of PRBCs will raise the hematocrit by approximately 3% and the hemoglobin by about 1g/dl.

A healthy pregnant client needs a hemoglobin concentration of at least 6 g/dl to maintain optimal cardiopulmonary function (Schorn & Phillippi, 2014). The decision to transfuse may depend on the quantity of blood lost, hemoglobin value, vital signs, or signs and symptoms. Even if vital signs are stable, tissues or organs may be starved for oxygen if blood volume is insufficient.

Tranexamic Acid (TXA)

TXA is an antifibrinolytic drug that inhibits the breakdown of clots and can make the victim's own hemostatic mechanisms more effective (Sentilhes et al., 2015). Long used for the prevention and treatment of bleeding in surgery and trauma, it is now used to prevent and decrease postpartum blood loss (Novikova, Hofmeyr, & Cluver, 2015). The World Maternal Antifibrinolytic Trial (WOMAN) concluded that TXA decreased the death due to bleeding in mothers with PPH by 20–30% without adverse effects (WOMAN Trial Collaborators, 2017). An IV infusion of 1 g TXA within the first hour of trauma or within 3hr of PPH can improve maternal outcomes (Murphy & Cullinan, 2020).

The 4 Cs: Thresholds of Blood Loss

The four key treatment thresholds of blood loss in a previously healthy pregnant or postpartum client can be remembered as the 4 Cs. A client who is small, thin, anemic, or hypertensive will likely deteriorate faster.

The first **C** is for **Compensated: Potential crisis.** When the client loses 500–1,000 ml of blood, the blood loss will probably be tolerated, but there is the potential for crisis if bleeding continues.

The second **C** is for **Challenged: Impending crisis.** With blood loss of 1,000–1,500 ml, the client can feel dizzy and experience palpitations. Heart rate and respirations are normal. Continued blood loss increases the risk of crisis.

The third **C** is for **Compromised: Actual crisis.** With blood loss of 1,500–2,000 ml, the client can display narrowed pulse pressure, heart rate over 100, respiratory rate 20–30, diaphoresis, weakness, faintness, and slightly decreased urine output.

The 4th **C** is for **Critical: Extreme crisis.** Blood loss of this magnitude holds the potential for severe crisis. When blood loss tops 2,000 ml, the client can display hypotension, narrowed pulse pressure, heart rate greater than 120, respiratory rate 30–40, pallor with cool extremities, restlessness, significantly decreased urine output. Blood loss greater than 2,500 ml may be accompanied by profound hypotension, heart rate over 140, respiratory rate over 40, and minimal to no urine output.

Distributive (Vasodilatory) Shock

Distributive or vasodilatory shock involves dilation of blood vessels throughout the body, which decreases circulation to the brain, heart, and kidneys and results in inadequate tissue perfusion (N. Smith, Lopez, & Silberman, 2023). Fluid leaks from capillaries into the surrounding tissues, causing edema while reducing intravascular volume. Anaphylactic shock, septic shock, and neurogenic shock are three of the most common kinds of distributive shock (Gaieski & Mikkelsen, 2023a).

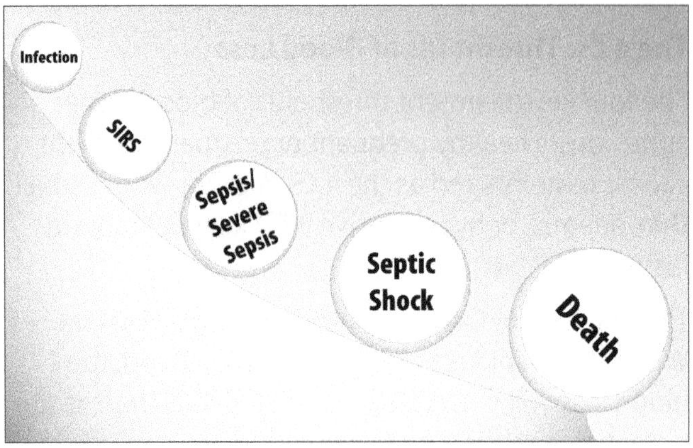

Figure 9-6. Infection can snowball quickly into septic shock and death.

Sepsis and Septic Shock

Sepsis, from the Greek *sepein*, "to rot" involves life-threatening organ dysfunction caused by an abnormal response to infection (Evans et al., 2021). Sepsis is a syndrome of systemic inflammatory response to pathogens or their byproducts, such as endotoxins or exotoxins, characterized by widespread tissue injury. It develops along a continuum, beginning with a localized infection and progressing through systemic inflammatory response, sepsis, severe sepsis, septic shock, multiorgan failure, and death.

Systemic inflammatory response syndrome (SIRS) is a generalized, whole-body response to localized infections or injuries (including ischemia, inflammation, and trauma) alone or in combination (Gaieski & Mikkelsen, 2023a). Sepsis is SIRS caused by infection (Duff, 2021). Severe sepsis is defined as sepsis plus at least one sign of organ dysfunction. Septic shock is defined as sepsis with circulatory, cellular, and metabolic dysfunction (with or without hypotension) that can be life-threatening (Gauer, Forbes, & Boyer, 2020).

In the United States, maternal sepsis is both rare and deadly. Maternal sepsis occurs in only 0.04% of births in the United States but plays a role in 23% of all maternal deaths (Hensley, Bauer, Admon, & Prescott, 2019). For each maternal death, another 50 mothers suffer life-threatening illness from sepsis (Gibbs et al., 2020).

Pathophysiology

In sepsis, proinflammatory compounds cascade into a cytokine storm that causes selective vasodilation and abnormal distribution of blood flow (Cunningham et al., 2022, ch. 50). Injured endothelium within the blood vessels leads to capillary leakage and accumulation of fluid within the interstitial space. Intravascular volume decreases because of vasodilation and capillary leakage, decreasing perfusion to organs and tissues. Inadequate volume within major blood vessels triggers the release of catecholamines such as adrenaline, which causes tachycardia to increase cardiac output. Leaky capillaries in the lungs can result in pulmonary edema and interfere with ventilation (Neviere, 2022).

Sepsis leads to coagulation abnormalities that can cause simultaneous widespread clotting in small vessels and profuse bleeding from various sites (Giustozzi et al., 2021). Lack of perfusion can cause tissue necrosis, organ failure, and death. Oxygen-deprived cells switch from aerobic to anaerobic metabolism, producing lactic acid that causes metabolic acidosis. Respiration increases to improve oxygenation and to expel lactic acid. Blood glucose initially rises in response to the release of catecholamines, then drops when the liver begins to malfunction.

Pregnancy causes physiologic changes to the immune system that can increase susceptibility to sepsis. Maternal sepsis can arise from local infections in the genital tract, kidney, lung, breast, gastrointestinal tract, or elsewhere, including wounds

Table 9-3

Symptoms Related to Blood Loss with PPH

Blood Loss ml	Blood Loss %	Systolic BP (mm Hg)	Signs and Symptoms
500–1,000 ml	10–15%	Normal	Possible palpitations, dizziness, pallor, tachycardia. Sometimes no sign or symptom.
1,000–1,500 ml	15–25%	Possibly slightly low	Probably weakness, sweating, pallor, tachycardia.
1,500–2,000 ml	25–35%	70–80	Restlessness, pallor, oliguria.
2,000 ml–3,000	35–45%	50–70	Collapse, air hunger, anuria.

Adapted from (1) "Massive Obstetric Haemorrhage," by J. Bonnar, 2000, *Baillière's Best Practice & Research, Clinical Obstetrics & Gynaecology, 14*(1), pp. 1–18. Copyright 2000 by Harcourt Publishers Ltd. (2) "Definitions and Classifications," by A. Coker and R. Oliver, in S. Arulkumaran, M. Karoshi, L. G. Keith, A. B. Lalonde, and C. B-Lynch (Eds.), *A Comprehensive Textbook of Postpartum Hemorrhage: An Essential Clinical Reference for Effective Management* (2nd ed., pp. 129–132), 2012, London, United Kingdom: Sapiens Publishing. Copyright by publisher.

from cesarean section or intrapartum vaginal trauma (Gibbs et al., 2020). In 2020, COVID-19 (SARS-CoV-2) emerged as a novel virus capable of causing severe pneumonia, septic shock, respiratory failure, and multiorgan failure (Ashokka et al., 2020).

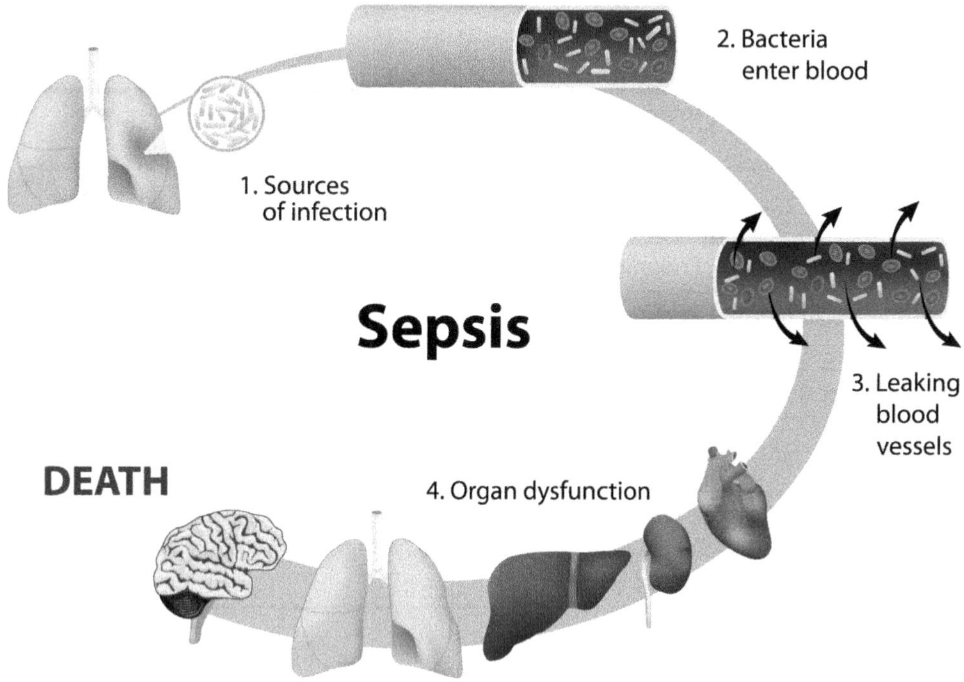

Figure 9-7. Sepsis begins as a localized infection that can progress through systemic inflammatory response, septic shock, multiorgan failure, and death (©designua/Adobe Stock).

Recognizing Sepsis

Because the signs and symptoms of sepsis are nonspecific and often resemble other conditions, recognizing sepsis and organ dysfunction can be challenging, especially during pregnancy. Clinical signs that would be suspicious for SIRS in a nonpregnant individual, for example, mild elevations of pulse, respiratory rate, and white blood cell (WBC) count, can be normal in a healthy pregnant client (Rojas-Suarez & Suarez Rueda, 2020). Because there is no specific test to diagnose sepsis and fever is not always present, it can be difficult to distinguish from certain noninfectious disorders such as PE, adrenal crisis, or severe hyperthyroidism. Signs and symptoms of sepsis can include malaise, nausea, vomiting, sweating, body aches, diarrhea, shaking chills, fever, tachycardia, tachypnea, mental status changes, or flushed, moist skin (Baldisseri, 2016). The clinical presentation can provide clues to the source of the infection. For example, coughing purulent sputum suggests pneumonia, whereas left flank pain and dysuria suggest pyelonephritis. Guidelines issued by California Maternal Quality Care Collaborative propose the following initial sepsis screen for all clients with suspected infection (positive if two or more criteria are met):

- Oral temperature below 96.8°F (36°C) or 100.4°F (38°C) or above.
- Heart rate greater than 110 bpm sustained for 15 min (A sustained maternal heart rate greater than 130 bpm is particularly concerning for end-organ injury.)
- Respiratory rate greater than 24 breaths per min sustained for 15 min.
- WBC count higher than 15,000/mm^3 or lower than 4,000/mm^3 or more than 10% immature neutrophils, a.k.a. bands (Gibbs et al., 2020).

If an abnormal value is detected, take a complete set of vital signs including oxygen saturation and take another complete set after 15 min (Gibbs et al., 2020). Although most pregnant clients with sepsis have an elevated heart rate and a temperature of 100.4°F (38.0°C) or higher, some remain afebrile (Gibbs et al., 2020). If the sepsis screen is positive, the California Maternal Quality Care Collaborative (CMQCC) recommends the following to assess for end-organ injury:

- Complete blood count (CBC), including percentage of bands and platelets.
- Coagulation status: PT/international normalized ratio (INR)/partial thromboplastin time (PTT).
- Comprehensive metabolic panel (specifically include bilirubin, creatinine).
- Venous lactic acid (may be elevated in labor).
- Urine output (place Foley catheter with urometer).
- Pulse oximetry.
- Mental status assessment (Gibbs et al., 2020).

The criteria for end-organ injury for diagnosis of maternal sepsis are in Table 9-5. Keep in mind that administering corticosteroids for fetal lung maturity can increase the WBC count. This elevation peaks 24 hr after dosing and returns to baseline values by 96 hr (Gibbs et al., 2020).

Management of Sepsis and Septic Shock

Pregnant clients with sepsis are at high risk for perinatal complications including PTB and fetal death, even when the infection is not intrauterine (Escobar, Echavarría, Zambrano, Ramos, & Kusanovic, 2020). The client with suspected sepsis requires rapid transfer to a hospital for emergency care. Critically ill clients frequently require admission to an intensive

Table 9-4
Leading Causes of Maternal Sepsis

Antepartum	Intrapartum / Immediate Postpartum	Postdischarge
Septic abortion	Intraamniotic infection (IAI) / Chorioamnionitis	Pneumonia/influenza
IAI/Chorioamnionitis	Endometritis	Pyelonephritis
Pneumonia/influenza	Pneumonia/influenza	Wound Infection / necrotizing fasciitis
Pyelonephritis	Pyelonephritis	Mastitis
Appendicitis	Wound Infection / necrotizing fasciitis	Cholecystitis

From *Improving Diagnosis and Treatment of Maternal Sepsis: A CMQCC Quality Improvement Toolkit* (p. 9), by R. Gibbs et al., 2020, Stanford, CA: California Maternal Quality Care Collaborative. Copyright 2019 by publisher.

care unit for ongoing management and reevaluation (Escobar et al., 2020; Evans et al., 2021).

For clients with sepsis and septic shock, survival decreases 7% with every hour antibiotic therapy is delayed (Escobar et al., 2020). Goals of treatment are to stabilize vital signs, avoid progression from sepsis to septic shock, and maximize tissue perfusion to limit cellular damage (Escobar et al., 2020). Treatment of sepsis and septic shock in pregnancy should follow the international Surviving Sepsis Campaign guidelines, which include infusion of 30 ml of crystalloids per kg of maternal weight within the first 3 hr—for example, 2.04 L for a 150-lb (68-kg) mother—and administration of broad-spectrum antimicrobials within the first hour after diagnosis (Evans et al., 2021; Niehaus & Baldisseri, 2020). Vasoactive agents such as dopamine, ephedrine, and norepinephrine are often necessary to maintain mean arterial pressure (MAP) above 65 mm Hg (Escobar et al., 2020). Pregnant clients with sepsis beyond the age of viability require frequent assessments of fetal wellbeing (Vaught, 2018). Consider administering betamethasone if the fetus is less than 37 weeks of gestation and birth is anticipated within 7 days (Vaught, 2018).

Serum lactate levels are monitored, and resuscitative strategies should be used to decrease lactate toward normal ranges. Blood cultures are collected, and broad-spectrum antimicrobial therapy may be discontinued in favor of an agent targeted specially at the pathogen once antibiotic susceptibility is defined (Escobar et al., 2020). For severe infections associated with sepsis and septic shock, antibiotic treatment is typically required for 7–10 days (Escobar et al., 2020).

Neurogenic Shock

Neurogenic shock is distributive shock that occurs after severe damage to the central nervous system, most commonly the brain or upper spinal cord (Gaieski & Mikkelsen, 2023a). In other forms of shock, the sympathetic nervous system compensates for low circulating volume by releasing epinephrine and norepinephrine (Johnson, Boyd, Grantham, & Eastwood, 2015). These neurotransmitters induce tachycardia, tachypnea, diaphoresis, and vasoconstriction. In a classic presentation of neurogenic shock, the victim is unable to activate the sympathetic nervous system (Hansebout & Kachur, 2018). Parasympathetic tone from the intact vagus nerve is largely unopposed, resulting in bradycardia (Johnson et al., 2015). Massive vasodilation and slowed heart rate result in sudden and severe hypotension. The skin is warm and flushed. Male victims can develop priapism—persistent erection of the penis due to vasodilation (Hansebout & Kachur, 2018).

Anaphylactic Shock

Anaphylaxis is an acute, potentially life-threatening, systemic allergic reaction caused by the sudden release of mast cell mediators (Campbell & Kelso, 2022). It most commonly results from immunoglobulin E (IgE)-mediated reactions to foods, drugs, and insect stings or from the direct release of mediators from mast cells and basophils in response to triggers such as exercise, contrast media, or latex (Gaieski & Mikkelsen, 2023a). It can involve urticaria (hives), hypotension, bronchospasm, and the rapid swelling of skin, mucosa, or submucosal tissues. Swelling can rapidly progress to airway obstruction and death. Anaphylactic symptoms appear during the first hour of exposure to the antigen, usually within 1–15 min. Rapid onset of symptoms heralds a more severe reaction. With severe anaphylaxis, a client can develop circulatory collapse, apnea, seizures, and coma within 1–2 min, and die soon after (Schatz & Dombrowski, 2023). Although anaphylaxis is rare in pregnancy, approximately three quarters of reactions occur while giving birth (McCall et al., 2020).

During pregnancy, labor, and birth, commonly administered medications can unexpectedly cause anaphylaxis. Antibiotics, especially penicillin, ampicillin, cefazolin, and ceftriaxone, are the most reported triggers of anaphylaxis in pregnant people (Schatz & Dombrowski, 2023). Anaphylaxis has been triggered by cervical ripening agents such as misoprostol, synthetic oxytocin, and medications used for anesthesia

(Schatz & Dombrowski, 2023). Strangely, there are case reports of breastfeeding implicated as a trigger of anaphylaxis, sometimes in conjunction with use of nonsteroidal antiinflammatory drugs (Shank, Olney, Lin, & McNamara, 2009).

Common signs and symptoms include

- **Skin:** Hives, redness, itching, swelling. Lesions are red and raised, may be small, or may become confluent with irregular borders and sometimes with central blanching.
- **Nose, throat, airway:** Congestion, sneezing, cough, hoarseness, laryngospasm, sensation of tightness in the throat. Upper-airway edema (including tongue or oropharynx swelling) can block the flow of air partially or completely. Stridor (high-pitched breathing sound) indicates narrowing of the upper airway. *Most anaphylactic deaths are due to complete airway obstruction.*
- **Eyes:** Itchy, red, tearing eyes.
- **Lungs:** Dyspnea, bronchospasm. Wheezing indicates bronchospasm or mucosal edema narrowing the lower airways.
- **Gastrointestinal tract:** Abdominal cramping, nausea, vomiting, or diarrhea.
- **Cardiovascular system:** Tachypnea, tachycardia, or hypotension. Hypotension is secondary to systemic vasodilation. When vascular tone is lost, compensatory tachycardia occurs. Increasingly permeable capillaries leak fluid into the interstitial space, causing edema with hypovolemia from third-spacing.
- **Mental status:** Anxiety, restlessness, tremor, decreased level of consciousness.
- **Systemic failure:** Cardiovascular collapse or respiratory arrest.

Table 9-5

Criteria for End-Organ Injury for Diagnosis of Maternal Sepsis
(A single criterion is sufficient for diagnosis)

Respiratory function	Acute respiratory failure as evidenced by acute need for invasive or noninvasive mechanical ventilation OR $PaO_2/FiO_2 < 300$
Coagulation status	Platelets <100 x 109/L, OR International normalized ratio (INR) >1.5 OR PTT >60 sec
Liver function	Bilirubin >2 mg/dl
Cardiovascular function	Persistent hypotension after fluid administration: SBP <85 mm Hg, OR Mean arterial pressure (MAP) <65 mm Hg OR >40 mm Hg decrease in SBP
Renal function	Creatinine >1.2 mg/dl OR Doubling of creatinine OR Urine output <0.5 ml/kg/hr (for 2 hr)
Mental status assessment	Agitation, confusion, or unresponsiveness
Lactic acid	2 mmol/L in the absence of labor (Lactic acid is not diagnostic in labor, but it is an important consideration for treatment.)

PaO_2 = Partial pressure of Oxygen in the alveoli; FiO_2 = Fraction of Inspired Oxygen; MAP = Mean Arterial Pressure.

Adapted from *Improving Diagnosis and Treatment of Maternal Sepsis: A CMQCC Quality Improvement Toolkit* (p. 14), by R. Gibbs et al., 2020, Stanford, CA: California Maternal Quality Care Collaborative. Copyright 2019 by publisher.

Management of Anaphylaxis

Anaphylaxis is life-threatening. Respiratory or cardiac arrest and death can occur within minutes of onset of symptoms (Campbell & Kelso, 2023). Do not attempt to treat severe reactions or to "wait and see." Activate EMS. The initial steps for management of anaphylaxis are the same regardless of whether the client is pregnant. Immediately remove the triggering agents if possible, support the airway, treat hypoxia with supplemental oxygen, aggressively infuse IV fluids, and give medications such as epinephrine and corticosteroids.

People with suspected anaphylaxis, pregnant or not, should receive intramuscular (IM) epinephrine immediately. *There are no absolute contraindications to the use of epinephrine for anaphylaxis of any severity* (Campbell & Kelso, 2023).

The 3 Bs of AFES

Breathing (hypoxia)

Blood pressure (hypotension)

Bleeding (coagulopathy)

Adapted from "AFE Emergency Stabilization Checklist: Breathing, Blood Pressure, Bleeding," by AFE Foundation, 2023 (https://amnioticfluidembolism.org/wp-content/uploads/2024/02/AFE-2023-EmergencyChecklist-1.pdf).

Epinephrine is most likely to be effective when administered in the early phases of anaphylaxis, before shock has developed; delays can increase the risk of death. The usual adult dose is 0.3 mg of 1:1,000 IM epinephrine injected into the mid-outer thigh and repeated every 5–15 min as needed (Gaieski & Mikkelsen, 2023b). If the client carries an epinephrine auto-injector (also known as an EpiPen®), remove the auto-injector from the carrier tube, remove the safety release, place the tip perpendicular against the middle of the outer thigh, and push until it clicks. Hold it to the thigh for 3 sec to inject the medication. Most clients with anaphylaxis respond to one or (occasionally) two doses of epinephrine when it is given shortly after symptoms occur (Campbell & Kelso, 2023).

Administer supplemental oxygen and bronchodilators if respiratory signs or symptoms persist after epinephrine is given, and assist respirations as indicated. Establish bilateral IV access with large bore catheters and rapidly infuse isotonic crystalloid solution (normal saline [NS] or lactated Ringer's [LR]). Infuse 1 L or more at a rapid rate if the client is unstable, or at a slower rate if vital signs are normal. Care provided by EMS and the hospital providers may include aggressive airway management including intubation or even cricothyrotomy as indicated, cardiac monitoring, large volumes of isotonic crystalloid solutions, vasopressors, nebulized albuterol (2.5 mg in 3 ml of NS) for bronchospasm, and methylprednisolone (1–2 mg/kg IV). H1 antihistamines such as cetirizine and diphenhydramine *do not* relieve upper- or lower-airway obstruction, hypotension, or shock, and in standard doses they do not inhibit mediator release from mast cells and basophils (Campbell & Kelso, 2023). They can, however, relieve itch and hives.

Amniotic Fluid Embolism Syndrome (AFES)

Amniotic fluid embolism (AFES) is a very rare but devastating complication in which a mother can experience cardiorespiratory collapse and DIC (Haftel & Chowdhury, 2023), usually during labor or within 30 min postpartum (Baldisseri & Clark, 2023). Although the pathophysiology of AFES is unclear, it is thought to occur when amniotic fluid enters the maternal circulation, causing the mother to respond to the foreign antigen material (e.g., bacteria, fetal skin or hair, or meconium) with a massive systemic inflammatory response and activation of the clotting cascade (Pacheco, Clark, Klassen, & Hankins, 2020). The condition presents abruptly, usually with a triad of first hypoxia and hypotension then coagulopathy. Whereas historically it was believed that AFES was caused by large volumes of particulate amniotic fluid entering the maternal circulation, it now appears that the incursion of even a very small amount of amniotic fluid can trigger the syndrome (Murphy & Cullinan, 2020). Because data suggest that AFES resembles anaphylaxis more than embolism, some authors recommend replacing the term with *anaphylactoid syndrome of pregnancy* and managing the condition accordingly (Clark, Hankins, Dudley, Dildy, & Porter, 1995; Haftel & Chowdhury, 2023; Murphy & Cullinan, 2020).

AFES is the second leading cause of peripartum maternal mortality in the United States and the number one cause of peripartum cardiac arrest (Haftel & Chowdhury, 2023). Survivors are at risk for permanent neurological injury, including persistent vegetative state or stroke. It occurs in 1 of 15,200 births in North America and in 1 of 53,800 in Europe (Murphy & Cullinan, 2020). Most cases of AFES occur during labor, immediately postpartum, or during cesarean section (Baldisseri & Clark, 2023). In exceedingly rare instances, AFES has been associated with medical or surgical abortion, miscarriage, amniocentesis, or trauma (Baldisseri & Clark, 2023). Risk factors include cesarean or instrumental vaginal birth; short, intense labor; age 35 years or greater; abnormal placenta attachment; eclampsia; induction of labor; uterine rupture; or polyhydramnios.

AFES is a clinical diagnosis based upon the characteristic signs and symptoms and exclusion of other potential causes of these findings (Baldisseri & Clark, 2023). Classic findings include

- A sense of impending doom, chills, nausea/vomiting, agitation, anxiety, or confusion immediately before collapse.
- Sudden cardiac and respiratory arrest.
- Low oxygen saturation, rapid breathing, difficulty breathing, pulmonary edema.
- Hypotension/cardiogenic shock.
- Arrhythmia.
- DIC with hemorrhage from IV access sites, uterus, wounds, bladder, and gastrointestinal tract.
- Rarely, tonic-clonic seizure or stroke (Baldisseri & Clark, 2023).

If AFES occurs in a community setting, call EMS and prepare for emergency transport. Treat as with shock or cardiac arrest (see "Cardiac Arrest in Pregnancy," below) until a paramedic or equivalent or a physician team assumes care. If the client survives the initial collapse, AFES is managed with supportive care in the intensive care unit.

In the hospital, management of unstable clients with AFES involves resuscitative efforts with simultaneous diagnostic evaluation. Standard basic and advanced cardiac life support interventions include manual chest percussions, airway management with supplemental oxygen and intubation, fluid resuscitation and arrhythmia management (Baldisseri & Clark, 2023). If shock persists, vasopressors may be used to maintain adequate BP. If the client has DIC or hemorrhage, immediate and rapid transfusion of blood products (usually through a massive transfusion protocol) can be lifesaving. If the client is pregnant with a viable fetus, giving birth can improve outcomes for both mother and infant (Baldisseri & Clark, 2023). Once the client is stabilized, the focus should be on maintaining a secure airway and hemodynamic stability, adequate oxygenation, and prevention of bleeding, usually within a hospital intensive care unit.

DIFFERENTIAL DIAGNOSES

Uterine atony, placental abruption, uterine rupture, preeclampsia/eclampsia, septic shock, PE, air embolism, myocardial infarction, stroke, anaphylaxis, drug reaction, and aspiration of gastric contents are leading suspects.

Cardiogenic Shock

Cardiogenic shock is failure of the heart to pump adequately, causing decreased cardiac output and inability to meet the metabolic requirements of the tissues. Cardiogenic shock can be related to cardiomyopathy (disease of heart muscle that weakens cardiac contractions), arrhythmia (faulty cardiac electrical impulses), or mechanical defects (issues like defective valves or ventricular septal defects that interfere with function). As the left heart fails, blood backs up and congests the pulmonary vasculature, causing pulmonary edema and tachypnea. If the right heart fails as well, jugular veins distend, the liver congests, and peripheral edema develops. Inadequate oxygen delivery leads to cellular damage, multiorgan failure, and death.

Cardiac output, the volume of blood pumped by the heart per minute, is calculated by multiplying the heart rate by stroke volume (the amount pumped per beat). Stroke volume is affected by blood volume, preload (blood returning to the heart), heart contractility (strength of heartbeat), afterload (the resistance the heart must overcome to eject blood). Cardiac output is typically 20% above baseline by 8 weeks of gestation, and it increases by almost 50% at term (Narvaez & Vrees, 2021).

Table 9-6

The Maternal Early-Warning Criteria

The Maternal Early-Warning Criteria
SBP (mm Hg) <90 or >160
DBP (mm Hg) >100
Heart rate (bpm) <50 or >120
Respiratory rate (breaths per min) <10 or >30
Oxygen saturation on room air, at sea level <95%
Oliguria, ml/hr for ≥2 hr—<35
Maternal agitation, confusion, or unresponsiveness
Client with preeclampsia reporting an unremitting headache or shortness of breath
A pregnant client meeting any of these criteria may be at risk for serious morbidity and mortality and should be evaluated immediately. This list is not exhaustive and does not replace clinical judgment.
Adapted from "The Maternal Early Warning Criteria: A Proposal from the National Partnership for Maternal Safety," by J. M. Mhyre et al., 2014, copublished by the *Journal of Obstetric, Gynecologic, & Neonatal Nursing, 43*(6), pp. 771–779, and *Obstetrics & Gynecology, 124*(4), 783–786. Copyright by Association of Women's Health, Obstetric and Neonatal Nurses.

During labor, cardiac output surges an additional 30% (Wenstrom, 2015). Cardiac output reaches a peak immediately postpartum when the involuting uterus autotransfuses about 500 ml from the uterine muscle to the systemic circulation, peripheral resistance increases, and extravascular fluid is mobilized (Wenstrom, 2015). Cardiac output and stroke volume increase by 59% and 71%, respectively, within 10 min after a term vaginal birth (Valente & Economy, 2023). Because of this process, heart failure is most likely to occur during labor or immediately postpartum, especially in the client with hypertension, valvular disease, arrhythmias, cardiomyopathies, amniotic fluid embolism, cocaine use, or ischemic heart disease. Cardiovascular disorders can develop for the first-time during pregnancy because of increased blood volume and cardiac output, decreased systemic vascular resistance, and physiologic anemia. Pregnancy can also exacerbate preexisting heart conditions.

Peripartum Cardiomyopathy

Cardiomyopathies are myocardial diseases associated with mechanical and/or electrical dysfunction (Cunningham et al., 2022, ch. 52). Peripartum cardiomyopathy is a condition of heart failure that develops late in pregnancy or within five months postpartum that affects 1 in 1,000–4,000 births in the United States (Cunningham et al., 2022, ch. 52). It carries a 25–50% risk of death, which is usually related to progressive

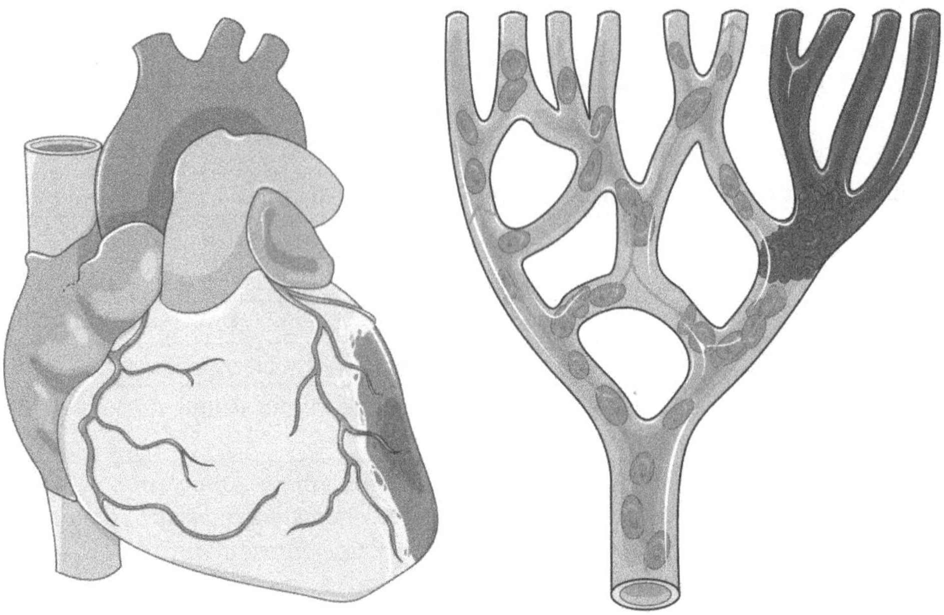

Figure 9-8. Myocardial infarction (MI) occurs when a blood clot blocks a vessel perfusing the heart. Signs and symptoms include discomfort in the anterior chest or epigastric area that sometimes radiates to the shoulders, arms, jaws, or back along with shortness of breath and nausea. Acute myocardial infarction is rare in pregnancy. MI is more likely to occur in mothers who are more than 35 years old, hypertensive, diabetic, or obese. Cigarette smoking and dyslipidemia are also risk factors. Left: "Myocardial Infarction—Anterolateral," by Servier Medical Art, 2016b (https://smart.servier.com/wp-content/uploads/2016/10/infarct4.png). CC BY 3.0. Right: "Thrombus Position and Consequences," by Servier Medical Art, 2016c (https://smart.servier.com/wp-content/uploads/2016/10/Infarctus2-562x680.png). CC BY 3.0.

congestive heart failure, arrhythmia, or thromboembolism (Deen, Albright, Chandrasekaran, & Stout, 2021). The cause is unknown, but genetic, inflammatory, hormonal, hemodynamic, and autoimmune influences may contribute (Tsang & Lang, 2022). Clinical signs include pulmonary edema, dyspnea, cough, orthopnea, tachycardia, and sometimes hemoptysis (Deen et al., 2021). Management goals for pregnant clients with heart failure are like those for those who are not pregnant; they include relief of symptoms, optimizing cardiac output, improving long-term outcomes, and treating precipitating factors (DeCara, Lang, & Davis, 2023).

Obstructive Shock

Obstructive shock can develop when perfusion is compromised because of a blockage that limits blood flow to or from the heart, such as tension pneumothorax, PE, or pericardial tamponade. The client with obstructive shock is unable to produce adequate cardiac output despite normal intravascular volume and myocardial function. Tension pneumothorax or pericardial tamponade can result from traumatic injury. A pregnant person is predisposed to PE by sluggish blood flow through the leg veins, venous pooling, and hypercoagulability. About 10% of maternal deaths are attributable to PE (Cunningham et al., 2022, ch. 55).

Shock Index (SI)

Heart Rate ÷ SBP.

≥0.9 indicates need for referral.

≥1.4 indicates urgent intervention in tertiary facility.

≥1.7 indicates high chance of adverse outcome.

(El Ayadi et al., 2016)

Easy SI

If the heart rate is greater than SBP, the client is at risk of severe shock and poor outcome. (Lai et al., 2016)

Recognizing and Managing Shock

Early recognition of shock can be lifesaving to the client, in hospital or out. Frequently assess and reassess every client to identify complications at their earliest presentation. Call EMS when your client shows signs of evolving hemodynamic compromise. Initiate emergency stabilization measures and support vital signs until EMS providers or hospital-based providers assume responsibility for care of the client.

Early Recognition

Most often, early warning signs of decompensation are recognizable for hours before life-threatening deterioration (Kyriacos Jelsma, & Jordan, 2011). Most maternal deaths can be prevented if the provider recognizes the early signs of clinical decline and takes appropriate action (Zuckerwise & Lipkind, 2017). Providers, however, are often slow to recognize hemorrhage, shock, hypertensive crisis, sepsis, venous thromboembolism, heart failure, and other acute critical illness.

The Maternal Early Warning Criteria tool (Table 9-6) proposed by the National Partnership for Maternal Safety can help providers to identify and respond to acute maternal illness at the earliest stages (Mhyre et al., 2014). The tool comprises a list of critical parameters that may indicate clinical decline. Although an isolated abnormal reading is not always cause for alarm, the midwife should reevaluate the client and consider transport if an abnormal value persists for two or more consecutive measurements, presents alongside other abnormal conditions, or reoccurs after resolution (Mhyre et al., 2014). A significantly abnormal value combined with risk factors or clinical signs of deterioration should be considered an emergency.

Shock Index

The shock index (SI) is a valuable bedside assessment that allows the clinician to quickly identify actual or potential shock by dividing the heart rate by SBP. If the numerical value for bpm is greater than the value for SBP, the SI is greater than 1 and hemodynamic compromise is likely (Borovac-Pinheiro, Pacagnella, Morais, & Cecatti, 2016; Le Bas, Chandraharan, Addei, & Arulkumaran, 2014; Nathan et al., 2015). In pregnancy and immediately postpartum, a value above 0.9 is concerning, and a value above 1 is significantly abnormal. For example, a client with a heart rate of 100 and an SBP of 90 has a SI of 1.1 (100 ÷ 90 = 1.1), indicating possible hypovolemia and early shock. An SI lower than 0.9 indicates the client is less likely to require massive resuscitation, and higher than 1.4 indicates the need for urgent intervention, stabilization, and transfer to tertiary care facility (Pandya & Mangalampally, 2018). An abnormal SI is often present long before alterations in vital signs indicate hypovolemia or sepsis. For the pregnant client with PPH, the SI is superior to the Maternal Early Warning Criteria in identifying need for intervention (Kohn, Dildy, & Eppes, 2018).

The basic steps of managing existing or impending shock are the same for each type of shock (AAOS, 2018).

- **Activate EMS immediately.**
- **Perform primary survey** using ABCDEF while taking a GOLDCART history, as appropriate. Stop any external bleeding. Assess for signs and symptoms of hemodynamic instability, including MAP below 65 mm Hg, a respiratory rate of 25 or higher, dyspnea, abnormal heart rate or rhythm, mental status changes, peripheral cyanosis, cold extremities, mottling, oliguria, or chest pain. Consider possible causes such as infection, bleeding, or a drug reaction. Quantify blood loss and determine the source with a thorough abdominal, vaginal, and rectal examination as indicated. Recall that blood loss can occur in multiple locations at once. For example, the client with a gushing laceration may also have an evolving hematoma.
- **Give supplemental oxygen** if the client is in respiratory distress or if the oxygen saturation is less than 95% (AAOS, 2018).

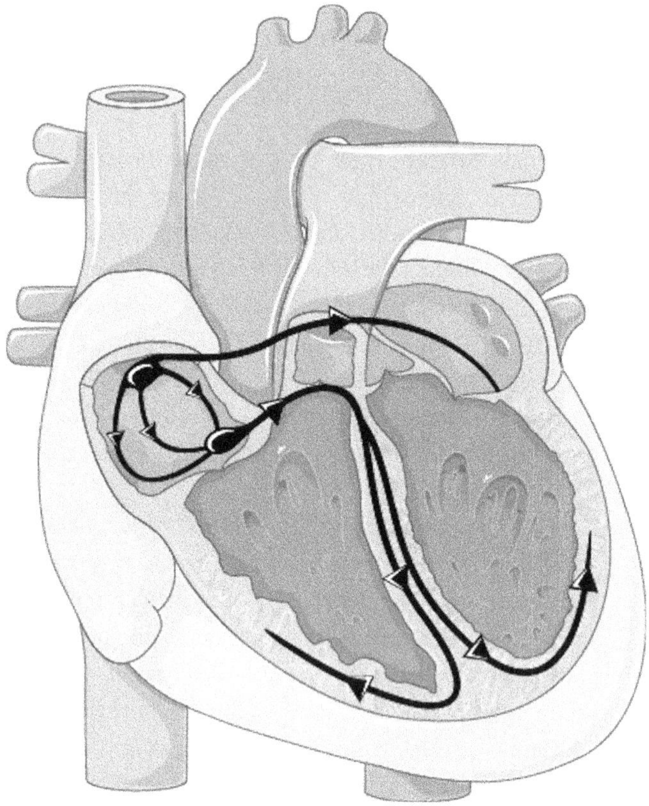

Figure 9-9. The conduction system of the heart consists of cardiac muscle cells and specialized conducting fibers that initiate impulses and move them rapidly through the heart. The sinus node, a cluster of cells in the upper part of the right atrial wall, is the heart's natural pacemaker. The AV node serves as a gate that slows the electrical signal before it passes to the ventricles. This delay ensures that the atria have a chance to contract fully before the ventricles are stimulated. After passing the AV node, the electrical current travels to the ventricles along special fibers embedded in the walls of the lower part of the heart. Arrhythmias occur when the pacemaker arises in a different part of the heart, or when the depolarizing impulse takes a different pathway. "Heart Conduction," by Servier Medical Art, 2016a (https://smart.servier.com/wp-content/uploads/2016/10/conduction_cardiaque.png). CC BY 3.0.

- **Re-evaluate** BP, heart rate, respiratory rate, peripheral oxygen saturation, and urine output every 10–15 min. Tachypnea, tachycardia, hypotension, low oxygen saturation, and air hunger can indicate low circulating volume (Belfort, 2023b). Progressively increasing heart rate and decreasing BP are presumed to be due to hypovolemia until proved otherwise (Belfort, 2023b).
- **Obtain IV or intraosseous access** for fluid replacement and medication administration. If access is IV, use large-bore (14 or 16 gauge) catheters at two different sites.
- **Protect from hypothermia.** Hypothermia less than 96.8°F (36°C) can decrease affinity of hemoglobin for

Fluid flows twice as fast through a 14-gauge IV catheter as it does through an 18-gauge.

oxygen, decreasing oxygen available to the tissues. Cooling can also cause arrhythmias by impairing electrical conduction in the heart. Warm IV fluids to body temperature by placing them in warm tap water. Cover the client with warm blankets and tuck hot water bottles in the armpits. Remove wet linens or clothing promptly. If the client is reasonably stable, keep the baby skin to skin.

- **Place in position of comfort** that yields the best vital signs for mother and fetus. Avoid supine positioning after 20 weeks of gestation.
- **Administer warmed crystalloid fluids.** Crystalloids are IV solutions with mineral salts or other small, water-soluble molecules. LR and 0.9% NS are crystalloid solutions commonly used in resuscitation. In shock, the purpose of crystalloid infusion is to stabilize the client until blood products are available. Crystalloid fluids stay briefly within the vasculature, then quickly extravasate into the tissues. About 60% of a bolus of NS diffuses out of the intravascular space within 20 min of infusion (AAOS, 2018). Although these fluids can maintain circulation in the short term, large infusions of crystalloid (more than 3–4 L) can decrease the oxygen-carrying capacity of the blood, cause acidosis and electrolyte derangement, impair coagulation, and cause third-spacing of fluid into the interstitial spaces (Belfort, 2023b; Schorn & Phillippi, 2014). One approach is to infuse crystalloids as a 250 ml bolus, followed by reassessment of vital signs. Boluses may be repeated to a maximum of four before reaching the hospital (AAOS, 2018). Consult with the receiving hospital for guidance.
- **Apply nonpneumatic antishock garments** (NASG) that compress the vasculature of the lower extremities, raising BP around vital organs. These are especially useful in low-resource settings and can improve outcomes in severe hypovolemic and distributive shock.
- **Rapidly transport** by ambulance to an appropriate facility.
- **Communicate and document.** Give the receiving provider an SBAR report. Document your care. Share records with the receiving facility.

Definitive Care for Clients with Shock

Successful management of the pregnant client with shock requires the expertise of a multidisciplinary team involving critical care, maternal-fetal medicine, respiratory care, nursing, and anesthesia specialists. The priority is to ensure a secure airway and adequate ventilation. If the client remains hypotensive despite the infusion of crystalloid fluids, vasopressor agents such as dopamine may be required. Blood products are necessary in the case of hemorrhage or coagulopathy. Cardiac monitoring should be initiated and cardiac dysfunction/arrhythmia should be managed in accordance with Advanced Cardiac Life Support guidelines (Murphy & Cullinan, 2020). Treatment is tailored to the etiology of shock. Whereas antibiotics are crucial in managing septic shock, epinephrine is the mainstay of treating anaphylaxis. In some cases, cesarean section can improve maternal hemodynamics and improve the infant's chance of survival. After stabilization the client is usually transferred to the ICU for continuing management.

Altered Level of Consciousness and Neurologic Emergencies

There are many medical emergencies or conditions that present with an alteration in mental status or level of consciousness. Syncope (fainting) or seizures can cause a transient loss of consciousness, followed by return to full consciousness. Head trauma, stroke, hypoxia, electrolyte or glucose imbalances, intoxicants, poisons, psychiatric disorders, and shock can cause an altered level of consciousness, as can many other conditions. Often the cause is unclear. A call to EMS with transport to an appropriate facility for definitive care is usually indicated for any change in mental status beyond simple fainting.

Headache in Pregnancy and Postpartum

Midwives often evaluate clients with headaches to determine whether the symptoms are benign or indicate a critical problem. Primary headaches, such as migraines and tension-type headaches are not associated with underlying medical problems. Secondary headaches are a symptom of some other condition (Ng, Cox, & Maiti, 2015). In a study involving severe headache lasting more than 24 hr in mothers up to 42 days postpartum (Stella, Jodicke, How, Harkness, & Sibai, 2007), etiologies were tension-type (39%), preeclampsia/eclampsia (24%), postdural puncture (16%), migraine (11%), pituitary hemorrhage/mass (3%), cerebral venous thrombosis (3%), and other (4%). A headache is the most frequent first symptom of COVID-19 and is usually severe, bilateral (80%), predominantly frontal (71%), crushing or tight (75%); and is usually associated with symptoms such as fever and congestion (García-Azorín et al., 2021).

Red-flag symptoms suggestive of a neurological emergency include (Nasr & Braksick, 2020)

- Thunderclap (reaches maximum intensity immediately)
- "Worst headache of my life"

- Drowsiness or depressed level of consciousness
- Worse with straining and Valsalva
- Stiff neck
- Accompanied by other neurological symptoms—seizures, weakness, vision loss
- Accompanied by other systemic symptoms—hypertension, peripheral edema
- A change in features from previous headaches
- New onset headache that awakens the client from sleep
- Headache related to trauma

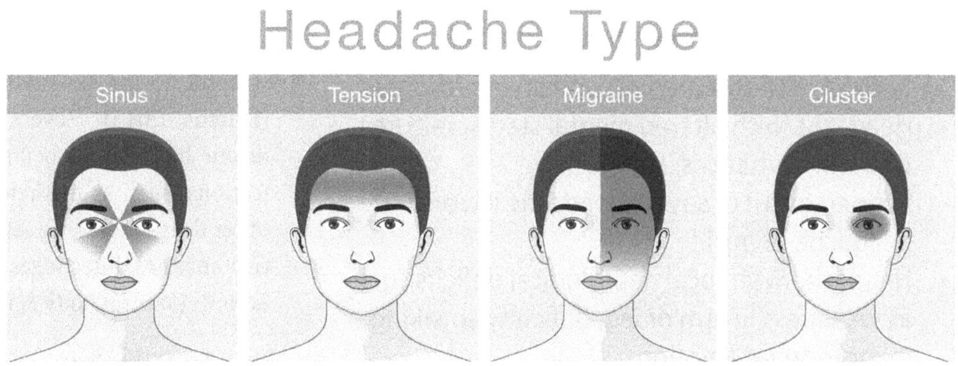

Figure 9-10. The location of the pain can provide clues to the type of headache (©logo3in1/Adobe Stock).

Preeclampsia/Hypertension

Somewhat common. **Dangerous!** Consider preeclampsia in any client over 20 weeks of gestation, in clients less than 20 weeks of gestation with a molar pregnancy, or in a postpartum client with headache (Lee, Guinn, & Hickenbottom, 2023). One third of pregnant clients beyond 20 weeks of gestation with a new or atypical headache and no prior significant headaches have preeclampsia (Lee et al., 2023; see also Chapter 10). Preeclampsia-related headache pain is usually experienced through the entire head and is mild to severe in intensity, constant, and throbbing. Blurred vision, light sensitivity, double vision, confusion, malaise, and nausea may be present. The client may have a scotoma (an abnormality in the field of vision surrounded by an area of normal vision), flickering lights in the visual field, or floaters.

Migraine

Common. Benign. Pain is usually unilateral, and of moderate intensity. Migraines are usually recurrent, with a throbbing or pulsating quality. They can be accompanied by nausea, vomiting, photophobia (light sensitivity), or phonophobia (noise sensitivity) and worsened by any physical activity. Migraines usually improve as pregnancy progresses.

Tension-Type Headache

Common. Benign. Tension-type headache is the most common headache in the general population, and the second-most prevalent disorder in the world (Taylor, 2022). The pain is usually mild to moderate intensity, bilateral, nonthrobbing, and without other associated features, but is sometimes severe, pulsing, or unilateral (Taylor, 2022). Pain is tight and bandlike and can be worse in the forehead and occiput. Tension-type headaches are often associated with tenderness and spasm in the muscles of the head, neck, or shoulders.

Sinus Headache

Possibly common. Benign. Sinusitis is commonly diagnosed as a cause for acute headache but does not usually cause recurrent headaches (Wippold, Whealy, & Kaniecki, 2023). Many clients complaining of a sinus headache turn out to have a migraine or tension-type headache when evaluated by a neurologist (Taylor, 2022). A client with suspected sinonasal headaches is best evaluated with nasal endoscopy (Wippold et al., 2023).

Cervicogenic Headache

Possibly common. Benign. Cervicogenic headaches occur when neck pain causes the head to hurt. These headaches appear to be caused by referred pain from the uppermost joints and muscle of the neck and sometimes follow neck trauma or whiplash injury (Watson, 2023). Cervicogenic headaches are unilateral, nonthrobbing, moderate to severe in intensity, and variable in duration (Watson, 2023). They radiate from occipital to frontal regions and often into the eye sockets; head movement makes them worse. They are often mistaken for sinus headaches.

Cluster Headaches

Uncommon. Cluster headaches are characterized by recurrent excruciating pain on one side of the head and around the eye. Associated symptoms include eye watering, nasal congestion, and eyelid edema. Symptoms persist for 15 min to 3 hr, then subside to recur frequently for weeks or months at a time, after which there are intervals of remission. Cluster headaches are poorly understood but involve the hypothalamus and the first branch of the trigeminal nerve.

Spinal Headache (Postdural Puncture Headache)

Somewhat uncommon. Benign. This condition occurs in people who have had epidural or spinal anesthesia. About

Danger signs associated with headache

Can indicate life-threatening underlying disorder

- Headache with altered mental status, seizures, visual disturbances, stiff neck
- Sudden onset of severe headache ("worst headache of my life")
- Headache with focal neurological deficits such as weakness in arm or leg, difficulty speaking, inappropriate emotion
- New onset of migraine-type headache
- Change in pain, pattern, or severity of usual headache
- Headache related to fever, head trauma, illicit drug use, toxic exposure, cough, exertion, sexual activity, or Valsalva maneuver
- Headache of new onset that interrupts sleep
- Headache unimproved by pain medication

Adapted from "Headache During Pregnancy and Postpartum," by M.-J. Lee, D. Guinn, and S. Hickenbottom, 2023, in V. A. Barss (Ed.), *UpToDate*. Copyright by UpToDate.

1–3% of clients obtaining an epidural block experience a "wet tap" in which the dura mater is punctured with a large-bore epidural needle (Hawkins & Bucklin, 2021). A spinal headache is thought to be caused by loss of cerebrospinal fluid, which causes intracranial structures to sag and sensory intracranial nerves to stretch when upright. The client complains of frontal or occipital pain. This headache usually develops within 72 hr of the procedure, and without treatment the pain usually resolves within a week (Bateman, Cole, Sun-Edelstein, & Lay, 2022). Pain worsens with standing or raising the head from the bed and improves with rest in a supine position. Oral analgesics and caffeine may be used to manage mild spinal headaches. With more severe or persistent pain, the anesthesiologist may consider placing an epidural blood patch (Hawkins & Bucklin, 2021). Approximately 20 ml of the client's own blood is injected into the epidural space near the site of the previous puncture. The injected blood clots over the dural hole and apparently seals off the leak, bringing rapid relief (Hawkins & Bucklin, 2021).

Reversible Cerebral Vasoconstriction Syndrome

Rare. **Can be dangerous.** Occurs as the result of a sudden constriction of the vessels that perfuse the brain. Onset is sudden and severe over multiple attacks, described as a "recurrent thunderclap headache" (Ng et al., 2015). Clients present with sudden, severe headaches that may be accompanied by confusion, agitation, visual disturbances, seizures, nausea, or vomiting. Forms that involve only a headache resolve spontaneously within 1–3 months, but rare catastrophic forms have led to stroke, brain edema, and death (Ducros, 2012). Reversible cerebral vasoconstriction syndrome has been associated with the use of ergonovine medications, such as methylergonovine (Methergine®), and with other drugs including selective serotonin reuptake inhibitors, triptans, nasal decongestants, cocaine, ecstasy, and amphetamines (Weerakkody & Gaillard, 2018).

Stroke (Cerebrovascular Accident)

Rare. **Dangerous!** Pregnancy-related stroke has an incidence of about 34 cases per 100,000 mothers (Grear & Bushnell, 2013). Stroke occurs when blood flow to the brain is stopped by blockage or rupture of a blood vessel. Ischemic stroke (comprising 87% of all strokes) occurs when the blood supply to the brain is obstructed, most commonly by a blood clot (American Stroke Association, n.d.). Headache can occur before, during, or after an ischemic stroke.

Hemorrhagic stroke involves the leaking or rupture of a cerebral artery, which decreases cerebral perfusion, increases intracranial pressure, and injures brain tissue. With intracerebral hemorrhage, headache can occur acutely when the stroke occurs or hours later as the hematoma expands and compresses sensitive intracranial structures (Ramzan & Mehla, 2023). Subarachnoid hemorrhage, usually caused by head trauma or the rupture of an aneurysm, involves bleeding within the subarachnoid space (between the meninges and the brain) into the cerebrospinal fluid. Most victims of subarachnoid hemorrhage have a severe headache at or near the time of the event, and about 10–43% experience a sentinel headache days or weeks beforehand due to aneurysm leakage (Ramzan & Mehla, 2023).

Stroke signs and symptoms are related to the part of the brain affected by the insult. Common findings are severe headache, abnormalities of vision and speech, unilateral weakness or numbness, eyelid and mouth drooping, unequal handgrips, paralysis, confusion, and memory loss. The headache pain of a subarachnoid hemorrhage is typically severe and sudden, peaking in seconds or minutes, often followed by vomiting, seizure, and loss of consciousness (Negro et al., 2017).

Brain Tumor

Very rare. **Usually dangerous.** Headache associated with brain tumor has a variable presentation related to tumor location, size, and rate of growth (Wippold et al., 2023). The headache may worsen with changes in body position, such as bending over, and be accompanied by nausea and vomiting (Wippold et al., 2023). Brain tumor headaches are usually accompanied by neurologic symptoms such as seizures, fatigue, cognitive dysfunction, or focal weakness.

Altered Level of Consciousness

The brain is the most metabolically active and perfusion-sensitive organ in the body and requires an uninterrupted supply of oxygen and nutrients to function (AAOS, 2018). Though it only represents about 2% of the total body weight, the brain receives about 15% of the cardiac output and metabolizes 25% of the body's glucose (AAOS, 2018). The brain is unable to store oxygen or glucose, and it requires robust blood flow to function effectively. A 3–5-sec interruption in blood flow can cause loss of consciousness (AAOS, 2018). When blood supply is diminished or disrupted, changes in mental status and vital signs can occur. There are many potential causes for altered level of consciousness or unresponsiveness in the pregnant client, including airway obstruction, shock, seizure, electrolyte or blood-glucose abnormality, hypoxia, substance abuse, poisoning, trauma, sepsis, or neurological disease.

Syncope in Pregnancy

Syncope, or fainting, is a brief loss of consciousness and postural tone that occurs when blood flow to the brain is temporarily reduced, usually by redistribution of blood volume, hypoglycemia, overheating, or a vagal response (Yarlagadda, Poma, Green, & Katz, 2010). Syncope may be associated with sudden hypotension, bradycardia, tachycardia, or arrhythmia. Victims of syncope usually have prodromal signs and symptoms (presyncope) for a short time before losing consciousness.

Presyncope or near syncope can last for seconds to minutes. Presyncope symptoms, like syncope itself, are caused by inadequate perfusion of the cerebrum (Whitledge, Ali, Basit, & Grossman, 2023). Presyncope can present as the beginning of a continuum that leads to syncope or it may resolve if the conditions that triggered the symptoms are corrected. The victim can experience lightheadedness; weakness; a sensation like a surge of heat; pale, sweaty skin; tachycardia; nausea; visual changes such as darkening, lightening, or tunnel vision; or auditory distortions (Benditt, 2022).

The client with symptoms of presyncope should immediately lie flat with the head at the level of the heart. If pregnant, the client should assume a side-lying position to avoid compression of the aorta and vena cava. Monitor vital signs and level of consciousness closely. If the client rests in this position for about 15 min, sipping water or juice and perhaps snacking, the symptoms should resolve. If they do not, the issue might be more serious than simple syncope.

To avoid syncope, the pregnant client should flex the leg muscles periodically during prolonged standing and sit for a minute before rising from a supine position. If BP trends in the low-normal range, instruct the client to drink fluids until the urine runs clear and to consume reasonable amounts of dietary salt. Prescription support stockings (waist-high are most effective) can reduce pooling of blood in the lower legs. Counsel the client to maintain optimal blood sugar with high protein snacks and to avoid simple carbohydrates and caffeine.

The client with a tendency toward presyncope or syncope can learn physical counterpressure maneuvers that can prevent syncope. Such maneuvers include leg crossing with tensing of the leg, abdominal, and buttock muscles; lowering the body into a squatting position; gripping opposing hands with fingers and pulling the arms hard in opposing directions; clenching the fist forcefully; or touching the chin to the chest and tightening the neck (Charlton et al., 2019). Although lower-body maneuvers are more effective, upper-body movements can be useful in tight spaces, such as an airplane seat with little leg room.

Orthostatic Syncope

Orthostatic syncope is related to autonomic dysfunction causing abnormal distribution of blood volume. When a healthy nonpregnant person stands, 500–1,000 ml of blood pools in the lower extremities, decreasing venous return to the heart and thereby decreasing cardiac output and BP (Palma & Kaufman, 2022). The body quickly responds with the baroreceptor reflex, which increases sympathetic tone and reduces parasympathetic outflow. Peripheral vascular resistance, venous return, and cardiac output increase, reversing the drop in BP until it is clinically insignificant.

In pregnancy, progesterone decreases vascular tone, which can increase the pooling of blood in dependent areas with prolonged standing or sudden change from supine to standing. In the second half of pregnancy, pressure from the gravid uterus can decrease blood flow through the vena cava when the person is supine or seated upright. Dehydration can increase this effect by reducing blood volume. When the ambient temperature is high, heat syncope can result from vasodilation, peripheral pooling, and volume depletion.

Postprandial orthostatic hypotension involves a decrease in BP 1–2 hr after a meal. It occurs most often in individuals with diabetes, those with autonomic disorders, and in the elderly. This condition is thought to result from impaired sympathetic and baroreceptor reflex function, abnormal rate of small intestinal nutrient delivery, gastric distension, and pooling of blood in the gastrointestinal tract (Trahair, Horowitz, & Jones, 2014).

Postural orthostatic tachycardia syndrome (POTS) is a disorder of the autonomic nervous system characterized by orthostatic intolerance. Symptoms can include palpitations, tachycardia, nausea, presyncope, syncope, and nonorthostatic issues, such as fatigue, cognitive issues ("brain fog"), headache, and gastrointestinal symptoms (Morgan, Smith, & Blitshteyn, 2022). The prevalence of

Table 9-7 **Symptoms Associated with Loss of Consciousness Can Aid Diagnosis**
Headache Think preeclampsia, stroke, hypoglycemia, carbon monoxide (CO) poisoning, trauma, tumor.
Chest pain Think arrhythmia or another cardiac event, pulmonary embolism (PE).
Shortness of breath Think PE, cardiac event, asthma, anaphylaxis.
Thirst Think heatstroke, shock.
Numbness Think spinal trauma, stroke.
Unilateral weakness or paralysis Think stroke, hypoglycemia.

POTS has increased since 2020 because it can follow a COVID-19 infection (Morgan, Smith, et al., 2022). Each person with POTS in pregnancy is unique in symptomatology, but most typically symptoms worsen in the first trimester, improve in the second trimester, and have a variable course in the third trimester and postpartum (Morgan, Chojenta, Tavener, Smith, & Loxton, 2018). During labor, pain can trigger autonomic instability. Individuals who have significant POTS symptoms at the time of conception tend to have a worsening of symptoms during pregnancy. Mild to moderate symptoms can stabilize or improve. Postpartum, about 50% of individuals experience improvement, possibly due in part to improved physical conditioning and incidental upper-body resistance training that naturally occurs when caring for a baby (Morgan, Smith, et al., 2022).

Vasovagal (Neurocardiogenic) Syncope

Vasovagal (neurocardiogenic) syncope is one of the most common causes of fainting in the pregnant and nonpregnant populations. A vagal response can be triggered by straining on the toilet; a hot, crowded environment; or emotional upset (Charan & Guttula, 2021). The trigger causes increased firing of the vagus nerve (increased parasympathetic activity), resulting in profound bradycardia—or even several seconds of asystole (Jeanmonod, Sahni, & Silberman, 2023). Simultaneously, decreased sympathetic activity promotes vasodilation and the pooling of blood. Cardiac output and blood pressure fall precipitously, and the person becomes dizzy or faints (Yarlagadda et al., 2010). Prodromal signs and symptoms (presyncope) typically develop over 1–5 min before the syncopal episode. When these symptoms occur, vasovagal syncope can be prevented by positioning the client in a side-lying position with the heart at the level of the head.

Convulsive Syncope

Convulsive syncope is a seizure-like reaction resulting from cerebral hypoperfusion that affects roughly 12% of clients presenting with syncope (Sheldon & Raj, 2020; Shmuely, Bauer, van Zwet, van Dijk, & Thijs, 2018). Tonic extension of the trunk and a salvo of involuntary myoclonic jerks commonly accompany neurocardiogenic syncope (Shmuely et al., 2018). Convulsive movements can be subtle or dramatic and sometimes can mimic an epileptic seizure. Convulsive syncope is usually brief (less than 20 sec), and the client usually recovers rapidly when placed in a side-lying position with the head at or lower than the level of the heart. After convulsive syncope, the client is alert and oriented, whereas an epileptic seizure is followed by a postictal episode of confusion or lethargy (Schachter, 2022). The client with syncope loses all body tone, but the person with seizure typically retains muscle tone throughout the episode. Whereas a person having a seizure sometimes demonstrates chewing movements, incontinence, lip-smacking, grasping, tongue-biting, or foaming from the mouth, the client with syncopal jerking displays none of these. Interestingly, up to 20–30% of clients with nonepileptic convulsive disorders are misdiagnosed with epilepsy (Siddiqi, Blackmore, & Siddiqi, 2020). Syncope can be distinguished from seizures with head-up tilt-table testing combined with EEG (Sheldon & Raj, 2020).

Cardiac Syncope

Cardiac syncope occurs when the heart is unable to pump enough blood to perfuse the brain. It is usually related to cardiopulmonary disease, such as arrhythmia, structural heart disease, acute myocardial infarction, cardiac valve disease, aortic dissection, cardiomyopathy, or PE that leads to insufficient perfusion of the brain (Albassam et al., 2019). People with diabetes, hypertension, and hyperlipidemia are at greater risk for heart damage, as are people who smoke (Mizrachi & Sitammagari, 2023). Undiagnosed congenital heart disease can be a concern for clients who have lived with minimal access to primary care.

In most instances, cardiac syncope occurs abruptly without nausea, dizziness, or other prodromal symptoms, although chest pain or palpitations can precede the event. It can occur in any posture, while lying in bed, and during effort when the cardiac output does not meet the increased demand (Albassam et al., 2019). After awakening, clients may have persistent cardiac symptoms, such as chest pain or an abnormal heart rate or rhythm.

Management of Syncope

Syncope is self-limiting. Like presyncope, syncope usually resolves quickly if the victim is positioned in a side-lying position with the head at the same level as, or lower than, the heart. Syncope can be artificially prolonged if the victim remains sitting upright. If the client remains unresponsive after being laid flat, the situation may be more serious than vasovagal syncope.

When syncope is associated with trauma, the victim requires prompt evaluation at a medical facility. Try to determine whether trauma caused loss of consciousness, or if the trauma was the result of syncope. If the client had chest pain while driving, then fainted and hit a tree, consider cardiac syncope along with any traumatic injuries. If syncope occurred after the chest struck the steering wheel in an MVC, loss of consciousness may be driven by internal bleeding or pericardial tamponade. If the client fainted, fell, and sustained a head injury (or fell, then fainted after striking the head), loss of consciousness may denote a neurologic emergency.

Syncope of Greatest Concern:

Call emergency medical services (EMS) for immediate transfer to emergency department

- Known or suspected structural heart disease
- Family history of sudden death at a young age
- Syncope during exertion
- Sudden syncope without prodromal symptoms
- Recent repetitive episodes of syncope
- Prolonged syncope (more than 1–2 min of unresponsiveness)
- Injury preceding or resulting from syncope
- Chest pain, difficulty breathing, tachycardia
- Persistent hypotension or bradycardia

DIFFERENTIAL DIAGNOSES

Seizure, transient ischemic attack/cerebrovascular accident, cardiac disease, arrhythmia.

Seizures

A seizure is a sudden surge of unusual electrical activity between brain neurons that can cause abnormal muscle tone, movements, behaviors, sensations, emotions, or states of awareness. Most seizures can be categorized as either focal, involving a specific region of the brain, or generalized, involving both sides of the brain simultaneously (Schachter, 2022). The location of the abnormal electrical activity in the brain and the amount of cortex that is involved determine the clinical presentation of the seizure. Focal seizures that begin in the occipital cortex can be perceived by the client as flashing lights. Seizures that involve the motor cortex cause rhythmic jerking movements of the face, arm, or leg on the side of the body opposite to the involved cortex (Schachter, 2022). A seizure that begins in the parietal cortex can cause distortion of spatial perception; a seizure that begins in the dominant frontal lobe can cause sudden speech difficulties. The individual might experience an aura at the onset of seizure activity involving confusion, twitching, distortions in hearing, vision, or spatial perception, or other altered bodily sensations or movements.

Generalized Tonic-Clonic Seizures (Grand Mal)

Generalized tonic-clonic seizures begin with sudden loss of consciousness with the eyes remaining open. The tonic phase involves sustained contraction of most body muscles, first in flexion and then in extension, for about 10–20 sec (Elmali, Auvin, Bast, Rubboli, & Koutroumanidis, 2020). The tonic contraction of the respiratory muscles can force air through the closed vocal cords, causing a strange, high-pitched scream (Elmali et al., 2020). The individual is unable to breathe and may become cyanotic. In the clonic phase, which usually lasts about 40–70 sec, the muscle tension transforms into a series of strong, rapid, full-body jerks and spasms that progressively decrease in strength and frequency until they cease. The post-ictal state includes a variable period of unconsciousness during which the person becomes quiet and breathing resumes, often deep and snoring. Consciousness returns gradually, accompanied by confusion or agitation. Bladder or bowel incontinence can occur as the seizure subsides.

Status Epilepticus

Status epilepticus is defined as a seizure with 5 min or more of continuous clinical seizure activity *or* recurrent seizures without return to consciousness between seizures (Wylie, Sandhu, & Murr, 2023). Although a short seizure does not usually cause lasting damage to the body, status epilepticus can deplete the brain of glucose and oxygen and cause systemic hypoxia, hypercapnia, blood-pressure changes, hyperthermia, and organ damage. About 16–20% of individuals having a first episode of generalized convulsive status epilepticus die as a result (Wylie et al., 2023).

Focal Seizures with Retained Awareness

The person who has focal seizures with retained awareness usually remains aware and alert throughout the episode and remembers the seizure. The seizure might manifest as the jerking or stiffening of a limb or one side of the face or body; visual or auditory changes; perceiving a strange smell, taste, or touch; memory or emotional disturbances; or sensations of hot or

Table 9-8
Differentiating Seizure from Syncope

Characteristic	Syncope	Seizure
Frequency	Common	Rare
Position of client before the event	Upright, standing or sitting	Any position
Trigger	Upright position; voiding or moving bowels; needle stick sight or of blood; warm, crowded environment	Flashing lights, missed anticonvulsant medication, lack of sleep, stress, viral illness
Prodromal signs and symptoms	Prodrome: Visual changes such as blurred, grayed, spotty, or tunnel vision, lightheadedness, sensation of heat or cold, sweating, heart pounding	Aura: Odd taste in mouth; seeing flashes of light or colors; auditory buzzing, ringing, or tones; perception of bad odor; dizziness, tingling, numbness, or pain; twitching
Onset	Slow, over several minutes	Sudden, within 1 min
Activity during event	Flaccid muscle tone; sometimes several uncoordinated clonic jerks occur at onset	Active movement, incontinence, lateral tongue biting
Duration	Usually less than 30 sec	Usually 1–3 min
Postictal confusion	Rapid return to orientation	Slow return to orientation, usually involves unresponsive period

Adapted from (1) *Nancy Caroline's Emergency Care in the Streets* (8th ed.), by American Academy of Orthopedic Surgeons, 2018, Burlington, MA: Jones & Bartlett Learning. Copyright by Jones & Bartlett Learning. (2) "IF IT'S NOT EPILEPSY . . . ," by P. E. M. Smith, 2001, *Journal of Neurology, Neurosurgery & Psychiatry, 70*, Suppl. 2, pp. ii9–ii14. Copyright by BMJ Publishing Group.

cold. After the seizure, the person may return to normal functioning or may experience postictal confusion or sleepiness.

Focal Seizures with Impaired Awareness

A person having a focal seizure with impaired awareness often appears awake but does not interact normally. Signs and symptoms include an unfocused gaze; repeating words or phrases; engaging in repetitive behaviors; remaining motionless; or displaying facial grimacing, gesturing, chewing, or lip-smacking (Schachter, 2022). Focal seizures can also involve the shaking of one hand, a metallic taste in the mouth, movement of every limb, or loss of consciousness (AAOS, 2018). Focal seizures with impaired awareness usually last less than 3 min, after which the victim enters the postictal phase and may experience sleepiness, confusion, or headache for up to several hours. The person is likely to remember the aura but not the events that occurred during and immediately after the seizure.

Psychogenic Nonepileptic Seizures

Psychogenic nonepileptic seizures are events resembling seizures or syncopal episodes that are not accompanied by pathological changes in brain activity. They are regarded as involuntary behavioral responses to internal or external triggers and are thought to be related to past trauma or maladaptive coping.

Etiology of Seizure

Across the lifespan, seizures affect about 8–10% of the population and account for 1–2% of all visits to the emergency department (Schachter, 2022). Epilepsy, a disorder of the brain that causes seizures, is diagnosed if a client has two or more unprovoked seizures occurring more than 24 hr apart. Seizures can also accompany head injury, substance use and withdrawal, stroke, severe hypoglycemia, brain infection, brain tumor, traumatic brain injury, electrolyte abnormalities, eclampsia, or other issues.

When a pregnant client is found seizing, the midwife's first thought is often eclampsia. Although it is important to consider this possibility, some pregnant people have preexisting seizure disorders and can have seizures at any time (McElrath & Gerard, 2023). During pregnancy, clients with epilepsy may experience more-frequent seizures, perhaps because of pregnancy-related hemodilution and increased blood volume, changes in serum-binding proteins, increases in life stressors, disturbed sleep, or hormone changes (McElrath & Gerard, 2023). Concerned about the risk of fetal malformations, pregnant clients sometimes take their anticonvulsant medications less frequently or at lower doses.

Management of Seizures

Most seizures resolve spontaneously within 1–2 min. Place the client in a side-lying position that minimizes the risk of injury from a fall or from contact with nearby objects. Do not place anything in the mouth of a seizing client. Have suction available to clear the airway if necessary and provide supplemental oxygen (Silverman et al., 2017).

- Summon EMS for transport. Give an SBAR report.
- ABCs and POP: Maintain an open airway.
- Clear the area of objects that can cause injury.
- Loosen any clothing that might compress the neck.
- Remove eyeglasses.
- Take vital signs and FHR after the seizure is over.
- Do not leave the client unattended.
- Give oxygen if pulse oximetry shows an oxygen saturation less than 94%.
- Avoid excessive sensory stimulation.
- If eclampsia is suspected, the midwife or EMS personnel can administer magnesium sulfate if local protocols allow.

Some clients with epilepsy consider seizures a commonplace event and refuse medical treatment after regaining consciousness. *Any* pregnant or postpartum client who has a seizure should be transported to the hospital. Seizures can be the first indication of eclampsia, stroke, or other serious problem. The hypoxia, electrolyte imbalance, and hyperthermia that sometimes accompany a seizure can be injurious to mother and baby.

Carbon Monoxide (CO) Poisoning

Carbon monoxide is an odorless, colorless gas formed by the incomplete combustion of organic compounds. CO intoxication is a leading cause of poison-related mortality and morbidity in industrialized countries. Although most cases of CO poisoning result from fire-related smoke inhalation, toxicity in pregnant people is usually due to accidental household exposure (Friedman & Stiller, 2016). CO toxicity can occur when exhaust systems malfunction, especially in poorly ventilated areas, or when equipment designed for the outdoors is used indoors. Possible sources include gas water heaters, kerosene space heaters, charcoal grills, propane stoves, and propane-fueled forklifts. When hurricanes cause power outages, it is not uncommon for people to develop CO toxicity from outdoor gasoline-powered backup generators placed too near HVAC equipment that draws the gas indoors. House fires generate CO along with other toxins, such as cyanide. Some suicides involve CO exposure. Fumes from some spray paints, solvents, degreasers, and paint removers are converted to CO in the liver. Smokers have baseline levels of carboxyhemoglobin around 10–15% and are more susceptible to toxic effects from other sources of CO (Manaker & Perry, 2023).

CO easily binds with maternal hemoglobin—its affinity is 240 times that of oxygen—and dissolves in the maternal blood

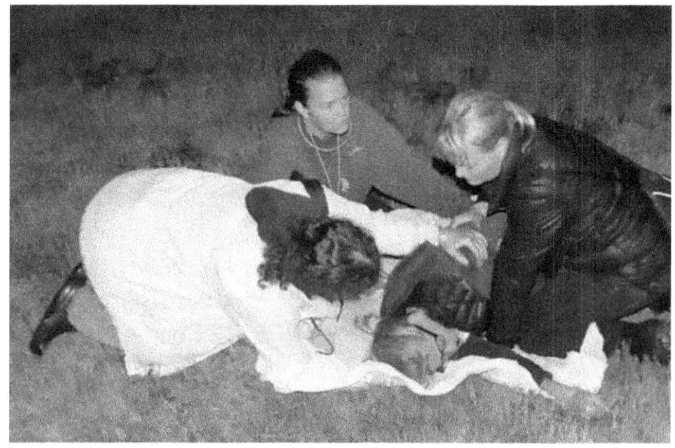

Figure 9-11. In a disaster-simulation drill, rescuers manage a seizing pregnant woman by rolling her to her side, removing her glasses, and protecting her from injury until the seizure subsides.

(Manaker & Perry, 2023). When the hemoglobin is saturated with CO, it cannot pick up oxygen, and the victim becomes hypoxic at the cellular level. The nervous system and heart are very susceptible to damage from CO poisoning, but other tissues can be affected.

CO diffuses across the placenta and binds even more readily with fetal hemoglobin. Levels of CO in fetal hemoglobin can become 10–15% higher in the fetus than in the mother and persist even after the mother begins to improve (Kosaki et al., 2021). Although fetuses exposed to mild or moderate CO poisoning usually develop normally, severe CO poisoning can lead to fetal limb malformation, microcephaly, hypotonia, persistent seizures, areflexia, and mental or motor disabilities, depending on the duration and severity of exposure and the stage of pregnancy when it occurs (Kosaki et al., 2021).

Victims of CO poisoning often overlook or fail to notice the symptoms, which can include headache, dizziness, nausea, flulike malaise, exertional dyspnea, chest pain, ventricular dysrhythmias, disorientation, lethargy, hallucinations, agitation, lack of coordination, abdominal pain, syncope, seizure, and coma. Cherry-red skin is a rare sign of severe toxicity; most CO poisoning victims are pale and cyanotic. Small infants may present with only vomiting and sometimes show symptoms before anyone else. Clients who present with these symptoms should be questioned about the use of gas- or oil-fueled appliances and the presence of similar symptoms in other household members, in pets, or in neighbors within the same building.

Emergency treatment priorities include stabilization of airway, breathing, and circulation; removal from the toxic environment; application of 100% oxygen; cardiac monitoring; and rapid transport. Give an SBAR report to convey information to the paramedic (or equivalent) or the receiving hospital. The pregnant client with high carboxyhemoglobin levels or serious symptoms can require treatment with hyperbaric oxygen at a regional facility. Hyperbaric oxygen accelerates the clearance of CO from the body, correcting hypoxia and preventing central nervous system damage (Kosaki et al., 2021).

Table 9-9

Sample GOLDCART History for Altered Level of Consciousness

(Information can be solicited from family or bystanders if the client cannot answer.)

General situation and history—Has this happened before? Is there a diagnosis? Has there been a recent illness? Is there any possibility of recent head injury? How many weeks pregnant are you? Do you have any health issues or pregnancy complications? How old are you? How many pregnancies have you had and how many babies? Is the baby moving?
Onset—When did the episode begin? What were you doing? Was the onset gradual or rapid? In what order did signs and symptoms appear? Did the episode follow the ingestion of any food, medication, or substance? Did you fall? Did you hit your head when you fell? Did an aura or prodrome precede loss of consciousness (consider seizure or syncope)? Was return to alertness relatively quick (probably syncope) or prolonged (consider seizure)? Did the light-headedness cause the fall (presyncope or syncope), or did you start to feel dizzy after the fall (trauma)?
Location—Where is your pain? Where do you have abnormal sensation or weakness? Does it start in one place and radiate to somewhere else? Where?
Duration—How long have you had symptoms? When was the onset? When did it change character?
Characteristics—Is the pain stabbing, shooting, or dull? Is the abnormal sensation tingly, prickly, itchy, or numb?
Associated symptoms—Any pain, weakness, headache, sweating, visual changes, numbness, shortness of breath, nausea, vomiting, fever, diarrhea, dizziness, or fainting?
Relieving/aggravating factors—Did you feel better or worse after eating? Did your symptoms improve when you changed position? Which position makes it better or worse?
Treatment—Have providers evaluated these symptoms previously? What did they recommend? Have you been following the recommendations? Have you been using alternative remedies? Has your condition changed since these treatments?

Heat-Related Illness

Like all warm-blooded animals, human beings must maintain body temperature within a narrow range to support normal functions. The body maintains normal temperature by balancing heat gains and losses. Processes such as skeletal muscle contraction and digestion generate heat. Dilating vessels on the skin increases heat loss, as does tachycardia (which speeds up blood flow), perspiration (especially when conditions allow it to evaporate rapidly), and respiration (which exchanges warm air for cool). When exposed to high temperatures, pregnant people, especially those in lower socioeconomic groups, are at risk for adverse pregnancy outcomes, including PTB and stillbirth (Chersich et al., 2020).

Extremes of heat can cause alteration in level of consciousness. Heat syncope can result from venous pooling and volume depletion. The client will usually make a full recovery if moved to a cool environment, allowed to rest in a side-lying position, and encouraged to take oral fluids.

Heat exhaustion can occur when someone in a warm ambient environment suffers excessive fluid loss with insufficient rehydration. Clients with heat exhaustion may show tachycardia; muscle weakness or cramps; thirst; anxiety; headache; nausea and vomiting; or hot, red skin. They usually recover after moving to a cool environment, resting in a side-lying position, and drinking at least 1 L of water or electrolyte beverage per hr. If recovery is not rapid or fetal heart tones are not reassuring, transport to a higher level of care.

Uncorrected, heat exhaustion can progress to heatstroke, a life-threatening systemic inflammatory reaction which can involve extreme hyperthermia, central nervous system dysfunction, and multiorgan failure (Epstein & Yanovich, 2019). Nonexertional heatstroke can develop during prolonged exposure to a hot environment with insufficient hydration. Exertional heatstroke can develop during heavy exercise on a hot, humid day. Core body temperature soars to 104.9°F (40.5°C) or higher, and sweating is no longer present. Respirations are rapid. Nausea, vomiting, hypotension, confusion, oliguria, loss of consciousness, or seizures can occur. Heatstroke requires rapid transport by ambulance, ice packs in the groin and axillae, rapid infusions of NS, and airway management as indicated by the client's condition.

Exercise-associated hyponatremia (EAH) can occur when athletes drink large amounts of water or sweat heavily without replacing electrolytes (Coffey et al., 2023), but it can develop during noncompetitive recreation or manual labor, commonly with high ambient temperature or insufficient air flow. It can occur up to 24 hr after prolonged exertion, as in endurance sports such as running or hiking (Grace, 2021). EAH is often associated with prolonged exertion (e.g., exercising for more than 4 hr), inadequate training or preparation, and high or low body mass index (BMI). Consider EAH in those who are aggressively hydrating with plain water who develop nausea and vomiting, headache, dizziness, confusion, headache, lethargy, seizures, anorexia, or coma (Klingert et al., 2022).

Other Etiologies of Altered Level of Consciousness

Trauma

Trauma, particularly when it involves hypoxia, shock, or head injury, can cause unconsciousness. Consider whether unconsciousness was caused by traumatic injury, or if a medical event such as hypoglycemia precipitated the trauma. If one pupil is dilated and unresponsive to light, suspect severe head injury or stroke. Cushing's triad (bradycardia, respiratory depression, and hypertension) can indicate elevated intracranial pressure secondary to head injury (E. R. Smith & Amin-Hanjani, 2019). Head injury is not usually associated with hypotension.

Diabetes

Individuals with diabetes can experience alterations in consciousness related to glucose levels, especially when insulin dependent, and can experience wide swings in blood sugar, from significantly hyperglycemic to seriously hypoglycemic, sometimes within a span of hours. Unstable blood glucose is most often seen in those who are learning to use insulin or who are noncompliant with treatment.

Hypoglycemia usually has a rapid onset and can be caused by too much insulin, inadequate food intake after insulin dose, exertion, malnutrition, sepsis, cancer (especially pancreatic), or hypothermia. Hypoglycemia can present with any of the following signs and symptoms:

- Fatigue
- Irregular or fast pulse
- Pale moist skin
- Shakiness
- Anxiety
- Irritability
- Tingling or numbness of the face or lips

Rarely, hypoglycemia can present similarly to stroke (especially in elderly people) with confusion, slurred speech, unilateral weakness or paralysis, and facial drooping.

Diabetic ketoacidosis (DKA) occurs when there is insufficient insulin to allow glucose to move from the blood into the cells. The cells become starved for glucose and begin to break down primary fats for energy, resulting in acidosis. DKA evolves over 12–48 hr. Symptoms of severe hyperglycemia are increased volume of urination, thirst, hunger, and fatigue, progressing to coma, deep respirations (Kussmaul), and acetone-scented breath. DKA is treated with insulin, IV fluids, careful attention to electrolytes (including calcium, phosphorus, potassium, and magnesium), and addressing the cause.

AVPU

Alert: Awake; eyes open; may be oriented to time, place, and person or disoriented.

Verbal: Appears asleep, but rouses when spoken to. Take note of any confusion or disorientation.

Painful stimuli: Not responsive to verbal stimulation but responds to painful stimuli. Pinch the fingernails or drag your knuckles over the sternum and observe the reaction. Purposeful responses include awakening, moaning, pushing you away, or withdrawing. Nonpurposeful responses to painful stimuli include decorticate posturing (arms flexed, legs extended) and decerebrate posturing (arms and legs extended), both of which can indicate grave neurological damage.

Unresponsive: Comatose, no response to any stimulus.

Poisoning

Poisoning can be accidental or intentional. Excessive alcohol consumption can cause a life-threatening coma. Sympathomimetics such as cocaine and methamphetamine can cause tachycardia, hypertension, dilated pupils, delirium, stroke, or cardiac arrest. Cholinergic substances found in pesticides (organophosphates, carbamates) and nerve agents (sarin, somin) cause headache, dizziness, bradycardia, weakness, coma, seizures, and SLUDGE (**S**alivation, **L**acrimation, **U**rination, **D**efecation, **G**astrointestinal upset, and **E**mesis). Atropine in large doses can reverse the effects.

A client with acute opiate toxicity from an overdose of heroin or prescription narcotic medications will have respiratory depression and pupils constricted to pinpoints. An IV drug abuser may have visible track marks. Naloxone 2 mg administered via nasal spray or very slowly by IV push will temporarily reverse the symptoms of opiate overdose and restore normal respiration.

Stroke

Suspect stroke in any client with altered level of consciousness. Associated symptoms include severe headache, vomiting,

Alert and Oriented x 4

Person—Knows one's own name.

Place—Knows location.

Time—Knows the date.

Purpose—Knows what was happening when the event occurred.

hemiparesis or hemiplegia, aphasia, unequal pupils, facial droop, slurred speech, drooling, unequal handgrips, seizures, incontinence, ataxia, vision problems, and vertigo.

Managing the Client with Altered Level of Consciousness

When a client develops an altered level of consciousness in a community setting, the midwife must rapidly evaluate and treat. Activate EMS to initiate transport to the hospital. Try to determine the etiology of the signs and symptoms and tailor management to your findings.

Initial Assessment

Use the chief complaint and information gained during the physical assessment to form a clinical impression and to guide management decisions. Respiration, pulse, mental status, skin color, temperature, and condition reflect the functioning of the respiratory, cardiovascular, and neurologic systems (AAOS, 2018). These critical systems maintain homeostasis as a tripod supports a camera. If one leg collapses, so will the others (AAOS, 2018).

The goals of management for the midwifery client with altered level of consciousness are to support vital functions, gather information about the possible causes, look for signs of trauma, and get the client to definitive care as rapidly as possible if the condition is serious. The information you gather at the scene can be invaluable to future providers. Do not delay transport to try determining a cause if the client is unstable.

GOLDCART History

Perform a GOLDCART history while simultaneously conducting a primary survey as detailed in chapter 4. When a client with altered mental status is unable to tell you what is wrong, you need to form your initial clinical impression from clues and signs. If an unresponsive pregnant client is not known to you, obtain history from witnesses or bystanders. Consider environmental clues such as unusual odors, others with similar symptoms in the vicinity, suicide notes, weapons, and drug containers or paraphernalia. Sometimes you will be unable to determine the cause of the client's symptoms.

Level of Consciousness, Motor Responses, and Reflexes

Use the mnemonic AVPU (**A**lert, **V**erbal, **P**ainful stimuli, **U**nresponsive) to categorize whether the client is alert, responds to verbal or painful stimuli, or is unresponsive. Wakefulness and awareness involve the coordinated activity of many areas of the brain. This network of brain structures is operative in people with spontaneous eye opening (Alert) or who open their eyes to the sound of a name being called (Verbal). If the client's eyes do not open to voice or a gentle shake, the provider can apply a painful stimulus (trapezius muscle squeeze, supraorbital pressure, mandibular pressure, or sternal rub) to test the level of cerebral function (Painful stimuli). A purposeful response such as a moan, defensive movements, or withdrawal indicates a higher level of cerebral function than a nonpurposeful or absent response. Decorticate posturing (arms bent inward on the chest, clenched fists, legs extended, feet turned inward) and decerebrate posturing (head is arched back with extension, adduction, and pronation of the arms, and extension of the legs) in response to painful stimuli can be an ominous sign of severe brain damage. A deeply unconscious client will have no response at all (Unresponsive).

Pupils

Assessing the reactivity of the pupils can determine whether altered mental status or coma has a metabolic or structural cause. If the pupils are unequal or not reacting to light, the problem may be structural, for example, a subarachnoid hemorrhage, tumor, stroke, or epidural hematoma (Mistovich et al., 2006). A client with altered mental status or coma from a metabolic etiology such as hypoglycemia, hypoxia, electrolyte imbalance, or drug overdose usually has equal pupils that react normally to light. Some people normally have unequal pupils (anisocoria). Although midposition fixed pupils are seen with severe sedative drug overdose or hypothermia, fixed dilated pupils may denote brain death. People who have overdosed with certain narcotics (morphine, heroin, codeine) usually have an altered mental status, slow or absent respirations, and pinpoint pupils.

Transfer Care

If the client is stable and alert, consult a physician or transfer care as indicated. Clients who are unresponsive or with significant mental status changes always require rapid transport to an appropriate facility, preferably by ambulance. If there is no trauma, move the unconscious client into the left lateral position to let secretions flow out of the mouth and to maximize placental perfusion. Call EMS and

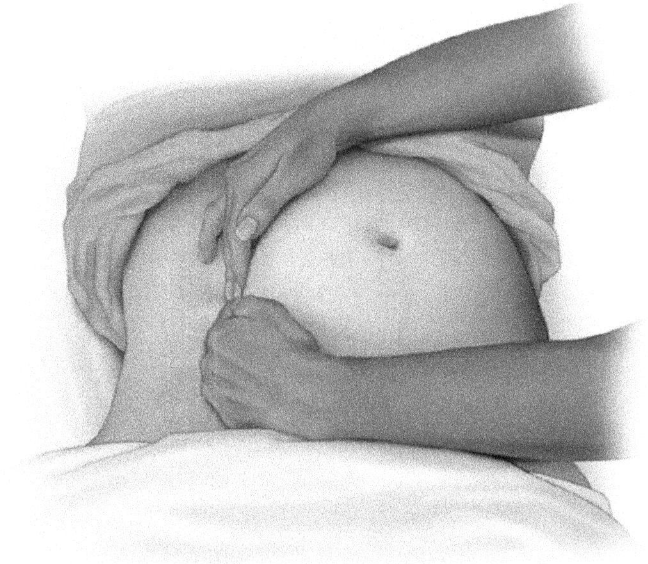

Figure 9-12. Left uterine displacement with two-handed technique. From "Maternal Cardiac Arrest: A Practical and Comprehensive Review," by F. M. Jeejeebhoy and L. J. Morrison, 2013, *Emergency Medicine International, 2013*, article 274814, fig. 2. CC BY 3.0.

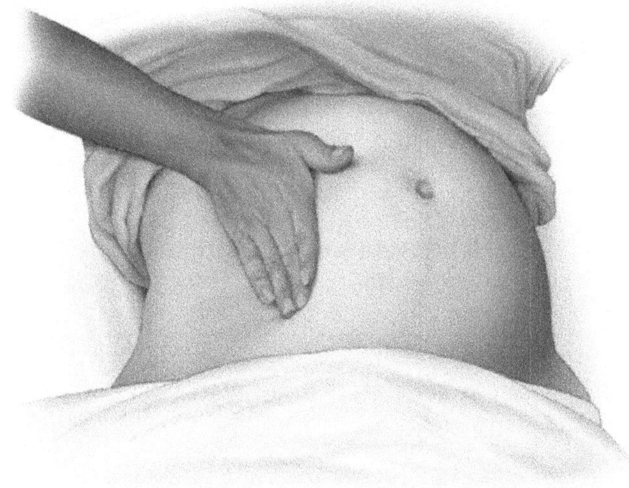

Figure 9-13. Left uterine displacement using one-handed technique. From "Maternal Cardiac Arrest: A Practical and Comprehensive Review," by F. M. Jeejeebhoy and L. J. Morrison, 2013, *Emergency Medicine International, 2013*, article 274814, fig. 3. CC BY 3.0.

stay by your client's side providing basic life support (see Chapter 4) while waiting for the ambulance to arrive. If there is trauma, manage as discussed earlier in this chapter. Frequently assess FHR. Start an IV line of NS or LR. If BP is low because of hypovolemia, institute appropriate fluid replacement.

Give an SBAR report to the EMS responder and, if possible, accompany your client to the hospital with records in hand. EMS management can include cardiac monitoring, IV fluid administration, high-flow oxygen, glucose testing, and perhaps medications such as naloxone. Throughout transport, perform reassessment, which includes rechecking and responding to vital signs and monitoring signs and symptoms.

At the hospital, providers will perform basic life support and attempt to discover or confirm a diagnosis. Clients with altered level of consciousness usually require urine and blood analysis and may also need computerized tomography or magnetic-resonance imaging to determine etiology. Clients suspected of infection of the central nervous system will undergo lumbar puncture so that cerebrospinal fluid can be evaluated. An electroencephalogram can be used to detect seizures. After the client has an accurate diagnosis, a plan should be made for definitive treatment.

Cardiac Arrest in Pregnancy

Cardiac arrest in pregnancy is a rare but catastrophic occurrence. Zelop & Brickner (2023) note that in the United States and United Kingdom, most cardiac arrests in pregnant people follow PE (29%), hemorrhage (17%), sepsis (13%), peripartum cardiomyopathy (8%), stroke (5%), preeclampsia-eclampsia (2.8%), or complications related to anesthesia (2%). Other causes include amniotic fluid embolism, myocardial infarction, preexisting cardiac disease, anaphylaxis, and trauma (Banayan et al., 2016; Zelop & Brickner, 2023).

Anatomical changes of pregnancy work against successful resuscitation of the pregnant client in cardiac arrest. Greater oxygen requirements and reduced chest compliance make ventilation more difficult. Flared ribs, raised diaphragm, increased body fat, and breast tissue enlargement make performing chest compression on a pregnant client challenging. Vomiting and subsequent aspiration are common.

When cardiac arrest occurs, follow American Heart Association (AHA) guidelines for adult cardiopulmonary resuscitation (CPR) with recommended modifications for the pregnant victim. Early and high-quality CPR, rapid transport, and rapid access to definitive care offer the best chance of a good outcome. These steps should involve multiple rescuers and are often performed simultaneously. EMS providers are well trained and equipped to manage a cardiac arrest, and paramedics (U.S.) and their equivalents can intubate and initiate Advanced Cardiac Life Support protocols.

1. **Recognize and Respond**—Make sure the scene is safe before approaching. Confirm unresponsiveness by tapping the victim's shoulder and shouting, "Are you all right?"
2. **Assess**—Health care professionals should take no more than 10 sec to check for a carotid pulse (Elmer, 2023). While doing so, the provider observes the client's

Table 9-10 **The Resuscitation CCAB**
Cervical spine/Control hemorrhage Consider restricting neck motion if there is trauma. Control hemorrhage.
Circulation Begin chest compressions following American Heart Association (AHA) guidelines. Push hard and fast at a rate of 100–120 compressions per min.
Airway Open the airway quickly with the head tilt-jaw thrust or head tilt-chin lift maneuver. Suction the airway when vomitus is present. Remove loose foreign bodies from the mouth. If you have an oral airway, you can insert it.
Breathing If the pregnant client is not breathing adequately, begin intermittent positive pressure using mouth-to-mouth or mouth-to-airway until a self-inflating bag and mask are available. Ventilate with the head and neck in a sniffing position without a pillow under the head. Continue ventilating with 100% oxygen via bag and mask. Apply cricoid pressure to block aspiration until the airway has been protected by a cuffed tracheal tube.
CCAB is a modification of the life support sequence recommended by the American Academy of Orthopedic Surgeons (2018). See also "Approaching the Victim" in Chapter 4.

respirations, and notes apnea or gasping, or if the client is pulseless. Lay rescuers should *not* check the victim's pulse and should assume the client is apneic if breathing is not evident (Kleinman et al., 2015).

3. **Activate** the emergency response system and call for an automated external defibrillator (AED).
4. **Lateral Uterine Displacement**—Ensure that the victim is on a firm surface—move the client to the floor or use a backboard if in bed. When the fundal height is greater than the umbilicus, supine positioning is likely to cause aortocaval compression. A left lateral tilt of the pregnant client from head to toe at an angle of 15–30° will usually relieve aortocaval compression while promoting effective chest compressions (Chu, Johnston, & Geohegan, 2020). The alternative is to displace the uterus laterally during resuscitative efforts and throughout postarrest care (Jeejeebhoy et al., 2015). To perform lateral uterine displacement, the provider stands to the left of the client, cups the uterus in two hands, and lifts the uterus upward and to the left off the maternal vessels (Figure 9-12). Alternatively, the provider can stand on the client's right (Figure 9-13) and push upward and to the left with one hand (Jeejeebhoy et al., 2015).
5. **Chest compressions**—Immediately start CPR. Chest compressions, applied with optimal rate, depth, and force without interruption, are the most essential element of CPR. After cardiac arrest, the lungs usually contain air and the pulmonary vessels and heart usually contain oxygenated blood. Compressions deliver this oxygen to the tissues.

   To perform compressions, place the heel of one hand in the center of the chest over the lower part of the sternum and the heel of their opposite hand on top of the first. This is the same hand position used for any adult victim. Straighten your arms and move your chest to a position directly over your hands, so you can use your body weight rather than your arm muscles to perform compressions. Continually reassess the rate and depth of your compressions to ensure that each one is optimally effective. Resuscitation is more likely to be successful if the depth is adequate and you allow full chest recoil between down-strokes (Elmer, 2023). Compress the chest at a rate of at 100–120 compressions per min with a depth of 2.0–2.5 in. (5–6 cm) with each downstroke. Allow the chest to recoil completely between downstrokes.

   When two or more rescuers are present, they should take turns doing chest compressions every 2 min, switching roles when the rhythm is assessed. Interruptions in chest compressions should be minimized except for certain interventions such as intubation or use of an AED. When compressions stop even briefly, perfusion pressure declines and client outcomes worsen. AHA uses the Bee Gees' song "Stayin' Alive" (Gibb, Gibb, & Gibb, 1977) to imprint the correct compression rate of about 100 bpm in the mind of the rescuer (Hafner, Jou, Wang, Bleess, & Tham, 2015; Hafner, Sturgell, Matlock, Bockewitz, & Barker, 2012; Kim et al., 2017; Tastan et al., 2017). This internal metronome for cardiac compressions is effective for laypeople and professionals alike (AHA, 2016a; Hafner, Jou, et al., 2015; Hafner, Sturgell, et al., 2012; Kim et al., 2017; Tastan et al., 2017).

   The next steps are of equal importance and should be initiated as soon as possible with several providers working together: airway management, ventilation, and defibrillation.
6. **Airway Management**—If spinal injury is suspected, place one hand on each side of the victim's head to restrict movement. Use the jaw-thrust maneuver to open

the airway by placing your thumbs on each cheekbone and your fingers under the lower jaw, then moving the lower jaw forward with your fingers while pressing with your thumbs. If there is no evidence of trauma, use the head-tilt chin-lift maneuver. Apply downward pressure to the client's forehead with one hand and lift the mandible below the chin with the other.

7. **Breathing support**—Give two breaths of normal ventilation volume. Attach high-flow oxygen if using mouth-to-mask or bag-mask ventilation (Link et al., 2015). If the uterus is very large, a pregnant client may need a smaller volume of air with each breath than a nonpregnant client (Zelop & Brickner, 2023). Immediately restart compressions. Continue cycles of 30 compressions and 2 breaths until EMS arrives or you are physically unable to continue.
8. **Advanced Airway**—Although there is inadequate evidence of improved survival or neurological outcome to recommend use of an advanced airway over a self-inflating bag resuscitator (Link et al., 2015), endotracheal (ET) intubation or supraglottic airway devices (SGA-laryngeal mask airway, laryngeal tube, or esophageal obturator airway) can protect against aspiration and gastric distension. Research disagrees on whether the use of an SGA device yields better outcomes than ET intubation (Link et al., 2015). Clearly, an SGA device is easier to use and requires much less training and practice. Perform bag-mask ventilation with 100% oxygen and suction the airway before placing an SGA or ET tube. If the victim has an advanced airway in place, deliver one breath every 6 sec to give 10 per min asynchronously while compressions continue.
9. **Defibrillate**—As soon as an AED becomes available, turn it on and follow prompts. The AED protocol is the same for a pregnant client as for any adult. Applying defibrillation and cardioversion shocks to the mother's chest passes minimal energy to the fetus and is considered safe throughout pregnancy (Zelop & Brickner, 2023). Follow the prompts and place one pad to the right of the sternum just below the clavicle and the other lateral to the cardiac apex midaxillary line, avoiding contact with breast tissue (Zelop & Brickner, 2023). Fetal monitors do not need to be removed before defibrillating the mother (Zelop & Brickner, 2023).
10. **IV/Intraosseous (IO) Access**—Rapid vascular access is necessary to administer drugs and fluids in critically ill clients. If personnel are available and time allows, place two large-bore IV catheters in the antecubital fossae. Because veins collapse during cardiac arrest, venous access can be difficult to obtain. IO access is a technique of inserting a needle into the medullary space or a bone and infusing fluids or medications directly into the highly vascularized bone marrow (Petitpas et al., 2016). IO access is quick, easy to learn and use, and effective. In adults and older children, IO access can be placed in the humeral head, proximal tibia, medial malleolus, sternum, distal radius, distal femur, and anterior-superior iliac spine (AHA, 2016b; de Vogel et al., 2011; Engels et al., 2016; Link et al., 2015).
11. **Medication Administration**—The advanced cardiac life support (ACLS) guidelines for pregnancy are the same as for the nonpregnant client. For the client in cardiac arrest, benefits outweigh risks if the medication restores circulation.
12. **Resuscitative Hysterotomy**—When cardiac arrest occurs in a hospital with a pregnant client and viable fetus, resuscitative hysterotomy (also known as a perimortem cesarean) is performed 4 min after cardiac arrest to improve survival of both mother and baby (Edelson et al., 2020; Zelop & Brickner, 2023). After the uterus is emptied, maternal cardiac output can increase by 60–80%, improving the chance for the mother's survival (Zelop & Brickner, 2023).

Experts disagree on the gestational age threshold at which to perform resuscitative hysterotomy. The age of neonatal viability is also controversial. Some newborns with immediate access to high-level neonatal intensive care can survive without deficits as early as 23–24 weeks of gestation (Guillén et al., 2015). Many hospitals provide full resuscitative care to infants 24 0/7 weeks of gestation and greater, and some provide full resuscitation for infants as young as 22 0/7 weeks of gestation. It is considered reasonable to perform perimortem hysterotomy for pregnancies at 20 weeks of gestation or later or with uterine size at or above the umbilicus to improve maternal survival regardless of whether the fetus is viable. (Zelop & Brickner, 2023). If the fetus is viable, perimortem hysterotomy can benefit the fetus as well.

Delivery should be performed at the site of resuscitation. The skin incision should be made by 4 min after cardiac arrest, and birth of the infant should occur by 5 min after onset—"the five-minute rule" (Zelop & Brickner, 2023). A vertical incision provides rapid access. Bleeding is often minimal because of poor perfusion. Chest compressions should continue without interruption. If the client is completely dilated and the fetus is at a low station, assisted vaginal birth with forceps or a vacuum device can be an appropriate alternative.

13. **Invasive CPR**—In a tertiary hospital, thoracotomy may be performed and open-heart massage initiated after 15 min of maternal cardiac arrest (Zelop & Brickner, 2023). Direct cardiac compression can provide near-normal perfusion of the brain and heart and improve chances of surviving cardiac arrest (Link et al., 2015).

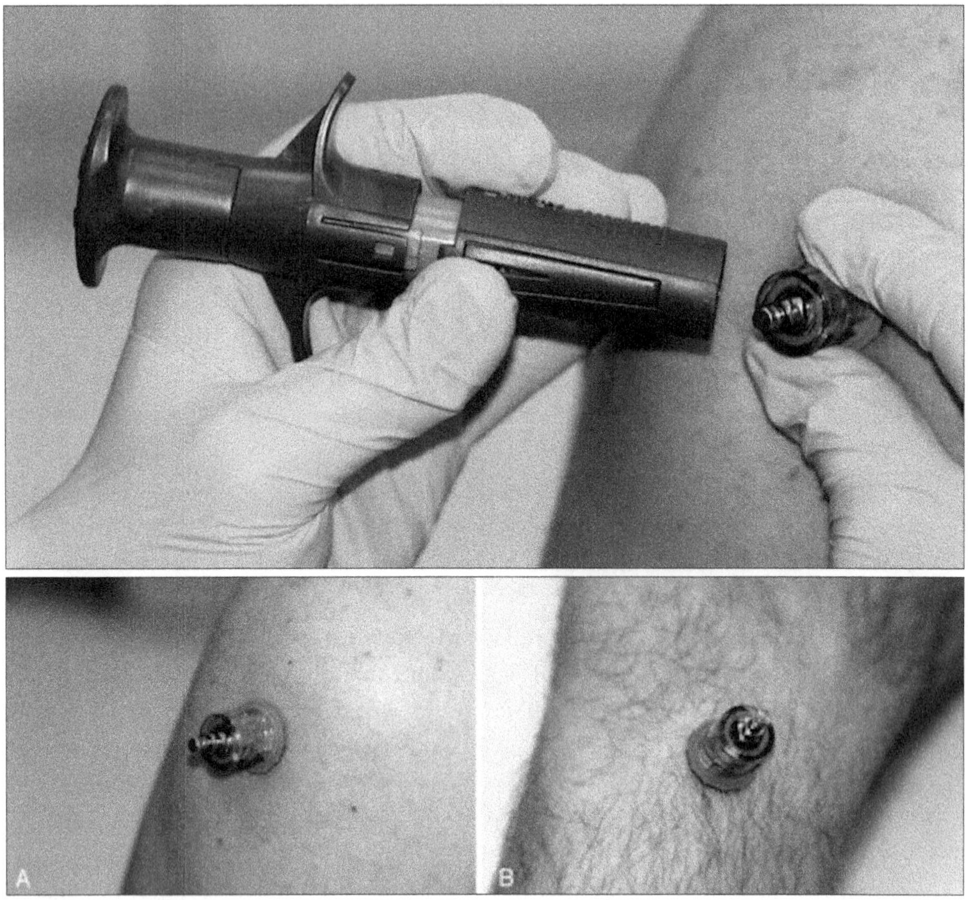

Figure 9-14. A disposable, spring-driven intraosseous (IO) access device (with an integrated trigger) approved by the U.S. Food and Drug Administration (A) into the humeral head on a cadaver; (B) into the proximal tibia. From "A Randomized Cadaver Study Comparing First-Attempt Success Between Tibial and Humeral Intraosseous Insertions Using NIO Device by Paramedics: A Preliminary Investigation," by L. Szarpak et al., 2016, *Medicine, 95*(20), fig. 1 [left] and fig. 3 [right]. CC BY 4.0.

Outcomes

In the nonpregnant client, brain damage can occur after 4–6 min of cardiac arrest (Zelop & Brickner, 2023). Pregnant people desaturate more quickly. Even if the cause of the cardiac arrest is survivable, the odds of successful resuscitation for the mother and fetus are low, even if everyone managing the case performed brilliantly. This is especially true if cardiac arrest occurs outside the hospital. The loss of a mother is devastating for any midwife. Any provider who experiences a maternal death should consider counseling to work through the inevitable difficult emotions that follow.

Topics for Discussion

1. You are waiting in a long checkout line in a busy department store when the pregnant shopper ahead of you crumples to the floor, jerks once, and lies still. What do you do?
2. Your client, Anna Rose E., 32 weeks pregnant, calls to report that she was in a minor car accident an hour ago. She was the unbelted driver in a compact car that hit a stopped car ahead of her at about 30 mph (48 kph). Both vehicles have significant damage but are not totaled. Her airbag deployed. Anna Rose tells you that everyone in both cars is "fine," but she has been having "more Braxton-Hicks contractions than usual" since the incident, and her abdomen is sore to the touch. What is your plan for Anna Rose?
3. Consuela and her baby Jorge had a home birth 2 days ago. When you arrive to conduct a postpartum assessment, you find Consuela moaning in her bed. Her partner Jennifer tells you that she came home from work this morning and found Consuela with a high fever, vomiting, shaking chills, and mild confusion. When you take Consuela's vital signs, her pulse is 120, her SBP is 100, and her temperature is 102°F (38.9°C). Her fundus is 2 cm above the umbilicus and very tender. What do you suspect? What do you do?
4. An hour after the baby is born, the house is filled with family members bearing gifts for the new arrival. You are helping the mother to latch the baby to the breast when you hear a crash. You spin around to see your client's sister having a grand mal seizure on the floor. What do you do?
5. Adeline Y., 34 weeks pregnant, calls at 11 p.m. complaining of a headache. Using the GOLDCART method, what questions would you ask her to assess her complaint?

References

Acar, B. S., & Meric, M. (2017). The effect of placenta location on the safety of pregnant driver and her fetus. *International Journal of Crashworthiness, 22*(2), 163–168. https://doi.org/10.1080/13588265.2016.1243609

AFE Foundation. (2023). AFE emergency stabilization checklist. Retrieved from https://amnioticfluidembolism.org/wp-content/uploads/2024/02/AFE-2023-EmergencyChecklist-1.pdf

Albassam, O. T., Redelmeier, R. J., Shadowitz, S., Husain, A. M., Simel, D., & Etchells, E. E. (2019). Did this patient have cardiac syncope? The rational clinical examination systematic review. *JAMA, 321*(24), 2448–2457. https://doi.org/10.1001/jama.2019.8001

Almuwallad, A., Cole, E., Ross, J., Perkins, Z., & Davenport, R. (2021). The impact of prehospital TXA on mortality among bleeding trauma patients: A systematic review and meta-analysis. *Journal of Trauma and Acute Care Surgery, 90*(5), 901–907. https://doi.org/10.1097/TA.0000000000003120

American Academy of Orthopedic Surgeons. (2018). *Nancy Caroline's emergency care in the streets* (8th ed.). Burlington, MA: Jones & Bartlett Learning.

American College of Obstetricians and Gynecologists Committee on Health Care for Underserved Women. (2012, reaffirmed 2022). *Intimate partner violence* (Committee Opinion 518). Retrieved from https://www.acog.org/clinical/clinical-guidance/committee-opinion/articles/2012/02/intimate-partner-violence

American College of Surgeons Committee on Trauma. (2018). *Advanced Trauma Life Support® student course manual* (10th ed.). Chicago, IL: American College of Surgeons.

American Heart Association. (2016a). *2016 hands-only CPR fact sheet*. Retrieved from http://cpr.heart.org/idc/groups/heart-public/@wcm/@ecc/documents/downloadable/ucm_487417.pdf

American Heart Association. (2016b). *ACLS provider manual: Supplementary material*. n.p.: Author. Retrieved from https://ahainstructornetwork.americanheart.org/idc/groups/ahaecc-public/@wcm/@ecc/documents/downloadable/ucm_481402.pdf

American Stroke Association. (n.d.). *Ischemic stroke (clots)*. Retrieved from https://www.stroke.org/en/about-stroke/types-of-stroke/ischemic-stroke-clots

Amezcua-Prieto, C., Ross, J., Rogozińska, E., Mighiu, P., Martínez-Ruiz, V., Brohi, K., . . . Thangaratinam, S. (2020). Maternal trauma due to motor vehicle crashes and pregnancy outcomes: A systematic review and meta-analysis. *BMJ Open, 10*(10). https://doi.org/10.1136/bmjopen-2019-035562

Ananth, C. V., & Kinzler, W. L. (2022). Acute placental abruption: Pathophysiology, clinical features, diagnosis, and consequences. In V. A. Barss (Ed.), *UpToDate*. Retrieved November 13, 2023, from https://www.uptodate.com/contents/acute-placental-abruption-pathophysiology-clinical-features-diagnosis-and-consequences

Antony, K. M., Racusin, D. A., Aagard, K., & Dildy, G. A., III. (2021). Maternal physiology. In M. B. Landon, H. L. Galan, E. R. M. Jauniaux, D. A. Driscoll, V. Berghella, W. A. Grobman, . . . A. G. Cahill (Eds.), *Gabbe's obstetrics: Normal and problem pregnancies* (8th ed., Kindle version, ch. 3). Philadelphia, PA: Elsevier.

Ashokka, B., Loh, M. H., Tan, C. H., Su, L. L., Young, B. E., Lye, D. C., . . . Choolani, M. (2020). Care of the pregnant woman with coronavirus disease 2019 in labor and delivery: Anesthesia, emergency cesarean delivery, differential diagnosis in the acutely ill parturient, care of the newborn, and protection of the healthcare personnel. *American Journal of Obstetrics & Gynecology, 223*(1), 66–74.e3. https://doi.org/10.1016/j.ajog.2020.04.005

Baldisseri, M. R. (2016). Shock and pregnancy. *Medscape*. Retrieved from https://emedicine.medscape.com/article/169450

Baldisseri, M. R., & Clark, S. L. (2023). Amniotic fluid embolism. In G. Finlay & V. A. Barss (Eds.), *UpToDate*. Retrieved November 13, 2023, from https://www.uptodate.com/contents/amniotic-fluid-embolism

Banayan, J., Rana, S., Mueller, A., Tung, A., Ramadan, H., Arany, Z., . . . Shahul, S. (2016). Cardiogenic shock in pregnancy: Analysis from the national inpatient sample: Medical complications of pregnancy related to hypertensive syndromes. *Pregnancy Hypertension, 6*(3), 220–221. https://doi.org/10.1016/j.preghy.2016.08.171

Bateman, B. T., Cole, N., Sun-Edelstein, C. & Lay, C. (2022). Post dural puncture headache. In M. Crowley, & R. P. Goddeau, Jr. (Eds.)., *UpToDate*. Retrieved November 13, 2023, from https://www.uptodate.com/contents/post-dural-puncture-headache

Belfort, M. A. (2023a). Overview of postpartum hemorrhage. In V. A. Barss (Ed.), *UpToDate*. Retrieved November 13, 2023, from https://www.uptodate.com/contents/overview-of-postpartum-hemorrhage

Belfort, M. A. (2023b). Postpartum hemorrhage: Medical and minimally invasive management. In V. A. Barss (Ed.), *UpToDate*. Retrieved November 13, 2023, from https://www.uptodate.com/contents/postpartum-hemorrhage-medical-and-minimally-invasive-management

Benditt, D. (2022). Syncope in adults: Clinical manifestations and initial diagnostic evaluation. In S. B. Yeon (Ed.), *UpToDate*. Retrieved November 13, 2023, from https://www.uptodate.com/contents/syncope-in-adults-clinical-manifestations-and-initial-diagnostic-evaluation

Bonanno, F. G. (2011). Clinical pathology of the shock syndromes. *Journal of Emergencies, Trauma and Shock, 4*(2), 233–243. https://doi.org/10.4103/0974-2700.82211

Bonnar, J. (2000). Massive obstetric haemorrhage. *Baillière's Best Practice & Research Clinical Obstetrics & Gynaecology, 14*(1). 1–18. https://doi.org/10.1053/beog.1999.0060

Borovac-Pinheiro, A., Pacagnella, R. C., Morais, S. S., & Cecatti, J. G. (2016). Standard reference values for the shock index during pregnancy. *International Journal of Gynecology & Obstetrics, 135*(1), 11–15. https://doi.org/10.1016/j.ijgo.2016.03.024

Brown, H. L., & Small, M. (2021). Trauma and related surgery in pregnancy. In M. B. Landon, H. L. Galan, E. R. M. Jauniaux, D. A. Driscoll, V. Berghella, W. A., Grobman, . . . A. G. Cahill (Eds), *Gabbe's obstetrics: Normal and problem pregnancies* (8th ed., Kindle version, ch. 32). Philadelphia, PA: Elsevier.

Burtch, R., Scott, C., Zimmerman, L., & Patel, A. (2016). Blood loss as a function of body surface area: Redefining parameters of obstetric blood loss. *Obstetrics & Gynecology, 128*(6), 1274–1280. https://doi.org/10.1097/AOG.0000000000001744

Campbell, R. L., & Kelso, J. M. (2022). Anaphylaxis: Acute diagnosis. In A. M. Feldweg (Ed.), *UpToDate*. Retrieved November 13, 2023, from https://www.uptodate.com/contents/anaphylaxis-acute-diagnosis

Campbell, R. L., & Kelso, J. M. (2023). Anaphylaxis: Emergency treatment. In A. M. Feldweg (Ed.), *UpToDate*. Retrieved November 13, 2023, from https://www.uptodate.com/contents/anaphylaxis-emergency-treatment

Charan, K. J., & Guttula, S. P. (2021). Syncope: A brief review. *Journal of Clinical and Pharmaceutical Research, 1*(3), 53–56. Retrieved from https://jcpr.in/index.php/journal/article/view/34

Charlton, N. P., Pellegrino, J. L., Kule, A., Slater, T. M., Epstein, J. L., Flores, G. E., . . . Swain, J. M. (2019). 2019 American Heart Association and American Red Cross focused update for first aid: Presyncope: An update to the American Heart Association and American Red Cross guidelines for first aid. *Circulation, 140*(24), e931–e938. https://doi.org/10.1161/CIR.0000000000000730

Chatrath, V., Khetarpal, R., & Ahuja, J. (2015). Fluid management in patients with trauma: Restrictive versus liberal approach. *Journal of Anaesthesiology Clinical Pharmacology, 31*(3), 308–316. https://doi.org/10.4103/0970-9185.161664

Chersich, M. F., Pham, M. D., Areal, A., Haghighi, M. M., Manyuchi, A., Swift, C. P., . . . Hajat, S. (2020). Associations between high temperatures in pregnancy and risk of preterm birth, low birth weight, and stillbirths: Systematic review and meta-analysis. *BMJ, 2020*, 371. https://doi.org/10.1136/bmj.m3811

Chu, J., Johnston, T. A., & Geohegan, J. (2020). Maternal collapse in pregnancy and the puerperium. *BJOG, 127*(5), e14–e52. https://doi.org/10.1111/1471-0528.15995

Clark, S. L., Hankins, G. D. V., Dudley, D. A., Dildy, G. A., & Porter, T. F. (1995). Amniotic fluid embolism: Analysis of the national registry. *American Journal of Obstetrics & Gynecology,172*(4, Pt. 1), 1158–1169. https://doi.org/10.1016/0002-9378(95)91474-9

Coffey, C. H., Casper, L. M., Reno, E. M., Casper, S. J., Hillis, E., Klein, D. A., . . . Keyes, L. E. (2023). First-trimester pregnancy: considerations for wilderness and remote travel. *Wilderness & Environmental Medicine, 34*(2), 201–210. https://doi.org/10.1016/j.wem.2022.12.001

Coker, A., & Oliver, R. (2012). Definitions and classifications. In S. Arulkumaran, M. Karoshi, L. G. Keith, A. B. Lalonde, & C. B-Lynch (Eds.), *A comprehensive textbook of postpartum hemorrhage: An essential clinical reference for effective management* (2nd ed., pp. 129–132). London, United Kingdom: Sapiens Publishing. Retrieved from https://www.glowm.com/pdf/PPH_2nd_edn_Chap-01.pdf

Collins, T. (2000). Understanding shock. *Nursing Standard, 14*(49), 35–39. https://doi.org/10.7748/ns2000.08.14.49.35.c2906

Colwell, C. (2023). Approach to shock in the adult trauma patient. In M. Ganetsky (Ed.), *UpToDate*. Retrieved November 13, 2023, from https://www.uptodate.com/contents/approach-to-shock-in-the-adult-trauma-patient

Cowley, R. A. (1975). A total emergency medical system for the state of Maryland. *Maryland State Medical Journal, 24*(7), 37–45.

Cunningham, F. G., Leveno, K. J., Dashe, J. S., Hoffman, B. L, Spong, C. Y., & Casey, B. M. (Eds.). (2022). *Williams obstetrics* (26th ed., Kindle version). New York, NY: McGraw-Hill.

D'Argent, L., Verelst, S., & Sabbe, M. (2020). Management of the pregnant trauma patient: A literature study. *Open Journal of Trauma, 4*(1), 038–046. https://doi.org/10.17352/ojt.000031

de Vogel, J., Heydanus, R., Mulders, A. G. M., Smalbraak, D. J. C., Papatsonis, D. N. M., & Gerritse, B. M. (2011). Lifesaving intraosseous access in a patient with a massive obstetric hemorrhage. *AJP Reports, 1*(2), 119–122. https://doi.org/10.1055/s-0031-1293514

DeCara, J. M., Lang, R. M., & Davis, M. B. (2023). Management of heart failure during pregnancy. In T. F. Dardas (Ed.), *UpToDate*. Retrieved November 13, 2023, from https://www.uptodate.com/contents/management-of-heart-failure-during-pregnancy

Deen, J., Albright, C. M., Chandrasekaran, S., & Stout, K. (2021). Heart disease in pregnancy. In M. B. Landon, H. L., Galan, E. R. M. Jauniaux, D. A. Driscoll, V. Berghella, W. A., Grobman, . . . A. G. Cahill (Eds), *Gabbe's obstetrics: Normal and problem pregnancies* (8th ed., Kindle version, ch. 42). Philadelphia, PA: Elsevier.

Deitchman, S. D., Ashkenazi, I., & Falk, H. (2020). Overview of blast injury. In D. Callaway & J. Burstein (Eds.), *Operational and medical management of explosive and blast incidents*. Cham, Switzerland: Springer. https://doi.org/10.1007/978-3-030-40655-4_1

Ducros, A. (2012). Reversible cerebral vasoconstriction syndrome. *Lancet Neurology, 11*(10), 906–917. https://doi.org/10.1016/S1474-4422(12)70135-7

Duff, W. P. (2021). Maternal and perinatal infection in pregnancy: Bacterial. In M. B. Landon, H. L., Galan, E. R. M. Jauniaux, D. A. Driscoll, V. Berghella, W. A., Grobman, . . . A. G. Cahill (Eds), *Gabbe's obstetrics: Normal and problem pregnancies* (8th ed., Kindle version, ch. 58). Philadelphia, PA: Elsevier.

Edelson, D. P., Sasson, C., Chan, P. S., Atkins, D. L., Aziz, K., Becker, L. B., . . . Topjian, A. A. (2020). Interim guidance for basic and advanced life support in adults, children, and neonates with suspected or confirmed COVID-19. *Circulation, 141*, e933–e943. https://doi.org/10.1161/CIRCULATIONAHA.120.047463

El Ayadi, A. M., Nathan, H. L., Seed, P. T., Butrick, E. A., Hezelgrave, N. L., Shennan, A. H., & Miller, S. (2016). Vital sign prediction of adverse maternal outcomes in women with hypovolemic shock: The role of Shock Index. *PLoS One, 11*(2), e0148729. https://doi.org/10.1371/journal.pone.0148729

Elmali, A. D., Auvin, S., Bast, T., Rubboli, G., & Koutroumanidis, M. (2020). How to diagnose and classify idiopathic (genetic) generalized epilepsies. *Epileptic Disorders, 22*(4), 399–420. https://doi.org/10.1684/epd.2020.1192

Elmer, J. (2023). Adult basic life support (BLS) for health care providers. In J. Grayzel (Ed.), *UpToDate*. Retrieved November 13, 2023, from https://www.uptodate.com/contents/adult-basic-life-support-bls-for-health-care-providers

Engels, P. T., Erdogan, M., Widder, S. L., Butler, M. B., Kureshi, N., Martin, K., & Green, R. S. (2016). Use of intraosseous devices in trauma: A survey of trauma practitioners in Canada, Australia and New Zealand. *Canadian Journal of Surgery, 59*(6), 374–382. https://doi.org/10.1503/cjs.011215

Epstein, Y., & Yanovich, R. (2019). Heatstroke. *New England Journal of Medicine, 380*(25), 2449–2459. https://doi.org/10.1056/NEJMra1810762

Escobar, M. F., Echavarría, M. P., Zambrano, M. A., Ramos, I., & Kusanovic, J. P. (2020). Maternal sepsis. *American Journal of Obstetrics & Gynecology MFM, 2*(3), 100149. https://doi.org/10.1016/j.ajogmf.2020.100149

Evans, L., Rhodes, A., Alhazzani, W., Antonelli, M., Coopersmith, C. M., French, C., . . . Levy, M. (2021). Surviving Sepsis Campaign: International guidelines for management of sepsis and septic shock 2021. *Critical Care Medicine, 49*(11), e1063–e1143. https://doi.org/10.1097/CCM.0000000000005337

Ferrada, P., Callcut, R. A., Skarupa, D. J., Duane, T. M., Garcia, A., Inaba, K., . . . AAST Multi-Institutional Trials Committee. (2018). Circulation first—The time has come to question the sequencing of care in the ABCs of trauma; an American Association for the Surgery of Trauma multicenter trial. *World Journal of mergency Surgery, 13*, 8. https://doi.org/10.1186/s13017-018-0168-3

Fowler, K. A., Leavitt, R. A., Betz, C. J., Yuan, K., & Dahlberg, L. L. (2021). Examining differences between mass, multiple, and single-victim homicides to inform prevention: findings from the National Violent Death Reporting System. *Injury Epidemiology, 8*(49). https://doi.org/10.1186/s40621-021-00345-7

Fowler, R., Pepe, P. E., Stevens, J., Ramirez, M. L., & Mell, H. (2018). Shock. In J. E. Campbell, R. L. Alson, & Alabama Chapter, American College of Emergency Physicians (Eds.), *International trauma life support for emergency care providers* (8th global ed., pp. 169–192). Harlow, United Kingdom: Pearson.

Friedman, P., & Stiller, R. J. (2016). Winter danger: Carbon monoxide poisoning during pregnancy: In the winter months, remain vigilant for CO poisoning, as the presenting signs are often nonspecific. *Contemporary OB/GYN, 61*(1), 27–30.

Gaieski, D. F., & Mikkelsen, M. E. (2023a). Definition, classification, etiology, and pathophysiology of shock in adults. In G. Finlay (Ed.), *UpToDate*. Retrieved November 13, 2023, from https://www.uptodate.com/contents/definition-classification-etiology-and-pathophysiology-of-shock-in-adults

Gaieski, D. F., & Mikkelsen, M. E. (2023b). Evaluation of and initial approach to the adult patient with undifferentiated hypotension and shock. In G. Finlay (Ed.), *UpToDate*. Retrieved November 13, 2023, from https://www.uptodate.com/contents/evaluation-of-and-initial-approach-to-the-adult-patient-with-undifferentiated-hypotension-and-shock

Galvagno, S. M., Jr., Nahmias, J. T., & Young, D. A. (2019). Advanced Trauma Life Support® update 2019. *Anesthesiology Clinics, 37*(1), 13–32. https://doi.org/10.1016/j.anclin.2018.09.009

García-Azorín, D., Sierra, Á., Trigo, J., Alberdi, A., Blanco, M., Calcerrada, I., . . . Peral, Á. L. G. (2021). Frequency and phenotype of headache in Covid-19: A study of 2194 patients. *Scientific Reports, 11*(1), 14674. https://doi.org/10.1038/s41598-021-94220-6

Gauer, R., Forbes, D., & Boyer, N. (2020). Sepsis: Diagnosis and management. *American Family Physician, 101*(7), 409–418.

Gibb, B., Gibb, R., & Gibb, M. (1977). Stayin' alive [Recorded by the Bee Gees]. On *Saturday night fever: The original movie soundtrack*. Baarn, Netherlands: PolyGram Records. (1977).

Gibbs, R., Bauer, M., Olvera, L., Sakowski, C., Cape, V. & Main, E. (2020). *Improving diagnosis and treatment of maternal sepsis: A CMQCC quality improvement toolkit*. Stanford, CA: California Maternal Quality Care Collaborative. Retrieved from https://www.cmqcc.org/sites/default/files/Sepsis Toolkit_FINAL.2_Errata_7.1.22.pdf

Giustozzi, M., Ehrlinder, H., Bongiovanni, D., Borovac, J. A., Guerreiro, R. A., Gąsecka, A., ... Parker, W. A. E. (2021). Coagulopathy and sepsis: Pathophysiology, clinical manifestations and treatment. *Blood Reviews, 50*. https://doi.org/10.1016/j.blre.2021.100864

Grace, Daniel. (2021). The management of hyperthermia and exercise-associated hyponatremia in low-resource and prehospital settings. *Current Medical Issues 19*(3), 165–170. Retrieved from https://journals.lww.com/cmii/fulltext/2021/19030/the_management_of_hyperthermia_and.8.aspx

Grear, K. E., & Bushnell, C. D. (2013). Stroke and pregnancy: Clinical presentation, evaluation, treatment and epidemiology. *Clinical Obstetrics and Gynecology, 56*(2), 350–359. https://doi.org/10.1097/GRF.0b013e31828f25fa

Greco, P. S., Day, L. J., & Pearlman, M. D. (2019). Guidance for evaluation and management of blunt abdominal trauma in pregnancy. *Obstetrics & Gynecology, 134*(6), 1343–1357. https://doi.org/10.1097/AOG.0000000000003585

Guillén, Ú., Weiss, E. M., Munson, D., Maton, P., Jefferies, A., Norman, M., ... Hansen, T. W. (2015). Guidelines for the management of extremely premature deliveries: A systematic review. *Pediatrics, 136*(2), 343–350. https://doi.org/10.1542/peds.2015-0542

Hafner, J. W., Jou, A. C., Wang, H., Bleess, B. B., & Tham, S. K. (2015). Death before disco: The effectiveness of a musical metronome in layperson cardiopulmonary resuscitation training. *Journal of Emergency Medicine, 48*(1), 43–52. https://doi.org/10.1016/j.jemermed.2014.07.048

Hafner, J. W., Sturgell, J. L., Matlock, D. L., Bockewitz, E. G., & Barker, L. T. (2012). "Stayin' Alive": A novel mental metronome to maintain compression rates in simulated cardiac arrests. *Journal of Emergency Medicine, 43*(5), e373–e377. https://doi.org/10.1016/j.jemermed.2012.01.026

Haftel, A., & Chowdhury, Y. S. (2023). Amniotic fluid embolism. In *StatPearls*. Treasure Island, FL: StatPearls Publishing. Retrieved November 13, 2023, from https://www.ncbi.nlm.nih.gov/books/NBK559107/

Hajduk, P., Nakamura, H., Ryan, S., & Puri, P. (2021). Fetal and birth trauma. In P. Puri (Ed.), *Pediatric surgery*, (pp. 453–471). Berlin, Germany: Springer. https://doi.org/0.1007/978-3-662-43559-5_138

Hanahara, K., Hitosugi, M., & Tateoka, Y. (2020). Education for appropriate seatbelt use required for early-phase pregnant women drivers. *Scientific Reports, 10*(1), 17609. https://doi.org/10.1038/s41598-020-74730-5

Hansebout, R. R., & Kachur, E. (2018). Acute traumatic spinal cord injury. In J. L. Wilterdink (Ed.), *UpToDate*. Retrieved November 13, 2023, from https://www.uptodate.com/contents/acute-traumatic-spinal-cord-injury

Hawkins, J. L., & Bucklin, B. A. (2021). Obstetric anesthesia. In M. B. Landon, H. L. Galan, E. R. M. Jauniaux, D. A. Driscoll, V. Berghella, W. A., Grobman, ... A. G. Cahill (Eds), *Gabbe's obstetrics: Normal and problem pregnancies* (8th ed., Kindle version, ch. 16). Philadelphia, PA: Elsevier.

Heck, J. L., Jones, E. J., Bohn, D., McCage, S., Parker, J. G., Parker, M., ... Campbell, J. (2021). Maternal mortality among American Indian/Alaska Native women: A scoping review. *Journal of Women's Health, 30*(2), 220–229. https://doi.org/10.1089/jwh.2020.8890

Hensley, M. K., Bauer, M. E., Admon, L. K., & Prescott, H. C. (2019). Incidence of maternal sepsis and sepsis-related maternal deaths in the United States. *JAMA, 322*(9), 890–892. https://doi.org/10.1001/jama.2019.9818

Hernandez, J. S., Alexander, J. M., Sarode, R., McIntire, D. D., & Leveno, K. J. (2012). Calculated blood loss in severe obstetric hemorrhage and its relation to body mass index. *American Journal of Perinatology, 29*(7), 557–560. https://doi.org/10.1055/s-0032-1310528

Hrvatin, I., & Rugelj, D. (2021, June 17). Risk factors for accidental falls during pregnancy—A systematic literature review. *Journal of Maternal-Fetal & Neonatal Medicine*. https://doi.org/10.1080/14767058.2021.1935849

Jacobs, L. M., Warshaw, A. L., & Burns, K. J. (2016). Empowering the public to improve survival in mass casualty events. *Annals of Surgery, 263*(5), 860–861. https://doi.org/10.1097/SLA.0000000000001517

Jeanmonod, R., Sahni, D., & Silberman, M. (2023). Vasovagal episode. In *StatPearls*. Treasure Island, FL: StatPearls Publishing. Retrieved January 29, 2024, from https://www.ncbi.nlm.nih.gov/books/NBK470277/

Jeejeebhoy, F. M., & Morrison, L. J. (2013). Maternal cardiac arrest: A practical and comprehensive review. *Emergency Medicine International, 2013*. https://doi.org/10.1155/2013/274814

Jeejeebhoy, F. M., Zelop, C. M., Lipman, S., Carvalho, B., Joglar, J., Mhyre, J. M., ... Page, R. L. (2015). Cardiac arrest in pregnancy: A scientific statement from the American Heart Association. *Circulation, 132*(18), 1747–1773. https://doi.org/10.1161/CIR.0000000000000300

Johnson, M., Boyd, L., Grantham, L., & Eastwood, K. (2015). *Paramedic principles and practice ANZ: A clinical reasoning approach*. Chatswood, NSW, Australia: Elsevier Australia.

Joseph, A. S. (2021). A modern trail of tears: The missing and murdered indigenous women (MMIW) crisis in the US. *Journal of Forensic and Legal Medicine, 79*. https://doi.org/10.1016/j.jflm.2021.102136

Kilpatrick, S. J. (2023). Initial evaluation and management of major trauma in pregnancy. In V. A. Barss (Ed.), *UpToDate*. Retrieved November 13, 2023, from https://www.uptodate.com/contents/initial-evaluation-and-management-of-pregnant-women-with-major-trauma

Kim, K. W., Kim, J. H., Choe, W. J., Kim, J. Y., Lee, S. I., Kim, K. T., ... Park, J. (2017). Effectiveness of 100 beats per minute music on cardiopulmonary resuscitation compression rate education: A manikin study. *Hong Kong Journal of Emergency Medicine, 24*(1), 12–17.

Klein, T. A., & Tadi, P. (2023). EMS scene safety. In *StatPearls*. Treasure Island, FL: StatPearls Publishing. Retrieved November 13, 2023, from https://www.ncbi.nlm.nih.gov/books/NBK557615/

Kleinman, M. E., Brennan, E. E., Goldberger, Z. D., Swor, R. A., Terry, B., Bobrow, B. J., ... Rea, T. (2015). Part 5: Adult basic life support and cardiopulmonary resuscitation quality: 2015 American Heart Association guidelines update for cardiopulmonary resuscitation and emergency cardiovascular care. *Circulation, 132*(18, Suppl. 2), S414–S435 https://doi.org/10.1161/CIR.0000000000000259

Klingert, M., Nikolaidis, P. T., Weiss, K., Thuany, M., Chlíbková, D., & Knechtle, B. (2022). Exercise-associated hyponatremia in marathon runners. *Journal of Clinical Medicine, 11*(22), 6775. https://doi.org/10.3390/jcm11226775

Kohn, J. R., Dildy, G. A., & Eppes, C. S. (2018). Shock index and delta-shock index are superior to existing maternal early warning criteria to identify postpartum hemorrhage and need for intervention. *Journal of Maternal-Fetal & Neonatal Medicine, 4*, 1–7. https://doi.org/10.1080/14767058.2017.1402882

Kosaki, Y., Maeyama, H., Nojima, T., Obara, T., Nakao, A., & Naito, H. (2021). Carbon monoxide poisoning during pregnancy treated with hyperbaric oxygen. *Clinical Case Reports, 9*(5), e04138. https://doi.org/10.1002/ccr3.4138

Krywko, D. M., Toy, F. K., Mahan, M. E., & Kiel, J. (2022). Pregnancy trauma. In *StatPearls*. Treasure Island, FL: StatPearls Publishing. Retrieved November 13, 2023 from https://www.ncbi.nlm.nih.gov/books/NBK430926/

Kyriacos, U., Jelsma, J., & Jordan, S. (2011). Monitoring vital signs using early warning scoring systems: A review of the literature. *Journal of Nursing Management, 19*(3), 311–330. https://doi.org/10.1111/j.1365-2834.2011.01246.x

Lai, W.-H., Wu, S.-C., Rau, C.-S., Kuo, P.-J., Hsu, S.-Y., Chen, Y.-C., ... Hsieh, C.-H. (2016). Systolic blood pressure lower than heart rate upon arrival at and departure from the emergency department indicates a poor outcome for adult trauma patients. *International Journal of Environmental Research and Public Health, 13*(6), 528. https://doi.org/10.3390/ijerph13060528

Lee, M.-J., Guinn, D., & Hickenbottom, S. (2023). Headache during pregnancy and postpartum. In V. A. Barss (Ed.), *UpToDate*. Retrieved November 13, 2023, from https://www.uptodate.com/contents/headache-during-pregnancy-and-postpartum

Lévesque, S., Boulebsol, C., Lessard, G., Bigaouette, M., Fernet, M., & Valderrama, A. (2021, June 15). Portrayal of domestic violence trajectories during the perinatal period. *Violence against Women, 28*(6–7), 1542–1565. https://doi.org/10.1177/10778012211014564

Link, M. S., Berkow, L. C., Kudenchuk, P. J., Halperin, H. R., Hess, E. P., Moitra, V. K., . . . Donnino, M. W. (2015). Part 7: Adult advanced cardiovascular life support: 2015: American Heart Association guidelines update for cardiopulmonary resuscitation and emergency cardiovascular care. *Circulation, 132*(18, Suppl. 2), S444–S464. https://doi.org/10.1161/CIR.0000000000000261

Lisonkova, S., Muraca, G. M., Potts, J., Liauw, J., Chan, W. S., . . . Lim, K. I. (2017). Association between prepregnancy body mass index and severe maternal morbidity. *JAMA, 318*(18), 1777–1786. https://doi.org/10.1001/jama.2017.16191

Ludermir, A. B., Lewis, G., Valongueiro, S. A., de Araújo, T. V. B., & Araya, R. (2010). Violence against women by their intimate partner during pregnancy and postnatal depression: A prospective cohort study. *Lancet, 376*(9744), 903–910. https://doi.org/10.1016/S0140-6736(10)60887-2

MacArthur, B., Foley, M., Gray, K., & Sisley, A. (2019). Trauma in pregnancy: A comprehensive approach to the mother and fetus. *American Journal of Obstetrics & Gynecology, 220*(5), 465–468e1. https://doi.org/0.1016/j.ajog.2019.01.209

Main, E., Martin, C., Romine, L., & Thomas, A. (2022). Definition, early recognition and rapid response to obstetric hemorrhage using triggers. In D. Lagrew, J. McNulty, C. Sakowski, V. Cape, E. McCormick, & C. H. Morton (Eds.), *Improving health care response to obstetric hemorrhage, v. 3.0: A CMQCC quality improvement toolkit* (pp. 93–103). Palo Alto, CA: California Maternal Quality Care Collaborative. Retrieved from https://www.cmqcc.org/sites/default/files/HEMToolkit_03252022 Errata 7.2022 (2).pdf

Manaker, S., & Perry, H. (2023). Carbon monoxide poisoning. In M. Ganetsky (Ed.), *UpToDate*. Retrieved November 13, 2023 from https://www.uptodate.com/contents/carbon-monoxide-poisoning

McCall, S. J., Bonnet, M.-P., Äyräs, O., Vandenberghe, G., Gissler, M., Zhang, W.-H., . . . Knight, M. (2020). Anaphylaxis in pregnancy: A population-based multinational European study. *Anaesthesia, 75*(11), 1469–1475. https://doi.org/10.1111/anae.15069

McElrath, T., & Gerard, E. E. (2023). Management of epilepsy during preconception, pregnancy, and the postpartum period. In J. F. Dashe (Ed.), *UpToDate*. Retrieved November 13, 2023, from https://www.uptodate.com/contents/management-of-epilepsy-during-preconception-pregnancy-and-the-postpartum-period

Mhyre, J. M., D'oria, R., Hameed, A. B., Lappen, J. R., Holley, S. L., Hunter, S. K., . . . D'alton, M. E. (2014). The maternal early warning criteria: A proposal from the National Partnership for Maternal Safety. Copublished in *Journal of Obstetric, Gynecologic, & Neonatal Nursing, 43*(6), 771–779, https://doi.org/10.1111/1552-6909.12504 and *Obstetrics & Gynecology, 124*(4), 783–786. https://doi.org/10.1097/AOG.0000000000000480

Mistovich, J. J., Krost, W. S., & Limmer, D. D. (2006). *Beyond the basics: Patient assessment.* https://www.emsworld.com/article/10322699/beyond-basics-patient-assessment

Mizrachi, E. M., & Sitammagari, K. K. (2023). Cardiac syncope. In *StatPearls*. Treasure Island, FL: StatPearls Publishing. Retrieved November 13, 2023, from https://www.ncbi.nlm.nih.gov/books/NBK526027/

Moise, K. J., Jr. (2022). Spontaneous massive fetomaternal hemorrhage. In V. A. Barss (Ed.), *UpToDate*. Retrieved November 13. 2023, from https://www.uptodate.com/contents/spontaneous-massive-fetomaternal-hemorrhage

Morgan, K., Chojenta, C., Tavener, M., Smith, A., & Loxton, D. (2018). Postural orthostatic tachycardia syndrome during pregnancy: A systematic review of the literature. *Autonomic Neuroscience, 215*, 106–118. https://doi.org/10.1016/j.autneu.2018.05.003

Morgan, K., Smith, A., & Blitshteyn, S. (2022). POTS and pregnancy: A Review of literature and recommendations for evaluation and treatment. *International Journal of Women's Health, 14*, 1831–1847. https://doi.org/10.2147/IJWH.S366667

Morris, B. D., III., & Hueppchen, N. A. (2021). Surgical disease and trauma in pregnancy. In B. Chou, J. L. Bienstock, & A. J. Satin (Eds.), *Johns Hopkins manual of gynecology and obstetrics* (6th ed., pp. 298–307). Philadelphia, PA: Wolters Kluwer.

Morrison, P. K., Pallatino, C., Fusco, R. A., Kenkre, T., Chang, J., & Krans, E. E. (2020). Pregnant victims of intimate partner homicide in the National Violent Death Reporting System database, 2003–2014: A descriptive analysis. *Journal of Interpersonal Violence, 37*(5–6), NP2652–NP2670. https://doi.org/10.1177/0886260520943726

Murphy, N. J., & Cullinan, B. (2020). Maternal resuscitation and trauma. In L. Leeman, L. Dresang, J. S. Quinlan, & S. R. Magee (Eds.), *Advanced life support in obstetrics: Provider manual* (9th ed., pp. 205–228). Leawood, KS: American Academy of Family Physicians.

Narvaez, J., & Vrees, R. (2021). Trauma in pregnancy: A clinical update for obstetrician-gynecologists. *Topics in Obstetrics & Gynecology, 41*(9), 1–7. https://doi.org/10.1097/01.PGO.0000753172.54103.b3

Nasr, D. M., & Braksick, S. A. (2020). Headache emergencies. In A. Rabinstein (Ed.), *Neurological emergencies: A practical approach* (pp. 49–66). Cham, Switzerland: Springer Nature.

Nathan, H. L., El Ayadi, A., Hezelgrave, N. L., Seed, P., Butrick, E., Miller, S., . . . Shennan, A. H. (2015). Shock index: An effective predictor of outcome in postpartum haemorrhage? *BJOG, 122*(2), 268–275. https://doi.org/10.1111/1471-0528.13206

National Association of Emergency Medical Technicians & American College of Surgeons, Committee on Trauma. (2020). *PHTLS: Prehospital trauma life support for first responders* (9th ed.). Burlington, MA: Jones & Bartlett Learning.

Negro, A., Delaruelle, Z., Ivanova, T. A., Khan, S., Ornello, R., Raffaelli, B., . . . Mitsikostas, D. D. (2017). Headache and pregnancy: A systematic review. *Journal of Headache and Pain, 18*(1), 1–20. https://doi.org/10.1186/s10194-017-0816-0

Neuman, J. E., & Promes, S. B. (2021). Trauma in pregnancy. In A. B. Wolfson et al. (Eds.), *Harwood-Nuss' clinical practice of emergency medicine* (7th ed., pp. 329–332). Philadelphia, PA: Wolters Kluwer.

Neviere, R. (2022). Pathophysiology of sepsis. In G. Finlay (Ed.), *UpToDate*. Retrieved November 13, 2023, from https://www.uptodate.com/contents/pathophysiology-of-sepsis

Ng, N., Cox, S., & Maiti, S. (2015). Headache in pregnancy: An overview of differential diagnoses. *Journal of Pregnancy and Child Health, 2*(130). https://www.omicsonline.org/open-access/headache-in-pregnancy-an-overview-of-differential-diagnoses-jpch.1000130.php?aid=37276

Niehaus, M. T., & Baldisseri, M. R. (2020). Sepsis in pregnancy. In R. Hyzy & J. McSparron (Eds.), Evidence-based critical care: A case study approach (2nd ed., pp. 767–770). Cham, Switzerland: Springer Nature.

Novikova, N., Hofmeyr, G. J., & Cluver, C. (2015). Tranexamic acid for preventing postpartum haemorrhage. *Cochrane Database of Systematic Reviews, 2015*(6). https://doi.org/10.1002/14651858.CD007872.pub3

One mass killing every 6.53 days: US shootings are on a record pace. (2023, April 21). *Guardian*. Retrieved from https://www.theguardian.com/us-news/2023/apr/21/us-mass-shooting-2023-alabama-tennessee-california

Ozsaker, E., Kaya, A., Alcan, A. O., van Giersbergen, M. Y., & Aktas, E. O. (2020). Forensic cases in the operating room: knowledge and practices of physicians and nurses. *Journal of PeriAnesthesia Nursing, 35*(1), 38–43. https://doi.org/10.1016/j.jopan.2019.06.010

Pacheco, L. D., Clark, S. L., Klassen, M., & Hankins, G. D. V. (2020). Amniotic fluid embolism: Principles of early clinical management. *American Journal of Obstetrics & Gynecology, 222*(1), 48–52. https://doi.org/10.1016/j.ajog.2019.07.036

Page, N., Roloff, K., Modi, A. P., Dong, F., & Neeki, M. M. (2020). Management of placental abruption following blunt abdominal trauma. *Cureus, 12*(9), e10337. https://doi.org/10.7759/cureus.10337

Palladino, C. L., Singh, V., Campbell, J., Flynn, H., & Gold, K. J. (2011). Homicide and suicide during the perinatal period: Findings from the National Violent Death Reporting System. *Obstetrics & Gynecology, 118*(5), 1056–1063. https://doi.org/10.1097/AOG.0b013e31823294da

Palma, J.-A., & Kaufman, H. (2022). Mechanisms, causes, and evaluation of orthostatic hypotension. In R. P. Goddeau, Jr. (Ed.), *UpToDate*. Retrieved November 13, 2023, from https://www.uptodate.com/contents/mechanisms-causes-and-evaluation-of-orthostatic-hypotension

Pandya, S., & Mangalampally, K. (2018). Critical care in obstetrics. *Indian Journal of Anaesthesia, 62*(9), 724–733. https://doi.org/10.4103/ija.IJA_577_18

Paterson-Brown, S. & Bamber, J. (2014). Prevention and treatment of haemorrhage. In M. Knight, S. Kenyon, P. Brocklehurst, J. Neilson, J. Shakespeare, & J. J. Kurinczuk (Eds.), *Saving lives, improving mothers' care—Lessons learned to inform future maternity care from the UK and Ireland Confidential Enquiries into Maternal Deaths and Morbidity 2009–2012* (pp. 45–55). Oxford, United Kingdom: National Perinatal Epidemiology Unit.

Petitpas, F., Guenezan, J., Vendeuvre, T., Scepi, M., Oriot, D., & Mimoz, O. (2016). Use of intra-osseous access in adults: A systematic review. *Critical Care, 20*, 102. https://doi.org/10.1186/s13054-016-1277-6

Petrone, P., & Marini, C. P. (2015). Trauma in pregnant patients. *Current Problems in Surgery, 52*(8), 330–351. https://doi.org/10.1067/j.cpsurg.2015.07.001

Petrosoniak, A., & Hicks, C. (2018). Resuscitation resequenced: A rational approach to patients with trauma in shock. *Emergency Medicine Clinics of North America, 36*(1), 41–60. https://doi.org/10.1016/j.emc.2017.08.005

Raja, A., & Zane, R. D. (2023). Initial management of trauma in adults. In J. Grayzel (Ed.), *UpToDate*. Retrieved November 13, 2023, from https://www.uptodate.com/contents/initial-management-of-trauma-in-adults

Ramzan, M., & Mehla, S. (2023). Migraine-associated stroke: Risk factors, diagnosis, and prevention. In R. P. Goddeau, Jr., & K. Eckler (Eds.), *UpToDate*. Retrieved November 13, 2023, from https://www.uptodate.com/contents/migraine-associated-stroke-risk-factors-diagnosis-and-prevention

Rogers, F. B., Rittenhouse, K. J., & Gross, B. W. (2015). The golden hour in trauma: Dogma or medical folklore? *Injury, 46*(4), 525–527. https://doi.org/10.1016/j.injury.2014.08.043

Rojas-Suarez, J. A., & Suarez Rueda, N. (2020). Maternal sepsis. In L. Leeman, L. Dresang, J. S. Quinlan, & S. R. Magee (Eds.), *Advanced life support in obstetrics: Provider manual* (9th ed., pp. 275–295). Leawood, KS: American Academy of Family Physicians.

Román-Gálvez, R. M., Martín-Peláez, S., Martínez-Galiano, J. M., Khan, K. S., & Bueno-Cavanillas, A. (2021). Prevalence of intimate partner violence in pregnancy: An umbrella review. *International Journal of Environmental Research and Public Health, 18*(2), 707. https://doi.org/10.3390/ijerph18020707

Royal College of Obstetricians & Gynaecologists. (2016). *Postpartum haemorrhage, prevention and management* (Green-top Guideline 52). Retrieved from https://www.rcog.org.uk/en/guidelines-research-services/guidelines/gtg52/

Sakamoto, J., Michels, C., Eisfelder, B., & Joshi, N. (2019). Trauma in pregnancy. *Emergency Medicine Clinics of North America, 37*(2), 317–338. https://doi.org/10.1016/j.emc.2019.01.009

Schachter, S. C. (2022). Evaluation and management of the first seizure in adults. In J. F. Dashe (Ed.), *UpToDate*. Retrieved November 13, 2023, from https://www.uptodate.com/contents/evaluation-and-management-of-the-first-seizure-in-adults

Schatz, M., & Dombrowski, M. P. (2023). Anaphylaxis during pregnancy and delivery. In A. M. Feldweg & V. A. Barss (Eds.), *UpToDate*. Retrieved November 13, 2023, from https://www.uptodate.com/contents/anaphylaxis-during-pregnancy-and-delivery

Schmidt, P., Skelly, C. L., & Raines, D. A. (2022). Placental Abruption. In *StatPearls*. Treasure Island, FL: StatPearls Publishing. Retrieved November 13, 2023, from https://www.ncbi.nlm.nih.gov/books/NBK482335/

Schorn, M. N., & Phillippi, J. C. (2014). Volume replacement following severe postpartum hemorrhage. *Journal of Midwifery & Women's Health, 59*(3), 336–343. https://doi.org/10.1111/jmwh.12186

Sentilhes, L., Lasocki, S., Ducloy-Bouthors, A. S., Deruelle, P., Dreyfus, M., Perrotin, F., . . . Deneux-Tharaux, C. (2015). Tranexamic acid for the prevention and treatment of postpartum haemorrhage. *British Journal of Anaesthesia, 114*(4), 576–587. https://doi.org/10.1093/bja/aeu448

Servier Medical Art. (2016a). *Heart conduction* [Graphic]. Retrieved from https://smart.servier.com/wp-content/uploads/2016/10/conduction_cardiaque.png

Servier Medical Art. (2016b). *Myocardial infarction—Anterolateral* [Graphic]. Retrieved from https://smart.servier.com/wp-content/uploads/2016/10/infarct4.png

Servier Medical Art. (2016c). *Thrombus position and consequences* [Graphic]. Retrieved from https://smart.servier.com/wp-content/uploads/2016/10/Infarctus2-562x680.png

Shank, J. J., Olney, S. C., Lin, F. L., & McNamara, M. F. (2009). Recurrent postpartum anaphylaxis with breast-feeding. *Obstetrics & Gynecology, 114*(2, Pt. 2), 415–416. https://doi.org/10.1097/AOG.0b013e3181a20721

Sheldon, R. S., & Raj, S. R. (2020). Seizures vs syncope: Distinguishing features for the clinic. In M. Brignole & D. G. Benditt (Eds.), *Syncope: An evidence-based approach* (2nd ed., pp. 69–81). Cham, Switzerland: Springer Nature.

Shmuely, S., Bauer, P. R., van Zwet, E. W., van Dijk, J. G., & Thijs, R. D. (2018). Differentiating motor phenomena in tilt-induced syncope and convulsive seizures. *Neurology, 90*(15), e1339–e1346. https://doi.org/10.1212/WNL.0000000000005301

Siddiqi, A. Z., Blackmore, D., & Siddiqi, Z. A. (2020). "Complex" vasovagal syncope: A zebra among horses. *Frontiers in Neurology, 11*, 1418. https://doi.org/10.3389/fneur.2020.550982

Silverman, E. C., Sporer, K. A., Lemieux, J. M., Brown, J. F., Koenig, K. L., Gausche-Hill, M., . . . Gilbert, G. H. (2017). Prehospital care for the adult and pediatric seizure patient: Current evidence based recommendations. *Western Journal of Emergency Medicine, 18*(3), 419–436. https://doi.org/10.5811/westjem.2016.12.32066

Smith, E. R., & Amin-Hanjani, S. (2019). Evaluation and management of elevated intracranial pressure in adults. In J. L. Wilterdink (Ed.), *UpToDate*. Retrieved November 13, 2023, from https://www.uptodate.com/contents/evaluation-and-management-of-elevated-intracranial-pressure-in-adults

Smith, J. F., & Wax, J. R. (2022). Uterine rupture: Unscarred uterus. In V. A. Barss (Ed.), *UpToDate*. Retrieved November 13, 2023, from https://www.uptodate.com/contents/uterine-rupture-unscarred-uterus

Smith, N., Lopez, R. A., & Silberman, M. (2023). Distributive shock. In *StatPearls*. Treasure Island, FL: StatPearls Publishing. Retrieved November 13, 2023, from https://www.ncbi.nlm.nih.gov/books/NBK470316/

Smith, P. E. M. (2001). If it's not epilepsy . . . *Journal of Neurology, Neurosurgery & Psychiatry, 70*(Suppl. 2), ii9-ii14. https://doi.org/10.1136/jnnp.70.suppl_2.ii9

Soma-Pillay, P., Catherine, N.-P., Tolppanen, H., & Mebazaa, A. (2016). Physiological changes in pregnancy. *Cardiovascular Journal of Africa, 27*(2), 89–94. https://doi.org/10.5830/CVJA-2016-021

Stella, C. L., Jodicke, C. D., How, H. Y., Harkness, U. F., & Sibai, B. M. (2007). Postpartum headache: Is your work-up complete? *American Journal of Obstetrics & Gynecology, 196*(4), 318.e1–e7. https://doi.org/10.1016/j.ajog.2007.01.034

Sterling, S. A., Jones, A. E., Coleman, T. G., & Summers, R. L. (2015). Theoretical analysis of the relative impact of obesity on hemodynamic stability during acute hemorrhagic shock. *Archives of Trauma Research, 4*(3), e22602. Retrieved from https://www.ncbi.nlm.nih.gov/pmc/articles/PMC4636541/

Szarpak, L., Truszewski, Z., Smereka, J., Krajewski, P., Fudalej, M., Adamczyk, P., & Czyzewski, L. (2016). A randomized cadaver study comparing first-attempt success between tibial and humeral intraosseous insertions using NIO device by paramedics: A preliminary investigation. *Medicine, 95*(20), e3724. https://doi.org/10.1097/MD.0000000000003724

Tastan, S., Ayhan, H., Unver, V., Cinar, F. I., Kose, G., Basak, T., . . . Iyigun, E. (2017). The effects of music on the cardiac resuscitation education of nursing students. *International Emergency Nursing, 31*, 30–35. https://doi.org/10.1016/j.ienj.2016.06.007

Taylor, F. R. (2022). Tension-type headache in adults: Pathophysiology, clinical features, and diagnosis. In R. P. Goddeau, Jr. (Ed.), *UpToDate*. Retrieved November 13, 2023, from https://www.uptodate.com/contents/tension-type-headache-in-adults-pathophysiology-clinical-features-and-diagnosis

Trahair, L. G., Horowitz, M., & Jones, K. L. (2014). Postprandial hypotension: A systematic review. *Journal of the American Medical Directors Association, 15*(6), 394–409. https://doi.org/10.1016/j.jamda.2014.01.011

Tsang, W., & Lang, R. M. (2022). Peripartum cardiomyopathy: Etiology, clinical manifestations, and diagnosis. In N. Parikh (Ed.), *UpToDate*. Retrieved November 13, 2023, from https://www.uptodate.com/contents/peripartum-cardiomyopathy-etiology-clinical-manifestations-and-diagnosis

Valand, P., Miles, J., & Pandya, A. N. (2020). The deleterious effects of war and conflict on the provision of health care for vulnerable populations and the potential effects of COVID-19 on vulnerable populations in conflict zones. *International Journal of Surgery: Global Health, 3*(6), e36. https://doi.org/10.1097/GH9.0000000000000036

Valente, A. M., & Economy, K. (2023). Maternal adaptations to pregnancy: Cardiovascular and hemodynamic changes. In V. A. Barss (Ed.), *UpToDate*. Retrieved November 13, 2023, from https://www.uptodate.com/contents/maternal-adaptations-to-pregnancy-cardiovascular-and-hemodynamic-changes

van Veelen, M. J., & Brodmann Maeder, M. (2021). Hypothermia in trauma. *International Journal of Environmental Research and Public Health, 18*(16), 8719. https://doi.org/10.3390/ijerph18168719

Vaught, A. J. (2018). Maternal sepsis. *Seminars in Perinatology, 42*(1), 9–12. https://doi.org/10.1053/j.semperi.2017.11.003

Wallace, M., Gillispie-Bell, V., Cruz, K., Davis, K., & Vilda, D. (2021). Homicide during pregnancy and the postpartum period in the United States, 2018–2019. *Obstetrics & Gynecology, 138*(5), 762–769. https://doi.org/10.1097/AOG.0000000000004567

Wallis, L. A., & Greaves, I. (2002). Injuries associated with airbag deployment. *Emergency Medicine Journal, 19*(6), 490–493. https://doi.org/10.1136/emj.19.6.490

Warner, R. L., Grabo, D. J., & Schwab, C. W. (2020). Care of the pregnant trauma patient. In A. B. Peitzman, D. M. Yealy, T. C. Fabian, & C. W. Schwab (Eds.), *The trauma manual: Trauma and acute care surgery* (5th ed., pp. 293–300). Philadelphia, PA: Wolters Kluwer.

Watson, J. C. (2023). Cervicogenic headache. In R. P. Goddeau, Jr. (Ed.), *UpToDate*. Retrieved November 13, 2023, from https://www.uptodate.com/contents/cervicogenic-headache

Weerakkody, Y., & Gaillard, F. (2018). Reversible cerebral vasoconstriction syndrome. *Radiopaedia*. Retrieved from https://radiopaedia.org/articles/reversible-cerebral-vasoconstriction-syndrome-2

Wei, S. H., Helmy, M., & Cohen, A. J. (2009). CT evaluation of placental abruption in pregnant trauma patients. *Emergency Radiology, 16*(5), 365–373. https://doi.org/10.1007/s10140-009-0804-z

Weinberger, S. E. (2023). Maternal adaptations to pregnancy: Dyspnea and other physiologic respiratory changes. In V. A. Barss (Ed.), *UpToDate*. Retrieved November 13, 2023, from https://www.uptodate.com/contents/maternal-adaptations-to-pregnancy-dyspnea-and-other-physiologic-respiratory-changes

Wenstrom, K. D. (2015). Cardiac disease. In J. T. Queenan, C. Y. Spong, & C. J. Lockwood (Eds.), *Protocols for high-risk pregnancies: An evidence-based approach* (5th ed., pp. 128–138). Oxford, United Kingdom: Blackwell Publishing. https://doi.org/10.1002/9781119001256.ch15

Whitledge, J. D., Ali, N., Basit, H., & Grossman, S. A. (2023). Presyncope. In *StatPearls*. Retrieved November 13, 2023, from https://www.ncbi.nlm.nih.gov/books/NBK459383/

Wippold, F. J., II, Whealy, M. A., & Kaniecki, R. G. (2023). Evaluation of headache in adults. In R. P. Goddeau, Jr. (Ed.), *UpToDate*. Retrieved November 13, 2023, from https://www.uptodate.com/contents/evaluation-of-headache-in-adults

WOMAN Trial Collaborators. (2017). Effect of early tranexamic acid administration on mortality, hysterectomy, and other morbidities in women with post-partum haemorrhage (WOMAN): An international, randomised, double-blind, placebo-controlled trial. *Lancet, 389*(10084), 2105–2116. https://doi.org/10.1016/S0140-6736(17)30638-4

World Health Organization and International Committee of the Red Cross. (2018). *Basic emergency care: Approach to the acutely ill and injured*. Geneva, Switzerland. Retrieved from https://shop.icrc.org/basic-emergency-care-approach-to-the-acutely-ill-and-injured-pdf-en

World Health Organization, Dept. of Reproductive Health and Research. (2011). *Intimate partner violence during pregnancy: Information sheet*. Retrieved from http://apps.who.int/iris/bitstream/handle/10665/70764/WHO_RHR_11.35_eng.pdf?sequence=1

Wu, Y., Chen, J., Fang, H., & Wan, Y. (2020). Intimate partner violence: A bibliometric review of literature. *International Journal of Environmental Research and Public Health, 17*(15), 5607. https://doi.org/10.3390/ijerph17155607

Wylie, T., Sandhu, D. S., & Murr, N. (2023). Status epilepticus. In *StatPearls*. Treasure Island, FL: StatPearls Publishing. Retrieved November 13, 2023, from https://www.ncbi.nlm.nih.gov/books/NBK430686/

Yarlagadda, S., Poma, P. A., Green, L. S., & Katz, V. (2010). Syncope during pregnancy. *Obstetrics & Gynecology, 115*(2, Pt. 1), 377–380. https://doi.org/10.1097/AOG.0b013e3181c4f550

Zelop, C. M., & Brickner, B. (2023). Sudden cardiac arrest and death in pregnancy. In V. A. Barss (Ed.), *UpToDate*. Retrieved November 13, 2023, from https://www.uptodate.com/contents/sudden-cardiac-arrest-and-death-in-pregnancy

Zuckerwise, L. C., & Lipkind, H. S. (2017). Maternal early warning systems—Towards reducing preventable maternal mortality and severe maternal morbidity through improved clinical surveillance and responsiveness. *Seminars in perinatology, 41*(3), 161–165. https://doi.org/10.1053/j.semperi.2017.03.005

Hypertensive Disorders of Pregnancy 10

Objectives

- Describe the typical clinical manifestations of chronic hypertension, gestational hypertension, and preeclampsia/eclampsia/HELLP syndrome.
- Explain the rationales of management for hypertensive disorders of pregnancy.
- Summarize the maternal and fetal effects of hypertension in pregnancy.
- Discuss the relationship between COVID-19 (SARS-CoV-2) infection and preeclampsia.
- Describe how the provider can assess the severity of chronic hypertension, gestational hypertension, and preeclampsia.

Composite Case Study

Maisie Leigh R., a 20-year-old gravida 1, para 0 (G1 P0), at 33 weeks of gestation, was training horses on a Colorado ranch. Because of her advanced pregnancy, she was no longer riding, but she felt safe doing groundwork with the yearlings. Maisie was fit and strong, and her pregnancy had been surprisingly uncomplicated except for a very mild case of COVID-19 at 20 weeks of gestation. She was therefore astonished and concerned when a sudden, severe headache caused her to stop working.

"Hi, Evelyn," Maisie began when her midwife answered the phone. "It's the strangest thing. I had no stamina today, I just felt wiped out. I couldn't keep working, so I stopped early for lunch and went inside hoping the air conditioning would revive me. But I kept feeling worse. I just vomited up my lunch. I have a nasty headache, and I never get headaches. When the headache started, my vision went all wonky. Like a window with spots of oil on it. I can't work anymore."

Evelyn Shepherd, CNM, a birth-center midwife with hospital privileges, ran through the GOLDCART line of questioning. She determined that the baby was moving normally and there were no signs of labor. Because the symptoms were consistent with preeclampsia, Evelyn met Maisie at the hospital to assess vital signs, evaluate laboratory studies, and monitor fetal well-being. Upon arrival at the hospital, Maisie's blood pressure was 190/110 mm Hg, and her urine protein/creatinine ratio was significantly elevated at 0.844. Her hematocrit was 40, suggesting hemoconcentration, but fortunately her platelets and liver enzymes were normal. Her serum creatinine was 0.96, significantly elevated above normal pregnancy values.

Dr. Wong ordered betamethasone 12 mg IM to encourage fetal lung maturation in anticipation of iatrogenic preterm delivery, Evelyn transferred Maisie's care to her backup physician, Kelsey Wong, D.O., in accordance with institutional protocols. Dr. Wong ordered intravenous labetalol to decrease Maisie's blood pressure and magnesium sulfate to decrease the risk of eclamptic seizure. The labetalol brought her blood pressure down to 144/94.

Because iatrogenic preterm delivery was necessary, Dr. Wong ordered betamethasone 12 mg IM to encourage fetal lung maturation. The fetal heart monitor showed a category I tracing with a baseline rate of 140, moderate variability, accelerations, and no decelerations. An ultrasound evaluation revealed a fetus with symmetric fetal growth restriction at the 6th percentile for growth and oligohydramnios with an amniotic fluid index of 4 cm. Doppler velocimetry values were mildly abnormal. The fetus scored a 6 of 10 on a biophysical profile. Dr. Wong consulted a maternal-fetal medicine specialist, and together they decided that the safest course of action was to induce labor.

Mother and fetus tolerated labor well. Maisie gave birth to a small but vigorous 3 lb 8 oz (1,600 g) boy named Michael, who was admitted to the neonatal intensive care unit (NICU) for prematurity. Shortly after giving birth, Maisie's symptoms improved, and 24 hr later the magnesium sulfate infusion was discontinued. She stayed in the hospital 4 days while her blood pressure stabilized. Maisie was followed closely through the postpartum period but had no further issues with hypertension. Michael was discharged from the NICU 6 weeks later in good health.

Hypertension in Pregnancy

Hypertensive disorders of pregnancy (HDP) affect 5–10% of pregnancies worldwide and are a leading cause of maternal death (Unger et al., 2020). Between 1987 and 2004, the United States had a 25% increase in preeclampsia, the most lethal of these conditions (Druzin, Shields, Peterson, Sakowski, et al., 2021, p. 8). The rate of preeclampsia increased further after the

2020 outbreak of COVID-19, because contracting this infection during pregnancy increases the risk of developing preeclampsia, preeclampsia with severe features, eclampsia, and HELLP—**H**emolysis, **E**levated **L**iver enzymes, **L**ow **P**latelets (Conde-Agudelo & Romero, 2021).

HDP are the most common indication for provider-initiated preterm birth (PTB) and are responsible for more than a third of iatrogenic PTBs (Ma'ayeh, Rood, Kniss, & Costantine, 2020). People with preeclampsia have five times the risk for hypertension later in life independent of other risk factors and double the risk for myocardial infarction, heart failure, stroke, peripheral arterial disease, kidney disease, and death related to these disorders (American College of Obstetricians & Gynecologists [ACOG], 2020a/2023). Their lifetime risk rises with the severity of preeclampsia and its reoccurrence in subsequent pregnancies (ACOG, 2020a/2023). HDP can develop, worsen, or persist in the first weeks postpartum, and are the leading cause of postpartum readmission in the United States (Bello, Miller, et al., 2018). Complications arising from HDP can be decreased or prevented when they are recognized and treated swiftly.

Blood-Pressure (BP) Measurement

In pregnancy, hypertension is defined as a sustained systolic blood pressure (SBP) ≥140 mm Hg or a sustained diastolic blood pressure (DBP) ≥90 mm Hg involving two readings taken at least 4 hr apart. Severe hypertension is defined as SBP of 160 mm Hg or higher, DBP of 110 mm Hg or higher, or both (ACOG, 2020a/2023). Severe hypertension should be confirmed sooner (within minutes) so the provider can initiate antihypertensive therapy without potentially harmful delay (ACOG, 2020a/2023). SBP of 160 mm Hg or higher is associated with higher risk of stroke (Reddy et al., 2020).

BP in pregnancy is dynamic, involving a circadian rhythm, seasonal variations, maternal activity, and the stage of pregnancy (Han et al., 2016). BP is higher in daytime (9 a.m.–6 p.m.) than at night (10 p.m.–3 a.m.) when systolic and DBP drop about 10–20% (Vijayvargia & Samariya, 2021). People with gestational hypertension and preeclampsia, however, tend to peak in the evening and overnight (Han et al., 2016).

In a healthy person, SBP and DBP fall in early pregnancy because of the decrease in systemic vascular resistance (Valente & Economy, 2023). BP rises through the third trimester but typically normalizes to prepregnant values by term (Valente & Economy, 2023). In labor, SBP and DBP increase 15–25% and 10–15%, respectively during each uterine contraction (Valente & Economy, 2023).

BP can be measured in a health care facility or at home using auscultatory or automated methods. The automated BP machines used widely in hospitals tend to underestimate both systolic and diastolic readings by as much as 10 mm Hg (Gabel & Peterson, 2021a). Although they are generally acceptable for clinical practice, a manual cuff should be used when the client is unstable and this margin of error would influence the management plan (Gabel & Peterson, 2021a). When you obtain a severe-range BP with an automated device or if there is a question about the accuracy of an electronic reading verify the reading manually (Gabel & Peterson, 2021a). Measurement by an automated device that can take multiple readings with the client sitting quietly alone in the examination room can be more accurate than one taken by a health care worker, especially for clients with white-coat hypertension (WCH).

Accurate BP measurement is of critical importance. The technique of measuring BP should be standardized. Place the client in a sitting or semirecumbent position, legs uncrossed, feet flat on the floor, back supported, and arm at heart level; this may require use of a pillow (Gabel & Peterson, 2021a). When the reading must be obtained while the client is recumbent, use the left lateral position with cuff at the level of the heart, which gives a reading similar to one taken with the client seated (August, 2023). The client should not talk, read, use a telephone or computer, or watch television (Han et al., 2016). Use of tobacco or caffeine 30 min before measurement can temporarily increase BP (ACOG, 2020a/2023).

Expose the client's bare arm and apply an appropriately sized cuff. Ensure that there is no air in the cuff when you fit it to the arm. The cuff should cover two-thirds of the distance between shoulder and elbow, and the bottom of the cuff should be 1–2 cm above the elbow (Han et al., 2016). A cuff that is too small will yield readings up to 30 mm Hg too high; an oversized cuff can measure 10–30 mm Hg too low (Gabel & Peterson, 2021a). BP measurements on one arm can differ by more than 10 mm Hg from those on the other. Take readings on both arms and use the arm with the higher initial reading for subsequent readings (Gabel & Peterson, 2021a). For upper-arm circumferences greater than 19.7 in. (50 cm), use the practicable but less accurate method of placing a cuff on the forearm and palpating for the appearance of the radial pulse at the wrist to measure SBP (Gabel & Peterson, 2021a).

Have the client sit for at least 5 min before you take BP. Any arm movement during measurement can invalidate the reading. Measure BP to the nearest 2 mm Hg (Gabel & Peterson, 2021a). If the initial BP is elevated, recheck in 10 min. Do not shift the client into a side-lying position to obtain a lower reading; this measurement would be inaccurate.

Home Blood-Pressure Monitoring

The American Heart Association (AHA) recommends home BP monitoring for pregnant clients with sustained hypertension or WCH (Pickering et al., 2008). At-home monitoring measures BP in the client's natural environment and might better reflect placental perfusion pressure than BP measurements in an office. Home monitoring can be lifesaving when it detects hypertension that might otherwise be missed. Home BP monitoring requires a client to assess BP at least twice daily for 3–7 days to rule out WCH, or indefinitely if the client is diagnosed with hypertension (Bello, Miller, et al., 2018). Make sure the cuff is the correct size and is a model approved for use in pregnancy (Bello, Woolley, et al., 2017; Tremonti, Beddoe, & Brown, 2017). Have the client bring the cuff to the prenatal visit and compare measurements to those of the equipment in the office. Instruct the client to call with elevated BP or severe headache, visual disturbances, epigastric pain, sudden weight gain, or malaise.

Categories of Hypertension

ACOG guidelines recognize three categories of HDP: gestational hypertension, chronic hypertension, and preeclampsia/eclampsia/HELLP syndrome (ACOG, 2020a/2023). Preeclampsia can also be superimposed upon chronic hypertension. Definitions of these conditions are as follows:

Chronic hypertension is a condition present before pregnancy or the 20th week of gestation. Hypertension that develops for the first time during pregnancy and persists after the postpartum period is also classified as chronic hypertension (ACOG, 2019).

Gestational hypertension is elevated BP after 20 weeks of gestation without proteinuria or other features of preeclampsia (August & Sibai, 2023a). Some people with gestational hypertension go on to develop preeclampsia. Some continue to have elevated BP after the postpartum period, changing the diagnosis to chronic hypertension.

Preeclampsia is a disorder caused by placental and maternal vascular dysfunction, characterized by new-onset hypertension and proteinuria or new onset of hypertension and end-organ dysfunction with or without proteinuria. Onset is usually after 20 weeks of gestation in a previously normotensive person. The condition resolves postpartum. Conditions that are widely considered variants of preeclampsia are as follows:

- **Eclampsia** is the term for grand mal seizures in a person with preeclampsia that are not caused by any other disorder.
- **HELLP syndrome** may be a subtype of preeclampsia with severe features though it occurs without proteinuria or hypertension in about 15% of cases (Sibai, 2023).
- **Preeclampsia superimposed on chronic hypertension** is diagnosed when a client with chronic hypertension develops worsening or resistant hypertension (especially acutely); new onset or sudden increase of proteinuria; and/or significant new end-organ dysfunction, such as visual disturbances, severe headache, or low platelets, after 20 weeks of gestation (ACOG, 2019).

In one analysis of nearly 4 million births, 11% of hospitalized mothers had a hypertension-related diagnosis (Fingar et al., 2017). Of these, 4.7% were diagnosed with preeclampsia, 3.8% with gestational hypertension, 1.7% with chronic hypertension, and 0.6% with unspecified hypertension (Fingar et al., 2017). Of those with preeclampsia, about 47% were diagnosed with mild or unspecified preeclampsia, 37% with preeclampsia with severe features or HELLP, 1.4% with eclampsia, and 15% with preeclampsia superimposed on chronic hypertension (Fingar et al., 2017).

Other Hypertensive Conditions

White-coat hypertension is a condition in which the client has elevated BP (140/90 mm Hg or higher) in a clinic or hospital but normal readings at home. Both ACOG and the International Society of Hypertension in Pregnancy (ISSHP) have recognized WCH as a valid diagnostic category in pregnancy (ACOG, 2019; Brown et al., 2018; Druzin & Shields, 2021a). For clients with WCH, the risk for having an infant that is preterm, small for gestational age, or in need of admission to the neonatal intensive care unit (NICU) is higher than for that of normotensive people, but lower than the risk for those with gestational hypertension (Johnson, Liu, Kalafat, Thilaganathan, & Khalil, 2020). Later in pregnancy, however, about 40% of clients with WCH develop gestational hypertension, and 8% of clients with WCH progress to preeclampsia (Druzin & Shields, 2021a). For the client with WCH, home monitoring provides more accurate assessment of BP than does an office examination (Brown et al., 2018; Brown, Mangos, Davis, & Homer, 2005; Townsend, O'Brien, & Khalil, 2016).

Masked hypertension is the opposite of WCH; BP is consistently normal in the office but elevated with home monitoring (Magee, Pels, et al., 2014). Risk factors include HDP in a previous pregnancy, diabetes, and smoking (Bello, Miller, et al., 2018). Masked hypertension and sustained hypertension entail comparable risk of cardiovascular events (Unger et al., 2020). The diagnosis is confirmed with BP monitoring at home and in the office.

Hypertensive Disorders of Pregnancy (HDP)

As shown above, the term *hypertensive disorders of pregnancy* encompasses a wide range of conditions from the chronic to the acute and from nonsevere to severe (Sibai, 2021). Often the clinical manifestations are similar when they have different underlying causes or etiologies. Although each disorder increases the risk of poor maternal and newborn outcomes, a

Table 10-1

Hypertensive Disorders of Pregnancy (HDP)

Chronic (preexisting) hypertension	
• Hypertension diagnosed or present before pregnancy or before 20 weeks of gestation. Hypertension first diagnosed during pregnancy that persists for at least 12 weeks postpartum is also considered chronic hypertension.	• Systolic blood pressure (SBP) ≥140 mm Hg, diastolic blood pressure (DBP) ≥90 mm Hg, or both. Ideally, this diagnosis is based on at least two elevated BP measurements taken at least 4 hr apart. In severe hypertension, the diagnosis can be confirmed in a shorter interval to facilitate timely treatment.
Gestational hypertension	
• New onset of SBP ≥140 mm Hg or DBP ≥90 mm Hg on at least two occasions 4 hr apart after 20 weeks of gestation in a previously normotensive client.	**And** • No proteinuria. • No severe features of preeclampsia (thrombocytopenia, renal insufficiency, elevated liver transaminases, pulmonary edema, or headache, confusion, or visual disturbances).
Preeclampsia	
• New-onset SBP ≥140 mm Hg or DBP ≥90 mm Hg on at least two occasions at least 4 hr apart after 20 weeks of gestation in a previously normotensive client **or** SBP ≥160 mm Hg or DBP ≥110 mm Hg confirmed within minutes to facilitate timely antihypertensive therapy. **And** • Proteinuria (≥300 mg from a 24-hr urine collection **or** extrapolated from a timed collection) **or** protein/creatinine ratio (PCR) ≥0.3 **or** urine dipstick reading ≥2+ when other quantitative methods are not available.	**Or,** in the absence of proteinuria, new-onset hypertension with new onset of any of the following: • Thrombocytopenia (platelet count <100,000/mcl). • Renal insufficiency (serum creatinine >1.1 mg/dl or doubling of baseline value in the absence of other renal disease). • Impaired liver function (liver transaminase levels at least twice the normal concentration). • Pulmonary edema. • Persistent headache, altered mental status, or visual disturbances.
Preeclampsia with Severe Features	
Any of these findings in a client with preeclampsia:	
• SBP ≥160 mm Hg or DBP ≥110 mm Hg on two occasions at least 4 hr apart (However, severe-range hypertension should be confirmed within a few minutes and anti-hypertension therapy should be started immediately upon confirmation). • Thrombocytopenia (platelet count <100,000/mcl). • Liver transaminase levels at least twice the normal concentration or severe, persistent right upper quadrant	(RUQ) or epigastric pain unresponsive to medication and not accounted for by alternative diagnoses, or both. • Renal insufficiency (serum creatinine >1.1 mg/dl or doubling of baseline value in the absence of other renal disease). • Pulmonary edema. • Persistent headache, altered mental status, or visual disturbances.

diagnosis of preeclampsia carries the greatest risk (Townsend et al., 2016). The community midwife must remain vigilant for signs and symptoms of hypertensive disorders and respond to them decisively if they occur.

Chronic Hypertension

Chronic hypertension is defined as BP at or above 140/90 mm Hg, documented before pregnancy or first recognized before 20 weeks of gestation. The diagnosis is also given when hypertension persists 12 or more weeks postpartum (ACOG, 2019). When a client presents for care in the second trimester, the diagnosis of chronic hypertension can be missed because of the normal physiologic decrease in BP between 13 and 19 weeks of gestation (Jeyabalan & Larkin, 2023). About 1–5% of pregnancies involve chronic hypertension, and the rate has been growing steadily, largely because of increasing maternal age and rising rates of obesity and diabetes (Shields, 2021a). Less commonly, hypertension can arise from a secondary cause such as pheochromocytoma, primary aldosteronism, Cushing syndrome, methamphetamine or cocaine use, or renal artery stenosis (Jeyabalan & Larkin, 2023). In a study of 152 million births in the National Hospital Discharge Survey, Ananth et al. (2019) found that chronic maternal hypertension in the United States increased more than 1,300% in the period 1970–2010, inclusive. Although the black-white disparity decreased markedly during the study period, by the end black mothers' rate

Hypertensive Disorders of Pregnancy (HDP) *continued*

<table>
<tr><th colspan="2">Eclampsia</th></tr>
<tr><td colspan="2">In a client with preeclampsia, generalized seizures not attributable to other causes.</td></tr>
<tr><th colspan="2">HELLP syndrome</th></tr>
<tr><td colspan="2">Hemolysis, elevated liver enzymes (to more than twice the upper limit normal concentrations), and low platelet count (hypertension and proteinuria are not always present).</td></tr>
<tr><th colspan="2">Chronic hypertension with superimposed preeclampsia</th></tr>
<tr><td colspan="2">Any of these findings in a client with chronic hypertension:</td></tr>
<tr><td>• Sudden increase in BP that was previously well-controlled or an escalation of antihypertensive therapy to control BP.</td><td>• New-onset proteinuria or sudden increase in proteinuria in a client with known proteinuria.</td></tr>
<tr><th colspan="2">Chronic hypertension with superimposed preeclampsia with severe features</th></tr>
<tr><td colspan="2">Any of these findings in a client with chronic hypertension and superimposed preeclampsia:</td></tr>
<tr><td>• SBP ≥160 mm Hg or DBP ≥110 mm Hg despite escalation of antihypertensive therapy.
• Thrombocytopenia (platelet count <100,000/mcl).
• Liver transaminase levels at least twice normal or severe, persistent RUQ, epigastric pain unresponsive to medication and not otherwise accounted for, or both.</td><td>• New-onset or worsening renal insufficiency.
• Pulmonary edema.
• Persistent headache, altered mental status, or visual disturbances.</td></tr>
<tr><td colspan="2">Adapted from (1) "Gestational Hypertension and Preeclampsia (Practice Bulletin 222)," by American College of Obstetricians and Gynecologists, 2020a/2023, Obstetrics & Gynecology, 135(6), e237–e260. Copyright 2020 by ACOG. (2) "Hypertensive Disorders in Pregnancy: Approach to Differential Diagnosis," by P. August and B. M. Sibai, 2023a, in V. A. (Ed.), UpToDate. Copyright by UpToDate.</td></tr>
</table>

of chronic hypertension was still 68% higher than that of white mothers.

BP occurs on a continuum; potential for harm increases with higher readings (Reddy et al., 2020). Criteria for hypertension were identical for the pregnant and nonpregnant until 2017, when AHA and the American College of Cardiology recommended lower diagnostic thresholds for hypertension in nonpregnant people to better identify and modify long-term cardiovascular risk (Jeyabalan & Larkin, 2023). They redefined *elevated blood pressure* as an SBP of 120–129 mm Hg and DBP below 80 mm Hg, *stage 1 hypertension* as an SBP of 130–139 mm Hg or DBP of 80–89 mm Hg, and *stage 2 hypertension* as an SBP of 140 mm Hg or higher or a DBP of 90 mm Hg or higher (Basile & Bloch, 2023; Carey & Whelton, 2018).

Although it is uncertain whether these lower thresholds should also be recommended in pregnancy, there is evidence that the risk of preeclampsia is greater in those with elevated BP or stage 1 hypertension than in normotensive pregnant people (Reddy et al., 2020; Wu et al., 2020). In addition, Reddy et al. (2020) found that 5%–8% of pregnant people with stage 1 hypertension develop preeclampsia; the baseline risk in normotensive people is 1%–2%. These subjects were also found to be at higher risk for PTB and adverse perinatal outcomes (Reddy et al., 2020). Revising criteria to apply lower thresholds for hypertension in pregnancy in accordance with the guidelines for nonpregnant people would increase identification of pregnancies at risk for HDP by 20% and would increase identification of pregnancies at risk for adverse neonatal outcomes by 3.8% (Jeyabalan & Larkin, 2023).

Chronic hypertension increases the risk for preeclampsia, placental abruption, postpartum hemorrhage, longer hospitalization, and need for planned or emergent cesarean section (Jeyabalan & Larkin, 2023). It also increases the risk of PTB, low birthweight, and NICU admission. Further, it appears to be associated with greater risk for congenital cardiac malformations, esophageal atresia, and hypospadias (Jeyabalan & Larkin, 2023). The risk of perinatal mortality is two to four times higher than that in pregnancies without chronic hypertension, even when adjusted for preeclampsia and birthweight (Jeyabalan & Larkin, 2023). Adverse pregnancy outcomes are more likely if hypertension is severe (SBP higher than 160 mm Hg) and/or end-organ damage develops (Bramham et al., 2014). Other maternal risks of chronic hypertension in pregnancy (Jeyabalan & Larkin, 2023) include

- Acute kidney failure—5.9 per 1,000 births
- Pulmonary edema—1.5 per 1,000 births
- In-hospital mortality—0.4 per 1,000 births
- Stroke/cerebrovascular complications—2.7 per 1,000 births
- Gestational diabetes—8.1%

Antepartum Management of Chronic Hypertension

Managing chronic hypertension in pregnancy involves balancing the risks of excessively high blood pressure (serious or fatal maternal cerebrovascular, cardiac, or renal events) against the risk of inadequate placental perfusion if BP becomes too low. Chronic hypertension requires careful evaluation by an obstetrician or maternal-fetal medicine (MFM) specialist early in pregnancy to evaluate risk for serious complications and determine whether antihypertensive medications are necessary. The Chronic Hypertension and Pregnancy (CHAP) Study (Tita et al., 2022), found that when the BP remains less than 140/90 mm Hg, pregnant people with chronic hypertension have a lower risk of preeclampsia with severe features, medically indicated PTB at less than 35 weeks of gestation, placental abruption, and fetal or neonatal death compared to when BP is higher than this threshold. As a result, ACOG and the Society for Maternal-Fetal Medicine [SMFM] have recommended that chronic hypertension in pregnancy should be treated with antihypertensive medications to achieve a target BP of less than 140/90, rather than the previously recommended threshold of 160/110 (ACOG, 2022; SMFM, 2022). People who are taking antihypertensive medications at conception should continue their treatment or change to an agent that is safer for pregnancy (ACOG, 2022; SMFM, 2022).

Because of the high risk of complications for the pregnant client with chronic hypertension, a physician should manage or comanage care. Consultation or comanagement by MFM specialists is prudent. Hospital birth should be planned. Management for the antepartum client with chronic hypertension includes (Jeyabalan & Larkin, 2023)

- Daily low-dose oral aspirin therapy (81 mg) is recommended after 12 weeks of gestation until giving birth to decrease the risk of developing preeclampsia (see below).
- A healthy diet and strict weight management are crucial; obesity is associated with higher BP.
- Baseline and ongoing evaluation should include BP, heart rate, cardiopulmonary auscultation, and evaluation for signs of cardiac dysfunction including cyanosis, liver enlargement, jugular venous distension, or pulmonary edema.
- Baseline laboratory studies should be obtained to evaluate kidney and liver function, including serum creatinine, liver transaminases, platelet count, and electrolytes and urine protein-creatinine ratio or 24-hr urine for protein.
- Transthoracic echocardiography or twelve-lead electrocardiogram should be considered for clients with longstanding or uncontrolled hypertension.
- Ultrasound studies can establish accurate dating and follow the growth of the fetus.
- Weekly or twice-weekly biophysical profiles or nonstress tests with amniotic fluid estimation are used to evaluate fetal wellbeing (ACOG, 2021/2024). These are usually started at 32 weeks of gestation but may be started sooner when the risk of fetal compromise is high.
- Discuss the signs and symptoms of preeclampsia and encourage the client to report any severe or persistent headache; visual disturbances; right-upper-quadrant (RUQ), chest, or epigastric pain; new onset of nausea or vomiting in the third trimester; new onset of shortness of breath; altered mental status; or vaginal bleeding.

Preeclampsia

Preeclampsia is a complex inflammatory syndrome that can affect multiple systems and have multiple causes (U.S. Preventive Services Task Force [USPSTF], 2021). It is usually associated with new-onset hypertension, most commonly near term, and resolves postpartum over a variable time (ACOG, 2020a/2023). About 90% of cases present after 34 weeks of gestation or postpartum (ACOG, 2020a/2023). Preeclampsia is thought to evolve from abnormalities in placental development or overactive inflammatory responses to normal placentation that lead to placental ischemia and maternal vascular dysfunction (USPSTF, 2021).

Preeclampsia is both common and serious, complicating up to 8% of pregnancies worldwide (ACOG, 2020a/2023). It is responsible for more than 500,000 fetal and neonatal deaths and more than 70,000 maternal deaths annually (Brown et al., 2018). In the United States, the rate of preeclampsia grew 25% between 1987 and 2004 (ACOG, 2020a/2023). Moreover, the client with a history of preeclampsia has an 18.2% risk of a cardiovascular event within 10 years; without preeclampsia, the risk is 1.7% (Folk, 2018).

Preeclampsia is the most dangerous of the HDP (Cunningham et al., 2022, ch. 40). Although most cases have good maternal, fetal, and newborn outcomes, it carries significant risk for serious maternal morbidity and mortality including abruption, pulmonary edema, myocardial infarction, blood-clotting abnormalities, brain hemorrhage, kidney failure, and liver dysfunction. Fetal risks include fetal growth restriction (FGR), preterm rupture of membranes, abnormal fetal heart rate (FHR) pattern, spontaneous or iatrogenic PTB, and fetal demise.

Pathophysiology

The abnormalities in uteroplacental circulation associated with preeclampsia develop very early in pregnancy, long before signs of disease. In normal pregnancies, the cytotrophoblast cells of the developing placenta extend through the uterine decidua and surface of the myometrium to penetrate the

Table 10-2
Risks of Chronic Hypertension in Pregnancy

Maternal	Fetal/Neonatal
• Severe hypertension • Superimposed preeclampsia • Abruption • Postpartum hemorrhage • Renal insufficiency/failure • Stroke • Myocardial infarction • Pulmonary edema • Death	• Fetal growth restriction (FGR) / small for gestational age • Preterm birth (PTB) • Congenital anomalies • Stillbirth • Neonatal death

maternal spiral arteries (August & Sibai, 2023b). To optimize blood flow for the developing fetus, these arteries transform from tight muscular channels to wide, curvy, low-resistance pipelines (August & Sibai, 2023b). In preeclampsia, this penetration is incomplete. As a result, maternal blood vessels remain narrow and unyielding, reducing blood flow to the developing placenta. A poorly perfused placenta releases substances into the maternal bloodstream that interfere with the function of endothelial cells. These substances damage and constrict blood vessels, particularly in the maternal kidney, brain, and liver, affecting organ function and causing systemic hypertension (Ali & Khalil, 2015).

Low placental perfusion can be both a cause and a result of abnormal placental development. Preeclampsia often follows conditions of maternal vascular insufficiency (such as hypertension, diabetes, and thrombophilia) and conditions that produce relative ischemia by increasing placental mass without increasing blood flow, such as hydatidiform mole, diabetes mellitus, and multiple pregnancy (Karumanchi, Lim, & August, 2023). Likewise, infection with COVID-19 can lead to systemic endothelial dysfunction and preeclampsia (Wei, Bilodeau-Bertrand, Liu, & Auger, 2021), especially in those with comorbidities such as obesity, diabetes, hypertension, and heart or lung disease (Villar et al., 2021). As gestation advances, this abnormal vasculature fails to meet the increasing demands for blood flow to the placenta, and the placenta develops ischemia.

Risk Factors

One third of people with preeclampsia are nulliparous, and most of the remainder are at higher-than-normal risk for the disease because of overweight/obesity, prior preeclampsia, chronic hypertension, multifetal pregnancy, chronic kidney disease, or diabetes (August & Sibai, 2023b). Obstructive sleep apnea is also a risk factor for preeclampsia. (Druzin & Shields, 2021a). In subsequent pregnancies after a diagnosis of preeclampsia, the rate of reoccurrence is approximately 25% (Bartal & Sibai, 2020). Preeclampsia in the second trimester carries a higher risk of reoccurrence (Bartal & Sibai, 2020).

Conde-Agudelo and Romero (2021) found that COVID-19 infection during pregnancy increases the risk of developing preeclampsia by 62%. Although asymptomatic and symptomatic COVID-19 infections alike increase the risk for preeclampsia, risk is higher with symptomatic infections (Conde-Agudelo & Romero, 2021; Papageorghiou et al., 2021). Preeclampsia tends to develop 3–4 weeks after diagnosis of COVID-19 infection (Conde-Agudelo & Romero, 2021).

A person with any of the following risk factors is considered at high risk and has at least an 8% chance of developing preeclampsia (ACOG & SMFM, 2021/2022):

- History of preeclampsia, especially when accompanied by an adverse outcome.
- Multifetal gestation.
- Chronic hypertension.
- Pregestational diabetes.
- Kidney disease.
- Autoimmune disease, including systemic lupus erythematosus and antiphospholipid syndrome.
- Combinations of multiple moderate-risk factors.

Some factors create a moderate risk for preeclampsia, and some increase risk more than others. These factors include (ACOG & SMFM, 2021/2022)

- Nulliparity.
- Obesity (BMI greater than 30).
- Mother or sister with preeclampsia.
- Lower income.
- Age 35 years or older.
- History of low birthweight or small-for-gestational-age baby, previous adverse pregnancy outcome.
- More than 10 years since last pregnancy.
- Assisted reproduction.
- Sub-Saharan African heritage, not because of biological propensities, but because of environmental, social, structural, and historical inequities that affect health exposures, access to health care, and the unequal distribution of resources (ACOG & SMFM, 2021/2022).
- Second or higher-numbered pregnancy with a new partner (Robillard et al., 2022).
- Lack of exposure to partner's sperm before conception from using barrier contraception or assisted reproduction technology (Robillard et al., 2022).

Prevention of Preeclampsia

Low-dose aspirin. For people at moderate to high risk of preeclampsia, daily low-dose aspirin (81 mg/day) can reduce the likelihood of developing the disease by 10–20% (August & Jeyabalan, 2023; USPSTF, 2021). Preeclampsia is a multifactorial system-wide syndrome involving inflammation throughout the body. Aspirin therapy decreases the activation of the immune system and oxidative stress and improves vascular function associated with preeclampsia. Low-dose aspirin therapy does not increase the risk of placental abruption or postpartum hemorrhage, nor does it increase mean blood loss (ACOG & SMFM, 2021/2022,). Consequently, ACOG and SMFM (2021) recommend low-dose aspirin prophylaxis for mothers at high risk of preeclampsia starting between 12 and 28 weeks of gestation (ideally 12–16 weeks) and continuing daily until giving birth. In people with chronic hypertension, low-dose aspirin seems less effective in preventing superimposed preeclampsia with severe features, FGR, or PTB (Banala et al., 2020).

Calcium supplementation. For pregnant people with nutritional deficiencies (especially in low-resource countries), calcium supplementation can reduce the incidence of preeclampsia (Hofmeyr, Lawrie, Atallah, & Torloni, 2018; Ives, Sinkey, Rajapreyar, Tita, & Oparil, 2020).

Of Potential Benefit

Exercise, especially during the first 20 weeks of gestation, appears to reduce the risk of preeclampsia without adverse fetal effects (Sorensen et al., 2003). To reduce the risk of preeclampsia, clients must perform at least 140 min per week of moderate-intensity exercise, enough to raise the heart rate and allow speaking but not singing (Davenport et al., 2018). Workouts of greater intensity appear to provide greater benefit than moderate-activity workouts (Sorensen et al., 2003).

Pravastatin (a medication used to improve serum cholesterol levels) appears to improve endothelial function and prevent injury from oxidation and inflammation. Its role in the prevention of preeclampsia is currently being studied (Costantine et al., 2021).

Metformin (a medication used to control blood sugar levels in people with diabetes) appears to reduce the incidence of preeclampsia. In one study of subjects without diabetes who had a BMI of more than 35, metformin therapy was associated with a 76% reduction in the incidence of preeclampsia, from 11.3% to 3.0% (Magee, Nicolaides, & Von Dadelszen, 2022; Syngelaki et al., 2016). More research is necessary to confirm benefit.

Clinical Presentation

Preeclampsia is usually diagnosed when a client between 20 weeks of gestation and 6 weeks postpartum experiences the new onset of hypertension with proteinuria or hypertension with dysfunction of major organs caused by abnormal perfusion, that is, end-organ dysfunction (ACOG, 2020a/2023). Preeclampsia can occur without proteinuria, and massive proteinuria (5 g/24 hr) does not necessarily indicate severe disease (August & Sibai, 2023b). Preeclampsia is more common at or near term. Although only 1.5% of pregnancies develop preeclampsia before 37 weeks of gestation, about half of these cases are severe (Shields, 2021b).

The clinical course of preeclampsia is unpredictable and potentially treacherous. One client presenting with subtle signs or symptoms of preeclampsia might progress to a life-threatening disease within hours; another might remain relatively stable for weeks. Preeclampsia usually resolves shortly after the baby is born, but delayed postpartum preeclampsia can develop as late as 42 days after giving birth (Al-Safi et al., 2011).

Preeclampsia with Severe Features

About 25% of preeclamptic clients have preeclampsia with severe features, which carries a higher risk of maternal/fetal morbidity and mortality (August & Sibai, 2023b). Preeclampsia with severe features is characterized by severe hypertension and/or one or more of the following nonspecific symptoms:

- Persistent and/or severe headache.
- Visual abnormalities such as new-onset photopsia (perceived flashes of light), scotomata (areas or islands of altered or absent vision in an otherwise normal visual field), cortical blindness, or blurred vision.
- Upper abdominal, retrosternal, or epigastric pain.
- Confusion, agitation.
- Difficulty breathing, orthopnea.
- Rarely, a client has symptoms of severe preeclampsia without hypertension (August & Sibai, 2023b).

The course of preeclampsia is variable. A stable client with nonsevere preeclampsia can develop severe features, HELLP syndrome, and/or eclampsia within hours (Druzin & Shields, 2021a). Rapid progression to severe preeclampsia is most common when preeclampsia develops before 34 0/7 weeks of gestation (Druzin & Shields, 2021a). Anyone with findings suggestive of severe preeclampsia requires urgent evaluation and prompt treatment to decrease BP (if it is elevated) and can require delivery (August & Sibai, 2023b; Druzin, Shields, Morton, & Peterson, 2021).

Postpartum Preeclampsia

Although most mothers with preeclampsia begin to improve as soon as they expel the placenta, for some, giving birth is not the cure. In about 5% of cases, the first signs of preeclampsia are recognized postpartum, typically within the first 48 hr after birth (August & Sibai, 2023b). Continue to assess clients for signs of preeclampsia and ask questions about symptoms that could suggest preeclampsia throughout the postpartum period. Most commonly, the client with postpartum preeclampsia presents with a severe headache and/or shortness of breath or malaise, usually accompanied by hypertension (Gabel & Peterson, 2021b).

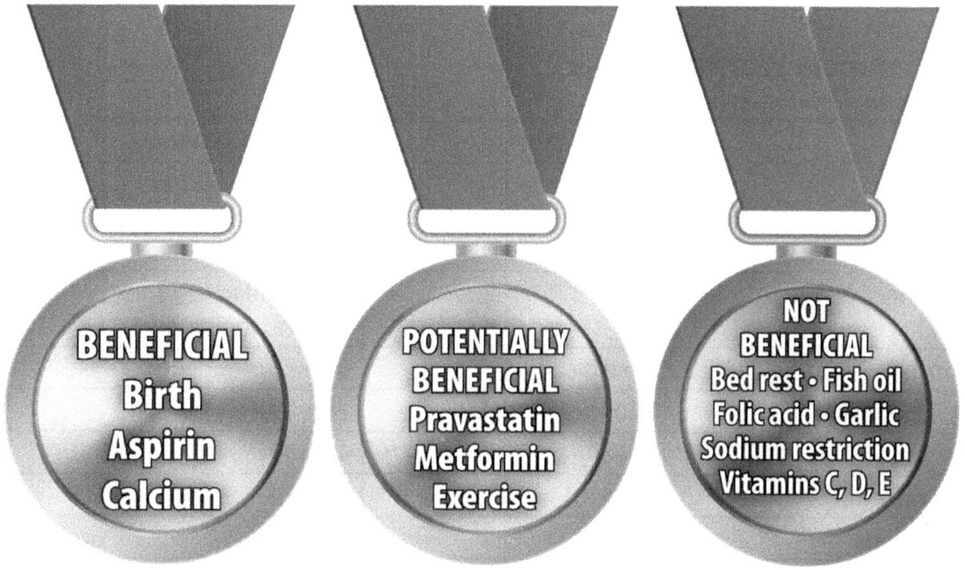
BENEFICIAL
Birth
Aspirin
Calcium
POTENTIALLY BENEFICIAL
Pravastatin
Metformin
Exercise
NOT BENEFICIAL
Bed rest • Fish oil
Folic acid • Garlic
Sodium restriction
Vitamins C, D, E

Figure 10-1. The only interventions proven to reduce the incidence of preeclampsia are calcium supplementation if dietary intake is insufficient and a daily low-dose aspirin tablet. People at high risk (for example, those with chronic hypertension) may be induced at 39 weeks of gestation to decrease the likelihood of preeclampsia. It appears that exercise and treatment with pravastatin or metformin can reduce the incidence of preeclampsia, but more studies are needed to confirm these findings. Bed rest; sodium restriction; fish oil; garlic, folic acid; and supplementation with vitamin C, D, or E have been proven ineffective in preventing preeclampsia. Adapted from "Preeclampsia—Pathophysiology and Clinical Presentations: JACC State-of-the-Art Review," by C. W. Ives, R. Sinkey, I. Rajapreyar, A. T. N. Tita, and S. Oparil, 2020, *Journal of the American College of Cardiology, 76*(14), p. 1699. Copyright by American College of Cardiology Foundation.

It is not fully understood why preeclampsia would develop or worsen postpartum, after the placenta is out. Disease onset does not appear to be related to retained placental fragments. It is possible that clients who develop postpartum preeclampsia have subclinical preeclampsia before giving birth and are slow to clear the associated inflammatory factors, and the disease process is exacerbated by postpartum fluid shifts (August & Sibai, 2023b).

Atypical Preeclampsia

Preeclampsia can occur without hypertension (especially with HELLP syndrome) or without proteinuria (August & Sibai, 2023b). In some cases of atypical preeclampsia, eclamptic seizure is the first manifestation of disease. In other cases, visual changes or severe headache are the presenting symptoms. Isolated gestational proteinuria can be an early sign of preeclampsia. Onset of preeclampsia before 20 weeks of gestation is rare and is usually related to renal disease, autoimmune disease, or molar pregnancy (ACOG, 2020a/2023).

HELLP Syndrome

HELLP syndrome is a critical form of preeclampsia with severe features associated with higher rates of maternal morbidity and mortality (ACOG, 2020a/2023). It is characterized by red-blood cell hemolysis, thrombocytopenia, and abnormal elevations in liver transaminases and develops in 1–2% of people with severe preeclampsia (Sibai, 2023). HELLP syndrome can be easy to miss. Up to 15% of HELLP cases do not involve hypertension or proteinuria (Sibai, 2023). Although it is mostly a third-trimester condition, some cases occur in the late second trimester, and 30% occur during the postpartum period (ACOG, 2020a/2023).

Signs and symptoms are as follows (Sibai, 2023):

- Proteinuria (86% or more)
- Hypertension (82–88%)
- RUQ/epigastric/substernal pain (40–90%)
- Nausea, vomiting (29–84%)
- Headache (33–61%)
- Visual changes (10–20%)
- Jaundice (5%)

Signs and symptoms usually have a rapid onset and can progress quickly to serious morbidity. The client with HELLP syndrome is at high risk of life-threating complications, including disseminated intravascular coagulation (DIC, 15–30%), pulmonary edema (8%), acute renal failure (3%), acute respiratory distress syndrome (1%), and stroke (1%) as well as placental abruption, acute kidney injury, subcapsular or intraparenchymal liver hematoma, and retinal detachment (Sibai, 2023). The risk of maternal death is about 1% (Druzin & Shields, 2021a).

Table 10-3

Preeclampsia Warning Signs

Watch for rapid changes in condition

Assess	Normal (Green)	Worrisome (Yellow)	Severe (Red)
Awareness	Alert/oriented	Agitated/confused Drowsy Difficulty speaking	Unresponsive
Headache	None	Mild headache Nausea, vomiting	Unrelieved headache Hyperreflexia
Vision	No difficulty	Blurred or impaired	Temporary blindness
SBP	100–139	140–159	≥160
DBP	50–89	90–109	≥110
Heart rate	61–110	110–120	>120
Respirations	11–24	<12 or 25–30	<10 or >30
Shortness of breath	Absent	Present	Present
Oxygen saturation	≥95%	<95%	<93%
Abdominal or chest pain	None	Nausea/vomiting Chest pain Abdominal pain	Nausea/vomiting Chest pain Abdominal pain
Fetal wellbeing	Category I Reactive NST	Category II Nonreactive NST FGR	Category III
Urine output	≥50 ml/hr	35–49 ml/hr	≤35 in 2 hr
Proteinuria	Dipstick Trace ≤300 mg/24 hr	≥300 mg/24 hr PCR >0.3 Dipstick 1+	≥300 mg/24 hr PCR >0.3 Dipstick 3+
Platelets	>139 k is normal >100 k of low concern	50–100 k	<50 k
Aspartate/alanine aminotransferase (ALT/AST)	<70	>70	>70
Creatinine	≤0.8	0.81–1.0	≥1.1

Adapted from "Preeclampsia Early Recognition Tool (PERT)," in M. L. Druzin, L. E. Shields, N. Peterson, C. Sakowski, V. Cape, and C. H. Morton (Eds.), *Improving Health Care Response to Hypertensive Disorders of Pregnancy: A California Maternal Quality Care Collaborative Quality Improvement Toolkit* (p. 193), 2021, Stanford, CA: California Maternal Quality Care Collaborative.

The diagnosis of HELLP is established when the following are present:

- Hemolysis, established by at least two of the following (Sibai, 2023):
  - Peripheral smear with schistocytes and burr cells.
  - Serum bilirubin 1.2 mg/dl or higher.
  - Lactate dehydrogenase (LDH) 2 or more times the upper limit of normal.
  - Severe anemia unrelated to blood loss.
- Elevated liver enzymes: aspartate aminotransferase (AST) or alanine aminotransferase (ALT) 2 or more times the upper limit of normal.
- Low platelets: below 100,000 cells/mcl.

Hepatic Complications

Rarely, marked elevations in liver enzymes (above 1,000–2,000 IU/L) with severe upper abdominal pain can indicate hepatic infarction or subcapsular hematoma of the liver. Hepatic infarction typically presents with markedly elevated liver enzymes, RUQ pain, and fever and can lead to liver failure and death (Sibai, 2021). Hepatic rupture is another rare but deadly complication of HELLP syndrome. The hematoma may remain contained beneath the Glisson capsule or rupture and hemorrhage into the peritoneal cavity (Sibai, 2021).

Profound hypovolemic shock in a previously hypertensive pregnant client with RUQ pain suggests rupture of a subcapsular hematoma of the liver, a surgical emergency that requires multidisciplinary treatment at a tertiary hospital. Hepatic rupture is usually accompanied by shoulder pain, shock, abdominal distension, rebound tenderness, DIC, and respiratory difficulty. Often there is fetal demise.

Overview of Management

Because severe maternal complications can develop quickly, clients with HELLP should be admitted to a tertiary center capable of providing maternal and NICU care (ACOG, 2020a/2023). Some authors suggest prompt birth regardless of gestational age (ACOG, 2020a/2023). Others recommend considering a course of antenatal steroids before proceeding to birth if the mother and fetus are stable before 34 0/7 weeks of gestation (Shields, 2021b). When birth is delayed, the client should be monitored closely with laboratory testing at least every 12-hr, continuous fetal monitoring, antihypertensive therapy as appropriate, and magnesium sulfate to prevent maternal seizures and for fetal neuroprotection in pregnancies below 32 0/7 weeks of gestation (ACOG, 2020a/2023). Signs and symptoms eventually resolve after giving birth, but HELLP can also persist or develop postpartum.

DIFFERENTIAL DIAGNOSES FOR PREECLAMPSIA / HELLP SYNDROME

Hyperthyroidism can present with hypertension and tachycardia (August & Sibai, 2023a).

Hyperparathyroidism can present with hypertension and hypercalcemia.

Recreational drugs such as cocaine, amphetamines, and phencyclidine (angel dust) can cause hypertension and tachycardia.

Gastroesophageal reflux and peptic ulcer disease may involve abdominal discomfort, but laboratory values will be normal, and pain may improve with antacid medications.

Hepatitis may involve RUQ pain and elevated liver enzymes. Serologic testing confirms the diagnosis.

Cholecystitis may present with RUQ, chest, or epigastric pain that radiates to the back. There is often fever and leukocytosis. Ultrasonography usually shows gallbladder abnormalities.

Pancreatitis may present with epigastric pain that radiates to the back and lipase or amylase readings up to three times or greater than the upper limit of normal.

Pheochromocytoma (a rare adrenal tumor that secretes epinephrine and norepinephrine) may present with hypertension, headache, sweating, palpitations, tremor, pallor, dyspnea, generalized weakness, and sometimes hyperglycemia.

Acute fatty liver of pregnancy (AFLP, inflammation and cell necrosis caused by fatty acids and their metabolites infiltrating the maternal liver) can present with many of the signs

First Thought, Worst Thought

What is the most likely cause of nausea and vomiting with RUQ/epigastric pain?

Gastroenteritis, cholecystitis

What is the worst it could be?

HELLP syndrome

and symptoms of HELLP syndrome, including hypertension, nausea and vomiting, abdominal pain, malaise, headache, elevated liver enzymes, and coagulopathy. Typically, serum fibrinogen level is below 300 mg/dl in AFLP and above 300 mg/dl in preeclampsia with severe features or HELLP unless there is also an abruption or major hemorrhage (August & Sibai, 2023a). The client with preeclampsia is afebrile; the client with AFLP may run a low-grade fever.

Antiphospholipid syndrome (an autoimmune thrombophilic condition) can present with hypertension, proteinuria, thrombocytopenia, and other signs of end-organ dysfunction. The pregnant client with antiphospholipid syndrome may develop severe preeclampsia, eclampsia, or placental insufficiency.

Mirror syndrome occurs when a person carrying a hydropic fetus and placenta develops generalized edema, often with lung involvement, that "mirrors" the edema of the fetus (Lockwood & Julien, 2022). Although it is a rare condition, mirror syndrome can develop in any pregnancy with fetal hydrops, including those with rhesus isoimmunization, congenital infection, twin-to-twin transfusion, structural anomalies, and fetal malignancies (Mathias & Rizvi, 2019). Mirror syndrome can mimic or coexist with preeclampsia, but there are dissimilarities (Mathias & Rizvi, 2019). In preeclampsia, the maternal hematocrit tends to increase (hemoconcentration); in mirror syndrome, hemodilution tends to decrease the hematocrit (Mathias & Rizvi, 2019). In preeclampsia, oligohydramnios is common; in mirror syndrome, polyhydramnios is likely.

Infection with COVID-19 appears to both mimic and increase the risk of preeclampsia (Abedzadeh-Kalahroudi, Sehat, Vahedpour, & Talebian, 2021). Headaches, malaise, and nausea are common manifestations of COVID-19. Pregnant people with COVID-19 often develop hypertension and kidney dysfunction that is very difficult to distinguish from preeclampsia (Farahani, Azadi, Hashemnejad, Agoushi, & Nirouei, 2021; Jayaram et al., 2021).

Migraine is characterized by recurrent headaches in people with normal laboratory test values. Migraine headaches are usually unilateral and tend to pulse or throb (Lee, Guinn, &

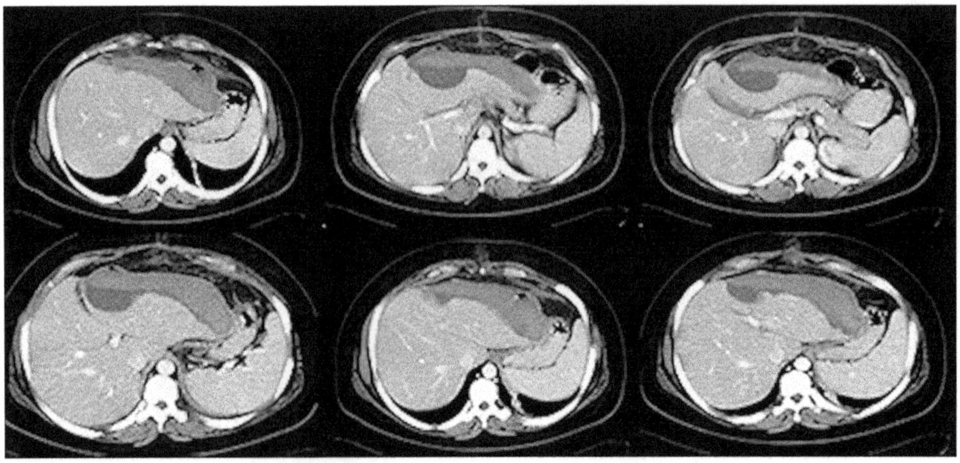

Figure 10-2. Hepatic rupture in HELLP syndrome. This case involved a 30-year-old woman, gravida 3, para 2 (G3 P2), at 38 weeks of gestation with a history of hypertension and obesity. She presented in labor and developed a sudden onset of pain in the RUQ that radiated to the right shoulder. Laboratory studies were consistent with HELLP syndrome. An emergency cesarean revealed a large amount of blood in the abdominal cavity from the rupture and active hemorrhage of a subcapsular hepatic hematoma involving the entire left lobe. She recovered and was discharged on the 13th postoperative day. From "Hepatic Rupture in HELLP Syndrome," by C. Moura et al., 2019, *Journal of Surgical Case Reports, 2019*, 10, fig. 2. CC-BY-NC 4.0.

Hickenbottom, 2023). Migraine headaches are often associated with irritability, difficulty concentrating, fatigue, insomnia, nausea, or sensitivity to light or sound. Sometimes there is an aura which involves shimmering lights or zigzags in the vision, tingling or numbness in one limb or on one side of the face, or even losing sight entirely in one or both eyes. These may be followed in minutes by scotomata (blurry or blind spots), numbness, or loss of sensation (Evans, 2014). Some atypical migraines can mimic stroke symptoms further by including weakness on one side of the body (hemiplegia). A migraine postdrome may involve fatigue, body aches and mental fogginess.

Unlike the symptoms of cerebral ischemic events, however, migraines usually begin slowly, spread or worsen over time, then gradually subside within 20–60 min. A person with migraine-related deficits typically regains function first in the areas first affected, then the other symptoms will resolve in order of occurrence. The client with cerebral ischemia usually presents with the simultaneous onset of multiple neurological symptoms that resolve more slowly or not at all.

Eclampsia

Eclampsia usually refers to new-onset, generalized tonic-clonic seizures or coma in a client with preeclampsia/HELLP syndrome (ACOG, 2020/2023a). Eclampsia is an expression of severe preeclampsia, not the endpoint of preeclampsia. People with eclampsia are at higher risk for placental abruption, HELLP, DIC, pulmonary edema, aspiration pneumonia, cardiopulmonary arrest, or acute renal failure, especially when the condition develops before 32 weeks of gestation (Bartal & Sibai, 2020). Eclampsia also greatly increases risk of serious morbidity including coma, status epilepticus, or total paralysis (Bartal & Sibai, 2020). Additionally, eclampsia can cause maternal hypoxic ischemic brain injury and seizure-related intracranial hemorrhage (Ghaly, Candido, Sauer, & Knezevic, 2012).

The pathogenesis of eclampsia is not well understood. Circulating factors related to preeclampsia, (e.g., vascular endothelial growth factor and placental growth factor) appear to increase the permeability of the blood-brain barrier (Bartal & Sibai, 2020). When the blood-brain barrier is disrupted, fluid, ions, and plasma protein can move into the sensitive brain tissue and cause swelling and damage (Bartal & Sibai, 2020). It is not clear whether the pathologic features in eclampsia are causes or effects of the convulsions. More than 50% of mothers with eclampsia have persistent neurocognitive dysfunction at 6 months postpartum. Some survivors show white-matter lesions on magnetic-resonance imaging (MRI) for years after giving birth, and others have poor vision for up to a decade (Nerenberg et al., 2017). Although eclampsia is the most common cause of pregnancy-associated intracranial hemorrhage, roughly 20–67% of these victims are found to have previously undetected cerebrovascular malformations (Ghaly et al., 2012).

About 59–70% of eclampsia cases occur antepartum, 20–30% occur intrapartum, and 20–30% occur postpartum (Bartal & Sibai, 2020; Berhan & Berhan, 2015). Eclampsia before 20 weeks of gestation is usually associated with a molar pregnancy (Norwitz, 2023a). About 90% of postpartum eclamptic seizures occur within 7 days after giving birth (Norwitz, 2023a). Eclampsia cannot be prevented with antihypertensive medications. Those who have experienced eclampsia have about a 2% risk of reoccurrence in future pregnancies (Bartal & Sibai, 2020).

Signs and Symptoms

Clinical signs and symptoms and results of laboratory evaluation cannot predict or exclude the development of eclampsia (Bartal & Sibai, 2020). Up to 40% of individuals with eclampsia do not show symptoms before onset of seizures, and in up to 60% of cases, convulsions are the first sign of preeclampsia (Bartal & Sibai, 2020). Before seizing, however, clients may develop marked edema, altered mental status, or any of the following (Bartal & Sibai, 2020):

- Proteinuria (86%).
- Hypertension (75%). About 25% of people with eclampsia do not have hypertension, especially when it occurs postpartum (Bartal & Sibai, 2020), and 20% of cases have nonsevere hypertension before developing seizures (Hastie et al., 2019).
- Headache (66%).
- Visual disturbances, e.g., diplopia (double vision), scotoma (partial loss of visual field or blind spot), photopsia (flashes of light in the field of vision), blurred vision, or transient cortical blindness (27%).
- RUQ or epigastric pain (25%).

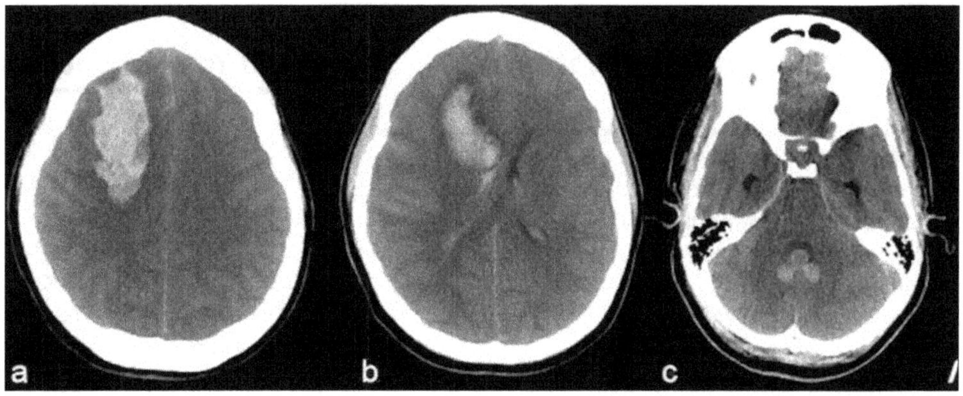

Figure 10-3. Preoperative computerized tomography (CT) cranial scans of an extremely lucky woman who survived eclampsia with a large cerebral hemorrhage. (a) Axial view showing dissecting hematoma in the right frontal lobe and extensive brain swelling. (b) Axial view showing extensive intraventricular hemorrhage, 1 cm midline shift, subarachnoid hemorrhage, and brain swelling. (c) Axial view showing ventricular hemorrhage. This case involved a 32-year-old G2P1 at 34 0/7 weeks of gestation. At her scheduled prenatal appointment, she had a BP of 150/90 without headache, proteinuria, or previous hypertension. She was sent to the maternity unit for evaluation. Laboratory studies did not show evidence of preeclampsia. Her BP rose to 180/110 and remained elevated despite administration of labetalol. About 10 hr after admission, she developed a diffuse headache, nausea, vomiting, and epigastric pain; but her liver enzyme and urine protein tests were normal. Suddenly, she developed a left-sided focal seizure, which progressed to generalized tonic–clonic seizures before she became unresponsive. Laboratory assessment showed HELLP syndrome. She was given a magnesium sulfate infusion and phenytoin for seizures and an emergency cesarean to give birth to an infant with Apgar scores of 8 and 10. Ninety minutes later, she displayed decerebrate posturing and nonreactive pupils. CT scans showed an intracerebral hematoma. She went into DIC and required 20 units of platelets and 4 units of fresh frozen plasma to correct the coagulopathy, then underwent right frontotemporal craniotomy to evacuate the hematoma. She was extubated on postoperative day 7, and after 3 weeks she was transferred to rehabilitation services for physical, occupational, and speech therapies. She regained full cognitive abilities, personality, and social activities within 6 months and did not require ongoing anticonvulsant therapy. From "Complete Recovery after Antepartum Massive Intracerebral Hemorrhage in an Atypical Case of Sudden Eclampsia," by R. F. Ghaly, K. D. Candido, R. Sauer, and N. N. Knezevic, 2012, *Surgical Neurology International, 3*, 65, fig. 1. CC-BY.

Clients with eclampsia usually present with tonic-clonic seizures, but some display partial seizures or subside into a coma without observed convulsions (Norwitz, 2023a). Coma can also result from a brain hemorrhage or brain swelling without hemorrhage. People with occipital-lobe seizures can experience auras and visual hallucinations before generalized convulsions (Garg, Kumar, & Malhotra, 2018).

At the onset of eclampsia, the client may suddenly lose consciousness or emit a strange scream. During the tonic phase, muscles of the arms, legs, chest, and back become rigid, and the individual usually becomes apneic and cyanotic (Norwitz, 2023a). After about 1 min, the muscles jerk and twitch for another 1–2 min. The client may foam at the mouth. Sputum may be bloody if the tongue is bitten. Some people with eclampsia experience multiple seizures in clusters (Garg et al., 2018). The postictal phase begins as the jerking movements subside. The client goes into a deep sleep with deep respirations, then over 10–20 min begins to awaken (Norwitz, 2023a). An individual emerging from the postictal state is often confused and groggy and sometimes complains of a headache.

Managing an Eclamptic Seizure

At the onset of seizure activity, call emergency medical services (EMS). When a client begins to seize, your priorities include preventing serious injury, ensuring a clear airway, maintaining adequate oxygenation, and preventing aspiration of saliva, blood, or vomited gastric contents. In the hospital, use bed rails, which should be padded, to keep the client safely in bed. In any setting, prevent falls, but do not hold the client down or try to restrain movement. Position the client in a lateral decubitus position.

Table 10-4
Acute Maternal Complications in Eclampsia

- Placental abruption (7–12%)
- Disseminated intravascular coagulation (DIC, 6.0–7.0%)
- Venous thromboembolism (VTE, 4.7%)
- Heart failure (3.0–9.5%)
- Pulmonary edema (3–12%)
- Acute renal failure (3.0–8.8%)
- Aspiration pneumonia (2–4%)
- Cerebrovascular disease (2–4%)
- Cardiomyopathy (1.0%)
- Cardiac arrest (0.5%)
- Death (up to 1%)

Adapted from "Eclampsia in the 21st Century," by M. F. Bartal and B. M. Sibai, 2020, *American Journal of Obstetrics & Gynecology, 226*, 2(Suppl.), table 2. Copyright by Elsevier.

Suction oral secretions as necessary. Give supplementary oxygen 8–10 L/min through a face mask but watch for secretions or vomit that can threaten the airway (Bartal & Sibai, 2020). Use pulse oximetry to monitor oxygen saturation. Although normal oxygenation usually returns after the convulsions resolve, hypoxia can develop in anyone with repetitive convulsions, aspiration pneumonia, or pulmonary edema (Bartal & Sibai, 2020).

After the clonic jerking has subsided, obtain intravenous (IV) access with a large-bore catheter. Start a loading dose of 4–6 g magnesium sulfate followed by a 1–2 g/hr maintenance dose if renal function is normal (Norwitz, 2023a). If you are unable to obtain IV access, give magnesium sulfate 10 g by the intramuscular (IM) route, 5 g in each buttock (Boushra, Natesan, Koyfman, & Long, 2022).

At least 3 min of fetal bradycardia is commonly observed during and immediately after seizure activity (Norwitz, 2023a). After the seizure resolves, the fetus may display variable or late heart rate decelerations, tachycardia, or minimal heart rate variability (Bartal & Sibai, 2020). Uterine contractions can become stronger and more frequent. These changes usually resolve within 3–10 min after the seizure stops and the mother returns to normal oxygenation (Bartal & Sibai, 2020). When an abnormal FHR pattern persists for more than 10–15 min despite interventions to improve maternal and fetal wellbeing or there is vaginal bleeding, suspect placental abruption (Norwitz, 2023a). Do not administer a fluid bolus to improve eclampsia-related FHR abnormalities; it increases the risk of pulmonary edema (Bartal & Sibai, 2020).

Table 10-5
If Your Client Has an Eclamptic Seizure

- Call emergency medical services (EMS).
- Do not attempt to restrain the client.
- Move the client to a safe place if there is danger of falling.
- Clear the area of dangerous objects and loosen any clothing that can compress the neck.
- If the client is wearing glasses, remove them.
- Do not force anything into the mouth.
- Ensure an open airway (suctioning may be necessary).
- Give oxygen to ensure adequate oxygenation.

After the seizure ends

- Attend to airway, breathing, and circulation and ensure that the placenta is optimally perfused (ABC-POP).
- Assess vital signs and auscultate lungs.
- Monitor FHR using a Doppler or fetoscope when continuous monitoring is unavailable.
- If breathing does not resume, support respiration.
- Position the client on the left side in the cardiopulmonary-resuscitation (CPR) recovery position.
- Do not leave the client unattended.
- Give an SBAR (**S**ituation, **B**ackground, **A**ssessment, **R**ecommendation) report to your backup physician (see "The SBAR Tool" in Chapter 4).
- If appropriate, assist EMS team in establishing intravenous (IV) access, initiating cardiac monitoring, administering medications, and preparing for transport. If possible, accompany the client to the hospital to support the client, assist the EMS team, and monitor the fetus *en route*.
- Start a loading dose of 4–6 g magnesium sulfate followed by a 1–2 g/hr maintenance dose if renal function is normal OR give 10 g IM if IV access is not available.
- Fax, copy, or bring records to the hospital.

Stabilization of Eclampsia

Eclampsia cannot be stabilized at home or in a birth center. Rapid transport to a suitable hospital with an advanced life support (ALS) provider can be lifesaving for mother and fetus. Ideally, the client with eclampsia should be managed in a tertiary-care facility with a NICU.

Eclampsia is an indication for prompt delivery at any gestational age (Norwitz, 2023a). Stabilizing the mother with antiseizure and antihypertensive medications can help the fetus recover from effects of maternal hypoxia, acidosis, and uterine tachysystole. Induction of labor can be a reasonable option if the mother and fetus are stable after an eclamptic seizure (Norwitz, 2023a), taking into consideration parity, gestational age, fetal position, and Bishop score. Persistent abnormal FHR is an indication for emergency cesarean section.

Newborns of mothers with eclampsia remote from term are at risk for having low birthweight and complications related to prematurity (Bartal & Sibai, 2020). Although iatrogenic prematurity poses challenges for the newborn, the risks of continuing the pregnancy for both mother and fetus greatly outweigh the risks of PTB. The perinatal death rate of eclampsia is about 5.6–11.8%, mostly due to placental abruption, FGR, or extreme prematurity (Bartal & Sibai, 2020).

At the hospital, goals of management include stabilizing the mother, preventing recurrent seizures, treating severe hypertension, and expediting birth. Magnesium sulfate is the drug of choice for preventing recurrent eclamptic seizures. Without it, about 10% of people with eclampsia have recurrent seizures (Norwitz, 2023a). Recurrent seizures can also indicate brain injury. Antihypertensive therapy should be administered for sustained SBP 160 mm Hg or higher or DBP 110 mm Hg or higher to prevent stroke, which is associated with 15–20% of mortality in people with eclampsia (Norwitz, 2023a).

Gestational Hypertension

Gestational hypertension affects 6–17% of healthy nulliparous individuals and 2–4% of multiparous mothers (Melvin & Funai, 2023). Although maternal outcomes are generally good, the condition is associated with long-term cardiovascular disease, including chronic hypertension, heart failure, and probably greater risk of stroke (Lo et al., 2020). The seizure risk for nonsevere gestational hypertension is less than 0.1% (Norwitz, 2023b).

Gestational hypertension is defined as the new onset of hypertension (SBP 140 or higher or DBP 90 or higher) at 20 weeks of gestation or greater over two readings in a previously normotensive client without proteinuria or new signs of end-organ dysfunction (ACOG, 2020a/2023). Readings should be obtained at least 4 hr apart. Gestational hypertension is deemed severe when SBP equals or exceeds 160 mm or DBP equals or exceeds 110 mm Hg. If BP is in the severe range, measure again within 15 min to avoid delaying the start of antihypertensive therapy.

Gestational hypertension is a provisional diagnosis for pregnant people with hypertension who do not have preeclampsia or chronic hypertension (Melvin & Funai, 2023). If the client develops proteinuria or new signs of end-organ dysfunction, the diagnosis changes to preeclampsia (Melvin & Funai, 2023). If the client has been diagnosed with gestational hypertension or preeclampsia and develops severe-range BP (SBP at or above 160 mm or DBP at or above 110 confirmed), the client meets the criteria for preeclampsia with severe features and should be treated immediately (Druzin & Shields, 2021b). Up to 50% of clients with gestational hypertension go on to develop preeclampsia 1–5 weeks after diagnosis, particularly when diagnosed before 34 weeks of gestation and if serum uric acid level is elevated (Melvin & Funai, 2023).

The client with gestational hypertension requires transfer of care or comanagement with a physician or MFM specialist. As with any hypertensive disorder, the client should plan to give birth in a hospital. Serial sonography to assess fetal growth, weekly antepartum testing, close monitoring of BP, and weekly laboratory studies are recommended (Druzin & Shields, 2021b). Mothers with gestational hypertension who develop severe-range BP have rates of FGR, PTB, abruption, and perinatal death similar to those of mothers with preeclampsia with severe features. In fact, some experts propose that gestational hypertension is an early stage of preeclampsia (ACOG, 2020a/2023). The client should be educated on the signs of preeclampsia and asked to call with any concerning findings or elevated readings from home BP monitoring.

Chronic Hypertension with Superimposed Preeclampsia

Chronic hypertension with superimposed preeclampsia is a condition wherein a pregnant client with chronic hypertension develops signs or symptoms of preeclampsia. About 20–50% of clients with chronic hypertension develop superimposed preeclampsia (ACOG, 2019). For those with end-organ disease or secondary hypertension, the rate of superimposed preeclampsia can be as high as 75% (ACOG, 2019). Superimposed preeclampsia tends to have an earlier onset and to be more severe than preeclampsia that develops in people without chronic hypertension. The risk is higher in those who are obese, those who smoke, those with a history of preeclampsia, and those with a baseline DBP at or above 100 mm Hg.

Superimposed preeclampsia may not have a straightforward presentation, but it is likely if previously well-controlled BP suddenly rises or when proteinuria suddenly appears or increases (Jeyabalan & Larkin, 2023). The diagnosis of superimposed preeclampsia with severe features is supported by the presence of any of the following (Jeyabalan & Larkin, 2023):

- Severely elevated SBP (160 mm Hg or higher) or DBP (110 mm Hg or higher) that remains high despite increasing antihypertensive therapy.
- Thrombocytopenia (platelet count less than 100,000/mcl).
- Elevated liver enzymes (two times the upper limit of the normal concentration).
- Severe persistent RUQ or epigastric pain unresponsive to medication and not explained by alternative diagnoses.
- New-onset or worsening renal insufficiency.
- Pulmonary edema.
- Severe headache.
- Visual disturbances.

Patient Intervention

When seizure begins

1. Call for help
2. Position patient in a left lateral decubitus position, head of bed down
3. Prevent maternal injury, side rails up, pad as appropriate
4. Establish open airway, maintain breathing, and have suction available
5. Provide oxygen

When seizure ends

1. Check and treat blood pressure per protocol
2. Obtain IV access: 1 or 2 large-bore IV catheters as soon as possible
3. Start magnesium loading dose

Medical Intervention

Magnesium Sulfate 4-6* grams IV loading dose over 20-30 minutes; followed by a 1-2 gram/hour maintenance dose if renal function is normal
*BMI >35 requires a 6 gram loading dose and 2 grams per hour maintenance dose

If patient has a recurrent seizure, give additional 2-4 grams of magnesium sulfate over 5 minutes*

If patient has a recurrent seizure after 2nd loading dose of magnesium sulfate, administer one of the following and notify anthesthesia

Medications

- Midazolam 1-2 mg IV; may repeat in 5-10 minutes **OR**
- Diazepam 5-10 mg IV slowly; may repeat q15 min to max of 30 mg **OR**
- Phenytoin 1,250 mg IV at a rate of 50 mg/minute
- Other medications have been used with the assistance of anesthesia providers such as:
  - Sodium thiopental
  - Sodium amobarbital
  - Propofol

Resolution

Resolution of seizure

1. Maintain magnesium sulfate infusion for at least 24-48 hours after the last seizure or after delivery, whichever is later
2. Assess for any signs of neurologic injury/focal deficit: head imaging should be considered if neurologic injury is suspected
3. Once the patient is stabilized preparations should be made for delivery; mode of delivery is dependent upon clinical circumstances surrounding the pregnancy

Discontinue therapy
For preeclampsia with severe features and eclampsia: 24-48 hours after delivery or after last seizure

NOTE: Administration beyond 24 hours may be indicated if the patient shows no signs of clinical improvement

*Monitor respiration and BP, EKG and signs of magnesium toxicity.

Figure 10-4. "Eclampsia Algorithm," in M. L. Druzin, L. E. Shields, N. Peterson, C. Sakowski, V. Cape, and C. H. Morton (Eds.), Improving Health Care Response to Hypertensive Disorders of Pregnancy*: A California Maternal Quality Care Collaborative Quality Improvement Toolkit* (p. 232), 2021. Stanford, CA: California Maternal Quality Care Collaborative. Copyright by publisher.

Table 10-6

Sample GOLDCART History for a Client with Signs and Symptoms of HDP

General situation and history—What symptoms are you having? How many weeks pregnant are you? Do you have any health issues or pregnancy complications? Have you ever had high blood pressure, either during pregnancy or when you were not pregnant? Have you taken your BP? What was the reading? Did you repeat it? How old are you? How many pregnancies and how many babies have you had? Have you felt the baby move normally?
Onset—How did your signs and symptoms begin? What were you doing? What time did it start? Was gradual or abrupt? Have you had this before? How did you feel before it started?
Location—Where is your pain or discomfort? Does it start in one place and radiate to somewhere else? Where?
Duration—What have you been doing since your signs and symptoms started? How have your symptoms changed?
Characteristics—Is the pain stabbing, shooting, crampy or dull? On a scale of 1–10, 10 being the worst pain you ever had and 1 being hardly there at all, what number would you give this pain? Where do you experience the pain?
Associated symptoms—Have you been having any issues with severe headaches, pain in your upper abdomen, chest pain, difficulty breathing, visual disturbances, or just feeling poorly? Has there been a sudden increase in your swelling with rapid weight gain? Any other pain, weakness, sweating, numbness, shortness of breath, nausea, vomiting, fever, diarrhea, dizziness, or fainting? Any bleeding or leaking fluid?
Relieving/aggravating factors—What makes it better or worse? Did your symptoms improve when you changed position?
Treatment—Have you used any medications, herbs, or remedies? What have you tried? Did they help?

Management of superimposed preeclampsia is similar to management of preeclampsia. Initial evaluation and monitoring should occur in a hospital. Severe disease develops rapidly in some cases. Eclampsia occurs in up to 2.4% of clients with superimposed preeclampsia (Jeyabalan & Larkin, 2023). In some cases, outpatient monitoring may be considered if there are no severe features, depending on gestational age and clinical characteristics (Jeyabalan & Larkin, 2023).

Management of the Client with Hypertension

Diagnosis, Transport, and Treatment

HDP can develop in previously healthy clients who are anticipating a home or birth-center birth. Even a modestly elevated, asymptomatic BP of 140/90 mm Hg can greatly increase the risk of poor outcomes for mothers and babies and can rapidly escalate to severe disease. Any pregnant client with confirmed BP at or above 160/110 mm Hg is having a hypertensive emergency. The presence of end organ symptoms such as headache, visual changes, or right upper quadrant pain can also indicate significant compromise.

Hypertension in Community Settings

Hypertension in labor or postpartum is usually the result of vasospasm and widespread inflammation occurring over weeks or months. Any client who develops severe-range hypertension (especially when associated with preeclampsia) is at risk for serious complications including placental abruption, pulmonary edema, myocardial infarction, stroke, acute respiratory distress syndrome, coagulopathy, renal failure, and retinal injury, especially if there are preexisting medical disorders (ACOG, 2020a/2023). If placental perfusion is marginally adequate at baseline, the fetus may have limited ability to compensate if the mother's condition worsens.

The Decision to Transfer

Appropriate client selection is key to achieving good outcomes in community settings. A high-risk pregnancy is at greater risk for maternal and newborn morbidity and mortality when birth occurs at home or in a birth center (Bastian, Keirse, & Lancaster, 1998; Bovbjerg, Cheyney, Brown, Cox, & Leeman, 2017; Cheyney et al., 2014). The community midwife is responsible for ongoing risk assessment to ensure that clients meet criteria for low-risk pregnancies, including absence of medical, obstetric, fetal, and/or neonatal conditions that would complicate labor, birth, or the postpartum period (AABC, 2017). It is important that the midwife and client discuss a plan for safe transport should complications arise. Hypertension is an absolute contraindication for birth in community settings except in an emergency (American Association of Birth Centers [AABC], 2017; American College of Nurse-Midwives [ACNM], 2016; National Institute for Health and Care Excellence [NICE], 2017). Under many state, local, and professional guidelines, clients with antepartum hypertension in a community setting require consultation or transfer of care, and those with hypertension in the intrapartum or postpartum period

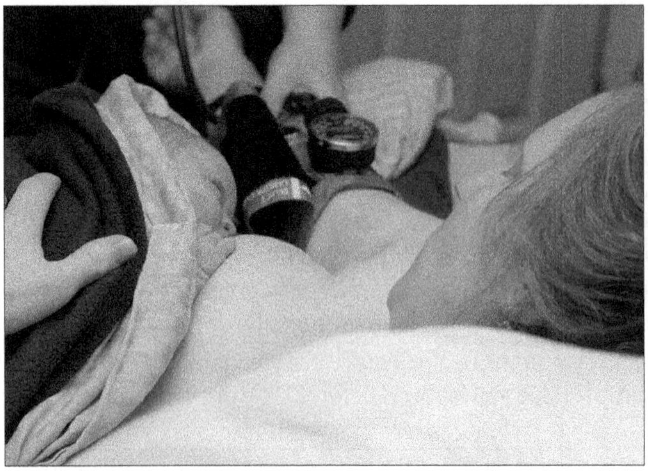

Figure 10-5. Maternal blood pressure (BP) must be monitored closely throughout the intrapartum and postpartum periods. The provider should obtain measurements with minimal disturbance to the bonding process.

require transport for hospital care (Kansas State Board of Healing Arts, 2021; MAWS Transport Guideline Cmte., 2011; Moore et al., 2018; ACNM, 2016).

Elevated BP in a previously healthy client can take both the midwife and the client by surprise. The client may have no symptoms and feel well. Often the client is emotionally invested in giving birth in a community setting and is disappointed or resistant to transfer. If the midwife does not have hospital privileges, transfer can mean not only a change of venue and the prospect of necessary interventions but also the loss of the trusted provider who has been the cornerstone of prenatal care.

Managing Transport

The midwife is a key player in orchestrating a safe transfer and addressing the client's concerns. Prepare the client for what will likely occur at the hospital and answer any questions. Acknowledge that transfer can be frightening and provide support as the client works through difficult emotions. Find positive things to say about the care that will be provided at the hospital to give your client confidence in the new care team. Explain the necessity of likely interventions such as IV medications, continuous fetal monitoring, and labor augmentation.

When a client develops new onset of hypertension in labor

- Initiate transport via EMS, preferably an ALS unit that can provide IV access, cardiac monitoring, or medications should they become necessary.
- Attend to airway, breathing and circulation and ensure the placenta is optimally perfused (ABC-POP). Obtain serial BP readings. Use a pulse oximeter to determine oxygen saturation. Assess for pulmonary edema.
- Monitor the fetus. If continuous monitoring is unavailable, auscultate FHR frequently and for longer than you would in intermittent auscultation. If an abnormal FHR pattern is present, place the mother in the position that yields the best FHR and optimizes uteroplacental perfusion. Usually left-lateral positioning improves both maternal BP and FHR.
- Call your collaborating physician and give an SBAR report.
- If appropriate, assist EMS in establishing IV access, initiating cardiac monitoring, administering medications, and preparing for transport. If possible, accompany the client to the hospital to provide support, assist the EMS team, and monitor the fetus *en route*. Fax or take records to the hospital.

Definitive Care

The goals of managing HDP include preventing seizures, controlling hypertension, and determining the management and timing of labor and birth (ACOG, 2020a/2023). Anyone with gestational hypertension or preeclampsia without severe features is at risk for developing severe-range BP during the intrapartum or postpartum period. Severe-range pressures should be treated promptly with antihypertensive medications. Symptoms and BP measurements should be monitored closely, and magnesium sulfate therapy (see below) should be initiated if the client meets the criteria for preeclampsia with severe features (ACOG, 2020a/2023). Upon arrival at the hospital, assessment and care usually proceed as follows:

First Steps

1. Perform a primary survey, obtain serial BPs. Confirm severe hypertension with a repeat BP assessment within 15 min.
2. Assess the fetus. Initiate continuous electronic fetal monitoring. Consider obtaining a biophysical profile or nonstress test with amniotic fluid estimation (ACOG, 2021/2024). Consider ordering a sonographic fetal growth assessment if growth has not been evaluated in the previous 3 weeks. Umbilical artery Doppler velocimetry is indicated if the fetus has growth restriction.
3. Establish IV access to facilitate administration of antihypertensive and anticonvulsant medications.
4. Administer antihypertensive therapy. If BP is confirmed in the severe range (SBP at or above 160 or DBP at or above 110), initiate treatment with antihypertensive medications promptly—within 30–60 min (ACOG, 2020a/2023). Immediate treatment with antihypertensive therapy can reduce the risk of stroke, abruption, congestive heart failure, myocardial ischemia, or renal injury/failure (ACOG, 2020a/2023). The agents used

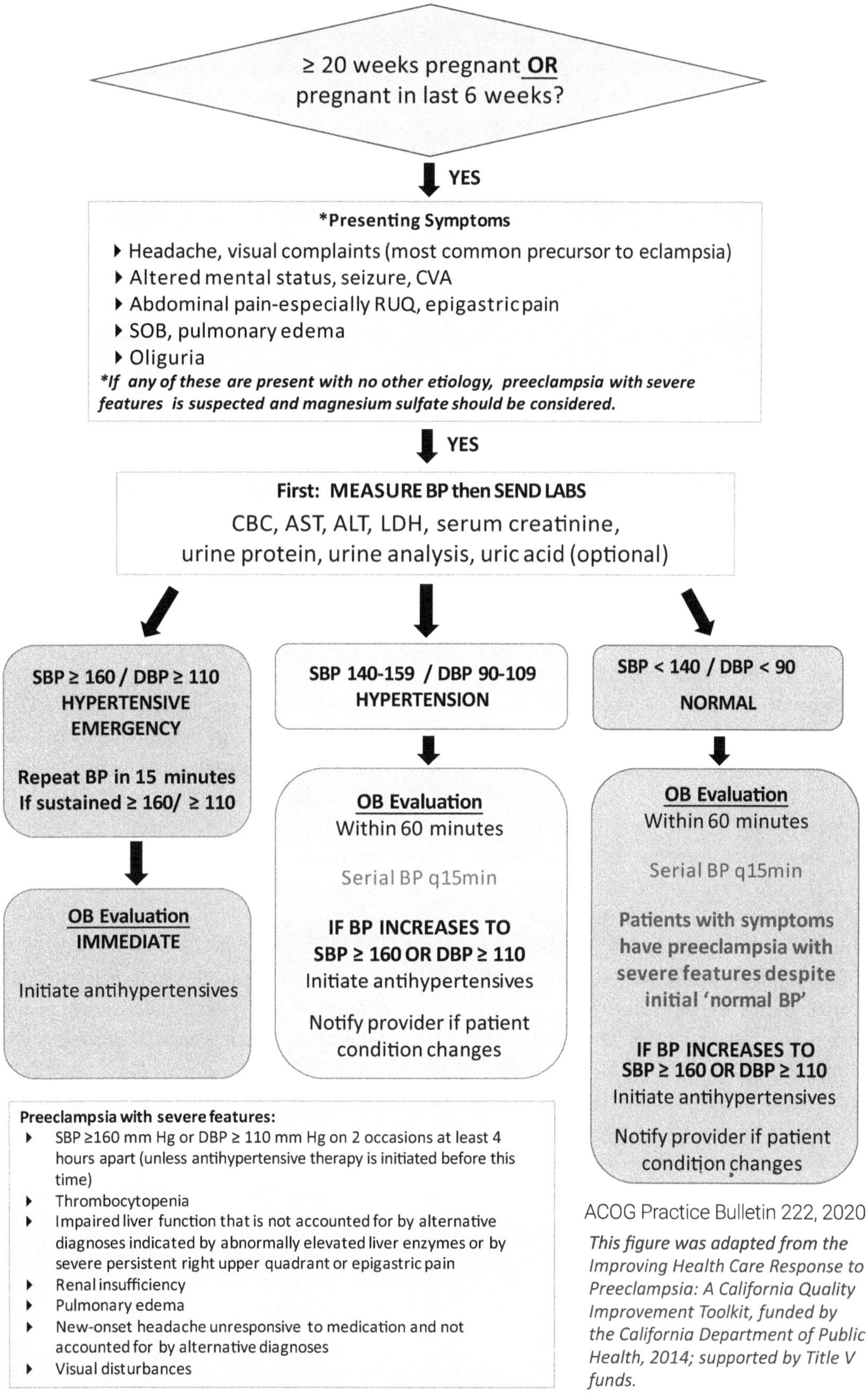

Figure 10-6. Acute diagnostic algorithm for HDP. "Acute Treatment Algorithm, Part 1," in M. L. Druzin, L. E. Shields, N. Peterson, C. Sakowski, V. Cape, and C. H. Morton (Eds.), *Improving Health Care Response to Hypertensive Disorders of Pregnancy: A California Maternal Quality Care Collaborative Quality Improvement Toolkit* (p. 195), 2021. Stanford, CA: California Maternal Quality Care Collaborative. Copyright by publisher.

or heart rate less than 50 beats/min), IV hydralazine, or oral nifedipine if venous access is not established. A Cochrane systematic review found no significant differences of efficacy or safety between hydralazine and labetalol or between hydralazine and calcium channel blockers (ACOG, 2020a/2023; Duley, Meher, & Jones, 2013). Oral labetalol is also an option. See Figure 10-7 for an antihypertensive treatment algorithm for hypertensive emergencies.

5. Administer seizure prophylaxis without delay, simultaneously with administration of antihypertensives. Magnesium sulfate ($MgSO_4$) is the drug of choice to prevent seizures in clients with preeclampsia with severe features or to prevent recurrent seizures in eclampsia (ACOG, 2020a/2023). Although its use is usually reserved for clients with preeclampsia with severe features, in some circumstances the provider and client may decide to use magnesium sulfate to prevent seizures in preeclampsia without severe features (ACOG, 2020a/2023). Although its exact mechanism is unknown, it apparently promotes dilation of constricted cerebral vessels, prevents disruption of the blood-brain barrier, and acts as a central anticonvulsant (Norwitz, 2023b). Magnesium sulfate is more effective than phenytoin or diazepam for controlling eclamptic seizures (ACOG, 2020a/2023).

The optimal dose is not well defined. Higher plasma concentrations of magnesium increase the potential for toxicity; lower concentrations risk being subtherapeutic. In the United States, the IV infusion rate of magnesium sulfate for seizure prophylaxis is usually a 4–6 g loading dose over 20–30 min followed by a maintenance dose of 1–2 g/hr (ACOG, 2020a/2023). For those requiring delivery, the infusion should continue through labor (through surgery if cesarean is required) and for 24 hr postpartum (ACOG, 2020a/2023). In prehospital or low-resource settings or in situations where IV access is unobtainable, magnesium sulfate can be administered by IM injection, first 10 g as a loading dose (5 g IM in each buttock), then 5 g every 4 hr (ACOG, 2020a/2023). This is a very painful injection; some providers mix the magnesium sulfate with 1 ml of xylocaine 2% solution to reduce discomfort.

About 25% of people receiving magnesium sulfate experience a decrease in BP, diaphoresis, flushing, and a sensation of warmth, probably related to peripheral vasodilation (Norwitz, 2023b). Some suffer nausea, vomiting, headache, muscle weakness, visual disturbances, or palpitations (Druzin, Shields, Peterson, & Lee, 2021). Magnesium sulfate is a smooth-muscle relaxant and central nervous system depressant, and an overdose can cause cardiopulmonary arrest. For this reason, the client on IV magnesium sulfate requires the use of an infusion pump and vigilant nursing care. The client loses deep tendon reflexes at a serum magnesium level of 9 mg/dl (7 mEq/L). Respiratory depression and cardiac arrest occur at 12 mg/dl (10 mEq/L) and 30 mg/dl (25 mEq/L), respectively (ACOG, 2020a/2023). Because magnesium sulfate is excreted through the kidneys, poor renal function increases the risk for toxicity. People at risk for impending respiratory depression can require aggressive airway management, including tracheal intubation; IV infusion of calcium gluconate 10% solution to reverse the effects; and IV furosemide to accelerate urinary excretion (ACOG, 2020a/2023).

Next Steps

Obtain Appropriate Laboratory Studies

Blood samples can be obtained when the IV line is started or samples can be drawn from another site. Laboratory tests together with history and physical examination can clarify whether the client is suffering from preeclampsia, gestational hypertension, chronic hypertension, or chronic hypertension with superimposed preeclampsia. These tests can also identify metabolic or hematologic abnormalities.

Blood Tests

The presentation of preeclampsia is variable, so the client may have any of the following characteristic abnormal findings on laboratory tests (August & Sibai, 2023b):

Complete Blood Count (CBC)

Anemia due to hemolysis. Red blood cells (RBCs) can become fragmented as they move through capillaries roughened by endothelial damage and filled with platelet-fibrin deposits.

Hemoconcentration due to third-spacing. The client with preeclampsia may have an unusually high hematocrit. Damaged blood vessels allow IV fluid to shift out of circulation and into the space between cells in tissues (interstitial space). Normally, hemodilution occurs throughout pregnancy and may

Facing page: Figure 10-7. "Acute Treatment Algorithm, Part 2: Antihypertensive Treatment Algorithm for Hypertensive Emergencies," in M. L. Druzin, L. E. Shields, N. Peterson, C. Sakowski, V. Cape, and C. H. Morton (Eds.), *Improving Health Care Response to Hypertensive Disorders of Pregnancy: A California Maternal Quality Care Collaborative Quality Improvement Toolkit* (p. 196), 2021. Stanford, CA: California Maternal Quality Care Collaborative. Copyright by publisher.

Treatment Recommendations for Sustained Systolic BP ≥ 160 mm Hg or Diastolic BP ≥ 110 mm Hg

*Antihypertensive treatment and magnesium sulfate should be administered simultaneously. If concurrent administration is not possible, antihypertensive treatment should be 1st priority.

*Labetalol IV as Primary Antihypertensive

Initial dose 20 mg labetalol IV

↓ Repeat BP in 10 minutes

SBP ≥ 160 or DBP ≥ 110 Give 40 mg labetalol IV

↓ Repeat BP in 10 minutes

SBP ≥ 160 or DBP ≥ 110 Give 80 mg labetalol IV

↓ Repeat BP in 10 minutes

SBP ≥ 160 or DBP ≥ 110 Give hydralazine 10 mg IV

↓ Repeat BP in 20 minutes

SBP ≥ 160 or DBP ≥ 110

Give hydralazine 10 mg IV ***and obtain emergent consultation*** from maternal-fetal medicine, anesthesia, internal medicine, or critical care for transfer of care or continuous IV infusion

*Hydralazine IV as Primary Antihypertensive

Initial dose: 5 - 10 mg hydralazine IV

↓ Repeat BP in 20 minutes

SBP ≥ 160 or DBP ≥ 110 Give hydralazine 10 mg IV

↓ Repeat BP in 20 minutes

If SBP ≥ 160 or DBP ≥ 110

Convert to labetalol pathway Give labetalol 20 mg IV per algorithm

↓ Repeat BP in 10 minutes

SBP ≥ 160 or DBP ≥ 110

Give labetalol 40 mg IV ***and obtain emergent consultation*** from maternal-fetal medicine, anesthesia, internal medicine, or critical care for transfer of care or continuous IV infusion

Nifedipine PO as Primary Antihypertensive

Initial dose: nifedipine 10 mg PO immediate release

↓ Repeat BP in 20 minutes

SBP ≥ 160 or DBP ≥ 110 Give nifedipine 20 mg PO

↓ Repeat BP in 20 minutes

SBP ≥ 160 or DBP ≥ 110 Give nifedipine 20 mg PO

↓ Repeat BP in 20 minutes

SBP ≥ 160 or DBP ≥ 110

Convert to labetalol 20 mg IV pathway ***and obtain emergent consultation*** from maternal-fetal medicine, internal medicine, anesthesia or critical care for transfer of care or continuous IV infusion

ACOG Practice Bulletin 203, 2019

Target BP: 130-150/80-100 mm Hg

Once BP threshold is achieved:
- Q10 min for 1 hr
- Q15 min for 1 hr
- Q30 min for 1 hr
- Q1hr for 4 hrs

*Intravenous hydralazine or labetalol should be given over 2 minutes. In the presence of sinus bradycardia or a history of asthma, hydralazine or nifedipine are preferred as initial agents. If maternal HR > 110, labetalol is preferred.

This figure was adapted from the Improving Health Care Response to Preeclampsia: A California Quality Improvement Toolkit, funded by the California Department of Public Health, 2014; supported by Title V funds.

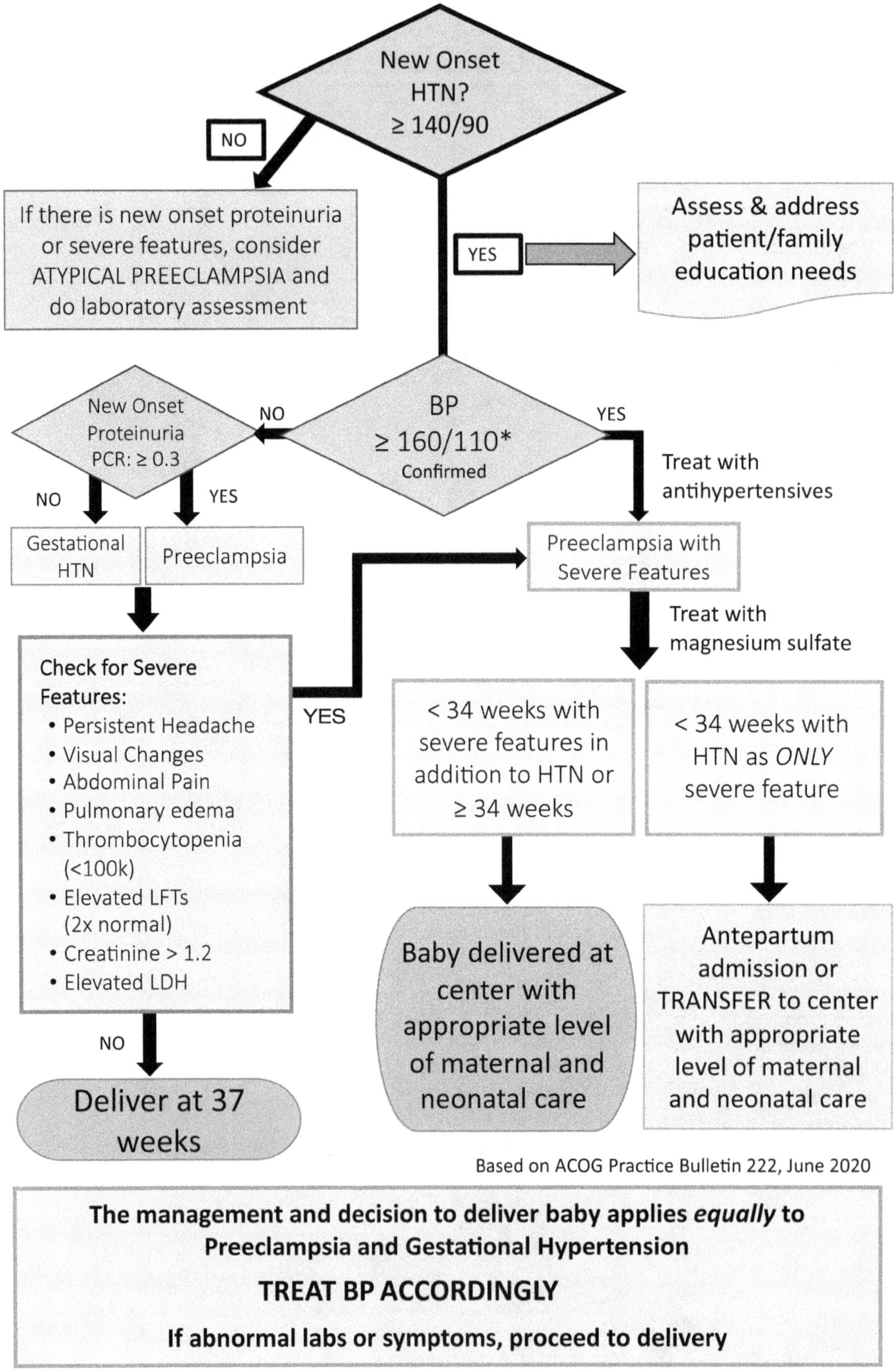

Figure 10-8. "Suspected Preeclampsia Algorithm," in M. L. Druzin, L. E. Shields, N. Peterson, C. Sakowski, V. Cape, and C. H. Morton (Eds.), *Improving Health Care Response to Hypertensive Disorders of Pregnancy: A California Maternal Quality Care Collaborative Quality Improvement Toolkit* (p. 178), 2021. Stanford, CA: California Maternal Quality Care Collaborative. Copyright by publisher.

cause physiologic anemia. Because people with hemoconcentration due to preeclampsia have lower intravascular volume, they have less tolerance for blood loss.

Low platelets. Activation of the coagulation cascade causes platelets to adhere to the damaged endothelial lining of blood vessels. This accelerated platelet consumption can cause thrombocytopenia. A platelet count less than 150,000/mcl occurs in roughly 20% of people with preeclampsia (August & Sibai, 2023b). A count less than 100,000/mcl can indicate that the disease is severe.

Abnormal cells on peripheral smear. If RBCs become traumatized while traveling through damaged, fibrin-choked blood vessels, a peripheral smear may show fragmented RBCs (schistocytes, burr cells).

Metabolic Panel

Elevated liver-enzyme levels (transaminases, AST, ALT): Liver chemistries are usually normal in preeclampsia, but the client with severe disease (especially HELLP syndrome) may develop elevated transaminase levels (defined as twice the upper limit of normal). Abnormal transaminases indicate reduced hepatic blood flow resulting from deposition of fibrin and microvesicular fat (abnormal fat within cells). This decreased perfusion leads to ischemia, tissue necrosis and, in severe cases, intrahepatic hemorrhage, subcapsular hematoma formation, or hepatic rupture (August & Sibai, 2023b).

Elevated serum creatinine concentration. In preeclampsia, serum creatinine concentration usually remains within the normal range for pregnancy or slightly elevated. With severe preeclampsia, serum creatinine concentration can increase sharply as a result of reduced intravascular volume and decreased glomerular filtration rate (GFR). In a normal pregnancy, plasma volume expansion and enhanced blood flow to the kidneys cause the GFR to increase, resulting in a physiologic decrease in serum creatinine. A creatinine level higher than 1.1 mg/dl or doubling of the serum creatinine concentration can indicate renal insufficiency. The most common cause of acute kidney injury in pregnancy is preeclampsia.

Coagulation Studies

Physiologic changes of pregnancy lead to a relative hypercoagulable state (that is, blood clots more readily). Prothrombin time (PT), partial thromboplastin time (PTT), and fibrinogen concentration are usually unaffected by preeclampsia unless there are additional complications such as HELLP or coagulopathy.

Decreased fibrinogen. Fibrinogen is a clotting factor protein (factor I) necessary for proper blood-clot formation. In the third trimester of a normal pregnancy, fibrinogen levels should be greater than 300 mg/dl (Belfort, 2023). A decrease in fibrinogen from the client's normal baseline is concerning even if the value remains in the range that would be normal for the nonpregnant client. A pregnant client with a fibrinogen level less than 200 mg/dl is at extreme risk for severe postpartum hemorrhage and DIC.

PT and activated partial thromboplastin time (aPTT) measure the time required for blood to clot. If preeclampsia affects blood clotting, PT and aPTT will increase.

Other Blood Tests

Increased lactate dehydrogenase level. LDH is an intracellular enzyme, found in the blood and other body tissues, that is involved with energy production in cells. High LDH levels may be a sign of tissue damage. LDH at or above 600 IU/L in preeclampsia may be caused by liver dysfunction (ischemic or necrotic tissues) or hemolysis (RBC destruction). Severely preeclamptic clients with LDH above 800 IU/L are more likely to develop eclampsia, abruption, hemolysis, HELLP syndrome, or DIC, and require admission to intensive care than people with normal LDH levels (Kharb, Bhandari, Singh, & Gupta, 2019).

Increased uric acid level. Uric acid is formed from the breakdown of protein in foods and the breakdown of cells. Normally, the kidneys filter this waste product from the bloodstream. If preeclampsia damages the kidneys, blood levels of uric acid can rise. Uric acid levels are often the earliest laboratory finding related to preeclampsia, but this test is not sensitive or specific for the diagnosis of preeclampsia or for predicting poor perinatal outcome (Sibai, 2021).

Urine Protein Measurements

Proteinuria occurs when disruption of the glomerular filtration barrier allows excess protein to be excreted into the urine. Protein should be measured in a clean-voided midstream collection. If the amniotic membranes are not intact or if there is lochia present, false positive readings can result, and a sample obtained via urinary catheter is required. As discussed previously, proteinuria in preeclampsia can be defined as any of the following (ACOG, 2020a/2023):

- 300 or more mg of protein in a 24-hr urine collection. This method is the most accurate for determining proteinuria.
- Random urine PCR 0.3 or higher.
- Protein 2+ or higher on a paper test strip dipped into a fresh, clean-voided midstream urine specimen (if other quantitative methods not available). Dipstick urinalysis tests have a high incidence of false negatives and false positives.

- Once proteinuria is documented with a 24-hr urine collection, it is unnecessary to reassess or quantify proteinuria. Beyond the diagnostic threshold, proteinuria does not affect perinatal outcomes or change management (ACOG, 2020a/2023).

If Preterm, Consider Corticosteroids

Abundant evidence confirms that antenatal corticosteroid therapy administered to clients at risk for PTB reduces the incidence and severity of respiratory distress syndrome, intraventricular hemorrhage, and necrotizing enterocolitis. It also decreases the risk of newborn death compared with unexposed preterm babies (Lee & Guinn, 2023). ACOG recommends administering a single course of corticosteroids between 24 0/7 weeks and 33 6/7 weeks of gestation and a single course between 34 0/7 weeks and 36 6/7 weeks to those who have not previously received antenatal corticosteroids in the current pregnancy if birth is likely to occur within 7 days (ACOG, 2017/2024). A single repeat course of antenatal corticosteroids should be considered for clients who are less than 34 0/7 weeks of gestation and at risk of PTB within 7 days if more than 2 weeks have passed since the first course (ACOG, 2017/2024). If maternal or fetal condition deteriorates, birth may be expedited, precluding administration of a full course. Antenatal corticosteroids can be considered at 22 0/7 weeks to 23 6/7 weeks of gestation after appropriate counseling if the family has decided to have the baby resuscitated (ACOG et al., 2021/2022). There is no evidence that antenatal steroids are beneficial below 22 weeks of gestation, so they are not recommended (ACOG et al., 2021/2022).

Consider Maternal Diagnostic Modalities

The client with chest pain requires an electrocardiogram and may need continuous cardiac monitoring. Imaging such as a chest x-ray or CT scan may be indicated for chest pain, abnormal lung sounds, low oxygen saturations, or difficulty breathing (Hauspurg & Jeyabalan, 2022). The client with suspected volume overload may require an echocardiogram.

A headache associated with altered consciousness, collapse, nausea or vomiting, a stiff neck, or photophobia suggests cerebral swelling or intracranial hemorrhage. The obstetrician may consult a neurologist to evaluate clients with neurologic deficits, abnormal neurologic examinations, visual disturbances, or severe, persistent headaches that do not respond to analgesics. A CT scan or MRI of the brain is often required.

Administer Fluids

When caring for a client with preeclampsia, the provider must ensure enough intravascular volume to perfuse the organs without overloading the cardiovascular system. Overhydration can cause fluid to escape from the intravascular compartment and collect in the interstitial space, causing generalized swelling and sometimes pulmonary or brain edema. For the client with severe preeclampsia, fluid balance should be closely monitored (August, 2023).

Total fluid intake is usually limited to 125 ml/hr unless clinical circumstances dictate a different management plan (Lucero, Champagne, & Gutierrez, 2021). A urinary catheter may be inserted for accurate measurement. Low urine output (oliguria) that does not respond to a 300 ml fluid challenge suggests renal insufficiency, which can be confirmed by elevated serum creatinine levels (August, 2023).

Determine Activity

The client with nonsevere preeclampsia who is not having acute complications can continue normal activity (ACOG, 2020b/2023; McCall, Grimes, & Lyerly, 2013). There is no evidence that bed rest improves outcomes for the client with HDP (ACOG, 2020b/2023; McCall et al., 2013). Moreover, prolonged bed rest and restricted physical activity increase the risk for venous thromboembolism (VTE), bone demineralization, and deconditioning and increase stress, inconvenience, and other hardships for the client and family. The client who is ill enough to remain in bed should have side rails up to prevent falls and use a sequential compression device to prevent VTE.

Childbirth Considerations and Timing

Recommendations for the timing of birth are as follows:

Gestational hypertension or preeclampsia without severe features: Birth is recommended by 37 weeks of gestation for clients with gestational hypertension or preeclampsia without severe features (ACOG, 2020a/2023). In general, birth should be expedited if fetal surveillance test results are abnormal, if there is rupture of membranes or vaginal bleeding, or if the client develops severe hypertension or end-organ dysfunction. Clients diagnosed at or after 37 weeks of gestation should proceed toward induction of labor (or cesarean if indicated) at the time of diagnosis.

Preeclampsia with severe features: Preeclampsia will grow increasingly severe if pregnancy progresses. For the client with severe-range BPs, expectant management before term benefits the fetus but risks the health of the mother (ACOG, 2019). When diagnosed at or beyond 34 weeks of gestation, birth is indicated by induction or cesarean section after the mother is stabilized (ACOG, 2020a/2023). When diagnosed before 34 weeks of gestation, expectant management with close in-hospital surveillance may be continued in some circumstances to provide neonatal benefit at the cost of higher maternal risk

(ACOG, 2020a/2023). Birth should *not* be delayed to allow for the administration of antenatal steroids in the late preterm period (ACOG, 2020a/2023). If maternal or fetal condition deteriorates, birth is expedited.

Superimposed preeclampsia without severe features: Recommendations include birth at 37 weeks of gestation and close maternal and fetal surveillance in the meantime.

Superimposed preeclampsia with severe features: Birth is recommended at the time of diagnosis if the client is more than 34 0/7 weeks of gestation. At any gestational age, proceed toward immediate birth after the mother is stabilized if any of the following are present: uncontrollable severe hypertension, eclampsia, pulmonary edema, DIC, new or increasing renal insufficiency, placental abruption, or abnormal fetal testing (ACOG, 2019). Expectant management with close surveillance in a hospital may be considered for clients less than 34 weeks of gestation.

Chronic hypertension: The recommended timing of birth varies with the clinical circumstances as follows (ACOG, 2019; Jeyabalan & Larkin, 2023):

- Clients with well-controlled chronic hypertension who do not require antihypertensive medication should give birth between 37 and 38 weeks of gestation.
- Clients well-controlled on antihypertensive medication should give birth between 37 and 39 weeks of gestation.
- Clients with severe hypertension that is difficult to control with medication should give birth between 34 0/7 and 36 6/7 weeks of gestation.

The mode of childbirth for the client with gestational hypertension or preeclampsia (with or without severe features) is determined by the usual obstetric considerations (ACOG, 2020a/2023). When the high potential for worsening disease is weighed against the likelihood of a lengthy induction of labor, cesarean section can be the best option for the client with severe features who is remote from term (ACOG, 2020a/2023). The probability of cesarean birth before 28 weeks of gestation can be as high as 97%; from 28 to 32 weeks of gestation, it can reach 65% (ACOG, 2020a/2023). There is evidence, however, that inducing labor and facilitating a vaginal birth in the client with preeclampsia with severe features remote from term does not worsen outcomes (ACOG, 2020a/2023).

Expectant Management

ACOG suggests that in-hospital expectant management can be considered for the client with preeclampsia with severe features before 34 0/7 weeks of gestation if mother and fetus are stable to allow the fetus to reach a higher gestational age (ACOG, 2020a/2023). In some cases of severe preeclampsia, birth may be delayed to allow for administration of antenatal steroids. In the late preterm period, the risks of expectant management (onset of severe hypertension, eclampsia, HELLP syndrome, placental abruption, FGR, and fetal death) must be balanced against the risk of PTB, higher rates of admission to the NICU, newborn respiratory complications, and neonatal death (ACOG, 2020a/2023). Maternal conditions that generally prohibit expectant management include (ACOG, 2020a/2023)

- Uncontrolled severe-range BP (persistent SBP at or above 160 mm Hg or DBP at or above 110 mm Hg, unresponsive to antihypertensive medication).
- Persistent headaches unresponsive to analgesics.
- Epigastric or RUQ pain that persists despite use of analgesics.
- Visual disturbances, loss of muscular strength, motor deficits, or altered mental status such as confusion, loss of memory, loss of alertness, disorientation, or poor judgment or thinking.
- Stroke.
- Chest pain / myocardial infarction.
- HELLP syndrome.
- Serum creatinine greater than 1.1 mg/dl or twice baseline.
- Pulmonary edema.
- Eclampsia.
- Suspected acute placental abruption or vaginal bleeding.

Fetal conditions that would prohibit expectant management include (ACOG, 2020a/2023)

- Abnormal fetal test results.
- Fetal death or bleak prognosis due to lethal anomaly or extreme prematurity.
- Persistent reversed end-diastolic flow in the umbilical artery on Doppler ultrasound.

Ambulatory management at home is sometimes an option for the client with gestational hypertension or preeclampsia without severe features if the fetus is stable and there is no preterm labor, vaginal bleeding, or preterm rupture of membranes (ACOG, 2020a/2023). Pregnant clients managed expectantly at home should be instructed to call with any concerning symptoms. They must be willing to monitor their BP at home and return for frequent fetal and maternal evaluations, which can include serial ultrasonic assessments for fetal growth, weekly nonstress tests and amniotic fluid indexes, weekly prenatal visits, and weekly laboratory tests for preeclampsia.

Any pregnant client reporting a severe headache unrelieved by acetaminophen, upper abdominal or chest pain, visual disturbances, decreased fetal movement, vaginal bleeding, or elevated BP on home monitoring requires reassessment in the labor and delivery unit. About 10–50% of clients who are diagnosed with gestational hypertension develop preeclampsia

Ibuprofen and other nonsteroidal antiinflammatory drugs given postpartum for pain management do not increase BP or prolong the duration of severe-range BP.

ACOG, 2020a/2023, 2021b; Blue et al., 2018; Penfield, McNulty, Oakes, & Nageotte, 2019; Premkumar, Ayala, Miller, Grobman, & Miller, 2021; Wang, Yang, Yu, & Man, 2020.

in 1–5 weeks (Melvin & Funai, 2023). Preeclampsia without severe features can progress to severe preeclampsia within days (ACOG, 2020a/2023).

Postpartum Hypertension

Whereas gestational hypertension and preeclampsia generally improve within 48 hr postpartum, in some cases these diseases can worsen postpartum, or arise as new conditions during the postpartum period (ACOG, 2020a/2023). About 60% of people who develop postpartum preeclampsia have no prior diagnosis of a hypertensive disorder of pregnancy (Hauspurg & Jeyabalan, 2022). Delayed-onset postpartum preeclampsia usually presents within the first 7–10 days after giving birth, but the literature documents (rarely) onset up to 3 months postpartum (Hauspurg & Jeyabalan, 2022). About 21% of eclampsia occurs after giving birth, and it may be the presenting symptom in up to 10–15% of clients with delayed postpartum preeclampsia (Hauspurg & Jeyabalan, 2022).

Headache is the most common symptom of postpartum preeclampsia, occurring in 60–70% of cases (Hauspurg & Jeyabalan, 2022). Danger signs include a headache that does not improve with the use of analgesic medications; thunderclap headaches that come on suddenly, severely, and unremittingly; or any headache associated with mental status changes, seizures, visual disturbances, or focal neurologic deficits.

DIFFERENTIAL DIAGNOSES

Consider migraine, postdural-puncture headache after spinal or epidural anesthesia, medication-related headache, cerebral venous thrombosis, and reversible cerebral vasoconstriction syndrome (Hauspurg & Jeyabalan, 2022). Other concerning symptoms include shortness of breath, upper abdominal pain, seizures, or chest pain.

Alarm Findings

Anyone who gives birth to a baby should be instructed about how to recognize alarm findings and when to call the provider. The Association of Women's Health, Obstetric, and Neonatal Nurses (AWHONN) developed the POST-BIRTH mnemonic to alert clients in the postpartum period to potential danger signs and to facilitate provider-client discussion (AWHONN, 2018). The mnemonic is as follows:

Call EMS if you have:

Pain in chest

Obstructed breathing or shortness of breath

Seizures

Thoughts of hurting yourself or someone else

Call your health care provider if you have:

Bleeding, soaking through 1 pad/hr, or blood clots the size of an egg or bigger

Incision that is not healing

Red or swollen leg that is painful or warm to touch

Temperature of 100.4°F (38°C) or higher

Headache that does not get better, even after taking medicine, or bad headache with vision changes

If you cannot reach your health care provider, call EMS or go to an emergency department.

Topics for Discussion

1. Nevaeh R., a 20-year-old primigravida at 39 0/7 weeks of gestation, is in labor at home. Upon your arrival her BP was 138/88, but now that she is in active labor, her systolic readings have been consistently in the 140s and 150s for the past 2 hr. What is your plan, and why?
2. Amanda Sue L, a 38-year-old G7 P5 arrives for her first appointment with you at 8 weeks of gestation. Her BP was 154/94. She feels well and has no symptoms. She tells you that she developed postpartum hypertension after her last birth, and she required labetalol therapy for about 3 months postpartum. About a year ago, when she was 6 months postpartum, she went to the emergency department for treatment of severe mastitis and found that her BP was 150/90. She did not have a follow-up appointment. What condition do you suspect? What are your next steps?
3. Ivy L., a 22-year-old primigravida arrived at her prenatal appointment complaining of extreme fatigue and nausea. She found a seat in the waiting room, then minutes later fell from her chair in a grand mal seizure. What do you do next?
4. You referred Kiki, a 28-year-old G2 P1 at 38 0/7 weeks of gestation, to the hospital for new-onset hypertension and a severe headache. She was diagnosed with preeclampsia with severe features. She called you in tears when the physician recommended immediate induction of labor. "I was planning a birth center birth! I don't want induction, continuous fetal monitoring, or any kind of medication!" she cried. What do you say?

References

Abedzadeh-Kalahroudi, M., Sehat, M., Vahedpour, Z., & Talebian, P. (2021). Maternal and neonatal outcomes of pregnant patients with COVID-19: A prospective cohort study. *International Journal of Gynecology & Obstetrics, 153*(3), 449–456. https://doi.org/10.1002/ijgo.13661

Al-Safi, Z., Imudia, A. N., Filetti, L. C., Hobson, D. T., Bahado-Singh, R. O., & Awonuga, A. O. (2011). Delayed postpartum preeclampsia and eclampsia: Demographics, clinical course, and complications. *Obstetrics & Gynecology, 118*(5), 1102–1107. https://doi.org/10.1097/AOG.0b013e318231934c

Ali, S. M. J., & Khalil, R. A. (2015). Genetic, immune, and vasoactive factors in the vascular dysfunction associated with hypertension in pregnancy. *Expert Opinion on Therapeutic Targets, 19*(11), 1495–1515. https://doi.org/10.1517/14728222.2015.1067684

American Association of Birth Centers. (2017). *Standards for birth centers* (12th ed.). Perkiomenville, PA: Author. Retrieved from https://cdn.ymaws.com/www.birthcenters.org/resource/resmgr/AABC-STANDARDS-RV2017.pdf

American College of Nurse-Midwives. (2016). Midwifery provision of home birth services (Clinical Bulletin 14). *Journal of Midwifery & Women's Health, 61*(1), 127–133. https://doi.org/10.1111/jmwh.12431

American College of Obstetricians and Gynecologists. (2017, corrected and reaffirmed 2024). *Antenatal corticosteroid therapy for fetal maturation* (Committee Opinion 713). Retrieved from https://www.acog.org/clinical/clinical-guidance/committee-opinion/articles/2017/08/antenatal-corticosteroid-therapy-for-fetal-maturation

American College of Obstetricians and Gynecologists. (2019). *Chronic hypertension in pregnancy* (Practice Bulletin 203). Retrieved from https://www.acog.org/clinical/clinical-guidance/practice-bulletin/articles/2019/01/chronic-hypertension-in-pregnancy

American College of Obstetricians and Gynecologists. (2020a, reaffirmed 2023). *Gestational hypertension and preeclampsia* (Practice Bulletin 222). Retrieved from https://www.acog.org/clinical/clinical-guidance/practice-bulletin/articles/2020/06/gestational-hypertension-and-preeclampsia

American College of Obstetricians and Gynecologists. (2020b, reaffirmed 2023). *Physical activity and exercise during pregnancy and the postpartum period* (Committee Opinion 804). Retrieved from https://www.acog.org/clinical/clinical-guidance/committee-opinion/articles/2020/04/physical-activity-and-exercise-during-pregnancy-and-the-postpartum-period

American College of Obstetricians and Gynecologists. (2021, reaffirmed 2024). *Antepartum fetal surveillance* (Practice Bulletin 229). Retrieved from https://www.acog.org/clinical/clinical-guidance/practice-bulletin/articles/2021/06/antepartum-fetal-surveillance

American College of Obstetricians and Gynecologists. (2022). *ACOG clinical guidance for the integration of the findings of the Chronic Hypertension and Pregnancy (CHAP) Study* (Practice Advisory). Retrieved from https://www.acog.org/clinical/clinical-guidance/practice-advisory/articles/2022/04/clinical-guidance-for-the-integration-of-the-findings-of-the-chronic-hypertension-and-pregnancy-chap-study

American College of Obstetricians and Gynecologists & Society for Maternal-Fetal Medicine. (2021, reaffirmed 2022). *Low-dose aspirin use for the prevention of preeclampsia and related morbidity and mortality* (Practice Advisory). Retrieved from https://www.acog.org/clinical/clinical-guidance/practice-advisory/articles/2021/12/low-dose-aspirin-use-for-the-prevention-of-preeclampsia-and-related-morbidity-and-mortality

American College of Obstetricians and Gynecologists, Society for Maternal-Fetal Medicine, Cahill, A. G., Kaimal, A. J., Kuller, J. A., & Turrentine, M. A. (2021, reaffirmed 2022). *Use of antenatal corticosteroids at 22 weeks of gestation* (Practice Advisory). Retrieved from https://www.acog.org/clinical/clinical-guidance/practice-advisory/articles/2021/09/use-of-antenatal-corticosteroids-at-22-weeks-of-gestation

Ananth, C. V., Duzyj, C. M., Yadava, S., Schwebel, M., Tita, A. T. N., & Joseph, K. S. (2019). Changes in the prevalence of chronic hypertension in pregnancy, United States, 1970 to 2010. *Hypertension, 74*(5), 1089–1095. https://doi.org/10.1161/HYPERTENSIONAHA.119.12968

Association of Women's Health, Obstetric, and Neonatal Nurses. (2018). *Save your life: Get care for these POST-BIRTH warning signs*. Retrieved from https://www.awhonn.org/wp-content/uploads/2020/02/pbwssylhandoutenglish.pdf

August, P. (2023). Treatment of hypertension in pregnant and postpartum patients. In V. A. Barss (Ed.), *UpToDate*. Retrieved November 14, 2023, from https://www.uptodate.com/contents/treatment-of-hypertension-in-pregnant-and-postpartum-patients

August, P., & Jeyabalan, A. (2023). Preeclampsia: Prevention. In V. A. Barss (Ed.), *UpToDate*. Retrieved November 14, 2023, from https://www.uptodate.com/contents/preeclampsia-prevention

August, P., & Sibai, B. M. (2023a). Hypertensive disorders in pregnancy: Approach to differential diagnosis. In V. A. Barss (Ed.), *UpToDate*. Retrieved November 14, 2023, from https://www.uptodate.com/contents/hypertensive-disorders-in-pregnancy-approach-to-differential-diagnosis

August, P., & Sibai, B. M. (2023b). Preeclampsia: Clinical features and diagnosis. In V. A. Barss (Ed.), *UpToDate*. Retrieved November 14, 2023, from https://www.uptodate.com/contents/preeclampsia-clinical-features-and-diagnosis

Banala, C., Moreno, S., Cruz, Y., Boelig, R. C., Saccone, G., Berghella, V., . . . Roman, A. (2020). Impact of the ACOG guideline regarding low-dose aspirin for prevention of superimposed preeclampsia in women with chronic hypertension. *American Journal of Obstetrics & Gynecology, 223*(3), 419.e1–419.E16. https://doi.org/\10.1016/j.ajog.2020.03.004

Bartal, M. F., & Sibai, B. M. (2020). Eclampsia in the 21st century. *American Journal of Obstetrics & Gynecology, 226*(2, Suppl.), s1237–s1253. https://doi.org/10.1016/j.ajog.2020.09.037

Basile, J., & Bloch, M. J. (2023). Overview of hypertension in adults. In J. P. Forman & K. Law (Eds.), *UpToDate*. Retrieved November 14, 2023, from https://www.uptodate.com/contents/overview-of-hypertension-in-adults

Bastian, H., Keirse, M. J. N. C., & Lancaster, P. A. L. (1998). Perinatal death associated with planned home birth in Australia: Population based study. *BMJ, 317*(7155), 384–388. https://doi.org/10.1136/bmj.317.7155.384

Belfort, M. A. (2023). Disseminated intravascular coagulation (DIC) during pregnancy: Clinical findings, etiology, and diagnosis. In V. A. Barss (Ed.), *UpToDate*. Retrieved November 14, 2023, from https://www.uptodate.com/contents/disseminated-intravascular-coagulation-dic-during-pregnancy-clinical-findings-etiology-and-diagnosis

Bello, N. A., Miller, E., Cleary, K., Wapner, R., Shimbo, D., & Tita, A. T. (2018). Out of office blood pressure measurement in pregnancy and the postpartum period. *Current Hypertension Reports, 20*(12), 101. https://doi.org/10.1007/s11906-018-0901-z

Bello, N. A., Woolley, J. J., Cleary, K. L., Falzon, L., Alpert, B. S., Oparil, S., . . . Shimbo, D. (2017). Accuracy of blood pressure measurement devices in pregnancy: A systematic review of validation studies. *Hypertension, 71*(2), 326–335https://doi.org/10.1161/HYPERTENSIONAHA.117.10295

Berhan, Y., & Berhan, A. (2015). Should magnesium sulfate be administered to women with mild pre-eclampsia? A systematic review of published reports on eclampsia. *Journal of Obstetrics and Gynaecology Research, 41*(6), 831–842. https://doi.org/10.1111/jog.12697

Blue, M. R., Murray-Krezan, C., Drake-Lavelle, S., Weinberg, D., Holbrook, B. D., Katukuri, V. R., . . . Mozurkewich, E. L. (2018). Effect of ibuprofen vs acetaminophen on postpartum hypertension in preeclampsia with severe features: A double-masked, randomized controlled trial. *American Journal of Obstetrics & Gynecology, 218*(6), 616.e1–616.e8. https://doi.org/10.1016/j.ajog.2018.02.016

Boushra, M., Natesan, S. M., Koyfman, A., & Long, B. (2022). High risk and low prevalence diseases: Eclampsia. *American Journal of Emergency Medicine, 58*, 223–228. https://doi.org/10.1016/j.ajem.2022.06.004

Bovbjerg, M. L., Cheyney, M., Brown, J., Cox, K. J., & Leeman, L. (2017). Perspectives on risk: Assessment of risk profiles and outcomes among women planning community birth in the United States. *Birth, 44*(3), 209–221. https://doi.org/10.1111/birt.12288

Bramham, K., Parnell, B., Nelson-Piercy, C., Seed, P. T., Poston, L., & Chappell, L. C. (2014). Chronic hypertension and pregnancy outcomes: Systematic review and meta-analysis. *BMJ, 348*, g2301. https://doi.org/10.1136/bmj.g2301

Brown, M. A., Magee, L. A., Kenny, L. C., Karumanchi, S. A., McCarthy, F. P., Saito, S., . . . Ishaku, S. (2018). Hypertensive disorders of pregnancy: ISSHP classification, diagnosis, and management recommendations for international practice. *Hypertension, 72*(1), 24–43. https://doi.org/10.1161/HYPERTENSIONAHA.117.10803

Brown, M. A., Mangos, G., Davis, G., & Homer, C. (2005). The natural history of white coat hypertension during pregnancy. *BJOG, 112*(5),601–606. https://doi.org/10.1111/j.1471-0528.2004.00516.x

Carey, R. M., & Whelton, P. K. (2018). Prevention, detection, evaluation, and management of high blood pressure in adults: Synopsis of the 2017 American College of Cardiology/American Heart Association hypertension guideline. *Annals of Internal Medicine, 168*(5), 351–358. https://doi.org/10.7326/M17-3203

Cheyney, M., Bovbjerg, M., Everson, C., Gordon, W., Hannibal, D., & Vedam, S. (2014). Outcomes of care for 16,924 planned home births in the United States: The Midwives Alliance of North America Statistics Project, 2004 to 2009. *Journal of Midwifery & Women's Health, 59*(1), 17–27. https://doi.org/10.1111/jmwh.12172

Conde-Agudelo, A., & Romero, R. (2021). SARS-COV-2 infection during pregnancy and risk of preeclampsia: A systematic review and meta-analysis. *American Journal of Obstetrics & Gynecology, 226*(1), 68–89.e3. https://doi.org/10.1016/j.ajog.2021.07.009

Costantine, M. M., West, H., Wisner, K. L., Caritis, S., Clark, S., Venkataramanan, R., . . . Mahmoud, S. A. (2021). A randomized pilot clinical trial of pravastatin versus placebo in pregnant patients at high risk of preeclampsia. *American Journal of Obstetrics & Gynecology, 225*(6), 666.e1–666.e15. https://doi.org/10.1016/j.ajog.2021.05.018

Cunningham, F. G., Leveno, K. J., Dashe, J. S., Hoffman, B. L., Spong, C. Y., & Casey, B. M. (Eds.). (2022). *Williams obstetrics* (26th ed. , Kindle version). New York, NY: McGraw-Hill.

Davenport, M. H., Ruchat, S.-M., Poitras, V. J., Jaramillo Garcia, A., Gray, C. E., Barrowman, N., . . . Mottola, M. F. (2018). Prenatal exercise for the prevention of gestational diabetes mellitus and hypertensive disorders of pregnancy: A systematic review and meta-analysis. *British Journal of Sports Medicine, 52*, 1367–1375. https://doi.org/10.1136/bjsports-2018-099355

Druzin, M. L., & Shields, L. E. (2021a). Diagnosis and classification. In M. L. Druzin, L. E. Shields, N. Peterson, C. Sakowski, V. Cape, & C. H. Morton (Eds.), *Improving health care response to hypertensive disorders of pregnancy: A California Maternal Quality Care Collaborative quality improvement toolkit* (pp. 26–34). Retrieved from https://www.cmqcc.org/resource/4616/download

Druzin, M. L., & Shields, L. E. (2021b). Gestational hypertension. In M. L. Druzin, L. E. Shields, N. Peterson, C. Sakowski, V. Cape, & C. H. Morton (Eds.), *Improving health care response to hypertensive disorders of pregnancy: A California Maternal Quality Care Collaborative quality improvement toolkit* (pp. 105–110). Retrieved from https://www.cmqcc.org/resource/4616/download

Druzin, M. [L.], Shields, L. E., Morton, C. H., & Peterson, N. (2021). Introduction. In M. L. Druzin, L. E. Shields, N. Peterson, C. Sakowski, V. Cape, & C. H. Morton (Eds.), *Improving health care response to hypertensive disorders of pregnancy: A California Maternal Quality Care Collaborative quality improvement toolkit* (pp. 11–13). Retrieved from https://www.cmqcc.org/resource/4616/download

Druzin, M. L., Shields, L. E., Peterson, N., & Lee, R. (2021). Preventing and managing eclamptic seizures. In M. L. Druzin, L. E. Shields, N. Peterson, C. Sakowski, V. Cape, & C. H. Morton (Eds.), *Improving health care response to hypertensive disorders of pregnancy: A California Maternal Quality Care Collaborative quality improvement toolkit* (pp. 126–136). Retrieved from https://www.cmqcc.org/resource/4616/download

Druzin, M. L., Shields, L. E., Peterson, N., Sakowski, C., Cape, V., & Morton, C. H. (Eds.). (2021). *Improving health care response to hypertensive disorders of pregnancy: A California Maternal Quality Care Collaborative quality improvement toolkit*. Retrieved from https://www.cmqcc.org/resource/4616/download

Duley, L., Meher, S., & Jones, L. (2013). Drugs for treatment of very high blood pressure during pregnancy. *Cochrane Database of Systematic Reviews*. https://doi.org/10.1002/14651858.CD001449.pub3

Evans, R. W. (2014). The clinical features of migraine with and without aura. *Practical Neurology*, 26–32. Retrieved from https://practicalneurology.com/articles/2014-apr/the-clinical-features-of-migraine-with-and-without-aura

Farahani, M., Azadi, K., Hashemnejad, M., Agoushi, A., & Nirouei, M. (2021). Ruled out of preeclampsia-like syndrome due to COVID-19: A case study. *Clinical Case Reports, 9*(12), e05195. https://doi.org/10.1002/ccr3.5195

Fingar, K. R., Mabry-Hernandez, I., Ngo-Metzger, Q., Wolff, T., Steiner, C. A., & Elixhauser, A. (2017). *Delivery hospitalizations involving preeclampsia and eclampsia, 2005–2014*. HCUP Statistical Brief, 222. Retrieved from https://www.hcup-us.ahrq.gov/reports/statbriefs/sb222-Preeclampsia-Eclampsia-Delivery-Trends.pdf

Folk, D. M. (2018). Hypertensive disorders of pregnancy: Overview and current recommendations. *Journal of Midwifery & Women's Health, 63*(3), 289–300. https://doi.org/10.1111/jmwh.12725

Gabel, K., & Peterson, N. (2021a). Accurate blood pressure measurement. In M. L. Druzin, L. E. Shields, N. Peterson, C. Sakowski, V. Cape, & C. H. Morton (Eds.), *Improving health care response to hypertensive disorders of pregnancy: A California Maternal Quality Care Collaborative quality improvement toolkit* (pp. 45–49). Retrieved from https://www.cmqcc.org/resource/4616/download

Gabel, K., & Peterson, N. (2021b). Nursing management and assessment of preeclampsia. In M. L. Druzin, L. E. Shields, N. Peterson, C. Sakowski, V. Cape, & C. H. Morton (Eds.), *Improving health care response to hypertensive disorders of pregnancy: A California Maternal Quality Care Collaborative quality improvement toolkit* (pp. 83–88). Retrieved from https://www.cmqcc.org/resource/4616/download

Garg, R. K., Kumar, N., & Malhotra, H. S. (2018). Posterior reversible encephalopathy syndrome in eclampsia. *Neurology India, 66*(5), 1316–1323. https://doi.org/10.4103/0028-3886.241364

Ghaly, R. F., Candido, K. D., Sauer, R., & Knezevic, N. N. (2012). Complete recovery after antepartum massive intracerebral hemorrhage in an atypical case of sudden eclampsia. *Surgical Neurology International, 3*, 65. Retrieved from https://surgicalneurologyint.com/surgicalint-articles/complete-recovery-after-antepartum-massive-intracerebral-hemorrhage-in-an-atypical-case-of-sudden-eclampsia/

Han, A., Helewa, M., Stones, W., Nathan, H., Miller, S., & Magee, L. A. (2016). Hypertension. In L. A. Magee, P. von Dadelszen, W. Stones, & M. Mathai (Eds.), *The FIGO textbook of pregnancy hypertension: An evidence-based guide to monitoring, prevention and management* (pp. 1–18). London, United Kingdom: Global Library of Women's Medicine.

Hastie, R., Brownfoot, F. C., Cluver, C. A., Walker, S. P., Hesselman, S., Tong, S., & Bergman, L. (2019). Predictive value of the signs and symptoms preceding eclampsia: A systematic review. *Obstetrics & Gynecology, 134*(4), 677–684. https://doi.org/10.1097/AOG.0000000000003476

Hauspurg, A., & Jeyabalan, A. (2022). Postpartum preeclampsia or eclampsia: Defining its place and management among the hypertensive disorders of pregnancy. *American Journal of Obstetrics & Gynecology, 226*(2, Suppl.), S1211–S1221. https://doi.org/10.1016/j.ajog.2020.10.027

Hofmeyr, G. J., Lawrie, T. A., Atallah, Á. N., & Torloni, M. R. (2018). Calcium supplementation during pregnancy for preventing hypertensive disorders and related problems. *Cochrane Database of Systematic Reviews*. https://doi.org/10.1002/14651858.CD001059.pub5

Ives, C. W., Sinkey, R., Rajapreyar, I., Tita, A. T. N., & Oparil, S. (2020). Preeclampsia—Pathophysiology and clinical presentations: JACC state-of-the-art review. *Journal of the American College of Cardiology, 76*(14), 1690–1702. https://doi.org/10.1016/j.jacc.2020.08.014

Jayaram, A., Buhimschi, I. A., Aldasoqi, H., Hartwig, J., Owens, T., Elam, G. L., & Buhimsci, C. S. (2021). "Who said differentiating preeclampsia from COVID-19 infection was easy?" *Pregnancy Hypertension, 26*, 8–10. https://doi.org/10.1016/j.preghy.2021.07.248

Jeyabalan, A., & Larkin, J. C. (2023). Chronic hypertension in pregnancy: Prenatal and postpartum care. In V. A. Barss (Ed.), *UpToDate*. Retrieved November 14, 2023, from https://www.uptodate.com/contents/chronic-hypertension-in-pregnancy-prenatal-and-postpartum-care

Johnson, S., Liu, B., Kalafat, E., Thilaganathan, B., & Khalil, A. (2020). Maternal and perinatal outcomes of white coat hypertension during pregnancy: A systematic review and meta-analysis. *Hypertension, 76*(1), 157–166. https://doi.org/10.1161/HYPERTENSIONAHA.119.14627

Kansas State Board of Healing Arts. (2021). *Kansas statutes annotated and Kansas administrative regulations relating to the practice of independent practice midwifery*. Retrieved from http://www.ksbha.org/documents/publications/PracticeHandbook_CNM-I.pdf

Karumanchi, S. A., Lim, K.-H., & August, P. (2023). Preeclampsia: Pathogenesis. In V. A. Barss (Ed.), *UpToDate*. Retrieved November 14, 2023, from https://www.uptodate.com/contents/preeclampsia-pathogenesis

Kharb, S., Bhandari, N., Singh, A., & Gupta, A. (2019). Lactate dehydrogenase and maternal and perinatal outcome in preeclamptic women. *Archives of Medicine and Health Sciences, 7*(2), 163. https://doi.org/10.4103/amhs.amhs_102_18

Lee, M.-J., & Guinn, D. (2023). Antenatal corticosteroid therapy for reduction of neonatal respiratory morbidity and mortality from preterm delivery. In V. A. Barss (Ed.), *UpToDate*. Retrieved November 14, 2023, from https://www.uptodate.com/contents/antenatal-corticosteroid-therapy-for-reduction-of-neonatal-respiratory-morbidity-and-mortality-from-preterm-delivery

Lee, M.-J., Guinn, D., & Hickenbottom, S. (2023). Headache during pregnancy and postpartum. In V. A. Barss (Ed.), *UpToDate*. Retrieved November 14, 2023, from https://www.uptodate.com/contents/headache-during-pregnancy-and-postpartum

Lo, C. C. W., Lo, A. C. Q., Leow, S. H., Fisher, G., Corker, B., Batho, O., . . . Oliver-Williams, C. (2020). Future cardiovascular disease risk for women with gestational hypertension: A systematic review and meta-analysis. *Journal of the American Heart Association, 9*(13), e013991. https://doi.org/10.1161/JAHA.119.013991

Lockwood, C. J., & Julien, S. (2022). Nonimmune hydrops fetalis. In V. A. Barss (Ed.), *UpToDate*. Retrieved November 14, 2023, from https://www.uptodate.com/contents/nonimmune-hydrops-fetalis

Lucero, J., Champagne, H., & Gutierrez, M. C. (2021). Fluid management in preeclampsia. In M. L. Druzin, L. E. Shields, N. Peterson, C. Sakowski, V. Cape, & C. H. Morton (Eds.), *Improving health care response to hypertensive disorders of pregnancy: A California Maternal Quality Care Collaborative quality improvement toolkit* (pp. 143–145). Retrieved from https://www.cmqcc.org/resource/4616/download

Ma'ayeh, M., Rood, K. M., Kniss, D., & Costantine, M. M. (2020). Novel interventions for the prevention of preeclampsia. *Current Hypertension Reports, 22*(2), 17. https://doi.org/10.1007/s11906-020-1026-8

Magee, L. A., Nicolaides, K. H., & Von Dadelszen, P. (2022). Preeclampsia. *New England Journal of Medicine, 386*(19), 1817–1832. https://doi.org/10.1056/NEJMra2109523

Magee, L. A., Pels, A., Helewa, M., Rey, E., von Dadelszen, P., & Audibert, F. (2014). Diagnosis, evaluation, and management of the hypertensive disorders of pregnancy: Executive summary. *Journal of Obstetrics and Gynaecology Canada, 36*(5), 416–438. https://doi.org/10.1016/s1701-2163(15)30588-0

Mathias, C. R., & Rizvi, C. (2019). The diagnostic conundrum of maternal mirror syndrome progressing to pre-eclampsia—A case report. *Case Reports in Women's Health, 23*, e00122. https://doi.org/10.1016/j.crwh.2019.e00122

MAWS Transport Guideline Committee & Ad Hoc Physician-Licensed Midwife Workgroup. (2011). *Planned out-of-hospital birth transport guideline*. Seattle, WA: Midwives Association of Washington State. Retrieved from https://www.washingtonmidwives.org/uploads/1/1/3/8/113879963/maws-ooh-transport-policy0211.pdf

McCall, C. A., Grimes, D. A., & Lyerly, A. D. (2013). "Therapeutic" bed rest in pregnancy: Unethical and unsupported by data. *Obstetrics & Gynecology, 121*(6), 1305–1308. https://doi.org/10.1097/AOG.0b013e318293f12f

Melvin, L. M., & Funai, E. F. (2023). Gestational hypertension. In V. A. Barss (Ed.), *UpToDate*. Retrieved November 14, 2023, from https://www.uptodate.com/contents/gestational-hypertension

Moore, T. L, Dove-Medows, E., Zaagman, A. U., Schumacher, G., Mitchell, C., Allswede, M., & Chu, B. S. (2018, October 30). *Re: Midwifery—General Rules (ORR#2018-031 LR)*. Retrieved from https://www.mha.org/Portals/0/Issues and Advocacy/combined-letter-midwife-rules-102018.pdf

Moura, C., Amaral, L., Mendes, J. Quintanilha, R., Bento, F. M., Leite, M. I., & Melo, A. (2019). Hepatic rupture in HELLP syndrome. *Journal of Surgical Case Reports, 2019*, 10, rjz277. https://doi.org/10.1093/jscr/rjz277

Nerenberg, K. A., Park, A. L., Vigod, S. N., Saposnik, G., Berger, H., Hladunewich, M. A., . . . Ray, J. G. (2017). Long-term risk of a seizure disorder after eclampsia. *Obstetrics & Gynecology, 130*(6), 1327–1333 https://doi.org/10.1097/AOG.0000000000002364

[NICE] National Institute for Health and Care Excellence. (2023). *Intrapartum care* (NICE Guideline NG235). Retrieved from https://www.nice.org.uk/guidance/ng235

Norwitz, E. R. (2023a). Eclampsia. In V. A. Barss (Ed.), *UpToDate*. Retrieved November 14, 2023, from https://www.uptodate.com/contents/eclampsia

Norwitz, E. R. (2023b). Preeclampsia: Antepartum management and timing of delivery. In V. A. Barss (Ed.), *UpToDate*. Retrieved November 14, 2023, from https://www.uptodate.com/contents/preeclampsia-antepartum-management-and-timing-of-delivery

Papageorghiou, A. T., Deruelle, P., Gunier, R. B., Rauch, S., García-May, P. K., Mhatre, M., . . . Villar, J. (2021). Preeclampsia and COVID-19: Results from the INTERCOVID prospective longitudinal study. *American Journal of Obstetrics & Gynecology, 225*(3), 289-e1–289.e17. https://doi.org/10.1016/j.ajog.2021.05.014

Penfield, C. A., McNulty, J. A., Oakes, M. C., & Nageotte, M. P. (2019). Ibuprofen and postpartum blood pressure in women with hypertensive disorders of pregnancy. *Obstetrics & Gynecology, 134*(6), 1219–1226. https://doi.org/10.1097/AOG.0000000000003553

Pickering, T. G., Miller, N. H., Ogedegbe, G., Krakoff, L. R., Artinian, N. T., & Goff, D. (2008). Call to action on use and reimbursement for home blood pressure monitoring: A joint scientific statement from the American Heart Association, American Society of Hypertension, and Preventive Cardiovascular Nurses

Association. *Hypertension, 52*(1), 1–9. https://doi.org/10.1161/HYPERTENSIONAHA.107.189011

Premkumar, A., Ayala, N. K., Miller, C. H., Grobman, W. A., & Miller, E. S. (2021). Postpartum NSAID use and adverse outcomes among women with hypertensive disorders of pregnancy: A systematic review and meta-analysis. *American Journal of Perinatology, 38*(1), 1–9. https://doi.org/10.1055/s-0040-1713180

Reddy, M., Rolnik, D. L., Harris, K., Li, W., Mol, B. W., Costa, F. D. S., . . . Palmer, K. (2020). Challenging the definition of hypertension in pregnancy: A retrospective cohort study. *American Journal of Obstetrics & Gynecology, 222*(6), 606.e1–606.e221. https://doi.org/10.1016/j.ajog.2019.12.272

Robillard, P.-Y., Dekker, G., Scioscia, M., & Saito, S. (2022). Progress in the understanding of the pathophysiology of immunologic maladaptation related to early-onset preeclampsia and metabolic syndrome related to late-onset preeclampsia. *American Journal of Obstetrics & Gynecology, 226*(2, Suppl.), S867–S875. https://doi.org/10.1016/j.ajog.2021.11.019

Shields, L. E. (2021a). Chronic hypertension in pregnancy. In M. L. Druzin, L. E. Shields, N. Peterson, C. Sakowski, V. Cape, & C. H. Morton (Eds.), *Improving health care response to hypertensive disorders of pregnancy: A California Maternal Quality Care Collaborative quality improvement toolkit* (pp. 100–104). Retrieved from https://www.cmqcc.org/resource/4616/download

Shields, L. E. (2021b). Severe hypertension or preeclampsia with severe features at <34 weeks of gestation. In M. L. Druzin, L. E. Shields, N. Peterson, C. Sakowski, V. Cape, & C. H. Morton (Eds.), *Improving health care response to hypertensive disorders of pregnancy: A California Maternal Quality Care Collaborative quality improvement toolkit* (pp. 111–120). Retrieved from https://www.cmqcc.org/resource/4616/download

Sibai, B. M. (2021). Preeclampsia and hypertensive disorders. In M. B. Landon, H. L. Galan, E. R. M. Jauniaux, D. A. Driscoll, V. Berghella, W. A. Grobman, . . . A. G. Cahill (Eds.), *Gabbe's obstetrics: Normal and problem pregnancies* (8th ed., Kindle version, ch. 27). Philadelphia, PA: Elsevier.

Sibai, B. M. (2023). HELLP syndrome (hemolysis, elevated liver enzymes, and low platelets). In V. A. Barss (Ed.), *UpToDate*. Retrieved November 14, 2023, from https://www.uptodate.com/contents/hellp-syndrome-hemolysis-elevated-liver-enzymes-and-low-platelets

Society for Maternal-Fetal Medicine. (2022). *Society for Maternal-Fetal Medicine statement: Antihypertensive therapy for mild chronic hypertension in pregnancy: The CHAP Trial*. Retrieved from https://els-jbs-prod-cdn.jbs.elsevierhealth.com/pb/assets/raw/Health Advance/journals/ymob/SMFM_Statement_CHAP_draft_April_2022.pdf

Sorensen, T. K., Williams, M. A., Lee, I. M., Dashow, E. E., Thompson, M. L., & Luthy, D. A. (2003). Recreational physical activity during pregnancy and risk of preeclampsia. *Hypertension, 41*(6), 1273–1280. https://doi.org/10.1161/01.HYP.0000072270.82815.91

Syngelaki, A., Nicolaides, K. H., Balani, J., Hyer, S., Akolekar, R., Kotecha, R., . . . Shehata, H. (2016). Metformin versus placebo in obese pregnant women without diabetes mellitus. *New England Journal of Medicine, 374*(5), 434–443. https://doi.org/10.1056/NEJMoa1509819

Tita, A. T., Szychowski, J. M., Boggess, K., Dugoff, L., Sibai, B., Lawrence, K., . . . Andrews, W. W. (2022). Treatment for mild chronic hypertension during pregnancy. *New England Journal of Medicine, 386*(19), 1781–1792. https://doi.org/10.1056/NEJMoa2201295

Townsend, R., O'Brien, P., & Khalil, A. (2016). Current best practice in the management of hypertensive disorders in pregnancy. *Integrated Blood Pressure Control, 9*, 79–94. https://doi.org/10.2147/IBPC.S77344

Tremonti, C., Beddoe, J., & Brown, M. A. (2017). Reliability of home blood pressure monitoring devices in pregnancy. *Pregnancy Hypertension, 8*, 9–14. https://doi.org/10.1016/j.preghy.2017.01.002

U.S. Preventive Services Task Force. (2021). Aspirin use to prevent preeclampsia and related morbidity and mortality: US Preventive Services Task Force recommendation statement. *JAMA, 326*(12), 1186–1191. https://doi.org/10.1001/jama.2021.14781

Unger, T., Borghi, C., Charchar, F., Khan, N. A., Poulter, N. R., Prabhakaran, D., . . . Schutte, A. E. (2020). 2020 International Society of Hypertension global hypertension practice guidelines. *Hypertension, 75*(6), 1334–1357. https://doi.org/10.1161/HYPERTENSIONAHA.120.15026

Valente, A. M., & Economy, K. (2023). Maternal adaptations to pregnancy: Cardiovascular and hemodynamic changes. In V. A. Barss (Ed.), *UpToDate*. Retrieved November 13, 2023, from https://www.uptodate.com/contents/maternal-adaptations-to-pregnancy-cardiovascular-and-hemodynamic-changes

Vijayvargia, N., & Samariya, M. (2021). Impaired circadian rhythm of blood pressure predicting adverse events in preeclampsia. *International Journal of Reproduction, Contraception, Obstetrics and Gynecology, 10*(2), 511–516. https://doi.org/10.18203/2320-1770.ijrcog20210005

Villar, J., Ariff, S., Gunier, R. B., Thiruvengadam, R., Rauch, S., Kholin, A., . . . Papageorghiou, A. T. (2021). Maternal and neonatal morbidity and mortality among pregnant women with and without COVID-19 infection: The INTERCOVID multinational cohort study. *JAMA Pediatrics, 175*(8), 1–10. https://doi.org/10.1001/jamapediatrics.2021.1050

Wang, B., Yang, X., Yu, H., & Man, X. (2020). The comparison of ibuprofen versus acetaminophen for blood pressure in preeclampsia: A meta-analysis of randomized controlled studies. *Journal of Maternal-Fetal & Neonatal Medicine, 35*(3), 592–597. https://doi.org/10.1080/14767058.2020.1720641

Wei, S. Q., Bilodeau-Bertrand, M., Liu, S., & Auger, N. (2021). The impact of COVID-19 on pregnancy outcomes: A systematic review and meta-analysis. *Canadian Medical Association Journal, 193*(16), E540–E548. https://doi.org/10.1503/cmaj.202604

Wu, D.-D., Gao, L., Huang, O., Ullah, K., Guo, M.-X., Liu, Y., . . . Huang, H.-F. (2020). Increased adverse pregnancy outcomes associated with stage 1 hypertension in a low-risk cohort: Evidence from 47 874 cases. *Hypertension, 75*(3), 772–780. https://doi.org/10.1161/HYPERTENSIONAHA.119.14252

Malpresentations and Cord Prolapse 11

Objectives

- Discuss the management of umbilical cord prolapse in community settings.
- Describe maternal and fetal conditions associated with a higher incidence of breech presentation.
- Explain why a mother with a pendulous maternal abdomen is at risk for labor dystocia and describe interventions to normalize the birth process in this situation.
- Describe how to facilitate labor progress for the client with a fetus who is in an occiput posterior position.
- Describe four maneuvers that the midwife may use to assist the birth of the aftercoming head of a breech baby in community settings.

Composite Case Study

Cordelia W., a 33-year-old gravida 3, para 2 (G3 P2), appeared to be very uncomfortable when she arrived at the birth center. She was clearly in the throes of hard labor, and there was a grunt in her breathing. Aaliyah Davis, CPM, supported her gently as she guided her to the birth room. Roger, Cordelia's burly husband, followed carrying an awkward collection—cooler, car seat, overnight bag, and water jug. As Cordelia came through the doorway, her water broke in a gush, and she dropped into a deep squat, pushing hard. Aaliyah stripped off Cordelia's underpants and saw, to her astonishment, two small feet beginning to emerge.

"It appears this little one is coming feet first," Aaliyah said calmly. "Roger, can you knock on that door and ask the secretary and nurse to come help me?" With a loud clatter, Roger dropped his load and sprinted to the adjacent office. Within moments, he returned with the two additional helpers as Aaliyah explained the situation to Cordelia. Aaliyah's instructions were calm and clear. "Ebony, can you please hand me that Doppler and call an ambulance? Kate, the birth equipment is all set up over there by the bed. Can you bring it closer and get vital signs?"

Roger held Cordelia in a supported squat beside the bed. The only sound was Cordelia's breathing as she involuntarily pushed. Aaliyah's hands defined a protected space around the emerging baby, poised but not touching, as the child slowly came into the light. The fetal legs emerged, following the normal sequence of breech birth. Then the pelvis appeared, followed by the umbilicus and both arms. At that point progress stopped, and Aaliyah became concerned. She used the shoulder press maneuver to encourage flexion of the fetal head, and the wet, slippery baby slid easily into her hands.

The baby girl looked stunned for a moment, then began to cry. Roger also looked stunned and began to cry. Aaliyah handed the baby to Cordelia and helped the new mother into bed, the umbilical cord still intact. The nurse and midwife dried the infant with soft blankets and performed a newborn assessment. The baby appeared healthy. Third stage labor was uneventful, and Cordelia's perineum was intact. By the time the ambulance arrived, mother and infant were stable, and transport was not required.

Malpresentations

The terms *malpresentation* and *malposition* are frequently interchanged, and different sources use different definitions. *Fetal malpresentation* is the term generally used when a fetal part other than the head is the first to descend into the pelvis (breech, shoulder) but is also widely used to describe compound, face, and brow presentations (American College of Obstetricians & Gynecologists [ACOG], 2014). *Fetal malposition* can be used to describe a suboptimal head position for a fetus in cephalic presentation, usually the occiput posterior (OP) or occiput transverse (OT) positions (Pilliod & Caughey, 2017). Asynclitism (fetal sagittal suture is tilted toward the sacrum or symphysis pubis) can also be considered a cephalic malposition. In this book, the term *malpresentation* denotes any fetal position associated with greater difficulty of labor or risk to the fetus.

For birth to occur, the fetus must pass through the bony pelvis. Ideally, the fetus finds the best fit in the intrauterine space by arranging the buttocks and flexed legs in the broad fundal cavity and the occiput oriented anteriorly in the narrower lower segment of the uterus. Labor with a malpresented fetus is usually slower and more difficult than normal labor, and maternal exhaustion is more likely to develop. Cervical dilation is usually slow and painful,

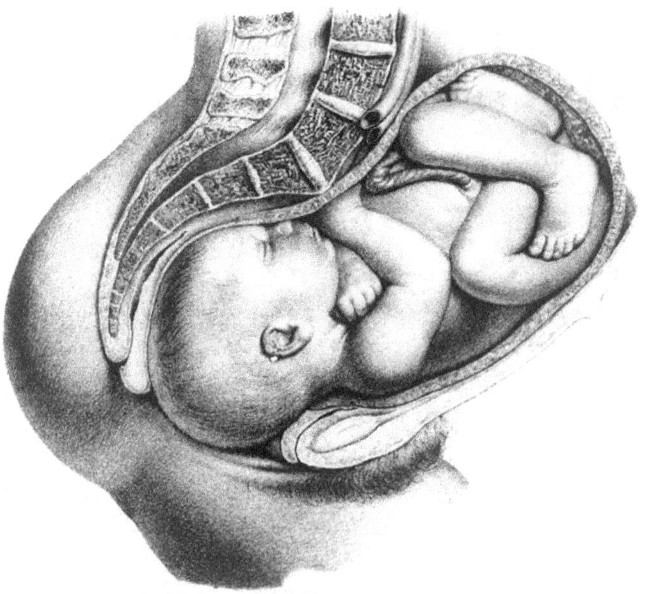

Figure 11-1. In the LOA fetus, flexion increases with descent. From *Atlas de l'Art des Accouchements* (plate 58, fig. 2), by A. Lenoir, M. See, and S. Tarnier, 1871, Paris, France: Victor Masson. In the public domain.

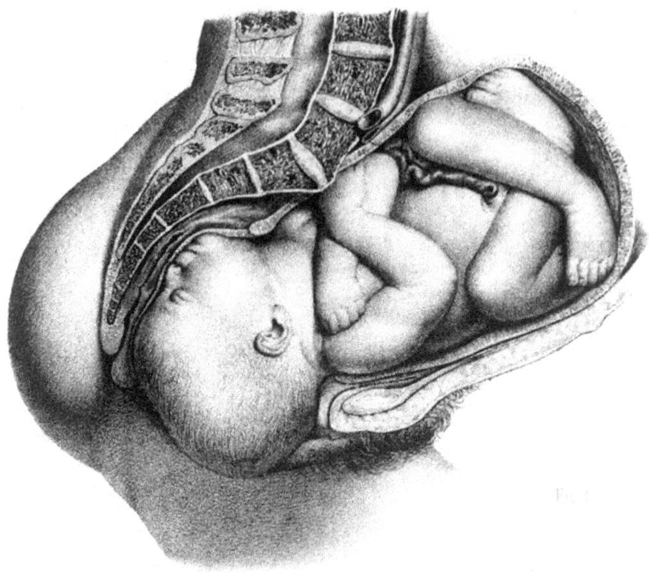

Figure 11-2. Extension in LOA position and crowning. From *Atlas de l'Art des Accouchements* (plate 59, fig. 1), by A. Lenoir et al., 1871, Paris, France: Victor Masson. In the public domain.

and the presenting part stays high. Neglected malpresentations can lead to obstructed labor and even uterine rupture. Greater effort is necessary to expel a malpresented fetus, and lacerations and atony are more likely to cause hemorrhage after the birth.

Maternal and Fetal Factors

Certain predisposing conditions can increase the likelihood of fetal malpresentation. Some of these are as follows (Mohammed & El-Chaâr, 2023a):

Maternal Factors

Contracted pelvis: A pelvis that is abnormally narrow in one or more of its diameters can interfere with the normal mechanism of labor and encourage malpresentation (Mohammed & El-Chaâr, 2023a). A contracted pelvic inlet can prevent the fetus from entering the pelvis or, if the fetus does engage, cause the presenting part to be deflexed, asynclitic, or nonvertex. Midpelvic contraction can prevent anterior rotation and force the fetus into OP position.

Pendulous maternal abdomen due to lax abdominal muscles, obesity, or lordosis can cause the uterus and fetus to lie forward on a horizontal plane (Kiran, Singh, & Sinha, 2015; Posner, 2023).

Neoplasms: Uterine fibroids or ovarian cysts can prevent the fetus from engaging.

Uterine anomalies such as an arcuate, bicornuate, or unicornuate uterus can result in a narrow or misshapen uterine chamber, causing the fetus to adopt an abnormal presentation. The nonpregnant horn of a bicornuate uterus can obstruct the descent of the fetus.

Fetal Factors

Fetal size: A fetus that is large in relation to the pelvic inlet sometimes adopts an abnormal presentation because it has too little room to move. A very small or preterm fetus often does so because it has too much.

Multiple gestation: Breech and transverse presentations are more common in multiple gestations.

Fetal anomalies: A fetus with congenital anomalies such as hydrocephaly and anencephaly or with abnormal tone is more likely to adopt an abnormal presentation.

Placenta previa: When the placenta implants across the cervix, the fetus cannot engage.

Abnormal volume of amniotic fluid: Polyhydramnios (excessive volume of amniotic fluid) allows the fetus too much freedom of movement, which can result in malpresentation. Oligohydramnios (low volume of amniotic fluid) can "shrink-wrap" the fetus, restricting movement and leading to persistent malpresentation.

Prelabor rupture of membranes can be the cause or effect of malpresentation. When there is a poor fit between the maternal pelvis and the presenting part, membranes are more likely to rupture before contractions begin. Rupture of membranes before the fetus has assumed an optimal orientation for birth can cause the fetus to descend in a malpresentation.

Mechanism of Normal Birth

Presentation is described by the fetal part that leads into the birth canal: face, brow, occiput (vertex), shoulder, limb, cord, or breech (frank, incomplete, complete). Rarely a hand or umbilical cord is the presenting part. Most commonly the fetus traverses the pelvis in a right or left occiput anterior (ROA/LOA) position—head down, back toward the mother's abdomen, and chin flexed to chest. This posture efficiently introduces the smallest diameter of the baby's head to the pelvis, simplifying birth.

The pelvic inlet is at a 90° angle to the pelvic outlet, forming a curved passage of bone and soft tissue with various diameters (Iversen, Kahrs, & Eggebø, 2021). The fetus must accommodate to pelvic features during descent by turning, flexing, extending, and restituting. At least half of these cardinal movements occur during the second stage of labor (Howard, 2021). The cardinal movements are as follows:

- **Engagement:** The widest part of the head descends below the pelvic inlet, the first bony obstacle to be negotiated (Eggebø & Hjartardottir, 2021). In primigravidas the fetus typically descends and engages before labor, but in multiparas the fetus can remain unengaged for most of labor.
- **Descent:** Uterine contractions cause descent to occur throughout labor, and voluntary bearing down encourages further descent in the second stage. The head typically enters the pelvis in a transverse position to conform to the shape of the pelvic inlet.
- **Flexion:** The fetal head is naturally flexed throughout gestation. As the fetal head descends, it encounters resistance from the muscles of the pelvic floor, increasing flexion. The occiput moves through the pelvis ahead of the forehead with the posterior (triangular) fontanel leading, and the baby's chin moves toward the chest. Flexion allows the smallest diameter of the head to move through the pelvis. When the head is not flexed, a wider diameter of fetal skull must negotiate the pelvic passage.
- **Internal rotation:** In most female adults, the midpelvis is widest from front to back, and the inlet is a transverse oval, widest from side to side (Garber & Dy, 2023). Both the outlet and the fetal head are anteroposterior ovals (Garber & Dy, 2023). To proceed through the pelvis, the fetal head must rotate internally 45° to face the mother's sacrum. Only the head makes this turn; the shoulders remain oblique.
- **Extension:** Extension occurs when contractions push the baby down onto the firm pelvic floor. Because the anterior wall of the pelvis (the symphysis pubis) is about 4–5 cm long and the posterior wall (the sacrum) is 10–15 cm, the occiput has a shorter path than the forehead (Garber & Dy, 2023). The nape of the neck reaches the pubic bone and pivots beneath it. The forehead advances across the sacrum and perineum, and the head is born. Then the fetus extends its head to follow the anatomic curve. At this point, the birth attendant observes perineal bulging, crowning, and then the birth of the head, facing the mother's anus.
- **Restitution:** When the baby's head is born, it faces the anus while the shoulders remain positioned diagonally inside the pelvis. As soon as the head is free, the baby's neck restitutes back 45° to realign with the shoulders.
- **External rotation:** The shoulders reach the pelvic floor and rotate internally to the anteroposterior orientation. The head rotates another 45° to follow the rotation of the shoulders.
- **Expulsion:** The anterior shoulder slides under the pubic bone and is born by lateral flexion. The posterior shoulder is born next, and the body should follow quickly.

The "Four Ps"

Successful childbirth involves interplay among the "four Ps": Passage, Passenger, Powers, and Psyche.

Passage

The birth passage comprises the bony pelvis and the overlying soft tissues. The female pelvis allows upright posture while providing the fetus a bony conduit to the outside world. The traditional model developed by Caldwell and Moloy (1933) proposes that the female pelvis occurs in any of four main types: gynecoid, anthropoid, android, and platypelloid, whereas males possess an android pelvis type. Evaluation of a large sampling of female pelvises using multidetector computerized tomography (CT) imaging, however, has revealed "an amorphous, cloudy continuum of shape variation" (Kuliukas, Kuliukas, Franklin, & Flavel, 2015, p. 490). Other research has demonstrated that males show similar pelvic variability and that differences among individuals are not as sex-specific as previously thought (Delprete, 2017).

There is an overall increase in pelvic capacity at both the inlet and the outlet from 20 to 32 weeks of gestation (Kjeldsen, Blankholm, Jurik, Salvig, & Maimburg, 2021). Each individual's unique internal dimensions determine whether a baby of a given size and orientation will fit. A tumor, a fibroid, an ovarian cyst, or a vaginal, uterine, or cervical septum can obstruct labor as can the resistance of the cervix and pelvic-floor muscles.

Maternal position and movement can affect the ability of the pelvis to expand. Rocking, swaying, stair climbing, and walking alter the relationship of the pelvic bones to one another and the shape of the pelvis continuously, possibly encouraging

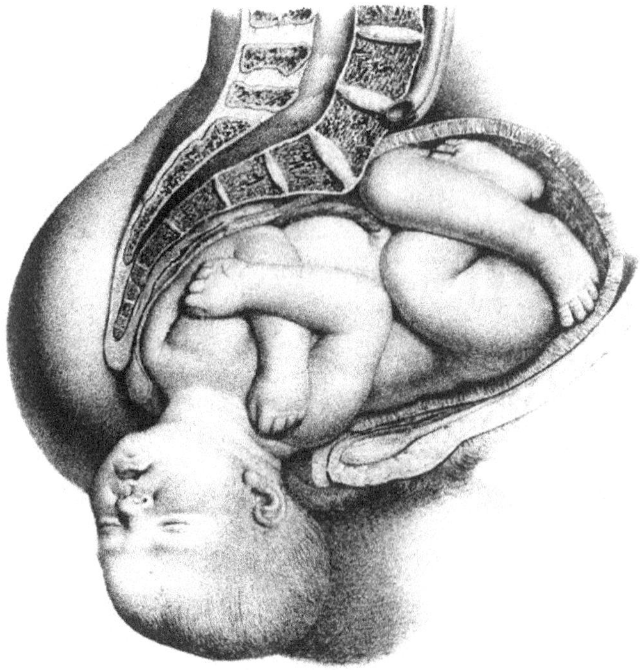

Figure 11-3. At birth, the extended head and neck restitute to align with the shoulders and trunk. From *Atlas de l'Art des Accouchements* (plate 59, fig. 2), by A. Lenoir et al., 1871, Paris, France: Victor Masson. In the public domain.

the fetus to descend (Simkin, Hanson, & Ancheta, 2017). Walking, standing, hands-and-knees, squatting, sitting upright, kneeling, and lateral positions can shorten the second stage of labor by a mean of 21.12 min (Berta, Lindgren, Christensson, Mekonnen, & Adefris, 2019).

Passenger

The size and position of the fetus are crucial to the success of labor and birth. Fetal position is influenced by uterine shape, available space, and maternal position and movement. Fetal position is voluntary to some extent, and a small alteration in posture such as a tilted or deflexed head can obstruct progress (Simkin et al., 2017). A stillborn infant, in contrast, lacks tone and tactile responsiveness and is more likely to assume a brow or face presentation. Although a healthy fetus is an active participant in the birth process, a preterm fetus with immature reflexes or a fetus with abnormal tone is often unable to make movements that facilitate birth. A fetus with hydrocephalus may be unable to engage, and one with a large axillary cystic hygroma may develop shoulder dystocia (Chawanpaiboon, Ciardelli, Chitty, & Pierro, 2002; Weiss, 1991).

Powers

The power of uterine contractions expels the fetus. Optimally strong, long, frequent, well-coordinated contractions hasten birth. If uterine activity is inadequate, vaginal birth will not occur. Maternal position influences the powers of labor.

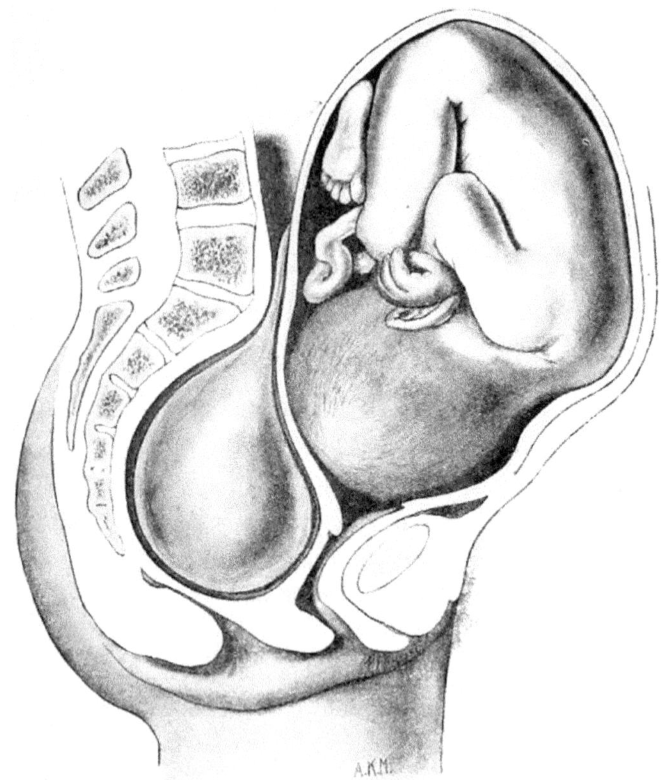

Figure 11-4. A large ovarian cyst can prevent the fetus from descending into the pelvis. From *Operative Midwifery* (2nd ed., p. 225), by J. M. Munro Kerr, 1911, New York, NY: William Wood. In the public domain.

Ambulation and upright positioning can improve the progress of cervical dilation, fetal head descent, and the frequency and duration of uterine contractions (Ibrahim, Said, & Elgzar, 2020). Hydration, movement, positioning, comforting touch, immersion in warm water, nipple stimulation, acupressure and warm compresses placed on the fundus can make contractions stronger and more effective (Simkin et al., 2017).

Psyche

The expectant mother's psychological state—self-concept, attitude, confidence, level of preparation, experience of pain, coping ability, reaction to circumstances, and social support—can all affect the course of labor. A confident, secure attitude can facilitate birth. A history of emotional trauma can create high levels of fear or anxiety during labor (Simkin et al., 2017). Suppressed memories of childhood trauma can surface unexpectedly during labor as panic, helplessness, or terror.

Cephalic Malpresentation

The presenting part is the part of the fetal body within or in closest proximity to the birth canal. A cephalic presentation occurs when the fetal head is the presenting part. Labor is most likely to progress without complications when the presentation is vertex, a cephalic presentation with the neck flexed with the chin against the chest and the posterior fontanel presenting (Cunningham et al., 2022, ch. 22). A cephalic malpresentation occurs when the fetus presents with a part of the head other than the vertex.

Signs and Symptoms

A difficult fit between fetus and mother can result from abnormal position, asynclitism, or an unfavorable relationship between the size of the fetal presenting part and the maternal pelvic passage. Suspect malpresentation when the laboring client's discomfort seems out of proportion to the strength of uterine contractions. Some clients complain of pain before a contraction is palpable and continue to feel pain afterwards (Mohammed & El-Chaâr, 2023b). Other clinical signs of actual or relative cephalopelvic disproportion frequently include

- PROM at term.
- Contractions that vary unpredictably in intensity, interval, or duration (Simkin et al., 2017).
- Contractions that occur in couplets or salvos followed by long intervals of uterine relaxation.
- Contractions that become less frequent in active labor.
- Deep back and/or rectal pain that does not subside between contractions.
- Uncontrollable urge to push before fully dilated, perhaps the body's attempt to make the head flex, then rotate (Chapman & Charles, 2018). There is no evidence to support or refute the traditional view that spontaneous pushing before complete dilation increases the risk of cervical trauma or other adverse maternal or fetal outcomes (Tsao, 2015).
- Fetus that remains at a high station during labor.
- Unengaged head before labor in a nulligravida.
- Slow progress in second-stage labor and vaginal gaping before the fetal head is visible.
- Cervix dangling like an empty sock in front of a head that is not well applied.
- Extreme molding of the head and significant caput succedaneum (edema of the scalp where the head contacts the cervix).

If the fetus has an asynclitic or OP head position in early labor, it is likely to rotate into a more favorable orientation over time. Only supportive care is needed if labor is progressing. If labor slows or stops and mother and baby are stable, transport may be necessary for oxytocic medication and/or epidural anesthesia, but probably not emergently. When in doubt, consult with a collaborating physician. If membranes are ruptured, the risk of intraamniotic infection increases with time and with each vaginal examination, particularly when the client carries Group B *Streptococcus* (GBS).

Table 11-1
Frequency of Malpresentations

Presentation	Frequency
Occiput posterior (OP)	1/19 births
Breech	1/33 births
Face	1/600–1/800 births
Brow	1/500–1/4,000 births
Transverse lie	1/833 births
Compound	1/1,500 births

Adapted from S. Julien and F. Galerneau, 2023, "Face and Brow Presentations in Labor," in V. A. Barss (Ed.), *UpToDate*. Copyright by UpToDate.

Prolonged Labor

Prolonged latent, first-stage, or second-stage labor can be a sign of malpresentation (H. Smith, Peterson, Lagrew, & Main, 2022). Uterine contractions can become inefficient, slowing dilation and leading to arrest of labor. Some cephalic malpresentations are compatible with vaginal birth, others are not. If labor slows or stops and mother and baby are stable, transport may be required for labor augmentation and/or epidural anesthesia. Slow progress in labor, however, is not necessarily an indication for cesarean section, especially in latent labor. Labor may require 6 hr or more to progress from 4 to 5 cm of dilation and 3 hr or more to progress from 5 to 6 cm (ACOG, 2024). Current ACOG guidance (ACOG, 2024) includes the following:

- Cervical dilation of 6 cm is considered the start of the active phase of labor.
- Active phase arrest of labor is defined as no progress in cervical dilation in clients who are at least 6 cm dilated with rupture of membranes despite 4 hr of adequate uterine activity or 6 hr of inadequate uterine activity with oxytocin augmentation.
- Prolonged second stage of labor is defined as
    - More than 3 hr of pushing in nulliparous clients.
    - More than 2 hr of pushing in multiparous clients.
- Providers should consider labor progress, clinical factors that may affect the likelihood of vaginal delivery, risks and benefits of available interventions, and client preference when second stage labor exceeds these limits. The provider may diagnose second-stage arrest earlier if there is a lack of fetal rotation or descent despite adequate contractions, pushing efforts, and time.
- In the latent phase, oxytocin should be administered for at least 12–18 hr after membrane rupture before diagnosing the client with a failed induction of labor. The decision to continue past 18 hr may be individualized according to clinical situation, client preference, and discussion of the risks and benefits.

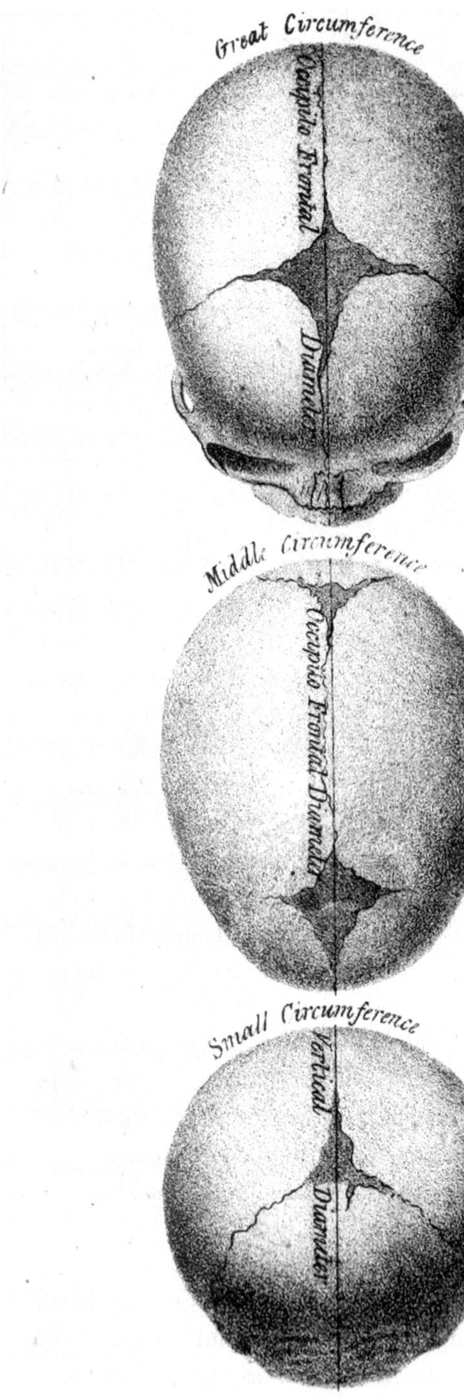

Figure 11-5. The importance of attitude. Fetal head circumference can decrease from large (top) to intermediate (center) to small (bottom) as a result of increasing flexion of the head. From *Midwifery Illustrated* (plate 25), by J. P. Maygrier (A. S. Doane, Trans.), 1834, New York, NY: Harper & Brothers. In the public domain.

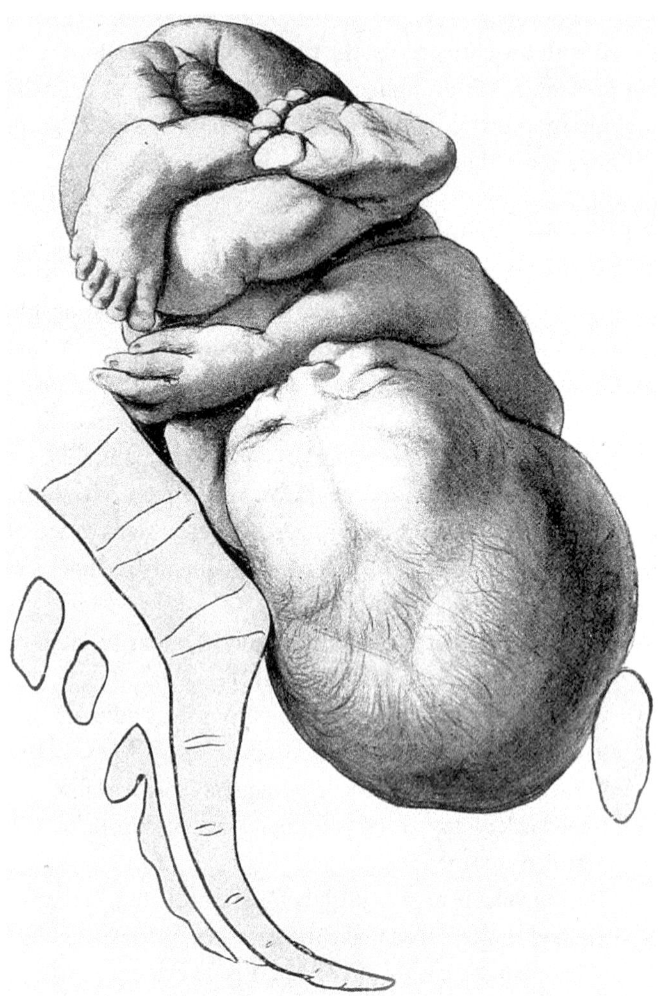

Figure 11-6. Hydrocephalus can prevent a fetus from descending into the pelvis. From *Operative Obstetrics, Including the Surgery of the Newborn* (p. 238, fig. 147) by E. P. Davis, 1911, Philadelphia, PA: W. B. Saunders. In the public domain.

Persistent Occiput Posterior

Occiput posterior (OP), a cephalic presentation with the fetal occiput directed toward the maternal sacrum, occurs in 15–20% of labors at onset and persists into the second stage in 5–8% (Elmore, McBroom, & Ellis, 2020). It appears that the rate of OP position in labor and birth has significantly increased over the past century: in 1896, the rate of OP position was given as 1 in 33 labors (Brothers, 1896), and 2% of these babies were born in OP position (Dorland, 1896). The OP position occurs twice as often among nulliparous individuals as in the multiparous (Barth, 2015). About 60% of OP positions are right occiput posterior (ROP—occiput oriented toward the right maternal sacroiliac joint), 30% are left occiput posterior (LOP—occiput oriented toward the left maternal sacroiliac joint), and 10% are direct occiput posterior—DOP, fetal occiput oriented over sacral midline (Barth, 2015). Rotation from OA to OP in second stage is rare, less than 5% (Barth, 2015).

A physiologically normal variant in the early part of labor, the OP position can become pathological when it leads to prolonged or arrested labor. The head of a fetus in OP position presents a larger diameter to the pelvis (due to deflexion) and is therefore less effective at dilating the cervix than its OA counterpart. Persistent OP position has been associated with higher rates of operative vaginal birth and cesarean section, postpartum hemorrhage, intraamniotic and postpartum infection, obstetric lacerations, and neonatal intensive care unit admissions (Elmore et al., 2020). In one study (Simpson, Chambers, Sharshiner, & Caughey, 2015), the rate of cesarean birth for nulliparous clients with fetuses in the OP position was 73.6% (compared to with 25% with OA) and 38.7% for multiparous clients with OP (compared with 7.5% OA). Although OP increases the risk of interventional birth overall, an OP baby with a smaller head circumference is more likely to accomplish spontaneous birth than one with a larger circumference (Yagel et al., 2017).

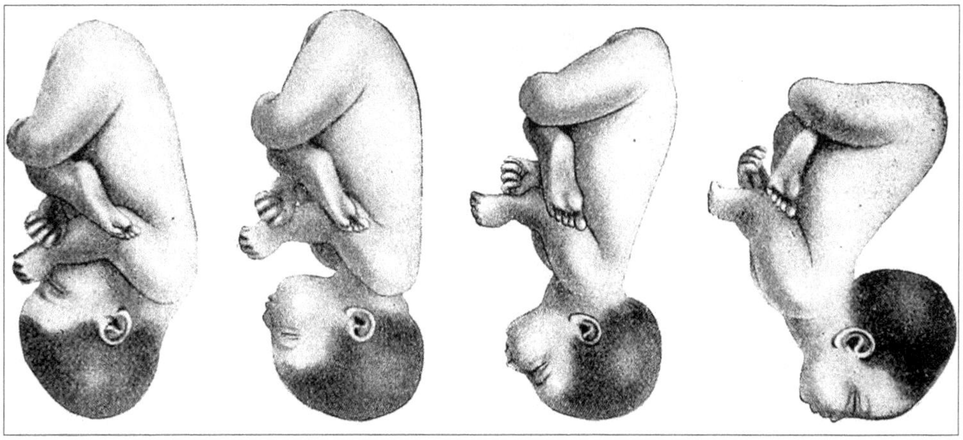

Figure 11-7. A fetus with a deflexed attitude presents a much larger diameter to the pelvis than one that is vertex with chin to chest. With the average brow presentation, the cervix must dilate to 13.5 cm to reach second stage. More important, the bony pelvis must accommodate this head diameter for birth to occur. From *Obstetrics: A Text-Book for the Use of Students and Practitioners* (3rd ed., p. 214, fig. 193–196), by J. W. Williams, 1912, New York, NY: Appleton. In the public domain.

Maternal factors that predispose to persistent OP position include a small pelvic outlet (particularly a narrow pubic arch), obesity, previous OP birth, gestational age 41 6/7 weeks or more, anterior placenta, and age greater than 35 years (Argani & Satin, 2022). A large fetus with a large head is more likely to remain in persistent OP position, have a longer second stage of labor, and have a higher risk of forceps or vacuum-assisted birth (Elmore et al., 2020). It appears that epidural anesthesia can increase the risk of persistent OP, presumably because the resulting relaxation of the pelvic musculature can inhibit physiologic rotation at the end of labor (Anim-Somuah, Smyth, Cyna, & Cuthbert, 2018; Argani & Satin, 2022).

OP fetal positioning can obstruct labor by creating relative cephalopelvic disproportion. Where there is good flexion (usually with LOP), the average OP fetus presents a 10.5 cm suboccipitofrontal diameter to the pelvic passage, which is 1 cm greater than the average diameter (9.5 cm) of a fetal head in the flexed occipitoanterior position (Mohammed & El-Chaâr, 2023a). If flexion does not occur (usually with ROP) the presenting diameter is occipitofrontal, which is 11.5 cm on average (Mohammed & El-Chaâr, 2023a). A fetus in OP position with a military attitude (partially deflexed) presents a diameter to the pelvis equivalent to that of a 4 lb 7 oz (2,000 g) increase in birthweight (Simpson et al., 2015).

Confirming the OP Position

When the fetus is OP, the occiput is in the posterior of the maternal pelvis, and the fetal brow is in the anterior. The fetus is in a vertical lie, roughly parallel to the mother's spine, head in or near the posterior pelvis, and back toward the maternal flank. The fetal back can be difficult to palpate. The buttocks and thighs are in the uterine fundus. The midwife sometimes feels many small parts through the abdominal wall. The abdomen can have a camel-back appearance with humps over the fetal head and buttocks and a concavity near the maternal umbilicus. Fetal heart tones (FHT) transmitted through the fetal scapula are more easily auscultated through the maternal flank on the same side as the fetal back, especially with a fetoscope (Mohammed & El-Chaâr, 2023a; H. Smith et al., 2022). Fetal heart sounds transmitted through the baby's chest may be loudest in the maternal lower abdomen (Mohammed & El-Chaâr, 2023a).

At the end of the first stage, a persistent anterior lip can develop with the OP or asynclitic baby if the narrow forehead (sinciput) does not keep the cervix retracted in the forepelvis (H. Smith et al., 2022). Cervical edema can result from uneven compression by the presenting part. Although the OP position by itself does not necessarily cause more painful labors or "back labor" (Lieberman, Davidson, Lee-Parritz, & Shearer, 2005), OP positioning increases the likelihood that the fetus will be a poor fit for the maternal pelvis, and any obstructed labor will be longer and more painful than one that proceeds unimpeded.

In advanced labor, OP positioning can be difficult to confirm by vaginal examination. The fetus that fits the pelvis imperfectly can develop thick caput that obscures suture and fontanel landmarks, and molding can distort the anatomy (H. Smith et al., 2022). The fetal posterior fontanel is triangular and found at the junction of the sagittal and lambdoid sutures. The anterior fontanel is diamond-shaped, larger, and located

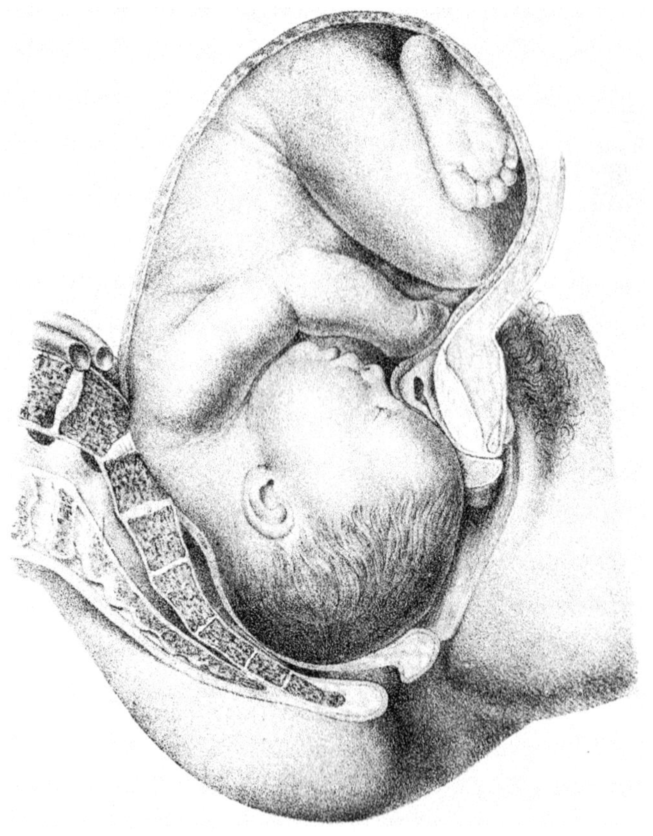

Figure 11-8. A well-flexed fetus in the OP position presents a suboccipitofrontal diameter to the pelvis with an average measurement of 10.5 cm, a centimeter greater than the presenting diameter of the average well-flexed occiput anterior baby. From *A Practical Treatise on Midwifery*... (plate XLIII), by F. J. Moreau (T. F. Betton, Trans.), 1844, Philadelphia, PA: Carey and Hart. In the public domain.

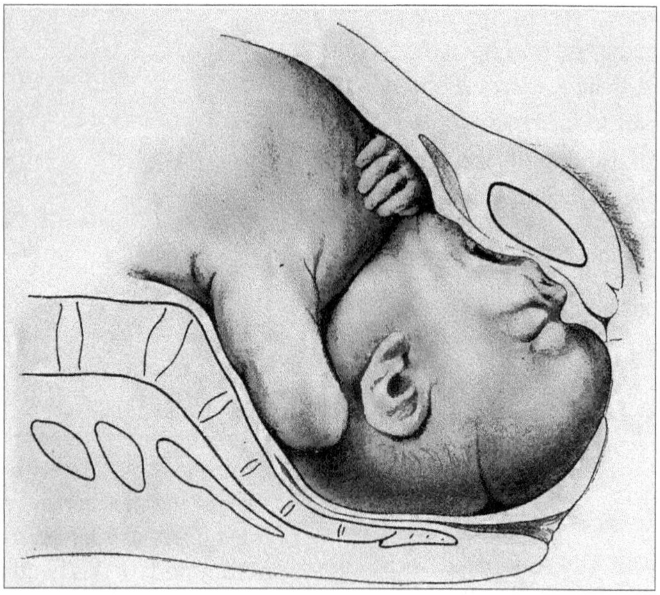

Figure 11-9. The partially extended head of an average-sized fetus in a deflexed OP-brow position presents with a mentovertical diameter of 13.5 cm, 4 cm greater than the diameter of a flexed occipitoanterior baby. In this illustration, an open fetal mouth pressed into the pubis and a posterior nuchal arm further impede progress. Although the fetal head is visible with maternal pushing, cesarean birth is necessary for this baby. From *Operative Obstetrics, Including the Surgery of the Newborn* (p. 123, fig. 18) by E. P. Davis, 1911, Philadelphia, PA: W. B. Saunders. In the public domain.

where the coronal suture intersects with the frontal suture and the sagittal suture. On cervical examination, when the posterior fontanel is oriented toward the right maternal posterior pelvis, the fetus is either ROP or ROT (right occiput transverse); when oriented toward the left maternal posterior pelvis, the fetus is LOP or LOT (left occiput transverse). If the fetus is ROP or LOP, the diamond-shaped anterior fontanel is to one side of the symphysis pubis at the front of the pelvis. The head typically enters the pelvis obliquely, with the sagittal suture to the right or the left of the midline (Mohammed & El-Chaâr, 2023a). Flexion is often suboptimal; when the attitude is not flexed, the anterior and posterior fontanels tend to be at the same station of descent.

The International Society of Ultrasound in Obstetrics and Gynecology recommends using transabdominal ultrasound to determine position of the fetal head and spine (Ghi et al., 2018). When the probe is placed in the suprapubic region, fetal orbits will be visible if the fetus is in an OP position (Eggebø & Hjartardottir, 2021; Ghi et al., 2018). Ultrasound also can identify asynclitism and poor flexion (Elmore et al., 2020). Spine position is highly predictive of birth position. In one study, when the fetal spine and occiput were both posterior in the first stage of labor, only 14% of cases rotated into an OA position at birth (Svelato et al., 2017).

If ultrasound is not available and the cervix is fully dilated, fetal position can be confirmed by inserting the fingers deeply into the vagina beyond the presenting part and palpating the fetal ear; the pinna points toward the posterior fontanel (Singh, 2019). Use caution to avoid disengaging the fetus. Sometimes reaching for the ear will increase flexion of the head and cause spontaneous rotation to occur (Hart & Walker, 2007).

Managing the OP Labor

Abram Brothers, a prominent New York physician, wrote in 1896 of OP labor, "If discovered early, the case should be left to nature, as spontaneous rotation of the occiput anteriorly will occur in the majority of cases" (Brothers, 1896, p. 98). The same recommendation holds true today: most OP babies rotate and proceed without incident. When labor is progressing and the fetal heart pattern is reassuring, watchful waiting and supportive care are the best strategy for managing a client with an OP labor (Argani & Satin, 2022).

Encourage the mother to ambulate and adopt positions and pursue activities that can encourage fetal rotation. Ensure that the client consumes fluids and nourishment and empties the bladder regularly. If the laboring client becomes exhausted during the latent phase of labor and nonpharmacological treatments are ineffective, consider facilitating therapeutic rest with medications such as diphenhydramine, doxylamine, or zolpidem (Hunter, 2015). Another regimen for therapeutic rest is morphine sulfate with promethazine, which reduces the need for subsequent induction of labor, increases client satisfaction, and does not increase the risk of poor perinatal outcomes (Maykin, Ukoha, Tilp, Gaw, & Lewkowitz, 2021).

Intact membranes give the fetus a pocket of lubricant in which to rotate. When the fetus is in a deflexed OP position, there is a tendency for water to break before labor, wedging the fetus in an undesirable position that can be difficult to change. While routine amniotomy is not recommended, in the setting of prolonged or delayed active-phase labor, artificial rupture of membranes can increase local prostaglandin levels and can increase the strength and frequency of uterine contractions (Mohammed & El-Chaâr, 2023b). Stronger contractions can facilitate rotation, flexion, and descent of the fetus.

Maternal Position Changes

A 2018 hospital-based study demonstrated that 50.8% of OP fetuses rotate to occiput anterior in labor if the mother is in a modified Sims' position lying with the fetal back toward the bed for at least 40 min/hr (Bueno-Lopez et al., 2018). Rotation occurred in only 21.7% of a random group allowed to choose other positions (Bueno-Lopez et al., 2018). About 85% of the Sims' group had vaginal births, but only 68.3% of the free-movement group did so (Bueno-Lopez et al., 2018).

Books such as *The Labor Progress Handbook* (Simkin et al., 2017) and *Optimal Foetal Positioning* (Sutton & Scott, 1996) and programs such as Spinning Babies®, developed by Gail Tully (https://spinningbabies.com) are in widespread use by midwives to alter pelvic dimensions, improve fetal position, and encourage effective labor. In 2021, a Miami hospital implemented Spinning Babies® training for nurses and physicians and reduced its cesarean section rate from 45.6% to 31.5% over a 6-month period (Barrera & Acosta, 2022). Limited evidence suggests that position changes and maternal activity can reduce the incidence of persistent OP position (Elmore et al., 2020; Liu, Chen, Yang, & Zhu, 2018). Other studies, however, show no benefit (Desbriere et al., 2013; Gupta, Sood, Hofmeyr, & Vogel, 2017; Le Ray et al., 2016; Lee, Munro, Oliver, & Flynn, 2021; Levy, Weingarten, Ali, Quist-Nelson, & Berghella, 2021; Mercier & Kwan, 2018; Mirzakhani, Karimi, Mohamadzadeh Vatanchi, Feroz Zaidi, & Mirzaei Najmabadi, 2020).

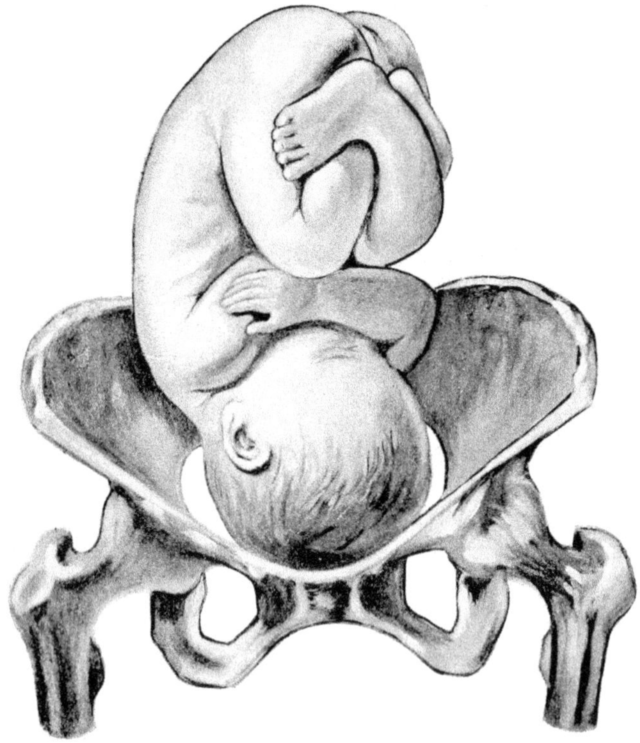

Figure 11-10. Right occiput posterior (ROP). The lie is vertical; the head is at or in the pelvis, the fetal back is in the right maternal flank, small parts are felt easily on the left maternal abdomen, the breech is in the fundus, and the cephalic prominence is on the left. From *The Principles and Practice of Obstetrics* (p. 175, fig. 199), by J. B. De Lee, 1914, Philadelphia, PA: W. B. Saunders. In the public domain.

Angelina Martinez Miranda, Naolí Vinaver, CPM, and Doña Irene Sotelo brought the traditional use of the rebozo (a multipurpose woven shawl common throughout Mexico) to midwives around the world through workshops and publication (Cohen & Thomas, 2015). Rebozo techniques for correcting fetal position involve draping the cloth around the mother's pelvis and using rocking movements from different angles to relax the pelvic musculature and ligaments, allowing the fetus greater freedom to complete the cardinal movements of birth (Cohen & Thomas, 2015). Rebozo techniques also decrease maternal pain and anxiety and enhance maternal satisfaction in labor (Mahmoud Mahmoud Saadoon, Yousif, & Fouad Mohammed, 2023).

Maternal positions such as knee-chest, lunging, hands-and-knees, kneeling, side-lying, squatting, pelvic rocking, or asymmetrical sitting have been used to correct persistent OP or asynclitic fetal positions (Elmore et al., 2020). Props such as bed stirrups, side tables, pillows, and peanut-shaped balls can promote relaxation of the pelvic floor, increase pelvic diameter,

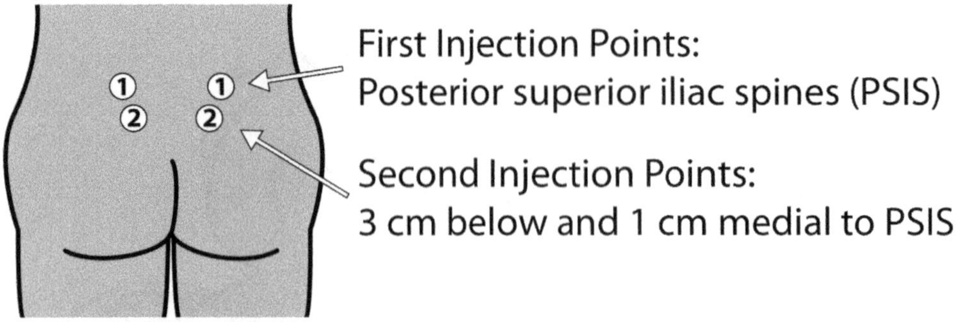

Figure 11-11. Sterile water injection sites for pain management. The standard technique involves injecting 0.1–0.3 ml of sterile water into four points surrounding the Michaelis rhomboid (Lee, Gao, et al., 2020). Intradermal and subcutaneous (SC) administrations appear equally effective (Almassinokiani et al., 2020). Two injections are given over the posterior-superior iliac spines, and two are given approximately 3 cm below and 1 cm medial to the posterior-superior iliac spines (Lee, Gao, et al., 2020). The injections cause blebs to form, ideally 3–4 mm in diameter (Lee, Gao, et al., 2020). Pain relief can last 10–180 min (NICE, 2023). Image adapted from "Impact on Caesarean Section Rates Following Injections of Sterile Water (ICARIS): A Multicentre Randomised Controlled Trial," by N. Lee et al., 2013, *BMC Pregnancy and Childbirth 13*, 105 (fig. 3). CC BY 2.0.

and encourage fetal rotation (Elmore et al., 2020). The double hip squeeze involves applying pressure to the anterior iliac crests with the intention of expanding the pelvic passage. Arching the back can make the fetus uncomfortable and encourage rotation (Leeman, 2020). If the abdomen is pendulous, the mother can hug it and lift, encouraging the long axis of the fetus to align with the pelvic inlet, relieving back pain, and possibly facilitating fetal rotation. Walcher's position, used historically to open the pelvis and promote rotation and descent, appears to benefit some people, but its effectiveness has not been formally studied. Walcher's position involves positioning the laboring client on the edge of the bed and dangling the legs so their weight can encourage the symphysis to open (Tully, 2016). It has also been achieved by placing the client supine with hips elevated on a stack of cushions (Kosmin, 2018).

Heat applied to the back, warm water immersion, and firm lower back massage can bring comfort and relaxation (Chapman & Charles, 2018). Intradermal or subcutaneous (SC) sterile water injections have been shown to be effective for management of low back pain in labor. The technique typically reduces pain by 30–50% without risk of adverse effects beyond brief but significant pain at the site of injection (Lee, Gao, et al., 2020). Sterile water injections appear to reduce pain by gating; that is, the pain of the injection overwhelms the pain referred there from the nerve plexus and viscera. Although Hutton, Kasperink, Rutten, Reitsma, and Wainman (2009) found that sterile water injections reduced the incidence of cesarean birth, others have found no such association (Derry, Straube, Moore, Hancock, & Collins, 2012; Lee, Gao, et al., 2020; National Institute for Health and Care Excellence [NICE], 2023).

Regardless of efficacy, the use of maternal position changes, ambulation, and other activities can enhance the mother's perception of control and participation. If the fetus moves into a more favorable position and is born vaginally, the mother can feel a sense of accomplishment and self-sufficiency. If the malposition persists and the use of a vacuum device, forceps, or cesarean section is necessary to accomplish the birth, the mother is likely to accept the need for intervention, knowing that other strategies were attempted and ultimately unsuccessful.

Manual and Digital Rotation of OP Fetus

Manual or digital rotation from the OP position to OA in the second stage of labor shortens labor and improves the rate of spontaneous birth (Barth, 2015; Bertholdt, Morel, Zuily, & Ambroise-Grandjean, 2022; Bertholdt, Piffer, Pol, Morel, & Guerby, 2021; Blanc et al., 2021; Broberg & Caughey, 2021; Elmore et al., 2020; Habek, Marton, Prka, & Luetić, 2017; Leeman, 2020; Masturzo et al., 2017; Os & Severinsson, 2017). The idea is to enhance the forces that naturally cause the fetus to flex and rotate (Leeman, 2020). To digitally rotate a fetus, insert your fingers to apply rotational force. In manual rotation, your whole hand grasps the fetal head.

ACOG and SMFM strongly recommend that providers consider manual rotation of the fetal head in the second stage of labor before moving to assisted vaginal birth or cesarean section (Blanc et al., 2021). There is good evidence for this recommendation. In one study, clients undergoing manual rotation were more likely to have a shorter second stage, were less likely to require operative delivery, and had babies with higher Apgar scores at 5 min (Blanc et al., 2021). In another study, manual rotation decreased cesareans from 79.4% to 10.2% in nulliparous clients; decreased cesareans in multiparous clients from 48.8% to 2.0%; decreased the rate of assisted vaginal births; and decreased the incidence of chorioamnionitis, endometritis, and 3rd- or 4th-degree perineal lacerations (Niu, Lee, Sharshiner, & Caughey, 2015). Conversely, in other research, the rate of successful rotation was 68%, but manual rotation did not decrease the rate of operative vaginal delivery or the rate of cesarean section (Verhaeghe et al., 2021). In hospital-based studies, the rate of successful rotation is higher for clients less than age 35,

For manual rotation, use your right hand for left positions and your left hand for right positions.

those who have previously given birth to two or more babies, and those with a body mass index (BMI) less than 28 kg/m^2 at the time of birth (Elmore et al., 2020). Manual rotation appears most effective when used on clients in spontaneous labor after fetal engagement (Elmore et al., 2020). There are no data on the use of manual rotation in community settings.

Advanced maneuvers such as digital or manual rotation should be attempted only by trained, experienced clinicians where local standards, protocols, and laws allow (Os & Severinsson, 2017). Midwives practicing in community settings or locations far from a hospital should weigh the benefits of hospital transfer before attempting manual rotation (Elmore et al., 2020). The manual rotation procedure can be very painful for the mother. Analgesia or epidural anesthesia can increase muscle relaxation and maternal comfort during the procedure. Ultrasound imaging, which is readily available in hospitals, can confirm the position of the fetal spine and occiput and help determine the direction of rotation in direct OP positions (Barth, 2015; Elmore et al., 2020).

Although lack of data makes the degree of risk unclear, digital and manual rotation appear to be reasonably safe and pose minimal risk of maternal or fetal injury (Elmore et al., 2020; Leeman, 2020). To obtain informed consent, discuss with the client the potential for maternal discomfort, fetal injury, and failure to accomplish rotation (Elmore et al., 2020). Abnormal fetal heart rate patterns due to cord compression can occur when the fetus is wrapped in or pressing on the umbilical cord. Cord prolapse is possible if the fetus is accidentally disengaged and more likely if there is polyhydramnios or a long cord. Discuss with the mother that if these complications occur in a community setting, delays in reaching definitive care could contribute to poor outcomes. Attempting manual rotation before full dilation may increase the incidence of cord prolapse, cervical lacerations, and abnormal fetal heart rate (FHR) patterns (Barth, 2015). Contraindications to digital and manual rotation include cord prolapse, abnormal bleeding, suspected fetopelvic disproportion, scarred uterus, fetal malformations, fetal blood coagulation abnormalities, abnormal FHR pattern, presentation of brow or face, suspected intrauterine infection, and concerns for maternal instability (Elmore et al., 2020).

Manual Rotation

Begin by confirming fetal position. Manual rotation is sometimes more successful when the procedure is performed with the fetal head at a higher station rather than wedged deeply into the pelvis (Broberg & Caughey, 2021). Ensure the

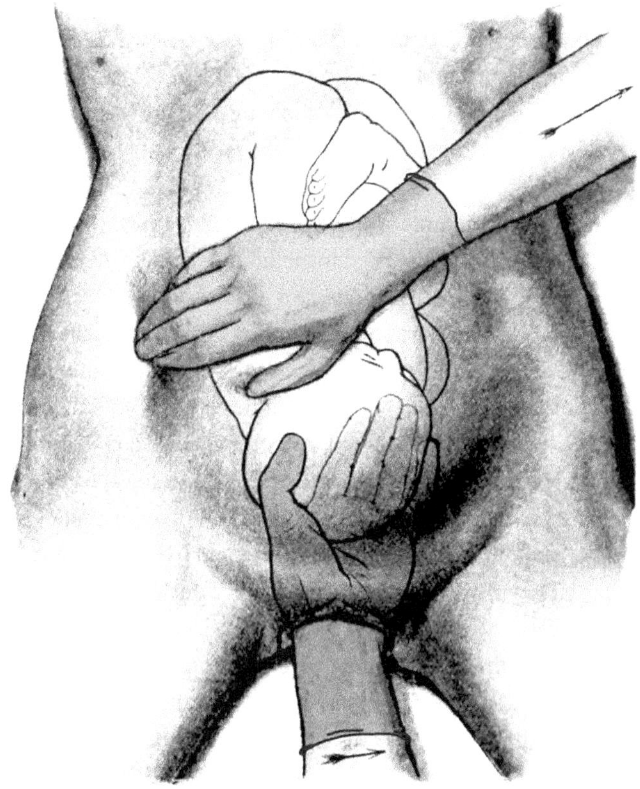

Figure 11-12. Manual rotation of the fetus from OP to OA is frequently performed by the same technique in favor more than a century ago. Adapted from *Operative Midwifery* (2nd ed., p. 30, fig. 15), by J. M. Munro Kerr, 1911, New York, NY: W. Wood. In the public domain.

cervix is completely dilated. Offer medication for pain management and relaxation where protocols allow. There are limited data about optimal positioning for manual or digital rotation; most research places the client in the lithotomy position (Barth, 2015; Blanc et al., 2021; Le Ray et al., 2016), although the procedure may be performed with the client in the lateral Sims' position or on hands and knees (Leeman, 2020). Monitor the FHR continuously throughout the procedure by whatever means is available. If decelerations or bradycardia occurs, stop immediately and initiate intrauterine resuscitation by placing the mother in whatever position most improves FHR and giving intravenous (IV) fluids.

For manual rotation from LOP in a dorsal position,

- Ensure the bladder is empty.
- Position the mother on hands and knees, side-lying, or in lithotomy position.
- Begin the process of rotation between contractions.
- Place your sterile, gloved right hand in the vagina, palm up, and spread four fingers evenly across the left side of the fetal occiput (Barth, 2015). The thumb may be placed on the opposite side of the head. Alternatively, you may grasp the occiput with the fingers over one ear and the thumb

over the other (Hart & Walker, 2007). Another approach is to place your hand in the posterior pelvis and cup the head in your palm like a baseball, applying pressure to create flexion. No study has compared the risks, benefits, or effectiveness of these techniques (Elmore et al., 2020).

- Carefully apply intermittent mild upward pressure to slightly displace the head to facilitate turning. CAUTION! Elevating the head can release a gush of fluid and cause the umbilical cord to prolapse (Yang et al., 2020). Upward pressure is risky in many clinical circumstances, such as a poorly engaged head or polyhydramnios.
- Ask the client to push with a contraction as you flex the fetal head and rotate the face toward the hollow of the sacrum with a counterclockwise motion like turning a doorknob. Your right hand will pronate (the movement used for closing a book). The mother's push should bring the baby down onto your hand and follow the natural mechanism for flexion and rotation along the short arc.
- Your left hand (or the hands of an assistant) is placed on the abdomen to guide the right fetal shoulder from the maternal left to right side to follow the rotation of the head (Leeman, 2020).
- If gentle force is ineffective, consider increasing flexion of the head to decrease the diameter (Barth, 2015). **Do not disengage the head from the pelvis.**
- Hold the fetal occiput in the OA position for several more contractions to reduce the risk of reverting to OP (Argani & Satin, 2022; Graham et al., 2014).

For manual rotations from right OP, perform the maneuver with your opposite hand and turn the fetus in the clockwise direction along the long arc.

Digital Rotation

Place the index and middle fingers of your hand over the occipital bone and your thumb over the parietal bone. Flex the head and use your index and middle fingers to rotate the head along the short arc (the direction requiring the least rotation) toward the occiput anterior (OA) position (Elmore et al., 2020). Alternatively, you can insert your index and middle fingers into the posterior fornix and place your fingertips into the lambdoid suture near the posterior fontanel (Barth, 2015). Use finger pressure to encourage flexion and rotate the head with a clockwise or counterclockwise movement while the mother pushes. Digital rotation is successful if the fetal occiput moves to OA within 45° of the midline (Graham et al., 2014). Remain in position and repeat the maneuver over three successive contractions or until the fetus remains in an OA position. If you are unsuccessful rotating the fetus in this direction, you may try encouraging rotation on the long arc (Broberg & Caughey, 2021).

Occiput Transverse (OT)

When a fetus is in an occiput transverse position, the occiput is oriented halfway between the sacral promontory and the pubic symphysis. On abdominal examination, the fetal back is palpated to the right or the left, toward the mother's flank. The small parts are felt on the opposite side of the back. The fetal buttocks are in the fundus. The fetal heart is loudest in the lower maternal abdomen. On digital vaginal examination, the fetal sagittal suture and fontanels are felt in the transverse diameter of the pelvis. When the posterior fontanel is on the mother's left side, the fetus is LOT; when the posterior fontanel is on the mother's right side, the fetus is ROT. If the head is flexed, the occiput is lower than the brow. On deep palpation, if one fetal ear is palpated underneath the pubic symphysis at 12 o'clock and another is palpable at 6 o'clock, the fetus is OT.

In a normal labor, the fetal head reaches 0 station in the transverse diameter (facing the side), then turns into the oblique to negotiate the midpelvis (Tully, 2020). About 80% of fetuses in the OT position rotate anteriorly to the occiput anterior position, about 10–15% rotate posteriorly to the OP position, and the rest remain OT (Caughey, 2023). If contractions or maternal pushing efforts are inadequate or if the pelvis is narrow front to back, the fetus may be unable to rotate (Caughey, 2023).

Persistent OT position is one that has continued 1 hr or longer in the second stage of labor (Caughey, 2023). All fetuses but the very smallest must rotate the head to an anteroposterior orientation before birth can occur. Transverse arrest occurs when the fetus is locked into the pelvis in an OT position and can go no farther (Caughey, 2023).

Management of Occiput Transverse

Manage persistent OT expectantly if FHT remain reassuring and the fetus continues to descend. In some cases, it is necessary to transfer the client to a hospital to augment ineffective contractions with oxytocin. Manual rotation can be performed by the trained provider during second-stage labor with the same technique used to rotate the OP fetus: nudging the fetus to a slightly higher station, flexing the head, and turning the fetal face toward the sacrum (Caughey, 2023). A hand on the abdomen gently encourages the fetal body to follow the rotation of the head (see above). One study, however, showed that planned prophylactic manual rotation of the OT fetus did not result in fewer operative births (De Vries et al., 2021).

In a hospital, a physician with sufficient expertise may use forceps to rotate the fetal head. Although the provider should not apply rotational forces with a vacuum extraction device, often the fetus rotates spontaneously with the downward/outward force that the device exerts (Caughey, 2023). If these

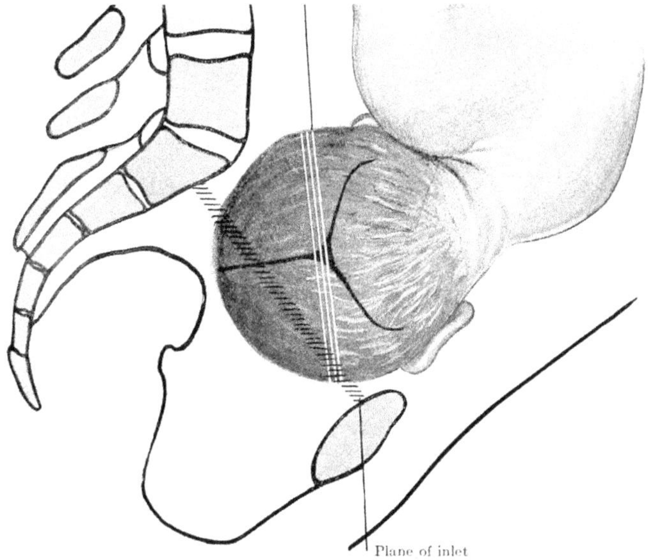

Figure 11-13. Anterior asynclitism occurs in a ROT fetus when the left fetal parietal bone enters the pelvis first, placing the sagittal suture nearer the sacral promontory than the pubic symphysis. From *The Principles and Practice of Obstetrics* (p. 182, fig. 207), by J. B. De Lee, 1914, Philadelphia, PA: W. B. Saunders. In the public domain.

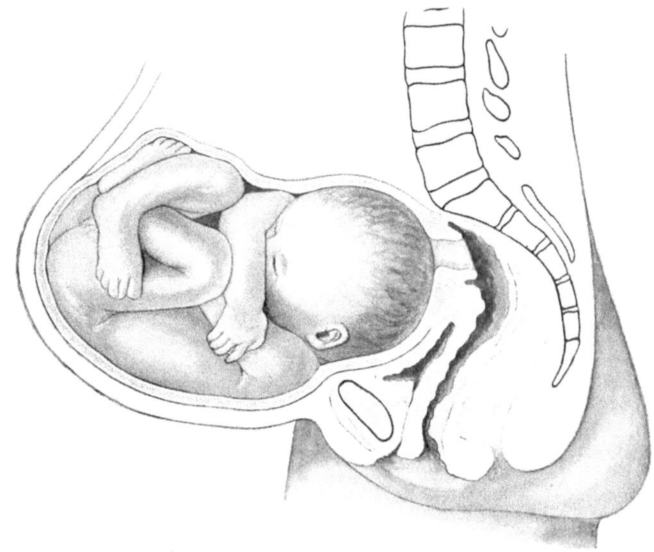

Figure 11-14. Malpresentation commonly occurs in mothers with pendulous abdomens. Poor maternal muscle tone, common in grand multiparas, causes the uterus to lie on a horizontal plane at right angles to the pelvic inlet. In this situation, labor contractions tend to drive the fetus into the sacrum rather than through the pelvic inlet. Lifting and supporting the abdomen with a pregnancy belt, a tied sheet, a rebozo, or the hands can encourage the fetus into a more vertical orientation. From *The Principles and Practice of Obstetrics* (p. 399, fig. 353), by J. B. De Lee, 1914, Philadelphia, PA: W. B. Saunders. In the public domain.

interventions are unsuccessful and vaginal birth is not possible, cesarean section is necessary.

Asynclitism

Asynclitism is an oblique malpresentation of the fetal head in labor. It occurs when either fetal parietal bone approaches the pelvic inlet ahead of the sagittal suture (Malvasi et al., 2015). The fetal occiput usually points to the maternal right or left. When the sagittal suture lies close to the sacral promontory, the examiner can palpate more of the anterior parietal bone and the condition is recognized as anterior asynclitism (Cunningham et al., 2022, ch. 22). Conversely, if the sagittal suture approaches the symphysis, more of the posterior parietal bone will be palpable and the condition is termed posterior asynclitism (Cunningham et al., 2022, ch. 22). With severe asynclitism, the ear may be palpable (Cunningham et al., 2022, ch. 22).

Ideally, the abdominal wall holds the pregnant uterus upright and encourages a vertical fetal lie at the onset of labor (Posner, 2023). A fetus, however, is seldom perfectly vertical when it enters the pelvis, and the maternal pelvis is often slightly crooked or tilted (Malvasi et al., 2015). Most fetuses start labor in an asynclitic OT or OA position (Malvasi et al., 2015). As labor progresses, the head straightens, and the sagittal suture becomes more centered.

A pendulous maternal abdomen can allow the fetus to lie nearly perpendicular to the pelvic inlet. In this situation, the fetus is most likely to enter the pelvis in anterior asynclitism. Instead of driving descent of the fetus, each contraction may propel the fetus into the opposite wall of the pelvic inlet or even upward and backward. Labor may fail to progress if the head abuts the bony walls and cannot advance.

Belly lifts or an abdominal binder can elevate the asynclitic fetus into a more vertical orientation and allow entry into the pelvis (Simkin et al., 2017). Pelvic rocking in forward-leaning positions, lunges, and rebozo techniques may encourage the process (Simkin et al., 2017). The Spinning Babies® program recommends managing asynclitism by performing side-lying releases (slow stretch to relax key pelvic musculature) on both sides of the mother's body, having the mother kneel and lean over a birth ball, side lunging, or resting with a peanut ball between the legs or ankles (Tully, 2020). If asynclitism is still present when the fetus is at a low station, it may prevent normal internal rotation and slow or stop labor. In this event, manual repositioning of the head to a synclitic orientation may facilitate vaginal birth. Persistent asynclitism sometimes necessitates the use of forceps, vacuum, or cesarean section (Habek et al., 2017).

Face Presentation

Face presentation occurs when the fetal face from forehead to mentum (chin) is the first part to enter the pelvis. Face presentation occurs in about 1 in 600–800 term singleton

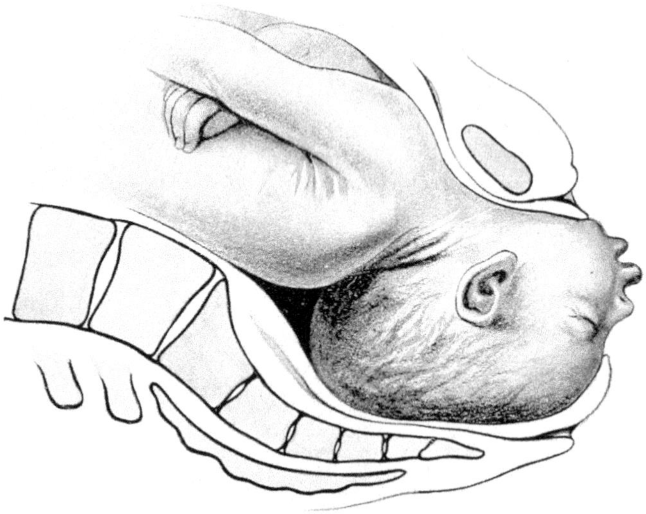

Figure 11-15. Mentum anterior face presentation. When the chin is anterior, the fetal neck pivots over the pubic bone, making room to clear the occiput. From *The Principles and Practice of Obstetrics* (p. 595, fig. 522), by J. B. De Lee, 1914, Philadelphia, PA: W. B. Saunders. In the public domain.

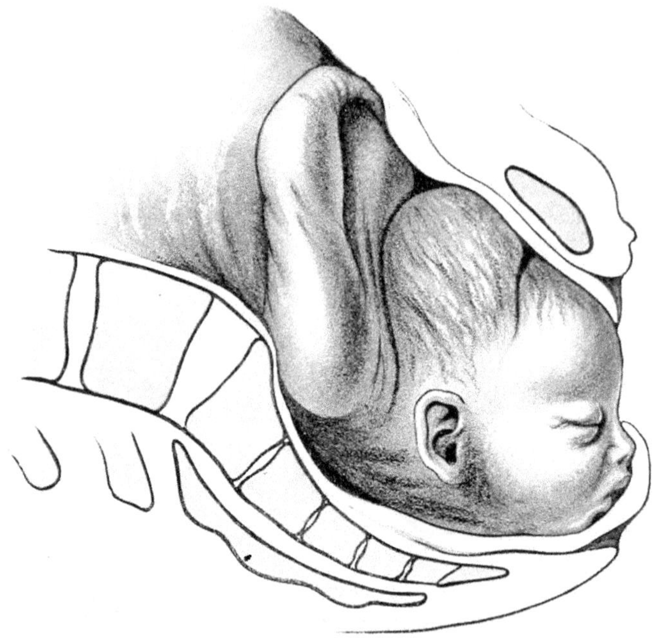

Figure 11-16. Mentum posterior face presentation, If the fetus is mentum posterior, the occiput usually impacts beneath the pubic bone as the fetus descends. The neck elongates until the back of the vertex is against the back, and the head cannot emerge. In this illustration, birth is further complicated by the position of the fetal arm and shoulder. From *The Principles and Practice of Obstetrics* (p. 597, fig. 525), by J. B. De Lee, 1914, Philadelphia, PA: W. B. Saunders. In the public domain.

births and is typically undiagnosed until complete dilation (Mohammed & El-Chaâr, 2023a). Approximately 70% of face presentations are mentum anterior or transverse, and about 30% are mentum posterior (Mohammed & El-Chaâr, 2023a). Many fetuses with face presentation begin labor in the brow position. During the process of engagement, the pressure of contractions and resistance from the maternal pelvis causes the fetal neck either to flex or to hyperextend until the occiput touches the back. Internal rotation occurs between the level of the ischial spines and ischial tuberosities, so that the chin is the actual presenting part.

As the face descends onto the perineum in a mentum anterior position, the fetal chin passes under the maternal symphysis pubis, the head is born by flexion and externally rotates, and the shoulders move into the usual position for birth. The rest of the birth proceeds as usual. Occasionally a previously vertex fetus suddenly adopts a face presentation just before birth, surprising the attendant with the crowning of the mouth, nose, and eyes.

Although more than 75% of mentum anterior fetuses can be born vaginally, the mentum posterior face presentation can only pass through the maternal pelvis if spontaneous rotation occurs or the fetus is very small (Julien & Galerneau, 2023). When a fetus descends in the mentum posterior face presentation, the head, neck, and shoulders attempt to enter the pelvis simultaneously. The hyperextended fetal neck is shorter than the maternal sacrum and is unable to extend further to follow the curve of Carus (Chapman & Charles, 2018). If the fetal mouth opens against the sacrum, it prevents further descent (Julien & Galerneau, 2023).

Face presentation is more common in the presence of certain fetal anomalies, including anencephaly, microcephaly, severe hydrocephalus, and anterior neck mass. Other risk factors include multiple nuchal cord loops, macrosomia, cephalopelvic disproportion, prematurity/low birthweight, macrosomia, contracted or platypelloid maternal pelvis, and previous cesarean birth (Julien & Galerneau, 2023). The multiparous client who has a pendulous abdomen or begins labor with an unengaged fetus has a greater risk of face presentation (Julien & Galerneau, 2023). Polyhydramnios can develop when the hyperextended neck constricts the esophagus, limiting fetal swallowing.

Managing Face Presentation

A persistent face presentation can be identified by Leopold's maneuvers. The cephalic prominence can be palpated on the same side as the fetal back with an indentation between them. More than 50% of face presentations are diagnosed on vaginal examination during the second stage of labor (Chapman & Charles, 2018). Upon digital examination, it is usually obvious that the fetus is not vertex; but the actual presentation can be unclear, especially if membranes are intact. Irregular, yielding, bumpy features are present where the midwife usually encounters skull bones and fontanels. Face presentation

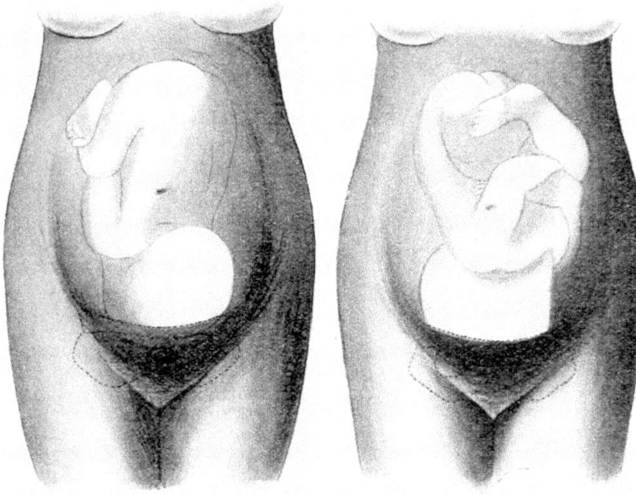

Figure 11-17. Recognizing a face presentation on abdominal examination: the light-colored areas are the firmest parts of the maternal abdomen. From *A Manual of Midwifery for Students and Practitioners* (p. 369), by H. Jellett, 1905, London, United Kingdom: Baillière, Tindall & Cox. In the public domain.

and frank breech can feel very similar on vaginal examination. Providers can mistake a mouth for an anus and malar bones or orbital ridges for fetal ischial tuberosities. In a face presentation, the mouth and orbital ridges form a triangle that can be lightly traced with the examining fingers, a hollow with two bumps above or below. In a frank breech, the ischial tuberosities and anus form a straight line, a hollow with bumps on each side (Hofmeyr, 2023c).

The mother should be transferred to the hospital if the fetus presents with a face in labor. Attempts at manual conversion of the mentum posterior face to a vertex or mentum anterior position are contraindicated and can result in uterine rupture, cord prolapse, or fetal cervical spine trauma (Julien & Galerneau, 2023). If the face presentation is mentum anterior or transverse and there are no other contraindications for vaginal delivery, labor is sometimes allowed to progress in a hospital with continuous fetal monitoring. Severe variable and late decelerations occur in 24–29% of labors in face presentation, and only 14% maintain normal FHR patterns (Julien & Galerneau, 2023).

Babies born in face presentation often have massive facial bruising and swelling. Facial, tracheal, and laryngeal trauma and edema can make ventilation difficult during resuscitation. These newborns often require endotracheal intubation. Swelling usually resolves within the first 24–48 hr after birth.

Brow Presentation

Brow presentation involves a fetal head extended midway between full flexion (vertex) and hyperextension (face). Most brow presentations are frontum anterior. Frontum transverse and frontum posterior positions are more likely to necessitate

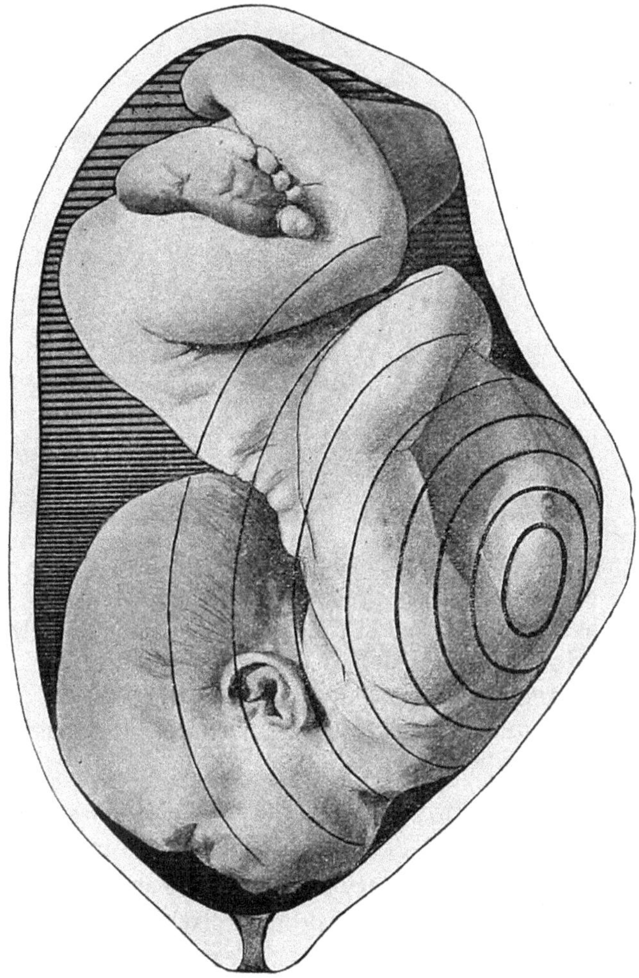

Figure 11-18. Site of the greatest intensity of heart sounds when the head is extended and the mentum is to the left. From *A Manual of Midwifery for Students and Practitioners* (p. 425), by H. Jellett, 1905, London, United Kingdom: Baillière, Tindall & Cox. In the public domain.

cesarean birth. Performing Leopold's maneuvers, you may feel an occipital prominence along the fetal back. On vaginal examination the forehead, anterior fontanel, supraorbital ridges, and bridge of the nose are palpable. The mouth, chin, and sagittal suture are out of reach. The presenting part can be very high and feel unusually large (Chapman & Charles, 2018).

Labor with a brow presentation is arduous, long, painful, and usually unsuccessful in achieving vaginal birth. If internal rotation does not occur, the mentoparietal diameter (typically measuring 13.5 cm) must pass through the pelvic inlet. Severe lacerations high into the vaginal fornices or into the rectum often accompany the birth of a fetus in brow presentation (Mohammed & El-Chaâr, 2023a).

Managing Brow Presentation

Some fetuses spontaneously convert to a face (30%) or OP (20%) presentation. Conversion to occiput anterior is

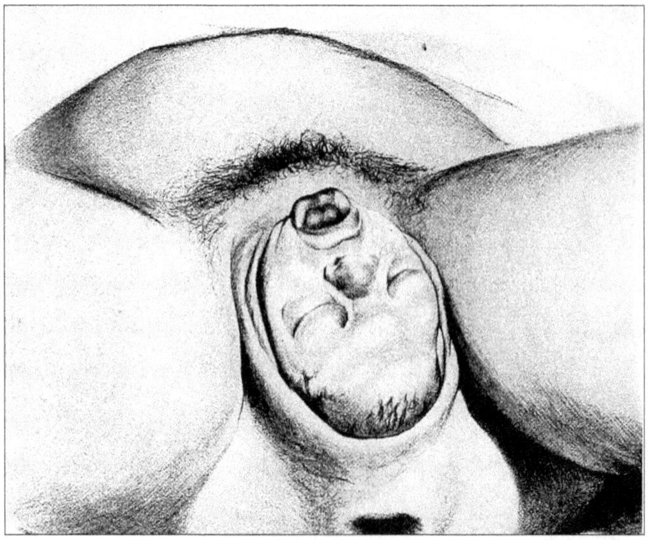

Figure 11-19. Face presentation on the perineum. A fetus in face presentation must negotiate the birth canal using its face as a dilating wedge. As a result, the face is often severely bruised and swollen at birth. From *Operative Obstetrics, Including the Surgery of the Newborn* (p. 132) by E. P. Davis, 1911, Philadelphia, PA: W. B. Saunders. In the public domain.

rare (Julien & Galerneau, 2023). The pelvic press during the second stage of labor and upright or squatting positions can improve the chance of vaginal birth (Chapman & Charles, 2018). Cephalopelvic disproportion is likely, and successful vaginal birth is possible only if the pelvis is roomy, the infant is small, and/or the infant is a macerated stillborn. Persistent brow presentation with obstructed labor is an indication for cesarean section.

Compound Presentation and Nuchal Arm

Compound presentation occurs when one or more fetal extremities are alongside the presenting part of the fetus. Most commonly, compound presentation involves a hand or arm alongside the fetal head. Compound presentations are more likely with any condition that prevents the fetus from completely filling the pelvic inlet with the presenting part, including prelabor rupture of membranes (PROM); induction of labor with an unengaged fetus; preterm labor; polyhydramnios; multiparity; contracted pelvis; pelvic masses; pendulous maternal abdomen; or multiple pregnancy (Mohammed & Tawagi, 2023). Obvious compound presentations, in which the hand is palpable alongside the head before birth, occur in about one of 500–1,000 births (Mohammed & Tawagi, 2023). An unknown number of others, undetected by digital examination in labor, correct spontaneously (Mohammed & Tawagi, 2023).

In a compound presentation, you can distinguish a hand from a foot by palpation: toes are all the same length, the big toe is not opposable, the foot is at right angles to the leg, and

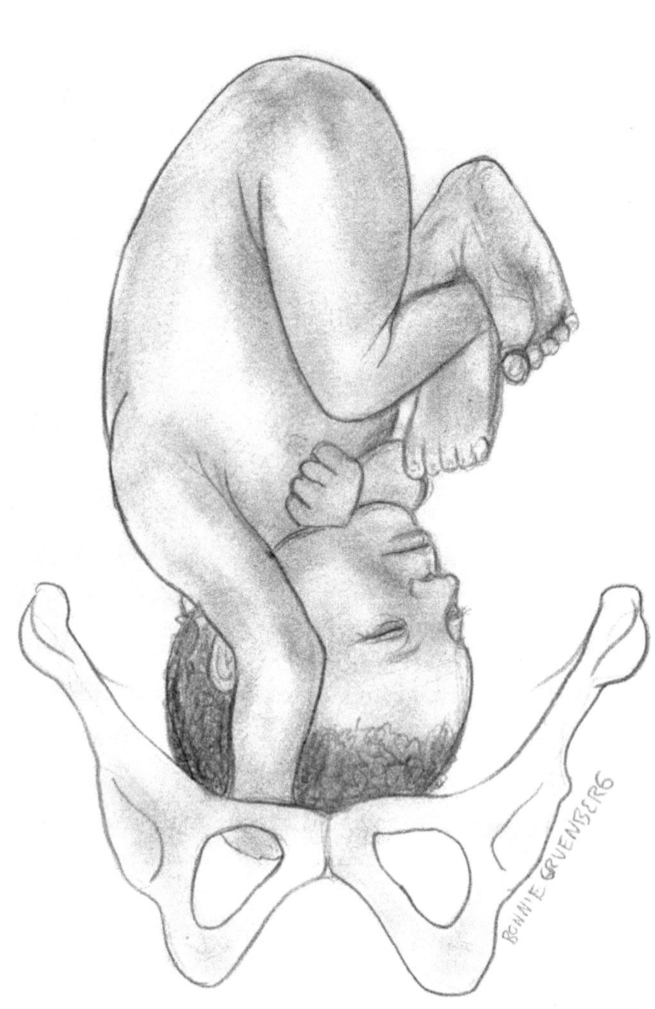

Figure 11-20. Compound presentation most commonly involves a hand or arm alongside the head.

the heel is prominent (Marshall & Raynor, 2014). A hand presentation occurs when the hand is the presenting fetal part, sometimes well ahead of the head. Occasionally, a fetal hand will grasp the examining fingers.

DIFFERENTIAL DIAGNOSES

Transverse lie with prolapsed arm or footling breech among others.

Managing Compound Presentation

Consider the possibility of compound presentation when the fetal head fails to engage or remains deviated from the midline in active labor, or with any arrest of labor in the active phase (Barth, 2021). A hand may be felt near the top of the fetal head, and fingers are sometimes palpated. Labor with a compound presentation is often long and difficult. Progress can stall or stop during the active phase or during pushing when the fetal hand becomes trapped between the head and the maternal sacrum (Barth, 2023). A compound foot is more likely to obstruct labor and is more commonly seen with preterm births (PTBs). Oxytocin augmentation is not recommended for obstructed labor because of the risk for uterine rupture (Barth, 2023).

Most sources agree that vaginal birth of a compound presentation involves some risk to mother and fetus. For this reason, transfer to the hospital may be advised for the client laboring in a community setting. The most common complication of compound and limb presentations is cord prolapse, which occurs in as many as 15–23% of cases (Barth, 2023; Mohammed & Tawagi, 2023). A limb trapped beside the head can (rarely) suffer irreversible circulatory compromise or become traumatized during birth (Kwok, Judkins, & Sherratt, 2015; Martinovski, Wilseck, & Mattson, 2015). Compound presentations can also cause extensive maternal lacerations. Even so, a large recent study concluded that compound presentation does not increase the risk of any major adverse obstetric or neonatal outcome (Haizler-Cohen et al., 2023).

If labor progresses normally, intervention is usually unnecessary for the vertex fetus with a compound hand (Cunningham et al., 2022, ch. 22; Mohammed & Tawagi, 2023). The fetus will often retract the limb as labor continues (Cunningham et al., 2022, ch. 22; Mohammed & Tawagi, 2023). Some providers gently pinch the fetal fingers between contractions to encourage retraction (Cunningham et al., 2022, ch. 22; Mohammed & Tawagi, 2023). Maternal position changes sometimes improve fetal positioning. Do not manipulate or attempt to manually reposition the prolapsed extremity (Barth, 2021). Seventy-five percent of fetuses with compound presentations involving the vertex and an upper extremity are born spontaneously (Barth, 2021). If the umbilical cord prolapses, a nonreassuring FHR pattern develops, or labor does not progress, a cesarean section might be required (Barth, 2021). Cesarean birth is also recommended for compound presentations involving fetal parts other than the vertex and a compound arm or hand (Barth, 2021).

Nuchal Arm

A nuchal arm is one draped around or alongside the neck with the hand at the nape or at the contralateral shoulder. Less commonly, the arm drapes around the posterior neck. Nuchal hands can present at the neck or cheek. Most fetuses that descend with a hand at the cheek, ear, or neck are born vaginally without any complications. Uncontrolled extension of the nuchal arm at birth can allow the sharp fetal elbow to cause a vaginal or perineal laceration.

Noncephalic Malpresentations

Gravity, fetal comfort, and the size and shape of the uterine cavity and pelvis greatly influence fetal lie (Strauss & Herrera, 2023). Noncephalic presentations are common early in

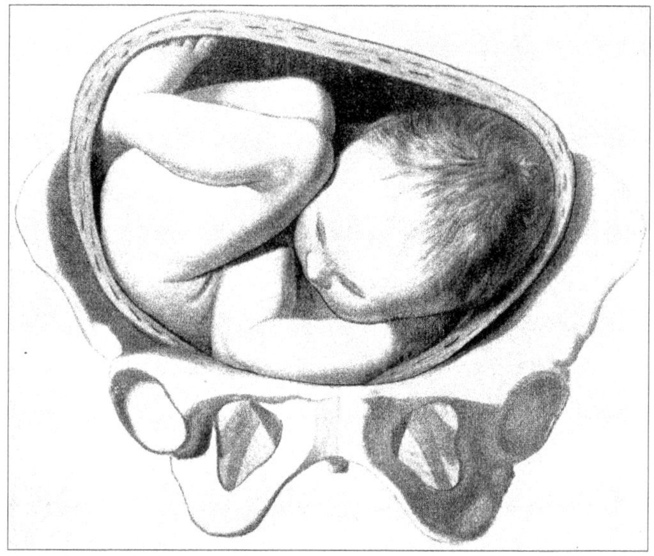

Figure 11-21. Transverse lie, back down. From *A Text-Book of Obstetrics* (7th ed., p. 285, fig. 237), by B. C. Hirst, 1912, Philadelphia, PA: W. B. Saunders. In the public domain.

pregnancy when the fetus has a comparatively larger pool of fluid in which to maneuver. By later pregnancy, the fetal pole with the greatest mass—the buttocks with flexed thighs—seems more comfortably accommodated in the uterine fundus unless placenta previa, uterine abnormalities, or uterine distension change internal dimensions. A longitudinal lie orients the fetal body axis along the line of gravity and provides greater room for fetal movement (Strauss & Herrera, 2023).

Transverse Lie

Transverse lie occurs when the long axis of the fetus is perpendicular to the long axis of the uterus. The fetal spine may be oriented "back-up" (dorsosuperior), presenting fetal small parts at the cervix, or "back-down" (dorsoinferior), presenting the fetal shoulder. A live fetus in transverse lie cannot be born vaginally, but most convert to a cephalic or breech presentation by the onset of labor (Strauss & Herrera, 2023). In resource-limited countries where ultrasound imaging, cesarean birth, and neonatal intensive care are often inaccessible, transverse lie in labor frequently results in sepsis, hemorrhage, stillbirth, and maternal death (Strauss & Herrera, 2023).

Most transverse lies are associated with premature birth, multiple gestations, placenta previa, contracted pelvis, uterine anomalies or tumors, polyhydramnios, fetal anomalies, or grand multiparity. Sometimes a transverse fetus with ruptured membranes prolapses a limb or its umbilical cord, creating a perinatal emergency. Maternal and perinatal mortality/morbidity with this complication are high in developing countries with limited resources, largely because the malpresented fetus obstructs labor and precipitates uterine rupture.

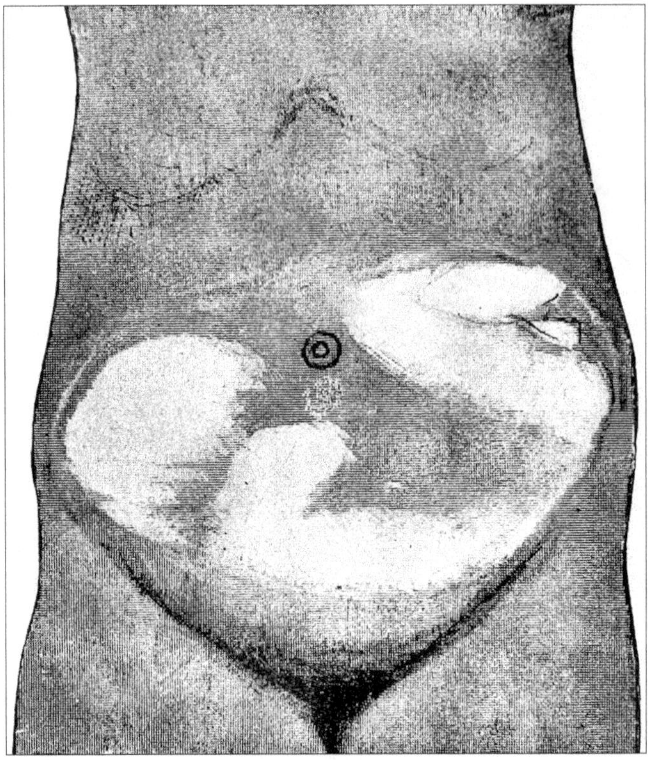

Figure 11-22. Abdominal palpation in transverse lie, back down. The lighter-colored areas represent fetal prominences that feel firmer to palpation. From *A Handbook of Midwifery* (p. 152), by W. R. Dakin, 1897, London, United Kingdom: Longmans, Green, & Co. In the public domain.

At 35–37 weeks of gestation, Leopold's maneuvers are about 70% accurate for distinguishing transverse lie (Strauss & Herrera, 2023). It can be more difficult to determine whether the fetal back is up or down. Fundal height may be lower than expected for gestational age. An ultrasound scan can clarify the exact fetal position and reveal maternal and fetal anatomical deviations influencing the malpresentation. Because the fetus will sometimes lie transverse if the placenta is across the cervix, do not perform a vaginal examination until placenta previa has been excluded.

Management of Transverse Lie

Ultrasound examination is necessary to confirm presentation, and, if not previously imaged during the pregnancy, to exclude major fetal malformation or abnormal placentation (Barth, 2021). The fetus in transverse lie may be turned to either a cephalic presentation via external version under tocolysis or born by cesarean section. After successful version, many fetuses spontaneously revert to transverse or turn to breech. If placenta previa is present, cesarean is necessary.

A transverse, oblique, or unstable lie persisting beyond 37 0/7 weeks of gestation is at risk for cord prolapse if the membranes rupture without a fetal part filling the pelvic inlet (Barth, 2021). Cord prolapse is 20 times more likely with an abnormal lie than it is with a cephalic presentation (Barth, 2021). If you suspect a transverse lie in labor, transport emergently.

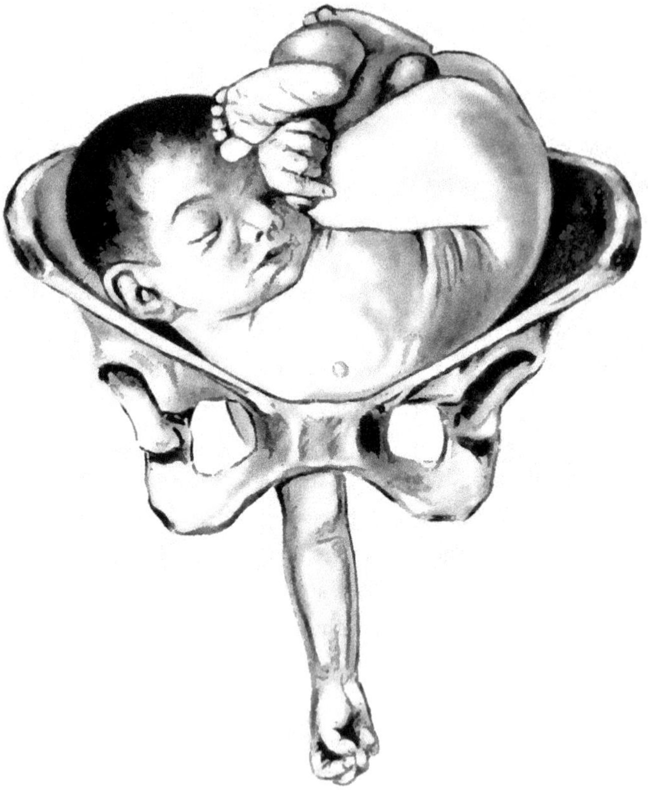

Figure 11-23. A transverse lie with a prolapsed arm is a dire emergency. From *The Principles and Practice of Obstetrics* (p. 617, fig. 546), by J. B. De Lee, 1914, Philadelphia, PA: W. B. Saunders. In the public domain.

Breech Presentation

Breech presentation (buttocks or feet at the cervix) is the most common of the noncephalic malpresentations. Breech presentation is considered normal until late in gestation and becomes a concern only during labor and birth. A fetus with normal anatomy, movement, amniotic fluid volume, and placental location usually orients to a head-down position near the end of pregnancy. Whereas 20–25% of fetuses under 28 weeks of gestation are breech, only 3–4% are breech at term (Hofmeyr, 2023a). About 5% of these term breech fetuses are discovered unexpectedly during labor (Sentilhes et al., 2020). About 25% of fetuses who are breech at 36 weeks of gestation spontaneously turn to cephalic presentation before birth (Hofmeyr, 2023a).

Maternal and fetal conditions that predispose to breech include (Hofmeyr, 2023a)

- Preterm gestation
- Either parent of fetus was term breech presentation
- Prior breech pregnancy
- Uterine abnormality

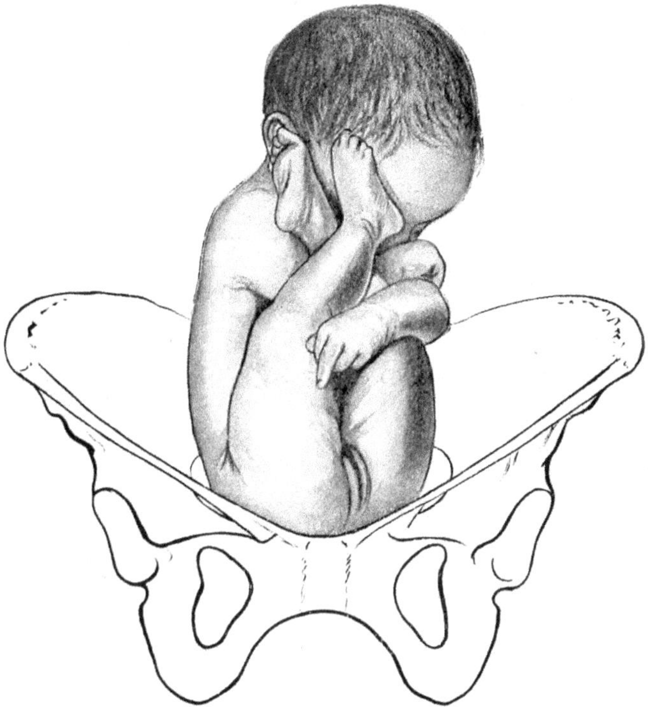

Figure 11-24. Term fetus in frank breech presentation. From *The Principles and Practice of Obstetrics* (p. 604, fig. 534), by J. B. De Lee, 1914, Philadelphia, PA: W. B. Saunders. In the public domain.

- Placenta previa or cornual placenta
- Grand multiparity
- Polyhydramnios or oligohydramnios
- Contracted maternal pelvis
- Fetal anomaly
- Extended fetal legs
- Multiple gestation
- Fetal neurologic impairment
- Maternal hypothyroidism
- Short umbilical cord
- Fetal growth restriction
- Fetal asphyxia
- Primiparity
- Female fetus
- Maternal anticonvulsant therapy
- Advanced maternal age

Frank Breech (50–70%)

With frank breech, the fetal buttocks enter the pelvis first. Hips are flexed, legs extended, and the feet are typically by the fetal head. The extended legs make it difficult for the fetus to somersault to vertex, and often it remains lodged in the frank breech position. Frank breech accounts for about half of all breech presentations and is most favorable for a vaginal birth.

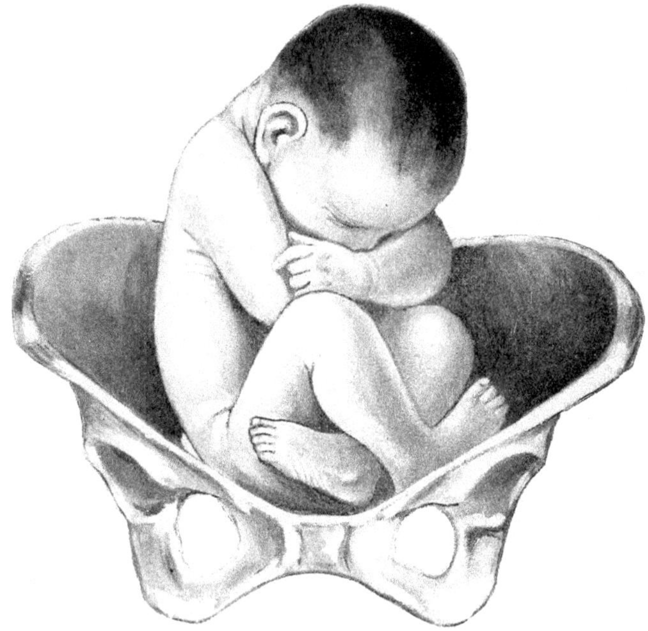

Figure 11-25. Complete breech presentation involves a fetus presenting with buttocks and thighs to the maternal pelvis. From *The Principles and Practice of Obstetrics* (p. 604, fig. 533), by J. B. De Lee, 1914, Philadelphia, PA: W. B. Saunders. In the public domain.

Complete Breech (5–10%)

The fetus in complete breech presentation sits cross-legged on the cervix. Both legs are bent, and the feet and buttocks are closest to the cervix. When compared to frank breech, vaginal birth of complete breech is at higher risk for cord prolapse, obstruction from a wedged leg, and birth asphyxia.

Incomplete Breech (10–40%)

The fetus in incomplete breech presentation has any combination of one or both hips extended. The fetus may present with one or both feet (footling breech), a knee, or (rarely) both knees (kneeling breech). Incomplete breech presentations create high risk for cord prolapse, labor obstruction, and adverse newborn outcomes, and are often considered a contraindication to planned breech vaginal birth.

Complications of Breech Presentation

Regardless of the mode of birth, perinatal morbidity and mortality for term fetuses in breech presentation is higher than for those in cephalic presentation (Sentilhes et al., 2020). The greatest risk occurs when breech presentation is associated with PTB, congenital anomalies, or birth trauma. More than 25% of fetuses presenting breech at birth are preterm (Floyd & Gimovsky, 2021). Vaginal breech birth puts the mother at higher risk for cervical, vaginal, or perineal lacerations. Cesarean birth, however, carries the usual risks associated with surgery and anesthesia and can

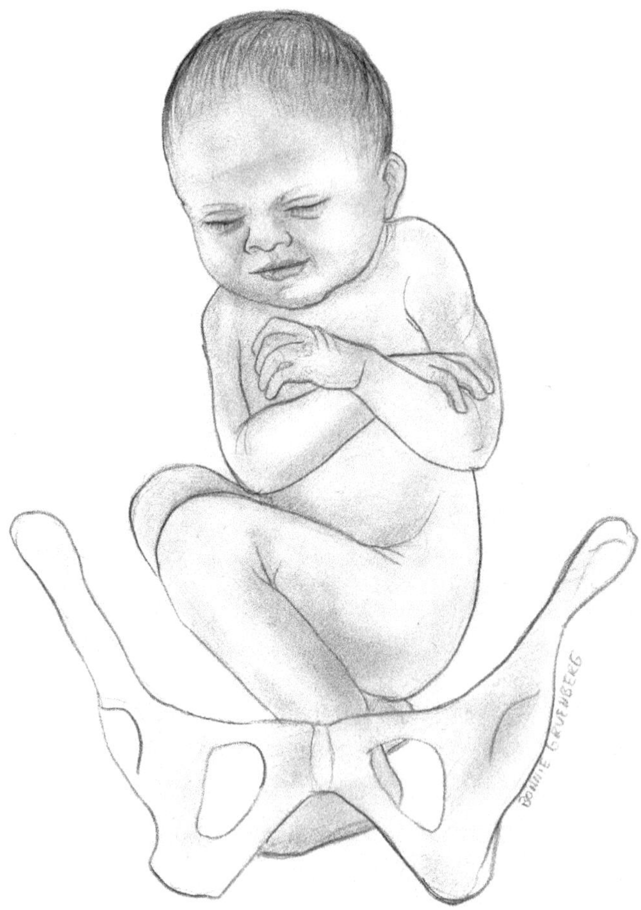

Figure 11-26. The double footling breech is a type of incomplete breech.

increase the risk of hemorrhage, abnormal placentation, and other complications in future pregnancies (Cunningham et al., 2022, ch. 28).

Congenital anomalies. Term fetuses in breech presentation at birth have a rate of congenital anomalies almost twice that of fetuses in cephalic presentation. These issues most commonly involve abnormalities of the hip, the central nervous system, the respiratory system, and the musculoskeletal system (Macharey, Gissler, Toijonen, Heinonen, & Seikku, 2021). Severe or lethal anomalies complicate up to 20% of preterm breech births and as much as 7% of term breech births (Floyd & Gimovsky, 2021).

Birth trauma. Injuries can occur in both vaginal and cesarean birth and most commonly involve fractures of the humerus, clavicle, or femur. The risk of traumatic injuries during vaginal or cesarean birth appears to be less than 1% (Sentilhes et al., 2020). When the fetal head is hyperextended before labor, vaginal breech birth can cause serious injury to the baby's spinal cord (Cunningham et al., 2014, ch. 28). Excessive stretching of the nerve roots from C5 to T1 nerve roots can lead to Erb (neonatal brachial plexus) palsy (Selcen, 2023). Aggressive vaginal examinations or

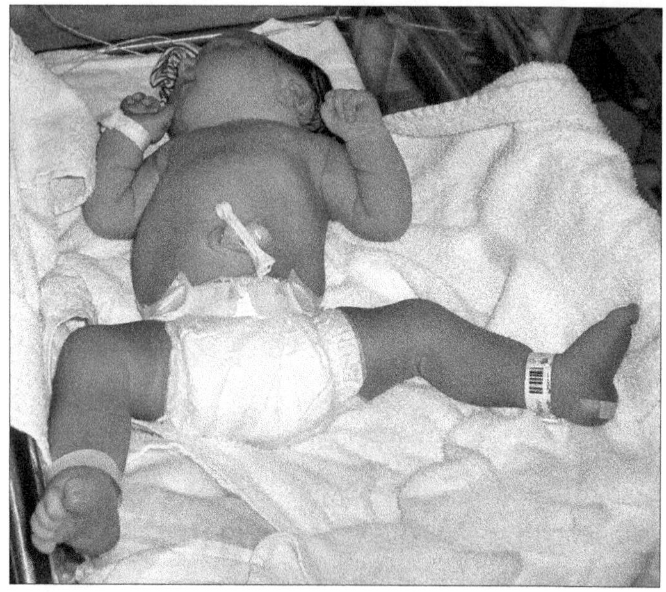

Figure 11-27. Breech birth is the main risk factor for developmental dysplasia of the hip, and the risk is higher in female babies. This baby is demonstrating abnormal abduction of the hips and thighs. Photograph shared with the author by baby's parents, printed with permission.

the pressures of birth can injure fetal testicles. The risk for asphyxia is also higher, especially with a vaginal birth of a nonfrank breech.

Cord prolapse occurs in about 1% of frank breech presentations but in more than 10% of footling breech presentations, because the irregular shapes of the presenting parts create gaps where the cord might fall through (Hofmeyr, 2023a).

Head entrapment occurs when the trunk births but the head remains in the pelvis. Though rare in term breech births, head entrapment can develop in up to 14% of preterm vaginal breech births (Impey, Murphy, Griffiths, & Penna, 2017). Whereas the flexed vertex fetus negotiates the bony pelvic corridor with the smallest and most moldable part of the head foremost, the breech fetus presents the narrow buttocks or lower limbs first, followed by the larger shoulders and the large and unmolded head. If the head cannot fit the pelvis, this fact may not become apparent until the body is born. The head of a preterm fetus is proportionately larger than that of a mature baby. If the body descends into the vagina before the cervix is fully dilated, the aftercoming head can become entrapped within the uterus.

Developmental hip dysplasia affects 2–27% of newborns presenting in the breech position at the end of pregnancy regardless of mode of birth (Shaw & Segal, 2016). The risk is highest for a female baby in a frank breech position. Screening for hip dysplasia at birth and at subsequent well-infant examinations includes performing Barlow and Ortolani tests and noting limb length discrepancy, asymmetric thigh or gluteal folds, and limited or asymmetric abduction (Shaw & Segal, 2016).

Assessing the Breech

The client who is carrying a breech fetus may report symptoms that suggest breech presentation. The kicking of fetal feet felt low in the pelvis can cause suprapubic cramping and bladder irritation. The fetal head can limit the movement of the diaphragm, causing the mother to feel short of breath. A mother with a fetus in breech presentation might report discomfort from something hard beneath her ribs

In breech presentations, the round, hard mass of the fetal head is usually palpable in the fundus. If you ballot it between your hands, it can be felt to move freely and independently from the fetal back. If there are feet in the fundus alongside the head, this rocking movement may be restricted. When the back is anterior and the fetus is well flexed, the head can tuck into the maternal flank and become difficult to palpate (Marshall & Raynor, 2014). Abdominal palpation is less accurate if the client is muscular or has a thick adipose layer.

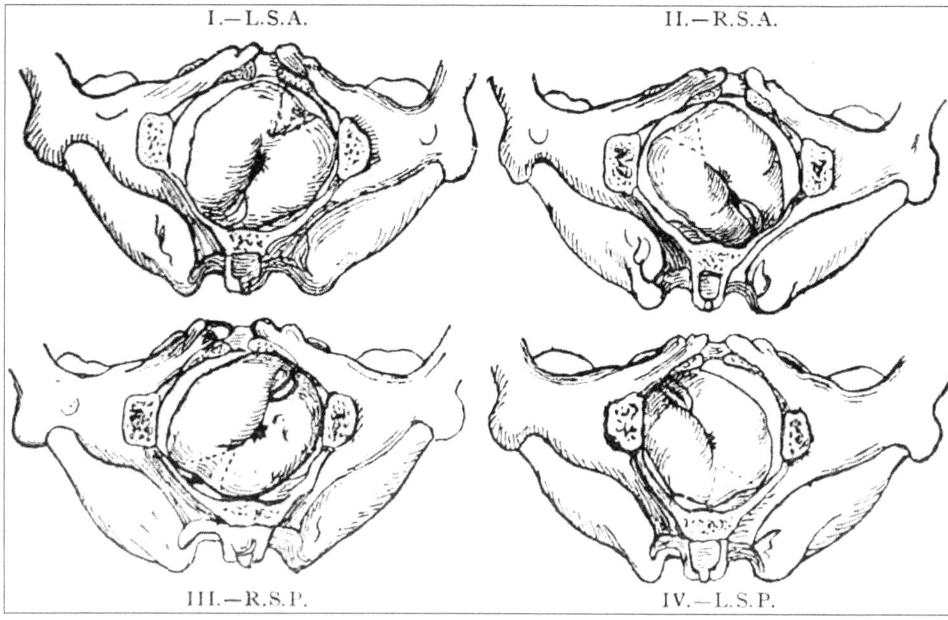

Figure 11-28. Four presentations of frank breech as felt in a vaginal examination. The contour is of two smooth hairless flexible swellings. The cleft between the buttocks leads to the anus, coccyx, and sacrum at one end and the fetal genitals at the other. Sometimes the anus contracts upon encountering the finger, and meconium is present. Illustration I depicts left sacral anterior; II, right sacral anterior; III, right sacral posterior; and IV, left sacral posterior. From *Practical Text-Book of Midwifery for Nurses and Students* (p. 171), by R. Jardine, 1899, New York, NY: Macmillan. In the public domain.

When your fingers trace the presenting part of a frank breech fetus from the suprapubic area along the fetal back to the fundus, you might feel an unbroken plane. The fetal pelvis may be palpated in the lower uterine segment as a tapered, irregular mass. When the fetal hips are balloted, the whole body moves, offering more resistance than when the head is balloted. The breech fetus does not usually engage in the pelvis before labor (Elfazari & El-Chaâr, 2023). An engaged frank breech fetus with head flexed into the maternal flank can be very difficult to distinguish from a well-engaged vertex fetus. With a vertex presentation, you might encounter a groove and hump where the neck joins the shoulders if the head is not deeply engaged.

The heart tones of an unengaged breech fetus can be heard most clearly above the umbilicus on the side of the fetal back. If the client is a multigravida with a pendulous abdomen, however, you may find heart tones above the umbilicus with a vertex fetus. As the fetus descends, heart tones move lower in the abdomen. A fetoscope, which allows direct auscultation of the fetal heart, is more accurate than a Doppler device for localizing the loudest fetal heart sounds.

On vaginal examination, the irregular mass of the breech feels more yielding than a rigid skull. The fit of presenting part to pelvis typically feels asymmetrical, and there are no sutures or fontanels. If the membranes are ruptured, the presenting part feels smooth, whereas the texture of fetal hair is often obvious when the head is presenting. The anus may be palpable as a depression between two bulges. As the fetus descends, it may expel thick, dark meconium into the vagina.

Breech presentation can be easily misidentified as vertex on antepartum and intrapartum examination, even if the provider is experienced. The yielding flesh of buttocks can feel very much like caput. A high station or a bulging bag of waters can impede assessment of the presenting part. The solid sacrum or hip of a frank breech can feel like the parietal bone of an asynclitic fetus on vaginal examination. About 8–10% of breech presentations are not recognized until labor (Ressl & O'Beirne, 2015; Stewart, 2017).

Antepartum sonography should be used to confirm any suspicion of breech presentation. Ultrasound evaluation can provide information such as fetal weight, the presence of fetal or uterine anomalies, umbilical cord length and whether it is wrapped around the fetus, abnormal placentation, and abnormalities of fluid volume. Ultrasound can also identify hyperextension of the fetal head or incomplete breech presentation that would contraindicate vaginal breech birth.

Noninvasive Breech Repositioning Interventions

Clinicians frequently use maternal postural interventions to encourage a breech baby to turn. Evidence is sparse for the efficacy of these interventions, but they are unlikely to cause harm and might be of benefit (Hofmeyr & Kulier, 2012; Impey et al., 2017). In one study, mothers carrying breech fetuses were instructed to lie on their right sides several times per day if the fetal backs were on the left side or lie on their left sides if the fetal backs were on the right side, beginning at 28–29 weeks of gestation (Shinmura et al., 2022). After 2 weeks, about 82% of fetuses had moved to cephalic presentations, compared to about 43% for the control group (Shinmura et al., 2022). Some studies show that maternal knee chest positioning can encourage spontaneous version to vertex (Kenfack et al., 2012; Tafazolifar, Kordi, Dadgar, Esmaily, & Mirteimouri, 2019); others show no benefit (Founds, 2005; C. Smith, Crowther, Wilkinson, Pridmore, & Robinson, 1999), and one suggested that knee-chest position *promotes* persistent breech position (Founds, 2006). The Spinning Babies® program makes specific recommendations, including forward-leaning inversions (mother kneels on couch, then carefully lowers upper body until first hands and then elbows are on the floor), standing sacral release (client's partner cups the sacrum while the mother moves), side-lying release, and rebozo techniques (Tully, 2019). In another technique, the mother lies flat on a firm surface, then the provider stacks pillows under the buttocks to achieve a modified bridge position, head low and back arched (Hunter, 2014). Fetal repositioning interventions are usually performed after 34 weeks of gestation 2–3 times daily, for at least 10 min per session (Hunter, 2014). Postural techniques appear to be more effective if they are performed when the fetus is active and the mother is well hydrated.

Acupuncture and moxibustion are techniques practiced in Traditional Chinese Medicine in accordance with the view that "life force" (*qi*) flows through the body along channels called meridians. Stimulating acupuncture points along the meridians with needles purportedly restores the flow of *qi* and thus a healthy balance. Moxibustion (which replaces needles with superficial burning mugwort) at the Zhiyin BL 67 energy point on the outer aspect of the fifth toenail reportedly encourages spontaneous version to cephalic position. Although some studies have found this an effective intervention (Coyle, Smith, & Peat, 2023; García-Mochón, Martín, Aranda-Regules, Rivas-Ruiz, & Vas, 2015; Rodrigues & Zorzim, 2017; Vas et al., 2009), others have not (Bue & Lauszus, 2016; Coulon et al., 2014; Sananes et al., 2016). One study showed synergistic benefit from acupuncture and moxibustion used together (Liao et al., 2021), and a Cochrane review found some evidence that moxibustion is most effective when used with either acupuncture or postural interventions (Coyle et al., 2023). Like postural techniques, moxibustion and acupuncture treatments appear harmless and worth trying.

External Cephalic Version (ECV)

ECV is a procedure involving the manual rotation of a fetus into a cephalic presentation by applying pressure to a pregnant client's abdomen (ACOG, 2018/2023). ACOG recommends that obstetric care providers offer ECV as an alternative to planned cesarean for mothers who have term singleton breech fetuses, desire a planned vaginal delivery of a vertex-presenting fetus, and have no contraindications (ACOG, 2018/2023). Clients who undergo successful ECV are more likely to achieve a vaginal birth, reducing cost of care, length of hospital stay, and postpartum complications such as endometritis, sepsis, and hemorrhage associated with persistent breech presentations (ACOG, 2018/2023). After a fetus is converted to vertex using ECV, however, the risk of cesarean birth for dystocia and abnormal FHR patterns is higher than that of the general obstetrical population (de Hundt, Velzel, de Groot, Mol, & Kok, 2014).

The success rate for ECV is about 58% overall (ACOG, 2020). The potential for success is greatest when the provider is experienced at ECV; the mother is multiparous; and the fetus has an unengaged presenting part, is in an oblique or transverse lie or complete breech presentation, has a nonanterior placenta, and is surrounded by adequate amniotic fluid (Cillard et al., 2021). Birthweight—actual or estimated by ultrasound—does not affect the success of ECV (Burgos et al., 2009). When undertaken in facilities with ultrasound, fetal monitoring and the capacity for emergency cesarean, ECV has about the same outcomes when performed by midwives or physicians (Beuckens et al., 2016; Hutton, 2016; Impey et al., 2017; Rijnders et al., 2008; Taylor & Robson, 2016; Walker et al., 2015). ECV reduces the occurrence of cesarean section by 43% without increasing the risk of adverse outcomes (ACOG, 2018/2023; Hofmeyr, Kulier, & West, 2015).

ECV is contraindicated in only 4% of breech presentations (Stewart, 2017). Absolute contraindications include placenta previa and previous classical cesarean section; concerns about fetal status, including nonreactive nonstress test or abnormal biophysical profile score; placental abruption; multifetal gestation before birth of first fetus; severe oligohydramnios; severe preeclampsia; significant fetal anomaly; known malformation of uterus; and breech with hyperextended head or arms above shoulders (Lerner, 2017). Relative contraindications include maternal hypertension, maternal obesity, fetal growth restriction, and low amniotic fluid volume (Hofmeyr, 2023b). There is limited data concerning ECV attempts on mothers who have a preexisting uterine scar or who undergo the procedure during the early stages of labor (ACOG, 2020/2023). The risks inherent in ECV must be weighed against the risk to mother and fetus if breech presentation persists. Adverse events have been associated with ECV, including placental abruption, labor, umbilical cord prolapse, rupture of membranes, fetal/neonatal demise, and fetomaternal hemorrhage, but these complications occur at rates from less than 1% (ACOG, 2020/2023) to about 7% (Dahl et al., 2021). Transient FHR abnormalities can occur during the procedure but usually resolve (ACOG, 2018/2023). Persistent breech presentation carries the risk of cord prolapse and the complications associated with breech birth for mother and baby.

Although the need for emergency cesarean after ECV occurs at a relatively low rate (1 in 200 to 1 in 550), ECV should be performed in a hospital able to perform immediate cesarean if fetal bradycardia develops (Skupski & Ghidini, 2016). ECV is generally performed at 37 weeks of gestation or later (ACOG, 2018/2023). Before performing ECV, the provider uses ultrasound to confirm fetal and placental location and exclude oligohydramnios. FHR monitoring or biophysical profile is used to determine fetal wellbeing before the procedure. The client should be counseled on the risks and benefits of the procedure. Establish IV access before the procedure in case intrauterine resuscitation or cesarean birth is required. Use of a tocolytic, usually terbutaline 0.25 mg subcutaneously (SC) 15–30 min before the procedure, relaxes the uterine muscle and increases the success rate of ECV (Magro-Malosso, Saccone, Di Tommaso, Mele, & Berghella, 2016). Spinal, epidural, or combined spinal-epidural anesthesia increases the success rate of version and may also reduce the force required for successful version, particularly in combination with tocolytic therapy (ACOG, 2020/2023). Fetal vibroacoustic stimulation can be used to shift the fetus into a position more favorable to version, such as from spine midline to spine lateral (Hofmeyr, 2023a).

ECV is performed by positioning the mother supine with a wedge under one hip tilting the uterus toward the provider. The provider lubricates the abdomen with ultrasound gel, manually disengages the breech from the pelvis, and presses the fetus into a forward or backward somersault. The ECV attempt should be abandoned if there is prolonged fetal bradycardia, discomfort to the client, or the procedure cannot be completed easily (ACOG, 2020/2023). After the procedure, the FHR is continuously monitored until it is stable and reactive. RhD-negative clients should receive RhD immune globulin immediately after ECV. ACOG recommends waiting for spontaneous onset of labor after successful ECV rather than proceeding with induction unless it is clinically indicated (ACOG, 2020/2023).

Factors Influencing the Success of External Cephalic Version (ECV)

ECV success rate increases with

- Transverse or oblique lie
- Multiparity
- Amniotic fluid index >18
- Breech unengaged
- Smaller fetus
- Normal maternal body mass index (BMI)
- Experienced clinician
- Placenta on posterior wall of uterus
- Complete (vs. footling) breech
- Tocolysis
- Neuraxial analgesia/anesthesia

ECV success rate decreases with

- Ruptured membranes
- Macrosomic fetus
- Relative oligohydramnios
- Maternal obesity
- Primigravida status
- Anterior placenta
- Tense maternal abdominal wall muscles
- Fetal head difficult to palpate
- Contracting or tense myometrium

Adapted from "External Cephalic Version: How to Increase the Chances for Success," by H. M. Lerner, 2017, *OBG Management, 29*(9), 26–32. Copyright by Frontline Medical Communications.

Mode of Birth

There are four approaches to planning birth of the term breech fetus:

- Perform external version before labor. If version is successful, the client may return home to await spontaneous labor, or the provider may offer induction of labor to encourage birth before the fetus reverts to breech. If the version is unsuccessful, cesarean birth should be planned (Hofmeyr, 2023b).
- Perform ECV before labor and plan for vaginal breech birth if version is not successful and the client is an acceptable candidate.
- Plan cesarean birth without attempting external version.
- Plan vaginal breech birth without attempting external version if the client is an acceptable candidate.

Vaginal Breech Birth

There is controversy surrounding the perceived safety of vaginal breech birth, due, in part, to a flawed trial in 2000. The Term Breech Trial (TBT) found that perinatal and neonatal mortality and serious morbidity were significantly higher for vaginal birth of breech infants than for planned cesarean section (Hannah et al., 2000). The findings of the TBT prompted ACOG and the Royal College of Obstetricians and Gynaecologists (RCOG) to recommend cesarean section for all term breech singleton pregnancies (Berhan & Haileamlak, 2016; Carbillon et al., 2020). Subsequently, the TBT was widely criticized for many shortcomings, including flawed study design; discrepancies in standard of care; large variations in clinical methods and in expertise of the provider; and lack of adherence to the inclusion criteria (Carbillon et al., 2020; Glezerman, 2006; Partridge, 2021; Walker, Dasgupta, Halliday, & Reitter, 2021). Most cases of neonatal death and neurodevelopmental delay included in the study appear unrelated to the type of birth, and analysis after 2 years showed no difference in outcomes between children born vaginally or surgically while participating in the trial (Glezerman, 2006).

Subsequently, a large prospective observational study in France and Belgium (PREMODA) concluded that in places where planned vaginal birth is a common practice, planned vaginal birth of singleton fetuses in breech presentation at term is a safe option for clients who meet strict selection criteria before and during labor (Goffinet, et al., 2006). Current evidence suggests that planned cesarean section at 39 weeks of gestation for a term breech fetus *slightly* reduces the risk of perinatal mortality from planned vaginal breech birth (Impey et al., 2017). This finding may be due to the prevention of stillbirths that might have occurred if the pregnancy had continued beyond 39 6/7 weeks of gestation, the avoidance of risks related to labor, or the greater risks of vaginal breech birth; but only the last factor is unique to breech presentation (Impey et al., 2017).

A 2018 ACOG guideline acknowledged that because most breech babies are born by cesarean in the United States, there are now fewer providers with the knowledge and skill to attend a vaginal breech birth (ACOG, 2018/2023). ACOG advises that "planned vaginal delivery of a term singleton breech fetus may be reasonable under hospital-specific protocol guidelines for both eligibility and labor management" (ACOG, 2018/2023). It further recommends that choice of birth route be made through shared decision-making with the client, taking into consideration the experience and comfort level of the provider, institutional guidelines, characteristics of the fetus, and the values and preferences of the client (ACOG, 2018/2023; Hofmeyr, 2023a).

In the United States, the cesarean birth rate for breech presentation is about 95%; in European countries, it is 70% or higher (Hofmeyr, 2023a). Limited data indicate that cesarean birth of breech fetuses improves perinatal outcomes slightly—more often when undertaken before labor begins (Hofmeyr, 2023a). However, Vlemmix et al. (2014), estimated that providers would need to perform 338 cesareans for breech presentation to prevent one perinatal death associated with breech vaginal birth. In France, one third of clients with a fetus in breech presentation at term undergo a trial of labor, and 70% of them have successful vaginal births (Sentilhes et al., 2020).

Perinatal mortality for breech babies is approximately 0.5/1,000 with cesarean section after 39 weeks of gestation, approximately 2.0/1,000 with planned vaginal breech birth, and about 1.0/1,000 with planned cephalic birth (Impey et al., 2017). In Norway, where one third of breech fetuses are birthed vaginally, Bjellmo et al. (2017) found that the neonatal mortality ranged between 0.7 and 1.0 per 1,000 live-born infants, regardless of mode of birth.

Most authorities consider vaginal breech birth safest when it occurs in a hospital with trained, supportive providers and facilities for immediate cesarean section (Bovbjerg, Cheyney, Brown, Cox, & Leeman, 2020; Chapman & Charles, 2018; Cheyney et al., 2014; Mehl-Madrona & Madrona, 1997; Zwerling, Shields, Meuchel, Cheng, & Caughey, 2017). Data from the Midwives Alliance of North America Statistics Project (MANA Stats) indicate that vaginal breech birth in a community setting carries higher risk of fetal/neonatal morbidity and a fetal/neonatal death rate of 16.8 out of 1,000 births (Bovbjerg et al., 2017). Similarly, Grünebaum, McCullough, Sapra, Arabin, and Chervenak (2017) noted that 1 in 168 planned home births was a breech birth and that home breech birth carries an elevated neonatal mortality rate of 127.52 in 10,000 births. In contrast, Fischbein's small studies of breech births in community settings showed good outcomes for well-chosen clients (Fischbein, 2015; Fischbein & Freeze, 2018).

Whereas some U.S. states prohibit midwives from attending planned breech births in community settings, others do not (Bovbjerg et al., 2017). The American College of Nurse-Midwives (ACNM, 2015) considers *planned* vaginal breech birth a high-risk procedure and suggests using a hospital, but it does not consider breech an absolute indication for transfer from home to hospital. It does, however, consider breech presentation identified in labor an indication for immediate transport (ACNM, 2015).

Vaginal breech birth is more likely to be successful if the client is in spontaneous labor and is carrying a term fetus that is anatomically normal, is in frank or complete breech presentation with a flexed head, has an estimated

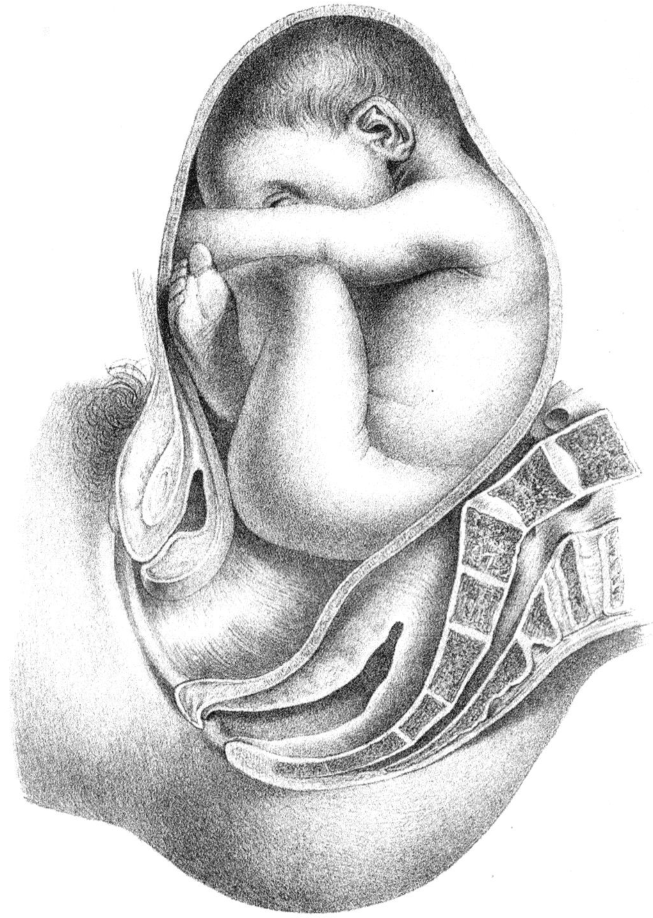

Figure 11-29. Fully dilated, membranes ruptured, breech at pelvic inlet. The mother is semireclining. She has a pendulous abdomen and the fetal head is in the fundus. From A Practical Treatise on Midwifery . . . (plate L), by F. J. Moreau (T. F. Betton, Trans.), 1844, Philadelphia, PA: Carey and Hart. In the public domain.

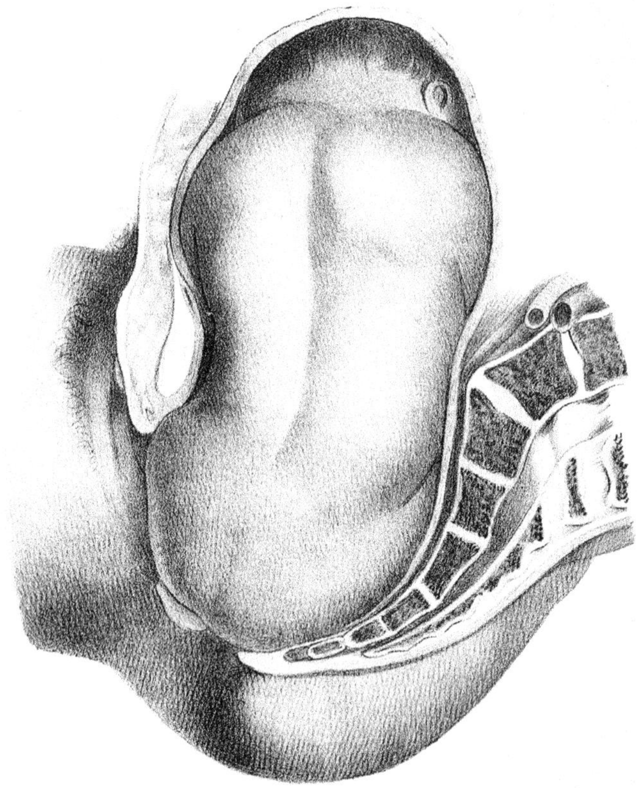

Figure 11-30. Breech descending left sacrum anterior. The breech has reached the pelvic outlet. The left hip is below the symphysis pubis and appears at the vulva. The right hip is cupped by the sacral cavity but remains on the same horizontal line as the left hip. In physiologic breech labor, the bitrochanteric diameter (about 10 cm) enters the pelvis in the transverse orientation, rotating in midpelvis and arriving at the pelvic outlet in the anterior-posterior position. From A Practical Treatise on Midwifery . . . (plate LI), by F. J. Moreau (T. F. Betton, Trans.), 1844, Philadelphia, PA: Carey and Hart. In the public domain.

weight of 5 lb 8 oz–8 lb 13 oz (2,500–4,000 g), and has a normal amniotic fluid volume (ACOG, 2018/2023). Safety is also improved if the provider is skilled in breech birth and if cesarean section is immediately available (ACOG, 2018/2023). Risk increases with hyperextended neck on ultrasound; incomplete breech presentation; or evidence of antenatal fetal compromise, such as a nonreactive NST or abnormal biophysical profile (Impey et al., 2017). Small, preterm, or growth-restricted fetuses weighing 2 lb 3 oz (1,000 g) or less are at greater risk of mortality: half the perinatal deaths in the TBT involved growth-restricted fetuses (Hofmeyr, 2023a). Fetuses weighing 8 lb 13 oz (4,000 g) or more are also at greater risk (Hofmeyr, 2023a). Risk of a poor newborn outcome appears higher in a pregnancy complicated by oligohydramnios, gestational diabetes, and nulliparity and with epidural anesthesia (Macharey, Gissler, Ulander, et al., 2017).

Some risks of vaginal breech birth may result from nonphysiologic labor management (Louwen, Daviss, Johnson, & Reitter, 2017). The technique of laying a pregnant mother supine for childbirth arose in the 1700s, promoted by barber-surgeons, apothecaries, and man-midwives (Dahlen, Homer, Leap, & Tracy, 2010). Medical tradition and provider convenience, not evidence, kept generations of mothers in the lithotomy position during birth.

Upright positioning for vaginal breech birth (standing, kneeling, or hands-and-knees) aligns the descending fetus with the curve of the birth canal, the forces of gravity, and the powers of expulsion (Farin et al., 2023; Walker, 2015). Supporting physiologic breech birth involves encouraging the client to remain upright and active through the first stage of labor, supporting spontaneous maternal movement during fetal descent, and promoting the position of choice for birth (Walker, 2015). An upright position for physiologic breech birth seems associated with a shorter second stage of labor,

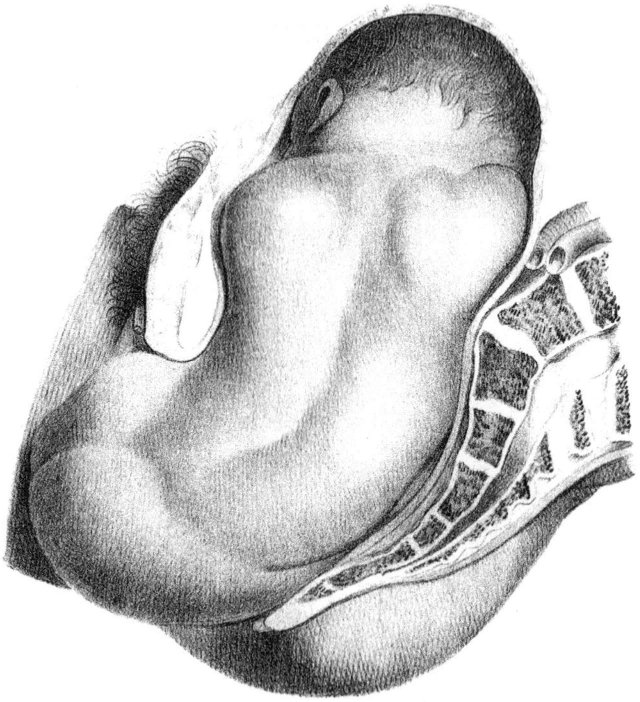

Figure 11-31. The breech has passed through the pelvic outlet and protrudes through the vulva. The left fetal hip was the first to emerge, passing beneath the pubic arch. The trunk curves with the presenting hip uppermost. The right hip must pass over the longer arc of sacrum, coccyx, and perineum. This mother is semisitting. From *A Practical Treatise on Midwifery*... (plate LII), by F. J. Moreau (T. F. Betton, Trans.), 1844, Philadelphia, PA: Carey and Hart. In the public domain.

less need for maneuvers, fewer maternal/neonatal injuries, and fewer cesareans than in supine vaginal birth (Bogner et al. 2015; Farin et al., 2023; Jennewein et al., 2017; Louwen et al., 2017; Wildschut, van Belzen-Slappendel, & Jans, 2017). Additionally, some mothers who complete a physiologic birth seem to bond more easily with their babies (Ebrahimi, Haratipour, Partash, & Bolbolhaghighi, 2021).

Mechanism of LSA Frank Breech Birth

There are three mechanisms of labor in breech presentations: birth of the buttocks and lower limbs, birth of the shoulders and arms, and birth of the head (Elfazari & El-Chaâr, 2023). In left sacrum anterior (LSA) frank breech birth, the sacrum is in the maternal left anterior quadrant, and the bitrochanteric diameter (the width from the outer points of the hips) is in the left oblique diameter of the pelvis (Elfazari & El-Chaâr, 2023). Physiologic breech birth usually occurs through a predictable series of fetal movements (Reitter, Halliday, and Walker 2020, p. 212):

- The fetal pelvis emerges with the sacrum transverse or oblique.

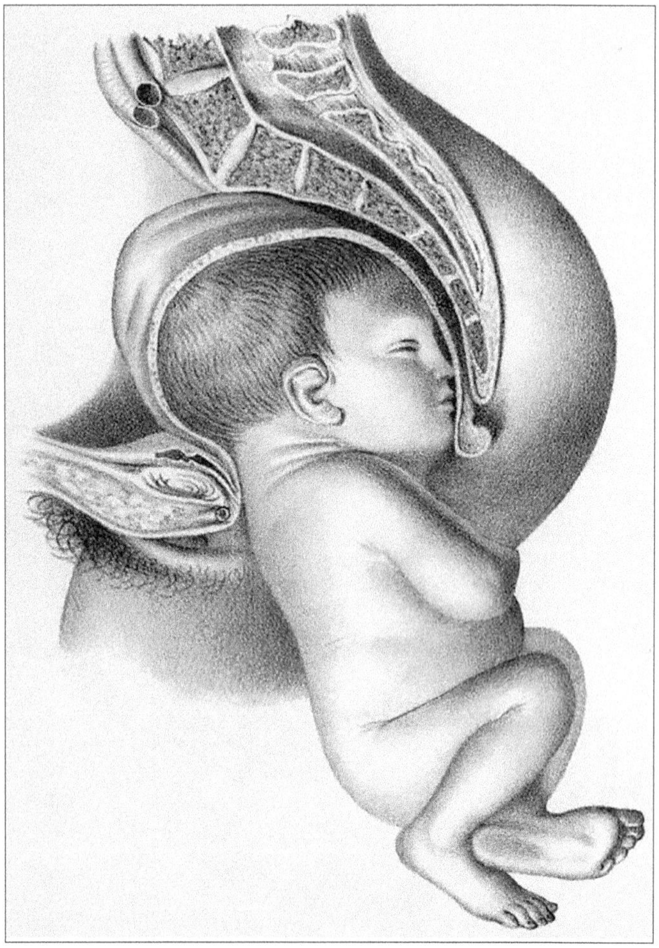

Figure 11-32. As the shoulders reach the pelvic inlet, they engage in an oblique diameter. As the left shoulder is born, the head rotates to bring the occiput behind the pubic symphysis, placing the face into the cavity of the sacrum. The mother is in an upright position. When the shoulders are free, the baby reflexively tightens the abdominal muscles, lifts the knees, and flexes the arms and head. From A Practical Treatise on Midwifery... (plate LIV), by F. J. Moreau (T. F. Betton, Trans.), 1844, Philadelphia, PA: Carey and Hart. In the public domain.

- The fetal sacrum rotates to orient toward the maternal pubis with descent front to back or "bum to tum" (a memorable term coined by Shawn Walker of the U.K.-based Breech Birth Network).
- Both extended fetal legs are born simultaneously by hip extension.
- From an extended position, the fetus performs a full-body recoil, flexing the hips and legs, adducting the arms, flexing the head, and resuming the position of flexion maintained during gestation.
- Flexed arms are born across the body elbow-first with the shoulders in the transverse diameter.
- The head is born by additional flexion and maternal pushing.

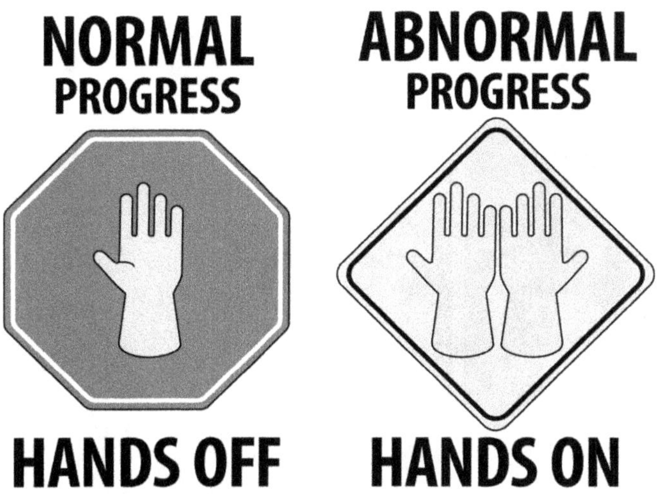

Figure 11-33. Normal breech: hands off; abnormal breech: hands on. If birth is proceeding physiologically, keep your hands off the breech but poised and ready. If birth is delayed or obstructed, hands-on intervention is necessary, but proceed with caution.

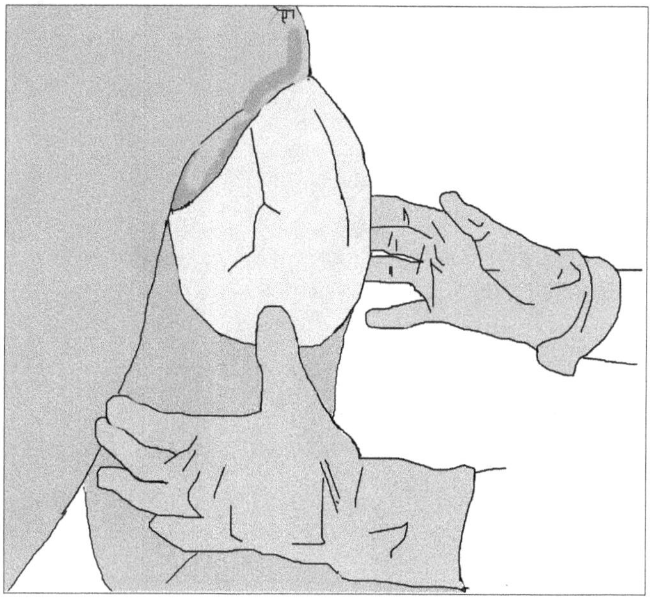

Figure 11-34. Protected-space technique. The provider keeps hands near (but not touching) the breech, safeguarding the birth process while anticipating both the need for maneuvers and the possibility of precipitous birth.

Birth of the Buttocks and Trunk

Engagement occurs when the baby's buttocks move through the pelvic inlet. Descent is often slow, but it should involve steady progress. The anterior buttock descends first. The fetus negotiates the curves of the pelvic passage by flexing at the waist. When it encounters the resistance of the pelvic floor, the anterior hip rotates forward, downward, and toward the midline, turning the fetal sacrum from the left anterior quadrant to the left transverse. The anterior buttock is born first, then the baby's anus, and finally the posterior buttock. The buttocks incline toward the mother's anus, and the anterior hip is born from under the symphysis. Meconium usually passes from the anus as the buttocks are born.

Birth of the Limbs and Shoulders

The legs normally spring free as the baby descends and are typically born simultaneously or nearly so. A sternal crease ("cleavage") visible on the chest indicates that the arms are not entrapped (Walker, 2015). Arms are usually born elbow-first, held across the torso with the shoulders in the transverse diameter (Reitter et al., 2020). By the time the fetal nipples and scapulae have emerged, the body has usually rotated to sacroanterior, putting the baby's buttocks in line with the mother's pubis, "front to back" (Reitter et al., 2020). The shoulders engage in the left oblique diameter of the pelvis. The anterior shoulder rotates beneath the symphysis, and the bisacromial diameter moves to an anterior-posterior orientation (Elfazari & El-Chaâr, 2023). The posterior shoulder is born, then the anterior shoulder emerges from under the symphysis.

Birth of the Head

When the shoulders are at the outlet, the head enters the pelvis with the occiput in the left anterior quadrant. The head remains flexed. When the head reaches the pelvic floor, it rotates internally until the brow is in the hollow of the sacrum and the occiput is under the symphysis (Elfazari & El-Chaâr, 2023). The baby's back is anterior, oriented toward the pubis. The head is born by flexion when the nape pivots under the symphysis and the chin, face, forehead, and occiput are born over the perineum.

Managing the Unexpected Breech Birth

The optimal way to gain expertise in breech birth is hands-on clinical experience. Because vaginal breech birth has become relatively uncommon, the next best way to get experience is by participating drills and simulations (Horasanlı, Demirbas, Cıcek, 2023; Lendahls & Oscarsson, 2017). Educational tools such as videos and written materials can also be helpful.

When breech is diagnosed in labor, call for help if there are others nearby who can assist and activate emergency medical services (EMS). If the baby is born safely before EMS arrives, you can cancel the request for an ambulance if assistance is not required. If you transfer to the hospital via ambulance, accompany the client to the hospital and monitor FHT *en route*. Prepare for birth, for neonatal resuscitation, and for postpartum hemorrhage. Ensure a warm environment for birth. Ask the ambulance driver to pull over if birth occurs *en route* to the hospital.

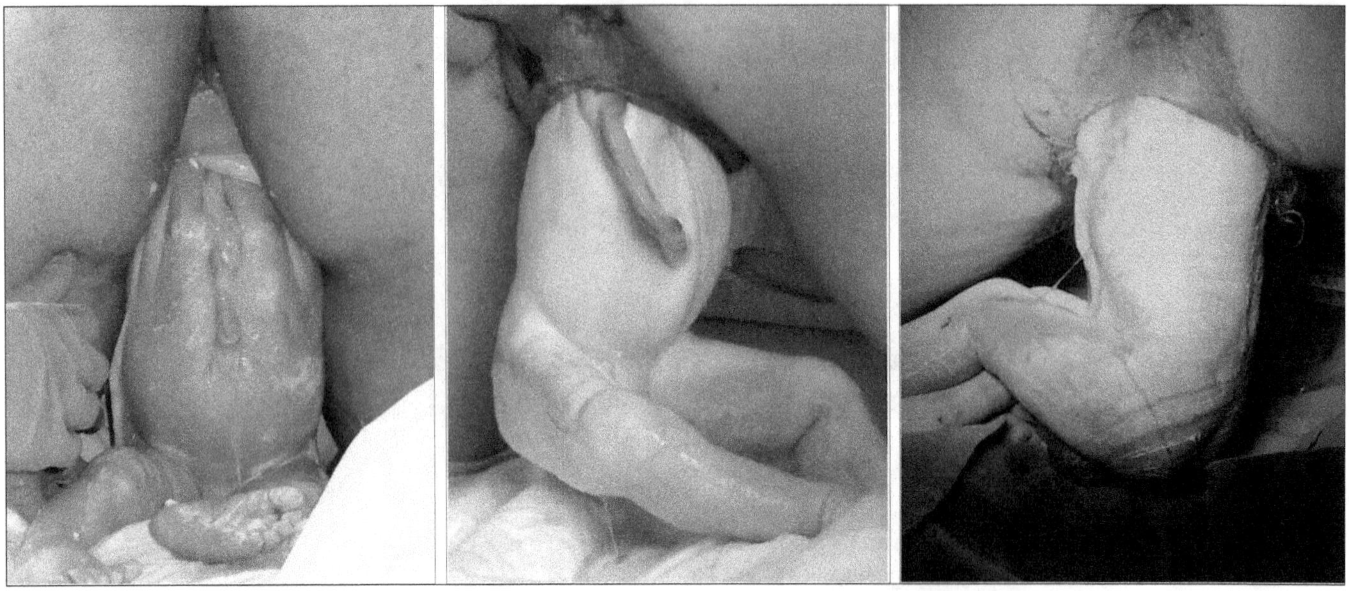

Figure 11-35. Physiologic breech birth. The crease between the nipples on the fetus to the left indicates that the arms are not trapped and will be born spontaneously. From "Practical Insight into Upright Breech Birth from Birth Videos: A Structured Analysis," by A Reitter, A. Halliday, and S. Walker, 2020, *Birth, 47*(2), p. 214. CC BY 4.0.

If birth is imminent, prepare to attend a breech birth. Spontaneous breech births usually proceed rapidly once the buttocks have descended past the ischial spines and onto the perineum (Reitter et al., 2020). In one study, most babies were born within 3 min of the birth of the fetal pelvis, even when assistive maneuvers were required (Reitter et al., 2020).

Birth is most likely to succeed when the mother is free to respond to the body's signals and the baby is free to adapt naturally to the forces of birth. The provider must respect the mechanism of normal birth but stand ready to restore it if birth is obstructed or delayed (Walker, 2015). Failure to interfere when the process becomes abnormal can endanger mother and baby. The principle of "Normal: hands off, abnormal: hands on" is especially important in managing the birth of an unexpected breech.

The midwife's role is the same in any physiologic birth: close evaluation of fetal wellbeing, extensive understanding of the natural mechanisms of birth, and readiness to respond to complications. Any interference with the natural mechanism increases the risk of difficulties that can threaten the life or wellbeing of the emerging infant. A hands-off approach encourages the fetus to maintain a position of flexion during the birth, simplifying birth. Unnecessary manipulation can cause the head to deflex and the arms to extend over the head.

The client who develops a strong urge to push should avoid bearing down until fully dilated. Pushing the fetus through a partially dilated cervix can cause the trunk to descend and allow the larger aftercoming head to become entrapped. With normal progress, the breech usually reaches the level of the ischial spines at 6 cm of dilation and reaches the pelvic floor at full dilation (Hofmeyr, 2023a). The breech may remain unengaged until dilation is complete and the amniotic sac has broken (Elfazari & El-Chaâr, 2023) or descend passively for up to 90 min before active pushing begins (Kotaska & Menticoglou, 2019). The pushing stage should take no more than 1 hr (Kotaska & Menticoglou, 2019).

Auscultate the FHR continuously or after each contraction in the second stage. Leave the amniotic membranes intact until they rupture naturally. When membranes rupture, auscultate FHT and consider performing a vaginal examination to check for cord prolapse (Chapman & Charles, 2018). Once the body is born, do not attempt to auscultate the FHR (Chapman & Charles, 2018). The cord is often compressed between the baby's head and maternal pelvis during birth of the arms, causing bradycardia (Chapman & Charles, 2018). The decision to intervene at this point should be based on lack of progress, not FHR (Chapman & Charles, 2018).

"Rumping" (the breech equivalent of crowning) occurs with a subtle rocking and shifting of the fetal buttocks (Ashwin & Anderson, 2017). As the baby emerges, use the protected space technique by poising your hands near the breech without touching it. Stand ready for immediate action if maneuvers are needed or if birth is precipitous.

Allow the breech to hang and to emerge at its own pace. Notice the baby's color, tone, and movements. A baby often appears pale and limp during a breech birth, but the umbilical cord should appear engorged and blue. Because handling the cord can cause cord vessels to spasm, do not check a pulse by pressing the cord or create slack by pulling down a loop (Chapman & Charles, 2018).

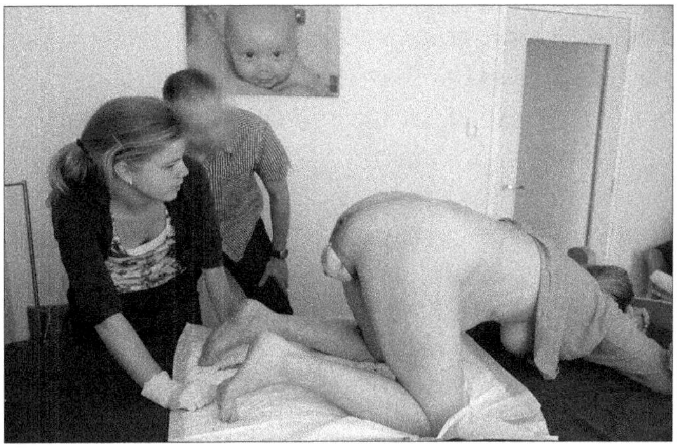

Figure 11-36. A community midwife arrives to evaluate a 34-year-old gravida 2, para 1 (G2 P1) at 38 5/7 weeks of gestation who had planned a hospital birth. The midwife finds her with irregular contractions, appearing calm and composed. Soon she instinctively adopts a knee-elbow position. Membranes rupture spontaneously, releasing meconium-stained fluid, and she begins to push uncontrollably. The midwife determines that she is fully dilated with a frank breech fetus. The parents decline transport to the hospital, believing that birth is imminent. Figures 11-36 through 11-42 from "The Art of Vaginal Breech Birth at Term on All Fours," by H. I. J. Wildschut, H. van Belzen-Slappendel, & S. Jans, 2017, *Clinical Case Reports, 5*(2), 182–186. CC-BY 4.0.

The baby's abdomen should be facing the mother's sacrum. The legs should release spontaneously, then the arms. Elbows visible at the perineum are reassuring, indicating that the arms are across the chest and not trapped above the head. As the body rotates, the arms are born. As the shoulders are born, a healthy baby flexes its legs toward the abdomen and brings its arms to its shoulders ("tummy crunch"). This action can cause the mother to instinctively change position from upright to horizontal, moving the pelvis around the baby's flexing head (Chapman & Charles, 2018).

If the baby's body and thighs are born easily and spontaneously, the head will probably follow without incident. Maternal perineal bulging and anal dilation is an indication that the head is properly positioned and birth is imminent. The fetal head enters the pelvis in the same diameter as it would in a vertex position (Chapman & Charles, 2018). When the shoulders have been born, the head is either in the maternal pelvis or needs maternal assistance to engage (Reitter et al., 2020). After the fetus vacates the uterus, contractions space out and the uterine muscle is no longer able to assist in the expulsion of the fetus (Reitter et al., 2020). Strong maternal effort is often needed to push the fetal head out.

The extraordinary photographs in Figures 11-36 through 11-42 document an unexpected home breech birth reported in Wildschut, van Belzen-Slappendel, Jans (2017).

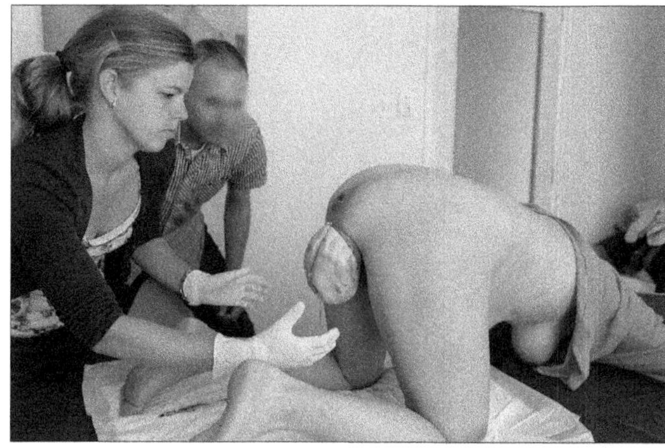

Figure 11-37. The midwife is calm and focused as she provides supportive care and reassurance. The fetal sacrum is in the anterior position.

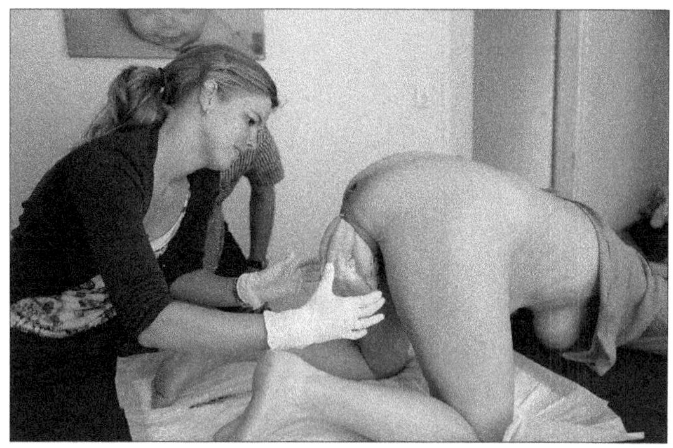

Figure 11-38. The midwife correctly keeps her hands near the breech but does not touch it, allowing mother and fetus to negotiate the process of birth without interference while standing ready to assist.

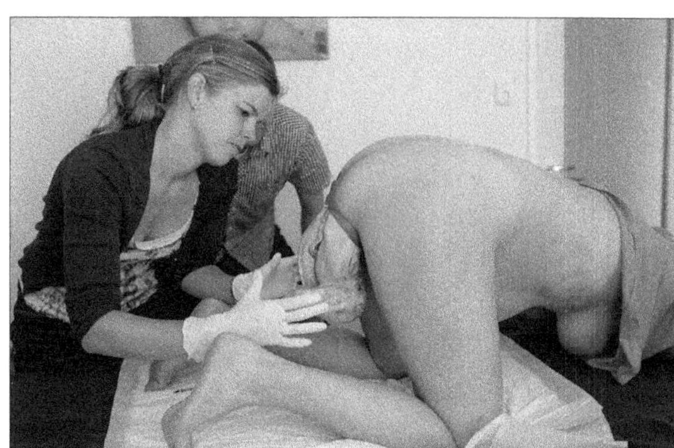

Figure 11-39. The fetus has released one leg, but there is no sign of the arms. The midwife is prepared to use Løvset's maneuver to release the arms.

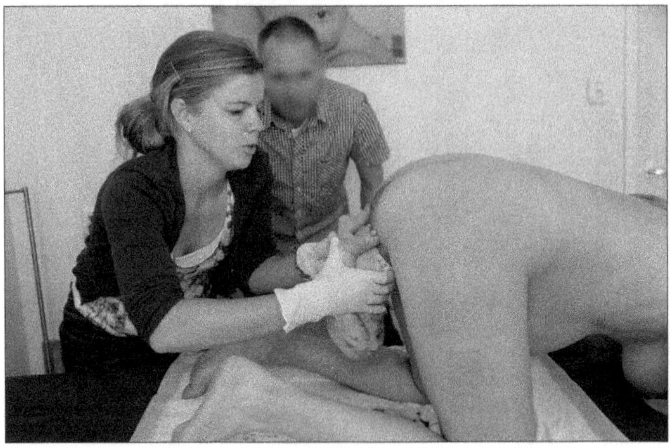

Figure 11-40. Gentle pressure below the clavicles causes the fetal head to flex and emerge (shoulder press maneuver).

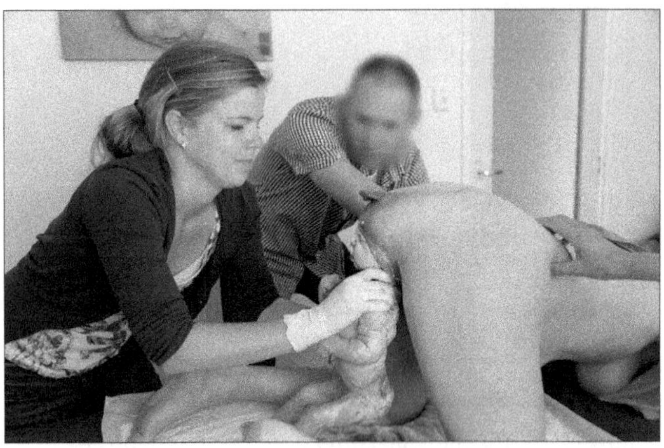

Figure 11-41. A meconium-stained baby with good tone enters the world.

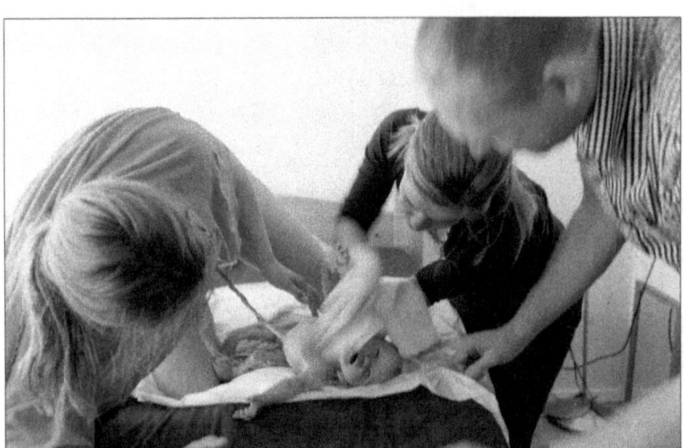

Figure 11-42. The midwife dries and stimulates the healthy baby while the parents get acquainted with the new arrival.

4 Rs to Restore the Natural Process of Breech Birth

- **R**estitute fetal back to anterior (Front to Back)
- **R**elease legs (Pinard)
- **R**otate shoulders and sweep arms (Løvset's, prayer hands, Louwen's 180° torque maneuver)
- **R**estore flexion to release head (shoulder press, Mauriceau-Smellie-Veit, Bracht)

Maneuvers for Abnormal Breech Birth

An RCOG guideline (Impey et al., 2017) recommends maneuvers to assist breech birth when there is evidence of poor fetal condition, if there is a delay of more than 5 min from birth of the buttocks to the head, or if there is a delay of more than 3 min from the umbilicus to the head. Reitter et al. (2020) suggest that for upright breech births, a delay of 90 sec or more at any point after rumping indicates that birth is unlikely to progress without intervention. Minor delays can often be corrected if the mother can move, change positions, and push (Reitter et al., 2020). When the mother is upright, gravity helps the baby descend, and natural fetal and maternal reflexes facilitate birth.

Prepare to intervene if the breech mechanisms do not progress as expected, and/or there is a delay that is not resolved by spontaneous maternal movement. Intervention is also frequently necessary if the fetus appears compromised. Most physiological breech interventions involve direct maneuvers that shift the baby into a cardinal movement or indirect maneuvers that move the mother to facilitate rotation. Breech Without Borders (n.d., 2020), a nonprofit organization dedicated to breech training, education, and advocacy, offers free instructional videos depicting the mechanism of breech birth and the application of interventional maneuvers as well as other valuable resources and information.

Birth of Trunk

The fetal pelvis is born with the fetal sacrum pointed toward a maternal hip. After the umbilicus emerges, the baby should rotate until its sacrum is in line with the mother's symphysis—think "front to back" or "bum to tum." If the fetal umbilicus points toward the maternal symphysis, birth is unlikely to progress, and intervention will become necessary. If delay occurs, grasp the fetal iliac crests and use rotation, not traction, to move the baby and restore the natural mechanism of breech birth.

Birth of the Legs

Pinard maneuver. Although legs are usually born spontaneously, the extended legs of a frank breech can sometimes impede the mechanism of birth. If they do not release with

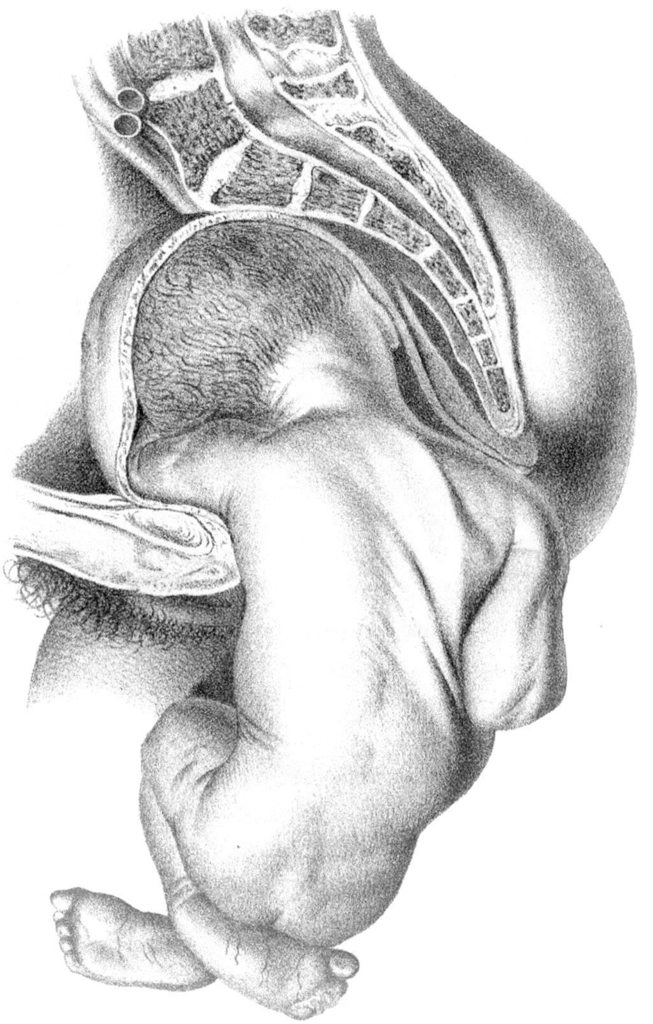

Figure 11-43. This baby has an arm up beside the head. If there is a delay with the birth at this point, the midwife will need to assist. From *A Practical Treatise on Midwifery*... (plate LIII), by F. J. Moreau (T. F. Betton, Trans.), 1844, Philadelphia, PA: Carey and Hart. In the public domain.

Table 11-2

Maneuvers to Restore the Natural Process of Breech Birth When There Is a Delay in Progress

Maneuver	Description
Front to back (*"bum to tum"*)	Keep baby's front to mother's back.
Pinard *(to release leg: press behind the knee)*	Use fingers behind knee to bring down leg.
Løvset's maneuver *(to release arms: half twist and dip)*	Place hands on fetal hips and rotate the fetus through 180° while keeping the back toward the maternal symphysis pubis. Dip downward and up to release arm, rotate in opposite direction, repeat. Sweep arms down if necessary.
Prayer hands *(to release arms: sandwich, lift and rotate)*	Sandwich the baby between palms, lift baby toward cervix, then rotate baby until the shoulders are in the transverse diameter.
Louwen's 180° torque maneuver *(to release arms: reverse shoulders, then face to sacrum to release arms)*	Turn impacted shoulder away from the maternal symphysis until baby faces the opposite direction. Then turn the baby back 90° until the baby faces the maternal sacrum.
Shoulder press/Frank's nudge *(to release head: press below clavicles, back toward pubis)*	Apply pressure to baby's torso just below the clavicles while gently directing baby's body toward the maternal pubis. May be combined with gluteal lift, wherein assistant lifts maternal buttocks up and out.
Mauriceau-Smellie-Veit maneuver *(to release head: chest on arm, fingers on cheekbones. Hand on back, fingers flex head)*	Place fetal chest on your forearm with the arms on either side. Place two fingers on baby's cheek bones. Place other hand over baby's shoulders with one or two fingers on the occiput. Help baby flex its head.
Bracht maneuver *(to release head: encircle hips and thighs, lift back)*	Encircle baby's hips and thighs and lower back with hands. Hold baby's back against maternal symphysis. Assistant applies suprapubic pressure to encourage head flexion.

maternal pushing and movement, use finger pressure in the fossa behind the knee to externally rotate and flex the leg with minimal disturbance to the mother (Reitter et al., 2020). Releasing the legs can also create space for the prayer hands maneuver (see below).

Birth of the Arms

In a vaginal breech birth, a nuchal arm is one that is abducted so it is trapped alongside or behind the fetal neck or head (Walker & Spillane, 2020). Winging of the scapulae (protruding from the back instead of lying flat) is a sign of extended arms (Malini, 2018). If the fetus has not assumed a sacroanterior (sacrum under the symphysis) position by the time it is born to the nipple line, one or both arms are probably extended, and maneuvers will be required to release them (Reitter et al., 2020; Walker, 2015; Walker & Spillane, 2020). Arm extraction can cause fetal shoulder dislocation or humerus fracture, but musculoskeletal injury is preferable to asphyxia from prolonged shoulder dystocia (Hofmeyr, 2023a).

In most breech births, the arms are crossed in front of the chest and emerge with the shoulders, which rotate into the anterior-posterior plane and emerge one at a time. Extended or nuchal arms can cause shoulder dystocia and arrest progress. The baby sometimes extends its arms if the provider gives inappropriate traction early in the birth process (Hofmeyr, 2023a).

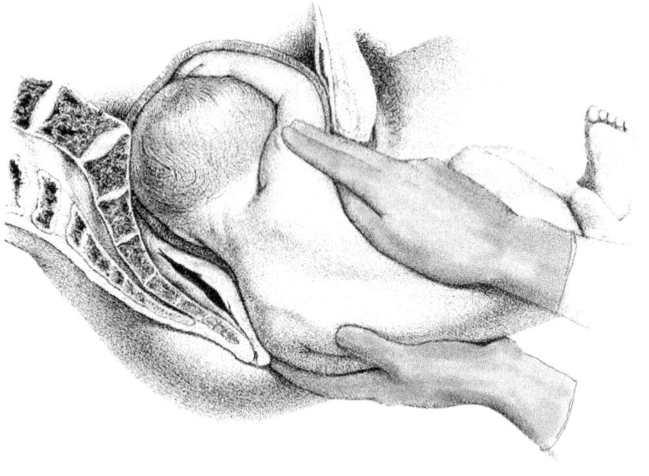

Figure 11-44. Bringing down the arm of the breech. Adapted from *Atlas de l'Art des Accouchements* (plate 86, fig. 1), by A. Lenoir, M. See, and S. Tarnier, 1871, Paris, France: Victor Masson. In the public domain.

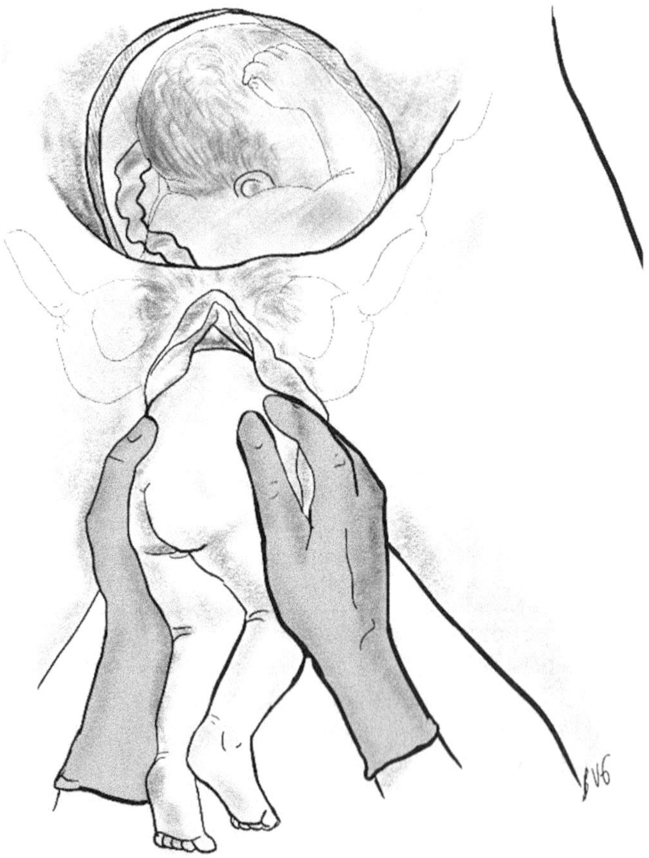

Figure 11-45. Løvset's maneuver (half twist and dip) is performed by placing the hands on the fetal hips and rotating the fetus through 180°. Dip downward and up to release the arm, rotate the baby in the opposite direction to release the contralateral arm. Sweep the arms down if necessary. Drawing by the author after *Atlas de l'Art des Accouchements* (plate 85, fig. 1), by A. Lenoir, M. See, and S. Tarnier, 1871, Paris, France: Victor Masson. Original in the public domain.

If the baby is right sacroanterior, the right arm is more likely to catch on the mother's pelvis, and if the baby is left sacroanterior, the left arm is more likely to impinge (Louwen et al., 2017, Appendix S1).

Løvset's maneuver is a method for rotating the fetus to assist with the birth of the arms. To release the anterior shoulder and arm, grasp the baby gently at the iliac crests with your thumbs over the sacrum. Rotate first in the direction in which the arm is pointing (Walker & Spillane, 2020). Rotate the fetus through 180°, then use light traction to dip the baby downward and up (Marshall, & Raynor, 2014). Some providers wrap the lower half of the baby in a towel to improve their grip (Barth, 2021). Reverse direction and rotate the fetus back 180°, then provide light traction once more to free the remaining arm. Finger pressure on the abdomen can damage internal organs.

If rotation alone fails to release the arm, advance a finger along the fetal scapula and over the shoulder, following the humerus to the antecubital fossa. With a beckoning motion of the fingers, sweep the baby's elbow in front of the face down toward the chest, and the arm should emerge. If the arms do not appear, apply pressure to the antecubital fossa until the wrist is accessible, then grasp it and sweep it down (Walker, 2015). If the arms are trapped behind the neck, try rotating the baby until the chest is facing the maternal symphysis pubis, then again attempt to sweep them down and extract them one by one (Hofmeyr, 2023a).

Prayer hands is another maneuver for freeing the shoulder and arms (Walker, 2018). Sandwich the baby between your palms with one on the baby's spine and the other on the abdomen. Your fingertips should be against the bony prominences of the shoulder girdle, and your palms should be flat to avoid injury to fragile abdominal organs (Walker, 2018). Elevate the baby slightly toward the cervix, then rotate the body until the chest aligns with the maternal pubis. The rotation should reposition the arms, which are still inside the mother. Keeping one hand on the fetal back, release an arm by sweeping it across the fetal face and down across the fetal torso under the maternal pubic arch (Walker & Spillane, 2020). Then rotate the fetus in the opposite direction until the back aligns with the mother's pubis and sweep the second arm down along the fetal torso.

Louwen's 180° torque maneuver also releases impacted arms by rotating the fetus. With the mother in an upright position, face the buttocks and place your fingers inside the vagina to contact the fetal shoulders. Without pulling, turn the impacted shoulder away from the maternal symphysis 180°, until the baby's abdomen faces the opposite direction (Louwen et al., 2017). Then turn the baby back 90° until it faces the maternal sacrum, in position for a physiologic descent.

Birth of the head

During a physiologic breech birth, a healthy baby facilitates head flexion just before birth by reflexively bringing its arms to its shoulders and its legs toward the abdomen, engaging its core muscles (Chapman & Charles, 2018). This movement often stimulates the mother to instinctively drop from an upright position to horizontal, moving her pelvis around the fetal head (Chapman & Charles, 2018). A hyperextended head, an incompletely dilated cervix, or unnecessary intervention by the provider can arrest birth of the head. If there is a delay in the birth of the head, the empty uterus sometimes enters the third stage of labor, causing the placenta to detach from the uterine wall with the head still unborn (Reitter et al., 2020).

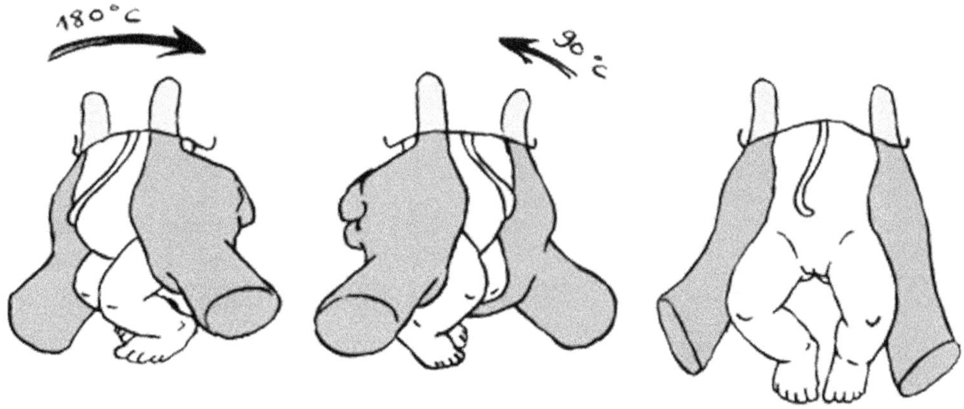

Figure 11-46. The "180° torque" maneuver moves the obstructed shoulder away from the maternal symphysis 180°, then back 90°. From "Does Breech Delivery in an Upright Position Instead of on the Back Improve Outcomes and Avoid Cesareans?" by F. Louwen, B.-A. Daviss, K. C. Johnson, and A. Reitter, 2017, *International Journal of Gynecology & Obstetrics, 136*(2), 151–161, fig. 1. CC BY-NC 4.0.

Whenever there is a delay in the birth process, a change in maternal position often helps. McRoberts' or Gaskin's maneuvers and running start or lunge positions can encourage physiologic release of the head by making more space in the pelvis (Shushan & Younis, 1992). Helping the mother move to hands-and-knees position, bringing the knees close together, and abducting the lower legs can open the outlet and create space for the fetal head (Shushan & Younis, 1992). Rocking or wiggling the hips can also facilitate birth. If the fetal hairline does not appear, the head has probably become deflexed, and maneuvers are required (Chapman & Charles, 2018).

Stay calm and act deliberately. Explore with your fingers to identify the problem. If dilation is incomplete, you can usually palpate cervical tissue restraining one or both sides of the head. If the head is hyperextended, you will feel only the triangular bottom of the jawbone at the top of the mother's sacrum (Walker, 2014b). The goal is to encourage the fetal head to flex and thus restore the normal process of birth. *Excessive traction or manipulation of a hyperextended head can occlude the vertebral arteries or dislocate the fetal neck, causing death* (Hofmeyr, 2023a).

Shoulder press (Frank's nudge) utilizes the bony structures of the pelvis to flex the head and complete the birth. If the head is deflexed in the midpelvis or if the chin is on or near the perineum, the baby's occiput is under the maternal pubic arch. Assist the mother to an all-fours or kneeling position. While facing the mother's buttocks, apply pressure to the baby's torso just below the clavicles while gently directing the baby's body straight back toward the maternal pubis (Louwen et al., 2017; Walker & Spillane, 2020). The pubic arch will push the occiput up and forward, causing the head to flex and descend into the curve of Carus (Walker, 2014b).

The gluteal lift is a maneuver to resolve soft tissue dystocia. If progress halts after the forehead is born, have your assistant lift the maternal buttocks up and out while you perform the shoulder press. This maneuver is especially effective if the perineum is tight or if the mother is obese (Walker, 2014b).

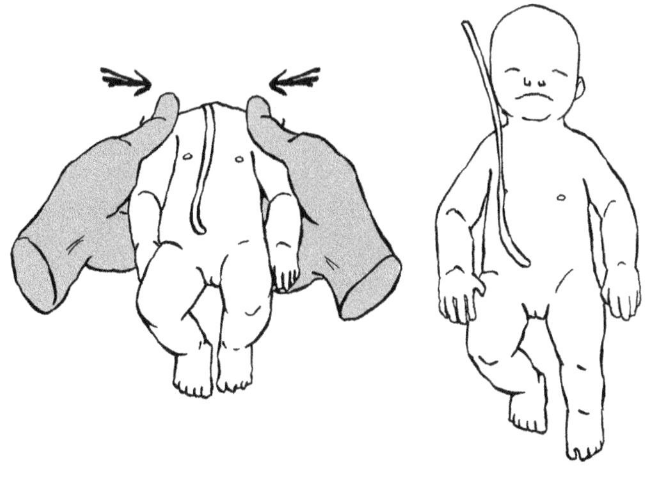

Figure 11-47. To perform Frank's nudge (shoulder press) maneuver, the provider presses below the baby's clavicles while directing the baby's body toward the mother's pubis. The head should flex and emerge easily. From "Does Breech Delivery in an Upright Position Instead of on the Back Improve Outcomes and Avoid Cesareans?" by F. Louwen, B.-A. Daviss, K. C. Johnson, and A. Reitter, 2017, International Journal of Gynecology & Obstetrics, 136(2), pp. 151–161, fig. 1. CC BY-NC 4.0.

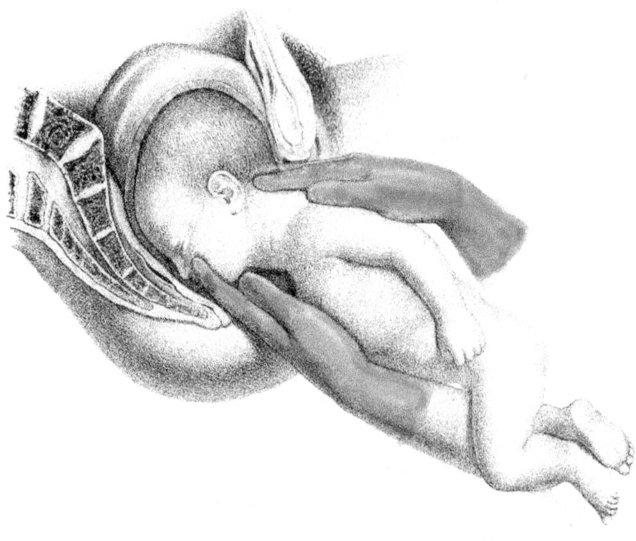

Figure 11-48. The Mauriceau-Smellie-Veit maneuver involves applying pressure to the fetal cheekbones and occiput to encourage head flexion. From *Atlas de l'Art des Accouchements* (plate 86, fig. 2), by A. Lenoir, M. See, and S. Tarnier, 1871, Paris, France: Victor Masson. In the public domain.

The Mauriceau-Smellie-Veit maneuver and its variants can increase head flexion to facilitate birth. Support the fetal trunk on your forearm and place two fingers gently on the baby's cheek bones. (Do not insert a finger in the mouth or use the jaw for leverage; to do so risks injury to the temporomandibular joint.) With your other hand, place your hand over the baby's shoulders with one or two fingers on the occiput. With pressure from both hands, help the baby to flex its head in a movement like nodding Yes (Chapman & Charles, 2018).

The Bracht Maneuver can encourage birth of the head if the client is semisitting or supine. Grasp the baby's hips (and the extended legs if frank breech) with both hands, fingers and thumbs encircling the lower back and thighs. Hold—do not push or press—the baby's back against the mother's symphysis. The object is to mimic the effect gravity would have had if the mother had chosen an upright position (Dunn, 2003). An assistant applies suprapubic pressure to encourage head flexion.

Head Entrapment

Head entrapment is a true emergency because it is usually accompanied by significant cord compression. It results from either a fetal body slipping through an incompletely dilated cervix or from cephalopelvic disproportion (Cunningham et al., 2022, ch. 28). Head entrapment is more likely if the fetus is footling breech or if the client begins to push before completely dilated. Preterm babies under 30 weeks of gestation have a risk of head entrapment as high as 14% due to their proportionately large heads and small, lean bodies (Kayem et al., 2008).

The shape of the fetal head can interfere with spontaneous birth. The head of the breech fetus can become distinctively long and narrow under intraabdominal pressure before labor. Elongation is more likely if the mother is nulliparous, the baby is large, the fluid volume is low, or the placenta is posterior (Walker, 2014a). An elongated head may encourage the fetal chin to catch on the sacral promontory, preventing flexion. Sometimes the aftercoming head must orient to the transverse diameter to come out (Walker, 2014a).

When the head is entrapped, the baby's best chance for survival is immediate transport to a hospital capable of managing obstetrical emergencies and neonatal intensive care. Guidelines in major textbooks recommend that EMS providers faced with breech head entrapment place two fingers into the vagina along each side of the baby's nose to provide an air channel for the baby (Robertson, Braude, Stonehocker, & Moreno, 2015), but this intervention is ineffective (Robertson et al., 2015). The head of the entrapped infant is generally within the uterus, not the vagina; if the head were on the pelvic floor, rapid delivery would occur (Robertson et al., 2015). It is also ineffective to perform chest compressions on a bradycardic or pulseless entrapped fetus (Robertson et al., 2015).

If the head of a breech baby does not emerge, transport immediately. Keep the baby's body warm. Avoid touching the cord unnecessarily. Position the mother in whatever position yields the best FHR.

In the hospital, an obstetrician can use Piper forceps to produce flexion of the fetal head and facilitate birth if the cervix is completely dilated (Barth, 2021). If forceps fail, the obstetrician may consider the Zavanelli maneuver: replacing the body of the fetus in the uterus and proceeding with cesarean section (Kotaska & Menticoglou, 2019). This procedure has yielded good outcomes in some cases, but it carries a high risk of maternal and fetal injury and fetal death (Hofmeyr, 2023a). Symphysiotomy (surgically dividing the cartilage of the pubic symphysis with a small incision) is practiced largely in regions where safe cesarean is unavailable and the mother's life is in danger (Hofmeyr, 2023a). It can cause long-term pain and disability for the mother. If the cervix is incompletely dilated, the obstetrician may attempt to widen the cervix surgically with Dührssen incisions, cutting the cervix at the 6, 2, and 10 o'clock positions (Hofmeyr, 2023a). This procedure carries many risks, including extension of the incision into the lower uterine segment and broad ligament, potentially damaging uterine vessels, ureter, and bladder and causing intractable hemorrhage (Hofmeyr, 2023a).

After Breech Birth

The breech baby is at higher risk for birth trauma and asphyxia. Be prepared to resuscitate the infant if necessary. Newborns born after abnormal fetal presentations should be examined by a pediatrician to screen for developmental dysplasia of the hip and other abnormalities.

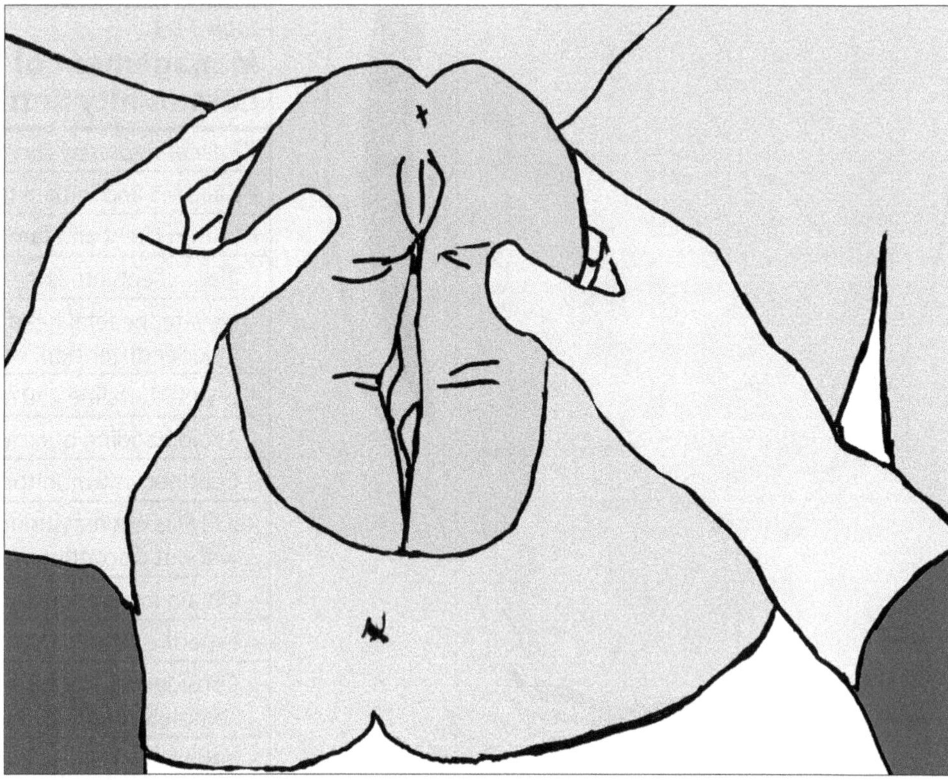

Figure 11-49. The Bracht maneuver encourages birth of the head by replicating the cardinal movements of spontaneous vaginal breech birth. The midwife gently grasps the body and extended legs of the fetus at the hips and holds them against the maternal symphysis. An assistant may give suprapubic pressure. The force of the uterine contractions expels the arms, shoulders, and head.

Umbilical Cord Presentations and Prolapse

Umbilical cord prolapse and the related conditions of funic presentation and occult cord prolapse carry a high risk of perinatal morbidity and mortality when they occur in labor. An overt cord prolapse (umbilical cord has extruded through the cervix and/or vagina) carries the highest risk of harm to the fetus. A funic (cord) presentation occurs when there is umbilical cord above the cervix but below the fetal presenting part. Compound cord presentation (occult umbilical cord prolapse) occurs when the cord is above the cervix and alongside the fetal presenting part (Wong, Kwan, Lau, Sin, & Leung, 2021). Any of these conditions can occur with or without ruptured membranes.

Funic (Cord) Presentation

Funic presentation occurs when the umbilical cord lies between the fetal presenting part and the cervix, with or without ruptured membranes. Funic presentation with intact membranes identified before 28 weeks of gestation usually resolves without intervention (Pagan et al., 2020). In the third trimester, funic presentation is rare and may spontaneously resolve by the time of labor (Aguiar, Cavaco Gomes, & Rodrigues, 2021).

Up to 38% of pregnancies with persistent funic presentation in the third trimester progress to cord prolapse (Petrikovsky, Terrani, Dillon, & Sichinava, 2021). If a funic presentation is diagnosed in the third trimester, Doppler studies and antenatal fetal surveillance are indicated (Pagan et al., 2020). Research is needed to determine whether scheduled cesarean section benefits the nonlaboring client with a funic presentation and a vertex fetus at term (Bush, Eddleman, & Belogolovkin, 2022).

In labor, the first sign of funic presentation might be deep variable FHR decelerations or intervals of fetal bradycardia. Upon vaginal examination, the cord may feel like a knobby, rubbery rope ahead of the presenting fetal part. If there is a bulging amniotic sac, it can be difficult to palpate cord through the cervix or distinguish a cord presentation from fetal fingers or ear. A cord pulse may be detectable, but *do not* compress the cord to verify pulsation. A funic presentation diagnosed in labor is an emergency because the FHR will probably become abnormal and the umbilical cord is likely to prolapse when membranes rupture (Aguiar et al., 2021).

Compound Cord Presentation (Occult Cord Prolapse)

Compound cord presentation, also known as occult cord prolapse, occurs when the cord slips down alongside, but not beyond, the presenting part (Wong, Kwan, et al.,2021). Because compound cord presentation may go unrecognized, it is probably underreported in the literature (Pagan et al., 2020). If the cord becomes compressed or the cord vessels begin to spasm, oxygen delivery to the fetus may be impaired. Evidence of fetal

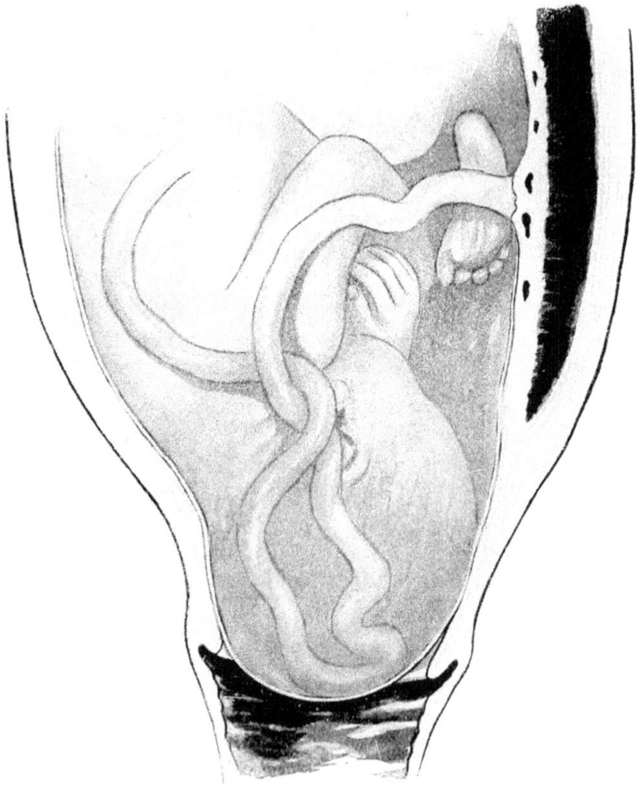

Figure 11-50. A funic or cord presentation occurs when the umbilical cord is the presenting part, often with intact amniotic membranes. From *The Principles and Practice of Obstetrics* (p. 628, fig. 554), by J. B. De Lee, 1914, Philadelphia, PA: W. B. Saunders. In the public domain.

compromise includes variable decelerations and bradycardia (Pagan et al., 2020). A compound cord presentation may not be palpable upon vaginal digital examination, and it is often a surprise finding at birth.

Umbilical Cord Prolapse

Umbilical cord prolapse is an unpredictable emergency that occurs when the cord slips through the cervix ahead of the fetal presenting part. The cord can be seen or felt on examination. Membranes may or may not be ruptured. If the cord develops a vasospasm or becomes compressed, umbilical cord prolapse can result in neonatal death, catastrophic neurological injury, or acute and long-term morbidity.

Umbilical cord prolapse occurs in 1–6 per 1,000 pregnancies (Wong, Kwan, et al., 2021). On average, the risk of death for babies with cord prolapse is approximately 1 in 14, but the risk of neonatal encephalopathy is relatively low, approximately 1 in 300 (Hehir, Hartigan, & Mahony, 2017). Cord prolapse has been described as an all-or-nothing complication, but most survivors are healthy and neurologically intact (Hehir et al., 2021). If the blood flow through the umbilical cord is sufficient, the newborn may remain unharmed, even if birth is delayed. Conversely, if blood flow is reduced by umbilical cord compression or vascular spasm, severe hypoxia or fetal death is likely (Ahmed & Hamdy, 2018; Hasegawa et al., 2017).

Table 11-3
Management of Cord Prolapse in the Community Setting

(Order of steps may vary)
• Call EMS and initiate transfer protocol.
• Inform client and family while intervening.
• Place client into knee-chest or modified Sims' position.
• Elevate the fetal head using manual pressure or bladder distension.
• Give terbutaline 250 mcg subcutaneously.
• Avoid handing or moving the cord.
• Continuously monitor FHR.
• If FHR is not reassuring, try changing maternal position without discontinuing head displacement.
• Obtain intravenous access.
• Expedite birth.
• Consider vaginal birth only if the client is multiparous, complete, and pushing.
• If the baby is born, prepare for resuscitation and postpartum hemorrhage.

Umbilical cord prolapse carries higher risk of perinatal injury and death when it occurs in community settings than when it occurs in a hospital (Ahmed & Hamdy, 2018; Lin, 2006). Survivors of umbilical cord prolapse in any setting are at risk for low 5-min Apgar scores, a need for assisted ventilation, low cord pH, meconium aspiration, and neonatal seizures. They also have greater (but still low) risks of neonatal encephalopathy and cerebral palsy (Ahmed & Hamdy, 2018).

In recent years, the incidence of umbilical cord prolapse has decreased overall, possibly due to the decrease in vaginal breech births, the increasing rate of cesarean birth, and the decreasing rate of grand multiparity (Hehir et al., 2021). In Ireland, for example, survival improved from 46% to 94% from 1940 to 2009 because of improvements in diagnosis, interventions that maintain cord perfusion during prolapse, improved neonatal management, and better preparation of providers through drills and simulations (Ahmed & Hamdy, 2018). Mortality remains as high as 27% in some African countries, however (Wong, Kwan, et al., 2021).

In most cases of umbilical cord prolapse, emergency cesarean birth is the preferred route of birth. Vaginal delivery is recommended only if birth is imminent and expected to proceed quickly (Ahmed & Hamdy, 2018; Bush et al., 2022; Cunningham et al., 2022, ch. 23; RCOG, 2014). In one study of hospital-based vaginal birth with cord prolapse, only 5% of babies born within 10 min had 5-min Apgar scores lower than 7 (RCOG, 2014). When vaginal birth took 20–30 min, 71% had 5-min Apgar scores less than 7 and required extensive resuscitation (RCOG, 2014).

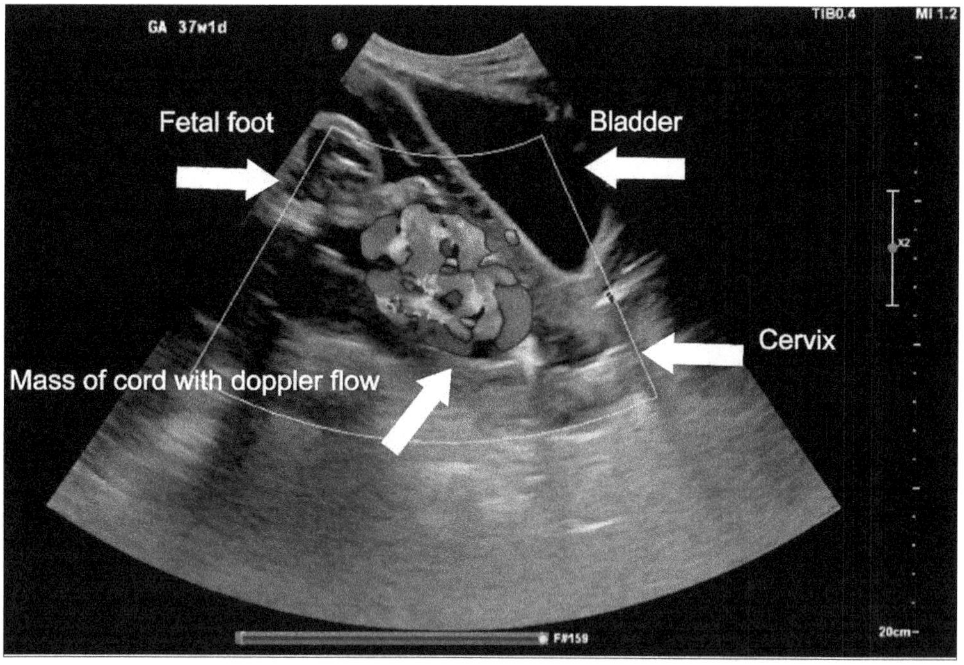

Figure 11-51. This woman was being induced for a medical complication of pregnancy at 37 weeks of gestation. Vertex presentation was verified with a bedside ultrasound scan upon arrival at the hospital. A cervical ripening balloon was placed, and was expelled into the vagina a few hours later. Sometime during the ripening process, the fetus changed position and the presentation could not be determined by Leopold's maneuvers or vaginal examination. A stat ultrasound showed a funic presentation, with the fetus in transverse lie and a fetal foot pushing the cord down into the cervix. Her cervix was 4 cm dilated, but the amnion was intact, preventing cord prolapse. She underwent urgent cesarean section. The baby was born with 9/9 Apgar scores. Author's case, used with permission.

Risk Factors

Maternal and fetal risk factors for cord prolapse include multiple gestation, grand multiparity, maternal uterine anomalies, uterine fibroids, polyhydramnios, and fetal presentation other than vertex, particularly breech and transverse lie (Pagan et al., 2020). Other risk factors include male fetal sex, umbilical cord length greater than 75 cm, minimal to absent coiling, low volume of Wharton's jelly, abnormal placentation, and marginal cord insertion (Pagan et al., 2020). Although preterm labor carries a higher risk of umbilical cord prolapse because of the smaller size of the fetus, higher likelihood of malpresentation, and greater amniotic fluid volume relative to fetal size, most cases of umbilical cord prolapse occur in term pregnancies (Ahmed & Hamdy, 2018). Further, cord prolapse can occur in pregnancies without risk factors (Ahmed & Hamdy, 2018).

Some authorities attribute almost 50% of umbilical cord prolapse cases to obstetric interventions; others found little correlation (Pagan et al., 2020). It is difficult to determine whether prolapse would have occurred spontaneously if the intervention had not been performed (Bush et al., 2022). Up to 57% of cases of umbilical cord prolapse occur within 5 min of membrane rupture, whether artificial or spontaneous (Pagan et al., 2020). Amniotomy undertaken with cervical dilation of 6 cm or less increases the risk of cord prolapse even when the fetus is well engaged (Kawakita, Huang, & Landy, 2018). Other interventions associated with cord prolapse include use of fetal scalp electrodes, intrauterine pressure catheters, manual rotation of the fetal head, and amnioinfusion (Bush et al., 2022). Cervical ripening balloons seem to increase the risk of cord prolapse only when filled with 150 ml of fluid (Hasegawa et al., 2017), as is common practice in Japan, but not with 60 ml or less, as in Western countries (Pagan et al., 2020).

Managing Umbilical Cord Prolapse

Although a visible or palpable umbilical cord in or hanging out of the vagina is diagnostic of overt cord prolapse, a nonreassuring fetal heart pattern is often the only evidence for compound cord presentation or funic presentation. Fetal bradycardia or variable decelerations are present in only 41–67% of cases of cord prolapse (Pagan et al., 2020). The cord may be palpable on vaginal examination or felt by the client if it is prolapsed, but compound cord presentation may not be diagnosed until birth, if at all. Prolapse can occur at any cervical dilation from minimal to complete, but it is most common at 5–6 cm and –1 to –2 station (Bush et al., 2022). Check the FHT and perform a digital vaginal examination, noting the presence of cord or limbs in the vagina. Check fetal presentation, station, and cervical dilation. If a tense, intact bag of waters is bulging into the vagina, sonographic imaging may be necessary to determine whether it contains a loop of umbilical cord (Wong, Kwan, et al., 2021).

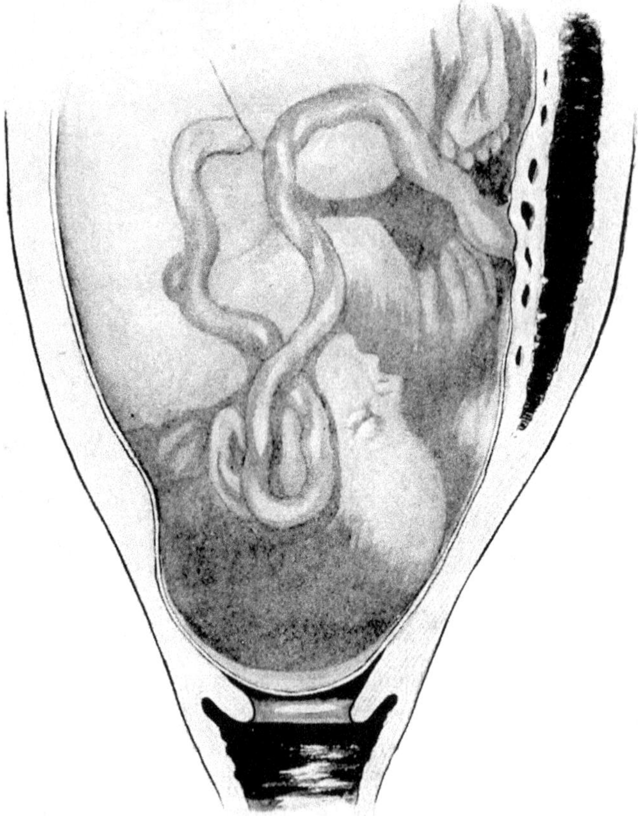

Figure 11-52. Compound cord presentation (occult cord prolapse) occurs when the cord is alongside the presenting fetal part. From *The Principles and Practice of Obstetrics* (p. 627, fig. 533), by J. B. De Lee, 1914, Philadelphia, PA: W. B. Saunders. In the public domain.

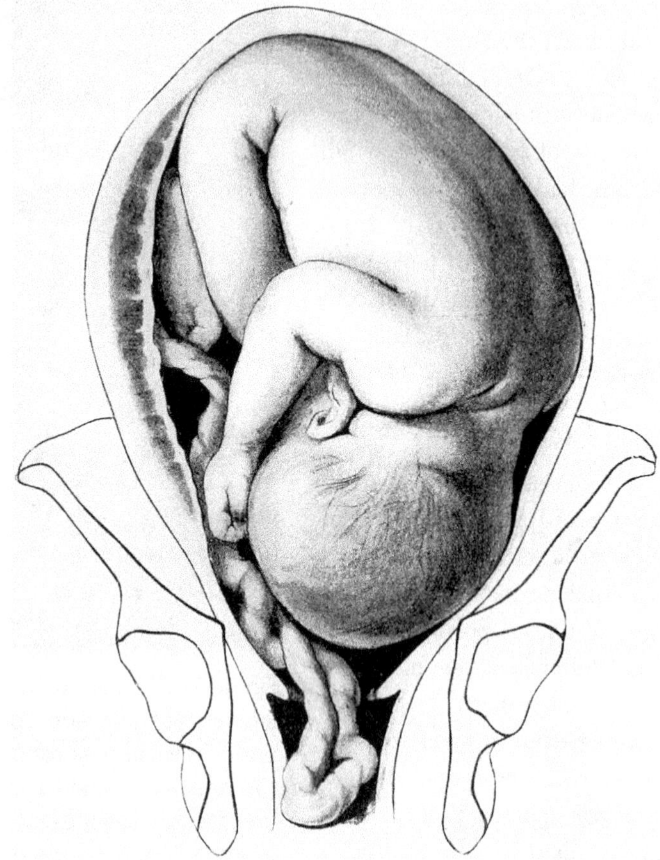

Figure 11-53. Umbilical cord prolapse occurs when the cord drops down ahead of the presenting part into or through the vagina. From *Operative Midwifery* (p. 132) by J. M. Munro Kerr, 1908, New York, NY: William Wood. In the public domain.

DIFFERENTIAL DIAGNOSES

Differential diagnoses for abnormal FHR patterns include maternal hypotension, uteroplacental insufficiency, umbilical cord compression, placental abruption, uterine rupture, abnormally frequent contractions, or vasa previa (Bush et al., 2022).

Get Help and Assign Tasks

If umbilical cord prolapse occurs at a home birth, have a family member or assistant call EMS immediately. At a freestanding birth center, convene all personnel present to assist. Activate emergency services and assign helpers to tasks such as faxing records and putting your telephone on speaker so you can give report to the receiving facility while taking care of the client.

Improve Oxygenation

Optimal fetal oxygenation is the goal, whether the baby is born vaginally or by cesarean section. Interventions to alleviate cord compression should be initiated immediately and until birth (Pagan et al., 2020). If the amniotic membranes are intact, take care to avoid accidental rupture (Wong, Kwan, et al., 2021).

Place the mother in the mother in the position that yields the best FHR. IV fluids expand intravascular volume and can improve perfusion of tissues. There is no evidence that maternal oxygen therapy improves umbilical artery pH or other neonatal outcomes. ACOG and RCOG discourage maternal oxygen supplementation for the management of an abnormal FHR tracing unless pulse oximetry shows the mother to be hypoxemic (ACOG Cmte. on Clinical Practice Guidelines—Obstetrics, Caughey, Gandhi, Kaimal, & Low, 2022/2023; Ahmed & Hamdy, 2018; Chatelet et al., 2022; RCOG, 2014).

Relieve Cord Compression

In most cases, you should use a combination of the following techniques to improve circulation through the umbilical cord:

Reposition the Mother

Immediately change maternal position to reduce pressure on the cord. The best position is the one that yields the best FHR. The knee-chest position is one of the most effective interventions for relieving cord compression (Wong, Kwan, et al., 2021). Turning the mother to knee-chest usually causes the fetus to shift toward the maternal diaphragm, sometimes retracting the cord, and may move the fetus out of your reach. In a moving ambulance, however, knee-chest may be challenging or unsafe to maintain.

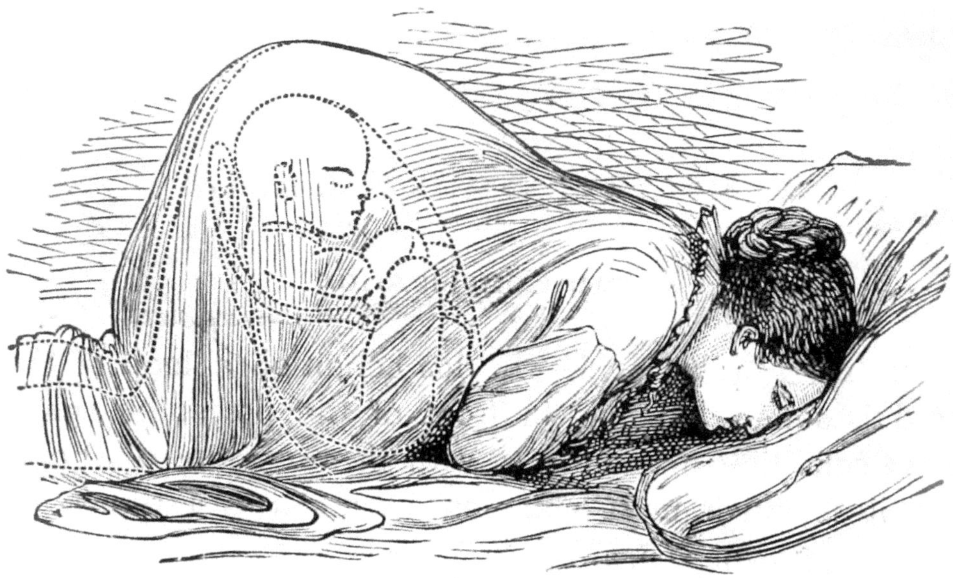

Figure 11-54. The knee-chest position tends to move the baby toward the maternal chest and navel and may cause the prolapsed cord to withdraw into the uterus. From *Practical Text-Book of Midwifery for Nurses and Students* (p. 202), by R. Jardine, 1899, New York, NY: Macmillan. In the public domain.

The Trendelenburg position is an alternative to knee-chest in which the head of the bed is tilted to about 15° below horizontal, so the maternal pelvis is higher than the head. In this position, gravity helps the fetus shift toward the uterine fundus (Wong, Kwan, et al., 2021). You may also elevate the maternal buttocks with a thick pillow or wedge (Wong, Kwan, et al., 2021). If necessary, a steeper Trendelenburg position (–30°) may be considered (Wong, Kwan, et al., 2021). You may also try modified Sims'/left lateral with pillows under the hip (Wong, Kwan, et al., 2021).

Manually Displace the Presenting Part

Elevating the presenting part greatly improves neonatal outcome (RCOG, 2014). Don sterile gloves, apply lubrication, and insert as much as your hand into the vagina as possible. The vaginas of most multiparous clients and many nulliparous ones can accommodate your entire hand during labor. Find the presenting part of the fetus and gently elevate it to relieve pressure on the cord. You will usually feel the fetus move entirely out of the pelvis into the upper uterine cavity. Once the fetus is disengaged, more loops of cord may prolapse (Wong, Kwan, et al., 2021). If you use arm strength alone to maintain fetal displacement, your muscles are likely to fatigue quickly. Try cupping your elbow in the palm of your free hand and leaning onto the internal arm, using your body weight to maintain pressure. *Avoid contact with the cord. Any pressure can cause the vessels within to spasm* (Boushra, Stone, & Rathbun, 2023).

It can be difficult to maintain elevation of the presenting part over a long and bumpy ambulance ride, and the situation could be potentially hazardous if the midwife chooses to forgo seat belt and shoulder harness to provide manual displacement in a moving vehicle. If FHT are reassuring after you displace the presenting part, RCOG (2014) advises that you may consider removing your hand from the vagina and maintaining displacement by applying continuous external suprapubic pressure upward or retrofilling the bladder (see below). Monitor FHR and let the rate and pattern guide your actions. Consider administering terbutaline (250 mcg SC) to weaken or stop uterine contractions. Each contraction forces the baby down toward the cervix and may increase cord compression while challenging the strength of anyone providing manual resistance.

You must maintain fetal displacement until the baby is delivered by cesarean section at the hospital. The surgical team will typically transfer the mother to the operating table with your hand still inserted in the vagina, quickly layer surgical drapes over both of you, and initiate general anesthesia. You should withdraw your hand only when the surgeon lifts the baby out of the abdomen from above.

Consider Retrofilling the Bladder

Another strategy for elevating the presenting part (by two stations) is to use the Vagos method of retrofilling the bladder (Kwan et al., 2021). The technique involves inserting an indwelling urinary catheter, infusing normal saline (NS) into the bladder, then clamping the catheter to retain the fluid (Kwan et al., 2021). Distending the bladder can also decrease uterine contractions and assist in relieving cord compression (Pagan et al., 2020).

Bladder filling seems to be a useful intervention only when the fetal presenting part is low in the pelvis (Kwan et al., 2021). If the fetus is already out of the pelvis, retrofilling the bladder is unlikely to change fetal station. Another

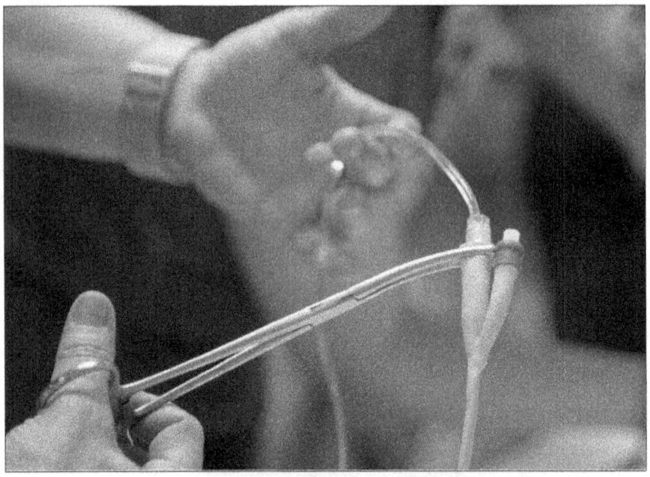

Figure 11-55. Attaching infusion tubing to a urinary catheter. Before retrofilling the bladder, use surgical clamps to attach the infusion tubing to the urinary catheter if the connectors are incompatible. Photograph by the author, taken at a Birth Emergency Skills Training Live Simulation Workshop. If this intervention were performed with a client, gloves would be used.

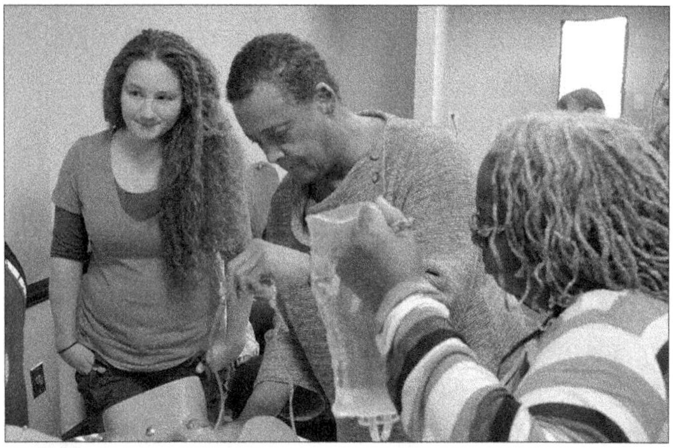

Figure 11-56. Infuse 500–750 ml of saline into the bladder while maintaining manual displacement of the presenting part. If the full bladder sustains the displacement, you may remove your hand. The preferred intervention is the one that yields optimal fetal heart tones (FHT). Photograph by the author, taken at a Birth Emergency Skills Training Live Simulation Workshop. If this intervention were performed with a client, gloves would be used.

disadvantage of this technique is the time needed to assemble the equipment, catheterize the bladder, about 2 min, and refill the bladder, a further 2–4 min (Wong, Kwan, et al., 2021). Bladder infusion should not delay transport, but it can often be accomplished while awaiting the ambulance. Save time by assembling the necessary equipment into a cord-prolapse kit beforehand. Ideally the bladder should be filled until it causes swelling above the pubis.

Technique for Bladder Retrofilling

- While you maintain manual pressure on the presenting part, your assistant should attach infusion tubing to a 1,000-ml bag of NS and prime the tubing.
- Catheterization can be accomplished with the client supine with pillows under the hips in modified Sims' position or in knee-chest, with or without the provider's hand in the vagina displacing the presenting part. Drain the bladder of urine using an indwelling (Foley) catheter (Chapman & Charles, 2018), then fill the catheter balloon with saline to hold it in place.
- Attach the infusion tubing to the urinary catheter. If the connectors are incompatible, you may be able to use a surgical clamp to attach them as shown in Figure 11-55.
- Use gravity or pressure on the bag of fluid to fill the bladder. If you roll the top of the IV fluid bag like a tube of toothpaste or squeeze it with a blood-pressure cuff, it will infuse faster. Fill the bladder to 500 ml, then close the roller clamp on the infusion set.
- Monitor FHT continuously. If the fetus remains bradycardic after the fluid infuses, allow more fluid to flow into the bladder to a maximum of 750 ml (Wong, Kwan, et al., 2021). Cross-clamp the catheter with a second surgical clamp and remove the infusion set.
- The bladder must be drained before birth. The client may experience uncomfortable fullness and bladder cramping *en route*, which can worsen during a long transport.

Stop Uterine Activity

If the mother is in active labor, tocolytic medication can be used to weaken or halt contractions, improving fetal oxygenation and making the mother more comfortable. Terbutaline 0.25 mg (250 mcg) SC is the agent of choice (Ahmed & Hamdy, 2018). The use of tocolytic medications can increase the risk of uterine atony and postpartum hemorrhage.

Consider Replacing the Cord

Vaginal replacement: The umbilical vessels may spasm if the cord becomes cool and dry. Some authorities recommend gently replacing any exposed cord back into the vagina and keeping it wet with moist gauze if this can be accomplished with minimal manipulation and compression (Bush et al., 2022; Marshall & Raynor, 2014).

Uterine replacement: Many experts advise against manually replacing the prolapsed cord into the uterus because of the risk of cord compression and subsequent bradycardia (Marshall & Raynor, 2014; RCOG, 2014). Others, including Barrett (1991) and Bush et al. (2022), note the potential for benefits such as improvement in the fetal heart pattern. If the client is distant from the hospital, or if severe FHR decelerations or bradycardia are unresponsive to all other interventions, then reduction of the cord into the uterus may be considered upon the advice of the collaborating physician (Pagan et al., 2020). Administer terbutaline before attempting cord replacement if the mother is in active labor. After the head is displaced from the pelvis, the cord is slipped over the widest part of the head and placed in the nuchal area (Bush et al., 2022). Once all the cord is in the uterus, the head is then gently guided toward the pelvis to block further escape of the umbilical cord (Bush et al., 2022). Attempt to replace the cord only if the prolapsed segment is short, cervical dilation is at least 4 cm, and the fetal presenting part is at or above −1 station (Wong, Kwan, et al., 2021). Abandon the attempt if not successful within 2 min (Wong, Kwan et al., 2021). You may have more success with the mother in knee-chest or Trendelenburg.

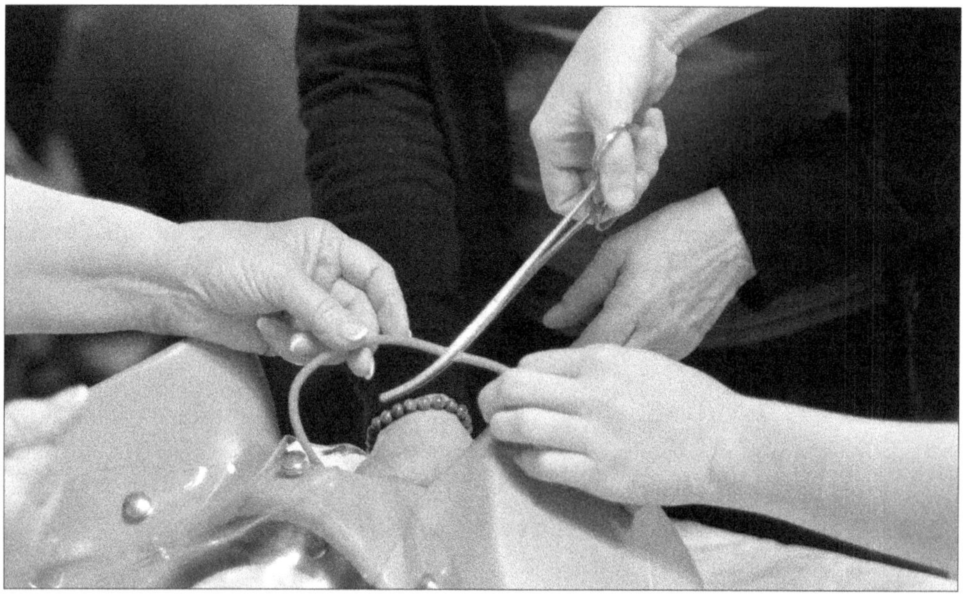

Figure 11-57. When 500–750 ml of fluid has been infused, cross-clamp the urinary catheter, disconnect the infusion kit, and secure it to the mother's leg. Photograph by the author, taken at a Birth Emergency Skills Training Live Simulation Workshop. If this intervention were performed with a client, gloves would be used.

Monitor FHR

Continuously monitor FHR with a Doppler device until birth is accomplished. Any fetus can deteriorate quickly and unpredictably and can suffer severe anoxic injury or death regardless of the time from prolapse to birth (Wong, Tse, et al., 2021). In one study (Wong, Tse et al., 2021), FHR was normal in 43.9% of cases, showed recurrent decelerations in 26.3%, and demonstrated persistent bradycardia in 29.8%. Intermittent cord compression during uterine contractions can result in variable or late decelerations or a combination of both (Wong, Tse, et al., 2021). Decelerations can sometimes be improved with an intervention such as changing maternal position or elevating the presenting part. Fetal bradycardia in the 90s suggests that the fetus is compensating for a partial disruption in gas exchange while maintaining adequate cardiac output (Wong, Tse, et al., 2021).

Severe fetal bradycardia is associated not only with cord compression, but also with umbilical vasospasm; FHR is unlikely to recover even if the cord compression is relieved (Wong, Tse et al., 2021). Bradycardia in the 60s or lower can indicate severe hypoxia or anoxia; profoundly depressed fetal cardiac output; and tissue acidemia leading to neurologic, cardiac, renal, or hepatic injury (Wong, Tse, et al., 2021). In a related study, researchers found that in cases of cord prolapse presenting with fetal bradycardia, the risk of severe acidosis (pH below 7) was 80% when bradycardia-to-birth interval was longer than 20 min, but only 17.2% when it was shorter (Wong, Kwan, et al. 2021). Prepare to resuscitate the infant in any case of cord prolapse.

Immediate Transport

Rapid transport to definitive care is critical for good outcomes. The fetus risks anoxia and death after only about 4 min of lost umbilical blood flow. Although there is general agreement among authorities that diagnosis-to-birth time of less than 20 min yields the best perinatal outcomes (Ahmed & Hamdy, 2018; Pagan et al., 2020; Wong, Tse, et al., 2021), the key determinants of fetal health appear to be the degree of cord compression and fetal condition before the event (Wong, Tse, et al., 2021). If the fetus was compromised before the prolapse, the interval from occlusion to damage is shorter. Research suggests that elevating the fetal presenting part and relieving cord compression are as important to a good outcome as the time to birth, perhaps more so (Khan, Naru, & Nizami, 2007).

Debriefing

Umbilical cord prolapse and emergency cesarean section can be traumatic for the provider, the client, the baby, and any support people present. It is helpful for the midwifery team, the ambulance crew, and the hospital team to debrief within a few days of the incident. In debriefing the family, include descriptions of what happened, steps taken to manage the problem and why they were necessary, and any implications for future births. People who experience trauma often have difficulty processing information in the first hours and days after the event. Over the postpartum period, give the client the opportunity to debrief, discuss, and express emotion.

Topics for Discussion

1. Explain the advantages of upright positioning for unexpected breech birth.
2. Kallie Jane M., G5 P4, has come to the birth center for a labor check. She says, "I'm not so sure this baby is in the right position." You do not have an ultrasound machine available. Describe how you would determine whether the fetus is transverse lie, breech, face presentation, or asynclitic and how you would manage each of these findings.
3. Describe the protected-space technique for breech birth.
4. Marianne W., G6 P5, is completely dilated with a persistently asynclitic fetus at –2 station. She has pushed an hour without descent. The FHT are normal. What options does the midwife have?
5. Margery J., G4 P3, has had a long, slow labor with a LOP fetus, but now is finally dilated to 10 cm and is –2 station. The FHT are normal. The first three pushes did not bring the baby any lower. What options does the midwife have?
6. Agnes C., G2 P1 at 40 0/7 weeks of gestation, is in active labor in the tub at your freestanding birth center. At her last cervical check an hour ago, she was 8 cm dilated. As she crests a strong contraction, her water breaks in a cloud of thick meconium fluid. As the water clears, you see a long blue umbilical cord floating in the water between her legs. What do you do?

References

Aguiar, T., Cavaco Gomes, J., & Rodrigues, T. (2021). Cord presentation in labour: Imminent risk of cord prolapse. *BMJ Case Reports, 14*(5), e243320. https://doi.org/10.1136/bcr-2021-243320

Ahmed, W. A. S., & Hamdy, M. A. (2018). Optimal management of umbilical cord prolapse. *International Journal of Women's Health, 10*, 459–465. https://doi.org/10.2147/IJWH.S130879

Almassinokiani, F., Ahani, N., Akbari, P., Rahimzadeh, P., Akbari, H., & Sharifzadeh, F. (2020). Comparative analgesic effects of intradermal and subdermal injection of sterile water on active labor pain. *Anesthesiology and Pain Medicine, 10*(2), e99867. https://doi.org/10.5812/aapm.99867

American College of Nurse-Midwives. (2015). Midwifery provision of home birth services (Clinical Bulletin 14). *Journal of Midwifery & Women's Health, 61*(1), 127–133. https://doi.org/10.1111/jmwh.12431

American College of Obstetricians and Gynecologists. (2014). *reVITALize obstetric data definitions* (version 1.0). Retrieved from https://www.acog.org/-/media/project/acog/acogorg/files/pdfs/publications/revitalize-ob.pdf?la=en&hash=-D9ECE1577C2A0B535F42C1B8DC492070

American College of Obstetricians and Gynecologists. (2018, reaffirmed 2023). *Mode of term singleton breech delivery* (Committee Opinion 745, interim update). Retrieved from https://www.acog.org/clinical/clinical-guidance/committee-opinion/articles/2018/08/mode-of-term-singleton-breech-delivery

American College of Obstetricians and Gynecologists. (2020, reaffirmed 2023). *External cephalic version* (Practice Bulletin 221). Retrieved from https://www.acog.org/clinical/clinical-guidance/practice-bulletin/articles/2020/05/external-cephalic-version

American College of Obstetricians and Gynecologists. (2024). First and second stage labor management (Clinical Practice Guideline 8). Obstetrics & Gynecology, 143(1), 144–162. Retrieved from https://www.acog.org/-/media/project/acog/acogorg/clinical/files/clinical-practice-guideline/articles/2024/01/first-and-second-stage-labor-management.pdf

American College of Obstetricians and Gynecologists Committee on Clinical Practice Guidelines—Obstetrics, Caughey, A., Gandhi, M., Kaimal, A. J., & Low, L. K. (2022, reaffirmed 2023). *Oxygen supplementation in the setting of category II or III fetal heart tracings* (Practice Advisory). Retrieved from https://www.acog.org/clinical/clinical-guidance/practice-advisory/articles/2022/01/oxygen-supplementation-in-the-setting-of-category-ii-or-iii-fetal-heart-tracings

Anim-Somuah, M., Smyth, R. M. D., Cyna, A. M., & Cuthbert A. (2018). Epidural versus non-epidural or no analgesia for pain management in labour. *Cochrane Database of Systematic Reviews*. https://doi.org/10.1002/14651858.CD000331.pub4

Argani, C. H., & Satin, A. J., (2022). Occiput posterior position. In V. A. Barss (Ed.), *UpToDate*. Retrieved November 14, 2023, from http://www.uptodate.com/contents/occiput-posterior-position

Ashwin, C., & Anderson, M. (2017). *Myles pocket reference for midwives* (E-Book). (n.p.): Elsevier Health Sciences.

Barrera, E., & Acosta, L. (2022). Spinning Babies® a professional development program for birth workers to reduce c-section rates. In *2022 SMH Best Practice Fair*. 8. Retrieved from https://scholarlycommons.baptisthealth.net/se-2022-smh-bpf/8

Barrett, J. M. (1991). Funic reduction for the management of umbilical cord prolapse. *American Journal of Obstetrics & Gynecology, 165*(3), 654–657. https://doi.org/10.1016/0002-9378(91)90303-9

Barth, W. H., Jr. (2015). Persistent occiput posterior. *Obstetrics & Gynecology, 125*(3), 695–709. https://doi.org/10.1097/AOG.0000000000000647

Barth, W. H., Jr. (2021). Malpresentations and malposition. In M. B. Landon, H. L. Galan, E. R. M. Jauniaux, D. A. Driscoll, V. Berghella, W. A. Grobman, . . . A. G. Cahill (Eds.). *Gabbe's obstetrics: Normal and problem pregnancies* (8th ed., Kindle version, ch. 17). Philadelphia, PA: Elsevier Health Sciences.

Barth, W. H., Jr. (2023). Compound fetal presentation. In V. A. Barss (Ed.), *UpToDate*. Retrieved November 14, 2023, from http://www.uptodate.com/contents/compound-fetal-presentation

Berhan, Y., & Haileamlak, A. (2016). The risks of planned vaginal breech delivery versus planned caesarean section for term breech birth: A meta-analysis including observational studies. *BJOG, 123*(1), 49–57. https://doi.org/10.1111/1471-0528.13524

Berta, M., Lindgren, H., Christensson, K., Mekonnen, S., & Adefris, M. (2019). Effect of maternal birth positions on duration of second stage of labor: Systematic review and meta-analysis. *BMC Pregnancy and Childbirth, 19*, 466. https://doi.org/10.1186/s12884-019-2620-0

Bertholdt, C., Morel, O., Zuily, S., & Ambroise-Grandjean, G. (2022). Manual rotation of occiput posterior or transverse positions: A systematic review and meta-analysis of randomized controlled trials. *American Journal of Obstetrics & Gynecology, 226*(6), 781–793. https://doi.org/10.1016/j.ajog.2021.11.033

Bertholdt, C., Piffer, A., Pol, H., Morel, O., & Guerby, P. (2021). Management of persistent occiput posterior position: The added value of manual rotation. *International Journal of Gynecology & Obstetrics, 157(3), 613–617.* https://doi.org/10.1002/ijgo.13874

Beuckens, A., Rijnders, M., Verburgt-Doeleman, G. H. M., Rijninks-van Driel, G. C., Thorpe, J., & Hutton, E. K. (2016). An observational study of the success and complications of 2546 external cephalic versions in low-risk pregnant women performed by trained midwives. *BJOG, 123*(3), 415–423. https://doi.org/10.1111/1471-0528.13234

Bjellmo, S., Andersen, G. L., Martinussen, M. P., Romundstad, P. R., Hjelle, S., Moster, D., & Vik, T. (2017). Is vaginal breech delivery associated with higher risk for perinatal death and cerebral palsy compared with vaginal cephalic birth? Registry-based cohort study in Norway. *BMJ Open, 7*(4), e014979. https://doi.org/10.1136/bmjopen-2016-014979

Blanc, J., Castel, P., Mauviel, F., Baumstarck, K., Bretelle, F., Haumonté, J. B., & D'Ercole, C. (2021). Prophylactic manual rotation of persistent occiput posterior to decrease operative delivery: A multicentric randomized trial. *American Journal of Obstetrics & Gynecology, 224*(2), S2. https://doi.org/10.1016/j.ajog.2020.12.105

Bogner, G., Strobl, M., Schausberger, C., Fischer, T., Reisenberger, K., & Jacobs, V. R. (2015). Breech delivery in the all fours position: A prospective observational comparative study with classic assistance. *Journal of Perinatal Medicine, 43*(6),707–713. https://doi.org/10.1515/jpm-2014-0048

Boushra, M., Stone, A., & Rathbun, K. M. (2023). Umbilical cord prolapse. In *StatPearls*. Treasure Island, FL: StatPearls Publishing. Retrieved from https://www.ncbi.nlm.nih.gov/books/NBK542241/

Bovbjerg, M. L., Cheyney, M., Brown, J., Cox, K. J., & Leeman, L. (2017). Perspectives on risk: assessment of risk profiles and outcomes among women planning community birth in the United States. *Birth, 44*(3), 209–221. https://doi.org/0.1111/birt.12288

Breech Without Borders. (n.d.). *Vaginal breech maneuvers*. Retrieved from https://www.breechwithoutborders.org/maneuvers/

Breech Without Borders. (2020). *Mechanics of breech birth*. Retrieved from https://www.breechwithoutborders.org/mechanics/

Broberg, J. C., & Caughey, A. B. (2021). A randomized controlled trial of prophylactic early manual rotation of the occiput posterior fetus at the beginning of the second stage vs expectant management. *American Journal of Obstetrics & Gynecology MFM, 3*(2), 100327. https://doi.org/10.1016/j.ajogmf.2021.100327

Brothers, A. (1896). *Infantile mortality during child-birth and its prevention*. Philadelphia, PA: P. Blakiston. Retrieved from https://archive.org/details/infantilemortali1896brot

Bue, L., & Lauszus, F. F. (2016). Moxibustion did not have an effect in a randomised clinical trial for version of breech position. *Danish Medical Journal, 63*(2), A5199. Retrieved from http://ugeskriftet.dk/files/scientific_article_files/2018-11/a5199.pdf

Bueno-Lopez, V., Fuentelsaz-Gallego, C., Casellas-Caro, M., Falgueras-Serrano, A. M., Crespo-Berros, S., Silvano-Cocinero, A. M., . . . Terré-Rull, C. (2018). Efficiency of the modified Sims maternal position in the rotation of persistent occiput posterior position during labor: A randomized clinical trial. *Birth, 45*(4), 385–392. https://doi.org/10.1111/birt.12347

Burgos, J., Melchor, J. C., Cobos, P., Centeno, M., Pijoan, J. I., Fernandez-Liebrez, L., & Martinez-Astorquiza, T. (2009). Does fetal weight estimated by ultrasound really affect the success rate of external cephalic version? *Acta Obstetricia et Gynecologica Scandinavica, 88*(1), 1101–1106. https://doi.org/10.1080/00016340903176792

Bush, M., Eddleman, K., & Belogolovkin, V. (2022). Umbilical cord prolapse. In V. A. Barss (Ed.), *UpToDate*. Retrieved November 14, 2023, from https://www.uptodate.com/contents/umbilical-cord-prolapse

Caldwell. W. E., & Moloy, H. C. (1933). Anatomical variations in the female pelvis and their effect in labour with a suggested classification. *American Journal of Obstetrics & Gynecology, 26*(4), 479–505. https://doi.org/10.1016/S0002-9378(33)90194-5

Carbillon, L., Benbara, A., Tigaizin, A., Murtada, R., Fermaut, M., Belmaghni, F., . . . Boujenah, J. (2020). Revisiting the management of term breech presentation: A proposal for overcoming some of the controversies. *BMC Pregnancy and Childbirth, 20*(1), 263. https://doi.org/10.1186/s12884-020-2831-4

Caughey, A. B. (2023). Occiput transverse position. In V. A. Barss (Ed.), *UpToDate*. Retrieved November 14, 2023, from http://www.uptodate.com/contents/occiput-transverse-position

Chapman, V., & Charles, C. (Eds.). (2018). *The midwife's labour and birth handbook* (4th ed.). Hoboken, NJ: John Wiley & Sons.

Chatelet, M., Lemoine, L., Balouet, P., Eudier, F., Saleh, A., Delomas, T., & Amiot, F. (2022). Umbilical cord prolapse in the prehospital setting: A case report. *Prehospital Emergency Care, 26*(2), 311–313. https://doi.org/10.1080/10903127.2021.1890285

Chawanpaiboon, S., Ciardelli, V., Chitty, L., & Pierro, A. (2002). Axillary cystic hygroma: A report of two cases. *Thai Journal of Obstetrics and Gynaecology, 14*(2), 163–167. Retrieved from https://tci-thaijo.org/index.php/tjog/article/download/88821/pdf_154

Cheyney, M., Bovbjerg, M., Everson, C., Gordon, W., Hannibal, D., & Vedam, S. (2014). Outcomes of care for 16,924 planned home births in the United States: The Midwives Alliance of North America Statistics Project, 2004 to 2009. *Journal of Midwifery & Women's Health, 59*(1), 17–27. https://doi.org/10.1111/jmwh.12172

Cillard, L., Verhaeghe, C., Spiers, A., Madzou, S., Descamps, P., Legendre, G., & Corroenne, R. (2021). External cephalic version: Predictors for success. *Journal of Gynecology Obstetrics and Human Reproduction, 50*(9), 102165. https://doi.org/10.1016/j.jogoh.2021.102165

Cohen, S. R., & Thomas, C. R. (2015). Rebozo technique for fetal malposition in labor. *Journal of Midwifery & Women's Health, 60*(4), 445–451. https://doi.org/10.1111/jmwh.12352

Coulon, C., Poleszczuk, M., Paty-Montaigne, M.-H., Gascard, C., Gay, C., Houfflin-Debarge, V., & Subtil, D. (2014). Version of breech fetuses by moxibustion with acupuncture: A randomized controlled trial. *Obstetrics & Gynecology, 124*(1), 32–39. https://doi.org/10.1097/AOG.0000000000000303

Coyle, M. E., Smith, C., & Peat, B. (2023). Cephalic version by moxibustion for breech presentation. *Cochrane Database of Systematic Reviews*. https://doi.org/10.1002/14651858.CD003928.pub4

Cunningham, F. G., Leveno, K. J., Dashe, J. S., Hoffman, B. L., Spong, C. Y., & Casey, B. M. (Eds.). (2022). *Williams obstetrics* (26th ed., Kindle version). New York, NY: McGraw-Hill.

Dahl, C. M., Zhang, Y., Ong, J. X., Yeh, C., Son, M., Miller, E. S., . . . Grobman, W. A. (2021). Patient characteristics associated with complications of external cephalic version. *American Journal of Obstetrics & Gynecology MFM, 3(5*), 100411. https://doi.org/10.1016/j.ajogmf.2021.100411

Dahlen, H. G., Homer, C. S. E., Leap, N., & Tracy, S. K. (2010). From social to surgical: Historical perspectives on perineal care during labour and birth. *Women and Birth, 24*(3), 105–111. https://doi.org/10.1016/j.wombi.2010.09.002

Dakin, W. R. (1897). *A handbook of midwifery*. London, United Kingdom: Longmans, Green, & Co. Retrieved from https://archive.org/details/handbookofmidwif00daki

Davis, E. P. (1911). *Operative obstetrics, including the surgery of the newborn*. Philadelphia, PA: W. B. Saunders. Retrieved from https://ia800306.us.archive.org/14/items/operativeobstetr00davi/operativeobstetr00davi.pdf

de Vries, B., Phipps, H., Kuah, S., Pardey, J., Matthews, G., Ludlow, J., . . . Hyett, J. A. (2021). Transverse position. Using rotation to aid normal birth-OUTcomes following manual rotation (The TURN-OUT Trial): A randomized controlled trial. *American Journal of Obstetrics & Gynecology MFM, 4*(1), 100488. https://doi.org/10.1016/j.ajogmf.2021.100488

de Hundt, M., Velzel, J., de Groot, C. J., Mol, B., & Kok, M. (2014). Mode of delivery after successful external cephalic version: A systematic review and meta-analysis. *Obstetrics & Gynecology, 123*(6), 1327–1334. https://doi.org/10.1097/AOG.0000000000000295

De Lee, J. B. (1914). *The principles and practice of obstetrics*. Philadelphia, PA: W. B. Saunders. Retrieved from https://archive.org/details/principlespracti00dele

Delprete, H. (2017). Pelvic inlet shape is not as dimorphic as previously suggested. *Anatomical Record, 300*(4), 706–715. https://doi.org/10.1002/ar.23544

Derry, S., Straube, S., Moore, R. A., Hancock, H., & Collins, S. L. (2012). Intracutaneous or subcutaneous sterile water injection compared with blinded controls for pain management in labour. *Cochrane Database of Systematic Reviews*. https://doi.org/10.1002/14651858.cd009107.pub2

Desbriere, R., Blanc, J., Le Dû, R., Renner, J. P., Carcopino, X., Loundou, A., & d'Ercole, C. (2013). Is maternal posturing during labor efficient in preventing persistent occiput posterior position? A randomized controlled trial. *American Journal of Obstetrics & Gynecology, 208*(1), 60-e1. https://doi.org/10.1016/j.ajog.2012.10.882

Dorland, W. A. N. (1896). *A manual of obstetrics*. Philadelphia, PA: W. B. Saunders.

Dunn, P. M. (2003). Erich Bracht (1882–1969) of Berlin and his "breech" manoeuvre. *Archives of Disease in Childhood—Fetal and Neonatal Edition, 88*(1), F76–F77. https://doi.org/10.1136/fn.88.1.F76

Ebrahimi, E., Haratipour, H., Partash, N., & Bolbolhaghighi, N. (2021). Non-physiological and physiological delivery method: Comparison of maternal attachment behaviors and anxiety. *Journal of Caring Sciences, 10*(1), 37–42. https://doi.org/10.34172/jcs.2021.011

Eggebø, T. M., & Hjartardottir, H. (2021). Descent of the presenting part assessed with ultrasound. *American Journal of Obstetrics & Gynecology*. https://doi.org/10.1016/j.ajog.2021.08.030

Elfazari, T., & El-Chaâr, D. (2023). Breech presentation. In G. D. Posner, A. Y. Black, G. Jones, & D. El-Chaâr (Eds.), *Oxorn-Foote human labor & birth* (7th ed., Kindle version, ch. 25). New York, NY: McGraw Hill.

Elmore, C., McBroom, K. & Ellis, J. (2020). Digital and manual rotation of the persistent occiput posterior fetus. *Journal of Midwifery & Women's Health, 65*(3), 387–394. https://doi.org/10.1111/jmwh.13118

Farin, A., Ceccaldi, P.-F., Tapie, L., Derisbourg, S., Desseauve, D., & Daelemans, C. (2023). Training for breech deliveries with the mother in an upright position: An innovative adaptation of a simulation model. *European Journal of Obstetrics & Gynecology and Reproductive Biology, 280*, 108–111. https://doi.org/10.1016/j.ejogrb.2022.11.015

Fischbein, S. J. (2015). "Home birth" with an obstetrician: A series of 135 out of hospital births. *Obstetrics & Gynecology International Journal, 2*(4), 00046. https://doi.org/10.15406/ogij.2015.02.00046

Fischbein, S. J., & Freeze, R. (2018). Breech birth at home: Outcomes of 60 breech and 109 cephalic planned home and birth center births. *BMC Pregnancy and Childbirth, 18*(1), 1–12. https://doi.org/10.1186/s12884-018-2033-5

Floyd, R. C., & Gimovsky, M. L. (2021). Breech presentation. In H. N. Winn, F. A. Chervenak, & R. Romero (Eds.), *Clinical maternal-fetal medicine online* (2nd ed., pp. 14.1–14.10). London, United Kingdom: CRC Press. Retrieved from https://www.taylorfrancis.com/chapters/oa-edit/10.1201/9781003222590-12/breech-presentation-randall-floyd-martin-gimovsky

Founds, S. A. (2005). Maternal posture for cephalic version of breech presentation: A review of the evidence. *Birth, 32*(2), 137–144. https://doi.org/10.1111/j.0730-7659.2005.00357.x

Founds, S. A. (2006). Clinical implications from an exploratory study of postural management of breech presentation. *Journal of Midwifery & Women's Health, 51*(4), 292–296. https://doi.org/10.1016%2Fj.jmwh.2005.11.010

Garber, A., & Dy, J. (2023). Normal mechanisms of labor. In G. D. Posner, A. Y. Black, G. Jones, & D. El-Chaâr (Eds.), *Oxorn-Foote human labor & birth* (7th ed., Kindle version, ch. 10). New York, NY: McGraw Hill.

García-Mochón, L., Martín, J. J., Aranda-Regules, J. M., Rivas-Ruiz, F., & Vas, J. (2015). Cost effectiveness of using moxibustion to correct non-vertex presentation. *Acupuncture in Medicine, 33*(2), 136–141. https://doi.org/10.1136/acupmed-2014-010696

Ghi, T., Eggebø, T., Lees, C., Kalachie, K., Rozenberg, P., Youssef, A., . . . Tutschek, B. (2018). ISUOG practice guidelines: Intrapartum ultrasound. *Ultrasound in Obstetrics & Gynecology, 52*(1), 128–139. https://doi.org/10.1002/uog.19072

Glezerman, M. (2006). Five years to the Term Breech Trial: The rise and fall of a randomized controlled trial. *American Journal of Obstetrics & Gynecology, 194*(1), 20–25. https://doi.org/10.1016/j.ajog.2005.08.039

Goffinet, F., Carayol, M., Foidart, J.-M., Alexander, S., Uzan, S., Subtil, D., . . . PREMODA Study Group. (2006). Is planned vaginal delivery for breech presentation at term still an option? Results of an observational prospective survey in France and Belgium. *American Journal of Obstetrics & Gynecology. 194*(4), 1002–1011. https://doi.org/10.1016/j.ajog.2005.10.817

Graham, K., Phipps, H., Hyett, J. A., Ludlow, J. P., Mackie, A., Marren, A., & De Vries, B. (2014). Persistent occiput posterior: OUTcomes following digital rotation: A pilot randomised controlled trial. *Australian and New Zealand Journal of Obstetrics and Gynaecology, 54*(3), 268–274. https://doi.org/10.1111/ajo.12192

Grünebaum, A., McCullough, L. B., Sapra, K. J., Arabin, B., & Chervenak, F. A. (2017). Planned home births: The need for additional contraindications. *American Journal of Obstetrics & Gynecology, 216*(4), 401.e1–401.e8. https://doi.org/10.1016/j.ajog.2017.01.012

Gupta, J. K., Sood, A., Hofmeyr, G. J., & Vogel, J. P. (2017). Position in the second stage of labour for women without epidural anaesthesia. *Cochrane Database of Systematic Reviews, 2017*(5). https://doi.org/10.1002/14651858.CD002006.pub4

Habek, D., Marton, I., Prka, M., & Luetić, A. (2017). Manual rotation in cases of the intrapartal arrest of fetal head. *European Journal of Obstetrics & Gynecology and Reproductive Biology, 219*, 66–67. https://doi.org/10.1016/j.ejogrb.2017.10.017

Haizler-Cohen, L., Fahimuddin, F. Z., Baxter, D., Sanghavi, K., Chornock, R. L., Saeed, H., . . . Mokhtari, N. (2023). Perinatal outcomes in pregnancies complicated by compound presentation at term. *American Journal of Obstetrics & Gynecology, 228*(1, Suppl.), S528. https://doi.org/10.1016/j.ajog.2022.11.903

Hannah, M. E., Hannah, W. J., Hewson, S. A., Hodnett, E. D., Saigal, S., & Willan, A. R. (2000). Planned caesarean section versus planned vaginal birth for breech presentation at term: A randomised multicentre trial. *Lancet, 356*(9239), 1375–1383. https://doi.org/10.1016/S0140-6736(00)02840-3

Hart, J., & Walker, A. (2007). Clinical rounds: Management of occiput posterior position. *Journal of Midwifery & Women's Health, 52*(5), 508–513. https://doi.org/10.1016/j.jmwh.2006.10.018

Hasegawa, J., Sekizawa, A., Arakaki, T., Ikeda, T., Ishiwata, I., Kinoshita, K., & Japan Association of Obstetricians and Gynecologists. (2020). Declined use of cervical ripening balloon did not reduce the incidence of umbilical cord prolapse in Japan. *Journal of Obstetrics and Gynaecology Research, 46*(8), 1349–1354. https://doi.org/10.1111/jog.14317

Hehir, M. P., Hartigan, L., & Mahony, R. (2017). Perinatal death associated with umbilical cord prolapse. *Journal of Perinatal Medicine, 45*(5), 565–570. https://doi.org/10.1515/jpm-2016-0223

Hirst, B. C. (1912). *A text-book of obstetrics* (7th ed.). Philadelphia, PA: W. B. Saunders. Retrieved from https://hdl.handle.net/2027/uva.x006070585

Hofmeyr, G. J. (2023a). Delivery of the singleton fetus in breech presentation. In V. A. Barss (Ed.), *UpToDate*. Retrieved November 14, 2023, from https://www.uptodate.com/contents/delivery-of-the-singleton-fetus-in-breech-presentation

Hofmeyr, G. J. (2023b). External cephalic version. In A. Chakrabarti (Ed.), *UpToDate*. Retrieved November 14, 2023, from https://www.uptodate.com/contents/external-cephalic-version

Hofmeyr, G. J. (2023c). Overview of breech presentation. In V. A. Barss (Ed.), *UpToDate*. Retrieved November 14, 2023, from https://www.uptodate.com/contents/overview-of-breech-presentation

Hofmeyr, G. J., & Kulier, R. (2012). Cephalic version by postural management for breech presentation. *Cochrane Database of Systematic Reviews*. https://doi.org/10.1002/14651858.CD000051.pub2

Hofmeyr, G. J., Kulier, R., & West, H. M. (2015). External cephalic version for breech presentation at term. *Cochrane Database of Systematic Reviews*. https://doi.org/10.1002/14651858.CD000083.pub3

Horasanlı, J. E., Demirbas, N., & Cıcek, S. (2023). Obstetric simulation training to breech delivery, shoulder dystocia, forceps, and vacuum experience. *Gynecology Obstetrics & Reproductive Medicine, 29*(1), 19–26. https://doi.org/10.21613/GORM.2022.1298

Howard, E. D. (2021). Evidence-based resources for the second stage of labor. *Journal of Perinatal & Neonatal Nursing, 35*(3), 201–203. https://doi.org/https://doi.org/10.1097/JPN.0000000000000584

Hunter, L. A. (2014). Vaginal breech birth: Can we move beyond the Term Breech Trial? *Journal of Midwifery & Women's Health, 59*(3), 320–327. https://doi.org/10.1111/jmwh.12198

Hunter, L. A. (2015). Complications during labor and birth. In, T. L. King, M. C. Brucker, J. Fahey, J. M. Kriebs, C. L. Gegor, & H. Varney, (Eds.), *Varney's midwifery* (5th ed., Kindle version, ch. 30). Burlington, MA: Jones & Bartlett.

Hutton, E. K. (2016). External cephalic version should be undertaken by midwives. *BJOG, 123*(3), 426. https://doi.org/10.1111/1471-0528.13821

Hutton, E. K., Kasperink, M., Rutten, M., Reitsma, A., & Wainman, B. (2009). Sterile water injection for labour pain: A systematic review and meta-analysis of randomised controlled trials. *BJOG, 116*(9), 1158–1166. https://doi.org/10.1111/j.1471-0528.2009.02221.x

Ibrahim, H., Said, H. & Elgzar, W. (2020). Effect of upright and ambulant positions versus lying down during the active first stage of labor on birth outcomes among nulliparous women: Randomized controlled clinical trial. *Frontiers of Nursing, 7*(3), 239–248. https://doi.org/10.2478/fon-2020-0035

Impey, L. W. M., Murphy, D. J., Griffiths, M., & Penna, L. K. (2017). Management of breech presentation. Green-Top Guideline 20b. *BJOG, 124*(7), e151–e177. https://doi.org/10.1111/1471-0528.14465

Iversen, J. K., Kahrs, B. H., & Eggebø, T. M. (2021). There are four, not seven cardinal movements in labor. *American Journal of Obstetrics & Gynecology MFM, 3*(6), 100436. https://doi.org/10.1016/j.ajogmf.2021.100436

Jardine, R. (1899). *Practical text-book of midwifery for nurses and students*. New York, NY: Macmillan. Retrieved from https://archive.org/details/practicaltextboo00jard

Jellett, H. (1905). *A manual of midwifery for students and practitioners*. London, United Kingdom: Baillière, Tindall & Cox. Retrieved from https://archive.org/details/b21932670

Jennewein, L., Brüggmann, D., Fischer, K., Raimann, F. J., Pfeifenberger, H. R., Agel, L., . . . Louwen. F. (2017). Learning breech birth in an upright position is influenced by preexisting experience—A FRABAT prospective cohort study. *Journal of Clinical Medicine, 10*(10), 2117. https://doi.org/10.3390/jcm10102117

Julien, S., & Galerneau, F. (2023). Face and brow presentations in labor. In V. A. Barss (Ed.), *UpToDate*. Retrieved November 14, 2023, from https://www.uptodate.com/contents/face-and-brow-presentations-in-labor

Kawakita, T., Huang, C.-C., & Landy, H. J. (2018). Risk factors for umbilical cord prolapse at the time of artificial rupture of membranes. *AJP Reports, 8*(2), e89-e94. https://doi.org/10.1055/s-0038-1649486

Kayem, G., Baumann, R., Goffinet, F., El Abiad, S., Ville, Y., Cabrol, D., & Haddad, B. (2008). Early preterm breech delivery: Is a policy of planned vaginal delivery associated with increased risk of neonatal death? *American Journal of Obstetrics & Gynecology, 198*(3), 289.e1–289.e6. https://doi.org/10.1016/j.ajog.2007.10.794

Kenfack, B., Ateudjieu, J., Ymele, F. F., Tebeu, P. M., Dohbit, J. S., & Mbu, R. E. (2012). Does the advice to assume the knee-chest position at the 36th to 37th weeks of gestation reduce the incidence of breech presentation at delivery? *Clinics in Mother and Child Health, 9*(1), 120601. Retrieved from https://pdfs.semanticscholar.org/bc6b/af529cabe1ab4fdf6a044d6cd20eb244d5a8.pdf

Khan, R. S., Naru, T., & Nizami, F. (2007). Umbilical cord prolapse—A review of diagnosis to delivery interval on perinatal and maternal outcome. *Journal of the Pakistan Medical Association, 57*(10), 487–491. Retrieved from https://jpma.org.pk/article-details/1221

Kiran, A., Singh, R. R., & Sinha, A. N. (2015). A clinical study of 100 cases of obstructed labour and its fetomaternal outcome. *Journal of Biology and Life Science, 6*(2), 141–147. https://doi.org/10.5296/jbls.v6i2.7564

Kjeldsen, L. L., Blankholm, A. D., Jurik, A. G., Salvig, J. D., & Maimburg, R. D. (2021). Pelvic capacity in pregnant women, identified using magnetic resonance imaging. *Acta Obstetricia et Gynecologica Scandinavica, 100*(8), 1454–1462. https://doi.org/10.1111/aogs.14168

Kotaska, A., & Menticoglou, S. (2019). Management of breech presentation at term (SOGC Clinical Practice Guideline 384). *Journal of Obstetrics and Gynaecology Canada, 41*(8), 1193–1205. https://doi.org/10.1016/j.jogc.2018.12.018

Kuliukas, A., Kuliukas, L., Franklin, D., & Flavel, A. (2015). Female pelvic shape: Distinct types or nebulous cloud? *British Journal of Midwifery, 23*(7), 490–496. https://doi.org/10.12968/bjom.2015.23.7.490

Kwan, A. H. W., Chaemsaithong, P., Wong, L., Tse, W. T., Hui, A. S. Y., Poon, L. C., & Leung, T. Y. (2021). Transperineal ultrasound assessment of fetal head elevation by maneuvers used for managing umbilical cord prolapse. *Ultrasound in Obstetrics & Gynecology, 58*(4), 603–608. https://doi.org/10.1002/uog.23544

Kwok, C.-S., Judkins, C.-L., & Sherratt, M. (2015). Forearm injury associated with compound presentation and prolonged labour. *Journal of Neonatal Surgery, 4*(3), 40–41. Retrieved from https://www.jneonatalsurg.com/ojs/index.php/jns/article/view/267/pdf

Le Ray, C., Lepleux, F., De La Calle, A., Guerin, J., Sellam, N., Dreyfus, M., & Chantry, A. A. (2016). Lateral asymmetric decubitus position for the rotation of occipito-posterior positions: multicenter randomized controlled trial EVADELA. *American Journal of Obstetrics & Gynecology, 215*(4), 511.e1–511.e7. https://doi.org/10.1016/j.ajog.2016.05.033

Lee, N., Gao, Y., Collins, S. L., Mårtensson, L. B., Randall, W., Rowe, T. M., & Kildea, S. (2020). Caesarean delivery rates and analgesia effectiveness following injections of sterile water for back pain in labour: A multicentre, randomised placebo controlled trial. *eClinicalMedicine, 25*. https://doi.org/10.1016/j.eclinm.2020.100447

Lee, N., Mårtensson, L. B., Homer, C., Webster, J., Gibbons, K., Stapleton, H., . . . Kildea, S. (2013). Impact on caesarean section rates following injections of sterile water (ICARIS): A multicentre randomised controlled trial. *BMC Pregnancy and Childbirth 13*, 105. https://doi.org/10.1186/1471-2393-13-105

Lee, N., Munro, V., Oliver, K., & Flynn, J. (2021). Maternal positioning with flexed hips to correct fetal occipito-posterior position in labour: A systematic review and meta-analysis. *Midwifery, 99*. https://doi.org/10.1016/j.midw.2021.103008

Leeman, L. M. (2020). Malpresentations, malpositions, and multiple gestation. In L. Leeman, L. Dresang, J. S. Quinlan, & S. R. Magee (Eds.), *Advanced life support in obstetrics: Provider manual* (9th ed., pp. 129–155). Leawood, KS: American Academy of Family Physicians.

Lendahls, L., & Oscarsson, M. G. (2017). Midwifery students' experiences of simulation-and skills training. *Nurse Education Today, 50*, 12–16. https://doi.org/10.1016/j.nedt.2016.12.005

Lenoir, A., See, M., & Tarnier, S. (1871). *Atlas de l'art des accouchements*. Paris, France: Victor Masson. Retrieved from https://www.google.com/books/edition/Atlas_de_l_art_des_accouchements_Continu/MBWK0w0wys0C?hl=&gbpv=1

Lerner, H. M. (2017). External cephalic version: How to increase the chances for success. *OBG Management, 29*(9), 26–32. Retrieved from https://cdn.mdedge.com/files/s3fs-public/Document/October-2017/obgm0290926.pdf

Levy, A. T., Weingarten, S., Ali, A., Quist-Nelson, J., & Berghella, V. (2021). Hands-and-knees posturing and fetal occiput anterior position: A systematic review and meta-analysis. *American Journal of Obstetrics & Gynecology MFM, 3*(4), 100346. https://doi.org/10.1016/j.ajogmf.2021.100346

Liao, J.-A., Shao, S.-C., Chang, C.-T., Chai, P. Y.-C., Owang, K.-L., Huang, T.-H., . . . Chen, Y.-C. (2021). Correction of breech presentation with moxibustion and acupuncture: A systematic review and meta-analysis. *Healthcare. 9*(6), 619. https://doi.org/0.3390/healthcare9060619

Lieberman, E., Davidson, K., Lee-Parritz, A., & Shearer, E. (2005). Changes in fetal position during labor and their association with epidural analgesia. *Obstetrics & Gynecology, 105*(5), 974–982. https://doi.org/10.1097/01.AOG.0000158861.43593.49

Lin, M. G. (2006). Umbilical cord prolapse. *Obstetrical & Gynecological Survey, 61*(4), 269–277. https://doi.org/10.1097/01.ogx.0000208802.20908.c6

Liu, L.-P., Chen, J.-H., Yang, Z.-J., & Zhu, J. (2018). Corrective effects of maternal extreme flexure and hip abduction combined with contralateral side-lying on persistent foetal occipito-posterior position. *International Journal of Nursing Practice, 24*(5), e12663. https://doi.org/10.1111/ijn.12663

Louwen, F., Daviss, B.-A., Johnson, K. C., & Reitter, A. (2017). Does breech delivery in an upright position instead of on the back improve outcomes and avoid cesareans? *International Journal of Gynecology & Obstetrics, 136*(2), 151–161. https://doi.org/10.1002/ijgo.12033

Macharey, G., Gissler, M., Toijonen, A., Heinonen, S., & Seikku, L. (2021). Congenital anomalies in breech presentation: A nationwide record linkage study. *Congenital Anomalies, 61*(4), 112–117. https://doi.org/1111/cga.12411

Macharey, G., Gissler, M., Ulander, V.-M., Rahkonen, L., Väisänen-Tommiska, M., Nuutila, M., & Heinonen, S. (2017). Risk factors associated with adverse perinatal outcome in planned vaginal breech labors at term: A retrospective population-based case-control study. *BMC Pregnancy and Childbirth, 17*(1), 93. https://doi.org/10.1186/s12884-017-1278-8

Magro-Malosso, E. R., Saccone, G., Di Tommaso, M., Mele, M., & Berghella, V. (2016). Neuraxial analgesia to increase the success rate of external cephalic version: A systematic review and metaanalysis of randomized controlled trials. *American Journal of Obstetrics & Gynecology, 215*(3), 276–286. https://doi.org/10.1016/j.ajog.2016.04.036

Mahmoud Mahmoud Saadoon, O. H., Yousif, A., & Fouad Mohammed, S. (2023). Effect of applying rebozo techniques on pain intensity and anxiety among primiparous women during the active phase of labor. *Egyptian Journal of Health Care, 14*(2), 476–486. https://doi.org/10.21608/ejhc.2023.297805

Malini, K. V. (2018). Breech presentation. In S. R. Kulkarni & K. Srinivas. (Eds.). (2018). *Ward rounds in obstetrics and gynecology* (pp. 26–40). New Delhi, India: Jaypee Brothers Medical Publishers. Retrieved from https://books.google.com/books?id=Ga52DwAAQBAJ&pg=PR13&lpg=PR13&dq

Malvasi, A., Barbera, A., Di Vagno, G., Gimovsky, A., Berghella, V., Ghi, T., . . . Tinelli, A. (2015). Asynclitism: A literature review of an often forgotten clinical condition. *Journal of Maternal-Fetal & Neonatal Medicine, 28*(16), 1890–1894. https://doi.org/10.3109/14767058.2014.972925

Marshall, J. E., & Raynor, M. D. (Eds.). (2014). *Myles' textbook for midwives* (16th ed., Kindle version). Edinburgh, United Kingdom: Elsevier Health Sciences.

Martinovski, M., Wilseck, Z. M., & Mattson, S. E. (2015). Neonatal compartment syndrome due to compound birth presentation. *Journal of Pediatric Surgery Case Reports, 3*(2), 79-81. https://doi.org/10.1016/j.epsc.2014.12.009

Masturzo, B., Farina, A., Attamante, L., Piazzese, A., Rolfo, A., Gaglioti, P., & Todros, T. (2017). Sonographic evaluation of the fetal spine position and success rate of manual rotation of the fetus in occiput posterior position: A randomized controlled trial. *Journal of Clinical Ultrasound, 45*(8), 472–476. https://doi.org/10.1002/jcu.22477

Maygrier, J. P. (1834). *Midwifery illustrated.* (A. S. Doane, Trans.). New York, NY: Harper & Brothers. Retrieved from https://collections.nlm.nih.gov/bookviewer?PID=nlm:nlmuid-67310750R-bk

Maykin, M. M., Ukoha, E. P., Tilp, V., Gaw, S. L., & Lewkowitz, A. K. (2021). Impact of therapeutic rest in early labor on perinatal outcomes: A prospective study. *American Journal of Obstetrics & Gynecology MFM, 3*(3), 100325. https://doi.org/10.1016/j.ajogmf.2021.100325

Mehl-Madrona, L., & Madrona, M. M. (1997). Physician- and midwife-attended home births: Effects of breech, twin, and post-dates outcome data on mortality rates, *Journal of Nurse-Midwifery, 42*(2), 91–98. Retrieved from http://www.azdhs.org/documents/licensing/special/midwives/committees/mspac/additional-resources/physician-midwife-attended-home-births.pdf

Mercier, R. J., & Kwan, M. (2018). Impact of peanut ball device on the duration of active labor: A randomized control trial. *American journal of Perinatology, 35*(10), 1006–1011. https://doi.org/10.1055/s-0038-1636531

Mirzakhani, K., Karimi, F., Mohamadzadeh Vatanchi, A., Feroz Zaidi, F., Mirzaei Najmabadi, K. (2020). The effect of maternal position on maternal, fetal and neonatal outcomes: A systematic review. *Journal of Midwifery and Reproductive Health, 8*(1), 1988–2004. https://doi.org/10.22038/jmrh.2019.38133.1423

Mohammed, R., & El-Chaâr, D. (2023a). Abnormal cephalic presentations. In G. D. Posner, A. Y. Black, G. Jones, & D. El-Chaâr (Eds.), *Oxorn-Foote human labor & birth* (7th ed., Kindle version, ch. 15). New York, NY: McGraw Hill.

Mohammed, R., & El-Chaâr, D. (2023b). Labor dystocia. In G. D. Posner, A. Y. Black, G. Jones, & D. El-Chaâr (Eds.), Oxorn-Foote human labor & birth (7th ed.; Kindle version, ch. 14). New York, NY: McGraw Hill.

Mohammed, R., & Tawagi, G. (2023). Compound presentations. In G. D. Posner, A. Y. Black, G. Jones, & D. El-Chaâr (Eds.), *Oxorn-Foote human labor & birth* (7th ed., Kindle version, ch. 27). New York, NY: McGraw Hill.

Moreau, F. J., (1844). *A practical treatise on midwifery: Exhibiting the present advanced state of the science.* (T. F. Betton, Trans.). Philadelphia, PA: Carey and Hart. Retrieved from https://archive.org/stream/b28270253

Munro Kerr, J. M. (1908). *Operative midwifery.* London, United Kingdom: Baillière, Tindall & Cox. Retrieved from https://wellcomelibrary.org/item/b21460668

Munro Kerr, J. M. (1911). *Operative midwifery: A guide to the difficulties and complications of midwifery practice* (2nd ed.). New York, NY: W. Wood. Retrieved from https://hdl.handle.net/2027/nnc2.ark:/13960/t2c832r3s

[NICE] National Institute for Health and Care Excellence. (2023). *Intrapartum care* (NICE Guideline NG235). Retrieved from https://www.nice.org.uk/guidance/ng235

Niu, B., Lee, V., Sharshiner, R., & Caughey, A. (2015). Manual rotation of fetuses in the occiput posterior position at delivery and adverse maternal outcomes.

American Journal of Obstetrics & Gynecology, 212(1), S83–S84. https://doi.org/10.1016/j.ajog.2014.10.180

Os, C., & Severinsson, E. (2017). How can manual rotation reduce vacuum, forceps and caesarean deliveries?—A review of the evidence. *Open Journal of Nursing, 7*, 68–85. https://doi.org/10.4236/ojn.2017.71007

Pagan, M., Eads, L., Sward, L., Manning, N., Hunzicker, A., & Magann, E. F. (2020). Umbilical cord prolapse: A review of the literature. *Obstetrical & Gynecological Survey, 75*(8), 510–518. https://doi.org/10.1097/OGX.0000000000000818

Partridge, B. (2021). Conceptual and ethical problems underpinning calls to abandon vaginal breech birth. *Women and Birth, 34*(2), e210-e215. https://doi.org/10.1016/j.wombi.2019.12.006

Petrikovsky, B., Terrani, M., Dillon, A., & Sichinava, L. (2021). Can cervical cerclage prevent umbilical cord prolapse in patients with funic presentation? *Journal of Diagnostic Medical Sonography, 37*(2), 109–112. https://doi.org/10.1177/8756479320972391

Pilliod, R. A., & Caughey, A. B. (2017). Fetal malpresentation and malposition: diagnosis and management. *Obstetrics and Gynecology Clinics of North America, 44*(4), 631–643. https://doi.org/10.1016/j.ogc.2017.08.003

Posner, G. D. (2023). Engagement, synclitism, asynclitism. In G. D. Posner, A. Y. Black, G. Jones, & D. El-Chaâr (Eds.), *Oxorn-Foote human labor & birth* (7th ed., Kindle version, ch. 8). New York, NY: McGraw Hill.

Reitter, A., Halliday, A., & Walker, S. (2020). Practical insight into upright breech birth from birth videos: A structured analysis. *Birth, 47*(2), 211–219. https://doi.org/10.1111/birt.12480

Ressl, B., & O'Beirne, M. (2015). Detecting breech presentation before labour: Lessons from a low-risk maternity clinic. *Journal of Obstetrics and Gynaecology Canada, 37*(8), 702–706. https://doi.org/10.1016/S1701-2163(15)30174-2

Rijnders, M., Herschderfer, K., Prins, M., van Baaren, R., van Veelen, A. J., Schönbeck, Y., & Buitendijk, S. (2008). A retrospective study of the success, safety and effectiveness of external cephalic version without tocolysis in a specialised midwifery centre in the Netherlands. *Midwifery, 24*(1), 38–45. https://doi.org/10.1016/j.midw.2006.07.009

Robertson, J. F., Braude, D. A., Stonehocker, J., & Moreno, J. (2015). Prehospital breech delivery with fetal head entrapment—A case report and review. *Prehospital Emergency Care, 19*(3), 451–456. https://doi.org/10.3109/10903127.2014.980476

Rodrigues, M. H., & Zorzim, V. I. (2017). Use of moxibustion and acupuncture in pregnant women with breech presentation: an integrative review. *Cogitare Enfermagem, 22*(1), 1–10. https://doi.org/10.5380/ce.v22i1

Royal College of Obstetricians and Gynaecologists. (2014). *Umbilical cord prolapse*. Green-top Guideline 50. Retrieved from https://www.rcog.org.uk/globalassets/documents/guidelines/gtg-50-umbilicalcordprolapse-2014.pdf

Sananes, N., Roth, G. E., Aissi, G. A., Meyer, N., Bigler, A., Bouschbacher, J. M., . . . Favre, R. (2016). Acupuncture version of breech presentation: A randomized sham-controlled single-blinded trial. *European Journal of Obstetrics & Gynecology and Reproductive Biology, 204*, 24–30. https://doi.org/10.1016/j.ejogrb.2016.07.492

Selcen, D. (2023). Neonatal brachial plexus palsy. In R. P. Goddeau, Jr. (Ed.), *UpToDate*. Retrieved November 14, 2023, from https://www.uptodate.com/contents/neonatal-brachial-plexus-palsy#!

Sentilhes, L., Schmitz, T., Azria, E., Gallot, D., Ducarme, G., Korb, D., . . . Verspyck, E. (2020). Breech presentation: Clinical practice guidelines from the French College of Gynaecologists and Obstetricians (CNGOF). *European Journal of Obstetrics & Gynecology and Reproductive Biology, 252*, 599–604. https://doi.org/10.1016/j.ejogrb.2020.03.033

Shaw, B. A., & Segal, L. S. (2016). Evaluation and referral for developmental dysplasia of the hip in infants. *Pediatrics, 138*(6), e20163107. https://doi.org/10.1542/peds.2016-3107

Shinmura, H., Matsushima, T., Okuda, N., Watanabe, A., Nagashima, A., Yamada, M., . . . Suzuki, S. (2022). Cephalic version by postural management in the lateral position without the knee-chest position for primiparous breech presentation: A retrospective cohort study. *Journal of Obstetrics and Gynaecology Research, 48*(3), 703–708. https://doi.org/10.1111/jog.15149

Shushan, A., & Younis, J. S. (1992). McRoberts maneuver for the management of the aftercoming head in breech delivery. *Gynecologic and Obstetric Investigation, 34*(3), 188–189. https://doi.org/10.1159/000292757

Simkin, P., Hanson, L., & Ancheta, R. (2017). The labor progress handbook: Early interventions to prevent and treat dystocia (4th Ed.). John Wiley & Sons.

Simpson, C. N., Chambers, C. N., Sharshiner, R., & Caughey, A. B. (2015). Effects of persistent occiput posterior position on mode of delivery. *Obstetrics & Gynecology, 125*, 82S–83S. https://doi.org/10.1097/01.AOG.0000463233.04675.ad

Singh, S. (2019). The second stage of labour. *International Journal of Reproduction, Contraception, Obstetrics and Gynecology, 8*(10), 4120–4129. https://doi.org/10.18203/2320-1770.ijrcog20194395

Skupski, D. W., & Ghidini, A. (2016). External cephalic version: Some tricks of the trade. *Birth, 43*(3), 189–192. https://doi.org/10.1111/birt.12242

Smith, C., Crowther, C., Wilkinson, C., Pridmore, B., & Robinson, J. (1999). Knee-chest postural management for breech at term: A randomized controlled trial. *Birth, 26*(2), 71–75. https://doi.org/10.1046/j.1523-536x.1999.00071.x

Smith, H., Peterson, N., Lagrew, D., & Main, E. (Eds.). (2022). *Toolkit to support vaginal birth and reduce primary cesareans: A quality improvement toolkit.* Stanford, CA: California Maternal Quality Care Collaborative. Retrieved from https://www.cmqcc.org/sites/default/files/Vbirth-Toolkit-with-Supplement_Final_11.30.22_2.pdf

Stewart, O. (2017). Malpresentations and malpositions. In M. Boyle (Ed.), *Emergencies around childbirth* (3rd ed., pp. 95–118). Boca Raton, FL: CRC Press.

Strauss, R. A., & Herrera, C. A. (2023). Transverse fetal lie. In V. A. Barss (Ed.), *UpToDate*. Retrieved November 14, 2023, from http://www.uptodate.com/contents/transverse-fetal-lie

Sutton, J., & Scott, P. (1996). *Understanding and teaching optimal foetal positioning* (2nd ed.). Tauranga, New Zealand: Birth Concepts.

Svelato, A., Ragusa, A., Alimondi, P., Di Tommaso, M., Marci, R., Barbagallo, V., . . . Perino, A. (2017). Occiput-spine relationship: Shoulders are more important than head. *European Review for Medical and Pharmacological Sciences, 21*(6), 1178–83. Retrieved from https://www.europeanreview.org/article/12387

Tafazolifar, M., Kordi, M., Dadgar, S., Esmaily, H., & Mirteimouri, M. (2019). The effect of knee-chest position on turning breech to cephalic presentation in pregnant women: Randomized clinical trial. *Iranian Journal of Obstetrics, Gynecology and Infertility, 21*(12), 57–64. https://doi.org/10.22038/ijogi.2019.12665

Taylor, P., & Robson, S. (2016). Midwifery-led ECV. *BJOG, 123*(3), 425. https://doi.org/10.1111/1471-0528.13822

Tsao, N. (2015). *Early pushing urge before full dilation: A scoping review* (Unpublished term paper). University of British Columbia, Vancouver. https://doi.org/http://dx.doi.org/10.14288/1.0108912

Tully, G. (2016). Opening the pelvic brim with Walcher's position. *Midwifery Today with International Midwife*, 117, 26–27. Retrieved from https://pubmed.ncbi.nlm.nih.gov/27192754/

Tully, G. (2019). *Helping your breech baby turn.* Bloomington, MN: Maternity House Publishing. Bloomington, IL. Retrieved from https://www.spinningbabies.com/product/helping-your-breech-baby-turn-ebook/

Tully, G. (2020). *Changing Birth on Earth: A midwife and nurse's guide to using physiology to avoid another unnecessary cesarean*. Bloomington, MN: Maternity House Publishing.

Vas, J., Aranda, J. M., Nishishinya, B., Mendez, C., Martin, M. A., Pons, J., . . . Perea-Milla, E. (2009). Correction of nonvertex presentation with moxibustion: A systematic review and metaanalysis. *American Journal of Obstetrics & Gynecology, 201*(3), 241–259. https://doi.org/10.1016/j.ajog.2008.12.026

Verhaeghe, C., Corroenne, R., Spiers, A., Descamps, P., Gascoin, G., Bouet, P.-E., . . . Legendre, G. (2021). Delivery mode after manual rotation of occiput posterior fetal positions. *Obstetrics & Gynecology, 137*(6), 999–1006. https://doi.org/10.1097/AOG.0000000000004386

Vlemmix, F., Bergenhenegouwen, L., Schaaf, J. M., Ensing, S., Rosman, A. N., Ravelli, A. C. J, . . . Kok, M. (2014). Term breech deliveries in the Netherlands: Did the increased cesarean rate affect neonatal outcome? A population-based cohort study. *Acta Obstetricia et Gynecologica Scandinavica, 93*(9), 888–896. https://doi.org/10.1111/aogs.12449

Walker, S. (2014a). Dolichocephaly—understanding 'breech head' molding [Web log post]. *The midwife, the mother and the breech.* Retrieved from https://breechbirth.org.uk/?s=understanding+'breech+head'+molding

Walker, S. (2014b). Shoulder press and gluteal lift [Web log post]. *The midwife, the mother and the breech.* Retrieved from https://breechbirth.org.uk/2014/06/15/shoulder-press-gluteal-lift/

Walker, S. (2015). Turning breech upside down: Upright breech birth. *MIDIRS Midwifery Digest, 25*(3), 325–330.

Walker, S. (2018). Rotational manoeuvre to release breech nuchal arms [Web log post]. *The midwife, the mother and the breech.* Retrieved from https://breechbirth.org.uk/tag/nuchal-arms/

Walker, S., Dasgupta, T., Halliday, A., & Reitter, A. (2021). Development of a core outcome set for effectiveness studies of breech birth at term (Breech-COS): A systematic review on variations in outcome reporting. *European Journal of Obstetrics & Gynecology and Reproductive Biology, 263*, 117–126. https://doi.org/10.1016/j.ejogrb.2021.06.021

Walker, S., Perilakalathil, P., Moore, J., Gibbs, C. L., Reavell, K., & Crozier, K. (2015). Standards for midwife practitioners of external cephalic version: A Delphi study. *Midwifery, 31*(5), e79–e86. https://doi.org/1016/j.midw.2015.01.004

Walker, S., & Spillane, E. (2020). Face-to-pubes rotational maneuver for bilateral nuchal arms in a vaginal breech birth, resolved in an upright maternal position: A case report. *Birth, 47*(2), 246–252. https://doi.org/10.1111/birt.12486

Weiss, B. D. (1991). Shoulder dystocia caused by axillary cystic hygroma. *Journal of Family Practice, 33*(5), 524, 528. Retrievd from https://cdn.mdedge.com/files/s3fs-public/jfp-archived-issues/1991-volume_32-33/JFP_1991-11_v33_i5_shoulder-dystocia-caused-by-axillary-cys.pdf

Wildschut, H. I. J., van Belzen-Slappendel, H., & Jans, S. (2017). The art of vaginal breech birth at term on all fours. *Clinical Case Reports, 5*(2), 182–186. https://doi.org/10.1002/ccr3.808

Williams, J. W. (1912). *Obstetrics: A text-book for the use of students and practitioners* (3rd ed.). New York: Appleton. Retrieved from https://archive.org/details/obstetricstextbo1912will/

Wong, L., Kwan, A. H. W., Lau, S. L., Sin, W. T. A., & Leung, T. Y. (2021). Umbilical cord prolapse: Revisiting its definition and management. *American Journal of Obstetrics & Gynecology, 225*(4), 357–366. https://doi.org/10.1016/j.ajog.2021.06.077

Wong, L., Tse, W. T., Lai, C. Y., Hui, A. S. Y., Chaemsaithong, P., Sahota, D. S., . . . Leung, T. Y. (2021). Bradycardia-to-delivery interval and fetal outcomes in umbilical cord prolapse. *Acta Obstetricia et Gynecologica Scandinavica, 100*(1), 170–177. https://doi.org/10.1111/aogs.13985

Yagel, O., Cohen, S. M., Lipschuetz, M., Bdolah-Abram, T., Amsalem, H., Kabiri, D., & Yagel, S. (2016). P17. 07: Persistent occiput posterior position: Impact of head circumference on obstetric outcomes. *Ultrasound in Obstetrics & Gynecology, 48*(Suppl. 1), 223. https://doi.org/Retrieved from https://obgyn.onlinelibrary.wiley.com/doi/full/10.1002/uog.16664

Yang, L., Yi, T., Zhou, M., Wang, C., Xu, X., Li, Y., . . . Meng, Z. (2020). Clinical effectiveness of position management and manual rotation of the fetal position with a U-shaped birth stool for vaginal delivery of a fetus in a persistent occiput posterior position. *Journal of International Medical Research. 48*(6). https://doi.org/10.1177/0300060520924275

Zwerling, B., Shields, M., Meuchel, L., Cheng, Y. W., & Caughey, A. B. (2017). The effect of birth location on neonatal and maternal morbidity/mortality for breech-presenting term fetuses. *American Journal of Obstetrics & Gynecology, 216*(1, Suppl.), S385. https://doi.org/10.1016/j.ajog.2016.11.390

Shoulder Dystocia 12

Objectives

- Name two differential diagnoses for shoulder dystocia.
- List four risk factors for shoulder dystocia.
- Describe the physiology of shoulder dystocia.
- Discuss risks, benefits, and efficacy of techniques for resolving shoulder dystocia.
- Discuss risks to mother and infant that follow shoulder dystocia.

Composite Case Study

Stella T., a 30-year-old gravida 3, para 2 (G3 P2) at 40 0/7 weeks of gestation arrived in the birth center almost crawling through the doorway. Her husband, Carlos, followed, unsure what he should do to help her. A contraction took hold, and Stella rocked on her hands and feet like a mother bear, her wails reverberating through the hall. Angela Curtiss, CPM, and her nurse Josephine had prepared the birth room in response to Carlos's frantic phone call: "I think my wife is gonna have the baby in the car! I'm driving as fast as I can!"

When the contraction ended, Angela and Josephine guided Stella into the birth room, noting the puddle of clear fluid where Stella had been crouching. Stella flung herself on the bed and Angela quickly assessed her. The fetal heart rate was 140, she was fully dilated, and the presentation was clearly vertex and left occiput anterior. "Great, Stella, you're complete! What position did you want to have your baby in? You were doing pretty good on all fours."

Another contraction began, and Stella swung off the bed into a supported squat, pushing involuntarily. "Well, it looks like we are going to have a baby," smiled Josephine as the head began to crown. Strangely, there was very little progress over the next few contractions. Little by little, the forehead squeaked out, then the eyebrows, the nose, and upper lip. Angela helped Stella to squat more deeply to make more room in her pelvis. The baby's chin finally emerged, then retracted snugly onto the perineum without restituting.

"Stella, I think this baby has tight shoulders. The head is out but you still have some work to do. We are going to keep trying different things until the baby is born." Working quickly, Angela helped Stella's hands to the floor into Gaskin's maneuver, then guided her into a lunge position. Stella pushed, but the baby did not move. Josephine put the phone on speaker and summoned an ambulance while readying resuscitation equipment and medications to manage a potential postpartum hemorrhage.

Angela asked Stella to crawl onto the bed on hands and knees. Stella pushed, but there was no progress. Angela inserted her fingers gently to determine whether the problem was a tight nuchal cord, impacted shoulders, or some other issue. She felt the shoulder wedged into the symphysis with little room to spare. Working quickly, Josephine helped Stella into McRoberts' position, and, standing on a stool, attempted to displace the fetal shoulder laterally with pressure on the left lower abdomen. The baby's head remained tightly applied to the perineum and was now turning deep purple.

Rapidly but methodically, Angela inserted her well-lubricated hand into the back of the vagina and, with difficulty, followed the posterior arm until she found the baby's hand caught behind its back. She brought the slippery arm around the front of the baby and swept it across the chest and out of the vagina. Stella pushed, and the chubby boy baby slid out easily about 2 min after the birth of the head. The baby was not breathing, had poor tone, and was unresponsive to the initial steps of neonatal resuscitation. Josephine handed Angela a resuscitation bag, and they ventilated the baby about 15 sec before he started to cry. His 5-min Apgar score was 9, and he had no apparent birth injuries. Josephine injected Stella with intramuscular oxytocin after the birth, and she did not hemorrhage Emergency medical services arrived to find mother and baby stable. Stella signed the EMS refusal-of-care release, arranged for her pediatrician to evaluate her baby after discharge from the birth center, and settled in for a peaceful recovery.

Understanding Shoulder Dystocia

Shoulder dystocia is widely defined as a cephalic vaginal birth that requires maneuvers beyond gentle downward traction to deliver the shoulders (American College of Obstetricians & Gynecologists [ACOG], 2017/2024; Rodis, 2023b; Royal College of Obstetricians & Gynaecologists [RCOG], 2012). Shoulder dystocia occurs in approximately 0.2–3.0%

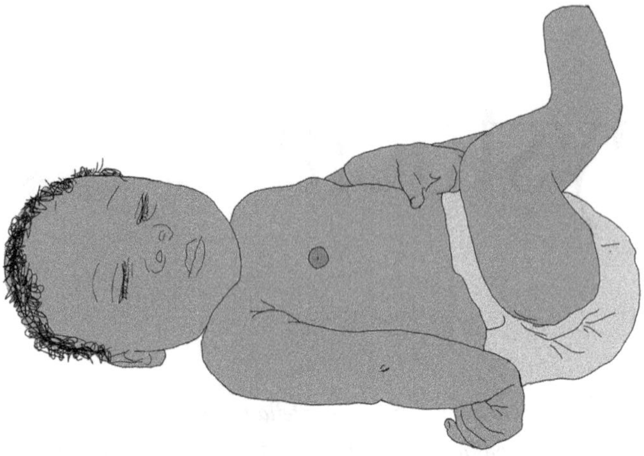

Figure 12-1, In the newborn, Erb palsy presents with the distinctive "waiter's tip" arm position. When the brachial plexus is injured, muscle imbalance adducts and internally rotates the shoulder, extends the elbow, and pronates the forearm. Often this damage is temporary.

of births and cannot be predicted by antenatal or intrapartum risk factors or by imaging studies (Rodis, 2023b). It occurs in any of three variations: when the anterior shoulder becomes impacted on the symphysis pubis, when the posterior shoulder becomes impacted on the sacral promontory, or both shoulders become impacted (ACOG, 2017/2024). Usually, the head is completely or partially delivered when shoulder dystocia is diagnosed. Once shoulder dystocia is recognized, expediting birth improves neonatal outcomes (ACOG Task Force on Neonatal Brachial Plexus Palsy, 2014/2019).

Pathophysiology

Normally, the fetal bisacromial diameter (the measurement between the most distal parts of the fetal shoulders) enters the pelvis obliquely, posterior shoulder first (Rodis, 2023a). The pelvis is wider in the oblique dimension than it is front to back, and the fetus gravitates toward the roomier angle (Rodis, 2023a). The head is born and restitutes as the shoulders rotate toward the anteroposterior (AP) position at the pelvic outlet. The anterior shoulder passes beneath the symphysis pubis slightly to the side of the midline and the body follows quickly.

Impaction of the shoulders can occur when the fetus enters the pelvis with the bisacromial diameter in the AP diameter of the inlet rather than in an oblique diameter (Amankwah, 2023). If the shoulders enter the pelvis in an AP orientation rather than obliquely or come through the pelvic inlet simultaneously, the anterior shoulder can lodge behind the symphysis pubis. The posterior shoulder can also become wedged on the sacral promontory. If the fetal head continues to descend, the neck elongates and the brachial plexus nerves, which supply motor function to the arm, can stretch or tear. The birth attendant can also cause brachial plexus injury by pulling or twisting the head or by applying lateral traction.

Risks

Even properly managed shoulder dystocia increases the risk of fetal and maternal injury. Maternal complications include postpartum hemorrhage in 11% and fourth-degree lacerations in 3.8% (ACOG, 2017/2024). Less commonly, maneuvers to resolve shoulder dystocia can cause maternal symphyseal separation, lateral femoral cutaneous neuropathy, cervicovaginal lacerations, urethral injury, bladder lacerations, and uterine rupture (Rodis, 2023a). The client who experiences shoulder dystocia out of hospital is at risk for severe postpartum hemorrhage, poor availability of full resuscitation for the infant, and long transport times to definitive care. About 5% of shoulder dystocias are associated with infant injury due to asphyxia or trauma (Rodis, 2023a).

Brachial plexus injury. The brachial plexus is a network that branches off the lower cervical and upper thoracic nerves (C5–8, T1) to innervate muscles and skin of the shoulder and arm (Selcen, 2023). Newborn brachial plexus palsy presents as a weak or paralyzed arm with a passive range of motion greater than the active (ACOG Task Force, 2014/2019). Erb palsy presents with the shoulder internally rotated, the elbow extended, and the forearm pronated (waiter's tip sign) illustrated in Figure 12-1. The condition develops when C-5 and C-6 nerve roots are excessively stretched. Klumpke's palsy presents with hand and medial forearm weakness and indicates damage to the C-8 and T-1 nerve roots. Stretching of the brachial plexus causes nerve damage that can be temporary or permanent. Most nerve injuries associated with shoulder dystocia gradually heal without deficit (Rodis, 2023a). Permanent brachial plexus damage occurs in 1–2 out of every 10,000 births (Burd, 2022).

Only about half of neonatal brachial plexus injuries follow shoulder dystocia, and 0.03–0.15% follow cesarean births (Selcen, 2023). The remainder follow vaginal births uncomplicated by shoulder dystocia. In a hands-on birth, the usual maneuvers of lowering and raising the fetal head direct the greatest force to the fetal shoulders parallel to the fetal spine (Lockwood, 2014). If a fetal shoulder impinges on the sacral promontory or if the anterior shoulder snags on the symphysis pubis, this maneuver can create substantial lateral traction. Furthermore, contractions of labor apply considerably more force than that typically applied by a birth attendant and can in themselves create enough lateral force to cause fetal injury (Lockwood, 2014). In the case of shoulder dystocia, the forces of labor alone can create up to 15.7% stretch on the brachial plexus, enough to cause injury to the newborn (Lockwood, 2014).

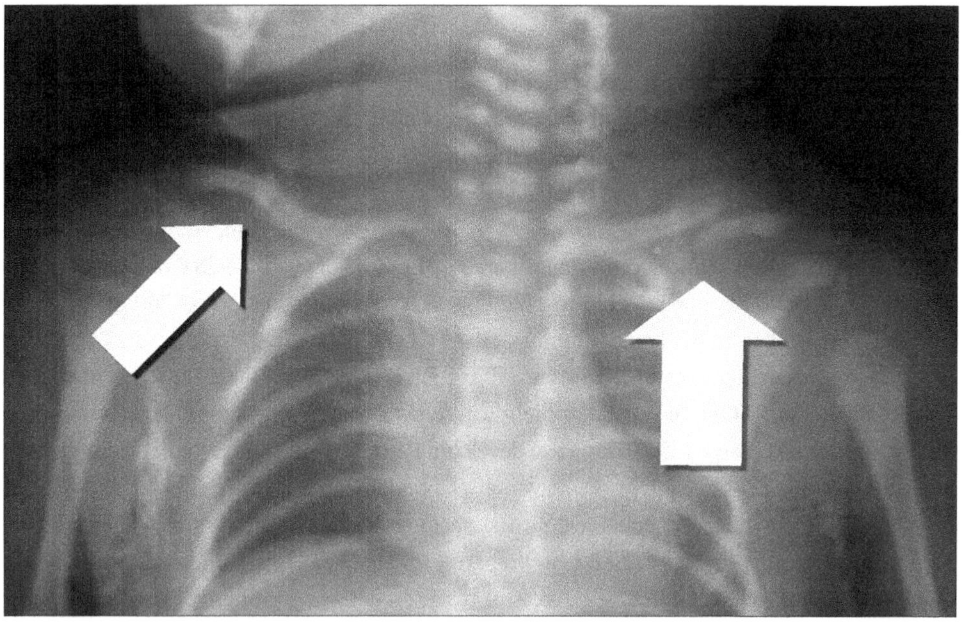

Figure 12-2. After shoulder dystocia, this infant presented with extensive subcutaneous emphysema of the neck, Erb palsy, and Moro reflexes absent bilaterally. A chest x-ray revealed bilateral clavicular fractures and air entrapped in the central part of the chest cavity. The paralysis resolved by the two-month checkup. From "Bilateral Clavicle Fracture in Two Newborn Infants," by A. Kanik, S. Sutcoglou, H. Aydinlioglu, E. Erdemit, and F. A. Ozer, 2011, *Iranian Journal of Pediatrics, 21*(4), p. 553. CC-BY-NC 3.0.

Clavicular fracture. The clavicle is the fetal bone most commonly fractured during vaginal birth, about 0.5% of vaginal births overall. (Kanik et al., 2011). The incidence of clavicular fracture is as high as 9.5% for births involving shoulder dystocia (Rodis, 2023a). Rarely, the provider may deliberately fracture one or both clavicles to resolve a severe shoulder dystocia.

A complete division of the clavicle is unusual; most fractures are of the greenstick type and can be asymptomatic at birth. By 7–10 days of life, a callus can be palpated along the healing bone. A complete fracture can present with irregularity and/or discoloration over the fracture site, decreased or abnormal movement of the affected arm, or absent Moro reflex on the affected side. Tenderness, crepitus, and deformity can be present at the site of injury, and the infant might cry in pain with passive movement of the arm. A displaced complete clavicular fracture can cause a pneumothorax.

Hypoxic ischemic encephalopathy (HIE). Neonatal HIE is a neurological syndrome that can occur after an event involving low oxygen and decreased blood flow to the brain (Victor, Rocha-Ferreira, Rahim, Hagberg, & Edwards, 2022). Even with optimal treatment, many infants with HIE die, and only 40% have normal neurologic outcomes (Wu, 2023). HIE due to shoulder dystocia is very rare, occurring in about 1 in 22,000 term vaginal births (Rodis, 2023b).

Perinatal death is a very rare complication occurring in no more than 0.35% of shoulder dystocias (Rodis, 2023b). Fatal shoulder dystocia can come as a complete surprise; often the fetal heart pattern is reassuring until the birth of the head. Although the risk of acidosis or HIE is very low if shoulder dystocia is of short duration (Leung et al., 2011), in almost half of deaths the head-body birth interval is less than 5 min (Hope et al., 1998). It is not clear why some fetuses deteriorate so quickly or why resuscitation does not revive them.

One hypothesis attributes these deaths to changes in intrauterine pressure, fetal circulation, and cerebral perfusion that follow the birth of the head (Kotaska & Campbell, 2014). In these cases, blood flow to the brain usually remains normal between uterine contractions as arterial blood circulates from the heart through the brain and then drains through veins into the fetal thorax. During a contraction, however, intrauterine pressure rises to 60–80 mm Hg above atmospheric pressure, and with maternal pushing it increases to more than 100 mm Hg above atmospheric pressure (Kotaska & Campbell, 2014). The fetal heart strongly pumps arterial blood into the head, but increased pressure on the fetal thorax occludes venous drainage. Intracranial pressure increases, and cerebral perfusion slows or stops, allowing anoxia and metabolic acidemia to develop quickly (Kotaska & Campbell, 2014).

It also appears that fetal hypovolemia plays a major role in poor outcomes after shoulder dystocia (Ancora, Meloni, Soffritti, Sandri, & Ferretti, 2020; Menticoglou & Schneider, 2016). During shoulder dystocia, the fetal thorax and the umbilical vein are vulnerable to compression. Circulation sometimes continues, however, through the firmer, high-flow umbilical arteries that carry blood to the placenta. When a significant amount of blood becomes trapped in the placenta, the fetus suffers relative hypovolemia. If the infant undergoes immediate cord clamping at birth, resuscitation may fail if volume is not replaced (Menticoglou & Schneider, 2016). The most intuitive and natural way to transfuse a newborn is to keep the cord unclamped and intact during resuscitation, maximizing oxygenation, decreasing acidosis, and infusing hemoglobin F, stem cells, and volume during the first critical interval (Mercer, Erickson-Owens, & Skovgaard, 2009). See also Chapter 13. If the cord must be clamped and cut quickly, milking or stripping the cord first can increase blood volume in the newborn.

Risk Factors

Although certain clinical conditions increase the risk of shoulder dystocia, it is not possible to predict which vaginal birth will be complicated by shoulder dystocia based on antepartum maternal characteristics or the intrapartum course (Mendez-Figueroa et al., 2021). In general, a client with one or more risk factors has less than a 1 in 10 chance of developing an actual shoulder dystocia (Rodis, 2023b). At least half of pregnancies complicated by shoulder dystocia have no risk factors (Rodis, 2023b). Obstetrical providers should be prepared to manage shoulder dystocia at every birth, regardless of the presence of risk factors. Any client with risk factors should receive personalized counseling on the risks of vaginal birth versus cesarean section and the risks and benefits of birth in a hospital or elsewhere.

Antepartum

Previous shoulder dystocia. A mother who has experienced shoulder dystocia has a likelihood of reoccurrence of at least 10% (Gherman, Gonik, & Ouzounian, 2021). The actual risk may be greater; this figure excludes mothers who chose cesarean birth to eliminate the possibility of reoccurrence (Gherman, Gonik, et al., 2021).

Diabetes. Clients with gestational or preexisting diabetes mellitus are several times more likely to experience shoulder dystocia than nondiabetic counterparts. The fetuses of diabetic mothers tend to have larger shoulders, more body fat, excessive fat accumulation in the abdominal and scapular regions, and thicker upper arms (Riskin & Garcia-Prats, 2023). Even a single elevated glucose value in a 75-g, 2-hr glucose tolerance test is associated with higher risk for macrosomia and shoulder dystocia (Rodis, 2023b). Well-controlled glucose alone does not necessarily reduce the risk. Outcomes seem to improve only when the client achieves mean glucose levels significantly lower than those of nondiabetic mothers (Rodis, 2023b).

Macrosomia. Some fetuses are too large to pass through the maternal pelvis. As birthweight increases, so does the incidence of shoulder dystocia because the trunk and chest grow larger relative to the head (Gherman, Gonik, et al., 2021). For example, the shoulders of a large fetus with a bisacromial diameter of 17 cm may be unable to even enter an average-sized pelvis, and an average-sized fetus with bisacromial diameter of 14 cm can encounter difficulty negotiating an unusually small pelvic inlet (Menticoglou, 2018). Although about half of all shoulder dystocia cases involve newborns with birthweight less than 8 lb 13 oz (4,000 g), the incidence of shoulder dystocia rises progressively when birthweight surpasses this threshold (Gherman, Gonik, et al., 2021). That said, most extremely large infants emerge without shoulder dystocia. The incidence for nondiabetic mothers has been reported (Beall, Spong, McKay, & Ross, 1998; Gherman, Gonik, et al., 2021) as 5.2% for neonates weighing 8 lb 13 oz–9 lb 6 oz (4,000–4,250 g), 9.1% for those 9 lb 6 oz–9 lb 15 oz (4,250–4,500 g), 14.3% for those 9 lb 15 oz–10 lb 8 oz (4,500–4,750 g), and 21.1% for those 10 lb 8 oz–11 lb (4,750–5,000 g). One large study gives a rate of 15.5% for newborns 11 lb (5,000 g) or greater (Øverland, Vatten, & Eskild, 2014).

Planned cesarean section is the only way to prevent shoulder dystocia. A policy of prophylactic cesarean for everyone suspected of carrying a large fetus, however, would lead to many unnecessary cesarean births of large and average-sized infants. Providers would need to perform 443 cesarean births for high-risk clients with diabetes and an estimated fetal weight greater than 9 lb 15 oz (4,500 g) to prevent one permanent brachial plexus injury (ACOG, 2017/2024). For the same fetal weight estimation in nondiabetic mothers, the ratio would be 3,695:1 (ACOG, 2017/2024). ACOG recommends that providers offer elective cesarean birth to all mothers carrying fetuses with an estimated weight 11 lb (5,000 g) or more and mothers with diabetes carrying fetuses 9 lb 15 oz (4,500 g) or more (ACOG, 2017/2024).

Fetal weight can be exceedingly difficult to accurately measure sonographically, by abdominal palpation, or by fundal height (Goetzinger, Odibo, Shanks, Roehl, & Cahill, 2014). Midwives using abdominal palpation tend to underestimate the weight of macrosomic fetuses (Kesrouani et al., 2017), while sonographic measurements tend to overestimate weight. In one study (Abramowicz & Ahn, 2022), about 50% of newborns of diabetic mothers with a sonographically estimated fetal weight 9 lb 6 oz (4,250 g) or greater had a birthweight of less than 8 lb 13 oz (4,000 g).

Postterm pregnancy. Postterm infants appear more likely to experience shoulder dystocia, probably because most fetuses grow with increasing gestational age (Floyd & Smeltzer, 2022).

Male sex. Shoulder dystocia is more likely to involve a male fetus, probably because males tend to weigh more (Burkhardt, Schmidt, Kurmanavicius, Zimmermann, & Schäffer, 2014). Fifty-one percent of all newborns and 70% of newborns greater than 9 lb 15 oz (4,500 g) are male (Rodis, 2023b).

Maternal obesity and high gestational weight gain. Mothers with a body mass index (BMI) of 30 kg/m^2 or higher at conception (Bracken & Langhe, 2021) and/or mothers who gain excessive weight during pregnancy (Kominiarek et al., 2018) are at higher risk for shoulder dystocia (Zhang, Wu, Li, & Zhang, 2018).

Advanced maternal age. Mothers over the age of 35 are more likely to experience shoulder dystocia (Heinonen, Saisto, Gissler, Kaijomaa, & Sarvilinna, 2021). This may be because they tend to have higher BMIs and are at higher risk for diabetes (Heinonen et al., 2021). Older mothers are more likely to be grand multiparas, and each successive infant tends to weigh 200 g more than the last up to the fifth birth (Rodis, 2023b).

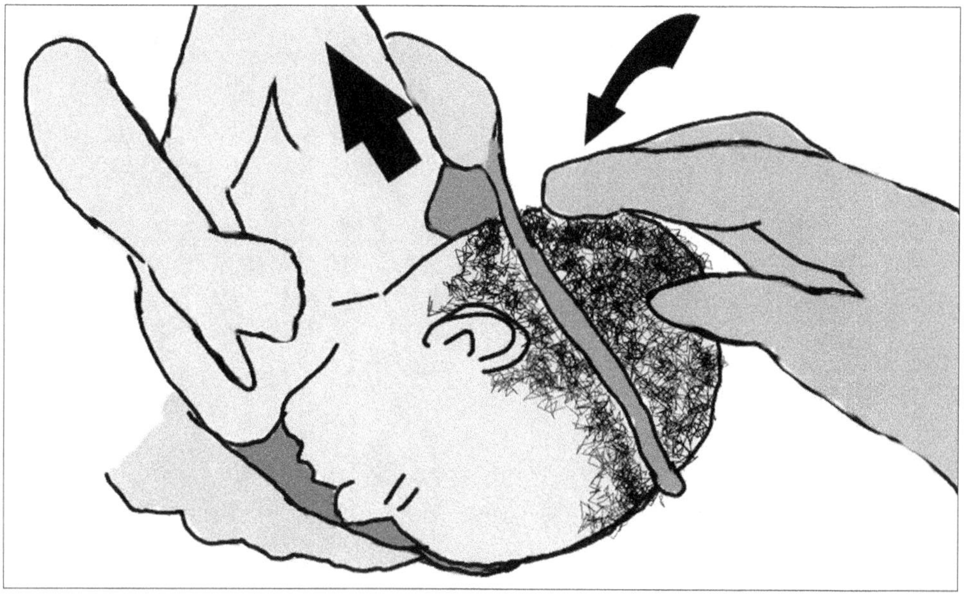

Figure 12-3. The pushback maneuver is the only maneuver that appears to prevent shoulder dystocia. The provider applies gentle resistance to the crowning head while the mother pushes, encouraging flexion and facilitating the rotation of the anterior shoulder from behind the symphysis. Adapted from "Prevention of Shoulder Dystocia: A Randomized Controlled Trial to Evaluate an Obstetric Maneuver," by O. Poujade et al., 2018, *European Journal of Obstetrics & Gynecology and Reproductive Biology, 227,* p. 53. Copyright by Elsevier.

Fetal hypertonus or hypotonus. A fetus with hypertonus or hypotonus appears more likely to experience shoulder dystocia. The hypertonic fetus (tight, elastic tone and limbs held unusually close to the body) can present fixed, unyielding shoulders to the maternal pelvis and have difficulty negotiating the bony passage. Causes of fetal hypertonus include inherited neuromuscular disorders or antenatal brain injuries, including those caused by hypoxia, congenital infection, intracranial hemorrhage, or placental/umbilical abnormalities (Hart, Sharma, Rittey, & Mordekar, 2015).

Conversely, a hypotonic fetus (weak, floppy tone, and limbs unfolded) is susceptible to malpresentations such as arms trapped behind the back, which can abduct and widen the shoulders and increase the risk of shoulder impingement. Fetal hypotonus is more common with inherited myopathy, neuromuscular junction disorder, or extreme prematurity. The fetus that dies *in utero* is at higher risk for shoulder dystocia due to lack of muscle tone (Kwan, Hui, Lee, & Leung, 2021). In one study of prelabor preterm stillbirths, the rate of shoulder dystocia was as high as 5% despite a median gestational age of 28 weeks and a proportionately large head (Gold, Mozurkewich, Puder, & Treadwell, 2016).

Intraamniotic infection (IAI, chorioamnionitis). Intrauterine infection can cause an underlying labor dystocia and longer second stage labor that appears to increase the risk of shoulder dystocia, particularly with the use of vacuum extraction (Palatnik et al., 2016).

Intrapartum

Greater than normal resistance between the fetal skin and vaginal walls, a fetal chest that is wider than the biparietal diameter, or rapid descent can disrupt rotation (ACOG, 2017/2024). Shoulder dystocia is more likely when second stage labor is precipitous or prolonged (Rodis, 2023b). Shoulder dystocia is more likely to occur with vaginal forceps or vacuum-assisted birth. It is unclear whether fetal shoulder malposition contributes to labor delays that necessitate operative delivery or operative delivery disrupts the normal mechanism of labor.

Prevention

Although numerous risk factors and associations for shoulder dystocia have been identified, ACOG still considers shoulder dystocia unpredictable and unpreventable (ACOG, 2017/2024), even for clients with multiple risk factors (Ouzounian et al., 2016). Risk factors are absent in at least half of births complicated by shoulder dystocia (Palatnik et al., 2016). Some risk-reducing strategies, however, seem beneficial.

The pushback maneuver, evaluated in a multicenter, randomized, single-blind trial, is the only intervention purported to reduce the occurrence of shoulder dystocia (Poujade et al., 2018). To use the pushback maneuver, place one hand gently on the crowning fetal head. While the mother pushes, provide enough resistance to maintain flexion and delay birth for 1–3 contractions. This resistance gives the fetal shoulders more time to enter the pelvic cavity, thereby encouraging the anterior shoulder to slip behind the symphysis pubis (Poujade et al., 2018). Closely monitor the

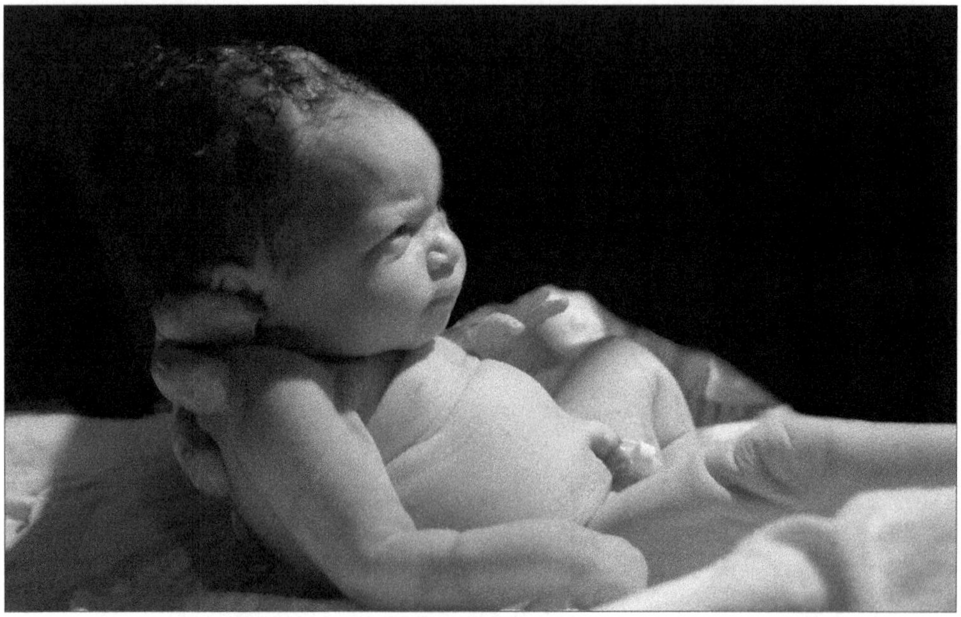

Figure 12-4. Amniotic band syndrome. This infant, 5 lb 8 oz (2,500 g), was found to have a right-arm motor deficit after operative delivery without shoulder dystocia. She was born to a primigravida after a long first stage and hours of pushing through a pelvis that appeared adequate. When the vacuum popped off her head twice, the obstetrician assisted her birth with forceps. The infant had abnormal rotation, abduction, and movement of her right arm. She was right occiput anterior, and her left shoulder was uppermost at birth. On a closer look, her right arm was hypoplastic, and there was an indentation across her right forearm. Her right arm had apparently been restrained by an amniotic band that restricted descent in labor. The band had not been identified on ultrasound. At one year of age, she was responding well to physical therapy and was likely to have normal use of her arm.

fetal heart rate (FHR) while using this maneuver. Poujade et al. (2018) found a significantly lower incidence of shoulder dystocia (1.5.%) than in the control group (3.8%) despite the inclusion of high-risk clients, such as those carrying macrosomic fetuses. There was, however, no difference in neonatal complications between the two groups.

Two-step technique: The provider who grasps the head as soon as it emerges and exerts downward traction can disrupt the rotation of the shoulders at the inlet, thereby encouraging the fetal shoulder to impinge on the maternal pelvis (Menticoglou, 2018). In about 20% of physiologic vaginal births, after the head is born, the shoulders do not move spontaneously through the inlet until the mother pushes with the next contraction (Menticoglou, 2018). Physiologic birth is supported when the midwife uses the two-step technique: (1) allow the head to deliver on one contraction, refrain from intervening while the uterus is uncontracted, and (2) allow the body to be born on the next contraction (Bottoms & Sokol, 1981; Downe & Marshall, 2014; Locatelli et al., 2011).

Between birth of the head and birth of the shoulders, the uterus is not contracting, the mother is not pushing, and the midwife's hands are usually off the head (Kotaska & Campbell, 2014). The head should be pinkish, and the FHR should be reassuring. In these circumstances, a head-to-body birth interval up to 4 min between contractions is common and safe (Kotaska & Campbell, 2014). *Do NOT wait for the next contraction if the head appears dark, pale, or blue: if the heart tones are abnormal; if there is a tight nuchal cord; or if there are other signs of complications.* Menticoglou (2018) suggests that the diagnosis of shoulder dystocia be made when the mother is unable to push the fetus out by her own efforts with the next contraction after the head is born.

Diet and lifestyle: Dietary and lifestyle modifications that reduce obesity before conception and limit weight gain during pregnancy can reduce the likelihood of macrosomia, potentially reducing shoulder dystocia (Rodis, 2023b). Induction of labor at 39 weeks of gestation can reduce the incidence of shoulder dystocia with fetal macrosomia related to diabetes, but not with nondiabetic fetal macrosomia (RCOG, 2012). Stringent control of gestational diabetes mellitus (GDM) can reduce the risk of macrosomia (Rodis, 2023b).

Maternal Positioning: Labor and birth in upright positions aligns the pelvic bones for maximal expansion and optimizes the fit between passenger and passage (Hanson, 2017). Sladek and colleagues, however, found that maternal position during birth does not affect the incidence of shoulder dystocia (Sladek, Bennett, Kaar, & Smith, 2017). There is evidence that giving birth in water decreases the incidence of shoulder dystocia (Cristina et al., 2022; Snapp, Stapleton, Wright, Niemczyk, & Jolles, 2020) and the likelihood of major postpartum hemorrhage (Cristina et al., 2022).

Avoid reducing the perineum: When the fetal head is slow to emerge, many providers use a technique of reducing the perineum over the fetal chin to allow the head to fully emerge. When the head is slow to expel, however, the issue is not with the soft tissue of the introitus but with the shoulders negotiating the bony pelvis (Poujade et al., 2018). Reducing the perineum does not benefit this process, and it can increase extension of the fetal head, interfering with the internal rotation of the fetal shoulders and possibly contributing to shoulder dystocia (Poujade et al., 2018).

Managing Shoulder Dystocia

Because shoulder dystocia can occur in the absence of risk factors, every birth attendant should stand ready to manage a shoulder dystocia in every birth. Conduct emergency drills regularly so that all team members know their roles and responsibilities. Resuscitation equipment should be set up and within reach. A warm, firm surface should be available for neonatal resuscitation. Place a stool at the bedside if you anticipate using McRoberts' maneuver so that the birth assistant might be in a better position to apply suprapubic pressure.

Responding to Shoulder Dystocia

Recognize Signs

Remember that in a physiologic two-step birth, the head can be born several minutes before a second contraction expels the shoulders. If the mother is not pushing, the face is pink and grimacing, and its head is resting normally on the perineum, a delay between birth of the head and the shoulders should not be considered shoulder dystocia. Auscultate heart tones while awaiting the next contraction.

In any birth, tune into clues that shoulder dystocia is developing. When the shoulders impinge on the bony pelvis, the neck elongates with each push until it reaches the perineum. It can be slow to emerge from brows to chin. When the head emerges completely, it retracts tightly against the perineum—"turtle sign." Whereas most fetuses spontaneously restitute to the right or left, the fetus with shoulder dystocia usually remains with the face oriented posteriorly, looking toward the mother's anus. The head begins to darken as it congests with blood secondary to impaired venous return. The usual maneuvers to accomplish birth fail to release the shoulders.

DIFFERENTIAL DIAGNOSES

While actual shoulder dystocia is comparatively rare, some fetuses require additional maternal effort to expel the shoulders because of maternal position, excessive adipose tissue, or a compound or nuchal limb. Other conditions can prevent birth of the shoulders, including fetal anomalies, Bandl's ring (pathologic circumferential constriction of part of the uterus), or amniotic bands. An umbilical cord that is very short or wrapped tightly around the fetal neck or body can cause a delay between the birth of the head and the shoulders. Maternal pelvic tumors or entanglement with a twin still *in utero* can also obstruct birth.

Finesse, Not Force

Using force alone to remove a turned key from a lock risks breaking the key. Using force alone to resolve a shoulder dystocia risks harm to the fetus.

Assume Leadership

When shoulder dystocia occurs, stay calm and remember that most obstructions resolve quickly with maternal position changes or fetal manipulation. If you suspect shoulder dystocia, calmly announce, "We have a shoulder dystocia" or other agreed-upon term. Have your postpartum hemorrhage medications and supplies readily available. Plan for neonatal resuscitation.

If a waterbirth was planned, ask the mother to exit the tub (Bartlett, 2017). Neonatal depression and postpartum hemorrhage often follow shoulder dystocia, and birth is easier to manage on a dry surface. Often, stepping out of the tub and climbing onto the bed dislodges the impinging shoulder.

Get Help

In a hospital, team members can include the obstetric provider, a pediatrician or neonatologist, one or more labor and delivery nurses, and a neonatal nurse. In a community setting where just one or two trained people are present, family members, doulas, and bystanders may be called upon to assist. Assign someone to call emergency medical services (EMS). If the infant is born quickly and all is well, you can cancel the call or decline EMS upon arrival. Encourage unnecessary people to leave the room. Remove clutter. Give a team member responsibility for recording times of maneuvers and interventions.

Prepare to Intervene

Engage the mother's cooperation and assume leadership. Instruct the mother in calm but urgent tones to push only when instructed to do so (Tharpe, Farley, & Jordan, 2021). Although open-glottis pushing is beneficial in routine births, shoulder dystocia requires strong pushing efforts timed with or after maneuvers.

Attempt interventions with a sense of urgency in rapid sequence and repeat as necessary. Resolving shoulder dystocia *does not* involve a linear progression from one maneuver to the next. *No maneuver is more likely to free the infant than any other* (Gittens-Williams, 2010; Nagpal, 2016). Managing shoulder dystocia usually involves performing many maneuvers in a very short time. Progress from the least invasive maneuvers to the most invasive whenever possible and continually reassess which interventions are of greatest benefit.

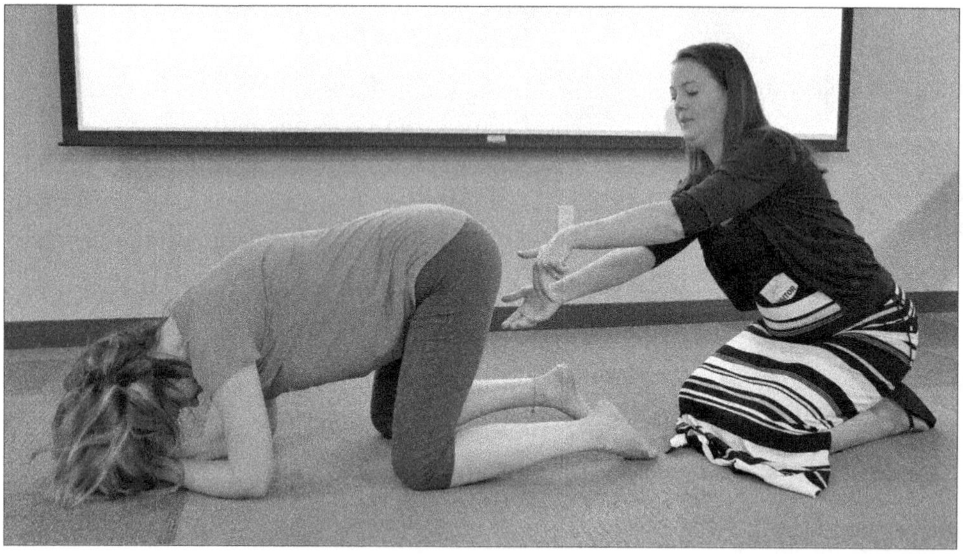

Figure 12-5. A student and instructor play "midwife and client" to practice Gaskin's maneuver in a Birth Emergency Skills Training workshop. Gaskin's maneuver may be used in preference to McRoberts' maneuver as the first intervention for a client with good mobility.

In one case, birth might occur quickly after a simple change in maternal position from side-lying to hands and knees. In another, you might need to move the client into McRoberts' position with suprapubic pressure, then attempt posterior axillary traction, then move the mother onto hands-and-knees, then attempt posterior axillary traction again, and then deliver the posterior arm to accomplish birth.

Routine Traction and External Maneuvers

When the fetal shoulders do not emerge spontaneously, the midwife should employ the least-invasive interventions—routine traction and external maneuvers—to facilitate birth. Routine traction involves guiding the baby to follow the normal mechanism of birth. External maneuvers involve moving the mother into positions that expand the pelvis or shift internal dimensions to enable birth.

Routine Traction

Initially, and between maneuvers, apply only gentle, brief, axial traction—that is, in line with the spine, without excessive downward or lateral force on the fetal neck—to ascertain whether the obstruction has been overcome (Crofts et al., 2008). Menticoglou (2018) discourages the use of *any* traction on the head to diagnose shoulder dystocia; if the mother cannot push the baby out on the next contraction after the head births, shoulder dystocia is evident. Traction *cannot* overcome the bony obstruction in true shoulder dystocia. The impaction can be resolved only by changing the orientation of the fetus or maternal pelvis, or by moving to surgical options. If the shoulders require more than gentle traction to deliver, immediately switch to other maneuvers to resolve the dystocia. When the obstruction is overcome, normal traction can facilitate birth (Rodis, 2023a).

Simulation studies have shown that providers, novice and expert alike, tend to use gentle traction initially, but apply greater force (in some cases excessive and extreme) as time passes, the shoulders remain undelivered, and anxiety mounts (Crofts et al., 2008; Walters et al., 2018). It is difficult, however, to determine how much force much is too much while applying traction. It is also difficult for an onlooker to accurately gauge the amount of force used by a provider (Walters et al., 2018).

Excessive pulling or pushing can cause serious injury to the infant. Nerve injury can occur when maternal or provider-applied forces stretch the brachial plexus beyond its limit (Singh, Shaji, Delivoria-Papadopoulos, & Balasubramanian, 2018). The infant can also suffer severe damage to the cervical spine (Saleh, Swanson, & Bragg, 2018), and there have been cases in which a live fetus was accidentally decapitated by excessive traction on the head (Habek, 2022; Vojtíšek, Kucerová, Duchanová, Krajsa, & Hejna, 2020).

Gaskin's Maneuver

Gaskin's maneuver involves assisting the mother to assume a position on hands and knees. Ina May Gaskin, CPM, introduced the maneuver to mainstream medicine in 1976, having learned it from a Belizean midwife who had observed the technique in Guatemala (Meenan, Gaskin, Hunt, & Ball, 1991). The elbows are extended, the knees are bent and against the floor or bed, and the abdomen is suspended (Zheng, Li, & Zhang, 2021). This is not the same as knee-chest, in which the client's chest is on the ground and hips are fully raised. Gaskin's maneuver has been shown to reduce the incidence of neonatal injury when compared to rotational maneuvers (Zheng et al., 2021). Whereas the dorsal lithotomy (flat on back) position limits pelvic expansion, Gaskin's maneuver can increase the AP diameter of the pelvic inlet by as much as 10 mm and increase the sagittal diameter by as much as 20 mm (Gobbo, Warren, & Hinshaw, 2020). Moreover, the sacrum can move freely when the client is on hands and knees, and gravity can provide an advantage. The act of changing position to hands and knees is often enough to resolve the obstruction. Apply gentle downward traction to the uppermost, posterior shoulder first, then upward traction to free the anterior shoulder (which rests against the symphysis pubis). Although medical texts often list this maneuver near the bottom of possible interventions for shoulder dystocia, for the mobile, unanesthetized mother giving birth outside a hospital, Gaskin's maneuver may be the most appropriate first choice.

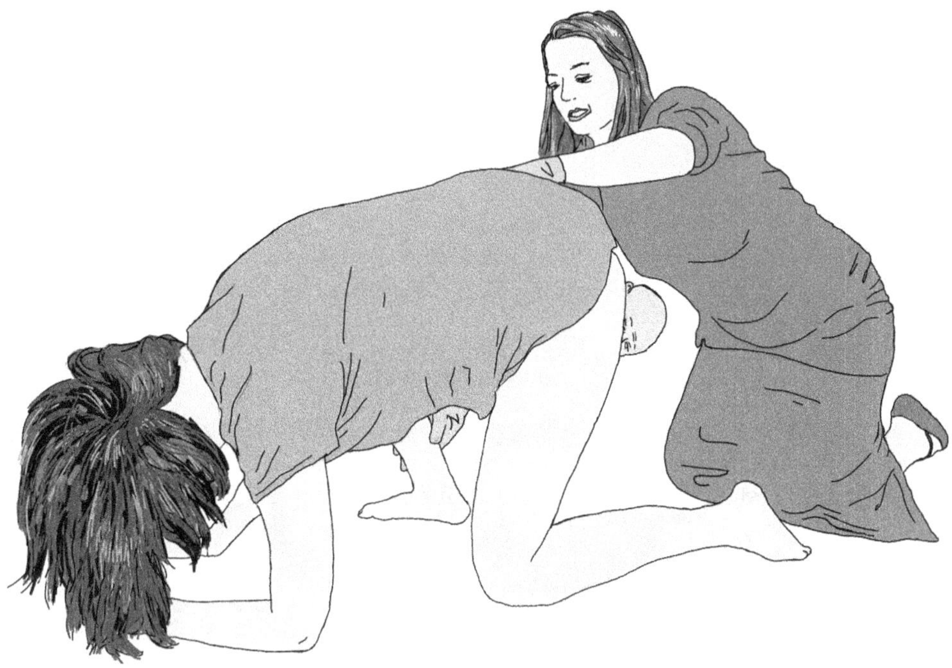

Figure 12-6. The running-start position. The midwife determines the location of the fetal back and moves the mother's leg forward on that side until the knee is by the armpit and the foot is flat on the floor.

Lunge (Running Start)

The lunge or "running start" position is a logical next step to expand pelvic diameters for the client in hands-and-knees position (Dahlke, Bhalwal, & Chauhan, 2017; Mercer & Erickson-Owens, 2009). Determine which of the mother's legs is on the same side as the fetal back. Grasp the leg near the ankle and physically bring it forward to position it. The knee should be by the armpit and the foot flat on the floor or mattress (Tully, 2012). Ensure that the forward leg remains close to the body and does not swing out to the side (Dixon & Cooke, 2019). Arching the back can beneficially flatten the lumbar curve. If this does not free the baby, the client can switch legs and perform the maneuver in reverse.

Squat

Squatting can increase pelvic capacity by about 30% (Carter, 1986), and it is a logical next step after the lunge for a freely mobile client (Hill & Cohen, 2016). When a mother squats deeply with feet flat on the floor, the pubic angle widens as the tuberosities are pulled up and apart (Carter, 1986). In fact, squatting has all the benefits of McRoberts' maneuver (see below) plus the advantages of gravity and maximal pelvic expansion (Gibb, 1995; Neill & Thornton, 2000).

McRoberts' Maneuver

McRoberts' maneuver is a technique to expand pelvic diameters by flexing the maternal thighs onto the abdomen (RCOG, 2012), which mimics a deep squatting position. McRoberts' maneuver increases the relative AP diameter of the pelvis by about 1 cm (Ansell [Irving], McAra-Couper, & Smythe, 2012), effecting ventral rotation of the symphysis pubis and flattening the sacral promontory until it no longer blocks the passage (Rodis, 2023a). It brings the pelvic inlet into alignment with the maximum expulsive force, increases pushing efficiency, and straightens lumbosacral lordosis (Rodis, 2023a). Many experts recommend this intervention as a safe, easy, and effective first step for resolving shoulder dystocia, especially for clients giving birth in supine or lithotomy position or clients with dense regional anesthesia (Cornthwaite, Crofts, Draycott, Siassakos, & Winter, 2015; Gobbo et al., 2020; Huntley & Smith, 2017; Rodis, 2023a; RCOG, 2012). McRoberts' position is effective in about 42% of cases (Rodis, 2023a)—some authorities say up to 90% (RCOG, 2012). McRoberts' also can make contractions almost twice as strong, causing an increase in uterine pressure (Buhimschi, Buhimschi, Malinow, & Weiner, 2001). Maternal Valsalva can further strengthen these contractions by about one third (Buhimschi et al., 2001).

To perform McRoberts' maneuver, remove any pillows from behind the client's back and lower the client into a supine position. Bring both legs back into a position of flexion and abduction until they rest on the abdomen, knees to nipples. The lumbar spine should be flat on the floor or bed. Use this maneuver in conjunction with suprapubic pressure (see below). When the client is in position, ask for a hard push. Provide gentle traction in direct alignment with the upper fetal spine with a downward slant no more than 45° below the horizontal plane (ACOG, 2017/2024) to assess whether the shoul-

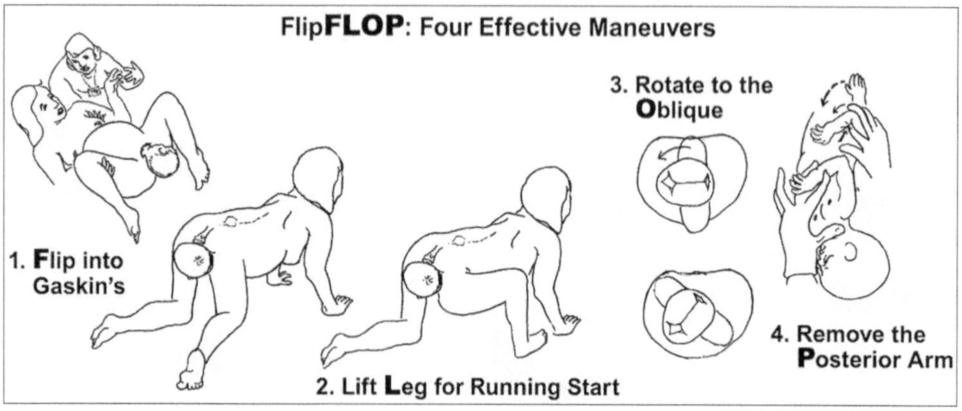

Figure 12-7. Countless midwives have used Gail Tully's FlipFLOP mnemonic to resolve shoulder dystocia. This memorable sequence helps midwives move from one maneuver to the next to accomplish birth. Graphic by Gail Tully, originator of Spinning Babies®, used with permission.

ders have been freed (RCOG, 2012; Rodis, 2023a). McRoberts' maneuver is most effective if there are two assistants helping to position the client's legs, and if the client grasps the underside of the thighs to retract the legs. Overzealous application of McRoberts' can potentially cause injury to the mother, such as symphyseal separation, sacroiliac-joint dislocation, lateral femoral cutaneous neuropathy, or transient dysfunction of the femoral nerve (ACOG, 2017/2024; Gherman, Ouzounian, Incerpi, & Goodwin, 1998). These same injuries can occur in the absence of shoulder dystocia, however (Scott, 2015).

The adipose layer of an obese client can interfere with assuming an effective McRoberts' position (Ansell [Irving], 2009). If the legs are not adequately flexed, the pelvis may not rotate enough to straighten the sacrum and open the pelvic outlet. The obese client sometimes has a panniculus (dense outpouching of subcutaneous fat over the lower abdomen) that can prevent effective suprapubic pressure (Ansell [Irving], 2009).

Suprapubic Pressure

McRoberts' maneuver is more effective when performed in conjunction with suprapubic pressure. An assistant to the midwife (preferably the strongest person available) stands on the side of the fetal back and applies moderately deep lateral suprapubic pressure with a fist or palm and locked elbows. Pressure should be applied on the soft tissue just above the pubic bone, not over the bone itself. Pressure should be aimed at the fetal shoulder, both downward to below the pubic bone and laterally toward the fetal face or sternum (ACOG, 2017/2024). This maneuver adducts the fetal shoulder toward the fetal chest or shifts it into an oblique orientation to help it move beneath the symphysis. A variation is to apply suprapubic pressure first and continue while bringing the client into McRoberts' position. Fundal pressure is always contraindicated because it can rupture the uterus or worsen the impaction.

While the client is in McRoberts' position and the assistant is applying suprapubic pressure, the midwife should grasp the fetal head between two hands and ask the mother for a very strong pushing effort. Keeping the neck in neutral alignment, gently guide the head downward, toward the mother's anus. This intervention helps help the posterior shoulder slip into the hollow of the sacrum, making room for the anterior shoulder to move beneath the pubis. The mother's expulsive efforts are the

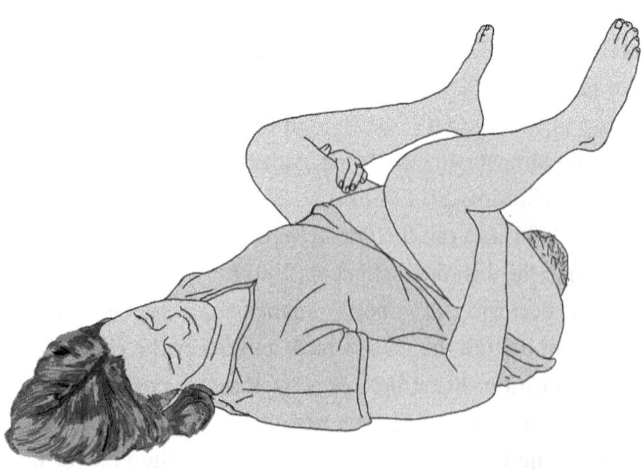

Figure 12-8. McRoberts' maneuver involves positioning the client supine with knees drawn toward the nipples, a position that increases the anteroposterior (AP) diameter of the pelvis about 1 cm, rotates the symphysis pubis ventrally, and flattens the sacral promontory.

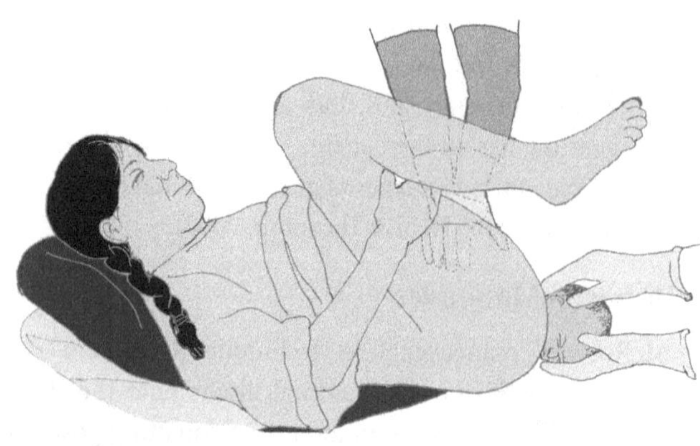

Figure 12-9. McRoberts' maneuver with suprapubic pressure can resolve almost half of all shoulder dystocia cases.

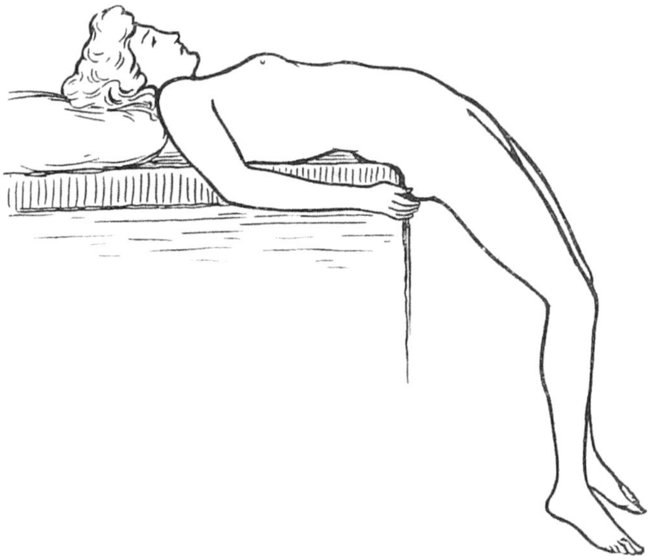

Figure 12-10. Walcher's position involves bracing the sacrum on a firm horizontal surface and allowing the legs to dangle. From A *Manual of Midwifery for Students and Practitioners* (p. 337), by H. Jellett, 1905, London, United Kingdom: Baillière, Tindall & Cox. In the public domain.

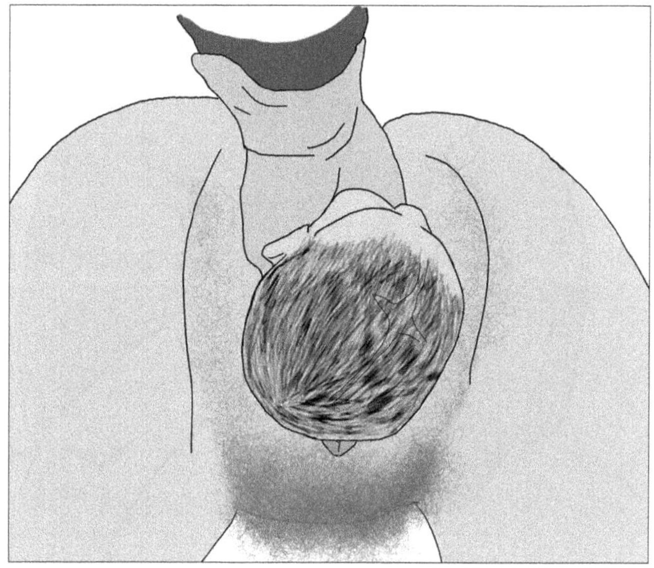

Figure 12-11. Internal maneuvers are most effective when performed with the entire hand in the vagina. To gain access, bring your fingertips together as if putting on a bracelet and work your hand into the posterior pelvis, where there is usually ample space.

force that delivers the infant. In most cases, this combination frees the fetus.

Walcher's Position

Walcher's position, first described by Arab physicians in the 11th century (Russell, 1982), involves positioning the client with the sacrum braced on a firm horizontal surface and letting the legs dangle. The weight of the legs causes the pelvis to hinge open, enlarging the AP diameter of the pelvic inlet. To use Walcher's position, help the client to a dorsal recumbent position and bring the hips to the side of the bed (Gherman, Gonik, et al., 2021). Drop the legs down toward the floor and allow them dangle or support them with a stool. Your assistant should apply suprapubic pressure directed at the back of the fetal shoulder, first toward the mother's spine, then angled toward the feet (Frye, 2013).

Leapfrog Maneuver

The leapfrog maneuver is essentially a combination of Walcher's and McRoberts' positions. Guide the mother into position with the hips at the edge of the bed. Grasp both lower legs to extend and lower them into Walcher's position while maintaining gentle support. Have your assistant apply suprapubic pressure and maintain it while you bring the mother's legs back into McRoberts' position (Gherman, Gonik, et al., 2021). The rationale is to disimpact the fetal shoulder from the symphysis by increasing the diameter of the inlet, then increasing the diameter of the outlet so the fetus will fit through. Often the baby comes out spontaneously when this maneuver is performed 1–3 times.

Internal Maneuvers

If maternal position changes fail to relieve the dystocia, move to direct manipulation of the fetus inside the vagina. Lubricate your gloved hand well and ask the mother's permission to proceed. Explain that turning the baby is invasive and uncomfortable but necessary. The best maneuver is the one that results in birth most quickly and with the least risk or trauma. Every case is unique. The art of midwifery is adapting evidence-based approaches to the situation at hand.

All internal maneuvers begin with the same action: inserting your entire hand posteriorly through the vaginal opening into the sacral hollow and assessing the probable cause of the obstruction. It is usually possible to insert your hand without cutting an episiotomy. It is easier to insert your hand if you bring the fingertips together, as if putting on a bracelet or reaching into a potato-chip tube (Crofts et al., 2008). If the posterior fetal shoulder is wedged behind the sacral promontory and the anterior shoulder is behind the pubic bone, you will feel a large, cavernous space in the vagina, which contains only the extremely stretched fetal neck.

Sweep your hand quickly but methodically around the fetus to determine the orientation of the shoulders in the pelvis. Determine whether the posterior shoulder is above, below, or at the sacral promontory and feel for cord, limbs, or fetal

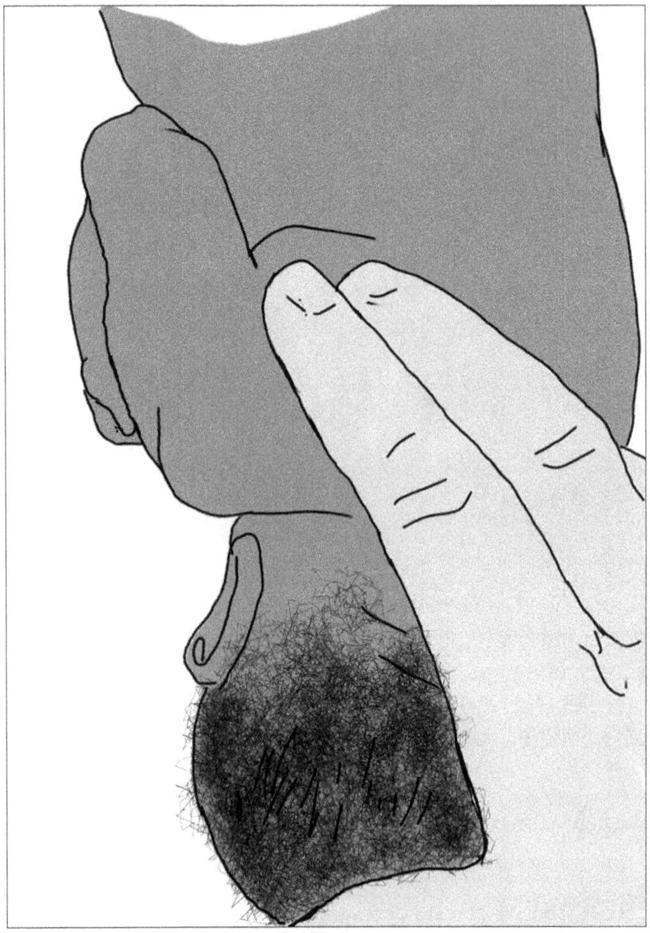

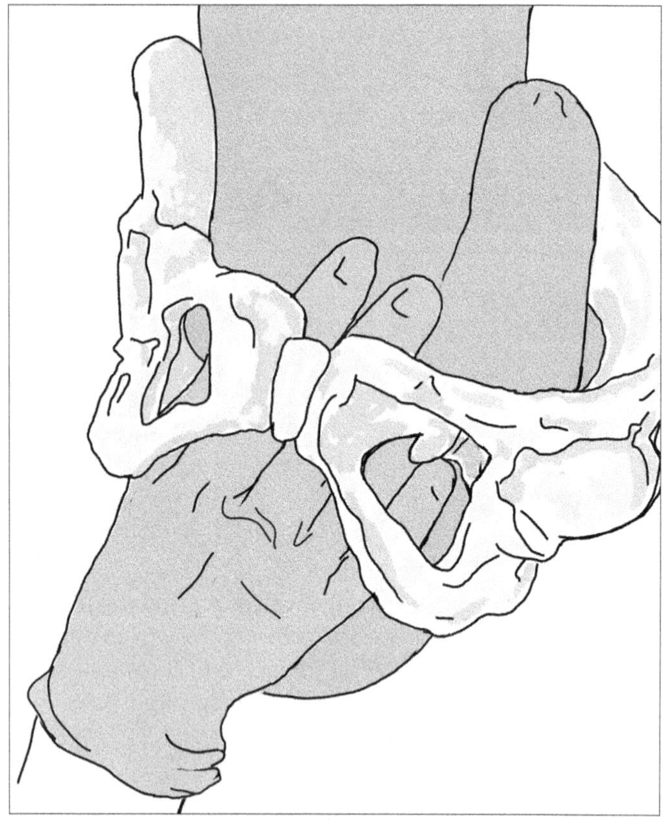

Figure 12-12. The Tharpe maneuver decreases the bisacromial diameter by folding the fetal shoulders inward.

malformations that may be preventing birth. Feel the bony architecture of the pelvis and consider the angles of pubis, sacrum, and sidewalls as they relate to the fetus. Careful exploration of the pelvis often reveals exactly what is needed to free the fetus. If you encounter a compound hand or arm, you can deliver it and resolve the obstruction. If the arm is not easily reachable, axillary adduction, traction, or rotation may be the appropriate first maneuver. If you find a tight nuchal cord, reduce it over the head, work it over the shoulders, or attempt to create slack. Leave it intact to continue the flow of oxygenated blood to the fetus (Rodis, 2023a).

Tharpe Maneuver

The Tharpe maneuver (Tharpe et al., 2021) decreases the fetal bisacromial diameter and encourages rotation. Folding the fetal shoulders toward the chest dislodges them from the symphysis or sacral promontory and reduces the width of the fetus. Nell Tharpe explains (personal communication, October 16, 2018):

> The right hand is inserted fully into the vagina, which is usually empty except for the greatly elongated neck. The fingers are used to follow the neck to the back, where the posterior axillary crease of the arm anterior to the midwife is palpated—without putting the fingers in the axilla. Traction is applied against the axillary crease using a downward and rotational motion. This spiraling motion typically brings the first shoulder into the pelvis and rotates the second shoulder to where it can spontaneously disimpact and be reached with the fingers of the left hand. The important thing is to avoid fingers in the axilla to prevent nerve damage.

If, once the shoulders are released, the baby does not readily birth as is common with big babies and tissue dystocia, then the fingers of each hand are placed against the posterior axillary creases bilaterally, and alternating pressure is applied to rotate the baby's shoulders one at a time from lateral toward the midline, keeping the baby's back toward the maternal symphysis while applying traction to keep the shoulders moving toward the vulva. This is similar to the Wood's Screw and Rubin's maneuvers; but rather than placing flat hands on the baby's chest and back, position the fingers against the axillary creases to keep the shoulders tucked in close.

Narrating the Examination

"When internal maneuvers are needed, be sure to tell the client and the maternity-care team what you are doing, feeling, and thinking. 'I'm putting my hand into the pelvis. I can feel the baby's anterior shoulder behind the symphysis. I feel the anterior crease. I am going to apply pressure. I can feel the shoulder moving . . .' This will help you to think systematically and keep everyone informed."

Nell Tharpe, personal communication, October 16, 2018.

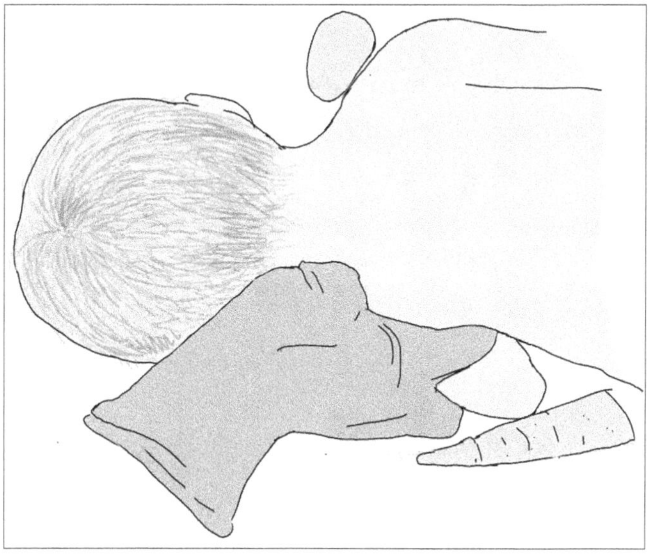

Figure 12-13. Posterior axillary traction. The grip for providing axillary traction is intuitive. Your index finger slides into the bony angle between the fetal torso and arm. Your thumb rests on the top of the shoulder, and your middle finger rests against the arm, ensuring that the force of traction is applied through the shoulder and not into the humerus. Do not dig your finger into the fetal axilla; this could cause nerve or vascular damage.

Posterior Axillary Traction

Posterior axillary traction is a simple internal maneuver that is effective in most circumstances and poses minimal risk to the infant (Ansell, Ansell, McAra-Couper, Larmer, & Garrett, 2019; Ansell [Irving] et al., 2012; Bothou et al., 2021). Use the hand on the same side of the body as the fetal back. For example, if the back of the head is pointing to the left, use your left hand (Menticoglou, 2018). If the Tharpe maneuver is performed first, the fingers are in position to perform axillary traction as an intuitive follow-up intervention.

The posterior shoulder is usually the most accessible part of the fetal torso. Upon entering the posterior vagina, follow the curve of the fetal neck until you feel the shoulder and slide your fingers over the scapula. Find the top of the axillary cleft lateral to the fetal scapula. Note that it makes a bony pouch that feels much like the gap between your forefinger and thumb. Slide one finger partially into the axilla, gaining purchase on the bony structures that give it strength. Digging into the soft tissue of the armpit can damage nerves or blood vessels (Gurewitsch & Allen, 2006). With one finger hooked onto the bony edge of the posterior axilla, your thumb on top of the shoulder, and one finger stabilizing the fetal arm against the torso, put pressure on the firm outer rim of the axilla. Pull in a continuous upward, outward motion along the curve of the maternal sacrum, shrugging and adducting the shoulder toward the fetal head and neck (Namak, Beck, Mertz, & Lord, 2016). If the posterior axilla is caught behind the sacral promontory, you may have to pull the axilla down to release it. This action can facilitate birth of the fetus because it adducts the shoulder (Namak et al., 2016). You can also apply axillary traction to the anterior shoulder (Namak et al., 2016)

Army Crawl

It can be helpful to provide axillary traction, then rotate the fetus until the posterior arm is uppermost. Perform the maneuver on the opposite axilla. If it does not free the baby, rotate the baby to the starting position and repeat axillary traction on the original arm. Work the baby out, first one axilla then the other,

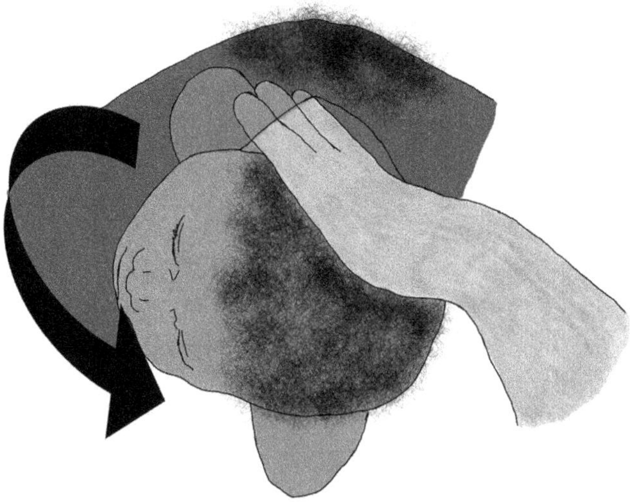

Figure 12-14. The Rubin maneuver involves entering the vagina posteriorly, then applying hand pressure to the back of the anterior or posterior fetal shoulder, whichever is more accessible, then rotating the shoulder toward the fetal face, causing the fetus to rotate.

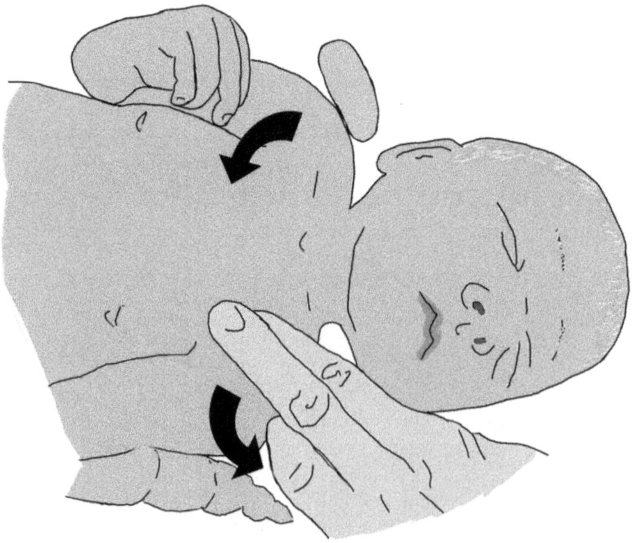

Figure 12-15. Woods' Screw. Woods' screw maneuver involves placing two fingers on the front of the fetal shoulders near the clavicles and applying pressure, which can cause the anterior shoulder to rotate through the pelvis, like a screw in a nut.

traction, turn, traction, turn, left, right, left, right. The fetus will advance like a soldier crawling low to avoid gunfire.

Rubin Maneuver

The Rubin maneuver adducts the fetal shoulder and rotates it out of AP orientation, allowing the posterior arm to enter the pelvis (Rodis, 2023a). If the fetal spine lies to the left, use your right hand; if it lies to the right, use your left. Insert one hand in the posterior vagina into the sacral hollow and work it into position against the back of the posterior fetal shoulder. Pressing on the shoulder rotates it anteriorly, toward the fetal face (Rodis, 2023a). After the shoulder is displaced into the wider oblique diameter, birth often occurs spontaneously when the mother pushes.

The Rubin maneuver can be combined with suprapubic pressure and/or McRoberts' maneuver. Alternatively, you can apply pressure to the back of the anterior shoulder if it is accessible (Rodis, 2023a). In a true shoulder dystocia, the anterior shoulder can be wedged so tightly behind the symphysis pubis that working a finger behind is difficult or impossible, and continued efforts can severely traumatize the mother's labia and urethral region (Ansell [Irving], 2009).

Woods' Screw

Woods' screw maneuver involves overcoming the bony obstruction of shoulder dystocia by displacing the fetal shoulders and initiating rotation (Woods, 1943). A screw, Woods noted, is strongly resistant to removal by direct pulling, but it comes out easily when turned (Woods, 1943). In a normal birth, after the head is born, the shoulders of a large fetus can be likened

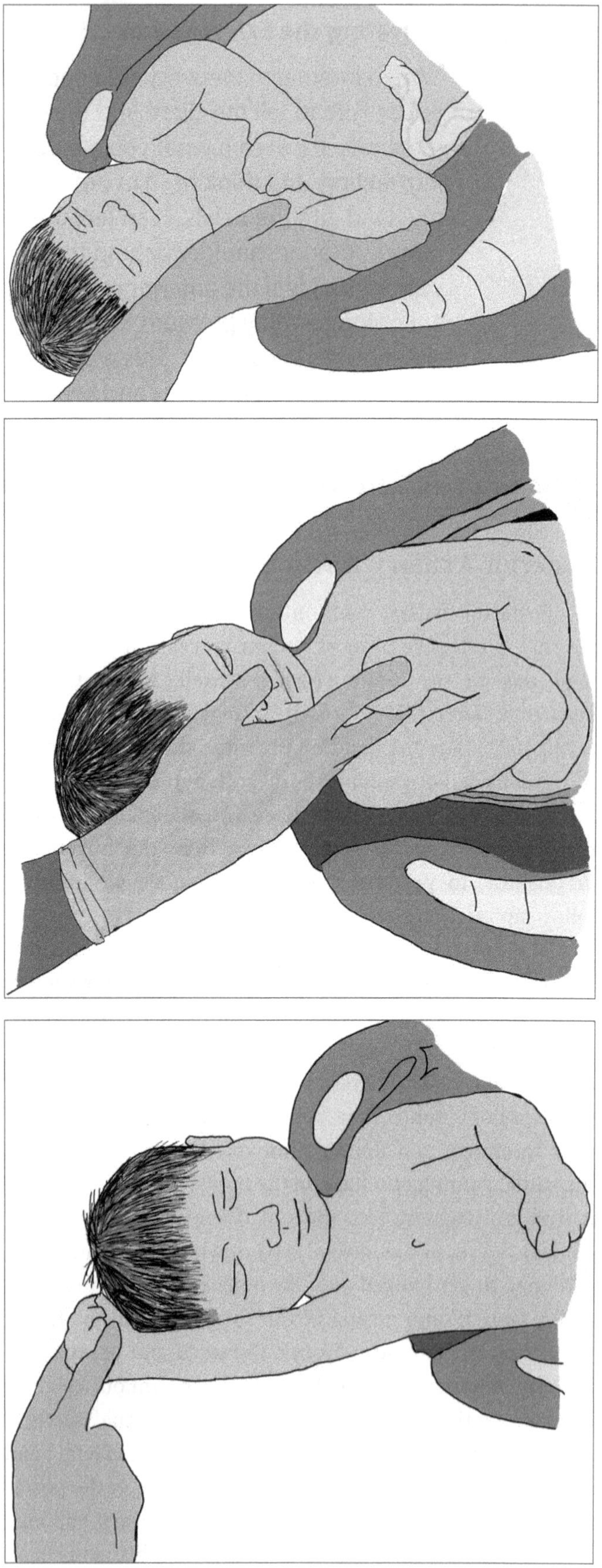

Figure 12-16. Delivering the posterior arm. Extracting the posterior arm is an effective maneuver for resolving shoulder dystocia.

to "a longitudinal section of a screw engaged in three threads, the "pubic thread," the "promontory thread," and the "coccyx thread" (Woods, 1943, p. 804). Woods compared shoulder dystocia to a screw with a crossed thread and the fetus to a bottle neck misaligned inside a twist-off cap (Woods, 1943). He wrote, "We cannot release safely the shoulders of a large baby with a 'crossed thread' unless we are able to correct the crossed thread attitude" (Woods, 1943, p. 797).

Woods' screw involves turning the fetus through the pelvis until the anterior shoulder advances from behind the pubic symphysis. Woods described using two fingers of the right hand to exert pressure on the clavicular surface of the posterior shoulder after it has passed the spines (Woods, 1943). Current recommendations include entering the vagina with the *entire hand*, the left hand if the fetal spine is to the mother's left (Rodis, 2023a). Maternal pushing provides the downward thrust needed to move the fetus. Press against the anterior surface of the posterior shoulder and turn the baby 180° counterclockwise (Rodis, 2023a). You can also combine the Rubin and Woods' maneuvers by placing one hand on the posterior aspect of the fetal shoulder and the other on the anterior aspect of the opposite shoulder. Pressure between the two hands can turn the baby clockwise or counterclockwise. Suprapubic pressure can be applied during Woods' maneuver.

Deliver Posterior Arm

Delivering the posterior arm is an extremely effective method for resolving shoulder dystocia. Hoffman et al. (2011), found it superior to other maneuvers, resolving the obstruction in 84.4% of cases, many of them after McRoberts' maneuver had failed, with a comparable rate of neonatal injury. Using a computer model, Grimm, Costello, and Gonik (2010) suggested that delivery of the posterior arm reduced expulsive force by 80% and anterior nerve stretch by 71%.

To deliver the posterior arm, insert your entire hand into the posterior vagina along the sacral curve. Find the posterior shoulder and follow it to the elbow. You can also use posterior axillary traction to bring the posterior shoulder lower for easier access to the arm. Flex the elbow across the fetal chest by applying pressure in the antecubital fossa, then grasp the wrist or hand and guide the arm gently across the fetal chest and out of the vagina. If the anterior shoulder is still wedged behind the symphysis, rotate the fetus and deliver the other arm. A major risk of this maneuver is inadvertent fracture of the baby's humerus if the upper arm is used for leverage or if the arm is drawn beyond its normal range of movement.

If the arm is trapped behind the fetus, remove your hand and insert your opposite hand for easier access to the fetal back. Follow the fetal back until you find the arm, then nudge it gently around to the front until it lies in front of the fetal chest (Gobbo et al., 2020). Withdraw your hand, then reinsert the opposite hand to the fetal chest and grasp the wrist. Sweep the arm over the chest and bring it out.

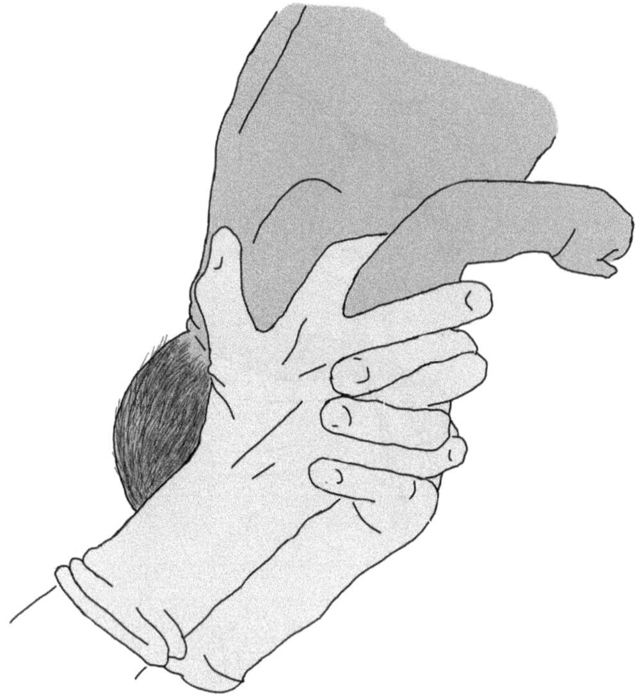

Figure 12-17. Menticoglou (2006) described a maneuver for providing axillary traction that can be described as the Armpit Finger Lock (AFL). Insert both hands into the vagina and approach the axilla from the front and back. Lock your hands together for strength and rotate or draw the fetus out. Menticoglou recommends using middle fingers across the axillae for strength, but some find the index fingers more intuitive and comfortable.

The Armpit Finger Lock (AFL/Menticoglou Maneuver)

Although extrication of the posterior arm usually resolves shoulder dystocia, it may not be feasible if the posterior arm is extended and pressed against the pelvic sidewall or is behind the fetal back (Barbieri, 2016). Thus Menticoglou (2006) advocated a technique that can be described as the AFL maneuver. Explain to the mother that you have been unable to free the baby and would like to try something that will probably be very uncomfortable. With permission, place the client in a dorsal position with the hips at the edge of the bed and the legs supported in a comfortable bent position. Get onto one knee and insert *both* hands into the vagina, clasped, index fingers extended, remaining fingers interlaced (Figure 12-17). Follow the fetal neck to the posterior shoulder (Menticoglou, 2006). It is often easier to access the posterior pelvis if an assistant supports the fetal head during the procedure. Place the right index or middle or finger (Namak et

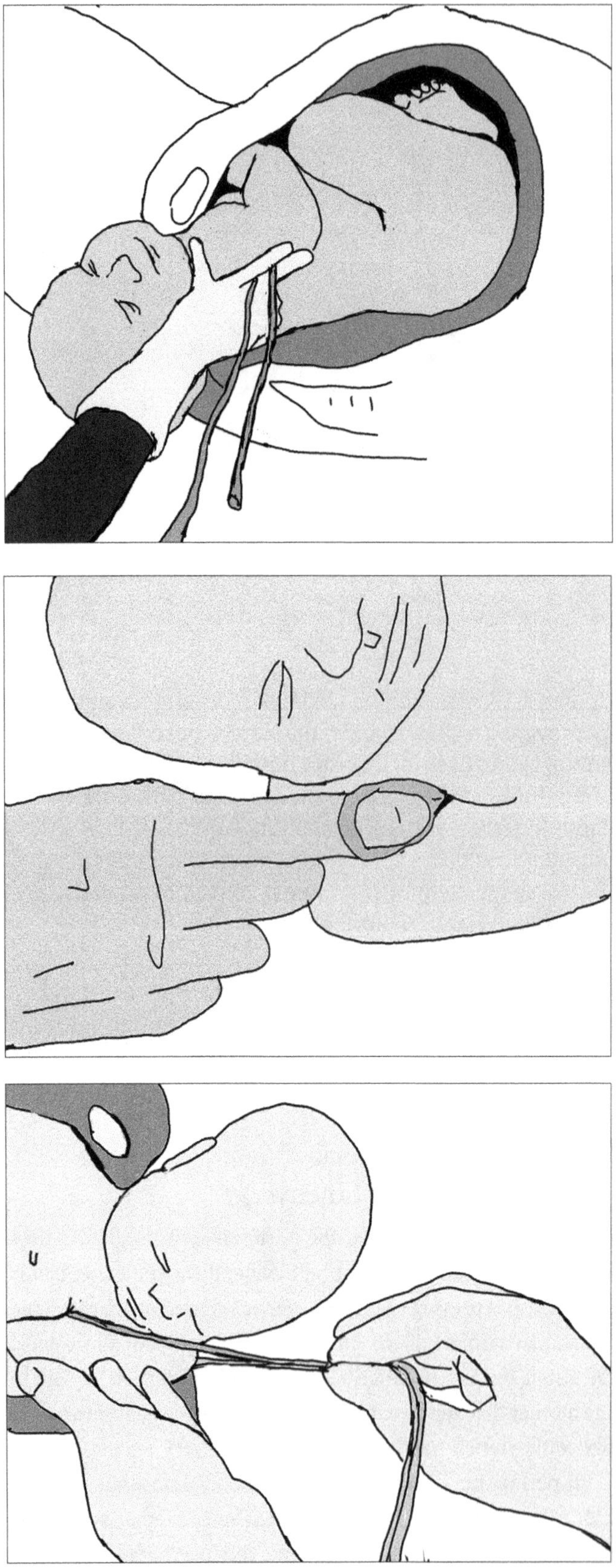

al., 2016) across the axilla from the mother's left side and the left middle or index finger across the axilla from the mother's right side, until the fingers of both hands overlap over the fetal axilla (Barbieri, 2016). Your remaining fingers are interlaced and are in the vagina below the fetal shoulder. Provide outward and downward traction on the posterior shoulder along the sacral curve. When the posterior shoulder is low in the pelvis, deliver the posterior arm, and the baby should come easily.

Posterior Axillary Sling Traction (PAST)

PAST involves passing a catheter through the fetal axilla, grasping both ends, and using traction to bring the shoulder into the sacral hollow (Cluver & Hofmeyr, 2009, 2015; Hofmeyr & Cluver, 2009). You may use a length of standard plastic medical tubing, such as intravenous (IV) infusion tubing, adult suction-catheter, or oxygen tubing. Fold the tubing in half over your fingertip and insert your hand into the vagina. Insert the loop of tubing between the posterior shoulder and the upper arm. Thread the catheter through the axilla and retrieve it with the fingers of your other hand. Apply slow, steady traction to the axilla laterally toward the side of the fetal back, then anteriorly along the pelvic curve. Have an assistant apply suprapubic pressure to adduct and disimpact the shoulder. The posterior shoulder will adduct and shrug toward the head and neck, reducing the width of the shoulder girdle. You can rotate the fetus a full 180° using this technique (Rodis, 2023a). PAST usually frees the posterior shoulder. If the posterior arm does not follow, it should be easy to reach after PAST creates room for manipulation (Cluver & Hofmeyr, 2015). Because the catheter sling keeps the arm close to the fetal torso, PAST can require less force than the AFL maneuver (Cluver & Hofmeyr, 2015).

Because the risk to the fetus is unclear, this maneuver should be reserved for intractable shoulder dystocias (Rodis, 2023a). One case study describes a difficult shoulder dystocia resolved by using a latex urinary catheter to perform PAST (McCarter, Theiler, & Rivera-Chiauzzi, 2021). The infant survived but sustained a circumferential left shoulder laceration that required debridement and surgical closure, probably a shearing injury caused by the stretch of the catheter. The child, however, had full use of the arm at one year of age.

Kwan et al. (2021) describe a difficult case involving a mother with uncontrolled diabetes, a previous cesarean, and a fetal demise who did not know she was pregnant until she began to crown on the toilet. After all other attempts to resolve

Figure 12-18. Posterior axillary sling traction (PAST) is an effective maneuver for resolving severe shoulder dystocia that requires less hand strength than the AFL maneuver. It involves threading a plastic catheter through the fetal posterior axilla and drawing the shoulder into the sacral hollow and out with lateral and anterior traction. Adapted from "Posterior Axilla Sling Traction for Shoulder Dystocia: Case Review and a New Method of Shoulder Rotation with the Sling," by C. A. Cluver and G. J. Hofmeyr, 2015, *American Journal of Obstetrics & Gynecology, 212*(6), pp. 784.e2–784.e3. Copyright by Elsevier.

the dystocia failed, the providers tied two long ribbon gauzes together, pushed the knot from the posterior axilla under the arm to the front of the body, grasped the knot with right-angle forceps, and pulled the gauze through the axilla to make a sling. Then they applied traction to the sling to simultaneously pull and rotate the posterior shoulder and free the baby. They found the ribbon gauzes easier to grasp than a rubber or plastic catheter.

Shoulder Shrug

The shoulder-shrug technique is a modification incorporating aspects of the AFL and PAST (Sancetta, Khanzada, & Leante, 2019). Insert your hand and grasp the posterior shoulder at the axilla using the thumb and index finger in a pincer grip (Sancetta et al., 2019). The tips of the fingers come together in the axillary fossa. Pull the axilla out toward the baby's head to retract (shrug) the shoulder toward the vaginal opening, against the baby's cheek. With the opposite hand, support the head in alignment with the spine and the retracted shoulder together as one unit. Keeping the retracted shoulder against the cheek, rotate this unit 180° in the direction the baby is facing. The impacted anterior shoulder will roll toward the baby's chest as it moves toward the posterior position. The shrugged shoulder should now be able to pass under the symphysis pubis, and the posterior shoulder should follow without delay. If this maneuver is unsuccessful, the provider can rotate the baby in the opposite direction.

Other Maneuvers and Measures

Measures to Increase Space in the Pelvis

These can be done at any point.

Empty Bladder

A full bladder can cause dystocia and/or postpartum hemorrhage and make suprapubic pressure difficult to perform (Rodis, 2023a). Routinely ensure that the client has an empty bladder at the time of birth. If there is a possibility that urine retention is obstructing birth, pass a catheter and drain the bladder.

Episiotomy

Because shoulder dystocia is a bone-on-bone obstruction and episiotomy opens soft tissue only, there is no evidence that episiotomy is useful in resolving shoulder dystocia (Sagi-Dain & Sagi, 2015). Episiotomy is only rarely necessary to gain access (Gurewitsch et al., 2004; RCOG, 2012; Sagi-Dain & Sagi, 2015). It is not usually difficult to work one's hands into a space that a baby's head had occupied shortly before. Moreover, it can be very difficult to cut an episiotomy when a large head is retracted into the perineum. Use of episiotomy to manage shoulder dystocia does not change the rate of brachial plexus palsy (Sagi-Dain & Sagi, 2015) or neonatal depression (Gurewitsch et al., 2004; Paris, Greenberg, Ecker, & McElrath, 2011), but it increases the rate of severe perineal injury nearly sevenfold (Gurewitsch et al., 2004). Additionally, postpartum hemorrhage is a concern after any shoulder dystocia, and episiotomy can increase maternal blood loss significantly.

In spite of the arguments against it, many authorities still recommend cutting a generous episiotomy or even a proctoepisiotomy (deliberate cutting through the vagina and rectum) to facilitate internal manipulation (ACOG, 2017/2024; Gobbo et al., 2020; Macones & Gherman, 2020; Rodis, 2023a) and deem it reasonable to cut an episiotomy before the birth of the head in the client at high risk for shoulder dystocia (Gobbo et al., 2020). In the HELPERR mnemonic (see "Mnemonics," below), episiotomy is the second consideration, after calling for help (Huntley & Smith, 2017). The midwife should weigh the evidence and consider the circumstances when deciding whether to cut an episiotomy.

Measures of Last Resort

Third-line surgical approaches to shoulder dystocia include the Zavanelli maneuver, abdominal rescue, symphysiotomy, and clavicular fracture (Mazhar & Nazir, 2016). They are usually performed by an obstetrician in a hospital after the aforementioned interventions have proven unsuccessful.

Zavanelli Maneuver (Gunn-Zavanelli-O'Leary Maneuver)

The Zavanelli maneuver is a last-resort measure that involves replacing the fetus in the uterine cavity (reversing the cardinal movements of labor) to allow birth by cesarean section (Ross & Beall, 2006). To perform the Zavanelli maneuver, the provider administers terbutaline or another tocolytic to stop contractions, rotates the head back to the position in which it emerged, flexes the head, and pushes the occiput back into the uterus as far as possible with the palm of the hand (Dharmasena, Berg, Hay, & Yoong, 2021). Although this maneuver is more straightforward on an anesthetized client, it is often surprisingly easy to accomplish without anesthesia, even after other maneuvers have failed (Rodis, 2023a). A cesarean section is performed immediately thereafter. The maneuver has been used for shoulder dystocia involving singletons, first twins with the second still unborn, conjoined twins, and stillborn fetuses (Sandberg, 1999). There is no data on the use of the Zavanelli maneuver performed in community settings.

Risks to the mother include infection, hemorrhage, and, uncommonly, trauma. Uterine rupture and bladder injury have been reported in the literature (Dharmasena et al., 2021).

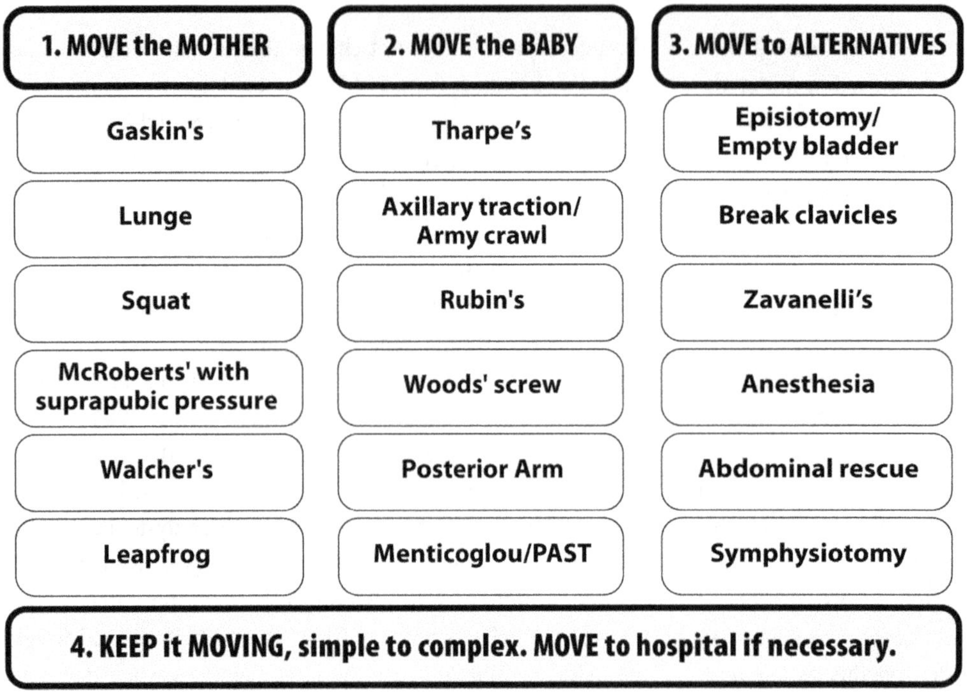

Figure 12-19. The mantra of shoulder-dystocia management is the four cardinal concepts: Move the mother. Move the baby. Move to alternatives. Keep it moving. The maneuvers within the first three categories offer many options to resolve the obstruction and can be applied in any sequence, ideally from simple to complex and from less invasive to more invasive, culminating in transport if the obstruction persists.

Neonatal outcomes are variable. Some infants do well, even when cesarean is delayed up to 70 min after replacement (Sandberg, 1999). Other infants suffer complications such as brachial plexus injuries; fractures of the clavicle, humerus and cervical spine; seizures; subarachnoid hemorrhage; HIE; cerebral palsy; delayed motor development; and intrauterine or neonatal death (Dharmasena et al., 2021). It cannot always be determined whether poor neonatal outcomes after Zavanelli's are attributable to replacing the fetus in the uterus, delay in birth, the manipulations undertaken before the Zavanelli maneuver was performed, or the shoulder dystocia itself (Dharmasena et al., 2021; Sandberg, 1999).

Labor typically ceases after the fetus is replaced (Sandberg, 1999). Rebirth while awaiting cesarean birth is extremely rare (Sandberg, 1999). While the Zavanelli maneuver can be quite uncomfortable for the unanesthetized mother, it is typically well tolerated by the mother with epidural anesthesia. One participant in an Internet forum reported being unaware that she was undergoing an emergency procedure until she felt a very strange sensation and thought, "Who just stuffed me with a cabbage?" (ChimChims, 2012).

General Anesthesia

General anesthetics can cause musculoskeletal and uterine relaxation. Under general anesthesia, normal downward traction can sometimes release severe shoulder dystocia (Lim, Gale, & Debroy, 2008). Oral or IV nitroglycerin can also be used to relax the uterus (Rodis, 2023a).

Abdominal Rescue (O'Leary Technique)

If the Zavanelli maneuver is unsuccessful, the physician may perform abdominal rescue by making a surgical incision into the uterus to gain access to the obstructing shoulder, then inserting a hand into the uterus to manually rotate the anterior shoulder to the oblique diameter while helping the posterior shoulder descend (O'Leary & Cuva, 1992). While the physician manipulates the fetus from above the symphysis, another provider should rotate the fetus in the vagina and try to deliver the posterior arm. There are case studies of good long-term outcomes from this procedure (Enekwe, Rothmund, & Uhl, 2012; O'Leary & Cuva, 1992).

Clavicular Fracture

If the shoulder is still impacted and the fetus is in danger of dying, the provider can intentionally fracture the fetal clavicle by applying upward pressure on the midportion of the fetal clavicle This intervention can collapse the shoulder girdle and hasten birth (Sahrphillips & Van Hoover, 2020). Iatrogenic clavicular fracture is now considered one of the last maneuvers to use (Gobbo et al., 2020). It can be very difficult to accomplish, and it carries the risk of pneumothorax and damage to the fetal subclavian vessels, which can cause life-threatening hemorrhage.

Symphysiotomy

Symphysiotomy is a rarely used surgical procedure that separates the pubic arch, facilitating birth. A physician incises the skin overlying the pubic symphysis and cuts into the joint with pivoting movements, dividing the fibers and supportive ligaments (Björklund, 2002) to create a small but permanent widening of the pubic arch (Enekwe et al., 2012; Rodis, 2023a). Although symphysiotomy effectively frees the baby, it can create lifelong pain and disability for the mother. Symphysiotomy is only undertaken when all other maneuvers have failed and cesarean is not available (Björklund, 2002; Enekwe et al., 2012; Rodis, 2023a).

Management in the Community Setting

Shoulder dystocia in a community setting is usually managed by a midwife with few trained assistants attending a mobile, healthy client some distance from a hospital. The optimal choice and order of maneuvers to resolve shoulder dystocia and prevent injury to mother and child are truly an expression of the art of midwifery. No study or experiment can directly compare the effectiveness of particular shoulder dystocia maneuvers or dictate their order of use (Ansell [Irving], 2009). A randomized trial, for example, would restrict providers to one maneuver or several in a fixed order; but managing shoulder dystocia, with clock ticking and lives at risk, requires the full range of options that the evolving crisis allows (Ansell [Irving], 2009).

Applying Maneuvers

As previously mentioned, shoulder-dystocia management is generally a progression from simple to complex and less invasive to more invasive, but each case is unique. Moving the mother into different positions is a good initial strategy. The provider may attempt each maneuver more than once before moving to the next intervention. The probability of success increases with the number of maneuvers tried (Rodis, 2023a). The fetus, however, is more likely to suffer injury during a prolonged dystocia requiring multiple maneuvers, probably resulting from issues related to the dystocia itself rather than the provider's interventions (Rodis, 2023a).

Apply your maneuvers smoothly by building slowly to a peak effort, avoiding high-intensity, short-duration interventions. Between maneuvers, briefly reevaluate the situation and strategize your next maneuvers. You can attempt a maneuver several times before moving to the next or backtrack and try one again. Often performing one maneuver facilitates the next. For example, axillary traction can bring the posterior shoulder low enough that the posterior arm is accessible.

Mnemonics

Mnemonics can give providers a structured framework to guide their actions as a learning tool. The mnemonic EMPOWERED reminds the community midwife to perform interventions in the order that makes the most sense in a particular clinical situation. The choice of interventions should be influenced by the client's weight, size, shape, position at diagnosis, physical surroundings, energy reserves, and ability to cooperate with maneuvers. If the client is lying in bed,

---

The **EMPOWERED** mnemonic for resolving shoulder dystocia. The first three steps are appropriate for all births.

Enable physiologic process.

Maintain calm.

Prepare for possible shoulder dystocia (maneuvers, resuscitation, and postpartum hemorrhage).

Obtain help if shoulder dystocia occurs; call emergency medical services (EMS).

Widen passage with external maneuvers (Gaskin's, lunge, McRoberts', suprapubic pressure, squat, Walcher's, leapfrog, empty bladder, episiotomy).

Execute internal maneuvers (Tharpe, axillary traction, army crawl, posterior arm, Rubin's, Woods', AFL/Menticoglou, PAST).

Record events.

Expedite transport.

Determine need for alternate or extreme measures.

McRoberts' with suprapubic pressure can be a prudent first step. Gaskin's, lunge, or supported squat can be preferable for the client on a birth stool. If a maneuver is not successful, try again or try something else.

The mnemonic **HELPERR**—HELPER in the Advanced Life Support Obstetrics® (ALSO) course (Gobbo et al., 2020)—is a widely used clinical tool that has guided providers' hands to resolve shoulder dystocia since the 1990s. **HELPERR** is an acronym for Call for **H**elp, **E**valuate for episiotomy, **L**egs (McRoberts' maneuver), **P**ressure (suprapubic), **E**nter vagina (rotary maneuvers), **R**emove posterior arm, **R**oll the client to hands and knees (Gobbo et al., 2020). The HELPERR mnemonic was developed primarily for use in hospitals, where mothers often give birth in lithotomy position with regional anesthesia and many trained assistants are at hand. Although providers have the freedom to implement the maneuvers in any sequence to fit the clinical situation, the mnemonic is often taught as a rigid, stepwise procession, giving the impression that performing maneuvers in the suggested order is the best practice (Ansell [Irving] et al., 2012).

Rapid Transport

If initial attempts to dislodge the baby fail, rapid transport is essential. Assign someone to call for EMS as soon as you suspect a shoulder dystocia. The client can always decline transport if the problem is resolved by the time the ambulance arrives. In most areas, transport by an advanced life support EMS squad is preferable to use of a private car if response times are short. U.S. paramedics and their peers elsewhere carry life-saving medications and equipment for IV infusions and newborn resuscitation, and they are trained to handle medical emergencies. They also offer additional experienced hands, a trained, experienced, undistracted driver, and lights and sirens that can part traffic snarls. The mother should have at least one large-bore IV line of crystalloid solution in anticipation of surgical procedures upon arrival at the hospital and the high likelihood of postpartum hemorrhage.

Call the labor and delivery unit at the receiving hospital and give a situation-background-assessment-recommendation (SBAR) report. Anyone can call for EMS, but ideally the midwife should make the SBAR report to the physician at the receiving hospital. Put your telephone on speaker so you can talk while you work to free the baby. Some midwives leave the telephone on speaker for continuous support and advice from the physician. The physician can notify the maternity care and neonatal intensive care units (NICUs) to prepare for your arrival. If you are at a birth center, a staff member may be able to fax records after you leave for the hospital. If you are at a home birth, take the chart so the hospital can make a copy.

Follow-Up

Although infants who have suffered significant shoulder dystocia sometimes require resuscitation, in one large hospital-based study, about 95% emerged without injury (Hoffman et al., 2011). The remainder suffered trauma and/or hypoxic injuries. A newborn who has gone through shoulder dystocia and/or resuscitation should be evaluated by a pediatrician soon after birth. Brachial plexus injuries can cause weakness, paralysis, or abnormal movement in one arm. Unintended clavicular fractures are not always detectable at birth without imaging studies. A study of non-anomalous term singleton hospital births to nulliparous mothers in California (2007–2011) found the rate of neonatal injury and death after shoulder dystocia significantly higher in low-volume and rural hospitals (Packer, Chaiken, Garg, & Caughey, 2021).

As soon as possible, have a brief preliminary conversation with the mother and any support people, explaining the problems that arose and what you did to solve them. The mother may be too physically or emotionally traumatized to process much of this information immediately after birth, so have a follow-up conversation within a few days to review the events in greater detail and assess the mother's emotional state. Ongoing conversations may be necessary to help the family process the events of the birth, especially if there was a poor outcome.

Documentation

In cases of shoulder dystocia, the attending midwife should carefully document each action and decision to preserve valuable clinical information for other providers and for protection against litigation (Zuckerwise et al., 2020). Standardized forms simplify the task of documenting a timeline; demonstrate that management was in line with the standards of care; improve the legibility, accuracy, and comprehensiveness of narrative notes; and can improve litigation defensibility (Zuckerwise et al., 2020). Documentation should be set down shortly after the event occurs so that it constitutes a contemporaneous medical note.

Antepartum

- Document risk factors for shoulder dystocia. Discuss these risk factors with the client and what it could mean for the client if a shoulder dystocia occurred out-of-hospital versus in-hospital. Discuss any concerns about transport distance and time and availability of full neonatal resuscitation. Document this conversation.
- Document the kind of screening test used for gestational diabetes (GDM) and the results. If the client declines screening, discuss potential consequences and document thoroughly. If the client has GDM, ensure that the chart contains detailed documentation of dietary counseling, blood-glucose logs, and medications. Thoroughly chart any conversations that occurred about the complications of poor glycemic control, including macrosomia.

Intrapartum

- Document estimated fetal weight (clinical or ultrasound) on the labor admission physical examination. Even if there is a large discrepancy between the estimated and actual weights, documentation verifies that fetal weight was considered in planning for birth and can be helpful if litigation ensues (Rodis, 2023a).
- Document the timeline of events and actions.
- Document the time of shoulder dystocia diagnosis and the position of the head at diagnosis.
- Describe the sequence, timing, duration, and results of each maneuver used.
- Document estimated force used in maneuvers in comparative terms such as *minimal*, *average*, and *maximal*.
- Document duration of shoulder dystocia in minutes and seconds.
- Document which shoulder was under the symphysis at diagnosis and birth.
- Describe the procedure, timing, and reason for episiotomy.

- Document the absence of fundal pressure.
- Document management of any ensuing postpartum hemorrhage and estimate blood loss.
- Document any maternal injury and the repair of any lacerations.
- Include the names of all personnel involved in the birth. Each provider involved should write a note. Collaborate while documenting and ensure that all notes agree regarding timeline and content.

Newborn

- Document birthweight and Apgar scores.
- Document any resuscitation needed and whether the cord was intact during resuscitation.
- Document carefully whether the infant was moving extremities.
- Document any signs of injury such as bruising or crepitus and any deviation from normal.

Follow-Up

- Document your conversations with the family about the events and outcomes.
- Document whether debriefing occurred and, if so, which providers were present.
- Document any follow-up regarding the condition of the newborn.

Topics for Discussion

1. At 37 0/7 weeks of gestation, Iris P. has multiple risk factors for shoulder dystocia, including poorly controlled GDM, estimated fetal weight of 8 lb 13 oz (4,000 g), and a history of shoulder dystocia. She has had full prenatal care with an obstetrician and would like to transfer into your home birth practice. She wants to give birth at home and lives 45 min from the nearest hospital, a community medical center where obstetricians take call from home. How would you discuss the risks of planning for birth at home versus hospital with her?
2. Bonita B., your midwifery apprentice, diagnosed a shoulder dystocia. Immediately, she began to pull hard on the baby's head and bend the neck laterally to release the shoulder. You stepped in and resolved the problem by using Gaskin's maneuver, then later advised her that her actions were inappropriate and could have seriously injured the baby. Bonita wants to know how her actions could have caused harm. What do you say?
3. Jeremy, a pregnant transgender man at 40 0/7 weeks of gestation, gave birth 30 min ago after a 4-min shoulder dystocia at a birth center. Dee, his midwife, successfully resuscitated the 4,500-g baby, who is breathing at a normal rate but is grunting and looking pale. The placenta has not yet delivered. What potential complications do you think Dee should consider, and how should Dee manage them if they occur? What concerns should Dee have regarding the newborn?
4. In resolving shoulder dystocia, why are external maneuvers preferred to internal maneuvers?
5. You resolve a shoulder dystocia by using Woods' screw maneuver, then delivering the posterior arm. The baby has limited movement of that arm and is unable to bring it to his mouth. What do you suspect is the problem? What are your next steps?

References

Abramowicz, J. S., & Ahn, J. T. (2022). Fetal macrosomia. In V. A. Barss (Ed.), *UpToDate*. Retrieved June 10, 2023, from https://www.uptodate.com/contents/fetal-macrosomia

Amankwah, Y. A. (2023). Shoulder dystocia. In G. D. Posner, A. Y. Black, G. Jones, & D. El-Chaâr (Eds.), *Oxorn-Foote human labor & birth* (7th ed., Kindle version, ch. 18). New York, NY: McGraw Hill.

American College of Obstetricians and Gynecologists. (2017, reaffirmed 2024). *Shoulder dystocia* (Practice Bulletin 178). Retrieved from https://www.acog.org/clinical/clinical-guidance/practice-bulletin/articles/2017/05/shoulder-dystocia

American College of Obstetricians and Gynecologists Task Force on Neonatal Brachial Plexus Palsy. (2014, reaffirmed 2019). Incidence of neonatal brachial plexus palsy. *Neonatal brachial plexus palsy*. Washington, DC: Author. Retrieved from https://www.acog.org/-/media/project/acog/acogorg/clinical/files/task-force-report/articles/2014/neonatal-brachial-plexus-palsy.pdf

Ancora, G., Meloni, C., Soffritti, S., Sandri, F., & Ferretti, E. (2020). Intrapartum asphyxiated newborns without fetal heart rate and cord blood gases abnormalities: Two case reports of shoulder dystocia to reflect upon. *Frontiers in Pediatrics, 8*. https://doi.org/10.3389/fped.2020.570332

Ansell, L., Ansell, D. A., McAra-Couper, J., Larmer, P. J., & Garrett, N. K. G. (2019). Axillary traction: An effective method of resolving shoulder dystocia. *Australian and New Zealand Journal of Obstetrics and Gynaecology, 59*(5), 627633. https://doi.org/10.1111/ajo.13029

Ansell (Irving), L. (2009). *Shoulder dystocia: Effective management of an obstetric emergency: A qualitative study* (Master's thesis). Auckland University of Technology, New Zealand. Retrieved from https://openrepository.aut.ac.nz/bitstream/handle/10292/814/AnsellL.pdf?sequence=4&isAllowed=y

Ansell (Irving), L., McAra-Couper, J., & Smythe, E. (2012). Shoulder dystocia: A qualitative exploration of what works. *Midwifery, 28*(4), e521–e528. https://doi.org/10.1016/j.midw.2011.05.007

Barbieri, R. L. (2016). Intractable shoulder dystocia: A posterior axilla maneuver may save the day. *OBG Management, 28*(4), 17–21. Retrieved from https://www.mdedge.com/obgyn/article/107793/obstetrics/intractable-shoulder-dystocia-posterior-axilla-maneuver-may-save-day

Bartlett, J. (2017). Water birth in the hospital setting. *International Journal of Childbirth Education, 32*(2), 19–25. Retrieved from https://icea.org/wp-content/uploads/2015/12/CBEd-Apr-FINAL.pdf?platform

Beall, M. H., Spong, C., McKay, J., & Ross, M. G. (1998). Objective definition of shoulder dystocia: A prospective evaluation. *American Journal of Obstetrics & Gynecology, 179*(4), 934–937. https://doi.org/10.1016/s0002-9378(98)70191-7

Björklund, K. (2002). Minimally invasive surgery for obstructed labour: A review of symphysiotomy during the twentieth century (including 5000 cases). *BJOG, 109*(3), 236–248. https://doi.org/10.1111/j.1471-0528.2002.01214.x

Bothou, A., Apostolidi, D. M., Tsikouras, P., Iatrakis, G., Sarella, A., Iatrakis, D., . . . Zervoudis, S. (2021). Overview of techniques to manage shoulder dystocia during vaginal birth. *European Journal of Midwifery, 5*, 48. https://doi.org/10.18332/ejm/142097

Bottoms, S. F., & Sokol, R. J. (1981). Mechanisms and conduct of labor. In L. Iffy & H. A. Kaminetzky (Eds.), *Principles and practice of obstetrics and perinatology* (pp. 815–837). New York, NY: John Wiley & Sons.

Bracken, O., & Langhe, R. (2021). Evaluation of maternal and perinatal outcomes in pregnancy with high BMI. *Irish Journal of Medical Science, 190*(4), 1439–1444. https://doi.org/10.1007/s11845-020-02456-4

Buhimschi, C. S., Buhimschi, I. A., Malinow, A., & Weiner, C. P. (2001). Use of McRoberts' position during delivery and increase in pushing efficiency. *Lancet, 358*(9280), 470–471. https://doi.org/10.1016/S0140-6736(01)05632-X

Burd, J. (2022). Shoulder dystocia. In V. Berghella (Ed.), *Obstetric evidence based guidelines* (4th ed., pp. 314–329). Boca Raton, FL: CRC Press. https://doi.org/10.1201/9781003102342

Burkhardt, T., Schmidt, M., Kurmanavicius, J., Zimmermann, R., & Schäffer, L. (2014). Evaluation of fetal anthropometric measures to predict the risk for shoulder dystocia. *Ultrasound in Obstetrics & Gynecology, 43*(1), 77–82. https://doi.org/10.1002/uog.12560

Carter, V. (1986). Another technique for resolution of shoulder dystocia. *American Journal of Obstetrics & Gynecology, 154*(4), 964. https://doi.org/10.1016/0002-9378(86)90499-0

ChimChims [Screen name]. (2012, March 26). Zavanelli maneuver—Baby pushed back inside after delivering head. Message posted to https://babyandbump.momtastic.com/threads/zavanelli-maneuver-baby-pushed-back-inside-after-delivering-head.927009/

Cluver, C. A., & Hofmeyr, G. J. (2009). Posterior axilla sling traction: A technique for intractable shoulder dystocia. *Obstetrics & Gynecology, 113*(2), 486–488. https://doi.org/10.1097/AOG.0b013e318190a2d6

Cluver, C. A., & Hofmeyr, G. J. (2015). Posterior axilla sling traction for shoulder dystocia: Case review and a new method of shoulder rotation with the sling. *American Journal of Obstetrics & Gynecology, 212*(6), 784e1–784.e7. https://doi.org/10.1016/j.ajog.2015.02.025

Cornthwaite, K., Crofts, J., Draycott, T., Siassakos, D., & Winter, C. (2015). *Training for obstetric emergencies: PROMPT and shoulder dystocia*. n.p.: The Health Foundation. Retrieved from http://patientsafety.health.org.uk/sites/default/files/resources/5.shoulder_dystocia-v3.pdf

Cristina, T., Mara, T., Arianna, S., Gennaro, S., Rosaria, C., & Pantaleo, G. (2022). Impact of waterbirth on post-partum hemorrhage, genital trauma, retained placenta and shoulder dystocia: A systematic review and meta-analysis. *European Journal of Obstetrics & Gynecology and Reproductive Biology. 276, 26–37.* https://doi.org/10.1016/j.ejogrb.2022.06.016

Crofts, J. F., Fox, R., Ellis, D., Winter, C., Hinshaw, K., & Draycott, T. J. (2008). Observations from 450 shoulder dystocia simulations: Lessons for skills training. *Obstetrics & Gynecology, 112*(4), 906–912. https://doi.org/10.1097/AOG.0b013e3181865f55

Dahlke, J. D., Bhalwal, A., & Chauhan, S. P. (2017). Obstetric emergencies: Shoulder dystocia and postpartum hemorrhage. *Obstetrics and Gynecology Clinics of North America, 44*(2), 231–243. https://doi.org/10.1016/j.ogc.2017.02.003

Dharmasena, D., Berg, L., Hay, A., & Yoong, W. (2021). The Zavanelli manoeuvre revisited: A review of the literature and a guide to performing cephalic replacement for severe shoulder dystocia. *European Journal of Obstetrics & Gynecology and Reproductive Biology, 266*, 63–73. https://doi.org/10.1016/j.ejogrb.2021.09.011

Dixon, L., & Cooke, H. (2019). Life-threatening emergencies. In S. Pairman, S. K. Tracy, H. G. Dahlen, & L. Dixon (Eds.). *Midwifery: Preparation for practice* (4th ed., book 2, pp. 943–992). Chatswood, NSW, Australia: Elsevier.

Downe, S., & Marshall, J. (2014). Physiology and care during the transition and second stage phases of labour. In J. Marshall & M. Raynor (Eds.), *Myles' textbook for midwives* (16th ed., pp. 367–394). Edinburgh, United Kingdom: Elsevier Health Sciences.

Enekwe, A., Rothmund, R., & Uhl, B. (2012). Abdominal access for shoulder dystocia as a last resort—A case report. *Geburtshilfe und Frauenheilkunde, 72*(7), 634–638. https://doi.org/10.1055/s-0032-1314962

Floyd, R. C., & Smeltzer, J. S. (2021). Shoulder dystocia. In H. N. Winn, F. A. Chervenak, & R. Romero (Eds.), *Clinical maternal-fetal medicine online*. https://doi.org/10.1201/9781003222590-11

Frye, A. (2013). *Holistic midwifery: A comprehensive textbook for midwives in homebirth practice, vol. II: Care of the mother and baby from the onset of labor through the first hours after birth* (2nd ed.). Portland, OR: Labrys Press.

Gherman, R., Gonik, B., & Ouzounian, J. (2021). Shoulder dystocia. In M. B. Landon, H. L. Galan, E. R. M. Jauniaux, D. A. Driscoll, V. Berghella, W. A. Grobman, . . . A. G. Cahill (Eds.), *Gabbe's obstetrics: Normal and problem pregnancies* (8th ed., E-Book, ch. 14). Philadelphia, PA: Elsevier.

Gherman, R. B., Ouzounian, J. G., Incerpi, M. H., & Goodwin, T. M. (1998). Symphyseal separation and transient femoral neuropathy associated with the McRoberts' maneuver. *American Journal of Obstetrics & Gynecology, 178*(3), 609–610. https://doi.org/10.1016/s0002-9378(98)70447-8

Gibb, D. (1995). The obstetrics. *Clinical Risk, 1*(2), 49–54. https://doi.org/10.1177/135626229500100202

Gittens-Williams, L. (2010). Contemporary management of shoulder dystocia. *Women's Health, 6*(6), 861–869. https://doi.org/10.2217/WHE.10.65

Gobbo, R. W., Warren, J. B., & Hinshaw, K. (2020). Shoulder dystocia. In L. Leeman, L. Dresang, J. S. Quinlan, & S. R. Magee (Eds.), *Advanced life support in obstetrics: Provider manual* (9th ed., pp. 129–155). Leawood, KS: American Academy of Family Physicians.

Goetzinger, K. R., Odibo, A. O., Shanks, A. L., Roehl, K. A., & Cahill, A. G. (2014). Clinical accuracy of estimated fetal weight in term pregnancies in a teaching hospital. *Journal of Maternal-Fetal & Neonatal Medicine, 27*(1), 89–93. Retrieved from https://www.ncbi.nlm.nih.gov/pmc/articles/PMC3929500/

Gold, K. J., Mozurkewich, E. L., Puder, K. S., & Treadwell, M. C. (2016). Complications associated with stillbirth delivery: A cross-sectional analysis. *Journal of Obstetrics and Gynaecology, 36*(2),208–212. https://doi.org/10.3109/01443615.2015.1050646

Grimm, M. J., Costello, R. E., & Gonik, B. (2010). Effect of clinician-applied maneuvers on brachial plexus stretch during a shoulder dystocia event: Investigation using a computer simulation model. *American Journal of Obstetrics & Gynecology, 203*(4), 339.e1,339.e5. https://doi.org/10.1016/j.ajog.2010.05.002

Gurewitsch, E. D., & Allen, R. H. (2006). Fetal manipulation for management of shoulder dystocia. *Fetal and Maternal Medicine Review, 17*(3), 239–280. https://doi.org/10.1017/S096553950600180X

Gurewitsch, E. D., Donithan, M., Stallings, S. P., Moore, P. L., Agarwal, S., Allen, L. M., & Allen, R. H. (2004). Episiotomy versus fetal manipulation in managing severe shoulder dystocia: A comparison of outcomes. *American Journal of Obstetrics & Gynecology, 191*(3), 911–916. https://doi.org/10.1016/j.ajog.2004.06.041

Habek, D. (2022). Intrapartal fetal decapitation after shoulder dystocia—A forensically acceptable or unacceptable complication? *Journal of Perinatal Medicine, 50*(4), 503–504. https://doi.org/10.1515/jpm-2021-0638

Hanson, L. (2017). Low-technology clinical interventions to promote labor progress. In P. Simkin, L. Hanson, & R. Ancheta, (Eds.), *The labor progress handbook: Early interventions to prevent and treat dystocia* (4th ed., pp. 231–259). Hoboken, NJ: John Wiley & Sons.

Hart, A. R., Sharma, R., Rittey, C. D., & Mordekar, S. R. (2015). Neonatal hypertonia—A diagnostic challenge. *Developmental Medicine & Child Neurology, 57*(7), 600–610. https://doi.org/10.1111/dmcn.12658

Heinonen, K., Saisto, T., Gissler, M., Kaijomaa, M., & Sarvilinna, N. (2021). Rising trends in the incidence of shoulder dystocia and development of a novel shoulder dystocia risk score tool: A nationwide population-based study of 800 484 Finnish deliveries. *Acta Obstetricia et Gynecologica Scandinavica, 100*(3), 538–547. https://doi.org/10.1111/aogs.14022

Hill, M. G., & Cohen, W. R. (2016). Shoulder dystocia: Prediction and management. *Women's Health, 12*(2), 251–261. https://doi.org/10.2217/whe.15.103

Hoffman, M. K., Bailit, J. L., Branch, D. W., Burkman, R. T., Van Veldhusien [*sic*], P., Lu, L., . . . Zhang, J. (2011). A comparison of obstetric maneuvers for the acute management of shoulder dystocia. *Obstetrics & Gynecology, 117*(6), 1272–1278. https://doi.org/10.1097/AOG.0b013e31821a12c9

Hofmeyr, G. J., & Cluver, C. A. (2009). Posterior axilla sling traction for intractable shoulder dystocia. *BJOG, 116*(13), 1818–1820. https://doi.org/10.1111/j.1471-0528.2009.02373.x

Hope, P., Breslin, S., Lamont, L., Lucas, A., Martin, D., Moore, I., . . . Settatree, R. (1998). Fatal shoulder dystocia: A review of 56 cases reported to the Confidential Enquiry into Stillbirths and Deaths in Infancy. *BJOG, 105*(12), 1256–1261. https://doi.org/10.1111/j.1471-0528.1998.tb10003.x

Huntley, M., & Smith, J. D. (2017). Management of shoulder dystocia using the HELPERR mnemonic. *British Journal of Midwifery, 25*(4), 240–244. https://doi.org/10.12968/bjom.2017.25.4.240

Jellett, H. (1905). *A manual of midwifery for students and practitioners*. London, United Kingdom: Baillière, Tindall & Cox. Retrieved from https://archive.org/details/b21932670

Kanik, A., Sutcuoglu, S., Aydinlioglu, H., Erdemir, A., & Ozer, E. A. (2011). Bilateral clavicle fracture in two newborn infants. *Iranian Journal of Pediatrics, 21*(4), 553–555. Retrieved from https://www.ncbi.nlm.nih.gov/pmc/articles/PMC3446140/

Kesrouani, A., Atallah, C., AbouJaoude, R., Assaf, N., Khaled, H., & Attieh, E. (2017). Accuracy of clinical fetal weight estimation by midwives. *BMC Pregnancy and Childbirth, 17*(1), 59. https://doi.org/10.1186/s12884-017-1242-7

Kominiarek, M. A., Saade, G., Mele, L., Bailit, J., Reddy, U. M., Wapner, R. J., . . . Tolosa, J. E. (2018). Association between gestational weight gain and perinatal outcomes. *Obstetrics & Gynecology, 132*(4), 875–881. https://doi.org/10.1097/AOG.0000000000002854

Kotaska, A., & Campbell, K. (2014). Two-step delivery may avoid shoulder dystocia: Head-to-body delivery interval is less important than we think. *Journal of Obstetrics and Gynaecology Canada, 36*(8), 716–720. Retrieved from https://www.jogc.com/article/S1701-2163(15)30514-4/pdf

Kwan, A. H. W., Hui, A. S. Y., Lee, J. H. S., & Leung, T. Y. (2021). Intrauterine fetal death followed by shoulder dystocia and birth by modified posterior axillary sling method: A case report. *BMC Pregnancy and Childbirth. 21*, 672. https://doi.org/10.1186/s12884-021-04126-4

Leung, T. Y., Stuart, O., Sahota, D. S., Suen, S. S. H., Lau, T. K., & Lao, T. T. (2011). Head-to-body delivery interval and risk of fetal acidosis and hypoxic ischaemic encephalopathy in shoulder dystocia: A retrospective review. *BJOG, 118*(4), 474–479. https://doi.org/10.1111/j.1471-0528.2010.02834.x

Lim, M.-N., Gale, A., & Debroy, B. (2008). Early resort to general anaesthesia in severe shoulder dystocia. *Journal of Obstetrics and Gynaecology, 28*(4), 436–437. https://doi.org/10.1080/01443610802163823

Locatelli, A., Incerti, M., Ghidini, A., Longoni, A., Casarico, G., Ferrini, S., & Strobelt, N. (2011). Head-to-body delivery interval using 'two-step' approach in vaginal deliveries: Effect on umbilical artery pH. *Journal of Maternal-Fetal & Neonatal Medicine, 24*(6), 799–803. https://doi.org/10.3109/14767058.2010.531307

Lockwood, C. J. (2014). Neonatal brachial plexus palsy: Is prevention possible? *Contemporary OB/GYN, 59*(7), 4–6.

Macones, G. A., & Gherman, R. (2020). Shoulder dystocia. In J. T. Queenan, C. Y. Spong, & C. J. Lockwood (Eds.), *Protocols for high-risk pregnancies: An evidence-based approach* (7th ed., pp. 581–586). Oxford, United Kingdom: Blackwell Publishing. https://doi.org/10.1002/9781119635307.ch56

Mazhar, S. B., & Nazir, A. (2016). Surgical management options for shoulder dystocia: Zavanelli maneuver, abdominal rescue, symphysiotomy, and cleidotomy. In A. Coomaraswamy, M. I. Shafi, G. W. Davila, & K. K. Chan (Eds.), *Gynecologic and obstetric surgery: Challenges and management options* (pp. 482–484). Oxford, United Kingdom: John Wiley & Sons. https://doi.org/10.1002/9781118298565.ch161

McCarter, A. R., Theiler, R. N., & Rivera-Chiauzzi, E. Y. (2021). Circumferential shoulder laceration after posterior axilla sling traction: A case report of severe shoulder dystocia. *BMC Pregnancy and Childbirth, 21*, 45. https://doi.org/10.1186/s12884-020-03526-2

Meenan, A. L., Gaskin, I. M., Hunt, P., & Ball, C. A. (1991). A new (old) maneuver for the management of shoulder dystocia. *Journal of Family Practice, 32*(6), 625–629.

Mendez-Figueroa, H., Hoffman, M. K., Grantz, K. L., Blackwell, S. C., Reddy, U. M., & Chauhan, S. P. (2021). Shoulder dystocia and composite adverse outcomes for the maternal-neonatal dyad. *American Journal of Obstetrics & Gynecology MFM, 3*(4), 100359. https://doi.org/10.1016/j.ajogmf.2021.100359

Menticoglou, S. (2018). Shoulder dystocia: Incidence, mechanisms, and management strategies. *International Journal of Women's Health, 10*, 723–732. https://doi.org/10.2147/IJWH.S175088

Menticoglou, S., & Schneider, C. (2016). Resuscitating the baby after shoulder dystocia. *Case Reports in Obstetrics and Gynecology, 2016*. https://doi.org/10.1155/2016/8674167

Menticoglou, S. M. (2006). A modified technique to deliver the posterior arm in severe shoulder dystocia. *Obstetrics & Gynecology, 108*(3), 755–757. https://doi.org/10.1097/01.aog.0000232505.65290.04

Mercer, J., Erickson-Owens, D., & Skovgaard, R. (2009). Cardiac asystole at birth: Is hypovolemic shock the cause? *Medical Hypotheses, 72*(4), 458–463. https://doi.org/10.1016/j.mehy.2008.11.019

Mercer, J. S., & Erickson-Owens, D. A. (2009). The midwifery view of shoulder dystocia. In J. A. O'Leary (Ed.), *Shoulder dystocia and birth injury: Prevention and treatment* (3rd ed., pp. 269–284). Totowa, NJ: Humana Press.

Nagpal, M. (2016). Shoulder dystocia. In A. Gandhi, N. Malhotra, J. Malhotra, N. Gupta, & N. Bora (Eds.), *Principles of critical care in obstetrics* (pp. 347–353). New Delhi, India: Springer. https://doi.org/10.1007/978-81-322-2692-5_33

Namak, S., Beck, K., Mertz, H., & Lord, R, (2016). Axillary digital traction maneuver: Shoulder dystocia management. *Journal of Family Medicine & Community Health, 3*(4), 1086–1090. Retrieved from https://www.jscimedcentral.com/FamilyMedicine/familymedicine-3-1086.pdf

Neill, A. M., & Thornton, S. (2000). Shoulder dystocia. *Obstetrician & Gynaecologist, 2*(4), 45–47. https://doi.org/10.1576/toag.2000.2.4.45

O'Leary, J. A., & Cuva, A. (1992). Abdominal rescue after failed cephalic replacement. *Obstetrics & Gynecology, 80*(3, Pt. 2), 514–516. Retrieved from https://journals.lww.com/greenjournal/Abstract/1992/09000/ABDOMINAL_RESCUE_AFTER_FAILED_CEPHALIC.54.aspx

Ouzounian, J. G., Korst, L. M., Sanchez, M., Chauhan, S., Gherman, R. B., Opper, N., & Wilson, M. L. (2016). Clinical risk factors do not predict shoulder dystocia.

Journal of Reproductive Medicine, 61(11–12), 575–580. Retrieved from https://pubmed.ncbi.nlm.nih.gov/30226711/

Øverland, E. A., Vatten, L. J., & Eskild, A. (2014). Pregnancy week at delivery and the risk of shoulder dystocia: A population study of 2,014,956 deliveries. *BJOG, 121*(1), 34–41. https://doi.org/10.1111/1471-0528.12427

Packer, C. H., Chaiken, S. R., Garg, B., & Caughey, A. B. (2021). 944 Neonatal outcomes among deliveries complicated by shoulder dystocia by hospital type. *American Journal of Obstetrics & Gynecology, 224*(2), S586-S587. https://doi.org/10.1016/j.ajog.2020.12.969

Palatnik, A., Grobman, W. A., Hellendag, M. G., Janetos, T. M., Gossett, D. R., & Miller, E. S. (2016). Predictors of shoulder dystocia at the time of operative vaginal delivery. *American Journal of Obstetrics & Gynecology, 215*(5), 624.e1–624.e5. https://doi.org/10.1016/j.ajog.2016.06.001

Paris, A. E., Greenberg, J. A., Ecker, J. L., & McElrath, T. F. (2011). Is an episiotomy necessary with a shoulder dystocia? *American Journal of Obstetrics & Gynecology, 205*(3), 217-e1–217.e3. https://doi.org/0.1016/j.ajog.2011.04.006

Poujade, O., Azria, E., Ceccaldi, P.-F., Davitian, C., Khater, C., Chatel, P., . . . Louton, D. (2018). Prevention of shoulder dystocia: A randomized controlled trial to evaluate an obstetric maneuver. *European Journal of Obstetrics & Gynecology and Reproductive Biology, 227,* 52–59. https://doi.org/10.1016/j.ejogrb.2018.06.002

Riskin, A., & Garcia-Prats, J. A. (2023). Infants of mothers with diabetes (IMD). In C. Armsby (Ed.), *UpToDate*. Retrieved June 10, 2023, from https://www.uptodate.com/contents/infants-of-mothers-with-diabetes-imd

Rodis, J. F. (2023a). Shoulder dystocia: Intrapartum diagnosis, management, and outcome. In V. A. Barss, (Ed.), *UpToDate*. Retrieved June 10, 2023, from https://www.uptodate.com/contents/shoulder-dystocia-intrapartum-diagnosis-management-and-outcome

Rodis, J. F. (2023b). Shoulder dystocia: Risk factors and planning birth of high-risk pregnancies. In V. A. Barss (Ed.), *UpToDate*. Retrieved June 10, 2023, from https://www.uptodate.com/contents/shoulder-dystocia-risk-factors-and-planning-birth-of-high-risk-pregnancies

Ross, M. G., & Beall, M. H. (2006). Cervical neck dislocation associated with the Zavanelli maneuver. *Obstetrics & Gynecology, 108*(3), 737–738. https://doi.org/10.1097/01.AOG.0000218694.07694.36

Royal College of Obstetricians and Gynaecologists. (2012). *Shoulder dystocia* (Green Top Guideline No. 42, 2nd ed.). London, United Kingdom: Author. Retrieved from https://www.rcog.org.uk/globalassets/documents/guidelines/gtg_42.pdf

Russell, J. G. B. (1982). The rationale of primitive delivery positions. *BJOG, 89*(9), 712–715. https://doi.org/10.1111/j.1471-0528.1982.tb05096.x

Sagi-Dain, L., & Sagi, S. (2015). The role of episiotomy in prevention and management of shoulder dystocia: A systematic review. *Obstetrical & Gynecological Survey, 70*(5), 354–362. https://doi.org/10.1097/OGX.0000000000000179

Sahrphillips, J. F., & Van Hoover, C. (2020). Maneuvering through a birth complicated by shoulder dystocia. *Journal of Midwifery & Women's Health, 65*(3), 395–403. https://doi.org/10.1111/jmwh.13087

Saleh, S., Swanson, K. I., & Bragg, T. (2018). Successful surgical repair and recovery in a 2-week-old infant after birth-related cervical fracture dislocation. *Journal of Neurosurgery: Pediatrics, 21*(1), 16–20. https://doi.org/10.3171/2017.7.PEDS17105

Sancetta, R., Khanzada, H., & Leante, R. (2019). Shoulder shrug maneuver to facilitate delivery during shoulder dystocia. *Obstetrics & Gynecology, 133*(6), 1178–1181. https://doi.org/10.1097/AOG.0000000000003278

Sandberg, E. C. (1999). The Zavanelli maneuver: 12 years of recorded experience. *Obstetrics & Gynecology, 93*(2), 312–317. https://doi.org/10.1016/S0029-7844(98)00340-8

Scott, K. M. (2015). Neural injury during pregnancy and childbirth. In C. M. Fitzgerald & N. A. Segal (Eds.), *Musculoskeletal health in pregnancy and postpartum: An evidence-based guide for clinicians* (pp. 93–114). Cham, Switzerland: Springer.

Selcen, D. (2023). Neonatal brachial plexus palsy. In R. P. Goddeau, Jr. (Ed.), *UpToDate*. Retrieved June 10, 2023, from https://www.uptodate.com/contents/neonatal-brachial-plexus-palsy

Singh, A., Shaji, S., Delivoria-Papadopoulos, M., & Balasubramanian, S. (2018). Biomechanical responses of neonatal brachial plexus to mechanical stretch. *Journal of Brachial Plexus and Peripheral Nerve Injury, 13*(1), e8–e14. https://doi.org/10.1055/s-0038-1669405

Sladek, S., Bennett, S., Kaar, J., & Smith, R. (2017). Does maternal position during delivery affect the incidence of neonatal shoulder dystocia? *Evidence-Based Practice, 20*(9), E5–E6. https://doi.org/10.1097/01.EBP.0000541828.78179.50

Snapp, C., Stapleton, S. R., Wright, J., Niemczyk, N. A., & Jolles, D. (2020). The experience of land and water birth within the American Association of Birth Centers *Perinatal Data Registry*, 2012–2017. *Journal of Perinatal & Neonatal Nursing, 34*(1), 16–26. https://doi.org/10.1097/JPN.0000000000000450

Tharpe, N. L., Farley, C. L., & Jordan, R. G. (2021). *Clinical practice guidelines for midwifery & women's health* (6th ed.). Burlington, MA: Jones & Bartlett Learning.

Tully, G. (2012). FlipFLOP: Four steps to remember. *Midwifery Today*, 103, 9–11. Retrieved from https://midwiferytoday.com/mt-articles/flipflop-four-steps-remember/

Victor, S., Rocha-Ferreira, E., Rahim, A., Hagberg, H., & Edwards, D. (2022). New possibilities for neuroprotection in neonatal hypoxic-ischemic encephalopathy. *European Journal of Pediatrics, 181,* 875–887 (2022). https://doi.org/10.1007/s00431-021-04320-8

Vojtíšek, T., Kucerová, Š. P., Duchanová, S., Krajsa, J., & Hejna, P. (2020). Traumatic decapitation of the fetus during birth: Criminalistic and forensic aspects. *American Journal of Forensic Medicine and Pathology, 41*(3), 234–237. https://doi.org/10.1097/PAF.0000000000000556

Walters, M., Eubanks, A., Weissbrod, E., Fischer, J., Staat, B., & Deering, S. (2018). Visual estimation of force applied during simulated deliveries complicated by shoulder dystocia. *American Journal of Perinatology Reports, 8*(4), e206–e211. https://doi.org/10.1055/s-0038-1673377

Woods, C. E. (1943). A principle of physics as applicable to shoulder delivery. *American Journal of Obstetrics & Gynecology, 45*(5), 796–804. https://doi.org/10.1016/S0002-9378(43)90948-2

Wu, Y. (2023). Clinical features, diagnosis, and treatment of neonatal encephalopathy. In J. F. Dashe (Ed.), *UpToDate*. Retrieved June 10, 2023, from https://www.uptodate.com/contents/clinical-features-diagnosis-and-treatment-of-neonatal-encephalopathy

Zhang, C., Wu, Y., Li, S., & Zhang, D. (2018). Maternal prepregnancy obesity and the risk of shoulder dystocia: A meta-analysis. *BJOG, 125*(4), 407–413. https://doi.org/10.1111/1471-0528.14841

Zheng, L., Li, H., & Zhang, H. (2021). Cohort study of use of the hands-and knees-position as the first approach to resolving shoulder dystocia and preventing neonatal birth trauma. *Gynecology and Obstetrics Clinical Medicine, 1*(3), 160–163. https://doi.org/10.1016/j.gocm.2021.08.001

Zuckerwise, L. C., Hustedt, M. M., Lipkind, H. S., Funai, E. F., Raab, C. A., & Pettker, C. M. (2020). Effect of implementing a standardized shoulder dystocia documentation form on quality of delivery notes. *Journal of Patient Safety, 16*(4), 259–263. https://doi.org/10.1097/PTS.0000000000000305

Fetal and Neonatal Health 13

Objectives

- Describe the possible causes and clinical significance of fetal heart rate (FHR) patterns:
  - Accelerations
  - Bradycardia
  - Tachycardia
  - Increased variability
  - Decreased/absent variability
  - Early decelerations
  - Variable decelerations
  - Late decelerations
- Describe how to perform basic newborn resuscitation using a self-inflating bag and mask.
- Discuss how to manage the infant with meconium-stained amniotic fluid.
- Explain the differences between primary and secondary apnea.
- Describe how to perform intrauterine resuscitation for the fetus in distress.

Composite Case Study

With a loud groan, Hawthorne G. pushed her son into the clear water of the deep birth tub and lifted him to the surface. The auburn-haired father leaned over the tub and laughed with sheer joy. The young mother met her husband's eyes and smiled. "We have a red-headed baby, Azure! Just like we hoped."

Rain Ellen, the midwife, immediately noticed the baby's lack of tone and pale, bluish color. She stimulated him by rubbing his back and flicking his feet. He gasped and arched his trunk but did not initiate respirations. Rain placed the stethoscope on the newborn's chest and heard a pulse of 80 beats per min (bpm) that was dropping. "Hawthorne, I need to help your baby start breathing, so we need to cut the cord and get him to dry land," said Rain as she placed the clamps.

Socorro, a birth-center nurse, had readied warm blankets and a resuscitation bag in the examination crib. Rain placed the well-formed full-term infant on the firm surface with a towel roll under his shoulders and opened his airway as Socorro dried his slippery body. Rain secured the resuscitation mask to the infant's face, ensuring that there were no air leaks. She squeezed the bag, but the chest did not rise. Rain adjusted the mask and repositioned the baby's head to open the airway. She tried again to ventilate the baby, but air did not enter the lungs. Using a bulb syringe, she cleared the infant's mouth. Gentle suctioning removed a large glob of sticky mucus that had been blocking his airway.

Rain reapplied the mask and began to ventilate the baby. Air entered the lungs easily as Rain squeezed the bag in a "Breathe-two-three. Breathe-two-three" rhythm. About 30 sec after resuscitation began, the baby was struggling against the mask and attempting to cry. Rain removed the mask and the baby screamed indignantly. The heart rate was now a normal 130 bpm and the baby was growing pinker with every wail.

After the mother had delivered the placenta and emerged from the tub, Socorro placed the baby skin-to-skin with Hawthorne and monitored him closely. He breastfed normally, and his blood glucose was a normal 66 mg/dl. Before discharge, Rain performed a newborn exam and critical congenital cardiac-defect screening, both of which were normal. Rain discussed danger signs and routine care with Hawthorne and Azure and made plans for a 48-hr home visit for reassessment, a metabolic-marker screen for the infant, and repetition of the critical congenital cardiac-defect screening.

Fetal Oxygenation

In labor, normal uterine contractions can reduce utero-placental perfusion by 60%, causing brief fetal and placental hypoxia (Turner, Mitchell, & Kumar, 2020). A normal term fetus with a healthy placenta compensates by reducing oxygen consumption and redirecting blood to the heart, brain, and adrenal glands at the peak of contractions. Between contractions, optimal perfusion resumes.

The healthy fetus can withstand these intervals of intermittent hypoxia without injury. An unhealthy fetus or one with an abnormal placenta, however, is predisposed to intrapartum hypoxia and is sometimes unable to tolerate even transient reductions in blood flow. There is great variability in the ability of a given fetus to tolerate the hypoxic stress of labor, and the individual threshold for injury is highly variable and unpredictable (G. J. Johnson et al., 2021).

Decreased oxygen delivery to the fetus can accompany

- Maternal compromise (hypoxia/anoxia, shock, hypertension, alkalosis);
- Inability of maternal or fetal blood to carry adequate oxygen (severe anemia, carbon monoxide poisoning);.
- Placental dysfunction (abruption, infarction);
- Uterine issues (rupture, tachysystole); or
- Fetal issues (arrhythmia, umbilical cord compression).

In the absence of a catastrophic event such as such as cord prolapse, placental abruption, or uterine rupture, intrapartum fetal compromise usually develops gradually (Turner et al., 2020 When hypoxia is significant, cardiac and vascular compromise can lead to an abnormal FHR, hypotension, widespread tissue ischemia, and acidosis. Uncorrected hypoxia can lead to death.

Neonatal Encephalopathy

Neonatal encephalopathy is a clinically defined syndrome of disturbed neurologic function in the infant 35 weeks of gestation or greater during the early neonatal period (American College of Obstetricians & Gynecologists [ACOG] & American Academy of Pediatrics [AAP], 2014/2019). It can result from a single insult (such as hypoxia-ischemia), multiple insults (such as infection plus hypoxia-ischemia), or combinations of acute and chronic disorders (Tan, 2023). If the condition is caused by multiple insults, a minor acute issue that would have been well-tolerated by a healthier baby can tip the balance to irreversible injury (Tan, 2023). The baby with neonatal encephalopathy can have an abnormal level of consciousness, such as hyperalertness, irritability, or lethargy; fewer spontaneous movements; respiratory or feeding difficulties; poor tone; abnormal posturing; or absent primitive reflexes; or seizures (Tan, 2023). At birth, the affected newborn usually has poor Apgar scores and a weak or absent cry (Tan, 2023).

Fetal growth restriction (FGR) is the strongest antepartum risk factor for neonatal encephalopathy (Tan, 2023). Other antepartum risk factors include severe preeclampsia, postdates pregnancy, and abnormal placental development (Tan, 2023). In labor, acute intrapartum events such as uterine rupture, placental abruption, cord prolapse, and maternal shock/death greatly increase the risk of neonatal encephalopathy (Tan, 2023). Other intrapartum risk factors include tight nuchal cord, persistent occiput posterior position, shoulder dystocia, operative vaginal birth, preeclampsia, intraamniotic infection (IAI), and prolonged rupture of membranes (Tan, 2023).

Although many authors use the terms *hypoxic ischemic encephalopathy (HIE)*, *neonatal encephalopathy*, and *birth asphyxia* interchangeably, HIE is "a cause-specific subset of neonatal encephalopathy" (ACOG & AAP, 2014/2019, p. xviii). HIE can involve cortical and white-matter injury, deep gray-matter lesions, arterial infarction, hemorrhage, developmental brain malformations, and other issues (Y. Wu, 2023). Suspected HIE is treated with therapeutic hypothermia, started within the first 6 hr after birth and continued for 72 hr. Treatment with both whole-body hypothermia and selective head cooling shortly after birth may protect neurons by reducing the cerebral metabolic rate. ACOG recommends using the term *neonatal encephalopathy* rather than *hypoxic ischemic encephalopathy* or *birth asphyxia* when discussing the situation with families, clinicians, and researchers because the first-named is based on clinically observable data rather than the presumed etiology of the disorder (ACOG & AAP, 2014/2019).

FHR Assessment

The fetal heart begins to beat about 28 days after fertilization, that is, at about 6 weeks after the last menstrual period. As gestation advances, the FHR pattern is an indirect indicator of fetal wellbeing, demonstrating not only cardiac status but also the healthiness of the nervous system, blood gases, and acid-base balance (D. A. Miller, 2022). Interpretation of FHR patterns is a fundamental skill of midwifery. Characteristics of the FHR can provide insight into whether the fetus is well-oxygenated or hypoxic, stressed or compensating. The principles underlying fetal heart monitoring are similar whether the provider uses an electronic fetal monitor, a Doppler, or a fetoscope. Many of the same patterns represented visually by a fetal monitor tracing can be recognized aurally on intermittent auscultation (IA). This chapter provides an overview of FHR interpretation. The reader is encouraged to pursue a more comprehensive program of study to develop expertise.

Electronic Fetal Monitoring (EFM)

EFM, known as cardiotocography *(CTG)* in Europe, can be performed either externally or internally. External monitoring of FHR can be used in the antepartum or intrapartum period.

External monitoring: Fetal heart tones (FHT) can be monitored externally using a Doppler ultrasound device which is attached to the maternal abdomen. The ultrasound waves detect the motion of the fetal heart and transmit information to create a complex wave form. This signal can be transmitted to the computer through wires or wirelessly.

Internal monitoring: A fetal electrocardiogram can be obtained by applying a bipolar spiral electrode to the fetal scalp. This method produces a clear signal with minimal artifact and accurate measurement of the variability between successive heartbeats. Electrode application is only used in the intrapartum period. Its use is typically delayed until after membranes have ruptured, but it can be applied through intact membranes if the fetal head is well applied to the cervix and there is adequate dilation (L. A. Miller, Miller, & Cypher, 2022). The cervix must be dilated sufficiently to allow placement, and the provider must be able to access and identify the fetal presenting part. Avoid placing an electrode when the mother has certain transmissible infections, such as human immunodeficiency virus or hepatitis, to decrease the risk of vertical transmission (Cahill, 2021).

Uterine activity: EFM also clarifies the relationship between the FHR and uterine contractions. A tocodynamometer ("toco") measures the duration and frequency of contractions but provides no information about the contraction strength. Each uterine contraction exerts pressure against a piston within a transducer which transmits information to the monitoring device (Kissler, Lowe, & Hernandez, 2020). Measuring contraction strength directly is possible with an intrauterine pressure catheter inserted into the uterine cavity. Uterine electromyography (electrohysterography or EHG), which involves recording electric signals from uterine muscle activity with electrodes placed on the maternal abdomen, is noninvasive and more accurate but is not commonly used in the United States (Maul, Maner, Olson, Saade, & Garfield, 2004). In the United States, a tracing is recorded on standard scaled paper, where a small square denotes 10 sec and a large square denotes 60 sec.

Table 13-1

Indications for Continuous Fetal Monitoring: NICE Guidelines

Maternal—Antenatal	**Fetal—Antenatal**
• EFM is in client's personalized care plan • Previous cesarean or other full-thickness uterine scar • Hypertension requiring medication • Rupture of membranes >24 hr before the onset of established labor • Any vaginal bleeding other than a show • Suspected intraamniotic infection (IAI) or sepsis • Preexisting diabetes (type 1 or 2); gestational diabetes requiring medication	• Noncephalic presentation / cord presentation • Small for gestational age (SGA); estimated fetal weight <10th percentile) with other high-risk features, e.g., abnormal Doppler scan results, reduced fluid volume or growth velocity • Advanced gestational age (more than 42 weeks at onset of established labor) • Oligohydramnios or polyhydramnios • Reduced fetal movements in the 24 hr before onset of regular contractions

Maternal—Intrapartum
• Contractions longer than 2 min or 5 or more in 10 min • Meconium • Single temperature ≥100.4°F (38°C) or two consecutive readings ≥99.5°F (37.5°C) 1 hr apart • Suspected IAI or sepsis • Client-reported pain differing from that normally associated with contractions • Fresh vaginal bleeding that develops in labor • Pulse >120 beats per min (bpm) on two occasions 20 min apart • Severe hypertension: single reading of either SBP ≥160 mm Hg or DBP ≥110 mm Hg, measured between contractions) • Hypertension: SBP ≥140 mm Hg or DBP ≥90 mm Hg on two consecutive readings 30 min apart, measured between contractions • Protein reading of 2+ on urinalysis **and** single SBP ≥140 mm Hg **or** DBP ≥90 mm Hg • Confirmed delay in the first or second stage of labor • Regional anesthesia • Oxytocin augmentation

Adapted from *Fetal Monitoring in Labour* (NICE Guideline NG229), by National Institute of Clinical Excellence (NICE), 2022 (https://www.nice.org.uk/guidance/ng229). Copyright 2023 by NICE.

Efficacy and Use

EFM arrived at the clinical bedside in the 1960s and immediately became the standard of care for everyone in labor in a hospital (Sartwelle, Johnston, Arda, & Zebenigus, 2021). Providers eagerly adopted the new technology with idealistic expectations of effectiveness (Mohan et al., 2021; Sartwelle et al., 2021), anticipating that if all fetuses were continuously monitored, quick intervention at the first sign of trouble could improve neonatal outcomes (Chuey, De Vries, Dal Cin, & Low, 2020). EFM did not undergo clinical trials before introduction and was introduced without well-defined parameters for use (Sartwelle et al., 2021). By the 1970s EFM had become routine, even though its use brought no improvement in acidemia, Apgar scores less than 4 at 5 min, neonatal intensive care unit (NICU) admission, neonatal encephalopathy, perinatal mortality, neurodevelopmental impairment after the first year of life, or cerebral palsy (Alfirevic, Gyte, Cuthbert, & Devane, 2017; Chuey et al., 2020; D. A. Miller, 2022). Fewer neonatal seizures occurred with the use of continuous electronic FHR monitoring, but long-term neurologic outcomes were the same as those with the use of IA (D. A. Miller, 2022).

Cerebral palsy is often the result of antepartum, rather than intrapartum, events (D. A. Miller, 2022). Most abnormal FHR patterns are not associated with fetal acidemia or hypoxemia, and most fetal acidemia or hypoxemia does not result in long-term neurologic damage (D. A. Miller, 2022). Most fetuses, including healthy ones, display abnormal FHR tracings at some point during labor, and it is not always possible to distinguish the fetus that is becoming compromised from the one that is not (Hill, Reed, Brown, & Newborn Brain Society, 2021). Although multiple late decelerations and decreased FHR variability (see below) correlate with greater risk of cerebral palsy, one study (Nelson, Dambrosia, Ting, & Grether, 1996) found cerebral palsy in just 0.19% of fetuses demonstrating these heart-rate abnormalities. False positive rates for continuous monitoring (classifying a healthy fetus as acidotic) as high as 99.8% have been reported (Devane et al., 2017).

Although continuous monitoring increases safety in some circumstances (for example, observing the effects of oxytocin infusion on fetal wellbeing and uterine activity during induced labor or when the mother or fetus has certain high-risk conditions), many hospitals continue to use this technology routinely for *all* labors (Maude, Skinner, & Foureur, 2016). One reason is that documented fetal heart status can be useful in legal defense. Another is that maternity units are frequently understaffed and intermittent monitoring requires nurses to spend more time at the bedside (L. A. Miller et al., 2022). Nonetheless, EFM remains the standard of care in most hospitals (ACOG, 2009/2021; Romano & Buxton, 2020). In the United States approximately 89% of people in labor have EFM (Chuey et al., 2020).

Intermittent Auscultation (IA)

IA is the periodic assessment of FHR using a fetoscope or a Doppler device (Read, 2018). It can be performed with a simple, inexpensive fetoscope in even the lowest-resource settings. IA is an essential midwifery skill that brings the provider into close physical contact with the mother at regular intervals, facilitating assessment of skin temperature and color, breathing characteristics, fetal movement, contractions, and maternal emotional state (Lewis & Downe, 2015). This closeness helps the midwife to identify complications at their earliest onset.

IA is used in preference to continuous fetal monitoring for mothers laboring in community settings. In fact, the Commission for the Accreditation of Birth Centers prohibits the use of EFM with laboring clients after admission to a birth center, though it does allow continuous EFM tracings before admission followed by handheld Doppler devices for IA afterwards (CABC, 2020). The American Association of Birth Centers (AABC) specifies that clients requiring continuous fetal monitoring should be promptly transferred to the appropriate level of care (AABC, 2017).

Whereas Doppler devices usually have a numerical display of FHR, auscultation with a fetoscope requires counting heartbeats while watching a clock. One method is to count heartbeats every 10–15 sec during the period of auscultation (Sholapurkar, 2022). Another method is to count in 6-sec intervals for 10 counts. Multiply each count by 10 to obtain a rate; for example, 14 beats in 6 sec equals 140 beats per min (bpm).

The provider using IA can document baseline FHR, the presence or absence of FHR decelerations and accelerations, the regularity of fetal heart rhythm, maternal pulse rate, the frequency and duration of contractions, uterine activity and tone, and fetal movements (Blix et al., 2019). The American College of Nurse-Midwives (ACNM, 2015) asserts that IA is unable to distinguish between types of deceleration or determine baseline variability. International Federation of Gynecology and Obstetrics (FIGO) guidelines, however, specify that a handheld Doppler that displays the FHR can be used to identify "even low variability" (Lewis & Downe, 2015, p. 11). It is not possible to measure FHR variability with a fetoscope.

ACOG recommends that intrapartum clients with high-risk pregnancies have electronic fetal heart-rate monitoring (EFM) but considers either continuous EFM or IA acceptable for low-risk clients (ACOG, 2009/2021). Internationally, evidence-informed fetal monitoring guidelines from major professional organizations favor IA over continuous EFM for low-risk clients (ACOG, 2019/2021; Lewis & Downe, 2015; Liston, Sawchuk, & Young, 2007; Maude et al., 2016; National Institute for Health & Care Excellence [NICE], 2022; Royal Australian and New Zealand College of Obstetricians & Gynaecologists, 2017). In the United Kingdom, NICE guidelines specify that the provider should *not* offer continuous EFM to clients at low risk of complications in established labor but should use IA instead (NICE, 2022). If a client chooses continuous monitoring, the client's wishes are to be respected.

There is no consensus on optimal frequency and duration of IA or parameters for interpreting and documenting findings, nor is there evidence of which high-risk conditions have better outcomes with the use of EFM (Romano & Buxton, 2020). In the United States, ACOG (2009/2021) recommends evaluating and documenting FHR at least every 15 min in the active phase of the first stage of labor and at least every 5 min in the second stage. ACNM (2015) supports monitoring every 15–30 min during the active phase, every 15 min during the latent phase of second stage labor, and every 5 min after pushing begins. In the United Kingdom, NICE guidelines recommend IA for at least 1 min every 15 min after a palpated contraction in the first stage of labor and for at least

1 min every 5 min in the second stage and specify that FHR be recorded as a single rate (NICE, 2022).

The FHR is usually monitored for at least 1 min after the end of the contraction or from the end of one contraction to the beginning of the next (Sholapurkar, 2022). Some guidelines recommend auscultating FHR after every contraction in second-stage labor (Blix et al., 2019). In Canada, guidelines recommend that the provider first establish the FHR baseline, then auscultate immediately after a contraction for 30–60 sec (Dore & Ehman, 2020). If a deceleration is heard or suspected immediately after a contraction, the provider can have the client change position before reassessing FHT by IA or initiate EFM (Dore & Ehman, 2020). If FHR decelerations are confirmed, continuous EFM is recommended (Dore & Ehman, 2020), and transport to a hospital is indicated for a nonreassuring FHR. Guidelines also note that when EFM is initiated in response to abnormal IA, it should remain in place for a minimum of 20 min. If the tracing and overall clinical picture remain normal, IA may be resumed (Dore & Ehman, 2020).

With any type of fetal monitoring, it is crucial to distinguish the maternal heart rate from that of the fetus. Mothers in labor often develop heart rates that equal or surpass those of their fetuses. The maternal heart rate should be documented regularly. In the second stage of labor, the Royal College of Obstetricians & Gynaecologists (RCOG) recommends palpating the maternal pulse every 15 min to differentiate between the heart rates (RCOG, 2015). If there is any question about whether the rate auscultated is maternal or fetal, apply a pulse oximeter to continuously monitor the mother's heart rate.

IA Technique

- Palpate the maternal abdomen before auscultating the FHR. Abdominal palpation allows the midwife to gather information about the fetal lie, position, presentation, and descent; the volume of amniotic fluid, contraction strength, duration, and effectiveness; and areas of tension or discomfort. Moreover, by touching a client mindfully, the midwife can obtain information at an intuitive level. These subtle undercurrents of knowing tend to coalesce at key moments, providing useful insights.
- Ask the client about fetal movement patterns over the last hours and days and about the last time movement was felt. Notice how the baby moves and responds to touch. Assess whether fetal movements seem overly restricted (possibly indicating low fluid and risk of cord compression) or overly expansive (possibly indicating polyhydramnios and greater risk of malpresentation).
- Place the fetoscope or Doppler at right angles to the fetal back just below the scapula for the strongest heart rate signal. Direct auscultation of the heart produces a soft clicking sound like the muffled ticking of a watch under a blanket.
- Palpate the mother's pulse to distinguish between the maternal and fetal rates.
- Determine the baseline by assessing the heart rate between contractions when the fetus is not moving.
- Evaluate periodic FHR changes by auscultating for accelerations and decelerations.

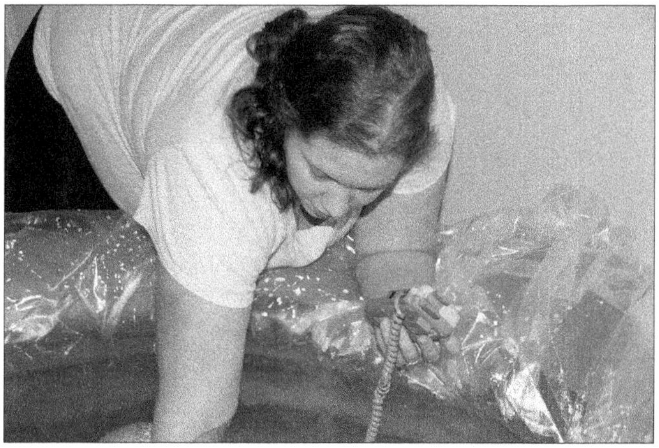

Figure 13-1. A midwife reaches into a birth pool to obtain fetal heart tones (FHT). Waterbirth is appropriate only for clients with normal fetal heart patterns.

Doppler Versus Fetoscope

Neonatal outcomes appear to be similar whether IA is performed with a Doppler device, with the abdominal transducer of an external fetal monitor, or with a fetoscope (Martis et al., 2017). A fetoscope amplifies the sound of the ventricular heart valves opening and closing. A Doppler device bounces ultra-high-frequency sound waves off the moving fetal heart valves and converts them to an electronic signal (L. A. Miller et al., 2022). Fetoscope use is more susceptible to human errors, whereas Doppler use is more susceptible to mechanical errors (Mdoe et al., 2018).

A fetoscope is inexpensive and suitable for use in low-resource areas. It allows direct auscultation of the fetal heart and provides useful information about fetal position. Fetoscope use, however, can interfere with maternal activities. The FHR is impossible to obtain if the mother is deep in a tub. It can be difficult to detect heart tones with a fetoscope if the client is obese, having strong contractions, has an anterior placenta, or is constantly changing position.

A Doppler device provides many advantages including (usually) a numerical readout and a speaker that makes the heart rate audible to everyone in the room. A Doppler allows the provider to auscultate heart tones with unobtrusive sensitivity and offer minimal disruption to the flow of labor,

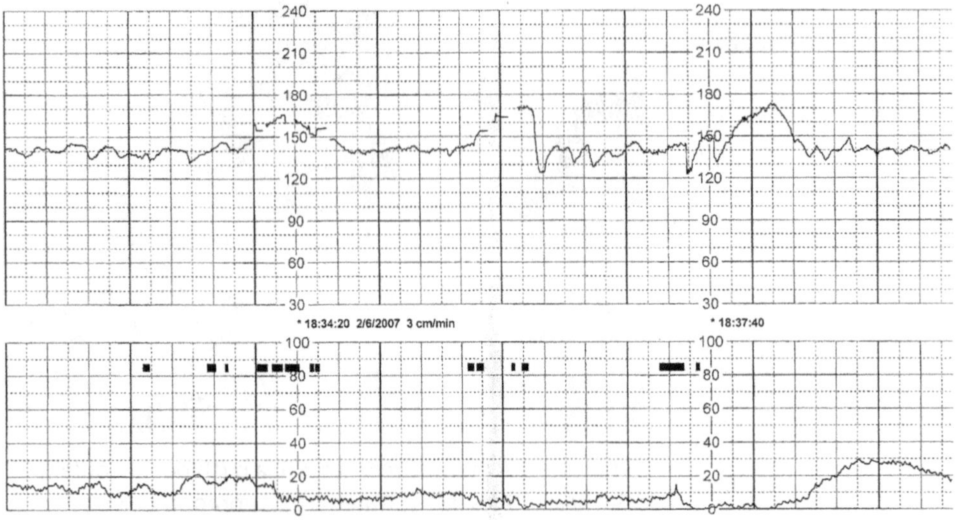

Figure 13-2. Heart tracing of a healthy fetus. The baseline is 145, and moderate variability and accelerations are present. Using criteria developed by the U.S. National Institute of Child Health and Human Development (NICHD) and others, this fetal heart tracing is category I (see "Classification of FHR Patterns," below). The short decelerations that follow the second acceleration and precede the third acceleration represent a Lambda pattern, a benign finding thought to indicate fetal blood pressure fluctuations due to cord stretch. Lambda patterns are common in early labor and are not associated with adverse outcomes or the development of abnormal heart-rate patterns.

no matter the activity or posture. In places without electricity, a wind-up Doppler device can be used. Interestingly, use of a Doppler device or a transducer is associated with a higher rate of cesarean sections due to presumed fetal distress when compared to a fetoscope (Martis et al., 2017).

FHR Pattern Characteristics

Midwives and other providers monitor fetuses during labor to determine whether they are well-oxygenated and to identify early signs of decompensation. FHR patterns provide potentially useful but sometimes ambiguous information about the fetal acid-base status at the time of observation. FHR patterns are categorized as baseline, periodic, or episodic. Whereas periodic patterns are related to uterine contractions, episodic patterns occur independently of contractions. FHR decelerations are abrupt or gradual in onset. FHR accelerations are abrupt in onset.

Baseline Fetal Heart Activity

Baseline fetal heart activity refers to elements such as rate, variability, and distinct FHR patterns such as sinusoidal or saltatory.

Rate

The normal range of the FHR baseline rate is 110–160 bpm. Vagal influence becomes progressively dominant as the fetus matures, causing the baseline FHR to gradually decrease (within the normal range) with advancing gestational age. When determining baseline rate, exclude segments that contain accelerations, decelerations, or intervals of marked FHR variability and segments of baseline that fluctuate more than 25 bpm. Take the average of the FHR over a 10-min interval and round to the nearest multiple of 5 (for example, 142 bpm = 140 bpm, 153 bpm = 155 bpm; Macones, Hankins, Spong, Hauth, & Moore, 2008). If there are not 2 min of baseline (not necessarily contiguous) in any 10-min interval, the baseline is indeterminate (Macones et al., 2008).

Abnormalities in Baseline Rate

Fetal Tachycardia

Fetal tachycardia is defined as a baseline heart rate greater than 160 bpm for at least 10 min. Tachycardia at rates greater than 180 carries a higher risk of neonatal morbidity (Lyons & McLaughlin, 2020). Causes of fetal tachycardia include (L. A. Miller et al., 2022)

- Elevated maternal temperature (fever, bathing in hot water).
- Acidemia (interruption of oxygen transfer from the environment to the fetus can lead to first hypoxemia and then to fetal metabolic acidemia).
- Infection.
- Medications/drugs (atropine, hydroxyzine, phenothiazines, terbutaline, albuterol, caffeine, theophylline, cocaine, methamphetamines).
- Fetal anemia.
- Maternal hyperthyroidism.
- Fetal arrhythmias (sinus tachycardia, supraventricular tachycardia, atrial fibrillation, atrial flutter, ventricular arrhythmia). Fetal supraventricular tachycardia, a disorder involving abnormal electrical pathways in the heart, usually presents with a regular FHR between 220 and 260 bpm and sometimes as high as 300 bpm, sustained or intermittent (Levine & Alexander, 2022).

Fetal Bradycardia

Fetal bradycardia is defined as a baseline heart rate less than 110 bpm for at least 10 min. Causes include fetal hypoxemia, maternal hypotension, medication effect, congenital heart block (as in maternal lupus or *Cytomegalovirus*), hypothermia, high vagal tone, and umbilical cord compression. Some normal fetuses, such as those in postdate pregnancies, have baseline bradycardia between 100 and 110 bpm (Ayres-de-Campos, Spong, Chandraharan, & FIGO Intrapartum Fetal Monitoring Expert Consensus Panel, 2015). Any FHR baseline less than 110 bpm requires continuous monitoring and thorough evaluation before it can be deemed a variation of normal (L. A. Miller et al., 2022).

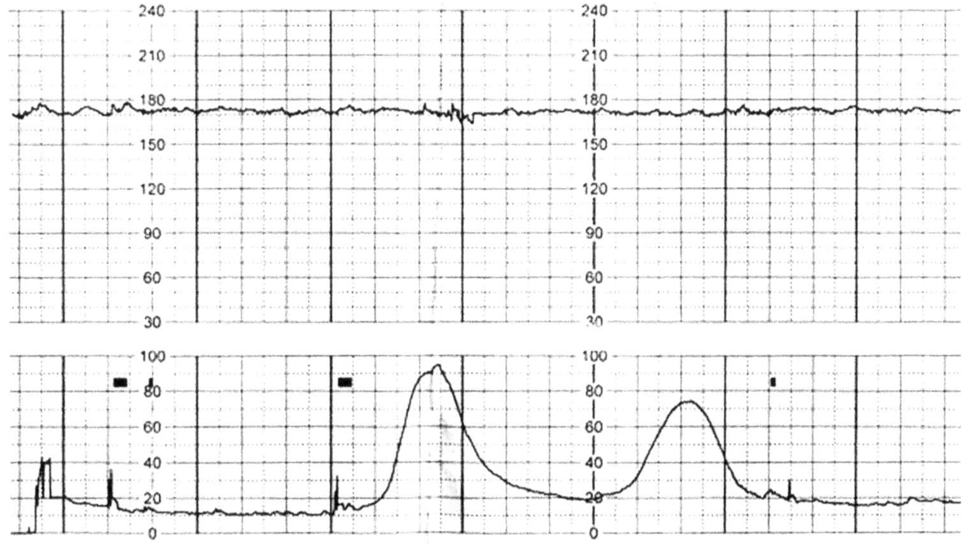

Figure 13-3. Fetal tachycardia in a mother with intraamniotic infection (IAI). The fetal tachycardia began about 2 hr before the mother became symptomatic.

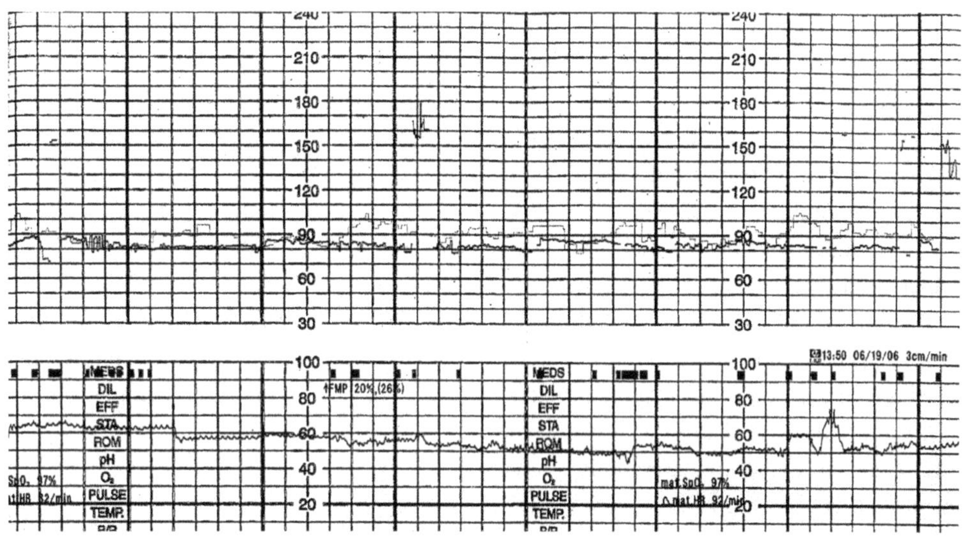

Figure 13-4. Fetal bradycardia due to heart block. This fetus had a rate in the 70s–80s for hours or days at a time from 27 to 34 weeks of gestation. At times the baseline rate would reach 60. The lighter line depicting a generally faster rate is the maternal pulse. Because the low rate was not related to hypoxia, and prematurity was a greater risk than the arrhythmia, preterm birth was not recommended. Fetuses with heart blocks tend to compensate for the slow rate by increasing contractile force and are often able to maintain acceptable cardiac output despite an alarmingly slow rate. This baby was born healthy at term and with no evidence of cardiac problems. The cause remained undetermined.

Baseline Variability

Variability is defined as beat-to-beat fluctuations in the FHR baseline rate with irregular amplitude and varying frequency. A variable baseline is caused by the push and pull between fetal sympathetic and parasympathetic influences which modify the baseline's waviness. Whereas the fetal vagus nerve lowers the heart rate, the sympathetic nervous system raises it. Their interplay results in constant adjustments in response to fetal environment. Heart-rate variability develops between 24 and 28 weeks of gestation with the maturation of the parasympathetic nervous system. Once the fetus has established a consistent pattern of normal FHR variability, absence of variability is concerning (D. A. Miller, 2022; L. A. Miller et al., 2022).

Baseline variability is depicted on an FHR monitor as irregular fluctuations in the baseline excluding accelerations and decelerations. Moderate variability is a reliable indicator of a normally oxygenated fetus and is characterized by oscillations of 6–25 bpm (Cunningham et al., 2022. ch. 24). For example, a healthy fetus with a baseline heart rate of 150 bpm might have fluctuations from 160 to 140 bpm, which would be charted as moderate variability of 20 bpm. A fetus with moderate variability is extremely unlikely to have fetal metabolic acidemia and ongoing hypoxic injury at the time it is observed (L. A. Miller et al., 2022).

Variability is charted as absent if no fluctuations are present, minimal if the amplitude range is 5 bpm or less, and marked if the amplitude range exceeds 25 bpm. Reduced baseline FHR variability is the single most reliable sign of fetal compromise (Cunningham et al., 2022. ch. 24). Minimal or

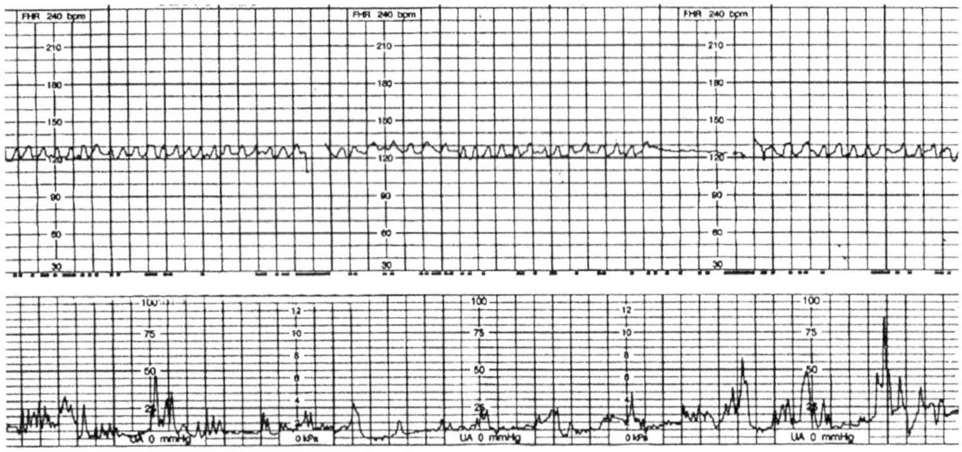

Figure 13-5. A sinusoidal pattern is often seen with severe fetal anemia. The uterine pattern of tachysystole and abnormal tracing is consistent with placental abruption. In this case, there was a fetomaternal hemorrhage.

absent variability can result from recurrent or sustained interruption in oxygen delivery, infection, extreme prematurity, cardiac arrhythmia, severe anemia, previous cerebral injury, or medications (narcotics, phenothiazines, barbiturates, and others). A fetus that is deeply asleep can have variability in the lower range of normal, but it usually remains above 5 bpm (Ayres-de-Campos et al., 2015).

Although absent or minimal variability accompanies fetal acidemia, it is associated with an umbilical cord pH less than 7.15 in only about 12–31% of cases (Cunningham et al., 2022. ch. 24). When FHR variability is minimal but decelerations are absent, fetal hypoxia is unlikely (Cunningham et al., 2022. ch. 24). Persistently absent variability within the normal baseline rate range and without decelerations can be seen after a fetal insult that has resulted in neurological damage (Cunningham et al., 2022. ch. 24). Marked variability is of uncertain clinical significance; it may represent a variant of normal (L. A. Miller et al., 2022) or an exaggerated autonomic response to intermittent hypoxia (Polnaszek et al., 2020).

Sinusoidal Pattern

A sinusoidal pattern is an undulating sine wave–like pattern showing steady amplitude and frequency (3–5 cycles per min) that persists for least 20 min (L. A. Miller et al., 2022). There are no accelerations and no variability, just a uniform oscillation of rate. A true sinusoidal pattern can occur with fetal intracranial hemorrhage, severe fetal asphyxia, or severe fetal anemia (such as that resulting from alloimmunization, fetomaternal hemorrhage, twin-to-twin transfusion syndrome, fetal parvoviral infection, or vasa previa with bleeding; Cunningham et al., 2022. ch. 24). Similar-appearing patterns can occur with IAI and after administration of narcotic analgesics.

Fetal Arrhythmia

Fetal arrhythmia is diagnosed in 1–3% of pregnancies (Yuan & Xu, 2020). It can be audible as an irregularity in the FHR that is subtle or pronounced, intermittent or continuous. It may sound as if the fetus had extra or absent heartbeats.

When an arrhythmia is detected antenatally, the client should be referred to a fetal cardiologist or maternal-fetal specialist for comprehensive evaluation. Diagnostic modalities may include two-dimensional ultrasound, M-mode sonography, pulsed-wave Doppler ultrasound, continuous electronic FHR monitoring, and other technology (Levine & Alexander, 2022). These specialists may recommend planning birth for the fetus with sustained arrhythmia in a hospital with continuous EFM during labor. EFM is unable to accurately monitor the fetus with a rate of 240 bpm or greater, however (L. A. Miller et al., 2022). Neonatal follow-up usually involves evaluation by a pediatrician or neonatologist. When a fetus develops a significant arrhythmia for the first time during labor in a community setting, transport to a hospital for continuous monitoring and for the availability of pediatric support at birth.

Periodic FHR Changes

Accelerations

Accelerations are transient escalations in FHR that follow movement, vaginal examinations, uterine contractions, fetal scalp stimulation, or sounds. Accelerations in FHR, whether spontaneous or in response to fetal scalp stimulation, indicate that the fetus is not acidemic (G. J. Johnson et al., 2021). Lack of accelerations, however, does not necessarily indicate compromise (D. A. Miller, 2022; L. A. Miller et al., 2022).

An acceleration moves from onset to peak in less than 30 sec. If the fetus is very active, accelerations can coalesce into a pattern that is difficult to distinguish from fetal tachycardia. A prolonged acceleration lasts 2 min or more, but less than 10 min. An elevated rate for longer than 10 min is considered a baseline change.

Decelerations

FHR decelerations are classified as early, late, variable, or prolonged. Early and late decelerations are gradual in onset and periodic in occurrence—that is, related to uterine contractions (L. A. Miller et al., 2022). Variable decelerations are abrupt in onset and may or may not be associated with contractions. Prolonged decelerations can be abrupt or gradual in onset and periodic or episodic in timing (L. A. Miller et al., 2022). Recurrent decelerations occur with at least 50% of uterine contractions in any 20-min segment. The depth of a deceleration is measured in bpm below the baseline to its lowest point (nadir).

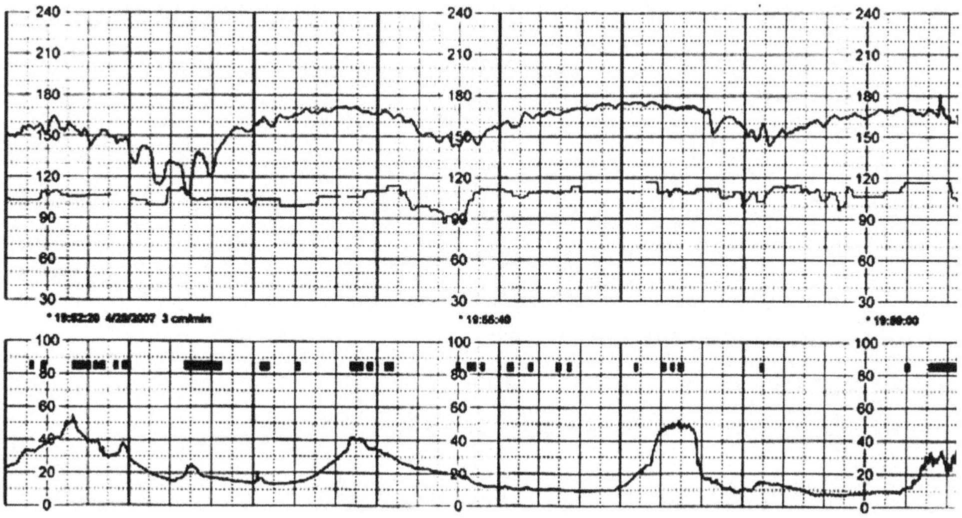

Figure 13-6. Late decelerations and fetal tachycardia that resulted in an emergency cesarean section. The mother was also tachycardic. The baby had Apgar scores of 3 and 9.

Early Decelerations

Early decelerations have a uniform shape: gradual onset (30 sec or more to nadir) at the start of the contraction, nadir at the peak of the contraction, and gradual resolution coinciding with the end of the contraction. On a fetal heart tracing, the deceleration appears to be the mirror image of the contraction. Early decelerations do not appear to be associated with fetal hypoxia, acidemia, or neurologic injury (D. A. Miller, 2022; L. A. Miller et al., 2022). They are widely believed to be associated with head compression, although recent research suggests otherwise (Lear et al., 2021).

Late Decelerations

A late deceleration of FHR usually begins after the onset of the uterine contraction, the nadir occurs after the peak, and the return to baseline occurs after the contraction has ended. The onset is gradual (onset to nadir 30 sec or more). Late decelerations indicate temporary interruption of oxygen transfer from the mother to the fetus during a contraction, resulting in transient fetal hypoxemia (L. A. Miller et al., 2022). If this reduction in oxygen delivery is recurrent or sustained, it can progress to acidemia. In most cases, when an acidemic fetus has late decelerations, the tracing also shows other FHR abnormalities such as fetal tachycardia, absent variability, and absent accelerations (L. A. Miller et al., 2022). Late decelerations can be caused by any condition that reduces blood flow to the fetus, including uterine tachysystole (more than five contractions in 10 min, averaged over a 30-min window), maternal hypotension, maternal hypertensive disorders, placental abruption, placenta previa, FGR, and IAI.

Variable Decelerations

A variable deceleration is a drop in the FHR that begins with the onset of the contraction and reaches a nadir in less than 30 sec. It lasts between 15 sec and 2 min and is 15 bpm or more in depth (Cunningham et al., 2022. ch. 24). Variable decelerations change in duration, intensity, and timing and reflect the fetal autonomic reflex response to compression of the umbilical cord. They are shaped like the letters *U*, *V*, or *W* on the fetal heart tracing and can be associated with contractions. Initially, pressure on the cord compresses the thin walled, yielding umbilical vein, reducing fetal venous return and triggering a reflex rise in heart rate—known informally as a "shoulder" (D. A. Miller, 2022; L. A. Miller et al., 2022). Continued pressure compresses the umbilical arteries, increasing fetal blood pressure (BP). The body compensates for this increase in BP by decreasing the heart rate, which manifests as a variable deceleration. As the compression decreases, this sequence occurs in reverse (D. A. Miller, 2022; L. A. Miller et al., 2022).

Prolonged Decelerations

A prolonged deceleration of the FHR is a gradual or abrupt decrease at least 15 bpm below the baseline lasting at least 2 min from onset to return to baseline. (A prolonged deceleration lasting 10 min or longer is considered a baseline change.) A

Variability classifications:

Absent: amplitude range undetectable

Minimal: amplitude range ≤5 bpm

Moderate (normal): amplitude range 6–25 bpm

Marked: amplitude range >25 bpm

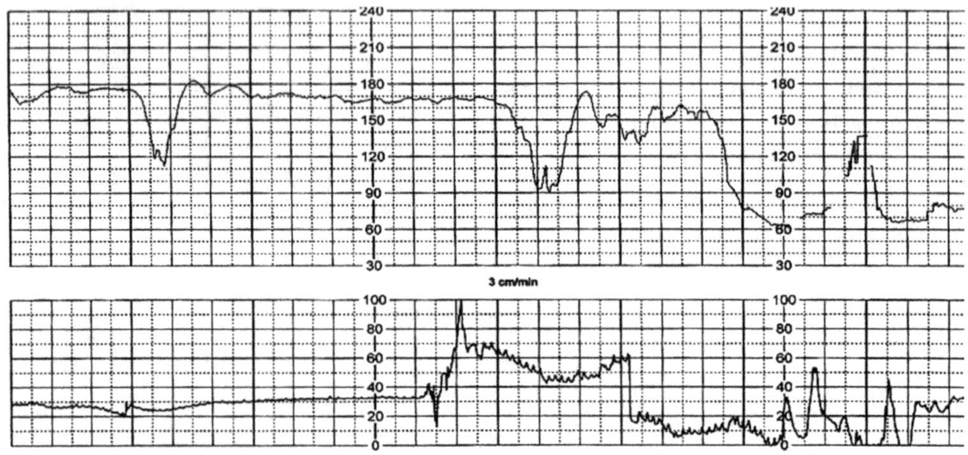

Figure 13-7. Variable fetal heart rate decelerations evolving to prolonged decelerations. These variable decelerations descend from a tachycardic baseline and were the result of a thin, tight nuchal cord. The baby was born vaginally just after this tracing was recorded, and Apgar scores were 8/9.

prolonged deceleration indicates interruption of oxygen transfer from the mother to the fetus. If this decrease in oxygen delivery is not corrected, the fetus can become increasingly hypoxemic and acidotic, then hypotensive and bradycardic (L. A. Miller et al., 2022). If this process is not interrupted, the fetus can go into cardiac arrest and die.

Classification of FHR Patterns

Interpretation of an FHR tracing includes assessment of baseline rate and variability; assessment of accelerations, decelerations, and sinusoidal pattern; assessment of uterine activity; and assessment of changes and trends (D. A. Miller, 2022; L. A. Miller et al., 2022). In 2008, the Eunice Kennedy Shriver National Institute of Child Health and Human Development (NICHD) convened a multidisciplinary panel of stakeholders to standardize nomenclature for EFM patterns (Robinson, 2008). The consensus was to adopt a three-tier system for the categorization of intrapartum EFM that has become the standard of care throughout the United States and elsewhere (Macones, 2022; Macones et al., 2008). FIGO and others have issued similar guidelines (Macones, 2022).

Category I FHR Tracing

Category I FHR tracings are normal. No action is required. If all the following criteria are present, it is likely the fetus has a normal acid-base balance at the time of the assessment.

Electronic Fetal Monitoring (EFM)

Category I FHR characteristics by EFM include (Macones et al., 2008)

- Baseline rate 110–160 bpm
- Moderate baseline FHR variability
- No late or variable decelerations
- Early decelerations present or absent
- Accelerations present or absent

Intermittent Auscultation (IA)

Category I FHR characteristics by auscultation include (ACNM, 2015):

- Normal FHR baseline between 110 and 160 bpm

AND

- Regular rhythm

AND

- Absence of FHR decreases or decelerations from the baseline
- Accelerations present or absent

Category II FHR Tracing

Category II FHR tracings are considered indeterminate. They do not meet criteria for either category I or III and are not predictive of abnormal fetal acid–base status (ACOG, 2009/2021).

EFM

Category II FHR tracings includes all FHR tracings not categorized as category I or category III. Examples of category II FHR characteristics by EFM can include any of the following (ACOG, 2009/2021; Macones et al., 2008):

Baseline rate

- Bradycardia accompanied by moderate baseline variability
- Tachycardia

Baseline FHR variability

- Minimal baseline variability
- Absent baseline variability with no recurrent decelerations
- Marked baseline variability

Accelerations

- Absence of induced accelerations after fetal stimulation

Periodic or episodic decelerations

- Recurrent variable decelerations accompanied by minimal or moderate baseline variability
- Prolonged deceleration more than 2 min but less than 10 min
- Recurrent late decelerations with moderate baseline variability

- Variable decelerations with other characteristics such as slow return to baseline, overshoots, or "shoulders"

IA

Category II FHR characteristics by auscultation include (ACNM, 2015)

- Irregular rhythm
- Presence of FHR decreases or decelerations from the baseline
- Tachycardia
- Bradycardia

Category III FHR Tracing

Category III tracings indicate that the acid-base balance of the fetus is probably abnormal at the time of the assessment.

EFM

Category III FHR characteristics by EFM can include (L. A. Miller et al., 2022):

- Absent variability with recurrent late decelerations
- Absent variability with recurrent variable decelerations
- Absent variability with bradycardia for at least 10 min
- Sinusoidal pattern for at least 20 min

IA

Under ACNM guidelines, category III FHR patterns are technically indistinguishable using IA because baseline variability cannot be determined with this technique (ACNM, 2015).

Managing Abnormal Fetal Heart Patterns in Community Settings

Monitor category I FHR tracings in a routine manner because these findings indicate the absence of fetal acidemia at the time of observation (Macones, 2022). Category II tracings are indeterminate and require close surveillance with consideration of the clinical circumstances and the characteristics of the fetal heart tracing over time. Under ACNM guidelines, when recurrent decelerations of the FHR are detected via IA, EFM is indicated to determine whether they are early, late, or variable decelerations (ACNM, 2015). NICHD criteria for EFM generated tracings can then be used to assign a diagnostic category of I, II, or III. Because continuous EFM is unavailable in most community settings, a category II FHR usually necessitates transfer to a hospital.

Assessment

If the fetal heart pattern seems abnormal, quickly reassess the client and consider the clinical situation. Is there a plausible explanation for your findings? An FHR of 165 with accelerations might be a result of maternal hyperthermia after a hot bath and may be resolved with hydration and a cooler environment. A new onset of FHR decelerations and rectal pressure in a multigravida in transition can indicate imminent birth. Sudden bradycardia coincident with spontaneous rupture of membranes is sometimes the first sign of umbilical cord prolapse.

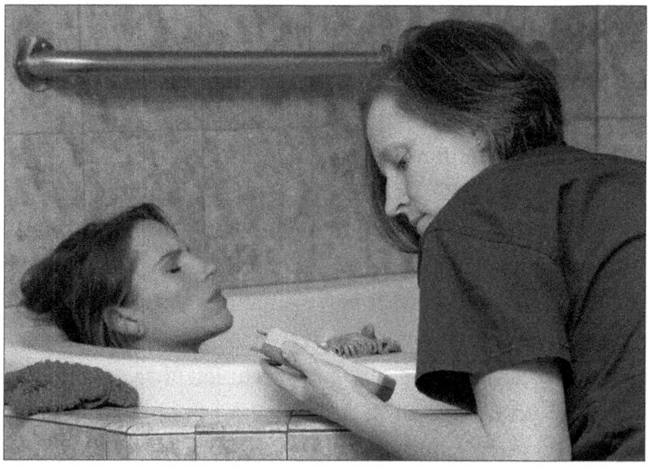

Figure 13-8. A midwife auscultates the fetal heart rate (FHR) with a hand-held Doppler device while a client relaxes in the tub. If the water is too hot, the fetus can become tachycardic. The probe of some units is waterproof, but the body of the device is not.

Compare the FHR with the maternal pulse to distinguish the two rates or apply a pulse oximeter to monitor the maternal heart rate in real time. Sometimes the fetal and maternal heart rates can be difficult to differentiate during labor. Fetal bradycardia can result in a rate within the normal maternal range. Pain, stress, shock, or fever can drive the maternal pulse into a rate within the ranges that would be considered normal for a fetus.

If you are uncertain about fetal wellbeing and there have been no spontaneous accelerations, consider vigorously stimulating the fetal scalp with your fingertips. If the fetus responds with an acceleration, the probability of acidosis is less than 10% (Macones, 2022). If no acceleration occurs in response to the stimulation, the probability of acidosis is about 50% (Macones, 2022).

Intrauterine Resuscitation

If you detect an abnormal FHR pattern, begin fetal resuscitation to improve perfusion and oxygenation while initiating rapid transport to a hospital capable of performing an emergency cesarean. In some cases, resuscitative measures resolve the abnormal pattern. Even if the abnormal pattern resolves, transfer to the hospital via ambulance is advisable unless birth is imminent, because recurrence of the abnormal rate is not predictable. Perform a digital examination to check for umbilical cord prolapse or rapid cervical dilation and fetal descent. Shift the mother's position to whatever position yields the best FHR pattern: side-lying, knee-chest, Trendelenburg, Fowler's, or knee-elbow (Macones, 2022).

If tachysystole is present (more than five contractions in 10 min, averaged over a 30-min window), consider tocolysis with subcutaneous terbutaline 0.25 mg to reduce the strength and frequency of contractions. Sometimes the FHR pattern improves if contractions are weaker, widely spaced, or absent. Hydration can improve placental perfusion if the mother is hypovolemic. Initiate an intravenous (IV) fluid bolus of 500–1,000 ml normal saline (NS) or lactated Ringer's solution. Use caution if the client's condition carries higher risk of volume overload (for example, if there are signs of preeclampsia).

ACOG no longer recommends the use of supplemental oxygen for intrauterine resuscitation in mothers with normal oxygen saturation (ACOG Cmte. on Clinical Practice Guidelines—Obstetrics, 2022/2023). Intrapartum oxygen supplementation does not improve umbilical artery pH, neonatal acidemia, admission to NICU, or any other meaningful clinical outcomes, and does not resolve category II FHR patterns (ACOG Cmte. on Clinical Practice Guidelines—Obstetrics, 2022/2023). Hyperoxygenation is associated with vasoconstriction, which has the potential to decrease placental oxygen delivery and tissue perfusion (Raghuraman, Wan, et al., 2018). Moreover, oxygen treatment has the potential to generate free oxygen radicals (Raghuraman, Wan, et al., 2018; Raghuraman, López, et al., 2020).

Documentation

If using IA, document the auscultated FHR along with information that puts it into context, such as contraction pattern, frequency and duration, maternal position, fetal baseline rate, and the presence of accelerations or decelerations. Document your assessments of the mother and fetus, any interventions, and any maternal–fetal responses to these interventions (L. A. Miller et al., 2022). Note how long you auscultated the FHR and whether the assessment was before, during, or after a contraction. Abnormal fetal heart patterns that are assessed numerically (tachycardia, bradycardia) can be documented as such, but avoid describing a deceleration as early, late, or variable if using IA (L. A. Miller et al., 2022).

Antepartum Fetal Surveillance

Antepartum fetal surveillance techniques based on evaluation of FHR patterns, sonography and umbilical artery Doppler velocimetry are routinely used to assess the risk of fetal death in pregnancies complicated by preexisting maternal conditions (e.g., chronic hypertension) and in those which complications have developed (e.g., FGR). The goals of antepartum surveillance are to identify fetuses at risk for injury due to abnormal oxygenation so that permanent injury or death might be avoided and to identify normally oxygenated fetuses to avoid unnecessary intervention (L. A. Miller et al., 2022). Antepartum surveillance is generally unable to prevent fetal deaths that occur from sudden catastrophic events such as placental abruption or umbilical cord prolapse (ACOG, 2021/2024).

Fetal Movement Assessment

The average human fetus makes about 30 gross movements per hr in periods of activity lasting about 40 min punctuated by quiet periods lasting about 20 min (Greenberg & Druzin, 2021). The mother can usually perceive about 70–80% of large fetal movements and few if any of fine movements such as limb flexion and extension, hand grasping, and sucking (Greenberg & Druzin, 2021). To evaluate fetal wellbeing, mothers are often instructed to note fetal activity daily and report to the provider if movements are fewer than usual or do not meet specific criteria. In one approach, maternal perception of 10 fetal movements in up to 2 hr is considered reassuring (ACOG, 2021/2024). In another, the mother counts movements for 1 hr three times a week; a reassuring result is when these "kick counts" equaled or exceeded that fetus's previously established baseline count (ACOG, 2021/2024).

It is unclear whether counting fetal movements improves perinatal outcomes (ACOG, 2021/2024). Prospective trials of fetal-kick counts for prevention of stillbirth have failed to conclusively show benefit (Greenberg & Druzin, 2021). One large meta-analysis showed no difference in stillbirth between the group that underwent counted movements and the group that did not; but there were increases in preterm birth, induction of labor, and cesarean section in the kick-count groups (Norman et al., 2018).

Nonstress Test (NST)

The NST is an evaluation performed in clients with complicated pregnancies who are not laboring in hope of improving fetal outcome. EFM is initiated, and the FHR is observed for an interval that is usually between 20 and 40 min (D. A. Miller, 2023). If FHR accelerations are noted in response to fetal movement or a uterine contraction, fetal wellbeing is confirmed (Aubin & El-Chaâr, 2023). The expectation is that if the tracing is abnormal, birth can be expedited. If the tracing is indeterminate, fetal wellbeing can be evaluated with further testing. Circumstantial evidence, longstanding convention, and medical-liability precedents have made the NST the standard for antepartum fetal assessment. There is, however, no convincing evidence from randomized trials that use of NSTs reduces fetal death or neurologic injury (D. A. Miller, 2023).

A normal result (reactive NST) is almost always associated with a neurologically intact and well-oxygenated fetus A reactive NST (normal or negative result) is characterized by at least two accelerations within a 20-min window, each lasting 15 sec or more and rising at least 15 bpm above baseline. Before 32 weeks of gestation, an FHR tracing is considered reactive if an acceleration is 10 bpm above baseline in amplitude and 10 sec in duration (Greenberg & Druzin, 2021). About 50% of NSTs are nonreactive between 24 and 28 weeks of gestation. That figure drops to about 15% between 28 and 32 weeks (Greenberg & Druzin, 2021).

Because healthy fetuses cycle in and out of quiet sleep, monitor FHR for at least 40 min before interpreting the test as nonreactive (Miller, 2023). Sometimes the fetus can have no heart rate accelerations for up to 80 min and still be normal (Greenberg & Druzin, 2021). A false-negative NST (one that yields a normal result less than 1 week before a fetal death) is exceedingly rare; a 1982 study yielded a false-negative rate of about 0.19% (L. A. Miller et al., 2022).

An abnormal result (nonreactive NST) is sometimes associated with a hypoxic/acidemic fetus. Although nonreactivity can be a sign of fetal hypoxemia, it can also be an effect of medication or maternal smoking or vaping before the test. It can also denote fetal immaturity, quiet fetal sleep, fetal neurologic or cardiac anomalies, or sepsis. A false positive is an abnormal result that prompts delivery but is not associated with fetal hypoxia (L. A. Miller et al., 2022). NSTs have a 50% false-positive rate (L. A. Miller et al., 2022).

External stimuli can be used to awaken a sleeping fetus and safely shorten the testing interval. Applying a vibroacoustic stimulation device (which produces buzzing and vibration) to the maternal abdomen may shorten average testing time almost 7 min and reduce the incidence of nonreactive NSTs by 40% (Espinoza, 2022). Increased fetal movement, increased number of accelerations, and improved variability have been observed with exposure to halogen light or to music, e.g., Mozart's "Turkish March" and Strauss's "Tritsch-Tratsch Polka" (Bolnick, Garcia, Fletcher, & Rayburn, 2006; Caridi, Bolnick, Fletcher, & Rayburn, 2004; Gebuza, Dombrowska, Kaźmierczak, Malgorzata, & Mieczkowska, 2017; Rahimikian, Rahiminia, Modarres, & Mehran, 2013).

Contraction Stress Test (CST)

The contraction stress test (CST), also known as the oxytocin challenge test, is a test used to identify fetuses with placental insufficiency (inadequate placental function, usually caused by inadequate blood flow). In all pregnancies, uterine contractions reduce blood flow to the placenta. This physiologic reduction in blood flow is well-tolerated by healthy fetuses. A fetus with inadequate placental reserve, however, typically has recurrent late decelerations in response to the hypoxia caused by uterine contractions (Greenberg & Druzin, 2021). These uterine contractions can be spontaneous or provoked by nipple stimulation or oxytocin infusion. The test is scored as follows (D. A. Miller, 2023):

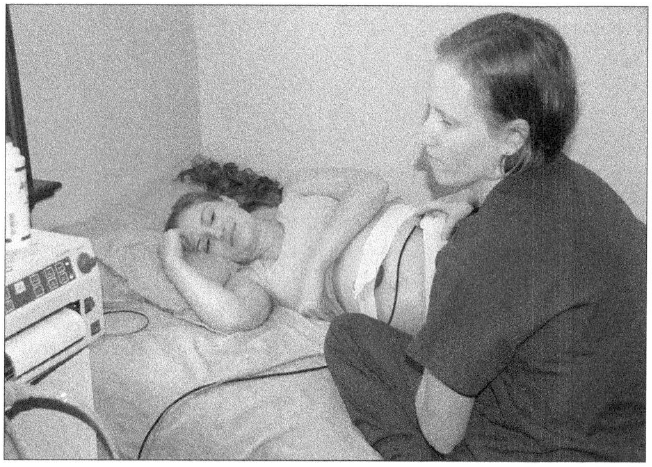

Figure 13-9. A midwife performs an NST on a client at 41 weeks of gestation in a birth center. Many freestanding birth centers have the capacity to perform NSTs, but the American Association of Birth Centers (AABC) prohibits the use of continuous EFM in labor.

Positive—A positive (abnormal) test has late decelerations after 50% or more contractions. The test is positive even if the contraction frequency is fewer than three in 10 min.

Negative—A negative (normal) test has no late decelerations or significant variable decelerations.

Equivocal—An equivocal-suspicious test has intermittent late decelerations or significant variable decelerations that do not meet the criteria for a positive test. An equivocal tachysystolic test has decelerations with contractions occurring more frequently than every 2 min or lasting longer than 90 sec.

Biophysical Profile (BPP)

The biophysical profile (BPP), a noninvasive method of antepartum assessment that uses ultrasound, is a dependable predictor of fetal wellbeing with a false-negative rate of 0.006% (L. A. Miller et al., 2022). The BPP evaluates five variables: acute central nervous system function is assessed through FHR reactivity via NST, and fetal movement, tone, and breathing are assessed via ultrasound. Adequacy of placental function is also evaluated sonographically by measuring the amniotic-fluid volume (L. A. Miller et al., 2022).

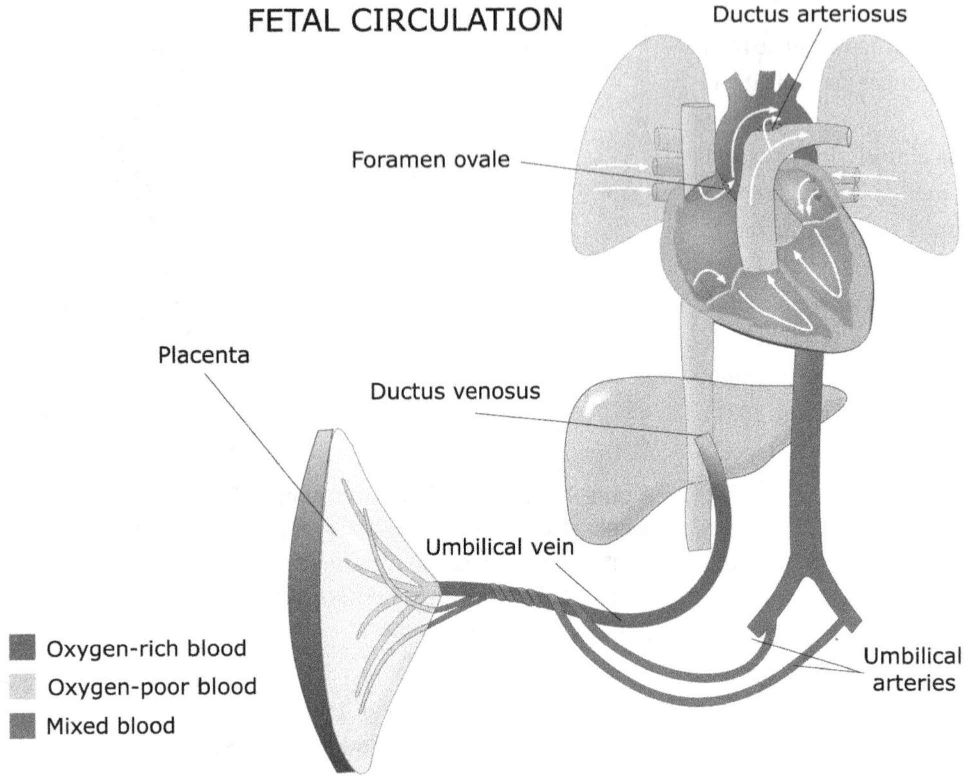

Figure 13-10. Deoxygenated blood leaves the fetus through two umbilical arteries, which arise from the internal iliac arteries. This blood courses through the umbilical cord into the placenta, where it offloads waste products and acquires oxygen and nutrients from the mother's blood. The umbilical vein carries oxygen-rich blood to the fetus and divides within the fetal abdomen. Part of this flow nourishes the liver while the majority moves on through the ductus venosus and flows through the inferior vena cava to the right atrium of the heart (©ellepigrafica/Adobe Stock).

Each normal parameter is assigned 2 points, and each abnormal finding is assigned 0 points. A biophysical profile score of 8–10 with normal amniotic fluid volume is considered normal. A score of 6 is suspicious and requires further testing (L. A. Miller et al., 2022). A fetus scoring less than 6 is potentially at risk for perinatal morbidity and mortality. Hospital management plans may include close surveillance or delivery of the infant and are based on clinical circumstances (L. A. Miller et al., 2022). Oligohydramnios (defined as an amniotic-fluid volume of 2 cm or less in the single deepest vertical pocket) requires further evaluation regardless of the composite score (ACOG, 2021/2024). The modified biophysical profile combines an NST with assessment of amniotic fluid volume only.

Umbilical Artery Doppler Velocimetry

Doppler sonography is a technique used to assess the vascular resistance in pregnancies complicated by fetal growth restriction. In growth-restricted fetuses, umbilical artery diastolic flow can be lower than normal. When FGR is severe, diastolic flow can be absent or even reversed. Such fetuses are at higher risk for stillbirth.

The Transition from Fetus to Neonate

A baby is more likely to die within the first four weeks of life than in any other period of childhood (Rozance & Wright, 2021). The risk of mortality is greatest in the first few days following birth. At birth, the fetal cardiopulmonary circuit must undergo profound changes necessary to maintain life outside the uterus. The newborn abruptly becomes responsible for thermoregulation, breathing, feeding, excreting, and maintaining homeostasis.

Fetal Circulation

Because the fetal lungs do not exchange gases, the fetal circulatory system has modifications to limit blood flow to the lungs and send blood instead to the placenta to pick up oxygen. The placenta has the lowest vascular resistance of any component of the fetal circulatory system and receives 40% of the fetal cardiac output, causing systemic pressure to remain low (Fernandes, 2021). The fluid-filled fetal lungs have high vascular resistance and receive significantly less cardiac output.

Deoxygenated blood leaves the fetus through two umbilical arteries and circulates through the placenta, where it offloads waste products such as carbon dioxide and acquires oxygen and nutrients from the mother's blood. Oxygen-rich blood returns to the fetus through the umbilical vein and splits into channels within the fetal abdomen. A small amount of this flow is directed to nourish the liver while the majority moves on through the ductus venosus and flows through the inferior vena cava to the right atrium of the heart.

The foramen ovale is an opening between the right and left atrium of the fetal heart that allows most of this enriched blood to bypass the lungs and proceed directly to the right and left ventricles and out the aorta (right-to-left shunt). This mechanism sends the most highly oxygenated blood to nourish the fetal heart and brain. Less-oxygenated blood returning from the fetal body via the vena cava moves to the right ventricle and mixes minimally with the oxygenated blood flowing from the ductus venosus (Fernandes, 2021). About 90% of right-ventricular output bypasses the lungs and is shunted through the ductus arteriosus to the descending aorta and from there to the umbilical arteries and the placenta.

Epithelial cells in the fetal airway produce fluid that fills the fetal lungs. Lung growth depends on the presence and volume of this fluid (Patterson et al., 2021). Fetal pulmonary vessels are tightly constricted, allowing only about 12% of the right-ventricular output to reach the lungs, just enough to let the lungs grow and develop (Murphy, 2005). Fetuses make breathing movements *in utero* from as early as 11 weeks of gestation, but these movements are not associated with significant movement of lung fluid (Rozance & Wright, 2021). This respiratory activity seems essential to the development of chest-wall and diaphragm muscles, and it plays a role in the regulation of lung fluid (Rozance & Wright, 2021). Late in pregnancy, fluid secretion in the fetal lungs decreases and absorption increases, but it is the first effective breaths at birth that drive the remaining alveolar fluid into the pulmonary vasculature (Fernandes, 2021). Pressure on the thorax during birth also squeezes fluid and mucus from the respiratory tract.

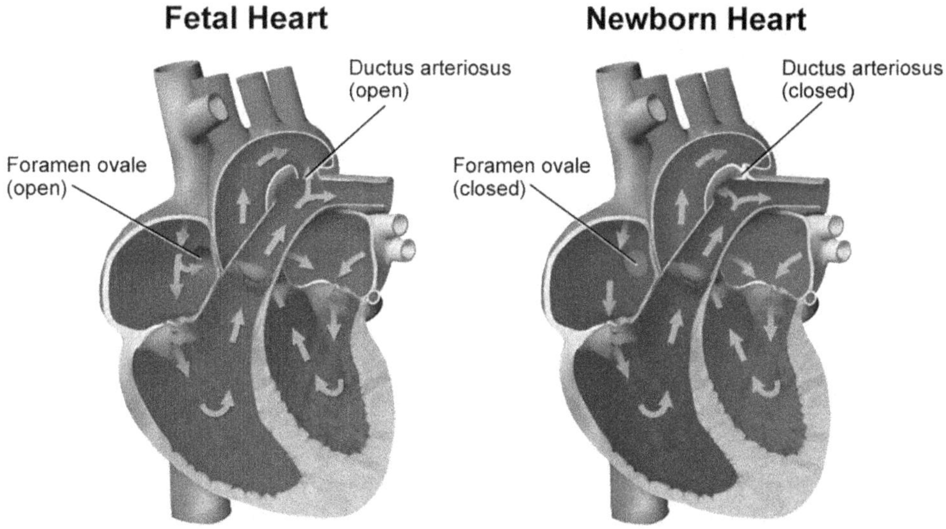

Figure 13-11. Fetal cardiac circulation utilizes shunts that largely bypass pulmonary circulation in favor of perfusing the placenta. "Neonatal Heart Circulation," by BruceBlaus, 2015 (https://commons.wikimedia.org/wiki/File:Neonatal_Heart_Circulation.png). CC BY-SA 4.0.

Neonatal Transition

Because the mother supports so many fetal metabolic needs, the fetus requires less oxygen and glucose than the newborn. Because the mother maintains the thermal environment, the baby does not need to burn fuel to stay warm. Oxygen consumption related to physiologic functions such as respiratory effort, gastrointestinal digestion and absorption, and kidney reabsorption are greatly reduced in the fetus. Fetal hemoglobin has much a greater affinity for oxygen than adult hemoglobin. Even so, fetal blood within the umbilical vein (the most-oxygenated blood in the fetal body) has an oxygen saturation of only 50–60% (Lara-Cantón et al., 2022). The blood in the inferior vena cava below the umbilicus is only about 25–40% saturated (Murphy, 2005).

In preparation for breathing, the fetal lungs must develop a thin air-blood barrier that allows gases to move into and out of the blood and surfactant that reduces surface tension and prevents the lungs from collapsing with every breath (Rozance & Wright, 2021). The first breath of air taken at birth marks a major anatomical and physiological transformation. In the minutes and hours that follow, the lungs must metamorphose into the primary organs of gas exchange and the circulatory system must remodel itself to create a new circulatory pathway (Mercer & Erickson-Owens, 2014). The physiologic events of neonatal transition appear to be most efficient when aeration of the lungs and increase in pulmonary blood flow occur before cord clamping (Brouwer et al., 2022; Kluckow & Hooper, 2015). The initial breath requires more effort than the breaths that follow. In the term infant, a surfactant within the alveoli reduces surface tension and prevents these small air sacs from

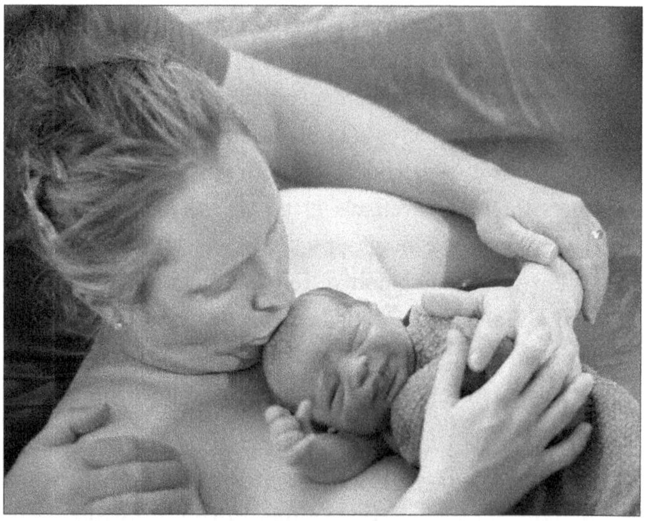
Figure 13-12. A healthy baby undergoes physiologic transition with an intact umbilical cord while she rests skin-to-skin with her mother and is caressed by her father in a birth tub.

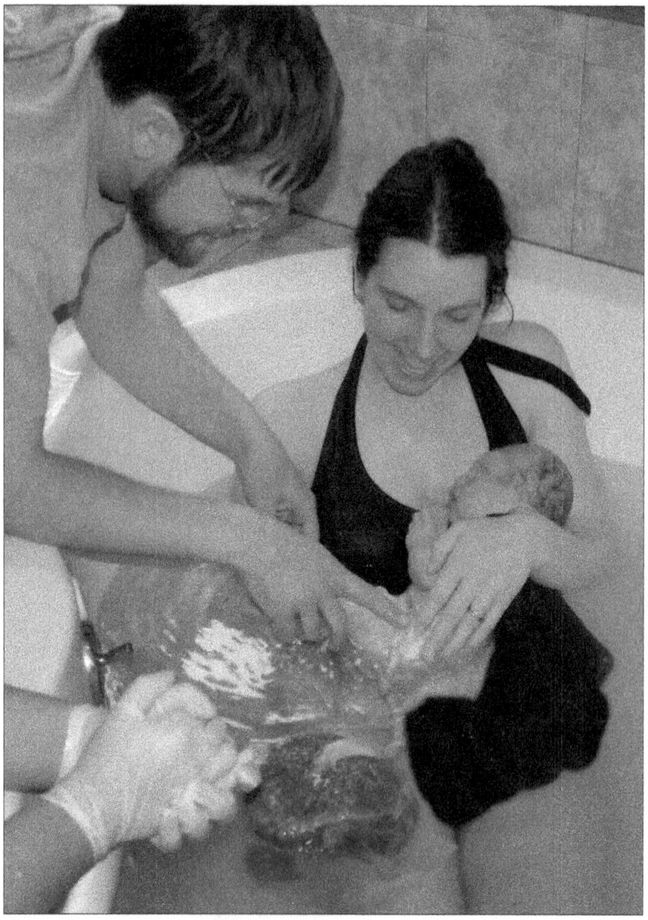

Figure 13-13. Physiologic third stage at a freestanding birth center. The placenta emerges with the unclamped cord still attached to the baby. The midwife stands by ready to assist but does not interfere. Interestingly, this birth was nearly bloodless.

collapsing with each exhalation, thus decreasing the work of breathing. Preterm infants may have so little pulmonary surfactant that they struggle to open their lungs with each breath.

Lung expansion and the oxygen in room air reduce pulmonary vascular resistance and pulmonary artery pressure, causing a dramatic increase in blood flow through the lungs. Oxygen floods the newborn's bloodstream in much greater quantities than was available *in utero*. The network of tiny blood vessels in the lungs progressively relaxes, creating a bed of low-resistance blood vessels that obtain oxygen from air-filled alveoli. As the baby breathes deeply or cries, more alveoli expand, and oxygen saturation climbs. A term newborn requires up to 10 min to reach an oxygen saturation of 90% (Weiner & Zaichkin, 2021). Alveolar fluid can persist for the first few hours postpartum, and complete relaxation of pulmonary vessels can take months (Weiner & Zaichkin, 2021).

By opening the vessels in the lungs before closing the placental circulation, the newborn smoothly exchanges one low-resistance vascular bed for another without decreasing blood volume.

It appears that contractions of the uterus help move blood from the placenta to the newborn while the cord is still intact, (Andersson & Mercer, 2021; Madar et al., 2021). The blood flows through the right heart, surges into the pulmonary vessels, picks up oxygen, and flows back to the heart. When the cord is clamped and the baby is separated from the vast network of placental blood vessels, systemic BP rises, increasing the flow of blood to the lungs. Increased vascular resistance and the massive surge in blood volume returning from the lungs raise pressure in the left atrium. At birth, the sudden increase in left-atrial pressure pushes the flap of the foramen ovale against the atrial septum, closing the 'right-left' shunt. This temporary closure occurs within minutes to hours of birth, but over time tissue proliferation seals the passage permanently (Murphy, 2005). The ductus arteriosus constricts but remains open for 24–48 hr after birth. Blood begins to circulate in the same pattern as it does in the adult.

Delayed Cord Clamping

The newborn clamp or tie was developed to prevent catastrophic blood loss when the cord is cut before the umbilical cord vessels are fully constricted. Delaying cord clamping until placental transfusion is complete increases the infant's hematocrit and iron stores, improves and stabilizes BP, improves respiratory function, and optimizes cerebral oxygenation (ACOG, 2020/2023). Infants who have delayed cord clamping reach a normal level of oxygen saturation significantly sooner than those with immediate cord clamping (Lara-Cantón et al., 2022). In preterm infants, delayed clamping improves transitional circulation and blood volume and decreases the incidence of necrotizing enterocolitis and intraventricular hemorrhage (ACOG, 2020/2023).

At birth, 40% of a term infant's blood volume is contained within the placenta and umbilical cord (Welsh, Elwell, Manister, & Gildersleeve, 2020). Delayed cord clamping allows the physiologic transfer of most of this blood into the body of the baby. The healthy term infant can gain 60–240 ml of volume through delayed cord clamping (Farrar et al., 2011).

The infant's position in relation to the undelivered placenta can facilitate or inhibit transfusion. Babies kept at or below the introitus can receive nearly the full volume of cord blood within 1–2 min. Those on the maternal abdomen may require 5 min to obtain the same amount (Andersson & Mercer, 2021; Mercer & Erickson-Owens, 2012). When the baby is 16–24 in. (40–60 cm) above the mother, placental transfusion ceases, and the effect is the same as immediate cord clamping (Katheria, Brown, Rich, & Arnell, 2017; Katheria, Lakshminrusimha, Rabe, McAdams, & Mercer, 2017). Umbilical cord milking can quickly provide a partial placental transfusion to a newborn that requires immediate resuscitation. Cord milking is typically accomplished by stripping the cord from the placental end to the baby over 2 sec, releasing to allow refill, and repeating 3–5 times (McAdams, Fay, & Delaney, 2018; Ortiz-Esquinas et al., 2020).

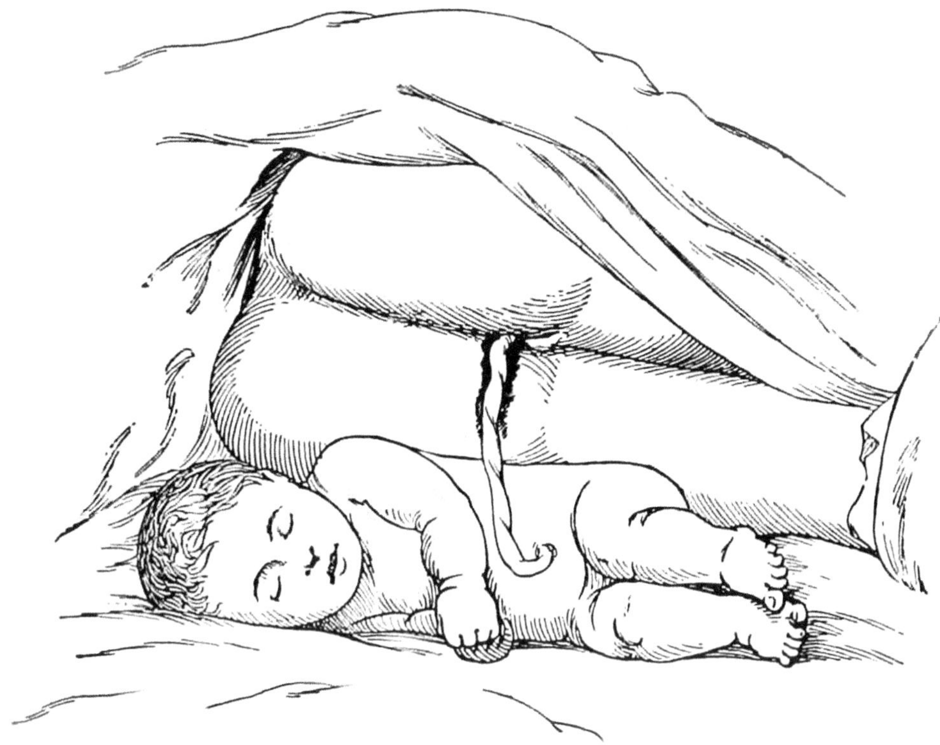

Figure 13-14. "The Position in Which the Child Should Be Placed after Birth," From *A Text-Book of Obstetrics* (2nd ed., p. 317), by B. C. Hirst, 1899, Philadelphia, PA; W. B. Saunders. In the public domain. Hirst disapproved of the practice of immediately cutting the cord and handing the baby to the nurse. He wrote (1899, p. 319) that it "does not take into account the fact that there remains a considerable quantity of fetal blood in the placenta; that it is an advantage to have all this blood, if possible, returned to the infantile body where it belongs, and that further, the depletion of the placenta renders its expulsion easier. The blood in the placenta will return to the child's body, if time is allowed for it." He also cites Pierre Budin, who in 1876 and 1886 demonstrated that an average of 3.2 oz (92 g) of blood was transferred to the infant when cord ligation was delayed 2.5 min.

Delayed cord clamping is nothing new. Erasmus Darwin, grandfather of Charles Darwin, wrote (1796, p. 235)

> Another thing very injurious to the child, is the tying and cutting the navel-string too soon; which should always be left till the child has not only repeatedly breathed, but till all pulsation in the cord ceases. As otherwise the child is much weaker than it ought to be; a part of the blood being left in the placenta, which ought to have been in the child; and at the same time the placenta does not so naturally collapse, and withdraw itself from the sides of the uterus, and is not therefore removed with so much safety and certainty.

Ventilation Before Cord Clamping

Ventilation of the lungs, opening of the pulmonary circuit, and closing of the placental circuit occur in a set interdependent sequence (Hooper et al., 2015; Lara-Cantón et al., 2022). By opening the vessels in the lungs before closing the placental circulation, the newborn smoothly exchanges one low-resistance vascular bed for another without decreasing blood volume, allowing the infant to equilibrate oxygen levels and pH through continuing placental exchange (Andersson & Mercer, 2021). This adaptation occurs over the first few minutes after birth only if the cord is intact.

With immediate cord clamping, the low-pressure placental vascular bed is eliminated before the pulmonary vessels dilate to form a new one (Niermeyer & Velaphi, 2013). Healthy newborns with spontaneous respirations are more likely to die or require admission for medical issues if the cord is clamped before or immediately after breathing starts (Ersdal, Linde, Mduma, Auestad, & Perlman, 2014). Cord clamping before respiration disrupts the physiologic transition by trapping much of the baby's blood volume in the placenta. With less blood volume and greater vascular tone, arterial pressure rises about 30% within four heartbeats, and cardiac output declines 30–50% (Hooper et al., 2015). Because the pulmonary vascular bed is constricted and blood volume is low, less blood returns to the left ventricle to be pumped to the body, further reducing cardiac output (Funai & Norwitz, 2023; Hooper et al., 2015). Additionally, just as cord compression causes variable decelerations in the fetus, clamping the cord can produce rapid and

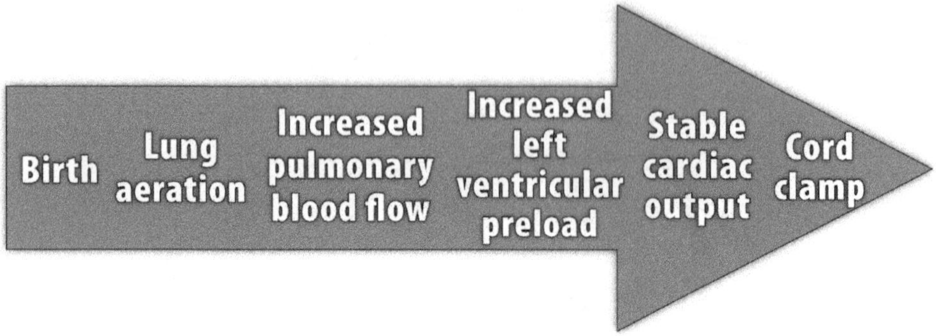

Figure 13-15. Physiologic sequence of events at birth leading to optimal cardiovascular function.

profound bradycardia in the nonbreathing newborn, sometimes to the point of necessitating resuscitation (Bhatt et al., 2013; Niermeyer & Velaphi, 2013). Immediate cord clamping also deprives the newborn of neuroprotective stem cells capable of quickly repairing injury to vital organs (Hutchon, 2015).

In preterm infants, cerebral hemorrhage can be triggered by fluctuations in blood flow to the brain. In a groundbreaking study involving preterm lambs, Bhatt and colleagues demonstrated ventilation before cord clamping increases pulmonary blood flow 8–10-fold and brings venous return and preload to the left ventricle of the heart without fluctuations in cardiac output (Bhatt et al., 2013). Blood returning from the lungs immediately replaces umbilical venous return as the primary source for left-ventricular preload while maintaining relatively stable cardiac output. Later research suggests that ventilation before cord clamping can reduce the risk of cerebral hemorrhage in preterm infants as well (Brouwer et al., 2022).

Relationship to Jaundice

Although a 2013 study reported a significant increase, 1.7%, in jaundice requiring phototherapy among infants with delayed cord clamping (McDonald, Middleton, Dowswell, & Morris, 2014), more recent research has shown no such association (Bennett, Munoz, Yao, & Singh, 2021; Bhoi, Mishra, & Rout, 2019; Carvalho et al., 2019; Rana, Ranneberg, Målqvist, Ashish, & Andersson, 2020; Shinohara & Kataoka, 2021; Yang, Duffy, Johnston, Fall, & Fitzmaurice, 2019). Some infants, however, develop higher levels of bilirubin, a compound created by the breakdown of red blood cells (RBCs), that are clinically insignificant (Fogarty et al., 2018; Yang et al., 2019). Delayed cord clamping can also cause polycythemia (elevated hemoglobin and hematocrit levels) in the first days of life, but not to the point of doing harm or requiring treatment (Fogarty et al., 2018; Qian et al., 2020). Overall, infants with delayed cord clamping are less likely to require admission to the NICU (Abdelmaksoud, Abdelraziq, Khashaba, & Diab, 2021; Korkut et al., 2021).

Timing

The ideal timing of cord clamping remains unknown but delay greater than 1 min appears beneficial (Andersson & Mercer, 2021). Although cord pulsations typically last 3–4 min (Di Tommaso et al., 2019), blood flow usually continues for about 5 min following birth, even after pulsations cease (Boere et al., 2015). In the first minute after birth, 50–70% of the placental transfusion volume moves into the baby (Chen, Li, Chang, Li, & Cui, 2018; Farrar et al., 2011; Yao, Moinian, & Lind, 1969). A study that compared immediate cord clamping with clamping delayed in 30-sec increments through 180 sec and until the end of cord pulsations (Chen et al., 2018) found statistically significant correlation between delays up to 90 sec and higher neonatal hematocrit at 24 hr.

ACOG, ACNM, AAP, the International Liaison Committee on Resuscitation, the European Resuscitation Council (ERC), and most other professional organizations in this field recommend delayed cord clamping for vigorous infants. The World Health Organization recommends a delay of approximately 1–3 min before cord clamping with all births while initiating essential neonatal care—unless the baby needs to be moved immediately for resuscitation (WHO, n.d.). Neonatal Resuscitation Program (NRP) and ACOG guidelines recommend delaying cord clamping at least 30–60 sec for most vigorous term and preterm infants; ERC recommends at least 1 min (Weiner & Zaichkin, 2021; Wyllie et al., 2015).

Physiologic cord management involves waiting for the cord to become pale and flat before clamping (Andersson & Mercer, 2021). Pulsations within the cord will no longer be palpable. If this stage is not reached by 3 min after birth, further delay may benefit the baby (Andersson & Mercer, 2021). Handle the cord gently; tension and compression can cause the vessels to spasm.

An infant born with a tight nuchal cord or after shoulder dystocia may be hypovolemic because of insufficient blood flow through the umbilical cord. Hypovolemia can cause sudden neonatal asystole, trigger an inflammatory cascade, or cause neurologic issues such as seizures, brain damage, or death (Mercer & Erickson-Owens, 2014). Delayed cord clamping can correct hypovolemia, increase red-cell count, and improve perfusion to all organs (Mercer & Erickson-Owens, 2014).

A tight nuchal cord should be ligated only in the extremely rare case that there is no other way to deliver the infant (Mercer & Erickson-Owens, 2014). The somersault maneuver can facilitate birth of the infant through a tight cord. The midwife holds the newborn's head close to the thigh or folds the baby up toward the symphysis (Mercer & Erickson-Owens, 2014). The body births, and the head stays next to the mother. The midwife unwinds the cord and places the baby on the mother or on the bed between the mother's legs, allowing placental blood to transfuse into the baby.

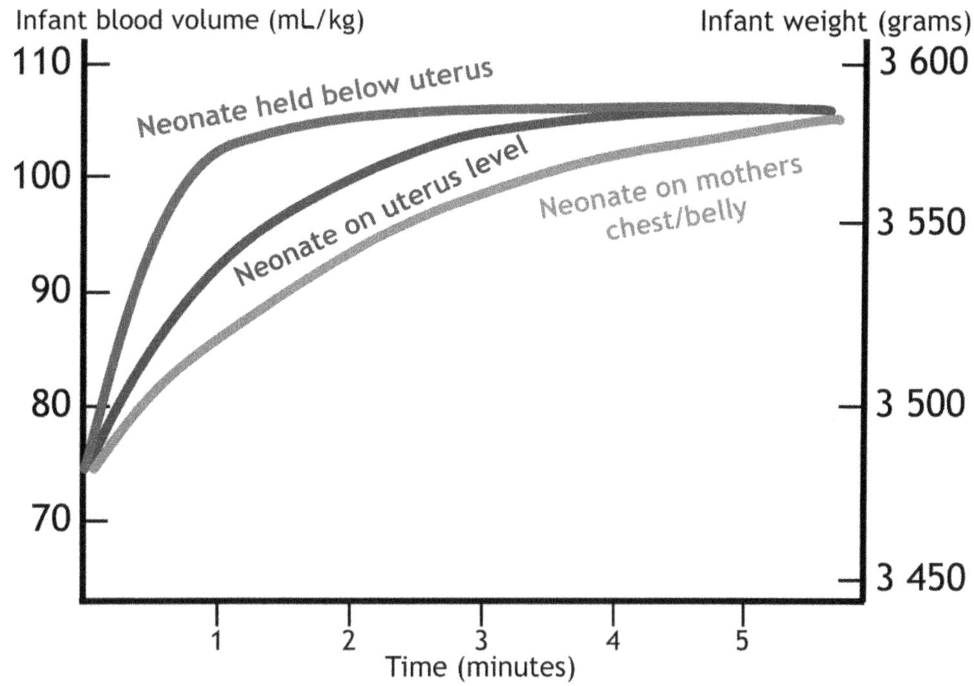

Figure 13-16. Most of the placental blood volume is transferred to the baby within 1–3 min of birth, but the transfusion often continues for 5 min or more, influenced by the baby's position in relation to the placenta. From "Cord Management of the Term Newborn," by O. Andersson, and J. S. Mercer, 2021, *Clinics in Perinatology, 48*(3), 447–470, fig. 3. CC BY 4.0.

Waterbirth Considerations

Waterbirth appears to be a safe option for low-risk, low-intervention births that gives comfort and relaxation to mothers and newborns alike (Bovbjerg, Cheyney, & Everson, 2016). Case studies in which infants born in the water experienced infection, water aspiration, and umbilical cord avulsion have caused widespread concerns about the safety of waterbirth (ACOG, 2016/2021; Pinette, Wax, & Wilson, 2004). Despite these concerns, there is strong evidence that waterbirth does *not* increase the risk of adverse neonatal outcomes over birth on land, including infectious or respiratory conditions (Bovbjerg, 2015; Bovbjerg et al., 2016; Burns, Boulton, Cluett, Cornelius, & Smith, 2012; Cluett, Burns, & Cuthbert, 2018; Geissbuehler, Stein, & Eberhard, 2004; Henderson et al., 2014; Lanier et al., 2021; Y. Liu et al., 2014; Lukasse, Rowe, Townend, Knight, & Hollowell, 2014; Shaw-Battista, 2017; Snapp, Stapleton, Wright, Niemczyk, & Jolles, 2020; Taylor, Kleine, Bewley, Loucaides, & Sutcliffe, 2016; Thoeni, Zech, Moroder, & Ploner, 2005; Valarezo, Powel, Benito, & Yates, 2019; Young & Kruske, 2013). In fact, analysis of data from the AABC Perinatal Data Registry from 2012 to 2017 showed that infants born in water in community settings (home or birth center) had a lower incidence of FHR abnormalities and shoulder dystocia and were less likely to need transfer to a higher level of care, require admission to a NICU, or experience respiratory complications when compared to infants born on dry land (Snapp et al., 2020). Their mothers had improved outcomes as well—fewer prolonged labors, genital lacerations, episiotomies, hemorrhages, and postpartum transfers (Snapp et al., 2020).

Umbilical cord avulsion (tearing or snapping of the umbilical cord) is a rare occurrence, but it appears to occur more often in waterbirths (Schafer, 2014). In several case studies, delays in discovering a torn or avulsed umbilical cord have caused neonatal hemorrhage (Schafer, 2014). Cord avulsion is most likely to occur when a baby with a short cord is brought rapidly to the surface. An infant with cord avulsion is a critical emergency; you must clamp the cord immediately before the baby exsanguinates. In every birth, in or out of water, evaluate the umbilical cord for bleeding that may indicate avulsion. Lowering the water level before birth and bringing the baby gently to the surface probably reduces the risk of cord avulsion (Snapp et al., 2020).

A few safety guidelines can minimize risk to the baby born in water:

- Keep the water temperature between 97.0°F and 100°F (36.1–37.7°C); measure hourly ("Model Practice Template for Hydrotherapy," 2017).
- When the baby is born, the head and body must be either entirely in the water or entirely out ("Model Practice Template," 2017). If the baby is resubmerged after it begins to breathe, there is a risk of aspiration or even drowning.

Contraindications for Waterbirth

- Maternal fever ≥100.4°F (38.0°C)
- Gestational age <37 weeks
- Abnormal vaginal bleeding
- Abnormal fetal heart pattern
- Active *Herpes simplex* lesion, hepatitis B or C, or human immunodeficiency virus (HIV)
- Musculoskeletal or mobility problems that prevent a quick exit from the tub
- Administration of sedating medications 1 hr or less before entering tub
- Pregnancy complications, medical conditions, or history of conditions that increase current risk (hypertension, history of postpartum hemorrhage or shoulder dystocia, et al.)

This list is not exhaustive: other maternal or fetal conditions can contraindicate waterbirth as well. Adapted from "A Model Practice Template for Hydrotherapy in Labor and Birth," 2017, *Journal of Midwifery & Women's Health, 62*(1), pp. 120–122. Copyright 2016 by American College of Nurse-Midwives.

- Guide the baby to the surface within 5–10 sec of birth.
- Avoid excessive tension on the cord. Keep cord clamps close at hand and investigate any unusual bleeding immediately following birth.
- Dry the baby's head. The baby will stay warm if skin-to-skin contact is maintained and the baby's lower extremities, abdomen, and chest remain under water.
- Delay cord clamping until pulsations cease and the cord turns white or until after delivery of the placenta ("Model Practice Template," 2017).
- If the baby needs resuscitative measures that cannot be conducted with the cord intact, clamp and cut the cord and move the baby to a warmed, flat surface. There is no advantage to moving the baby to a position higher than the mother, such as the edge of the tub, with the cord attached because the placental transfusion can stop if the baby is more than 16 in. (40 cm) above the mother (Katheria, Brown, Rich, et al., 2017; Katheria, Lakshminrusimha, et al., 2017).
- If a nuchal cord prevents birth and cannot be reduced, try the somersault maneuver. If this maneuver fails, have the client stand so you can double-clamp and cut the cord out of the water. *Never clamp or cut a nuchal cord underwater.* The client should remain standing for birth ("Model Practice Template," 2017).
- The baby may remain with the mother in the tub if both mother and baby are stable. Remove the newborn from the tub for assessment if the heart rate is greater than 160 bpm or less than 100 bpm, if the baby's body temperature is 100.4°F (38°C) or higher or lower than 97.0°F (36°C), or if there are signs of respiratory distress ("Model Practice Template," 2017).

Neonatal Resuscitation in Community Settings

The International Liaison Committee on Resuscitation was organized in 1992 to provide a forum in which principal international resuscitation organizations can reach consensus on the science of resuscitation. In the United States, the prevailing standard for newborn resuscitation is the Neonatal Resuscitation Program (NRP), an educational offering of the American Heart Association and AAP. Research shows that NRP training improves effectiveness of resuscitation, builds the confidence of providers, and improves 5-min Apgar scores (Fernandes, 2023).

AAP, however, considers home birth less safe than birth in a hospital or freestanding birth center and supports provision of care *only* by midwives who are certified by the American Midwifery Certification Board (Watterberg & Cmte. on Fetus and Newborn, 2020). Consequently, NRP guidelines are largely specific to the care of newborns born in hospitals attended by a team of providers that may include neonatologists, obstetricians, midwives, nurses, and anesthesiologists (Lane, 2014).

The only providers eligible to become NRP instructors are physicians, registered nurses, nurse practitioners, respiratory-care practitioners, and physician assistants with experience in intrapartum obstetrics (AAP, 2022). Yet all birth attendants are expected to meet the standard of care whether the birth is planned for hospital, birth center, or home (Wyllie et al., 2015). Although AAP offers an Essentials option for NRP providers (Lessons 1–4), the North American Registry of Midwives (NARM) requires that certified professional midwives complete NRP Advanced Provider curriculum (Lessons 1–11) and attend an instructor-led training event (NARM, 2021).

In accordance with NRP recommendations that one qualified birth attendant should assume sole management of the infant at a low-risk birth, most planned community births are staffed by one midwife and one assistant, both trained in neonatal resuscitation (Lane, 2014). NRP guidelines stipulate, however, that two dedicated, trained attendants are required in the event of intrapartum complications, including shoulder dystocia and category II FHR patterns (Weiner & Zaichkin, 2021). Many of these complications are unpredictable. NRP also specifies that two attendants must be present and committed exclusively to the care of the infant for any higher-risk births, such as those involving gestational age of 41 weeks or more and suspected fetal macrosomia (Weiner & Zaichkin, 2021). Most community midwifery practices lack the staff and resources to provide three or more attendants at every birth (Lane, 2014).

NRP guidelines recommend use of equipment such as an oxygen blender, electrocardiography (ECG), and radiant warmer, and recommend use of continuous positive airway pressure (CPAP) in some circumstances (Weiner & Zaichkin, 2021). Although some community midwives carry compressed air and oxygen blenders, the majority carry only oxygen and can deliver either room air, 100% oxygen, or an unmeasured mixture of the two to the infant. Not every midwife carries CPAP equipment. Many rely on bulb syringes, filtered mucus-trap catheters or portable battery-powered units for suctioning.

In a community setting, any baby needing significant resuscitation requires transportation to a hospital. At least one provider must remain to care for the mother if emergency medical services (EMS) regulations or policies prohibit transporting a mother, infant, and midwife in the same ambulance. Paramedics (U.S.) and their counterparts have the training and equipment to intubate, obtain IV access, and give resuscitative medication to the newborn in the field, but often they have little experience with intubating infants. In some areas, a basic life-support crew that cannot perform these tasks is the first or only EMS response.

Uncontrolled ambient temperatures present special challenges to resuscitation. Extreme cold or heat in the midwife's vehicle, for example, can reduce the efficacy or shelf life of medications. Infants risk serious hypothermia when full resuscitation is performed throughout a long transport (Carmichael, McCullough, & Kempley, 2007). Heated infant transport mattresses function optimally at ambient temperatures 66°–82°F (19°–28°C). They will not work if left in the cold for a long time, and they can become dangerously hot if exposed to excessive heat.

Table 13-2

Neonatal Resuscitation Equipment Used in Home Birth

Keep equipment accessible in a designated area.

Airway equipment

- Self-inflating bag—500 ml with 40-cm pop-off valve
- Round soft silicone masks sized for the preterm and term infant
- Stethoscope
- Advanced airway kit, laryngeal mask airway (LMA), or endotracheal (ET) intubation supplies
- Suctioning devices with catheters, such as mucus traps with filters or mechanical suction
- 5-ml syringes
- Nasogastric tubes—sizes 6 French Gauge (FG), 8 FG, and 10 FG
- Hypoallergenic tape
- Latex-free gloves
- Small gauze squares

Intravascular access equipment

- Supplies for placing intraosseous (IO) access or umbilical venous catheter
- Normal saline (NS)

Medications

1:10,000 (0.1 mg/ml) epinephrine

Additional items

- Self-warming transport mattress
- Plastic wrap or bag for unexpected premature infant
- Plastic or fleece hats
- Heating pad or hot water bottle for warming blankets (never use on the infant!)
- Towels
- Good portable light and spare batteries
- Sterile packs of scissors and at least 3 umbilical clamps
- Sharps disposal container
- Clock/watch with a seconds display
- Record-keeping charts
- Identification bracelets

Adapted from (1) "Equipment Used in Homebirth," by Resuscitation Council UK, 2011 (https://www.resus.org.uk/library/quality-standards-cpr/equipment-used-home-birth). Copyright 2014–2020 by author. (2) "Closing the Theory–Practice Gap: Intrapartum Midwifery Management of Planned Homebirths," by S. Vedam, M. Goff, and V. Nolan-Marnin, 2007, *Journal of Midwifery and Women's Health, 52*(3), 291–300. Copyright by American College of Nurse-Midwives.

Resuscitating the Infant

Within 30 sec after birth, about 85% of term newborns breathe spontaneously (Weiner & Zaichkin, 2021). Another 10% begin to breathe with drying and stimulation. About 5% of term neonates require positive-pressure ventilation (PPV), 2% require intubation, and 1–3 infants per 1,000 births require chest compressions or emergency medications (Weiner & Zaichkin, 2021). The foundation of neonatal resuscitation is the effective ventilation of the infant's lungs (Weiner & Zaichkin, 2021). Whereas adult cardiac arrest is usually a result of heart disease or trauma, newborn cardiac arrest is usually a result of inadequate gas exchange, either before birth from failed placental respiration or after birth from failure to breathe. Worldwide, up to two thirds of newborn deaths could be prevented by low-technology care such as keeping infants warm and promptly aerating their lungs (Castle, 2018).

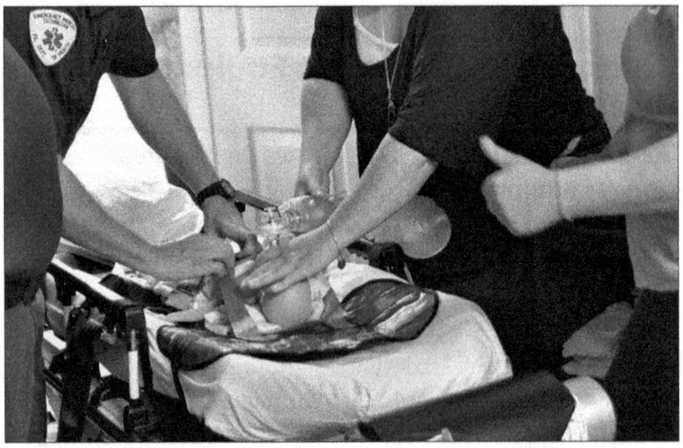

Figure 13-17. A nurse gives the thumbs-up as a midwife and an emergency medical services (EMS) responder practice neonatal resuscitation in an emergency drill. The midwife's hand position on the mask is incorrect, however—her fingers should contact the newborn's mandible, not cover the face—underscoring the need for frequent practice. The participants should also be wearing gloves. Providers of various disciplines who practice together tend to work better together in actual emergencies.

Table 13-3

Conditions that Increase the Risk for a Depressed Newborn

Maternal conditions: Extremes of maternal age, seizure disorder, diabetes mellitus, hypertension, substance abuse, previous history of stillbirth. **Fetal conditions:** Prematurity, postmaturity, congenital anomalies, macrosomia, anemia, isoimmunization, FGR, or multiple gestation. **Antepartum conditions:** Placenta previa, placental abruption, oligohydramnios, polyhydramnios. **Birth complications:** Transverse lie or breech presentation; IAI; meconium-stained or foul-smelling amniotic fluid; abnormal FHR pattern; shoulder dystocia; maternal administration of a narcotic shortly before birth; vacuum, forceps, or cesarean birth.
Adapted from "Neonatal Resuscitation in the Delivery Room," by C. J. Fernandes, 2023, in C. Armsby (Ed.), *UpToDate*. Copyright by UpToDate.

All community midwives and their ancillary staff should undergo extensive training in neonatal resuscitation and refresh their learning at frequent intervals. A comprehensive program that readies the midwife to resuscitate newborns is beyond the scope of this book. What follows is an overview of neonatal resuscitation techniques as they pertain to community settings. Midwives should seek additional training with hands-on practice in neonatal resuscitation before attending any birth and refresh skills at least every two years to maintain proficiency.

Preparing for Resuscitation

Neonatal resuscitation can be stressful for even the most seasoned midwife. The provider who memorizes the steps of resuscitation and mentally rehearses them on the way to every birth is likely to find that events flow more smoothly and are likely to lead to a successful outcome. In every birth, ensure that the equipment needed for successful resuscitation is in working order and laid out for easy access (see Table 13-2). To decrease the risk of neonatal hypothermia, set the room temperature at 74–77°F (23–25°C) and turn off any fans (Weiner & Zaichkin, 2021). Ensure that emergency contact numbers are accessible and ensure that team members know what roles they will play in an emergency. Although the need for resuscitation sometimes comes as a surprise, certain maternal, fetal, and intrapartum risk factors are predictably associated with a depressed infant (see Table 13-3).

Before birth occurs in a community setting, consider the antepartum and intrapartum issues that could affect the wellbeing of the infant. These resuscitation considerations are represented by the mnemonic GRAND:

Gestational age: All planned births in community settings should involve term fetuses. Preterm infants, however, are sometimes unexpectedly born outside a hospital, usually because of poor pregnancy dating. In other cases, ambiguous signs of preterm labor go unrecognized until the infant arrives. Preterm infants are much more vulnerable to hypothermia, hypoglycemia, respiratory difficulty, and other issues than term newborns and require special considerations during resuscitation and transport. Post-term infants are at higher risk of meconium aspiration syndrome (MAS).

Risk factors: Maternal and fetal risk factors such as those listed in Table 13-3 increase the likelihood that a neonate will need resuscitation or special care. For example, if the mother has diabetes or the fetus is growth restricted, there is a higher risk of hypoglycemia in the infant.

Amniotic fluid: Newborns born through abnormal amniotic fluid (e.g., meconium-stained, grossly bloody, foul-smelling) are more likely to require resuscitation.

Number of infants: Surprise multiples increase the need for resuscitation and complicate logistics. For example, twins require two sets of resuscitation equipment and additional care providers.

Distance: Before every birth, consider how long it may take to transport a newborn from the site of birth. Which hospitals are closest? If the hospital has a NICU, what level of care does it offer? If the site of birth is remote, is helicopter

Resuscitation Considerations: Think GRAND

Gestational age

Risk Factors

Amniotic fluid

Number of infants

Distance from definitive care

First Thought, Worst Thought:

What is the most likely cause of a depressed newborn?

Primary apnea—transient poor tone and apnea with good heart rate (resolves with stimulation, drying and repositioning).

What is the worst it could be?

Severely hypoxic or anoxic infant, brain damage, or stillbirth.

transport to a tertiary facility possible? What is the typical time for ambulance response, and is it affected by traffic or time of day? Is your local EMS staffed by EMTs, paramedics (or their non-U.S. equivalents), or both?

Apnea at Birth

Apnea in a newborn is classed as primary or secondary, and it can begin before, during, or after birth. In response to severe hypoxia, either *in utero* or after birth, FHR and tone decrease, and the baby initiates gasping respirations. If severe hypoxia continues, the fetus will stop breathing efforts (Goldsmith & Martin, 2019). This is primary apnea. Most newborns that fail to breathe spontaneously at birth are in primary apnea and will respond to drying, warmth, and stimulation by initiating respirations. Intrauterine resuscitation can correct primary apnea in the fetus (Kluckow & Hooper, 2015).

Continued severe hypoxia causes loss of consciousness and failure of the neural centers in the brainstem that control respiratory drive (Wyllie et al., 2015). This condition is termed secondary apnea. If the baby does not breathe deeply at birth, the lung vessels remain constricted and blood continues to flow through the fetal circuit, largely bypassing the lungs. The fetal heart muscle shifts into anaerobic metabolism and becomes less efficient, beating at about half the usual rate (Wyllie et al., 2015). Arterioles in the intestines, kidneys, muscles, and skin constrict to prioritize perfusion of the brain, heart, and liver. Over time, compensatory mechanisms begin to fail, causing organ damage and death (Wyllie et al., 2015).

A fetus can pass through primary apnea *in utero* and be in secondary apnea at birth. No amount of stimulation can initiate spontaneous breathing in the baby with secondary apnea. If an infant does not respond immediately to back rubs and brisk toweling, aggressive resuscitation is necessary and may include bag-mask ventilation, intubation, IV volume replacement, and cardiopulmonary resuscitation (CPR).

Most infants that are depressed at birth revive if their lungs are ventilated. Effective aeration of the lungs is most likely to reverse hypoxic decline if initiated early (Weiner & Zaichkin, 2021). Over the span of a few minutes, inflation of the lungs and oxygenation should cause the alveoli to expand and the pulmonary vasculature to dilate. If the infant still has adequate circulation, oxygenated blood will perfuse the heart muscle and heart rate will increase. Oxygenated blood will flow to the brain, and the respiratory center will begin to function. The baby will begin to breathe spontaneously and regain consciousness.

If persistent hypoxia has caused the heart muscle to fail, chest compressions and ventilation must be provided to transport oxygen from the lungs to the heart muscle. Within a minute or two, the heart muscle is usually oxygenated enough to maintain circulation. Occasionally the heart requires medication to restore circulation.

Resuscitation with Intact Umbilical Cord

As discussed above, evidence suggests that delaying umbilical cord clamping until respirations are established promotes a physiologic transition at birth (Ashish et al., 2022; Bhatt et al., 2013; Blank et al., 2018; Hooper et al., 2015; Katheria, Brown, Faksh, et al., 2017; Katheria, Poeltler, et al., 2016; Mercer, Erickson-Owens, & Skovgaard, 2009; Niermeyer & Velaphi, 2013). The compromised fetus has an even greater need for optimal oxygenation and cardiac output while making the transition to newborn (Katheria, Lakshminrusimha, et al., 2017). Resuscitation with the umbilical cord intact, standard practice for most home-birth midwives, appears to combine proven benefits of delayed cord clamping with lifesaving resuscitative measures (Andersson & Mercer, 2021; Fulton, Stoll, & Thordarson, 2016; Mercer & Erickson-Owens, 2014). Although NRP guidelines state there is currently insufficient evidence to recommend neonatal resuscitation with an intact cord (Weiner & Zaichkin, 2021), available data suggest that infants that are resuscitated while attached to the placental circulation intact have better oxygen saturation, better Apgar scores, and better outcomes (Andersson et al., 2019; Andersson & Mercer, 2021; Mercer, Nelson, & Skovgaard, 2011).

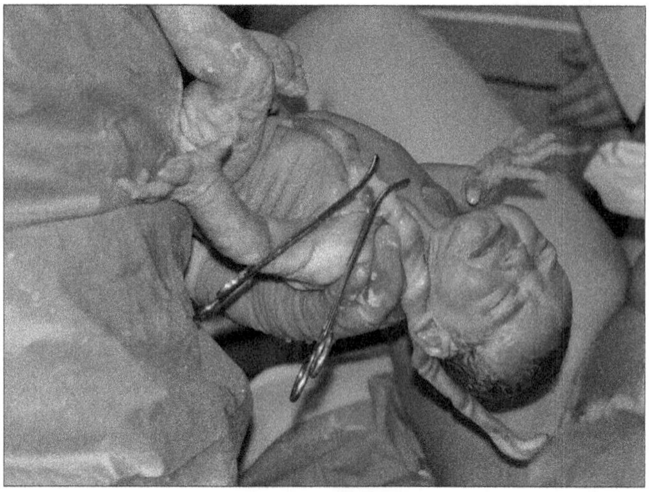

Figure 13-18. Immediate cord clamping puts the newborn at great disadvantage by interrupting the transfusion of blood, stem cells, and other substances from the placenta, and it is especially risky before the onset of respirations. Despite its drawbacks, the practice remains commonplace at many North American hospitals. Note the engorged blood vessels in the length of cord between the clamp and the placenta containing blood that would have transferred into the baby if cord clamping had been delayed.

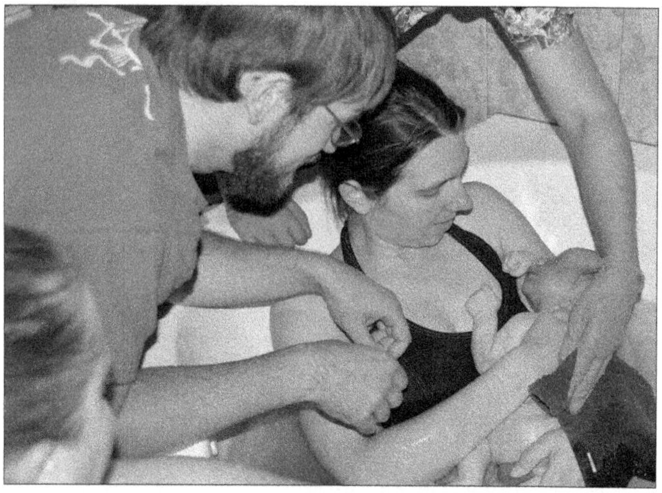

Figure 13-19. The first step of neonatal resuscitation in a community setting is to stimulate the baby with the umbilical cord still attached. This newborn was healthy but was not breathing effectively and showed central cyanosis about 20 sec after birth. Rubbing him with a washcloth encouraged effective respirations, and no further assistance was needed.

In community settings, the recommended technique for resuscitation with an intact umbilical cord is to place the baby between the mother's legs on a clean, warm, dry surface (van Rheenen & Brabin, 2006). In the hospital, however, culture, protocols, and lack of training can create barriers to resuscitation with an intact cord (Fulton et al., 2016). In British Columbia, 78% of midwives sampled had performed intact-cord resuscitation at planned home births but never in the hospital (Fulton et al., 2016). Some hospitals in Europe and elsewhere have begun to integrate intact-cord neonatal resuscitation into practice by using a mobile resuscitation trolley (Katheria, Sorki, et al., 2018; Mercer & Erickson-Owens, 2014). The trolley provides a warm, secure platform for resuscitation on which suction, oxygen blender, pulse oximeter, and CPAP devices are easily mounted. The trolley easily supports the infant during vaginal or cesarean birth while placental circulation remains intact.

Initial Steps of Resuscitation for a Full-Term Baby

During the "golden minute," the first minute after birth, assess the baby to determine whether resuscitation is needed. The following recommendations are derived largely from Weiner and Zaichkin's *Textbook of Neonatal Resuscitation* (2021), widely considered the standard of care in the United States, with changes to increase their relevance to birth in community settings.

The Vigorous Newborn

The initial steps of neonatal care include providing warmth, drying, tactile stimulation, positioning to open the airway, and clearing secretions from the airway if necessary (Weiner & Zaichkin, 2021). Immediately after birth, rapidly assess the infant:

- Is the baby breathing or crying?
- Is the baby well-flexed and with good color?
- Does the baby appear full-term?

If all three answers are yes, the baby is vigorous and the initial steps can be performed skin to skin on the mother's chest or abdomen. Mother-baby skin contact is a crucial regulator of the neonatal autonomic nervous system, promotes breastfeeding, hastens expulsion of the placenta, reduces bleeding, maintains warmth, reduces stress levels, and forges a vital bond between mother and child (Boundy et al., 2016; Chi Luong, Long Nguyen, Huyn Thi, Carrara, & Bergman, 2016; Dehghani, Movahed, Dehghani, & Nasiriani, 2015; Widström, Brimdyr, Svensson, Cadwell, & Nissen, 2019). All newborns benefit, but skin-to-skin contact is particularly advantageous for preterm infants in low-resource areas without NICUs and incubators (Charpak et al., 2005).

The baby should be dried with warm towels, and mother and baby should be covered with dry blankets for warmth. At a home birth, blankets can be warmed with a heating pad or hot water bottle. *Caution! Never use a heating pad or hot water bottle directly on the baby. Severe burns can result.* A newborn should never be in contact with a surface hotter than skin temperature. Replace the wet linen beneath the baby with dry to reduce heat loss. If the room is unavoidably cold, consider covering the baby with a sheet of food-or medical-grade plastic wrap or bag, then covering with a warm blanket, taking care to guard against suffocation (Weiner & Zaichkin, 2021).

If necessary, stimulate the baby to breathe by rubbing the back or the foot. The newborn who remains skin to skin with the mother may not cry much. If the baby is breathing and growing pinker, the heart rate is above 100, and tone is normal, the baby does not need to cry and should not be stimulated further (Harper, 2014). Wipe secretions from the baby's mouth and nose with a cloth as necessary. Bulb suctioning is used when the infant has trouble clearing secretions. The vigorous baby born through meconium-stained fluid is managed in the same way as any other vigorous newborn and does not require additional suctioning (Weiner & Zaichkin, 2021). While the baby is skin to skin, monitor breathing, tone, activity, color, and temperature to determine whether additional interventions are required.

Table 13-4
The Five Criteria of the Apgar Score

	Score of 0	Score of 1	Score of 2
Skin color (Appearance)	Cyanotic or pale all over	Blue extremities, body pink (acrocyanosis)	No cyanosis, body and extremities pink
Heart rate (Pulse)	**Absent**	**<100 bpm**	**≥100 bpm**
Reflex irritability (Grimace)	No response to stimulation	Grimace on suction or with stimulation	Cries spontaneously or with stimulation
Muscle tone (Activity)	None, flaccid tone	Some flexion of extremities	Flexed extremities, active movement.
Respiratory effort (Respiration)	Absent respirations	Weak, irregular, gasping respirations	Strong, robust cry or normal breathing

Assess initial Apgar scores at 1 and 5 min of life. If the Apgar score is less than 7 at 5 min, continue to assess and score every 5 min up to 20 min. A 5-min Apgar score of 7–10 is considered reassuring, a score of 4–6 is moderately abnormal, and a score of 0–3 is low in the term infant and late-preterm infant. Although the Apgar score does not predict individual neonatal mortality or neurologic outcome, in general infants with low 5-min Apgar scores are at higher risk for death and cerebral palsy. Most infants with low Apgar scores, however, do not develop cerebral palsy.

Adapted from "The Apgar Score," by American Academy of Pediatrics Committee on Fetus and Newborn and American College of Obstetricians and Gynecologists Committee on Obstetric Practice, 2015, *Pediatrics, 136*(4), 819–822. Copyright by American Academy of Pediatrics.

The Nonvigorous Newborn

If a rapid assessment shows the infant to be nonvigorous, proceed with resuscitation. Perform the initial steps as follows:

Provide Warmth and Dry the Infant

It is critical to ensure that the baby does not develop cold stress. During resuscitation, there is a high risk that the infant will become hypothermic. Hypothermia increases the baby's metabolic rate and oxygen consumption, which can cause or worsen hypoxemia, which in turn can cause or worsen pulmonary vasoconstriction (Karlsen, 2019). It can also increase the baby's glucose consumption, which can lead to hypoglycemia (Karlsen, 2019).

Use warmed towels or blankets to warm, dry, and stimulate the infant for the first 30 sec after birth with the cord intact. When linens become saturated, replace them. Rub the back or feet. Preterm infants less than 32 weeks of gestation do not need to be dried; instead, they should be covered immediately in plastic wrap to reduce heat loss (Weiner & Zaichkin, 2021).

NRP specifies that if resuscitation is needed, the umbilical cord should be cut and the baby taken to a radiant warmer to guard against heat loss (Weiner & Zaichkin, 2021). As previously discussed, initiating resuscitation with an intact umbilical cord, however, is the standard of care for most community midwives (Andersson & Mercer, 2021; Fulton, Stoll, & Thordarson, 2016; Mercer & Erickson-Owens, 2014). Delayed cord clamping keeps the baby close to the mother and allows a transfusion of oxygenated blood from the placenta while resuscitation begins (Katheria, Lakshminrusimha, et al., 2017). If the mother is in the tub or other location that limits intervention, clamp and cut the cord and move the infant to a warm, dry, stable surface for resuscitation. When clamping the cord of a nonvigorous baby, always place the clamp about 6 in. (15 cm) from the infant's body to ensure sufficient length to facilitate placement of an umbilical venous catheter should it become necessary. If the mother is in the tub or other location that limits intervention, clamp and cut the cord

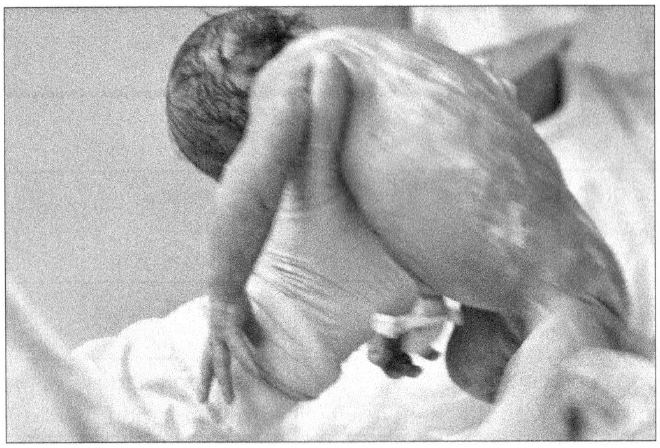

Figure 13-20. After a cesarean birth, this nonvigorous baby displayed poor tone and apnea and was moved to a radiant warmer for resuscitation. Unfortunately, the umbilical cord was clamped close to the infant's abdomen. The cord clamp of a nonvigorous baby should always be placed 6 in. (15 cm) from the body to facilitate umbilical venous catheter insertion should it become necessary.

and move the infant to a warm, dry, stable surface for resuscitation. Always place the clamp about 6 in. (15 cm) from the infant's body to ensure sufficient length to facilitate placement of an umbilical venous catheter should it become necessary.

The baby's body temperature must be kept between 97.7°F (36.5°C) and 99.5°F (37.5°C). Use of a TransWarmer® infant transport mattress (a gel-filled, self-heating device that provides up to 2 hr of warming) or equivalent neonatal thermal mattress is an effective way to maintain the infant's optimal temperature throughout resuscitation, from the birth bed to the NICU bed. It is very useful for maintaining warmth for preterm infants during transport when used in conjunction with plastic wrap (Chawla, Amaram, Gopal, & Natarajan, 2011; Langan, Watson, O'Connor, Moore, & Patton, 2020; Y.-Q. Liu et al., 2018). Protect the TransWarmer® from ambient cooling or heating; to provide optimal warmth it must be at room temperature when activated.

Stimulate the Baby

If drying the baby does not stimulate the onset of spontaneous breathing, gently rub the baby's back, trunk or extremities or flick the feet.

Open and Clear the Airway

Position the baby supine with the neck neural or extended slightly in the "sniffing" position, looking toward the ceiling. Hyperextension or flexion of the neck can close the airway. Placing a small, rolled towel under the baby's shoulders can help maintain the correct position for an open airway. This technique is especially useful if the infant has a large occiput due to molding, edema, or prematurity (Weiner & Zaichkin, 2021).

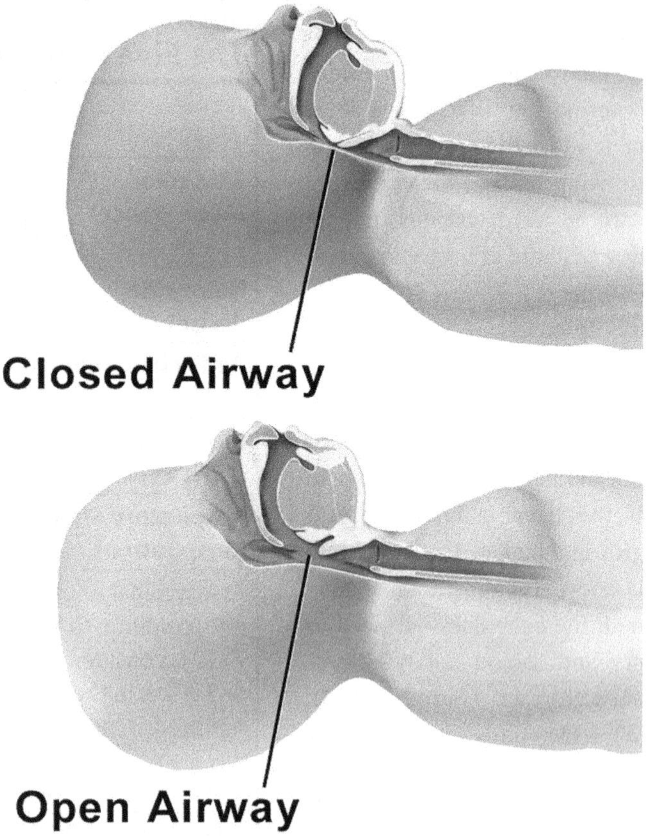

Figure 13-21. A baby's airway opens when the head is in a neutral or sniffing position. Hyperextension or flexion can block the flow of air. "CPR Infant Closed vs Open Airway," by BruceBlaus, 2016 (https://commons.wikimedia.org/wiki/File:CPR_Infant_Closed_vs_Open_Airway.png). CC BY-SA 4.0.

Clear the airway if the baby is not breathing or has poor tone, if secretions are blocking the airway, or the baby cannot clear its own airway. Gently suction the mouth, then the nose, with a bulb syringe or DeLee mucus extractor (Vedam et al., 2007). If the baby has copious secretions coming from the mouth, turn the head to the side to allow the fluids to collect in the cheek, then suction (Weiner & Zaichkin, 2021). Some midwives carry battery-operated suction machines. If using a suction catheter, set the control until negative pressure reads 80–100 mm Hg when the tubing is occluded (Weiner & Zaichkin, 2021). Call EMS if the baby remains nonvigorous after the first 30 sec of stimulation.

Current NRP guidelines maintain that the nonvigorous infant born through meconium-stained fluid should be managed using the same steps of newborn care described here. Routine laryngoscopy and deep suction are no longer recommended because it does not improve infant outcomes. Intubation and tracheal suction are only necessary if the lungs do not inflate with PPV, airway obstruction is suspected, and other attempts to correct the problem have failed (Weiner & Zaichkin, 2021).

Evaluate the Infant's Response

Over the next 30 sec, assess the baby to determine if additional resuscitation is needed. If the baby is apneic or has gasping respirations, immediately initiate PPV (see "If Adequate Breathing Is Absent . . ." below) and call for help. Continued tactile stimulation of an apneic or gasping baby and delay of PPV beyond the first minute of life worsens neonatal outcomes (Weiner & Zaichkin, 2021).

If the baby is breathing, assess the heart rate with a stethoscope along the left side of the baby's chest (Weiner & Zaichkin, 2021). You can tap your finger in rhythm with the baby's heartbeat so that other team members will know the heart rate. Count the beats in 6 sec intervals and multiply the number of beats by 10 by putting zero at the end of the total, then announce the beats per min to your team members. You can also assess the heart rate using the handheld Doppler ultrasound monitor used for FHR assessment (Weiner & Zaichkin, 2021). A pulse oximeter can accurately calculate the heart rate of a healthy baby but may not function if the infant is not perfusing normally (Weiner & Zaichkin, 2021). In the hospital, electrocardiography (ECG) is the most accurate method for evaluating the baby's heart rate. Checking a pulse by feeling for cord pulsations is no longer recommended because it is less accurate (Weiner & Zaichkin, 2021).

If there are adequate respirations, the infant's heart rate should remain above 100 bpm (Weiner & Zaichkin, 2021). If the baby is crying or breathing adequately and the heart rate is over 100 bpm, keep the baby skin to skin with the mother and observe closely for signs of decompensation. If the heart rate remains less than 100 bpm, initiate PPV even if the baby is breathing (Weiner & Zaichkin, 2021).

If the Infant Shows Central Cyanosis, Use Pulse Oximetry and Give Oxygen

Some healthy infants have central cyanosis (blue lips, tongue or torso) for a few minutes after birth (Weiner & Zaichkin, 2021), and acrocyanosis (blue hands and feet) can persist up to 48 hr (Eichenwald, 2022). If the baby is breathing and has a heart rate over 100 but has persistent central cyanosis, place a pulse oximeter on the right hand or wrist to measure the oxygen saturation. A pulse oximeter estimates the percentage of hemoglobin that is carrying oxygen. When oxygenated blood leaves the heart through the aorta, it nourishes the heart muscle via the coronary arteries first, then the brain, and then the rest of the body (Weiner & Zaichkin, 2021). In most neonates,

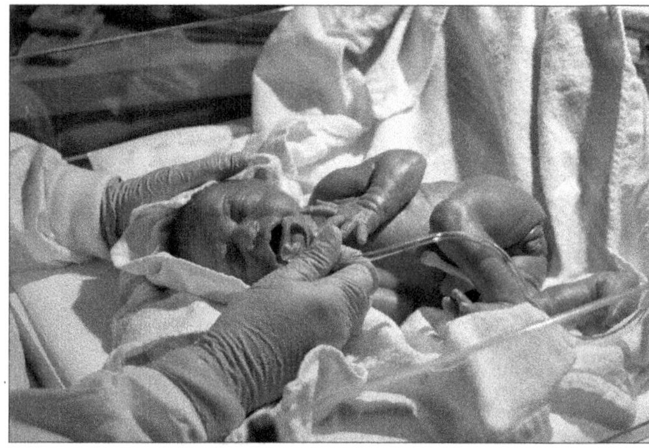

Figure 13-22. A nurse uses oxygen tubing to provide blow-by oxygen to a preterm infant shortly after birth. This baby was born in a hospital and is under a radiant warmer.

the artery supplying blood to the right arm branches from the aorta before the ductus arteriosus (preductal) and carries the most oxygen-rich blood in the body. Therefore, a pulse oximeter on the right hand or wrist usually reflects the oxygen saturation of the blood that is perfusing the baby's heart and brain. The left arm and both legs may have a lower oxygen saturation.

Because visual assessment of cyanosis is unreliable, NRP guidelines specify that oxygen should be given if the infant's preductal oxygen saturation is less than the targeted range for the infant's age in minutes (Weiner & Zaichkin, 2021). A chart of target preductal oxygen saturation measurements for the first 10 min of life is found below in Table 13-5. If, for example, a baby displays central cyanosis at 6 min of age and a pulse oximeter applied to the right wrist shows an insufficient oxygen saturation of 70%, oxygen should be given. At 10 min of age, if the baby's oxygen saturation reflects the normal value of 85–95%, oxygen should be gradually discontinued until the baby maintains this percentage on room air. A healthy baby breathing room air sometimes takes more than 10 min to reach oxygen saturation of 90% or greater (Weiner & Zaichkin, 2021).

In a hospital, the percentage of oxygen is usually regulated with the use of a blender. If an oxygen blender is not available, turn on the oxygen source and attach oxygen tubing or a mask. If the baby is breathing spontaneously, hold the oxygen tubing or mask close to the nose and mouth. As the baby improves, you can decrease the amount of oxygen reaching the baby by moving the oxygen farther away until the baby is able to maintain normal oxygen saturation on room air (Weiner & Zaichkin, 2021). Do not administer free-flow oxygen through the mask of a self-inflating bag; the flow is likely to be inadequate.

If a breathing baby with a pulse greater than 100 has difficulty maintaining normal saturation on 100% oxygen or the breathing remains labored, CPAP may be indicated (Weiner & Zaichkin, 2021). CPAP is provided by a flow-inflating bag

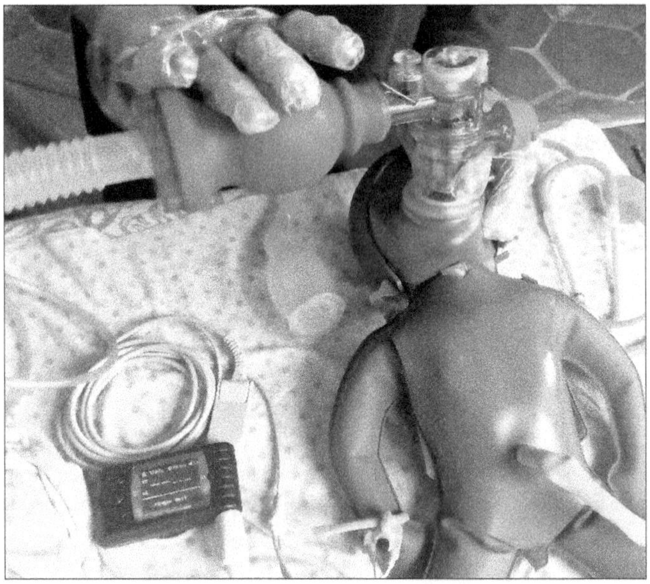

Figure 13-23. Correct technique for positive-pressure ventilation (PPV) involves encircling the mask with thumb and index finger and placing the remaining three fingers under the bony angle of the jaw to lift the jaw gently up toward the mask. Note the pulse oximeter on the baby's right wrist. Photograph by Andrea Dixon.

or T-piece resuscitator, equipment not always carried by community midwives. A self-inflating bag will not work.

If Adequate Breathing Is Absent, Start PPV

Ventilation of the lungs is the single most crucial and effective intervention in resuscitation of a newborn (Weiner & Zaichkin, 2021). Effective ventilation can be achieved with a flow-inflating bag, a self-inflating bag, or with a T-piece. The self-inflating bag reinflates when released and does not require a compressed gas source. It is commonly used in community practices and in resource-limited areas. Without a reservoir, it only delivers up to 40% oxygen, but with a reservoir, it can deliver up to 100% oxygen. The flow-inflating bag, or anesthesia bag, is filled by compressed gas from a tank or other source. This bag might be an option at a birth center but is unlikely to be used for home births due to the need for compressed air. This bag requires a tight face-mask seal, but it gives a better feel for lung compliance. A pressure manometer must be used to reduce risk of overinflating the lungs. A T-piece ventilator works similarly to the flow-inflating bag but has an adjustable flow-control valve that optimizes inflation pressure and inspiratory time. It requires a compressed-gas source. Use

Ventilation of the lungs is the most important step in neonatal resuscitation and usually revives a compromised newborn.

Table 13-5
Target Preductal Oxygen Saturation after Birth

1 min	60–65%	3 min	70–75%	5 min	80–85%
2 min	65–70%	4 min	75–80%	10 min	85–95%

care when storing resuscitation equipment; ventilation bags degrade and become useless with age or exposure to excessive heat in parked vehicles.

When PPV is necessary, it should be started without delay within 1 min of birth. Initiate PPV if the baby is gasping or apneic or if the pulse is less than 100 bpm (Weiner & Zaichkin, 2021). In addition, a trial of PPV is an option if the baby is breathing, the heart rate is 100 bpm or higher, but the oxygen saturation remains persistently low despite free-flow O_2 or CPAP (Weiner & Zaichkin, 2021).

Infants 35 weeks of gestation or more should be resuscitated on room air (21% oxygen). Premature infants less than 35 weeks of gestation should be resuscitated with 21–30% oxygen using an oxygen blender if available (Weiner & Zaichkin, 2021). At least two providers are needed for PPV. In a hospital a radiant warmer is used to provide warmth during ventilation of the infant. In a community setting, the infant is ideally placed on a self-warming infant transport mattress to prevent hypothermia. Position yourself at the head of the baby. With light downward hand pressure, seal the mask evenly on the infant's face without air leakage. A correctly sized mask covers the tips of the chin, mouth, and nose without putting pressure on the eyes. Hold the mask so that your little, ring, and middle fingers extend over the mandible like the letter E, and the thumb and index fingers form a C-shape over the mask. Gently lift the jaw up toward the mask to maintain an airtight seal.

Compress the bag until the chest rises, taking care not to overinflate the lungs. The first breath requires more pressure than the breaths that follow, and some premature infants have more lung resistance than term infants. If the chest does not rise, check mask size and positioning for air leaks and equipment for proper functioning. Ventilate 40–60 times per min. You are likely to maintain the correct rate if you repeat to yourself "BREATHE . . . two . . . three . . . BREATHE . . . two . . . three . . . " as you ventilate, compressing the bag every time you say "BREATHE," then allowing the baby to exhale while you finish the count (Weiner & Zaichkin, 2021). Attach a pulse oximeter, if available, to the right hand/wrist to observe for rising oxygen saturation. If you must provide PPV for more than a few minutes or the stomach appears distended, insert an orogastric or nasogastric tube to vent the stomach.

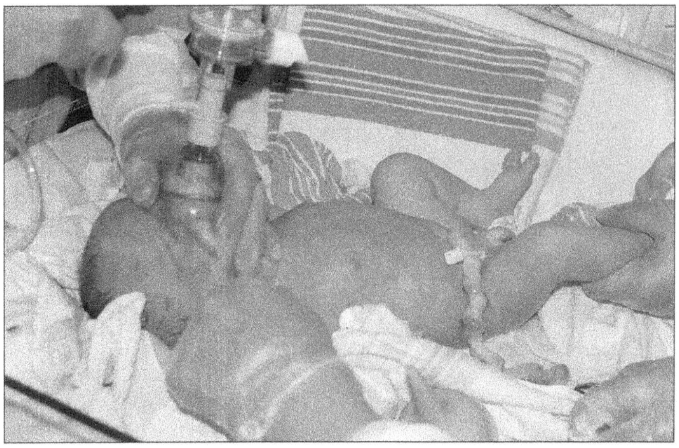

Figure 13-24. PPV will effectively resuscitate the vast majority of infants. This provider's technique is incorrect, however. The fingers should not cross the baby's neck or press into soft tissue.

Reevaluate

After 15 sec of PPV, evaluate the heart rate with a stethoscope. If PPV was started because the baby's heart rate was less than 100 bpm, the rate should begin to increase within 15 sec of effective ventilation.

- **If the heart rate is increasing**, continue PPV and check the baby's response again at 30 sec after initiating PPV.
- **If the heart rate does not increase**, check to be sure the baby's chest is moving with each respiration.
- **If the chest is moving**, continue to ventilate and assess the baby's heart rate again after another 15 sec of PPV.
- **If the chest is NOT moving,** start the ventilation corrective steps. NRP uses the mnemonic MR SOPA for the six corrective ventilation steps (Weiner & Zaichkin, 2021):

M: Mask adjustment
R: Reposition the head
S: Suction mouth and nose
O: Open the mouth
P: Pressure increase to maximum 40 cm H2O for term infants and 30 cm H2O in preterm infants.
A: Alternative airway—endotracheal (ET) tube or laryngeal mask (see "Consider Inserting an Alternative airway," below)

A carbon dioxide (CO_2) detector can be used during the ventilation corrective steps (MR SOPA) or to confirm ET tube placement. If ventilation is effective, the baby's lungs will release carbon dioxide. A CO_2 detector inserted between the mask and the PPV device should turn yellow when the baby exhales. A CO_2 detector may be inaccurate in infants with poor cardiac output, such as those in cardiac arrest.

Reevaluate After 30 Sec

After 30 sec of effective PPV (as indicated by a rising heart rate or chest movement), reassess the heart rate.

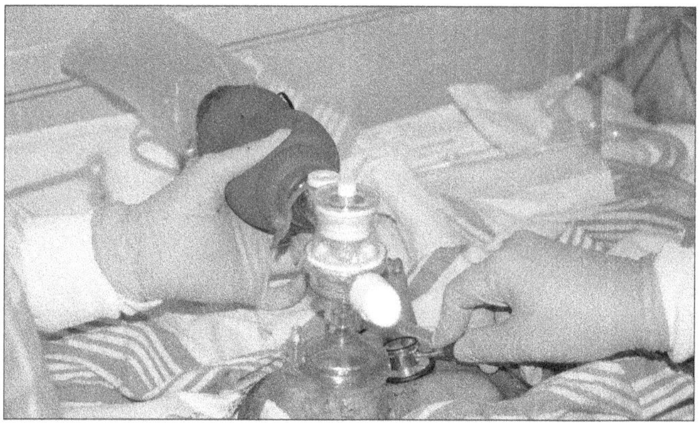

Figure 13-25. After 15 sec of PPV, reevaluate the heart rate with a stethoscope.

- **If the heart rate is at least 100 bpm**, continue ventilating at 40–60 breaths per min while watching the baby's heart rate, chest movement, and respiratory effort (Weiner & Zaichkin, 2021). When the heart rate remains consistently greater than 100 bpm, gradually decrease the rate and pressure of PPV while watching for the baby to maintain sustained effective respirations. Do not be too quick to discontinue PPV. After PPV is discontinued, monitor the newborn's oxygen saturation and respiratory effectiveness, effort, and rate. The baby working to breathe may benefit from free-flow oxygen or CPAP. Titrate oxygen delivery to meet the target saturation range indicated in Table 13-5 (Weiner & Zaichkin, 2021).
- **If the heart rate is greater than 60 bpm, but less than 100 bpm *and increasing*** continue to support respirations with PPV (40–60 breaths per min).
- **If the heart rate is at least 60 bpm, but less than 100 bpm and *not increasing* after 30 sec of PPV that moves the chest,** reassess your ventilation technique and rate and revisit the steps in MR SOPA (Weiner & Zaichkin, 2021). Assess for breath sounds on both sides of the chest. In the hospital, cardiac monitoring would be initiated.

Consider Inserting an Alternative airway

Consider inserting an alternative airway if the first five steps of MR SOPA are unsuccessful in achieving ventilation of the lungs, if the heart rate does not improve with PPV, or if PPV is used for more than a few minutes. ET intubation and the LMA are equally effective at securing the airway of the newborn, and both are vastly superior to PPV via face mask (Trevisanuto et al., 2015). Although ET is a difficult procedure that carries a high risk of adverse outcomes if performed improperly (Byrne, Patel, Johnson, & Wetzel, 2017; Sawyer et al., 2017), a trained provider can safely and easily place an LMA in a single attempt within 19–35 sec (Byrne et al., 2017; Wanous, Wey, Rudser, & Roberts, 2017). Any midwife who intends to perform neonatal

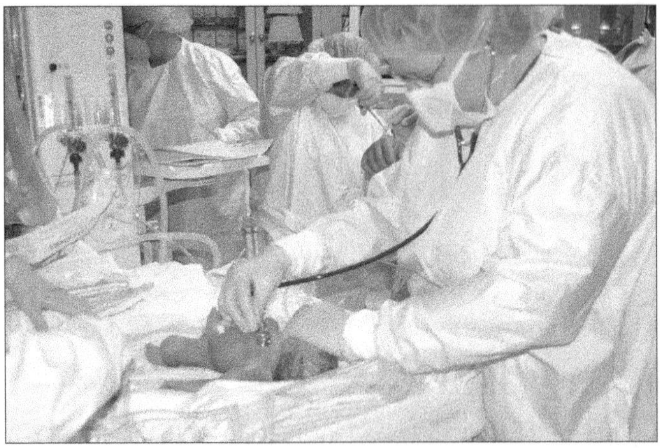

Figure 13-26. A nurse reassesses the heart rate of a newborn while giving supplemental oxygen. This baby was gasping and had poor tone shortly after cesarean birth. After 30 sec of PPV, the baby began to cry and draw up his knees. Supplemental oxygen was continued for several minutes, after which the baby was able to maintain adequate respirations without assistance.

resuscitation should complete a comprehensive training program that provides instruction in the placement of alternative airways. This text provides an overview, not a substitute for actual training.

Laryngeal Mask Airway (LMA)

Ease of use and effectiveness make the LMA an excellent choice for securing the airway of a baby born in a community setting. Manufacturers have produced many variations of the device, but the basic design is an airway tube attached to a small, supple mask with a (generally inflatable) cuff. The mask is inserted into the infant's mouth and advanced into the throat until it makes a seal over the entrance to the trachea, a.k.a. glottis (Weiner & Zaichkin, 2021). When the cuff is inflated, the PPV device is attached to the airway tube and air is directed into the newborn's trachea. The laryngeal mask is especially useful for newborns with anomalies involving the mouth, lip, tongue, palate, or neck that make it difficult to ventilate with a face mask or achieve intubation.

Weiner & Zaichkin (2021) note that the LMA device is designed for use in infants weighing 4 lb 7 oz–11 lb (2,000–5,000 g). Some LMA devices have inflatable masks, soft gel masks, or ports that admit an orogastric tube to decompress the stomach. Because laryngeal masks differ, become familiar with the manufacturer's instructions for the device you are likely to use.

To place an LMA, wear gloves and use clean technique.

1. Remove the LMA from the package and examine it to make sure it is undamaged. Attach a syringe to the inflation port and completely deflate the cuff surrounding the mask. You may lubricate the back of the LMA with a water-soluble lubricant.

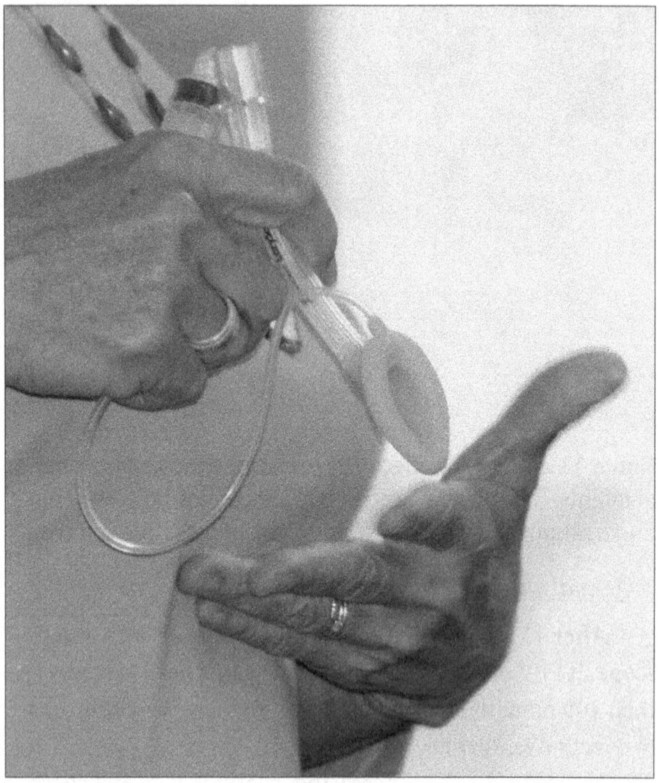

Figure 13-27. For providers who do not often perform neonatal resuscitation, the LMA is faster, easier, and safer to use than an ET tube.

2. Move the baby's head into the "sniffing" position and stand at the head. Hold the LMA as you would hold a pencil. The mask opening should face toward the baby's tongue and chin. The flat bottom of the mask, which has no opening, faces the baby's palate.
3. Carefully open the newborn's mouth and insert the tip of the mask with the opening against the baby's tongue and the closed bottom against the baby's palate. Advance the LMA inward (Weiner & Zaichkin, 2021). The device should easily move into position and seat itself in the desired location. When you feel resistance, stop.
4. Inflate the LMA if your device requires it. Inject just enough air into the inflation port to seal the airway. The pilot balloon should be softly inflated but easily compressible. The optimal volume of air differs from mask to mask, but it is usually 2–4 ml.
5. Place a CO_2 detector on the airway tube and attach a PPV device. Secure in place.
6. Check placement. If the lungs are ventilated and the baby is exchanging gases, the CO_2 detector will turn yellow within 8–10 breaths. The newborn's heart rate will rise, the chest wall will move, and you will hear equal breath sounds with a stethoscope. Leakage of air through the

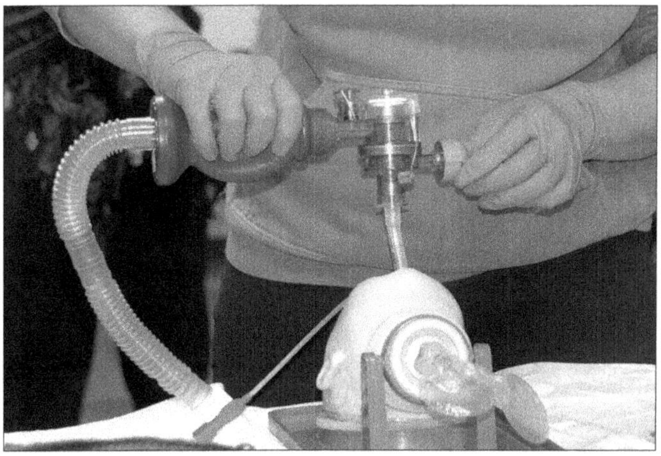

Figure 13-28. A midwife practices ventilating the lungs of a neonatal mannequin through an LMA. Photograph taken during a Birth Emergency Skills Training workshop.

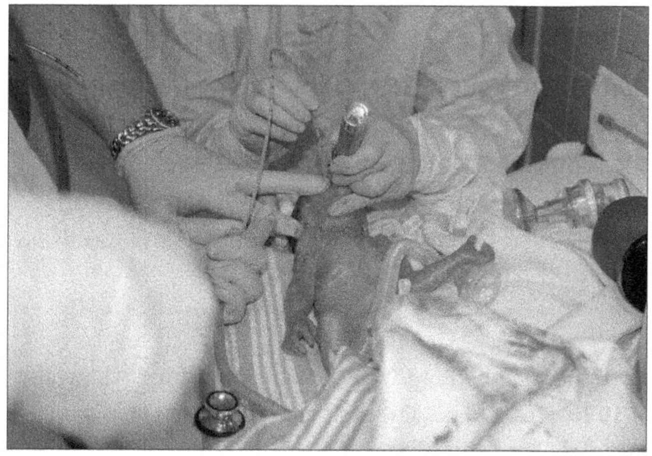

Figure 13-29. Intubation of a preterm infant born via cesarean section is skillfully performed by the neonatal team of an urban hospital.

infant's mouth can indicate incorrect placement (Weiner & Zaichkin, 2021).

7. If necessary, lubricate a size 5F or 6F gastric tube and introduce it through the gastric drain port. Attach a syringe and draw gently to aspirate air and stomach contents.
8. The baby can breathe and cry with the device in place. If the baby begins to breathe effectively and has a heart rate over 100 bpm, the device may be removed. If you need to remove the LMA, suction secretions first, then deflate the mask if indicated.

Endotracheal (ET) Intubation

ET intubation is a complex task that creates the risk of significant injury to the infant when performed by a provider unskilled in the technique. ET is advised if the infant's heart rate remains less than 100 bpm and is not increasing after PPV with an LMA or face mask (Weiner & Zaichkin, 2021). The NRP guidelines strongly recommend intubation of the trachea before starting chest compressions (Weiner & Zaichkin, 2021).

1. Use birthweight and gestational age to determine the proper size laryngoscope blade. Use a straight Miller laryngoscope blade, size 1 for a term infant, size 0 for a preterm infant. Size 00 is sometimes used for an early preterm infant.
2. Use birthweight and gestational age to determine the proper sized ET tube. A baby greater than 34 weeks of gestation and greater than 4 lb 6.5 oz (2,000 g) will need a 3.5-mm internal diameter (ID) ET tube. A preterm infant 28–34 weeks and 2 lb 3 oz–4 lb 6.5 oz (1,000–2,000 g) needs a 3.0-mm ID ET tube. A small preterm infant less than 28 weeks and below 2 lb 3 oz (1,000 g) needs a 2.5-mm ID ET tube.
3. Place the baby supine with the body lying straight and the neck slightly extended in the sniffing position.
4. Hold the laryngoscope in your left hand between the thumb and the first two or three fingers so the blade hangs down like an *L* shape. Insert the blade in the midline and slide it over the tongue and oropharynx until the tip reaches the space between the tongue and the epiglottis (vallecula).
5. Lift the laryngoscope to allow visualization of the vocal cords without levering off the upper gums. As you look into the laryngoscope, the epiglottis should appear as a triangular structure at the top of your view. The vocal cords should look like pale curtains flanking the dark tracheal opening. Visualization should be easier if an assistant provides gentle pressure on the cricoid cartilage with thumb and forefinger. If you see only the esophagus, your blade is too deep. Pull back slightly and the epiglottis should drop into view.
6. When you see the vocal cords, hold the ET tube with your right hand and introduce the tube through the right side of the baby's mouth. Wait for the vocal cords to open and slip the ET tube between them, advancing until the vocal cords are situated between the marked guide lines on the tube. Hold the tube firmly against the newborn's hard palate while you remove the laryngoscope, taking care not to dislodge the tube.
7. Secure the tube.
8. Attach your PPV equipment and ventilate the baby.
9. Limit each intubation attempt to no more than 30 sec (Weiner & Zaichkin, 2021).

A rapid increase in heart rate, chest rise, and detection of exhaled carbon dioxide confirms successful placement of the ET tube. A neonatal stethoscope placed in each axilla accurately verifies equal breath sounds. There should be minimal air leak

A and B before C

Do NOT start chest compressions until the lungs have been ventilated. If the chest is not moving with PPV, the lungs have not been ventilated and chest compressions are not yet required. Chest compressions are reserved for cases where effective ventilation fails to raise the baby's heart rate.

from the mouth. The CO_2 detector should turn yellow after 8–10 breaths unless CO_2 levels are too low to detect because the infant has low cardiac output or abnormal lung function. If you are sure the tube is correctly placed, secure it with tape or a commercial stabilization device.

If the heart rate is still below 60 bpm, reevaluate the effectiveness of CPR and make sure the ET tube is still in the trachea. If the endotracheal tube is in the esophagus, the CO2 detector will not change color, and you may hear gurgling if you auscultate over the baby's stomach as air is forced into it. Unrecognized accidental placement of an ET tube in the esophagus can kill the baby. "When in doubt, pull it out."

The Longest Minute . . .

Continue compressions and ventilation for a full 60 sec before reassessing the newborn's heart rate. It may be the longest minute of your life.

Provide Chest Compressions

Provide chest compressions if the infant's heart rate remains less than 60 bpm despite at least 30 sec of PPV with chest movements. Newborns who do not respond to ventilation are usually hypoxemic, acidotic, and have insufficient blood flow through their coronary arteries (Weiner & Zaichkin, 2021). Heart function becomes depressed, and the heart is unable to beat effectively until coronary blood flow is restored. Providing rhythmic chest compressions while ventilating the lungs circulates and oxygenates the blood and restores perfusion to the heart muscle. Once the heart beats normally again, it can resume perfusing vital organs including the brain. When the brain is well oxygenated, spontaneous respirations should resume.

Before starting chest compressions, consider inserting an alternative airway if not already in place, ensure the lungs are being effectively ventilated, and increase oxygen to 100%. Stand at the infant's head to give chest compressions. Imagine a line drawn between the baby's nipples and place your thumbs just below it on the center of the baby's sternum, avoiding the ribs and the xyphoid process. Encircle the torso with your hands with your fingertips under the baby's back. Compressions should be on the lower third of the sternum, approximately one third the depth of the chest. Always keep your thumbs in contact with the sternum throughout the cycles of compression and release but allow the chest to expand under your hands during the release phase.

If the heart rate is below 60 bpm or if the extremities are cool, the pulse oximeter may fail to read.

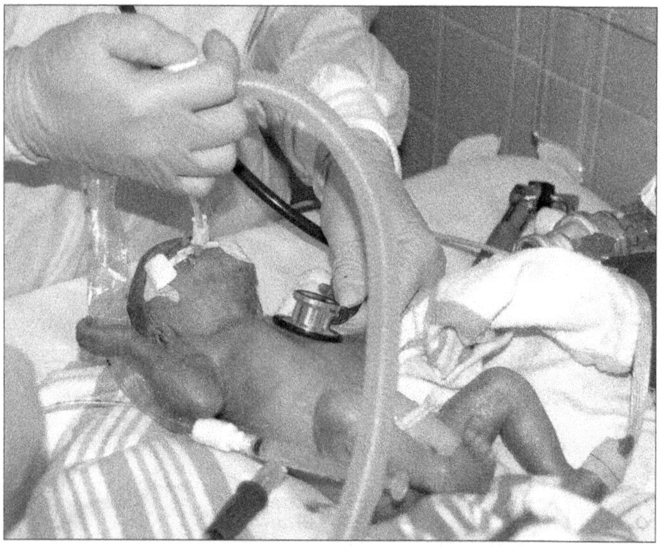

Figure 13-30. After 60 sec of compressions with ventilation, recheck the infant's heart rate. If it is greater than 60 bpm, discontinue compressions and resume ventilation at 40–60 breaths per min.

The ventilation should be administered after every third compression, yielding a total of 30 breaths and 90 compressions every minute. Whoever gives compressions should repeat the words "One-and-Two-and-Three-and-BREATHE-and-One-and. . . ." The baby is ventilated during the "breathe-and" beat of the rhythm, and exhalation occurs during the next downward stroke (Weiner & Zaichkin, 2021).

When providing CPR to an adult, it is easier for the rescuer to maintain the correct compression rate if keeping the beat of the Bee Gees' hit song "Stayin' Alive" (105 bpm; Gibb, Gibb, & Gibb, 1977). Realizing that a different mental metronome was required to keep pace with the faster neonatal rate, Roehr et al. (2014) found that compressing to the beat of "SOS" by ABBA (Ulvaeus, Andersson, & Andersson, 1975) significantly improved the ability of providers to deliver a rate of 120 bpm during mannequin drills. Further research is needed to determine whether "SOS" would provide a useful internal metronome for providers resuscitating infants.

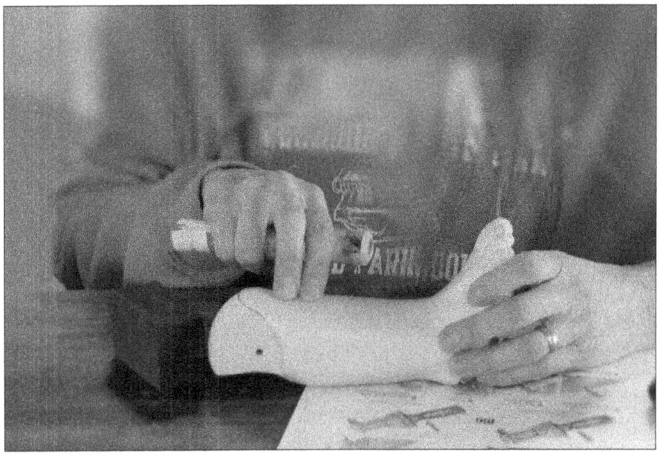

Figure 13-31. A midwife locates landmarks for IO needle placement on a model of a neonatal lower limb. The optimal site is approximately 2 cm below and 1–2 cm medial to the tibial tuberosity. Photograph by Cathy Saunders.

Continue the rhythm of compression and ventilation for a full 60 sec, then stop to check the heart rate (Weiner & Zaichkin, 2021). NRP recommends using an electronic cardiac monitor (ECG) to assess the newborn's heart rate while compressions continue. If you are transporting via advanced-life-support ambulance, the paramedic or equivalent will use an ECG monitor. At a home birth, a stethoscope provides the most accurate assessment. A pulse oximeter cannot give a reliable reading if the baby is in cardiac arrest.

- **If the heart rate is 60 bpm or above,** stop chest compressions and resume PPV at 40–60 breaths per min: "BREATHE-two-three, BREATHE-two-three."
- **If the heart rate remains below 60 bpm**, resume compressions with ventilation and confirm that CPR is effective. If both ventilations and compressions are adequate and the heart rate is not rising, epinephrine is required.

Establish Vascular Access

Consider obtaining IV access if the baby's heart rate remains less than 60 bpm *and* you have already provided at least 30 sec of effective PPV *and* you have given an additional 60 sec of chest compressions with PPV using 100% oxygen. The next step in the NRP resuscitation algorithm calls for giving epinephrine. Although epinephrine can be given directly into an ET tube, vascular access facilitates the administration of multiple doses without interrupting ventilation. Vascular access is also necessary if volume replacement is required for a hypovolemic infant.

Umbilical Vein Cannulation

NRP guidelines recommend the umbilical IV catheter as the first-line method for obtaining intravascular access on a newborn, and it is the preferred method in a hospital. The midwife can acquire training for this procedure through the NRP or S.T.A.B.L.E.® certification courses. A description of this potentially difficult procedure is beyond the scope of this text.

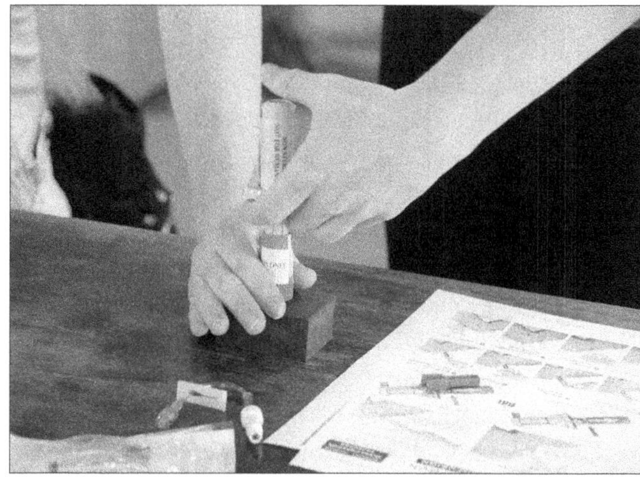

Figure 13-32. A spring-loaded IO insertion device is quick and easy for trained providers to use.

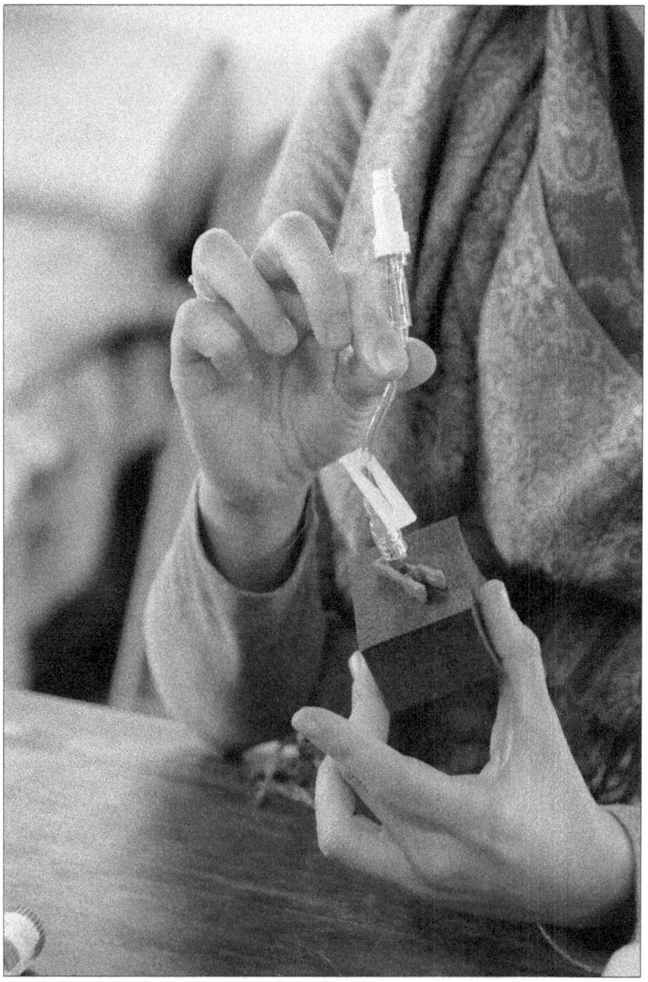

Figure 13-33. During a training session, a midwife inserts an IO needle into a foam block, secures it with a clip, and attaches infusion tubing in well under 1 min.

Intraosseous (IO) Access

IO access allows for the infusion of fluids and medications and/or blood products into the bone marrow. The marrow cavity (intramedullary space) within larger bones is highly vascular and noncollapsible, and it has a direct connection to the venous system (Schwindt et al., 2022). An IO needle is inserted through the skin and into the flat part of a large bone, penetrating the bone marrow cavity (Weiner & Zaichkin, 2021). Fluids and medications administered via IO reach the central circulation almost as fast as when infused through a central line (DeBoer, Russell, Seaver, & Vardi, 2008). The provider can use the IO needle to administer any medications or fluids that would be infused into an umbilical venous catheter.

Compared to the umbilical IV catheter, the IO needle is much simpler, quicker, and safer for providers who do not often perform newborn resuscitation (Abe, Blum, & Yamamoto, 2000; Byrne et al., 2017; Rajani, Chitkara, Oehlert, & Halamek, 2011; Scrivens et al., 2019). The overall complication rate is only about 1% (Byrne et al., 2017). Complications usually involve preterm infants and include osteomyelitis, skin infection, skin necrosis, subcutaneous abscess, fat embolism, and fractures (Ellemunter, Simma, Trawöger, & Maurer, 1999), as well as compartment syndrome, which if severe can require amputation of the leg (Suominen, Nurmi, & Lauerma, 2015). In one study of simulated resuscitation, procedure time was shortened by 106 sec when participants used a laryngeal mask and IO needle instead of an ET tube and umbilical catheter, enough to influence the outcome of resuscitation (Byrne et al., 2017).

Manufacturers market a variety of IO devices that can be inserted manually or using a battery-operated drill. Learn to perform the procedure safely, skillfully, and quickly through hands-on instruction, and read the package insert on the model you will be using before you need to resuscitate a baby. As in any procedure, every provider must conform to local standards of practice and legal protocols.

To insert an IO device:

1. Find the insertion site on the surface of the lower leg, approximately 2 cm below and 1–2 cm medial to the tibial tuberosity (Weiner & Zaichkin, 2021).
2. Prepare the insertion site with antibacterial solution.
3. Position the IO needle perpendicular to the skin and advance the device through the skin to the periosteum, then pop through the bone cortex into the marrow space. Single-use spring-loaded devices make placement easier. If placing the needle by hand, use strong downward pressure with a twisting motion. If your model requires the use of a bone drill to gain access, hold downward pressure while depressing the trigger. You will feel a change in resistance when you gain access to the marrow.
4. Remove the stylet according to manufacturer's instructions.
5. Secure the needle. Stabilization is crucial. Slight movements of the IO needle can dislodge it or enlarge the point of insertion (DeBoer et al., 2008).
6. Connect a prefilled infusion set to the hub of the needle, open the stopcock, flush the needle with 3–5 ml of NS to open the bone marrow space, and infuse the medication or fluid.
7. After each administration of fluid or medication, palpate the soft tissue surrounding the device for swelling and extravasation that would indicate that the device is no longer in place (DeBoer et al., 2008). Because fluid in the extravascular space accumulates at the lowest point, palpate the posterior surface of the leg for edema (DeBoer et al., 2008). Compartment syndrome can occur when fluids are trapped within the layers of nonexpandable fascia surrounding each group of muscles and the surrounding nerves and blood vessels.

Administer Epinephrine

Epinephrine is a cardiac and vascular stimulant that constricts the peripheral vessels and increases blood flow to the coronary arteries (Weiner & Zaichkin, 2021). Administer epinephrine if the infant's heart rate remains less than 60 bpm *and* you have already provided at least 30 sec of effective PPV *and* you have given an additional 60 sec of chest compressions with PPV using 100% oxygen. By this stage of resuscitation, an advanced airway and IV access should already be in place.

- Use a 1:10,000 concentration of epinephrine (0.1 mg/ml). Rapidly give 0.02 mg/kg (0.2 ml/kg) of epinephrine via the IV or IO route. Follow with a 3-ml flush of NS. You can repeat the dose every 3–5 min.
- If there is no intravascular access, one dose of epinephrine may be administered into the ET tube. The recommended dose for ET administration is higher than the intravascular/intraosseous route: give 0.1 mg/kg (1 ml/kg) then follow with several positive-pressure breaths.
- Continue compressions and ventilation with 100% oxygen for 1 full minute. The heart rate should improve to 60 bpm or higher. If the heart rate remains less than 60 bpm, continue compressions and ventilation. Consider other issues such as pneumothorax or hypovolemia.

Consider Intravascular Volume Expanders

Consider administering IV fluids to expand blood volume if the baby has not responded to the steps of resuscitation and there is a risk factor for acute hypovolemia such as suspected abruption, umbilical cord prolapse, or tight nuchal cord. To give a volume expander, draw 10 ml/kg NS into a 30–60-ml syringe and infuse via the IV or IO vascular access.

Discontinuing Resuscitative Efforts

Most newborns with no detectable heart rate after 20 min of resuscitation do not survive. There are, however, rare case reports of infants who had no heart rate for longer and recovered without severe disabilities (Weiner & Zaichkin, 2021). NRP guidelines deem it reasonable to consider discontinuing resuscitative efforts after 20 min if there is a persistent absence of heart rate through all applicable steps of resuscitation (Weiner & Zaichkin, 2021). Take into account how long the heart rate has been absent, whether all necessary interventions have been executed, gestational age, the presence of significant congenital anomalies, the preferences of the family, the views of team members, and the accessibility of postresuscitative resources such as neonatal intensive care and therapeutic hypothermia (Weiner & Zaichkin, 2021). Before discontinuing resuscitation, consult the receiving pediatrician or your collaborating physician or ask the EMS responders to contact their medical control for guidance.

Table 13-6
Newborn Conditions Requiring Prompt Consultation

- Malformations affecting function
  Examples: Cleft palate, imperforate anus, diaphragmatic hernia
- Musculoskeletal concerns
  Examples: Clavicle or arm fracture, limb malformation
- Features suggesting syndrome (one or more minor abnormalities or one major abnormality)
  Examples: Webbed digits, ear abnormalities, abnormal red reflex, unusual facial features
- Cardiac Conditions
  Examples: Central cyanosis, murmurs, abnormal cardiac sounds, abnormal critical congenital heart defect (CCHD) test
- Respiratory conditions
  Examples: Slow or rapid respirations, retractions, abnormal lung sounds, abnormal pulse oximetry reading
- Nerve injuries
  Examples: Brachial plexus palsy, facial palsy
- Head injuries
  Examples: Cephalohematoma, skull fracture, suspected subgaleal or intracranial hemorrhage
- Abdominal wall defects
  Examples: Gastroschisis, omphalocele
- Neural tube defects
  Examples: Meningocele, encephalocele, spinal abnormality
- Infection
  Examples: Sepsis, conjunctivitis, umbilical cord infection
- Neurologic abnormality
  Examples: Seizure, abnormal tone or posture
- Genitourinary defects
  Examples: Ambiguous genitalia, hypospadias

Timing of consultation is influenced by stability of infant and potential for issue to affect normal function such as breathing, circulation, feeding, elimination, temperature regulation, and metabolism. Adapted from "Neonatal Care," by P. J. Reis and T. Bell, in J. Phillippi and I. Kantrowitz-Gordon (Eds.), *Varney's Midwifery* (7th ed., Kindle versionm ch. 39), 2024, Burlington, MA: Jones & Bartlett Learning. Copyright by publisher.

Postresuscitation Care

The infant who has required resuscitation is at risk of further decompensation after vital signs have returned to normal. Compromised newborns tend to compensate for a time, then become gravely ill, at which point they become extremely difficult to resuscitate. Any newborn who has required PPV for more than 30–60 sec should be transported to a facility capable of managing an acutely ill neonate (Weiner & Zaichkin, 2021). Additionally, any infant with respiratory distress, tachypnea, persistent central cyanosis, hypoglycemia, hypothermia, fever, poor tone, difficulty feeding, or other signs of abnormal transition requires immediate transport via ambulance to an appropriate facility for evaluation.

Abnormal Neonatal Conditions

Most infants born at home and in freestanding birth centers are healthy. The initial evaluation performed by the midwife includes an assessment of respiratory rate; breathing effort; heart rate; color of lips, mouth and trunk; temperature; and a complete physical examination. A baby must also demonstrate the ability to feed, void, and stool normally to be considered healthy.

Some infants seem normal at birth but develop signs of abnormal transition. Others develop issues later in the weeks following birth. Whereas newborns in a hospital typically receive close observation for 24–48 hr after birth, the community midwife typically monitors mother and infant for only a few hours postpartum. The baby with abnormal vital signs, glucose metabolism, or temperature may compensate for hours, then suddenly deteriorate and require increasing levels of support to remain stable.

The community midwife is responsible for identifying any deviations from normal and determining appropriate follow-up. Danger signs include abnormal breathing (evidenced by grunting, nasal flaring, retractions, central cyanosis, persistently low oxygen saturation, or abnormal respiratory rate), abnormal tone, difficulty feeding (vomiting, inability to initiate or sustain sucking), lethargy, seizure activity, abnormal heart rate or heart sounds, or jaundice that is excessive or appears in the first 24 hr after birth. If the findings are questionable, call the baby's pediatrician, neonatologist, or other authority for advice. Always err on the side of caution. If you suspect the baby is experiencing a potentially serious complication, call EMS and arrange for safe transport to a hospital with a NICU capable of managing the baby's issues.

AHH! Mnemonic: Abnormal Breathing, Hypothermia, and Hypoglycemia

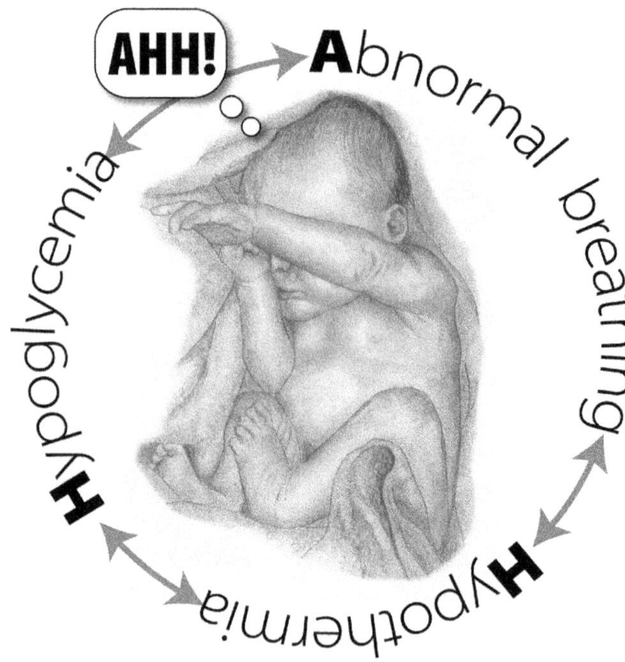

Figure 13-34. The mnemonic AHH! Abnormal breathing, Hypothermia, and Hypoglycemia are three common interrelated complications frequently encountered by midwives in community settings. The infant with abnormal breathing, hypothermia, or hypoglycemia can present with nonspecific signs including irritability, tremors, tachypnea, grunting, seizures, lethargy, floppiness, cyanosis, apnea, poor suck or refusal to feed, and temperature instability. A baby who develops any of these conditions is at risk of developing the others.

Abnormal breathing, **H**ypoglycemia, and **H**ypothermia are interrelated conditions in the neonate. Any of these three conditions can be a cause or result of any of the others. Hypoglycemia can disturb central nervous system function, resulting in tachypnea, apnea, or respiratory distress, and affect metabolic processes, resulting in hypothermia. Hypothermia can increase oxygen consumption, respiratory rate, pulmonary vasoconstriction, and respiratory distress. The newborn with abnormal breathing or cold stress uses glucose at an accelerated rate and can become hypoglycemic. Because glucose is the primary energy source for the brain, hypoglycemia can cause lethargy, coma, or failure of the respiratory drive. Because insufficient oxygen reduces the baby's ability to burn brown fat for heat production, infants that require resuscitation are at risk for hypothermia. Signs and symptoms for these conditions often overlap; the newborn with any of these problems can present with nonspecific signs including respiratory distress; pale, mottled, or cyanotic skin; lethargy; hypotonia; and inability to feed effectively.

Abnormal Breathing

Respiratory distress, the most common cause of newborn admission to a NICU, can develop unexpectedly, even in the infant that appeared to be healthy and vigorous at birth. Infants with uncorrected breathing abnormalities can deteriorate rapidly into respiratory failure (Karlsen, 2019). Fairly common causes of abnormal breathing include (Hermansen & Mahajan, 2015) transient tachypnea of the newborn (TTN), respiratory distress syndrome, pneumonia, sepsis, pneumothorax, and persistent pulmonary hypertension. Less common causes include congenital heart defects, airway malformations, and inborn errors of metabolism (IEM).

Listen to the heart and lungs and count the respiratory and heart rates. The normal respiratory rate for a newborn is 30–60 breaths per min (Fraser, 2019). Infants normally have irregular breaths, ranging from shallow and fast to deep and slow, interspersed with short pauses. There should be clear, equal breath sounds, and the lips, tongue, and gums should be pink. The mucous membranes of the mouth readily show cyanosis in any infant and can be used to assess those with darkly pigmented skin.

A baby that is having trouble breathing often presents with distinctive physical signs. Retractions are an abnormal inward movement of the chest wall as the infant inhales. Retractions can be intercostal (depressions between the ribs during inspiration), subcostal (depressions below the rib cage), suprasternal (depression above the sternum at the base of the throat) or substernal (depression below the sternum at the solar plexus).

Nasal flaring is the baby's attempt to draw in more air by increasing the size of the airway. Grunting respirations indicate that the baby is trying to compensate for collapsed alveoli by partially closing the vocal cords to trap air in the small airways. Grunting is more likely to indicate a serious issue if it is associated with nasal flaring, cyanosis, or retractions, or if it appears for the first time several hours after birth (Karlsen, 2019). Other possible findings associated with abnormal breathing include:

- Tachypnea (respiratory rate more than 60 breaths per min)
- Bradypnea (respiratory rate less than 30 breaths per min) or apnea
- Difficulty maintaining normal O_2 saturation, cyanosis
- Tachycardia, bradycardia
- Decreased activity, lethargy, hypotonia, difficulty waking
- Poor suck or refusal to feed
- Hypoglycemia /transient hyperglycemia
- Temperature instability

Abnormal breathing can quickly deteriorate to apnea. Any baby with the signs listed above requires prompt transport by ambulance to a facility with a level III NICU. Contact the neonatologist *en route* and give an SBAR report. Gasping respirations are ineffective and indicate impending cardiopulmonary arrest. Manage the gasping baby by immediately supporting respirations with PPV. If the heart rate is low and not rising, consider an LMA or ET (Karlsen, 2019).

If the baby shows signs of respiratory distress, attach a pulse oximeter to the right hand or wrist. NRP program specifies that the baby's oxygen saturation should be 85–95% after 10 min of life. The S.T.A.B.L.E program advises that after 24 hr of age, this percentage should rise to 95–99% (Karlsen, 2019). If a baby's oxygen saturation is persistently less than 90–95% when the baby is 1–24 hr old and there are no other signs of respiratory distress, contact the pediatrician and ask for advice. Take a glucose reading and assess temperature. Try to put a clinical picture together so you can report your findings accurately to the pediatrician.

A newborn in respiratory distress is usually uninterested in breastfeeding because energy resources are directed into doing the work of breathing. Do not try to feed a baby who is having difficulty breathing. Infants with labored respirations have uncoordinated sucking, swallowing, and breathing reflexes, and there is a risk that the baby will aspirate stomach contents into the lungs (Karlsen, 2019).

Meconium Aspiration Syndrome (MAS)

MAS occurs when the fetus passes meconium into the amniotic fluid, breathes it in, and develops lung disease that results in hypoxia and acidosis after birth. In the United

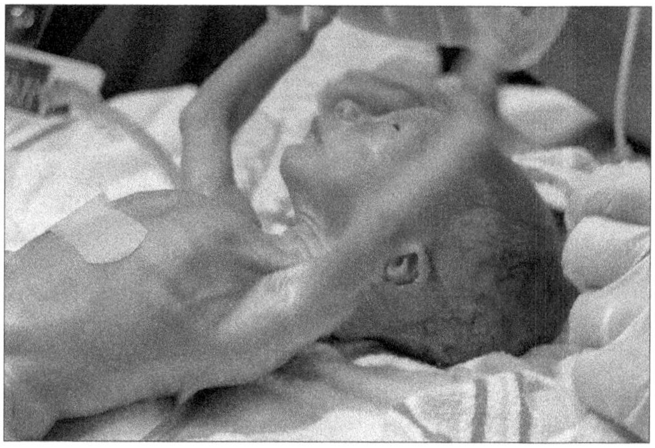

Figure 13-35. Retractions. This term newborn had developed undetected asymmetric FGR *in utero*. Shortly after birth, he had labored breathing with intercostal, substernal, and suprasternal retractions. He required admission to the NICU and several weeks of stabilization before he was ready to discharge home.

States, MAS occurs in 0.1–0.4% of live births, affecting about 2–10% of infants born through meconium-stained amniotic fluid (Garcia-Prats, 2023). The severity of MAS ranges from mild respiratory distress to respiratory failure (Garcia-Prats, 2023).

Meconium begins to form in the fetal intestines during the first trimester and is made from the residue of desquamated cells from the intestine and skin, gastrointestinal mucin, swallowed globs of fetal hair and vernix caseosa, amniotic fluid, and intestinal secretions (Garcia-Prats, 2023). Before 16 weeks of gestation, the fetus passes meconium freely into the amniotic fluid. Around 20 weeks of gestation, the anal sphincter becomes functional, and meconium generally remains within the intestines until the fetus is mature. Because passage of meconium *in utero* often represents fetal maturity, postdates pregnancy is a risk factor for MAS (Hermansen & Mahajan, 2015; Ward & Caughey, 2022).

Hypoxia can cause fetal gasping that allows aspiration of meconium *in utero* (Garcia-Prats, 2023). Depressed neonates are especially likely to draw meconium into the lungs with their first breath. Aspirated meconium can cause pulmonary disease through airway obstruction, chemical irritation, surfactant inactivation, or inflammation. Most cases of severe MAS are probably related to pathologic intrauterine processes such as chronic asphyxia and infection rather than the aspiration of meconium itself (Garcia-Prats, 2023).

Infants with MAS can show tachypnea, cyanosis, retractions, abdominal breathing, grunting, or nasal flaring. As the lungs overinflate, the anterior-posterior diameter of the chest may increase, giving the baby a barrel-chested appearance (Garcia-Prats, 2023). Fine and coarse crackles are often heard on auscultation of the lungs. Infants with MAS are more likely to suffer pneumothorax and persistent pulmonary hypertension.

Twenty to 33% of infants born through meconium-stained amniotic fluid are nonvigorous at birth, probably because meconium passage is associated with pathologic intrauterine processes, such as chronic hypoxia and infection, that place stress on the fetus (Garcia-Prats, 2023). Although it appears that thick, particulate meconium fluid produces worse neonatal outcomes than thin staining, the amount of support the baby will need at birth is unpredictable (Khatun, Parvin, & Naurin, 2019; Mohammad, Jamal, Sohaila, & Ali, 2018). Transfer the mother with meconium-stained fluid to a hospital with a NICU if this can be safely accomplished before birth. In current NRP guidelines, the initial steps of resuscitation for the baby born through meconium-stained fluid are the same as for any other baby. Suctioning is performed if there is an airway obstruction, but routine deep tracheal suctioning is no longer recommended (Weiner & Zaichkin, 2021). Be especially vigilant for other signs of fetal compromise and for newborn deterioration. The newborn with suspected MAS, like any newborn with respiratory distress, should be immediately transported to a hospital with a NICU.

Transient Tachypnea of the Newborn (TTN)

TTN occurs when delayed resorption and clearance of fetal alveolar fluid results in pulmonary edema (K. E. Johnson, 2021). Prematurity, cesarean birth, maternal diabetes, and maternal asthma are risk factors. The affected baby usually develops tachypnea within 2 hr of birth, sometimes with cyanosis, retractions, and grunting. With pediatrician-led hospital care, TTN usually resolves within 12–24 hr, or occasionally as long as 72 hr (K. E. Johnson, 2021). The presentation of TTN is very similar to that of other more severe conditions, such as pneumonia, sepsis, cardiac disease, and respiratory distress syndrome (K. E. Johnson, 2021).

Congenital Heart Defects

Congenital heart defects (CHD) are the most common congenital abnormality, occurring in about 1% of infants (Altman, 2022; Oster, 2023). Of these, approximately 25% have a critical congenital heart defect (CCHD), defined as one requiring surgery or catheter-based intervention in the first year of life (Oster, 2023). In the first hours or days after birth, up to 30% of infants with CCHD show no signs or symptoms (Oster, 2023). Other infants have abnormal murmurs or heart rhythms or develop shock, cyanosis, tachypnea, and/or pulmonary edema shortly after birth. Some critical defects are asymptomatic until the ductus arteriosus closes a few days after birth and the infant experiences catastrophic decline (Oster, 2023).

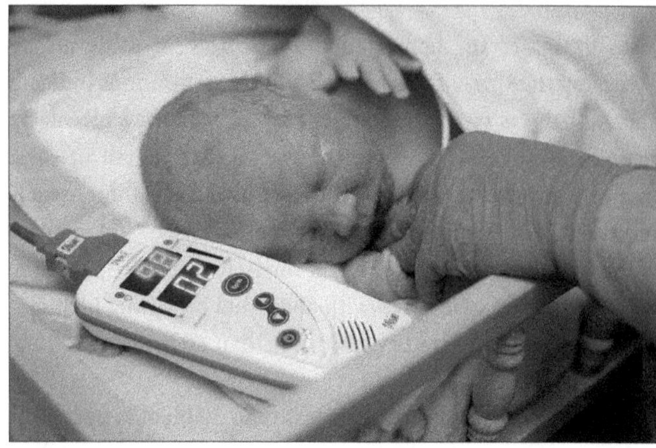

Figure 13-36. A birth-center nurse performs initial pulse-oximeter screening for CCHD on a newborn with facial bruising at 4 hr of age. This assessment should be repeated when the baby is 2 or 3 days old. A portable pulse oximeter can save lives in a community or low-resource setting.

Infants with CCHD undiagnosed in the early neonatal period can suffer mortality as high as 30% (Oster, 2023).

About 73% of CCHD are detected by antenatal ultrasound (Oster, 2023). In populations such as the Amish that frequently decline routine ultrasound examinations during pregnancy and routine pediatric care during childhood, these defects can remain undiagnosed until the child becomes critically ill (K. K. Miller et al., 2016). Delay in diagnosis increases the risk of morbidity and mortality for the child.

Worldwide, pulse oximetry is commonly used as a screening method for CCHD in newborns (Narayen, Blom, Bourgonje, et al., 2016). AAP recommends pulse oximetry screening between 24 and 48 hr of age (AAP, 2021). If CCHD screening is performed too early, a false positive is more likely. If it is performed too late, the defect may not be discovered until the child is compromised. Besides revealing heart defects, CCHD screening can also detect noncardiac complications such as sepsis and respiratory compromise, increasing early recognition and referral for treatment. Despite these benefits, one study found that in the state of Michigan, CCHD screenings were performed on fewer than half the babies born at home or in birth centers (Withrow, Fussman, Thompson, & Kleyn, 2019).

Infants born in community settings are usually under a midwife or nurse's direct care for 3–6 hr after birth, then remain with the parents until a provider reevaluates them 2–3 days later (K. Wu & Stapleton, 2017). Because CCHDs are often asymptomatic in the early neonatal period, there is a risk that a baby with an undiagnosed heart anomaly will be evaluated as normal at birth, then die suddenly a short time later. One approach is to screen the infant born in a community setting twice, once in the first hours of life and again on day 2 or 3 (Narayen, Blom, Bourgonje, et al., 2016; Narayen, Blom, Van

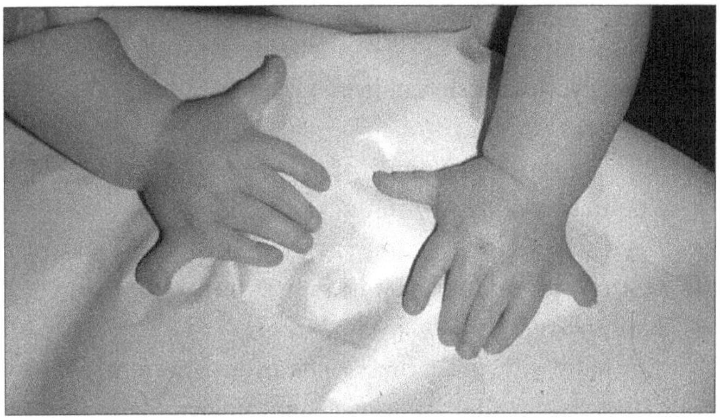

Figure 13-37. Bilateral polydactyly with short fingers in a child with Ellis-van Creveld (EvC) syndrome, a type of dwarfism common among the Old Order Amish of Pennsylvania. EvC is associated with high incidence of severe congenital heart defects Often, the child has pulmonary hypoplasia and does not have enough lung tissue to survive. People with this condition have six fingers on each hand and sometimes six toes on each foot, short limbs, and a normal torso that seems disproportionately long. From "Ellis-Van Creveld Syndrome," by G. Baujat and M. Le Merre, 2007, *Orphanet Journal of Rare Diseases*, 2, 27. CC BY 2.0.

Geloven, et al., 2018; Williams et al., 2021). The early screening improves identification of a serious heart defect before discharge but increases the risk of false positives. Some of these false positives indicate the presence of other abnormal conditions such as infection.

Every community midwife should carry a pulse oximeter that is adaptable for maternal or infant use. Hand-held pulse oximeters are portable, reliable, widely available, and largely affordable. Smartphone-compatible pulse oximeters are an effective, economical option for some low-resource settings (Huizing et al., 2017).

To screen for CCHD with a pulse oximeter, measure oxygen saturation in the newborn's right hand (preductal reading) and either foot (postductal). The device can malfunction if there is interference from other electrical or electronic devices, ambient light, poor probe attachment, poor perfusion, and/or hemoglobinopathy (Oster, 2023). Try warming the baby's extremity before placing the probe to improve blood flow to the site. False-positive rates are greater at high altitude (Oster, 2023).

A positive (failed) screen can include (Centers for Disease Control, 2023)

- Any oxygen-saturation measurement less than 90% in initial or repeat screen

OR

- Oxygen saturation less than 95% in the right hand and either foot on three measurements, separated by 1 hr

OR

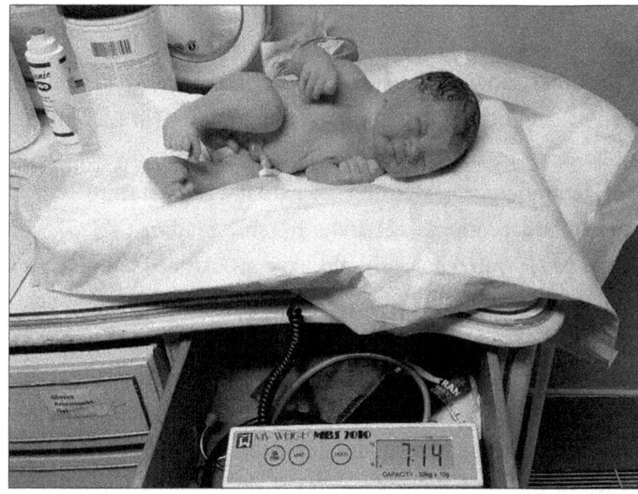

Figure 13-38. Exposed to the air. To prevent hypothermia, neonates should be protected from cold and drafts. Skin exposure to the air during weighing and physical assessment should be as brief as possible.

- An absolute difference in oxygen saturation more than 3% between the right hand and foot on three measurements at 1-hr intervals

A baby that fails CCHD screening requires immediate evaluation by a pediatrician, pediatric cardiologist, or neonatologist to determine the cause of hypoxemia and exclude life-threatening conditions. Most infants with a positive screen require an echocardiogram. Those with a CCHD identified on echocardiography require urgent consultation with a pediatric cardiologist and/or transfer to an appropriate facility (Oster, 2023).

Because pulse oximetry can fail to identify certain CCHDs, it can miss as many cases as it detects (Oster, 2023). Although an asymptomatic infant with a normal test is somewhat reassuring, in some circumstances a child with a CCHD can have a negative screen. Remain alert for signs of undiagnosed heart disease in every newborn examination.

Certain disease syndromes are characterized by severe heart defects. Ellis-van Creveld (EvC) syndrome is a type of dwarfism seen in as many as 1 in 200 births among the Old Order Amish of Pennsylvania but is rare in the population at large (K. K. Miller et al., 2016). Heart defects occur in more than half of infants with EvC (usually atrial septal defects or lack of an atrial septum), and many of these children also have pulmonary hypoplasia as well. Children with EvC who have a normal heart, lungs, and chest have a normal life expectancy. If a couple has a child with EvC, odds are 1 in 4 that they will have another.

Hypothermia

Routine care at birth involves conserving the infant's body heat. Newborn hypothermia can contribute to neonatal mortality and morbidity in any birth setting (Mullany, 2010). Environment and internal physiologic processes determine the newborn's ability to regulate body temperature (Fraser, 2021). Although a rectal temperature can accurately assess deep body temperature, obtaining an axillary temperature is less invasive and produces accurate, reliable readings (Nadkarni et al., 2021). A newborn should have an axillary temperature from 97.7° to 99.5°F (36.5°–37.5°C), inclusive (McKee-Garrett, 2023). WHO (1997) classifies newborn hypothermia as mild, core temperature 96.8°–97.6°F (36°–36.4°C); moderate, 89.6°–96.6°F (32°–35.9°C); or severe, less than 89.6°F (32°C). Hypothermia increases neonatal mortality by 400% in the first 5 days of life, and every 1.8F° (1C°) decrease of a newborn's body temperature increases the mortality risk by 80% (Beletew, Mengesha, Wudu, & Abate, 2020).

Infants are extremely vulnerable to heat loss in the early neonatal period, especially if preterm or small for gestational age (SGA). Neonates readily lose body heat because they have a high ratio of surface area to body mass and limited subcutaneous fat. Growth-restricted newborns can have significant difficulty balancing heat loss with heat production.

The newborn has limited ability to generate heat by shivering, and instead produces heat by metabolizing brown fat, a process unique to newborns. By about 26 weeks of gestation, a fetus begins to build stores of brown fat in the neck, scapula, axillae, and mediastinum and around the kidneys and adrenal glands (Fraser, 2021). Brown fat can generate more energy than any other body tissue (Fraser, 2021). Once a baby depletes the stores of brown fat, they are not replaced. Infants who have undergone prolonged resuscitation or a period of hypoxia may be unable to metabolize brown fat to stay warm.

The highest risk of hypothermia occurs shortly after birth. The temperature of a newborn who is not dried and warmed can fall 3.6–7.2F° (2–4C°) in the first 10–20 min (Champlain Maternal Newborn Regional Program [CMNRP], 2013). A baby exposed to cold uses compensatory mechanisms to conserve and generate heat. Blood vessels constrict in the arms, legs, and skin to keep warm blood in the core of the body. The arms and legs are drawn in toward the trunk to reduce exposed surface area (Karlsen, 2019). The baby becomes restless, moving the limbs and crying to generate warmth.

When infants become hypothermic, metabolic oxygen and glucose consumption increase. A baby already in respiratory distress may be unable to meet the increased demand for oxygen. Hypoxemia can trigger or worsen pulmonary vasoconstriction. If glucose stores become exhausted, hypoglycemia can develop. Signs and symptoms of neonatal hypothermia are nonspecific and can indicate other serious conditions, but include (CMNRP, 2013)

- Bluish extremities and cool, mottled, or pale skin
- Hypoglycemia, transient hyperglycemia
- Tachycardia, bradycardia
- Rapid or slowed breathing, apnea
- Respiratory distress, grunting, retractions
- Decreased activity, lethargy, hypotonia, difficulty waking
- Central cyanosis, low oxygen saturation
- Poor suck or refusal to feed

Any baby with any of these signs and symptoms requires evaluation by a pediatrician or neonatologist. Symptoms of hypothermia can mimic or coexist with symptoms of other conditions such as respiratory distress, hypoglycemia, sepsis, metabolic disorders, or CCHD. Failure to rapidly refer an unstable baby to definitive care can result in profound damage or death.

Preventing hypothermia is much easier than managing the resulting cascade of problems. Keep the infant in a thermal neutral zone (the environmental temperature that allows staying warm with the least expenditure of energy). The ideal method for maintaining warmth is to place the baby skin-to-skin with the mother and cover both with a blanket. Infants who breastfeed within 1 hr after birth are less likely to become hypothermic than those with delayed breastfeeding (Beletew et al., 2020). The preterm infant or any baby born into an unavoidably cool environment should be covered with food-grade plastic wrap, then with a blanket. Be mindful of drafts, air currents, and the potential for radiant heat loss near cold windows. Avoid placing the baby on cool surfaces such as a metal scale. Use a neonatal thermal mattress or maternal skin-to-skin positioning to maintain warmth if the baby requires transportation to the hospital. Dress the newborn and wrap in blankets if a transport device is used. Lay the baby on a prewarmed surface in a warm room (or keep the baby skin to skin) when conducting the newborn assessment. Skin-to-skin contact can be used to rewarm a newborn experiencing mild hypothermia (CMNRP, 2013). If the baby's temperature remains low despite breastfeeding and skin-to-skin contact, consult the pediatrician or neonatologist and transport to the hospital for evaluation and rewarming.

Hypoglycemia

Neonatal hypoglycemia, a preventable cause of brain damage, affects 5–15% of all infants and about half of at-risk infants (Edwards & Harding, 2021). Hypoglycemia can be asymptomatic or present with nonspecific symptoms, and if uncorrected can lead to neurologic injuries (Dani & Corsini, 2020). The fetus stores sugar as glycogen in the liver, heart, lung, and skeletal muscle, but is inefficient at concerting it to glucose.

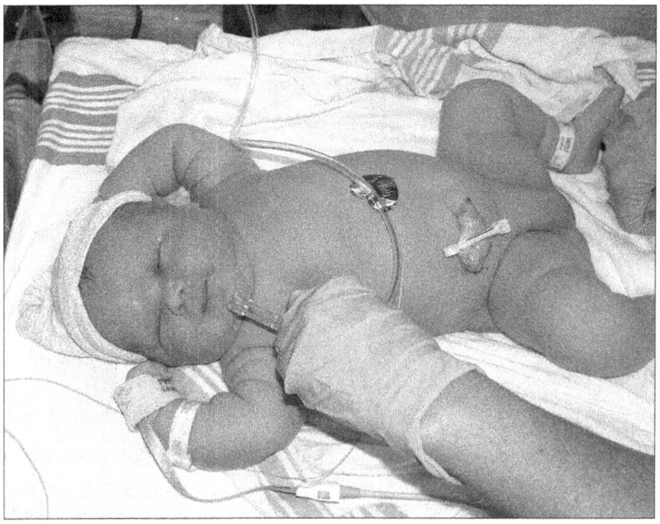

Figure 13-39. Macrosomia. This 12-lb girl was born at 37 0/7 weeks of gestation to a client with uncontrolled diabetes and limited prenatal care. Infants of mothers with uncontrolled diabetes are at high risk of neonatal hypoglycemia, cardiac defects and other congenital anomalies, respiratory distress, birth trauma, jaundice, stillbirth, and neonatal death.

Table 13-7
Risk Factors That Predispose a Newborn to Hypoglycemia

- Large size for gestational age (LGA) with or without maternal diabetes
- Perinatal stress (maternal preeclampsia or hypertension, FHR abnormalities, hypothermia, hypoxia, sepsis, CHD, perinatal hypoxia or asphyxia)
- Resuscitation following birth
- Small for gestational age (SGA)
- Premature or postmature birth
- Mother with diabetes
- Certain congenital syndromes
- Delayed start of feeding
- Maternal treatment with antidepressants, tocolytics, or beta blockers
- Maternal substance abuse
- Family history of genetic hypoglycemia

Adapted from "Neonatal Hypoglycemia: Presenting Pattern and Risk Factors of Neonatal Hypoglycemia," by S. A. Bhand, F. Sheikh, A. R. Siyal, M. A. Nizamani, and M. Saeed, 2014, *Professional Medical Journal, 21*(4), 747. Copyright by Professional Medical Journal.

The mother provides most of the glucose needed to meet fetal energy demands. After the cord is cut, the mother no longer supplies glucose, and the baby begins to break down glycogen. If glycogen stores are inadequate, if there is excessive insulin in the baby's blood (a condition that sometimes accompanies maternal diabetes), or if glucose consumption is abnormally high, the baby may not be able to maintain adequate glucose levels (Abramowski, Ward, & Hamdan, 2022).

The Infant at Risk for Hypoglycemia

A newborn's risk of neonatal hypoglycemia varies with the clinical situation and individual characteristics. A chronically stressed fetus that uses most or all of the placentally transferred glucose for survival and growth has little or no stored glycogen for transitioning to extrauterine life (Karlsen, 2019). Preterm and SGA infants may also have inadequate glycogen stores that deplete quickly after birth. When the mother is using mood-stabilizing medications such as tricyclic antidepressants, serotonin-norepinephrine reuptake inhibitors, and selective serotonin reuptake inhibitors, the risk of neonatal hypoglycemia is as high as 34%, depending on the drug (Wackernagel et al., 2020). When an infant has been subjected to perinatal asphyxia, hypoglycemia increases the risk of poor neurologic outcomes (Wackernagel et al., 2020).

Maternal Diabetes

The newborn of a mother with diabetes (Type 1, Type 2, or gestational) is at risk of hypoglycemia in the first days of life. The fetus obtains glucose from the mother's bloodstream through placental transfer. When a mother has abnormally high blood-glucose levels, the fetal blood-glucose level is also elevated. The fetus increases insulin production to metabolize this extra glucose. When the cord is clamped at birth, maternal glucose transfer stops, but the newborn's insulin level can remain abnormally elevated. These infants are at risk of a precipitous drop in glucose 1 hr or more after birth (Karlsen, 2019). Sometimes their insulin levels do not adjust to extrauterine life for days, during which they are at risk for episodes of severe hypoglycemia. Some newborns require intensive blood-glucose management for at least 2–3 days after birth. Mothers with poorly controlled diabetes or who require medication (such as insulin or metformin) should plan birth at a hospital with a NICU to address the many greater risks to themselves and to their infants (Goyal et al., 2020).

Although prenatal glucose testing involves diagnostic thresholds that determine the presence or absence of diabetes, impaired glucose tolerance is a continuum. A mother deemed nondiabetic after glucose screening can have daily blood-glucose levels that fluctuate into the abnormal range, increasing the amount of glucose transferred to the fetus. Many mothers with subclinical impaired glucose tolerance have large-normal or macrosomic infants at risk of hypoglycemia after birth (Ju, Rumbold, Willson, & Crowther, 2008).

Symptomatic Hypoglycemia

Most newborns with hypoglycemia remain asymptomatic, even when blood-glucose concentrations are very low (Rozance, 2023). Signs of hypoglycemia are nonspecific and resemble the signs of respiratory distress, hypothermia, and other complications. These include

- Jitteriness, tremors, myoclonic jerks, exaggerated Moro reflex, seizures
- Diaphoresis, clammy skin
- Irritability, high-pitched cry
- Temperature instability, hypothermia
- Tachycardia, bradycardia
- Tachypnea, slowed breathing, apnea
- Respiratory distress, grunting, retractions
- Decreased activity, lethargy, hypotonia, difficulty waking
- Cyanosis, low oxygen saturation
- Poor suck or refusal to feed

A baby with any of these findings requires prompt evaluation by a pediatrician or neonatologist. Signs of hypoglycemia can mimic or coexist with those of other conditions such as hypothermia, respiratory distress, sepsis, metabolic disorders, or CHD. Prompt transport to the nearest facility capable of managing an unstable neonate can be lifesaving. When in doubt, transport.

Caring For the At-Risk Infant

Severe hypoglycemia can quickly be fatal for the infant born in a community setting (Schuppener & Corliss, 2020). The at-risk infant, like all newborns, should be encouraged to feed as soon as possible after the birth. Feeding at the breast stabilizes neonatal glucose levels more effectively than feedings of formula or expressed breastmilk (Wackernagel et al., 2020). Skin-to-skin contact and free access to the breast has been shown to promote safe glucose stabilization in the first hours after birth, even for infants of mothers with diet-controlled diabetes (Dalsgaard, Rodrigo-Domingo, Kronborg, & Haslund, 2019). Ensure that the infant is alert and sucking strongly, rhythmically, and effectively.

In general, newborns at risk of hypoglycemia should feed by 1 hr of age and undergo blood-glucose screening about 30 min after the feeding (Adamkin & Cmte. on Fetus and Newborn [CFN], 2011). Healthy infants have a drop in glucose over the first 2 hr after birth, sometimes to as low as 30 mg/dl, whether they are fed with breastmilk, formula, or both (Wight & Academy of Breastfeeding Medicine [ABM], 2021). There is no absolute numerical threshold of blood-glucose concentration or duration of hypoglycemia that can accurately predict poor neurodevelopmental outcome, and there is no fixed glucose level below which the baby will show clinical signs (Adamkin & CFN, 2011; Rozance, 2023). Thus, there is no consensus on when to screen infants and what concentration of glucose requires therapeutic intervention in the asymptomatic infant (Rozance, 2023).

Bedside reagent test-strip glucose analyzers are inexpensive and practical, but they can be unreliable (especially if the glucose levels are very low), and they are susceptible to sample or user error (Adamkin & CFN, 2011; Narvey & Marks, 2019). Most guidelines are based on plasma glucose concentrations. These can be 15% or more higher than glucose concentrations measured in whole blood, which are used in point-of-care glucose analyzers (Rozance, 2023). For neonates at risk of hypoglycemia, AAP recommends maintaining a blood-glucose level greater than 40 mg/dl in the first 4 hr after birth and greater than 45 mg/dl in hours 4–24 of life in high-risk neonates (Adamkin, 2017; Adamkin & CFN, 2011; Dani & Corsini, 2020). The S.T.A.B.L.E. Program considers neonatal glucose levels stable if they are 50–110 mg/dl (Karlsen, 2019). Recommended management can include continued skin-to-skin positioning with frequent suckling (or feeding expressed colostrum or infant formula), interval reassessment of blood-glucose levels or transport to a higher level of care (Wight & & ABM, 2021). Infants born in community settings are often discharged home as early as 2–4 hr after birth. In the absence of close surveillance, hypoglycemia can develop undetected. Longer surveillance and short-interval follow-up may be prudent for neonates with risk factors. Instruct the parents to offer feedings at 2–3-hr intervals and tell them how to recognize signs of a compromised infant. Discuss any concerns regarding timing of discharge with a pediatrician or neonatologist.

Neonatal Hyperbilirubinemia

Hyperbilirubinemia (excess bilirubin in the blood) is common in the first week of life. It can be mild and transient or severe and serious. Physiologic jaundice is a common and usually benign transitional occurrence in newborns, occurring in about 60% of term infants and 80% of preterm infants in the first week of life (Rohan, 2021). Pathologic hyperbilirubinemia is one of the most common reasons for readmission of newborns in the first 2 weeks after birth (Rohan, 2021).

Pathophysiology

Three aspects of newborn physiology cause bilirubin levels to rise during the first few days after birth:

- The fetus compensates for the low-oxygen intrauterine environment by developing high hematocrit and high concentration of hemoglobin. Fetal hemoglobin has a different composition from the adult form and attaches

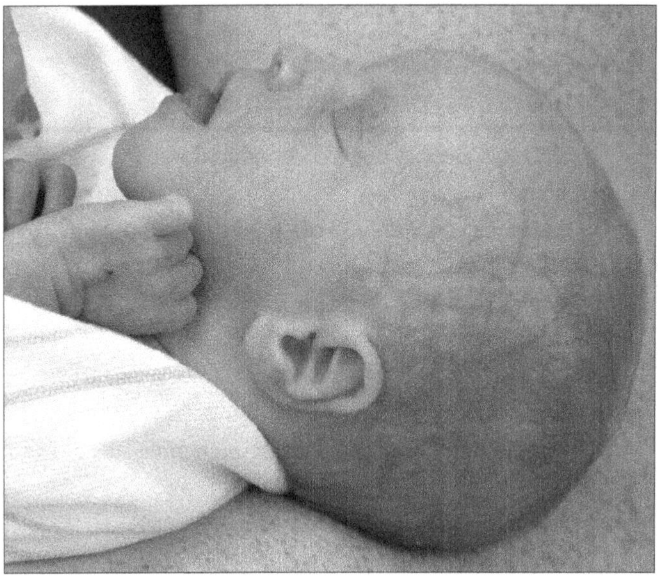

Figure 13-40. An infant born with growth restriction is at higher risk of jaundice necessitating phototherapy. This baby required weeks of care in the neonatal intensive care unit (NICU) for management of issues that included jaundice and hypoglycemia. After her difficult beginning she grew to be a healthy and highly intelligent child.

to oxygen more strongly. After birth, the baby obtains oxygen in abundance directly from the air. Surplus fetal RBCs break down so that adult hemoglobin can replace fetal hemoglobin.

- The breakdown of hemoglobin releases unconjugated (indirect) bilirubin into the blood stream. This unconjugated bilirubin must be converted to a conjugated (direct) water-soluble form so that the newborn can excrete it through urine and stool (Reis & Bell, 2024). The metabolic pathway that conjugates bilirubin in the liver is immature in the newborn (Reis & Bell, 2024). Unconjugated bilirubin is often released faster than the liver can process it.
- Intestinal bacteria break conjugated bilirubin down further so that it can be excreted (Reis & Bell, 2024). The newborn is born with a gastrointestinal tract that is essentially sterile. In the first days of life, conjugated bilirubin is reabsorbed and recirculated through the enterohepatic system more than it would be in an older baby with established gut flora (Reis & Bell, 2024).

Hyperbilirubinemia can develop when the mother produces antibodies that cross the placenta and destroy fetal blood cells (isoimmunization). Hemolysis related to isoimmunization can be fatal for the fetus or infant, and it often involves anti-C, anti-D (rhesus/Rh), anti-E, and anti-K (Kell) antibodies. If mother has a positive antibody screen or has not undergone prenatal antibody screening, the infant's blood type should be determined as soon as possible using either cord or peripheral blood and the infant should have a direct antiglobulin test (Kemper et al., 2022).

Table 13-8
Newborn Hyperbilirubinemia

Physiologic jaundice
Jaundice is detectable at 2–4 days after birth
Total bilirubin rises slowly and peaks at day 3 or 4 of life at less than 13 mg/dl
Hyperbilirubinemia
Jaundice is detectable during first 24 hr after birth
Total bilirubin rises quickly, up to more than 5 mg/dl/24 hr; it peaks at more than 13 mg/dl
Visible jaundice persists after one week of life
Newborn may have risk factors such as cephalohematoma, ABO blood group or RhD incompatibility, or polycythemia
Breast milk insufficiency jaundice
Jaundice appears in first week after birth
Total bilirubin levels can rise to more than13 mg/dl
Exclusively breastfed: feeds poorly, weight loss and signs of dehydration, infrequent urine output
Delayed meconium passage
Breast milk jaundice
Jaundice appears after first week of life and persists for up to 12 weeks
Mildly elevated bilirubin levels that do not rise
Feeds well, normal weight gain, normal urine output

Adapted from "Neonatal Care," by P. J. Reis and T. Bell, in J. Phillippi and I. Kantrowitz-Gordon (Eds.), *Varney's Midwifery* (7th ed., Kindle version, ch. 39), 2024, Burlington, MA: Jones & Bartlett Learning. Copyright by publisher.

Jaundice related to ABO incompatibility is usually mild and is most common when the mother has type O blood and the baby has type A or type B. About 12–15% of pregnancies have risk factors for ABO incompatibility, but only 3–4% of newborns have a positive direct Coombs test (Whitehurst, 2020). Symptomatic ABO hemolytic disease is very rare, developing in fewer than 1% of newborns.

There are two main categories of feeding-related hyperbilirubinemia. Jaundice related to suboptimal intake typically peaks on days 3–5 after birth and is related to poor feeding and dehydration, often accompanied by excessive weight loss (Kemper et al., 2022). It is more likely to develop in the baby who breastfeeds fewer than 8–12 times per day in the first week of life or who has ineffective milk transfer with nursing. Once termed "breastfeeding jaundice," AAP now describes this condition as suboptimal intake jaundice because it is associated with inadequate milk intake rather than with breastfeeding and can occur in bottle-fed infants as well (Kemper et al., 2022). In contrast, breast milk jaundice syndrome involves high levels

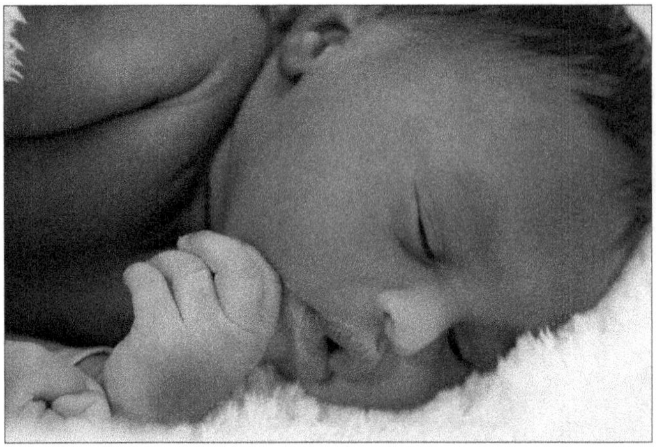

Figure 13-41. Because it can be difficult to visually identify jaundice in dark-skinned infants, hyperbilirubinemia can be missed by providers who do not assess the gums and the sclerae of the eyes.

Table 13-9
Risk Factors for Pathologic Hyperbilirubinemia

- Gestational age less than 37 completed weeks (high risk)
- Gestational age 37 0/7–38 6/7 weeks (medium risk)
- Jaundice in the first 24 hr
- Maternal-fetal blood type incompatibility
- Maternal age ≥25 years
- Male sex
- Delayed meconium passage
- Certain metabolic diseases involving hemolysis
- Sepsis
- Congenital hypothyroidism
- Birth trauma such as bruising or cephalohematoma
- Previous sibling received phototherapy
- Exclusive breastfeeding, particularly if ineffective
- Excessive weight loss

of unconjugated bilirubin that persist despite adequate breast milk intake and weight gain. It usually presents at about three to five days of life, peaks within 2 weeks of gestational age, and declines to normal levels over 3–12 weeks (Wong & Bhutani, 2022). Although hyperbilirubinemia is generally mild and usually does not require treatment, it should be monitored closely (Kemper et al., 2022).

Glucose-6-phosphate dehydrogenase (G6PD) deficiency, a genetic disorder that causes hemolytic anemia and jaundice in infants, is not uncommon in people of Mediterranean, Middle Eastern, Arab, Southeast Asian, and sub-Saharan African descent (Kemper et al., 2022). A newborn with G6PD deficiency can develop a sudden, extreme, and unpredictable increase in bilirubin (Kemper et al., 2022). Less common but serious causes of pathological neonatal jaundice include sepsis, rubella, toxoplasmosis, occult hemorrhage, hemolytic disease, bile duct abnormalities, and biliary atresia.

Assessment

Every newborn has a rise in bilirubin levels shortly after birth. As levels of unconjugated bilirubin climb, bilirubin begins to shift out of the bloodstream into the tissues. Jaundice can be detected by blanching the newborn's skin with the pad of your finger, revealing the underlying color. Jaundice usually first appears in the face, sclera of the eyes, and oral mucous membranes and moves down the trunk and into the extremities with increasing bilirubin levels. The characteristic yellowness that indicates jaundice is usually visible when the total serum bilirubin (TSB) level exceeds 5–6 mg/dl (Olusanya, Kaplan, & Hansen, 2018). Visual assessment *cannot* determine the severity of hyperbilirubinemia in a baby with significant jaundice (Kemper et al., 2022); but an infant with no visible jaundice or only slight yellowing of the face is very unlikely to have significant hyperbilirubinemia (Kemper et al., 2022).

Bilirubin can be accurately measured using a venous blood sample or a point-of-care transcutaneous meter. A transcutaneous bilirubinometer is a noninvasive device that estimates a newborn's transcutaneous bilirubin (TcB) level by means of a light and is valid when TSB is less than 15 mg/dl (Kemper et al., 2022). AAP recommends that all newborns be screened for elevated bilirubin using either TSB or TcB before discharge from the hospital and at the newborn pediatric visit (Kemper et al., 2022).

The Bhutani nomogram is a standardized bilirubin calculator that assesses risk in consideration of gestational age at birth, risk factors, number of hours since birth, and bilirubin values and offers recommendations for management based on the degree of risk (Reis & Bell, 2024). In a healthy newborn, total bilirubin plasma levels peak 48–92 hr after birth with values between 7 mg/dl and 9 mg/dl (Reis & Bell, 2024). Hyperbilirubinemia is defined as a total bilirubin level that is higher than the 95th percentile on the Bhutani nomogram in infants 35 weeks of gestation or more (Reis & Bell, 2024). The nomogram and an online tool for calculating an infant's bilirubin levels can be found at https://bilitool.org/

Unconjugated bilirubin is highly neurotoxic and can cause permanent brain damage. Jaundice is diagnosed as pathologic when bilirubin levels are significantly elevated, when onset of jaundice occurs before 24 hr of age, when bilirubin is rising rapidly, when jaundice persists longer than 2 weeks, or when the baby is producing dark urine that stains the clothing (Ullah, Rahman, & Hedayati, 2016). Serious signs of jaundice-related illness include poor feeding, dark urine, light stools, vomiting, lethargy, and shrill cries with arching bodies.

About 2% of term infants develop severe hyperbilirubinemia with levels exceeding 20 mg/dl (Muchowski, 2014). A total bilirubin level that is higher than 25–30 mg/dl carries the risk of bilirubin-induced neurologic dysfunction (BIND), which can occur when bilirubin binds to brain tissue (Reis & Bell, 2024). Acute bilirubin encephalopathy (ABE) is evidenced by cerebral symptoms such as irritability, high-pitched cry, hypertonia or hypotonia, seizures, and possibly death if not treated (Reis & Bell, 2024). Kernicterus, permanent cerebral damage resulting from ABE (Reis & Bell, 2024), can be prevented with phototherapy, IV immunoglobulins, or exchange transfusion to reduce the levels of serum bilirubin (Wolf et al., 2020). Kernicterus has become rare in term infants with the advent of phototherapy, but the rate of bilirubin neurotoxicity has not changed in preterm infants (Kemper et al., 2022; Qattea, Farghaly, Elgendy, Mohamed, & Aly, 2022).

Table 13-10

Common Causes of Neonatal Seizures by Age

First Day of Life	Second Day of Life	Day 3 to 6 Months
• Anoxia/hypoxia • Trauma • Intracranial • hemorrhage • Drugs • Infection • Hypoglycemia/ • hyperglycemia • Pyridoxine deficiency	• Sepsis • Trauma • Inborn errors of metabolism (IEM) • Hypoglycemia • Hypocalcemia • Hyponatremia/hypernatremia • Hyperphosphatemia • Drug withdrawal • Congenital anomalies or developmental brain disorders • Hypertension • Benign familial neonatal seizures	• Hypocalcemia • Infection • Hyponatremia/ hypernatremia • Drug withdrawal • IEM • Hyperphosphatemia • Congenital anomalies or developmental brain disorders • Hypertension • Benign idiopathic neonatal seizures

Adapted from "A Practical Approach to Emergencies in the Neonatal Period," by A. Mata-Peréz, M. Soto-Martínez, and A. Yock-Corrales, 2016, *Journal of Neonatal Biology, 5*(1), 1000213, table 4.

Treatment

Frequent feedings to promote the growth of intestinal flora and encourage the passage of meconium can hasten the resolution of physiologic jaundice. Decisions to initiate phototherapy or perform other interventions are guided by the gestational age, the level of bilirubin in relation to the hour of age, and the presence of risk factors for bilirubin neurotoxicity (Kemper et al., 2022). The baby with significantly elevated serum bilirubin is usually treated with phototherapy. When a baby's skin is exposed to light at a blue to blue-green wavelength, the bilirubin turns soluble and becomes more easily excreted in the bile or the urine. Although jaundice necessitating phototherapy usually requires hospital admission, phototherapy may be continued at home (Anderson, Kandasamy, & Kilcullen, 2022). If bilirubin levels are extremely high and there is an immediate risk of neurologic damage, an exchange transfusion can be used to remove bilirubin and, in some cases, to remove circulating antibodies and damaged RBCs. The procedure involves incrementally removing the infant's blood and replacing it with fresh donor blood or plasma.

Infection

Neonates are highly susceptible to infection, but do not react to pathogens in obvious ways as do older children and adults. Some neonates do not develop fever in response to infection. In others, temperature above 100.4°F (38°C) indicates a potentially life-threatening condition. About 12–28% of all febrile newborns presenting to a pediatric emergency room have significant bacterial illness (Ishimine, 2009). Symptoms of infection may be vague and nonspecific, and it may be difficult to pinpoint the source. Whereas a toddler may have inflammation at the site of an infection, a newborn may not.

The infant can contract infection through the umbilical stump, skin, mucous membranes, circumcision site, or internal systems such as the respiratory, gastrointestinal, and urinary tracts. Early-onset newborn sepsis occurs within the first week of life, usually within the first 72 hr (Rohan, 2021). Neonatal sepsis can begin *in utero* from the ascent of bacteria after rupture of membranes, and it is especially likely after prolonged rupture of the amniotic membranes. It can also occur when pathogens such as *Cytomegalovirus* or *Toxoplasma gondii* cross the placenta. Infants with sepsis often have nonspecific symptoms such as lethargy, poor feeding, irritability, poor tone, respiratory distress, apnea, tachycardia or bradycardia, hypoglycemia, hypothermia, jaundice, rashes, seizures, or vomiting. They may appear pale or mottled. Late-onset sepsis presents beyond 3–7 days of age and is usually related to exposure to pathogens during or shortly after birth. Late-onset septicemia can involve pneumonia or meningitis (Rohan, 2021). Unrecognized sepsis can decline quickly into septic shock. Any infant with abnormal vital signs or other signs of illness needs prompt evaluation at a facility capable of managing serious compromise.

Congenital TORCH infections are a group of diseases that affect the fetus and the newborn that have overlapping signs and symptoms. The acronym TORCH refers to **T**oxoplasmosis; **O**ther (e.g., syphilis, HIV, enterovirus, parvovirus, and varicella); **R**ubella; **C**ytomegalovirus; and **H**erpes simplex virus. Any of them can be life-threatening in the newborn.

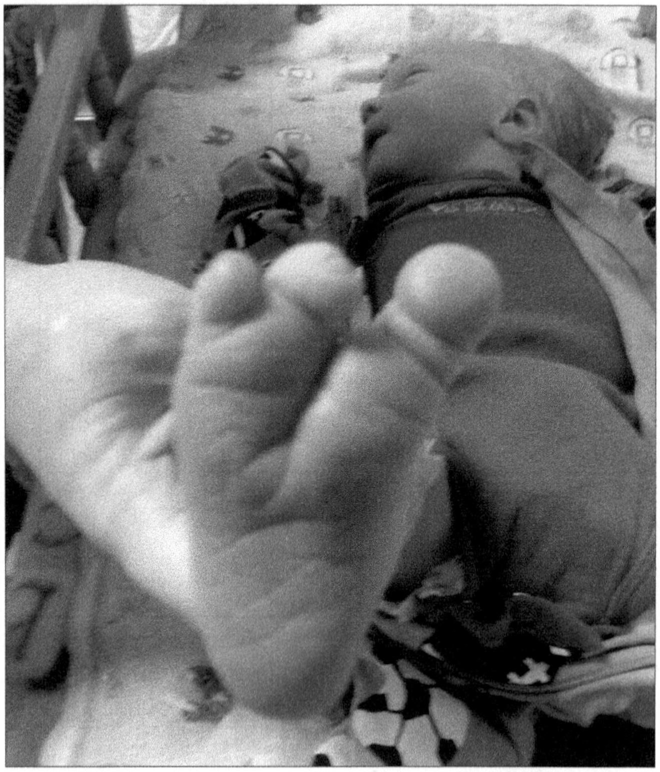

Figure 13-42. An infant born with a noticeable physical anomaly can have other abnormalities of structure or function.

Neonatal Seizures

A seizure is the equivalent of an electrical storm in the brain, resulting in an alteration of behavior or function. Newborn seizures can be related to neonatal encephalopathy; structural brain injuries including ischemic and hemorrhagic stroke; metabolic issues (most often glucose and electrolyte abnormalities); or central nervous system or systemic infections (Shellhaas, 2023). Mothers who overdilute commercial baby formula or make their own can cause the newborn to develop hyponatremia which can manifest as seizures. Any seizure in a newborn is clinically significant. Seizures in the neonate often indicate underlying disease capable of causing permanent brain damage.

Because the brain of the newborn is too immature to sustain organized seizure activity, neonatal seizures manifest as lip smacking; sucking; alterations in tone such as rigidity; swimming or bicycling movements; grimacing; alterations in breathing patterns; or abnormal facial, tongue, or eye movements. These usually occur while the infant is unconscious. Status epilepticus is defined by seizures lasting more than 30 consecutive minutes or two more consecutive seizures without an interval of consciousness between them. Epilepsy is the susceptibility to recurrent seizures. An epileptic syndrome involves a specific set of signs and symptoms characterized by neurologic and encephalographic anomalies.

Jitteriness

Jitteriness involves a tremulous, back-and-forth oscillation of the infant's limbs, usually observed as an excessive response to stimulation such as touch or loud noise. Mild jitteriness can occur in healthy infants, but severe jitteriness sometimes results from drug withdrawal, hypocalcemia, hypoglycemia, or neonatal encephalopathy, any of which can also produce seizures (Nguyen, Kaplan, & Wilfong, 2021). Whereas seizures are characterized by unconsciousness, the jittery infant is usually awake, and no associated autonomic disturbance is present (Nguyen et al., 2021). The movement can be decreased by removing the stimulus or flexing the limbs. Seizures usually involve the eyes. Jitteriness is not associated with ocular movement.

Inborn Errors of Metabolism (IEM)

IEM are uncommon metabolic disorders that often go unrecognized without targeted testing, such as congenital hypothyroidism, galactosemia, maple syrup urine disease, phenylketonuria, and many others. Most involve defects of genes that code for enzymes that convert certain substances into others. Individually, IEM are rare. Most occur in fewer than 1 per 100,000 births (Raghuveer, Garg, & Graf, 2006). Taken together, however, IEM are more common, 1 in 1,500 births (Raghuveer et al., 2006). Most of these diseases are carried on recessive genes and are more prevalent in closed communities where consanguinity is high, including the Amish, Old Order Mennonites, some Jewish groups, and certain Native Americans (Patay, 2005). For example, although maple syrup urine disease is extremely rare overall, with an incidence of 1 in 185,000 and a carrier frequency of 1 in 215,

1 in 10 Old Order Mennonites in Wisconsin is a carrier (Kuhl et al., 2017). Although tandem mass spectrometry testing for IEM is mandated in many areas, any given newborn may be tested for as few as seven or as many as 40 IEM, determined by the location of birth (Raghuveer et al., 2006). More than 1,000 IEM have been identified by researchers, and it is likely that there are many others that remain unrecognized. Babies who pass newborn metabolic screens can be afflicted by disorders not included on the panel (Ferreira, van Karnebeek, Vockley, & Blau, 2019).

The infant with IEM may begin to show signs days or weeks after birth. Although signs and symptoms can depend on the disorder, infants with metabolic disorders often present with lethargy, poor feeding, vomiting, tachypnea, or seizures. As the illness progresses, danger signs can include (Raghuveer et al., 2006)

Abnormal tone: Hypotonia, hypertonia

Abnormal posture: Fisting, arching backward

Abnormal Movements: Tongue-thrusting, lip-smacking, myoclonic jerks

Abnormal level of consciousness: Lethargy, coma

Laboratory studies sometimes show abnormalities such as elevated plasma ammonia levels, hypoglycemia, and metabolic acidosis. The infant may have an unusual odor, e.g., boiled cabbage in cases of tyrosinemia, fish in methylcrotonylglycinuria, or sweaty feet in glutaric aciduria type 2 (Mohamed, 2011). The child with maple syrup urine disease, as the name implies, has urine that smells like maple syrup or fenugreek.

Diarrhea

A newborn with diarrhea can very quickly become dehydrated, develop electrolyte imbalances, and lapse into hypovolemic shock. Diarrhea can result from bacterial infection, food intolerance, or other things, but it is usually viral. Assessment of diarrhea can be difficult. An infant with diarrhea has very frequent stools that are usually green, full of mucus (or specks of blood), and foul-smelling. Bowel movements are sometimes so liquid that they leave a water ring in the diaper. Diarrhea can be accompanied by fever or irritability. Signs of dehydration include insufficient quantity of urination, dry mouth, lethargy, and sunken eyes and fontanels. Diarrhea is rare in a baby who is exclusively breastfed. A breastfed baby normally has as many as 6–10 moist, semiliquid, yellow, often large stools every day. Inexperienced parents often confuse this with diarrhea.

Vomiting

Vomiting is associated with many different conditions of the newborn. Life-threatening problems can appear very similar to mild viral gastroenteritis or significant gastroesophageal reflux. Vomiting can indicate obstruction in the gastrointestinal tract, high intracranial pressure (as may occur with intraventricular hemorrhage), or infection. Although it is not unusual for neonates to swallow maternal blood during birth and then regurgitate red or brown mucus, bloody emesis can indicate a life-threatening problem.

Bilious vomiting (vomiting green bile) indicates a functional or anatomical intestinal obstruction. Malrotation is a congenital anomaly which occurs when the intestines do not rotate into their normal position during early fetal development, creating an unfixed length of bowel that can later twist on itself. Malrotation is fairly rare but is usually diagnosed in the first month of life in an infant that appears healthy at birth. Symptoms include bilious vomiting, feeding problems, lethargy, and sometimes shock.

New parents sometimes confuse vomiting with "spitting up" or regurgitation, a sudden reflux of stomach contents mixed with mucus that can appear copious and often occurs after burping. Spitting up often occurs after overfeeding or placing the infant flat after a large meal. Spitting up occurs less often if the infant is fed before it is screaming with hunger, if the infant is kept upright while feeding, and if the infant is not overfed.

Topics for Discussion

1. Meredith G. presented to her routine prenatal appointment at 39 0/7 weeks of gestation. When Christina, her midwife, auscultated the FHR, the rhythm was distinctly irregular. This was a new finding. How does Christina explain this finding to Meredith? What are Christina's next steps?
2. Dennie is questioned by a physician about why she performed artificial ventilation with the umbilical cord intact rather than cutting it and moving the infant to a resuscitation bed. How could she answer the question?
3. Describe how to place an LMA in an apneic newborn.
4. Malcolm, a certified nurse-midwife with a rural home-birth practice, visited his client Elise in her mountain cottage for a follow-up visit. Upon assessment, two-day-old infant Stefan was very sleepy and hard to wake, and he had significant jaundice from his head to his legs. What questions should Malcolm ask Elise? What are Malcolm's next steps?
5. Baby Lucy has been skin to skin with her mother for the hour since birth, snuggled under cozy fleece blankets. She mouthed at the breast but never latched. Now her core temperature is 97°F (36°C), and her tone is somewhat floppy. What should the midwife do next?

References

Abdelmaksoud, S. R., Abdelraziq, H. E., Khashaba, R. A., & Diab, A. M. (2021). Delayed cord clamping in infants of diabetic mothers: Laboratory and clinical outcomes. *Journal of Child Science, 11*(1), e74–e79. https://doi.org/10.1055/s-0041-1726460

Abe, K. K., Blum, G. T., & Yamamoto, L. G. (2000). Intraosseous is faster and easier than umbilical venous catheterization in newborn emergency vascular access models. *American Journal of Emergency Medicine, 18*(2), 126–129. https://doi.org/10.1016/S0735-6757(00)90001-9

Abramowski, A., Ward, R., & Hamdan, A. H. (2022). Neonatal hypoglycemia. In *StatPearls*. Treasure Island, FL: StatPearls Publishing. Retrieved October 30, 2023, from https://www.ncbi.nlm.nih.gov/books/NBK537105/

Adamkin, D. H. (2017). Neonatal hypoglycemia. *Seminars in Fetal & Neonatal Medicine, 22*(1), 36–41. https://doi.org/10.1016/j.siny.2016.08.007

Adamkin, D. H., & Committee on Fetus and Newborn. (2011). Postnatal glucose homeostasis in late-preterm and term infants. *Pediatrics, 127*(3), 575–579. https://doi.org/10.1542/peds.2010-3851

Al Wattar, B. H., Honess, E., Bunnewell, S., Welton, N. J., Quenby, S., Khan, K. S., . . . Thangaratinam, S. (2021). Effectiveness of intrapartum fetal surveillance to improve maternal and neonatal outcomes: A systematic review and network meta-analysis. *Canadian Medical Association Journal, 193*(14), E468–E477. https://doi.org/10.1503/cmaj.202538

Alfirevic, Z., Gyte, G. M. L., Cuthbert, A., & Devane, D. (2017). Continuous cardiotocography (CTG) as a form of electronic fetal monitoring (EFM) for fetal assessment during labour. Cochrane Database of Systematic Reviews. https://www.cochranelibrary.com/cdsr/doi/10.1002/14651858.CD006066.pub3/full

Altman, C. A. (2022). Identifying newborns with critical congenital heart disease. In C. Armsby (Ed.), *UpToDate*. Retrieved June 25, 2023, from https://www.uptodate.com/contents/identifying-newborns-with-critical-congenital-heart-disease

American Academy of Pediatrics. (2021). *Program to Enhance the Health & Development of Infants and Children (PEHDIC): Newborn screening: Critical congenital heart defects*. Retrieved from https://ww w.aap.org/en-us/advocacy-and-policy/aap-health-initiatives/PEHDIC/Pages/Newborn-Screening-for-CCHD.aspx

American Academy of Pediatrics. (2022). *NRP instructor*. Retrieved from https://www.aap.org/en-us/continuing-medical-education/life-support/NRP/Pages/Instructor.aspx

American Academy of Pediatrics Committee on Fetus and Newborn & American College of Obstetricians and Gynecologists Committee on Obstetric Practice. (2015). The Apgar score. *Pediatrics, 136*(4), 819–822. https://doi.org/10.1542/peds.2015-2651

American Association of Birth Centers. (2017). *Standards for birth centers* (12th ed.). Perkiomenville, PA: Author. Retrieved from https://www.birthcenters.org/resource/resmgr/AABC-STANDARDS-RV2017.pdf

American College of Nurse-Midwives. (2015). Intermittent auscultation for intrapartum fetal heart rate surveillance. *Journal of Midwifery & Women's Health. 60*(5), 626–632. https://doi.org/10.1111/jmwh.12372

American College of Obstetricians and Gynecologists. (2009, reaffirmed 2021). *Intrapartum fetal heart rate monitoring: Nomenclature, interpretation, and general management principles* (Practice Bulletin 106). Retrieved from https://www.acog.org/clinical/clinical-guidance/practice-bulletin/articles/2009/07/intrapartum-fetal-heart-rate-monitoring-nomenclature-interpretation-and-general-management-principles

American College of Obstetricians and Gynecologists. (2016, reaffirmed 2021). *Immersion in water during labor and delivery* (Committee Opinion 679). Retrieved from https://www.acog.org/clinical/clinical-guidance/committee-opinion/articles/2016/11/immersion-in-water-during-labor-and-delivery

American College of Obstetricians and Gynecologists. (2019, reaffirmed 2021). *Approaches to limit intervention during labor and birth* (Committee Opinion 766). Retrieved from https://www.acog.org/clinical/clinical-guidance/committee-opinion/articles/2019/02/approaches-to-limit-intervention-during-labor-and-birth

American College of Obstetricians and Gynecologists. (2020, reaffirmed 2023). *Delayed umbilical cord clamping after birth* (Committee Opinion 814). Retrieved from https://www.acog.org/Clinical/Clinical-Guidance/Committee-Opinion/Articles/2020/12/Delayed-Umbilical-Cord-Clamping-After-Birth

American College of Obstetricians and Gynecologists. (2021, reaffirmed 2024). *Antepartum fetal surveillance* (Practice Bulletin 229). Retrieved from https://www.acog.org/clinical/clinical-guidance/practice-bulletin/articles/2021/06/antepartum-fetal-surveillance

American College of Obstetricians and Gynecologists & American Academy of Pediatrics (2014, reaffirmed 2019). *Neonatal encephalopathy and neurologic outcome* (2nd ed.). Washington, DC: American College of Obstetricians and Gynecologists. Retrieved from https://www.acog.org/-/media/project/acog/acogorg/clinical/files/task-force-report/articles/2014/neonatal-encephalopathy-and-neurologic-outcome.pdf

American College of Obstetricians and Gynecologists Committee on Clinical Practice Guidelines—Obstetrics. (2022, reaffirmed 2023). *Oxygen supplementation in the setting of category II or III fetal heart tracings* (Practice Advisory). Retrieved from https://www.acog.org/clinical/clinical-guidance/practice-advisory/articles/2022/01/oxygen-supplementation-in-the-setting-of-category-ii-or-iii-fetal-heart-tracings

Anderson, C. M., Kandasamy, Y., & Kilcullen, M. (2022). The efficacy of home phototherapy for physiological and non-physiological neonatal jaundice: A systematic review. *Journal of Neonatal Nursing, 28*(5), 312–326. https://doi.org/10.1016/j.jnn.2021.08.010

Andersson, O., & Mercer, J. S. (2021). Cord management of the term newborn. *Clinics in Perinatology, 48*(3), 447–470. https://doi.org/10.1016/j.clp.2021.05.002

Andersson, O., Rana, N., Ewald, U., Målqvist, M., Stripple, G., Basnet, O., . . . Ashish, K. C. (2019). Intact cord resuscitation versus early cord clamping in the treatment of depressed newborn infants during the first 10 minutes of birth (Nepcord III)—A randomized clinical trial. *Maternal Health, Neonatology and Perinatology, 5*, 15. https://doi.org/10.1186/s40748-019-0110-z

Ashish, K. C., Budhathoki, S. S., Thapa, J., Niermeyer, S., Gurung, R., Singhal, N., & Nepal Neonatal Network. (2022). Impact of stimulation among non-crying neonates with intact cord versus clamped cord on birth outcomes: observation study. *BMJ Paediatrics Open, 5*(1), e001207. https://doi.org/10.1136/bmjpo-2021-001207

Aubin, S. L., & El-Chaâr, D. (2023). Fetal health surveillance in labor. In G. D. Posner, A. Y. Black, G. Jones, & D. El-Chaâr (Eds.), *Oxorn-Foote human labor & birth* (7th ed., Kindle version, ch. 12). New York, NY: McGraw Hill.

Ayres-de-Campos, D., Spong, C. Y., Chandraharan, E., & FIGO Intrapartum Fetal Monitoring Expert Consensus Panel. (2015). FIGO consensus guidelines on intrapartum fetal monitoring: Cardiotocography. *International Journal of Gynecology & Obstetrics, 131*(1), 13–24. https://doi.org/10.1016/j.ijgo.2015.06.020

Baujat, G., & Le Merre, M. (2007). Ellis-Van Creveld syndrome. *Orphanet Journal of Rare Diseases, 2*, 27. https://doi.org/10.1186/1750-1172-2-27

Beletew, B., Mengesha, A., Wudu, M., & Abate, M. (2020). Prevalence of neonatal hypothermia and its associated factors in East Africa: A systematic review and meta-analysis. *BMC Pediatrics, 20*(1), 1–14. https://doi.org/10.1186/s12887-020-02024-w

Bennett, C., Munoz, J. L., Yao, M., & Singh, K. (2021). Effects of delayed cord clamping on neonatal hyperbilirubinemia in pre-gestational diabetes at term.

Journal of Maternal-Fetal & Neonatal Medicine, 35(25):7267–7275. https://doi.org/10.1080/14767058.2021.1946785

Bhand, S. A., Sheikh, F., Siyal, A. R., Nizamani, M. A., & Saeed, M. (2014). Neonatal hypoglycemia;; Presenting pattern and risk factors of neonatal hypoglycemia. *Professional Medical Journal, 21*(4), 745–749. https://doi.org/10.29309/TPMJ/2014.21.04.2312

Bhatt, S., Alison, B. J., Wallace, E. M., Crossley, K. J., Gill, A. W., Kluckow, M., . . . Hooper, S. B. (2013). Delaying cord clamping until ventilation onset improves cardiovascular function at birth in preterm lambs. *Journal of Physiology, 591*(8), 2113–2126. https://doi.org/10.1113/jphysiol.2012.250084

Bhoi, S., Mishra, N. R., & Rout, S. (2019). Duration of cord clamping and physiological jaundice in newborn: A case–control study. *Indian Journal of Child Health, 6*(4), 186–188. https://doi.org/10.32677/IJCH.2019.v06.i04.010

Blank, D. A., Badurdeen, S., Kamlin, C. O. F., Jacobs, S. E., Thio, M., Dawson, J. A., . . . Davis, P. G. (2018). Baby-directed umbilical cord clamping: A feasibility study. *Resuscitation, 131*, 1–7. https://doi.org/10.1016/j.resuscitation.2018.07.020

Blix, E., Maude, R., Hals, E., Kisa, S., Karlsen, E., Nohr, E. A., . . . Kaasen, A. (2019). Intermittent auscultation fetal monitoring during labour: A systematic scoping review to identify methods, effects, and accuracy. *PLoS ONE 14*(7), e0219573. https://doi.org/10.1371/journal.pone.0219573

Boere, I., Roest, A. A., Wallace, E., Ten Harkel, A. D. J., Haak, M. C., Morley, C. J., . . . Te Pas, A. B. (2015). Umbilical blood flow patterns directly after birth before delayed cord clamping. *Archives of Disease in Childhood—Fetal and Neonatal Edition, 100*(2), F121–F125. https://doi.org/10.1136/archdischild-2014-307144

Bolnick, J. M., Garcia, G., Fletcher, B. G., & Rayburn, W. F. (2006). Cross-over trial of fetal heart rate response to halogen light and vibroacoustic stimulation. *Journal of Maternal-Fetal & Neonatal Medicine, 19*(4), 215–219. https://doi.org/10.1080/14767050500526131

Boundy, E. O., Dastjerdi, R., Spiegelman, D., Fawzi, W. W., Missmer, S. A., Lieberman, E., . . . Chan, G. J. (2016). Kangaroo mother care and neonatal outcomes: A meta-analysis. *Pediatrics, 137*(1), e20152238. https://doi.org/10.1542/peds.2015-2238

Bovbjerg, M. (2015). Waterbirth: An integrative analysis of peer-reviewed literature. *Journal of Midwifery & Women's Health, 60*(6), 787. https://doi.org/10.1111/jmwh.12399

Bovbjerg, M. L., Cheyney, M., & Everson, C. (2016). Maternal and newborn outcomes following waterbirth: The Midwives Alliance of North America statistics project, 2004 to 2009 cohort. *Journal of Midwifery & Women's Health, 61*(1), 11–20. https://doi.org/10.1111/jmwh.12394

Brouwer, E., Knol, R., Kroushev, A., Van Den Akker, T., Hooper, S. B., Roest, A. A., & Te Pas, A. B. (2022). Effect of breathing on venous return during delayed cord clamping: An observational study. *Archives of Disease in Childhood—Fetal & Neonatal Edition, 107*(1), 65–69. https://doi.org/10.1136/archdischild-2020-321431

BruceBlaus [Screen name]. (2015, November 12). Neonatal heart circulation [Graphic]. Retrieved from https://commons.wikimedia.org/wiki/File:-Neonatal_Heart_Circulation.png

BruceBlaus [Screen name]. (2016, October 3). CPR infant closed vs open airway [Graphic]. Retrieved from https://commons.wikimedia.org/wiki/File:CPR_Infant_Closed_vs_Open_Airway.png

Burns, E. E., Boulton, M. G., Cluett, E., Cornelius, V. R., & Smith, L. A. (2012). Characteristics, interventions, and outcomes of women who used a birthing pool: A prospective observational study. *Birth, 39*(3), 192–202. https://doi.org/10.1111/j.1523-536X.2012.00548.x

Byrne, B. J., Patel, R. S., Johnson, C. S., & Wetzel, E. A. (2017). Which airway and vascular access procedures should new neonatal resuscitation program trainees be taught? *Open Journal of Pediatrics & Neonatal Care, 2*(2), 31–37. Retrieved from https://web.archive.org/web/20220615120348/http://scireslit.com/Pediatrics/OJPNC-ID17.pdf

Cahill, A. G. (2021). Intrapartum fetal evaluation. In M. B. Landon, H. L. Galan, E. R. M. Jauniaux, D. A. Driscoll, V. Berghella, W. A. Grobman, . . . A. G. Cahill (Eds.), *Gabbe's obstetrics: Normal and problem pregnancies* (8th ed., Kindle version, ch. 15). Philadelphia, PA: Elsevier.

Caridi, B. J., Bolnick, J. M., Fletcher, B. G., & Rayburn, W. F. (2004). Effect of halogen light stimulation on nonstress testing. *American Journal of Obstetrics & Gynecology, 190*(5), 1470–1472. https://doi.org/10.1016/j.ajog.2004.02.031

Carmichael, A., McCullough, S., & Kempley, S. T. (2007). Critical dependence of acetate thermal mattress on gel activation temperature. *Archives of Disease in Childhood—Fetal and Neonatal Edition, 92*(1), F44-45. https://doi.org/10.1136/adc.2006.096297

Carvalho, O. M. C., Augusto, M. C. C., Medeiros, M. Q., Lima, H. M. P., Viana, A. B., Jr., Araujo, E., Jr., & Carvalho, F. H. C. (2019). Late umbilical cord clamping does not increase rates of jaundice and the need for phototherapy in pregnancies at normal risk. *Journal of Maternal-Fetal & Neonatal Medicine, 32*(22), 3824–3829. https://doi.org/10.1080/14767058.2018.1473367

Castle, N. (2018). Neonatal and maternal resuscitation. In V. Chapman & C. Charles (Eds.), *The midwife's labour and birth handbook* (4th ed., pp. 339–352). Hoboken, NJ: John Wiley & Sons.

Centers for Disease Control and Prevention. (2023). *Critical congenital heart defects screening methods*. Retrieved from https://www.cdc.gov/ncbddd/heartdefects/hcp.html

Champlain Maternal Newborn Regional Program. (2013). *Newborn thermoregulation: Self-learning module*. Retrieved from http://www.cmnrp.ca/uploads/documents/Newborn_Thermoregulation_SLM_2013_06.pdf

Charpak, N., Gabriel Ruiz, J., Zupan, J., Cattaneo, A., Figueroa, Z., Tessier, R., . . . Worku, B. (2005). Kangaroo mother care: 25 years after. *Acta Paediatrica, 94*(5), 514–522. https://doi.org/10.1111/j.1651-2227.2005.tb01930.x

Chawla, S., Amaram, A., Gopal, S. P., & Natarajan, G. (2011). Safety and efficacy of Trans-warmer mattress for preterm neonates: Results of a randomized controlled trial. *Journal of Perinatology, 31*(12), 780–784. https://doi.org/10.1038/jp.2011.33

Chen, X., Li, X., Chang, Y., Li, W., & Cui, H. (2018). Effect and safety of timing of cord clamping on neonatal hematocrit values and clinical outcomes in term infants: A randomized controlled trial. *Journal of Perinatology, 38*, 251–257. https://doi.org/10.1038/s41372-017-0001-y

Chi Luong, K., Long Nguyen, T., Huyn Thi, D. H., Carrara, H. P., & Bergman, N. J. (2016). Newly born low birthweight infants stabilise better in skin-to-skin contact than when separated from their mothers: A randomisedcontrolled trial. *Acta Paediatrica, 105*(4), 381–390. https://doi.org/10.1111/apa.13164

Chuey, M., De Vries, R., Dal Cin, S., & Low, L. K. (2020). Maternity providers' perspectives on barriers to utilization of intermittent fetal monitoring. *Journal of Perinatal & Neonatal Nursing, 34*(1), 46–55. https://doi.org/10.1097/JPN.0000000000000453

Cluett, E. R., Burns, E., & Cuthbert, A. (2018). Immersion in water during labour and birth. *Cochrane Database of Systematic Reviews*. https://doi.org/10.1002/14651858.CD000111.pub4

Commission for the Accreditation of Birth Centers. (2020). *Indicators of compliance with standards for birth centers* (reference ed. 2.2). St. Paul, MN: Author. Retrieved from https://www.birthcenteraccreditation.org/go/get-cabc-indicators/

Cunningham, F. G., Leveno, K. J., Dashe, J. S., Hoffman, B. L., Spong, C. Y., & Casey, B. M. (Eds.). (2022). *Williams obstetrics* (26th ed., Kindle version). New York, NY: McGraw-Hill.

Dalsgaard, B. T., Rodrigo-Domingo, M., Kronborg, H., & Haslund, H. (2019). Breastfeeding and skin-to-skin contact as non-pharmacological prevention of neonatal hypoglycemia in infants born to women with gestational diabetes; A Danish quasi-experimental study. *Sexual & Reproductive Healthcare, 19*, 1–8. https://doi.org/10.1016/j.srhc.2018.10.003

Dani, C., & Corsini, I. (2020). Guidelines for management of neonatal hypoglycemia: Are they actually applicable? *JAMA Pediatrics, 174*(7), 638–639. https://doi.org/10.1001/jamapediatrics.2020.0632

Darwin, E. (1796). *Zoonomia; or, the laws of organic life* (Vol. II). London, United Kingdom: J. Johnson. Retrieved from https://ia801204.us.archive.org/13/items/zoonomiaorlawsof11darw/zoonomiaorlawsof11darw.pdf

DeBoer, S., Russell, T., Seaver, M., & Vardi, A. (2008). Infant intraosseous infusion. *Neonatal Network, 27*(1), 25–32. https://doi.org/10.1891/0730-0832.27.1.25

Dehghani, K., Movahed, Z. P., Dehghani, H., & Nasiriani, K. (2015). A randomized controlled trial of kangaroo mother care versus conventional method on vital signs and arterial oxygen saturation rate in newborns who were hospitalized in neonatal intensive care unit. *Journal of Clinical Neonatology, 4*(1), 26–31. https://doi.org/10.4103/2249-4847.151163

Devane, D., Lalor, J. G., Daly, S., McGuire, W., Cuthbert, A., & Smith, V. (2017). Cardiotocography versus intermittent auscultation of fetal heart on admission to labour ward for assessment of fetal wellbeing. *Cochrane Database of Systematic Reviews*. https://doi.org/10.1002/14651858.CD005122.pub5

Di Tommaso, M., Carotenuto, B., Seravalli, V., Magro-Malosso, E. R. M., Pinzauti, S., Torricelli, M., & Petraglia, F. (2019). Evaluation of umbilical cord pulsatility after vaginal delivery in singleton pregnancies at term. *European Journal of Obstetrics & Gynecology and Reproductive Biology, 236*, 94–97. https://doi.org/10.1016/j.ejogrb.2019.03.008

Dore, S., & Ehman, W. (2020). Fetal health surveillance: Intrapartum consensus guideline. *Journal of Obstetrics and Gynaecology Canada, 42*(3), 316–348.e9. https://doi.org/10.1016/j.jogc.2019.05.007

Edwards, T., & Harding, J. E. (2021). Clinical aspects of neonatal hypoglycemia: A mini review. *Frontiers in Pediatrics, 8*. https://doi.org/10.3389/fped.2020.562251

Eichenwald, E. C. (2022). Approach to cyanosis in the newborn. In C. Armsby (Ed.), *UpToDate*. Retrieved June 25, 2023, from https://www.uptodate.com/contents/approach-to-cyanosis-in-the-newborn

Ellemunter, H., Simma, B., Trawöger, R., & Maurer, H. (1999). Intraosseous lines in preterm and full term neonates. *Archives of Disease in Childhood—Fetal and Neonatal Edition, 80*(1), F74–F75. https://doi.org/10.1136/fn.80.1.F74

Ersdal, H. L., Linde, J., Mduma, E., Auestad, B., & Perlman, J. (2014). Neonatal outcome following cord clamping after onset of spontaneous respiration. *Pediatrics, 134*(2), 265–272. https://doi.org/10.1542/peds.2014-0467

Espinoza, J. (2022). Antepartum fetal monitoring. In O. A. Olutoye (Ed.), *Anesthesia for maternal-fetal surgery* (pp. 119–136). Cambridge, United Kingdom: Cambridge University Press.

Farrar, D., Airey, R., Law, G. R., Tuffnell, D., Cattle, B., & Duley, L. (2011). Measuring placental transfusion for term births: Weighing babies with cord intact. *BJOG, 118*(1), 70–75. https://doi.org/10.1111/j.1471-0528.2010.02781.x

Fernandes, C. J. (2021). Physiologic transition from intrauterine to extrauterine life. In C. Armsby (Ed.), *UpToDate*. Retrieved October 30, 2023, from https://www.uptodate.com/contents/physiologic-transition-from-intrauterine-to-extrauterine-life

Fernandes, C. J. (2023). Neonatal resuscitation in the delivery room. In C. Armsby (Ed.), *UpToDate*. Retrieved October 30, 2023, from https://www.uptodate.com/contents/neonatal-resuscitation-in-the-delivery-room

Ferreira, C. R., van Karnebeek, C. D. M., Vockley, J., & Blau, N. (2019). A proposed nosology of inborn errors of metabolism. *Genetics in Medicine, 21*(1), 102–106. https://doi.org/10.1038/s41436-018-0022-8

Fogarty, M., Osborn, D. A., Askie, L., Seidler, A. L., Hunter, K., Lui, K., . . . Tarnow-Mordi, W. (2018). Delayed vs early umbilical cord clamping for preterm infants: A systematic review and Meta-analysis. *American Journal of Obstetrics & Gynecology, 218*(1), 1–18. https://doi.org/10.1016/j.ajog.2017.10.231

Fox, D., Coddington, R., & Scarf, V. (2022). Wanting to be 'with woman', not with machine: Midwives' experiences of caring for women being continuously monitored in labour. *Women and Birth 35*(4), 387–393. https://doi.org/10.1016/j.wombi.2021.09.002

Fraser, D. (2019). Chest and Lung Assessment. In E. P. Tappero & M. E. Honeyfield (Eds.), *Physical assessment of the newborn: A comprehensive approach to the art of physical examination* (6th ed., Kindle version, ch. 6). New York, NY: Springer.

Fraser, D. (2021). Newborn adaptation to extrauterine life. In K. R. Simpson, P. A. Creehan, N. O'Brien-Abel, C. K. Roth, & A. J. Rohan (Eds.), *AWHONN's Perinatal Nursing* (5th ed., pp. 564–578). Philadelphia, PA: Wolters Kluwer.

Fulton, C., Stoll, K., & Thordarson, D. (2016). Bedside resuscitation of newborns with an intact umbilical cord: Experiences of midwives from British Columbia. *Midwifery, 34*, 42–46. https://doi.org/10.1016/j.midw.2016.01.006

Funai, E. F., & Norwitz, E. R. (2023). Labor and delivery: Management of the normal first stage. In V. A. Barss (Ed.), *UpToDate*. Retrieved June 25, 2023, from https://www.uptodate.com/contents/labor-and-delivery-management-of-the-normal-first-stage

Garcia-Prats, J. A. (2023). Meconium aspiration syndrome: Pathophysiology, clinical manifestations, and diagnosis. In C. Armsby (Ed.), *UpToDate*. Retrieved June 25, 2023, from https://www.uptodate.com/contents/meconium-aspiration-syndrome-pathophysiology-clinical-manifestations-and-diagnosis

Gebuza, G., Dombrowska, A., Kaźmierczak, M., Malgorzata, G. & Mieczkowska, E. (2017). The effect of music therapy on the cardiac activity parameters of a fetus in a cardiotocographic examination. *Journal of Maternal-Fetal & Neonatal Medicine, 30*(20), 2440–2445. https://doi.org/10.1080/14767058.2016.1253056

Geissbuehler, V., Stein, S., & Eberhard, J. (2004). Waterbirths compared with landbirths: An observational study of nine years. *Journal of Perinatal Medicine, 32*(4), 308–314. https://doi.org/10.1515/JPM.2004.057

Gibb, B., Gibb, R., & Gibb, M. (1977). Stayin' alive [Recorded by the Bee Gees]. On *Saturday night fever: The original movie soundtrack* [CD]. Baarn, Netherlands: PolyGram Records.

Goldsmith, J. P., & Martin, G. J. (2019). Neonatal resuscitation. In J. P. Phelan (Ed.), *Critical care obstetrics* (6th ed., pp. 193–214). Oxford, United Kingdom: John Wiley & Sons.

Goyal, S., Kortsmit, K., Cox, S., D'Angelo, D. V., Romero, L., Henderson, Z. T., & Barfield, W. D. (2020). Prevalence of home births and associated risk profile and maternal characteristics, 2016–2018. *Obstetrics & Gynecology, 136*(6), 1195–1203. https://doi.org/10.1097/AOG.0000000000004129

Greenberg, M. B., & Druzin, M. L. (2021). Antepartum fetal evaluation. In M. B. Landon, H. L. Galan, E. R. M. Jauniaux, D. A. Driscoll, V. Berghella, W. A. Grobman, . . . A. G. Cahill (Eds.), *Gabbe's obstetrics: Normal and problem pregnancies* (8th ed., Kindle version, ch. 27). Philadelphia, PA: Elsevier.

Harper, B. (2014). Birth, bath, and beyond: The science and safety of water immersion during labor and birth. *Journal of Perinatal Education, 23*(3), 124–134. https://doi.org/10.1891/1058-1243.23.3.124

Henderson, J., Burns, E. E., Regalia, A. L., Casarico G., Boulton M. G., & Smith, L. A. (2014). Labouring women who used a birthing pool in obstetric units in Italy: Prospective observational study. *BMC Pregnancy and Childbirth, 14*, 17. https://doi.org/10.1186/1471-2393-14-17

Hermansen, C. L., & Mahajan, A. (2015). Newborn respiratory distress. *American Family Physician, 92*(11), 994–1002. Retrieved from http://www.aafp.org/afp/2015/1201/p994.html

Hill, M. G., Reed, K. L., Brown, R. N., & Newborn Brain Society Guidelines and Publications Committee. (2021, June). Perinatal asphyxia from the obstetric standpoint. *Seminars in Fetal & Neonatal Medicine, 26*(4), 101259. https://doi.org/10.1016/j.siny.2021.101259

Hirst, B. C. (1899). *A text-book of obstetrics* (2nd ed.). Philadelphia, PA: W. B. Saunders. Retrieved from https://archive.org/details/atextbookobstet05hirsgoog/

Hooper, S. B., te Pas, A. B., Lang, J., van Vonderen, J. J., Roehr, C. C., Kluckow, M., . . . Polglase, G. R. (2015). Cardiovascular transition at birth: A physiological sequence. *Pediatric Research, 77*(5), 608–614. https://doi.org/10.1038/pr.2015.21

Huizing, M. J., Villamor-Martinez, E., Chavagne, I. A., Vanagt, W. Y., Spaanderman, M. A., & Villamor, E. (2017). Reliability and validity of a smartphone-paired pulse oximeter for screening of critical congenital heart defects in newborns. *Neonatology, 112*(4), 324–329. https://doi.org/10.1159/000477294

Hutchon, D. J. (2015). Ventilation before umbilical cord clamping improves physiological transition at birth or "Umbilical cord clamping before ventilation is established destabilizes physiological transition at birth." *Frontiers in Pediatrics, 3*, 29. https://doi.org/10.3389/fped.2015.00029

Ishimine, P. (2009). Approach to the infant with fever. In G. Q. Sharieff & M. McCollough. (Eds.), *Neonatal and infant emergencies* (pp. 105–121). Cambridge, United Kingdom: Cambridge University Press.

Johnson, G. J., Salmanian, B., Denning, S. G., Belfort, M. A., Sundgren, N. C., & Clark, S. L. (2021). Relationship between umbilical cord gas values and neonatal outcomes: Implications for electronic fetal heart rate monitoring. *Obstetrics & Gynecology, 138*(3), 366–373. https://doi.org/10.1097/AOG.0000000000004515

Johnson, K. E. (2021). Transient tachypnea of the newborn. In C. Armsby (Ed.), *UpToDate*. Retrieved June 25, 2023, from https://www.uptodate.com/index.html#!/contents/transient-tachypnea-of-the-newborn

Ju, H., Rumbold, A. R., Willson, K. J., & Crowther, C. A. (2008). Borderline gestational diabetes mellitus and pregnancy outcomes. *BMC Pregnancy and Childbirth, 8*, 31. https://doi.org/10.1186/1471-2393-8-31

Karlsen, K. (2019). *The S.T.A.B.L.E. Program: Post-resuscitation/pre-transport stabilization care of sick infants: Guidelines for neonatal healthcare providers* (6th ed., Kindle version). Park City, UT: S.T.A.B.L.E. Program.

Katheria, A. C., Brown, M. K., Faksh, A., Hassen, K. O., Rich, W., Lazarus, D., . . . Finer, N. N. (2017). Delayed cord clamping in newborns born at term at risk for resuscitation: A feasibility randomized clinical trial. *Journal of Pediatrics, 187*, 313–317.e1. https://doi.org/10.1016/j.jpeds.2017.04.033

Katheria, A. C., Brown, M. K., Rich, W., & Arnell, K. (2017). Providing a placental transfusion in newborns who need resuscitation. *Frontiers in Pediatrics, 5*, 1. https://doi.org/10.3389/fped.2017.00001

Katheria, A. C., Lakshminrusimha, S., Rabe, H., McAdams, R., & Mercer, J. S. (2017). Placental transfusion: A review. *Journal of Perinatology, 37*(2), 105–111. https://doi.org/10.1038/jp.2016.151

Katheria, A., Poeltler, D., Durham, J., Steen, J., Rich, W., Arnell, K., . . . Finer, N. (2016). Neonatal resuscitation with an intact cord: A randomized clinical trial. *Journal of Pediatrics, 178*, 75–80e3. https://doi.org/10.1016/j.jpeds.2016.07.053

Katheria, A. C., Sorki, S., Hassen, K., Faksh, A., Ghorshi, Z., & Poeltler, D. (2018). Acceptability of bedside resuscitation with intact umbilical cord to clinicians and patients' families in the United States. *Frontiers in Pediatrics, 6*, 100. https://doi.org/10.3389/fped.2018.00100

Kemper, A. R., Newman, T. B., Slaughter, J. L., Maisels, M. J., Watchko, J. F., Downs, S. M., . . . Russell, T. L. (2022). Clinical practice guideline revision: Management of hyperbilirubinemia in the newborn infant 35 or more weeks of gestation. *Pediatrics, 150* (3), e2022058859. https://doi.org/10.1542/peds.2022-058859

Khatun, M., Parvin, R., & Naurin, S. (2019). Prediction of perinatal outcome with meconium-stained liquor. *Ibrahim Cardiac Medical Journal, 9*(1–2), 67–73. https://doi.org/10.3329/icmj.v9i1-2.53996

Kissler, K. J., Lowe, N. K., & Hernandez, T. L. (2020). An integrated review of uterine activity monitoring for evaluating labor dystocia. *Journal of Midwifery & Women's Health, 65*(3), 323–334. https://doi.org/10.1111/jmwh.13119

Kluckow, M., & Hooper, S. B. (2015). Using physiology to guide time to cord clamping. *Seminars in Fetal & Neonatal Medicine, 20*(4), 225–231. https://doi.org/10.1016/j.siny.2015.03.002

Korkut, S., Oğuz, Y., Bozkaya, D., Türkmen, G. G., Kara, Ö., Uygur, D., & Oğuz, Ş. S. (2021). Evaluation of the effects of delayed cord clamping in infants of diabetic mothers. *American Journal of Perinatology, 38*(3), 242–247. https://doi.org/10.1055/s-0039-1695799

Kuhl, A., van Calcar, S., Baker, M., Seroogy, C. M., Rice, G., & Schwoerer, J. S. (2017). Development of carrier testing for common inborn errors of metabolism in the Wisconsin Plain population. *Genetics in Medicine, 19*(3), 352–356. https://doi.org/10.1038/gim.2016.104

Lane, P. (2014). *Neonatal resuscitation training for health care providers in the home birth and birth center setting: A proposal for improving neonatal outcomes* (Doctoral dissertation). Frontier Nursing University, Hyden, KY. Retrieved from http://believemidwiferyservices.com/wp-content/uploads/2012/10/Neonatal-Resuscitation-Training-for-Health-Care-Providers-in-the-Home-Birth-and-Birth-Center-Setting.pdf

Langan, M., Watson, C., O'Connor, T., Moore, Z., & Patton, D. (2020). What is the effectiveness of combining warming mattresses and plastic bags versus plastic bags only for thermoregulation in preterm infants? A systematic review. *Journal of Neonatal Nursing, 26*(1), 30–36. https://doi.org/10.1016/j.jnn.2019.09.006

Lanier, A. L., Wiegand, S. L., Fennig, K., Snow, E. K., Maxwell, R. A., McKenna, D. (2021). Neonatal outcomes after delivery in water. *Obstetrics & Gynecology, 138*(4), 622–626 https://doi.org/10.1097/AOG.0000000000004545

Lara-Cantón, I., Badurdeen, S., Dekker, J., Davis, P., Roberts, C., te Pas, A., & Vento, M. (2022). Oxygen saturation and heart rate in healthy term and late preterm infants with delayed cord clamping. *Pediatric Research*. https://doi.org/10.1038/s41390-021-01805-y

Lear, C. A., Westgate, J. A., Bennet, L., Ugwumadu, A., Stone, P. R., Tournier, A., & Gunn, A. J. (2021). Fetal defenses against intrapartum head compression—Implications for intrapartum decelerations and hypoxic-ischemic injury. *American Journal of Obstetrics & Gynecology*. https://doi.org/10.1016/j.ajog.2021.11.1352

Levine, J. C., & Alexander, M. E. (2022). Fetal arrhythmias. In V. A. Barss (Ed.), *UpToDate*. Retrieved June 25, 2023, from https://www.uptodate.com/contents/fetal-arrhythmias

Lewis, D., & Downe, S. (2015). FIGO consensus guidelines on intrapartum fetal monitoring: Intermittent auscultation. *International Journal of Gynecology & Obstetrics, 131*(1), 9–12. https://doi.org/10.1016/j.ijgo.2015.06.019

Liston, R., Sawchuck, D., & Young, D. (2007). Fetal health surveillance: Antepartum and intrapartum consensus guideline (SOGC Clinical Practice Guideline 197, electronic version). *Journal of Obstetrics and Gynaecology Canada, 29*(9, Suppl. 4), S3–S56. Retrieved from https://www.glowm.com/pdf/Fetal health surveillance antepartum and intrapartum Consensus Guideline.pdf

Liu, Y., Liu, Y., Huang, X., Du, C., Peng, J., Huang, P., & Zhang, J. (2014). A comparison of maternal and neonatal outcomes between water immersion during labor and conventional labor and delivery. *BMC Pregnancy Childbirth, 14*, 160. https://doi.org/10.1186/1471-2393-14-160

Liu, Y.-Q., Lei, M. J., Liu, T. T., Li, Y. F., Cui, C. Y., Ni, L. J., & Jin, C. D. (2018). Efficacy and safety of the heated gel mattress for prevention of hypothermia in preterm infants during intra-hospital transport: A meta-analysis. *TMR Integrative Nursing, 2*(3), 132–140. https://doi.org/10.12032/TMRIN20180717

Lukasse, M., Rowe, R., Townend, J., Knight, M., & Hollowell, J. (2014). Immersion in water for pain relief and the risk of intrapartum transfer among low risk nulliparous women: Secondary analysis of the Birthplace national prospective cohort study. *BMC Pregnancy and Childbirth, 14*, 60. https://doi.org/10.1186/1471-2393-14-60

Lyons, P., & McLaughlin, N. (2020). Fetal heart rate monitoring. In P. Lyons & N. McLaughlin (Eds.), *Obstetrics in family medicine: A practical guide* (3rd ed., pp. 197–201). Cham, Switzerland: Humana Press. https://doi.org/10.1007/978-3-030-39888-0_27

Macones, G. (2022). Intrapartum category I, II, and III fetal heart rate tracings: Management. In V. A. Barss (Ed.), *UpToDat*e. Retrieved June 25, 2023, from https://www.uptodate.com/contents/intrapartum-category-i-ii-and-iii-fetal-heart-rate-tracings-management

Macones, G. A., Hankins, G. D., Spong, C. Y., Hauth, J., & Moore, T. (2008). The 2008 National Institute of Child Health and Human Development workshop report on electronic fetal monitoring: Update on definitions, interpretation, and research guidelines. *Obstetrics & Gynecology, 112*(3), 661–666. https://doi.org/10.1097/AOG.0b013e3181841395

Madar, J., Roehr, C. C., Ainsworth, S., Ersdal, H., Morley, C., Rüdiger, M., . . . Wyllie, J. P. (2021). European Resuscitation Council guidelines 2021: Newborn resuscitation and support of transition of infants at birth. *Resuscitation, 161*, 291–326. https://doi.org/10.1016/j.resuscitation.2021.02.014

Martis, R., Emilia, O., Nurdiati, D. S., & Brown, J. (2017). Intermittent auscultation (IA) of fetal heart rate in labour for fetal well-being. *Cochrane Database of Systematic Reviews*. https://doi.org/10.1002/14651858.CD008680.pub2

Mata-Peréz, A., Soto-Martínez, M., & Yock-Corrales, A. (2016). A practical approach to emergencies in the neonatal period. *Journal of Neonatal Biology, 5*(1), 1000213. https://www.walshmedicalmedia.com/open-access/a-practical-approach-to-emergencies-in-the-neonatal-period-2167-0897-1000213.pdf

Maude, R. M., Skinner, J. P., & Foureur, M. J. (2016). Putting intelligent structured intermittent auscultation (ISIA) into practice. *Women and Birth, 29*(3), 285–292. https://doi.org/10.1016/j.wombi.2015.12.001

Maul, H., Maner, W. L., Olson, G., Saade, G. R., & Garfield, R. E. (2004). Non-invasive transabdominal uterine electromyography correlates with the strength of intrauterine pressure and is predictive of labor and delivery. *Journal of Maternal-Fetal & Neonatal Medicine, 15*(5), 297–301. https://doi.org/10.1080/14767050410001695301

McAdams, R. M., Fay, E., & Delaney, S. (2018). Whole blood volumes associated with milking intact and cut umbilical cords in term newborns. *Journal of Perinatology, 38*(3), 245–250. https://doi.org/10.1038/s41372-017-0002-x

McDonald, S. J., Middleton, P., Dowswell, T., & Morris, P. S. (2014). Effect of timing of umbilical cord clamping of term infants on maternal and neonatal outcomes. *Evidence-Based Child Health, 9*(2), 303–397. https://doi.org/10.1002/ebch.1971

McKee-Garrett, T. M. (2023). Assessment of the newborn infant. In C. Armsby (Ed.), *UpToDate*. Retrieved October 30, 2023, from https://www.uptodate.com/contents/assessment-of-the-newborn-infant

Mdoe, P. F., Ersdal, H. L., Mduma, E., Moshiro, R., Kidanto, H., & Mbekenga, C. (2018). Midwives' perceptions on using a fetoscope and Doppler for fetal heart rate assessments during labor: A qualitative study in rural Tanzania. *BMC Pregnancy and Childbirth, 18*(1), 103. https://doi.org/10.1186/s12884-018-1736-y

Mercer, J. S., & Erickson-Owens, D. A. (2012). Rethinking placental transfusion and cord clamping issues. *Journal of Perinatal & Neonatal Nursing, 26*(3), 202–217. https://doi.org/10.1097/JPN.0b013e31825d2d9a

Mercer, J. S., & Erickson-Owens, D. A. (2014). Is it time to rethink cord management when resuscitation is needed? *Journal of Midwifery & Women's Health, 59*(6), 635–644. https://doi.org/10.1111/jmwh.12206

Mercer, J., Erickson-Owens, D., & Skovgaard, R. (2009). Cardiac asystole at birth: Is hypovolemic shock the cause? *Medical Hypotheses, 72*(4), 458–463. https://doi.org/10.1016/j.mehy.2008.11.019

Mercer, J. S., Nelson, C. C., & Skovgaard, R. L. (2011). Umbilical cord clamping: Beliefs and practices of American nurse-midwives. *Journal of Midwifery & Women's Health, 45*(1), 58–66. https://doi.org/10.1016/s1526-9523(99)00004-5

Miller, D. A. (2022). Intrapartum fetal heart rate monitoring: Overview. In V. A. Barss (Ed.), *UpToDate*. Retrieved October 30, 2023, from https://www.uptodate.com/contents/intrapartum-fetal-heart-rate-monitoring-overview

Miller, D. A. (2023). Nonstress test and contraction stress test. In A. Chakrabarti (Ed.), *UpToDate*. Retrieved October 30, 2023, from https://www.uptodate.com/contents/nonstress-test-and-contraction-stress-test

Miller, K. K., Vig, K. S., Goetz, E. M., Spicer, G., Yang, A. J., & Hokanson, J. S. (2016). Pulse oximetry screening for critical congenital heart disease in planned out of hospital births and the incidence of critical congenital heart disease in the Plain community. *Journal of Perinatology, 36* (12), 1088–1091. https://doi.org/10.1038/jp.2016.135

Miller, L. A., Miller, D., & Cypher, R. L. (2022). *Mosby's pocket guide to fetal monitoring: A multidisciplinary approach* (9th ed., e-book). St. Louis, MO: Elsevier.

A model practice template for hydrotherapy in labor and birth. (2017). *Journal of Midwifery & Women's Health, 62*(1), 120–126. https://doi.org/10.1111/jmwh.12587

Mohamed, S. (2011). Recognition and diagnostic approach to acute metabolic disorders in the neonatal period. *Sudanese Journal of Paediatrics, 11*(1), 20–8. Retrieved from https://www.ncbi.nlm.nih.gov/pmc/articles/PMC4949777/

Mohammad, N., Jamal, T., Sohaila, A., & Ali, S. R. (2018). Meconium stained liquor and its neonatal outcome. *Pakistan Journal of Medical Sciences, 34*(6), 1392–1396. https://doi.org/10.12669/pjms.346.15349

Mohan, M., Ramawat, J., La Monica, G., Jayaram, P., Fattah, S. A., Learmont, J., . . . Lindow, S. (2021). Electronic intrapartum fetal monitoring: A systematic review of international clinical practice guidelines. *AJOG Global Reports, 1*(2), 100008. https://doi.org/10.1016/j.xagr.2021.100008

Muchowski, K. E. (2014). Evaluation and treatment of neonatal hyperbilirubinemia. *American Family Physician, 89*(11), 873–878. Retrieved from http://www.aafp.org/afp/2014/0601/p873.pdf

Mullany, L. C. (2010). Neonatal hypothermia in low-resource settings. *Seminars in Perinatology, 34*(6), 426–433. https://doi.org/10.1053/j.semperi.2010.09.007

Murphy, P. J. (2005). The fetal circulation. *Continuing Education in Anaesthesia Critical Care & Pain, 5*(4), 107–112. https://doi.org/10.1093/bjaceaccp/mki030

Nadkarni, K. P., Mayo, Z., Laux, J. P., McRea, A., Angelillo, D., Meitzen, R., . . . Lohr, J. A. (2021). Axillary thermometry demonstrates greater reliability compared with rectal thermometry in healthy neonates. *Clinical Pediatrics, 60*(6–7), 298–303. https://doi.org/10.1177/00099228211005293

Narayen, I. C., Blom, N. A., Bourgonje, M. S., Haak, M. C., Smit, M., Posthumus, F., . . . te Pas, A. B. (2016). Pulse oximetry screening for critical congenital heart disease after home birth and early discharge. *Journal of Pediatrics, 170*, 188–192.e1. https://doi.org/10.1016/j.jpeds.2015.12.004

Narayen, I. C., Blom, N. A., van Geloven, N., Blankman, E. I., van den Broek, A. J., Bruijn, M., . . . te Pas, A. B. (2018). Accuracy of pulse oximetry screening for critical congenital heart defects after home birth and early postnatal discharge. *Journal of Pediatrics*, 197, 29–35.e1. https://doi.org/10.1016/j.jpeds.2018.01.039

Narvey, M. R., & Marks, S. D. (2019). The screening and management of newborns at risk for low blood glucose. *Paediatrics & Child Health, 24*(8), 536–554. https://doi.org/10.1093/pch/pxz134

Nelson, K. B., Dambrosia, J. M., Ting, T. Y., & Grether, J. K. (1996). Uncertain value of electronic fetal monitoring in predicting cerebral palsy. *New England Journal of Medicine, 334*(10), 613–618. https://doi.org/10.1056/NEJM199603073341001

Nguyen, T. T., Kaplan, P. W., & Wilfong, A. (2021). Nonepileptic paroxysmal disorders in infancy. In J. F. Dashe, (Ed.), *UpToDate*. Retrieved October 30, 2023, from https://www.uptodate.com/contents/nonepileptic-paroxysmal-disorders-in-infancy

[NICE] National Institute for Health and Care Excellence. (2022). *Fetal monitoring in labour* (NICE Guideline NG229). Retrieved from https://www.nice.org.uk/guidance/ng229

Niermeyer, S., & Velaphi, S. (2013). Promoting physiologic transition at birth: Re-examining resuscitation and the timing of cord clamping. *Seminars in Fetal & Neonatal Medicine, 18*(6), 385–392. https://doi.org/10.1016/j.siny.2013.08.008

Norman, J. E., Heazell, A. E. P., Rodriguez, A., Weir, C. J., Stock, S. J., Calderwood C. J., . . . Whyte, S. (2018). Awareness of fetal movements and care package to reduce fetal mortality (AFFIRM): A stepped wedge, cluster-randomised trial. *Lancet, 392*(10158),1629–1638. https://doi.org/10.1016/S0140-6736(18)31543-5

North American Registry of Midwives. (2021). *NARM NRP policy update May 2021*. Retrieved from https://narm.org/2021/05/narm-nrp-policy-update-may-2021/

Olusanya, B. O., Kaplan, M., & Hansen, T. W. (2018). Neonatal hyperbilirubinaemia: A global perspective. *Lancet Child & Adolescent Health, 2*(8), 610–620. https://doi.org/10.1016/S2352-4642(18)30139-1

Ortiz-Esquinas, I., Rodríguez-Almagro, J., Gómez-Salgado, J., Arias-Arias, Á., Ballesta-Castillejos, A., & Hernández-Martínez, A. (2020). Effects of cord milking in late preterm infants and full-term infants: A systematic review and meta-analysis. *Birth, 47*(3), 259–269. 41. https://doi.org/10.1111/birt.12500

Oster, M. (2023). Newborn screening for critical congenital heart disease using pulse oximetry. In C. Armsby (Ed.), *UpToDate*. Retrieved October 30, 2023, from https://www.uptodate.com/index.html#!/contents/newborn-screening-for-critical-congenital-heart-disease-using-pulse-oximetry

Patay, Z. (2005). Metabolic disorders. In P. Tortori-Donati, A. Rossi, & R. Biacheri (Eds.), *Pediatric neuroradiology: Brain* (pp. 543–721). Berlin, Germany: Springer.

Patterson, J., North, K., Dempsey, E., Ishoso, D., Trevisanuto, D., Lee, A. C. C., & Kamath-Rayne, B. D. (2021). Optimizing initial neonatal resuscitation to reduce neonatal encephalopathy around the world. *Seminars in Fetal & Neonatal Medicine, 26*(4), 101262. https://doi.org/10.1016/j.siny.2021.101262

Pinette, M. G., Wax, J., & Wilson, E. (2004). The risks of underwater birth. *American Journal of Obstetrics & Gynecology, 190*(5), 1211–1215. https://doi.org/10.1016/j.ajog.2003.12.007

Polnaszek, B., López, J. D., Clark, R., Raghuraman, N., Macones, G. A., & Cahill, A. G. (2020). Marked variability in intrapartum electronic fetal heart rate patterns: Association with neonatal morbidity and abnormal arterial cord gas. *Journal of Perinatology, 40*(1), 56–62. https://doi.org//10.1038/s41372-019-0520-9

Qattea, I., Farghaly, M. A. A., Elgendy, M., Mohamed, M. A., & Aly, H. (2022). Neonatal hyperbilirubinemia and bilirubin neurotoxicity in hospitalized neonates: Analysis of the US Database. *Pediatric Research, 91*, 1662–1668. https://doi.org/10.1038/s41390-021-01692-3

Qian, Y., Lu, Q., Shao, H., Ying, X., Huang, W., & Hua, Y. (2020). Timing of umbilical cord clamping and neonatal jaundice in singleton term pregnancy. *Early Human Development, 142*. https://doi.org/10.1016/j.earlhumdev.2019.104948

Raghuraman, N., López, J. D., Carter, E. B., Stout, M. J., Macones, G. A., Tuuli, M. G., & Cahill, A. G. (2020). The effect of intrapartum oxygen supplementation on category II fetal monitoring. *American Journal of Obstetrics & Gynecology, 223*(6), 905.e1–905.e7. https://doi.org/10.1016/j.ajog.2020.06.037

Raghuraman, N., Wan, L., Temming, L. A., Woolfolk, C., Macones, G. A., Tuuli, M. G., & Cahill, A. G. (2018). Effect of oxygen vs room air on intrauterine fetal resuscitation: A randomized noninferiority clinical trial. *JAMA Pediatrics, 172*(9), 818–823. https://doi.org/10.1001/jamapediatrics.2018.1208

Raghuveer, T. S., Garg, U., & Graf, W. D. (2006). Inborn errors of metabolism in infancy and early childhood: An update. *American Family Physician, 73*(11), 1981–1990. Retrieved from https://www.aafp.org/afp/2006/0601/p1981.html

Rahimikian, F., Rahiminia, T., Modarres, M., & Mehran, A. (2013). Comparison of halogen light and vibroacoustic stimulation on nonreactive fetal heart rate pattern. *Iranian Journal of Nursing and Midwifery Research, 18*(2), 112. Retrieved from https://www.ncbi.nlm.nih.gov/pmc/articles/PMC3748565/

Rajani, A. K., Chitkara, R., Oehlert, J., & Halamek, L. P. (2011). Comparison of umbilical venous and intraosseous access during simulated neonatal resuscitation. *Pediatrics, 128*(4), e954–e958. https://doi.org/10.1542/peds.2011-0657

Rana, N., Ranneberg, L. J., Målqvist, M., Ashish, K. C., & Andersson, O. (2020). Delayed cord clamping was not associated with an increased risk of hyperbilirubinaemia on the day of birth or jaundice in the first 4 weeks. *Acta Paediatrica, 109*(1), 71–77. https://doi.org/10.1111/apa.14913

Read, B. (2018). Fetal heart rate monitoring in labour. In V. Chapman & C. Charles (Eds.), *The midwife's labour and birth handbook* (4th ed., pp. 61–74). Hoboken, NJ: John Wiley & Sons.

Reis, P. J., & Bell, T. (2024). Neonatal care. In J. Phillippi & I. Kantrowitz-Gordon (Eds.), *Varney's midwifery* (7th ed., Kindle version, ch. 39). Burlington, MA: Jones & Bartlett Learning.

Resuscitation Council UK. (2011). Equipment used in homebirth. Retrieved from https://www.resus.org.uk/library/quality-standards-cpr/equipment-used-homebirth

Robinson, B. (2008). A review of NICHD standardized nomenclature for cardiotocography: The importance of speaking a common language when describing electronic fetal monitoring. *Reviews in Obstetrics and Gynecology, 1*(2), 56–60. Retrieved from https://www.ncbi.nlm.nih.gov/pmc/articles/PMC2505172/

Roehr, C. C., Schmölzer, G. M., Thio, M., Dawson, J. A., Dold, S. K., Schmalisch, G., & Davis, P. G. (2014). How ABBA may help improve neonatal resuscitation training: Auditory prompts to enable coordination of manual inflations and chest compressions. *Journal of Paediatrics and Child Health, 50*(6), 444–448. https://doi.org/10.1111/jpc.12507

Rohan, A. J. (2021). Newborn adaptation to extrauterine life. In K. R. Simpson, P. A. Creehan, N. O'Brien-Abel, C. K. Roth, & A. J. Rohan (Eds.), *AWHONN's Perinatal Nursing* (5th ed., pp. 651–688). Philadelphia, PA: Wolters Kluwer.

Romano, A. M., & Buxton, M. (2020). A multimethod improvement project to strengthen intermittent auscultation practice among nurse-midwives and nurses. *Journal of Midwifery & Women's Health, 65*(3), 362–369. https://doi.org/10.1111/jmwh.13113

Royal Australian and New Zealand College of Obstetricians and Gynaecologists. (2019). *Intrapartum fetal surveillance: Clinical guideline* (4th ed.). East Melbourne, Australia: Author. Retrieved from https://ranzcog.edu.au/wp-content/uploads/2022/05/Intrapartum-Fetal-Surveillance.pdf

Royal College of Obstetricians and Gynaecologists. (2015). *Intermittent auscultation: Key recommendations*. Retrieved from https://www.rcog.org.uk/en/guidelines-research-services/audit-quality-improvement/each-baby-counts/ebc-2015-report/fetal-monitoring/intermittent-auscultation/recommendations-intermittent-auscultation/

Rozance, P. J. (2023). Pathogenesis, screening, and diagnosis of neonatal hypoglycemia. In C. Armsby (Ed.), *UpToDate*. Retrieved October 30, 2023, from https://www.uptodate.com/contents/pathogenesis-screening-and-diagnosis-of-neonatal-hypoglycemia

Rozance, P. J., & Wright, C. J. (2021). The neonate. In M. B. Landon, H. L. Galan, E. R. M. Jauniaux, D. A. Driscoll, V. Berghella, W. A. Grobman, . . . A. G. Cahill (Eds.), *Gabbe's obstetrics: Normal and problem pregnancies* (8th ed., Kindle version, ch. 23). Philadelphia, PA: Elsevier.

Sartwelle, T. P., Johnston, J. C., Arda, B., & Zebenigus, M. (2021). Electronic fetal monitoring in the twenty-first century: Language, logic and Lewis Carroll. *Clinical Ethics, 16*(3), 213–221. https://doi.org/10.1177/1477750920971800

Sawyer, T., Foglia, E., Hatch, L. D., Moussa, A., Ades, A., Johnston, L., & Nishisaki, A. (2017). Improving neonatal intubation safety: A journey of a thousand miles. *Journal of Neonatal-Perinatal Medicine, 10*(2), 125–131. https://doi.org/10.3233/NPM-171686

Schafer, R. (2014). Umbilical cord avulsion in waterbirth. *Journal of Midwifery & Women's Health, 59*(1), 91–94. https://doi.org/10.1111/jmwh.12157

Schuppener, L. M., & Corliss, R. F. (2020). Infant death following home birth: A case report of fatal neonatal hypoglycemia. *Journal of Forensic Sciences, 65*(3), 995–998. https://doi.org/10.1111/1556-4029.14247

Schwindt, E., Pfeiffer, D., Gomes, D., Brenner, S., Schwindt, J.-C., Hoffmann F., & Olivieri, M. (2022). Intraosseous access in neonates is feasible and safe—An analysis of a prospective nationwide surveillance study in Germany. *Frontiers in Pediatrics, 10*. https://doi.org/10.3389/fped.2022.952632

Scrivens, A., Reynolds, P. R., Emery, F. E., Roberts, C. T., Polglase, G. R., Hooper, S. B., & Roehr, C. C. (2019). Use of intraosseous needles in neonates: A systematic review. *Neonatology, 116*(4), 305–314. https://doi.org/10.1159/000502212

Shaw-Battista, J. (2017). Systematic review of hydrotherapy research: Does a warm bath in labor promote normal physiologic childbirth? *Journal of Perinatal & Neonatal Nursing, 31*(4), 303–316. https://doi.org/10.1097/JPN.0000000000000260

Shellhaas, R. (2023). Clinical features, evaluation, and diagnosis of neonatal seizures. In J. F. Dashe, (Ed.), *UpToDate*. Retrieved October 30, 2023, from https://www.uptodate.com/contents/clinical-features-evaluation-and-diagnosis-of-neonatal-seizures

Shinohara, E., & Kataoka, Y. (2021). Prevalence and risk factors for hyperbilirubinemia among newborns from a low-risk birth setting using delayed cord clamping in Japan. *Japan Journal of Nursing Science, 18*(1), e12372. https://doi.org/10.1111/jjns.12372

Sholapurkar, S. L. (2022). Intermittent auscultation (surveillance) of fetal heart rate in labor: A progressive evidence-backed approach with aim to improve methodology, reliability and safety. *Journal of Maternal-Fetal & Neonatal Medicine, 35*(15), 2942–2948. https://doi.org/10.1080/14767058.2020.1811664

Snapp, C., Stapleton, S., Wright, J., Niemczyk, N., & Jolles, D. (2020). The experience of land and water birth within the American Association of Birth Centers perinatal data registry, 2012–2017. *Journal of Perinatal & Neonatal Nursing, 34*(1), 16–26. https://doi.org/10.1097/JPN.0000000000000450

Suominen, P., Nurmi, E., & Lauerma, K. (2015). Intraosseous access in neonates and infants: Increased risk of compartment syndrome and leg amputation. *Resuscitation, 96* (Suppl. 1), 131–132. https://doi.org/10.1016/j.resuscitation.2015.09.313

Tan, S. (2023). Etiology and pathogenesis of neonatal encephalopathy. In J. F. Dashe (Ed.), *UpToDate*. Retrieved October 30, 2023, from https://www.uptodate.com/contents/etiology-and-pathogenesis-of-neonatal-encephalopathy

Taylor, H., Kleine, I., Bewley, S., Loucaides, E., & Sutcliffe, A. (2016). Neonatal outcomes of waterbirth: A systematic review and meta-analysis. *Archives of Disease in Childhood—Fetal and Neonatal Edition, 101*(4), F357–F365. https://doi.org/10.1136/archdischild-2015-309600

Thoeni, A., Zech, N., Moroder, L., & Ploner, F. (2005). Review of 1600 water-births. Does water birth increase the risk of neonatal infection? *Journal of Maternal-Fetal & Neonatal Medicine, 17*(5), 357–361. https://doi.org/10.1080/14767050500140388

Trevisanuto, D., Cavallin, F., Nguyen, L. N., Nguyen, T. V., Tran, L. D., Tran, C. D., . . . Moccia, L. (2015). Supreme laryngeal mask airway versus face mask during neonatal resuscitation: A randomized controlled trial. *Journal of Pediatrics, 167*(2), 286–291.e1. https://doi.org/10.1016/j.jpeds.2015.04.051

Turner, J. M., Mitchell, M. D., & Kumar, S. S. (2020). The physiology of intrapartum fetal compromise at term. *American Journal of Obstetrics & Gynecology, 222*(1), 17–26. https://doi.org/10.1016/j.ajog.2019.07.032

Ullah, S., Rahman, K., & Hedayati, M. (2016). Hyperbilirubinemia in neonates: Types, Causes, clinical examinations, preventive measures and treatments: A narrative review article. *Iranian Journal of Public Health, 45*(5), 558–568. Retrieved from https://www.ncbi.nlm.nih.gov/pmc/articles/PMC4935699/

Ulvaeus, B., Andersson, B., & Andersson, S. (1975). SOS [Recorded by ABBA]. On *ABBA* [CD]. New York, NY: Atlantic Records. (1974).

Valarezo, V., Powel, J. E., Benito, C., & Yates, J. (2019). Outcomes of water immersion during the second stage of labor. *Obstetrics & Gynecology, 133*, 54S. https://doi.org/10.1097/01.AOG.0000559003.81801.6b

van Rheenen, P. F., & Brabin, B. J. (2006). A practical approach to timing cord clamping in resource poor settings. *BMJ, 333*(7575), 954–958. https://doi.org/10.1136/bmj.39002.389236.BE

Vedam, S., Goff, M., & Nolan-Marnin, V. (2007). Closing the theory–practice gap: Intrapartum midwifery management of planned homebirths. *Journal of Midwifery & Women's Health, 52*(3), 291–300. https://doi.org/10.1016/j.jmwh.2007.02.013

Wackernagel, D., Gustafsson, A., Edstedt Bonamy, A.-K., Reims, A., Ahlsson, F., Elfving, M., . . . Hansen Pupp, I. (2020). Swedish national guideline for prevention and treatment of neonatal hypoglycaemia in newborn infants with gestational age ≥35 weeks. *Acta Paediatrica, 109*(1), 31–44. https://doi.org/10.1111/apa.14955

Wang, J., Tao, E., Mo, M., Ding, W., Yuan, J., Wang, M., . . . Zheng, H. (2021). Perinatal risk factors influencing neonatal hypoxic ischemic encephalopathy in southern China: A case–control study. *American Journal of Perinatology, 38*(Suppl. 1), e182–e186. https://doi.org/10.1055/s-0040-1708884

Wanous, A. A., Wey, A., Rudser, K. D., & Roberts, K. D. (2017). Feasibility of laryngeal mask airway device placement in neonates. *Neonatology, 111*(3), 222–227. https://doi.org/10.1159/000450691

Ward, C., & Caughey, A. B. (2022). The risk of meconium aspiration syndrome (MAS) increases with gestational age at term. *Journal of Maternal-Fetal & Neonatal Medicine, 35*(1), 155–160. https://doi.org/10.1080/14767058.2020.1713744

Watterberg, K., & Committee on Fetus and Newborn. (2020). Providing care for infants born at home. *Pediatrics, 145*(5), e20200626. https://doi.org/10.1542/peds.2020-0626

Weiner, G. M., & Zaichkin, J. (Eds.). (2021). *Textbook of neonatal resuscitation* (8th ed.). Itasca, IL: American Academy of Pediatrics.

Welsh, S., Elwell, J., Manister, N. N., & Gildersleeve, R. K. (2020). Implementing delayed umbilical cord clamping in cesarean birth using a novel method: A pilot study of feasibility and safety. *Journal of Midwifery & Women's Health, 65*(1), 109–118. https://doi.org/10.1111/jmwh.13075

Whitehurst, R. M. (2020). ABO incompatibility. In T. L. Gomella, F. G. Eyal, & F. Bany-Mohammed (Eds.), *Gomella's neonatology: Management, procedures, on-call problems, diseases, and drugs* (8th ed.). New York, NY: McGraw-Hill. Retrieved from https://accesspediatrics.mhmedical.com/content.aspx?bookid=2762&sectionid=234452607

Widström, A. M., Brimdyr, K., Svensson, K., Cadwell, K., & Nissen, E. (2019). Skin-to-skin contact the first hour after birth, underlying implications and clinical practice. *Acta Paediatrica, 108*(7), 1192–1204. https://doi.org/10.1111/apa.14754

Wight, N. E., & Academy of Breastfeeding Medicine. (2021). ABM clinical protocol #1: guidelines for glucose monitoring and treatment of hypoglycemia in term and late preterm neonates, revised 2021. *Breastfeeding Medicine, 16*(5), 353–365. https://doi.org/10.1089/bfm.2021.29178.new

Williams, K. B., Horst, M., Hollinger, E. A., Freedman, J., Demczko, M. M., & Chodhury, D. (2021). Newborn pulse oximetry for infants born out-of-hospital. *Pediatrics, 48*(4), e2020048785. https://doi.org/10.1542/peds.2020-048785

Withrow, E., Fussman, C., Thompson, K., & Kleyn, M. (2019). Evaluation of pulse oximetry screening rates among the midwife-attended out-of-hospital birth community in Michigan. *Journal of Midwifery & Women's Health, 64*(4), 421–426. https://doi.org/10.1111/jmwh.12958

Wolf, M. F., Childers, J., Gray, K. D., Chivily, C., Glenn, M., Jones, L., . . . Greenberg, R. G. (2020). Exchange transfusion safety and outcomes in neonatal hyperbilirubinemia. *Journal of Perinatology, 40*, 1506–1512 https://doi.org/10.1038/s41372-020-0642-0

Wong, R. J., & Bhutani, V. K. (2022). Unconjugated hyperbilirubinemia in neonates: Etiology and pathogenesis. In C. Armsby (Ed.), *UpToDate*. Retrieved October 30, 2023, from https://www.uptodate.com/contents/unconjugated-hyperbilirubinemia-in-neonates-etiology-and-pathogenesis

World Health Organization. (1997). *Thermal protection of the newborn: A practical guide*. Report WHO/RHT/MSM/97.2. Geneva, Switzerland: World Health Organization. Retrieved from https://apps.who.int/iris/bitstream/handle/10665/63986/WHO_RHT_MSM_97.2.pdf

World Health Organization. (n.d.). *Optimal timing of cord clamping for the prevention of iron deficiency anaemia in infants*. Retrieved from https://www.who.int/elena/titles/full_recommendations/cord_clamping/en/

Wu, K., & Stapleton, R. (2017). Newborn discharge timing. In B. J. Snell & S. L. Gardner (Eds.), *Care of the well newborn* (Kindle version, ch. 7). Burlington, MA: Jones & Bartlett.

Wu, Y. (2023). Clinical features, diagnosis, and treatment of neonatal encephalopathy. In J. F. Dashe (Ed.), *UpToDate*. Retrieved October 30, 2023, from https://www.uptodate.com/contents/clinical-features-diagnosis-and-treatment-of-neonatal-encephalopathy

Wyllie, J., Bruinenberg, J., Roehr, C. C., Rüdiger, M., Trevisanuto, D., & Urlesberger, B. (2015). European Resuscitation Council guidelines for resuscitation 2015, Section 7: Resuscitation and support of transition of babies at birth. *Resuscitation, 95*, 249–263. https://doi.org/10.1016/j.resuscitation.2015.07.029

Yang, S., Duffy, J. Y., Johnston, R., Fall, C., & Fitzmaurice, L. E. (2019). Association of a delayed cord-clamping protocol with hyperbilirubinemia in term neonates. *Obstetrics & Gynecology, 133*(4), 754–761. https://doi.org/10.1097/AOG.0000000000003172

Yao, A. C., Moinian, M., & Lind, J. (1969). Distribution of blood between infant and placenta after birth. *Lancet. 294*(7626), 871–873. https://doi.org/10.1016/s0140-6736(69)92328-9

Young, K., & Kruske, S. (2013). How valid are the common concerns raised against water birth? A focused review of the literature. *Women and Birth, 26*(2), 105–109. https://doi.org/10.1016/j.wombi.2012.10.006

Yuan, S. M., & Xu, Z. Y. (2020). Fetal arrhythmias: Prenatal evaluation and intrauterine therapeutics. *Italian Journal of Pediatrics 46*(1), 21. https://doi.org/10.1186/s13052-020-0785-9

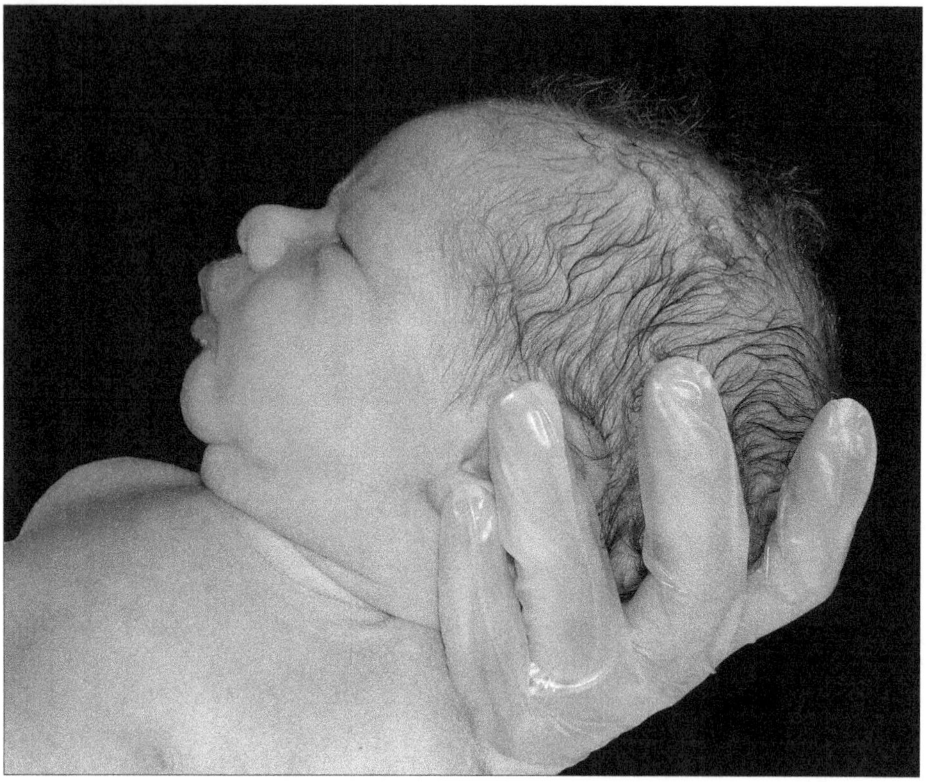

Preterm Birth and the Low-Birthweight Infant 14

Objectives

- Discuss how diagnosis is established for preterm prelabor rupture of the membranes (PPROM).
- Identify risk factors and warning signs of preterm labor (PTL).
- Discuss the risks and benefits of interventions for PTL, including antibiotics, tocolytics, corticosteroids, cerclage, alpha-hydroxyprogesterone, and serial cervical-length assessments.
- Describe how to safely transport a preterm infant to a higher level of care.

Composite Case Study

Agnes L., a 25-year-old gravida 1, para 0 (G1 P0) at 28 weeks of gestation, called her midwife, Teale, to report mild cramping, like a menstrual period. "It's very mild, barely there at all. I wouldn't even call except I'm getting a slimy discharge and I'm wondering if I have BV again." Teale agreed that Agnes should come to the office to be evaluated.

When she arrived, Agnes told Teale that she had been feeling "off" since last night, with more fatigue than usual. Teale measured Agnes's fundal height at 29 cm and palpated the fetus as vertex. The fetal heart rate was a steady 150. On sterile speculum exam, something white and shiny filled the vagina, and at first Teale could not comprehend what she was seeing. In the next moment, she realized with horror that she was looking at the bulging amniotic sac.

"Agnes, it appears you are in preterm labor," said Teale gently. "We need to call an ambulance and transport you to a hospital that can care for preterm babies." While waiting for emergency medical services, Teale explained the likely course of events and answered Agnes's questions while starting an intravenous infusion. She called the receiving hospital's transfer line and was placed in a conference call with the obstetrician, the certified nurse-midwife, the neonatologist, and the maternity charge nurse. The hospital approved the transfer and assigned her to room 312. Teale confirmed that she would fax the prenatal records to the maternity department. When the crew loaded Agnes onto the stretcher, Teale grabbed her birth bags and hopped into the ambulance. En route, *Teale monitored the fetal heart rate and strategized with the paramedic about how they might manage the birth if the baby was born* en route. *Teale considered giving terbutaline before departing but decided against it because Agnes was not having palpable contractions.*

At the hospital, Agnes underwent an ultrasound examination which determined that Agnes was dilated to about 6 cm. The amniotic sac had hourglassed through the partially dilated cervix and filled the vagina. The hospital team treated Agnes with steroids to accelerate fetal lung development and reduce the likelihood of fetal cerebral hemorrhage. The obstetrician ordered magnesium sulfate for fetal neuroprotection and a course of antibiotics. The team opted not to start tocolysis, because Agnes was not contracting.

After three days of little change, Agnes's amniotic membranes spontaneously ruptured at 28 3/7 weeks of gestation. She swiftly moved into active labor and gave birth to baby boy. The nurses showed Agnes how to use a breast pump and encouraged her to spend time in the neonatal intensive care unit to bond with her son. Agnes was unspeakably sad when she was discharged from the hospital and had to leave her baby behind, but the NICU staff helped her participate in infant care during her daily visits. The infant faced many challenges during the three months he spent in the NICU but was later discharged home without significant health issues.

Preterm Labor and Birth

Preterm labor (PTL) is defined as the presence of uterine contractions with progressive effacement and dilation of the cervix before 37 completed weeks of gestation. About 15 million preterm infants are born every year worldwide. Global rates of preterm birth (PTB) range from 5% in parts of Europe to 18% in parts of Africa (Mandy, 2022b). Most PTB spontaneously follows PTL, preterm prelabor rupture of membranes, or (rarely) cervical insufficiency. About 30–35% of PTB, however, is iatrogenic, occurring in the absence of spontaneous labor or rupture of membranes, usually in response to maternal or fetal complications (Valencia, Mol, & Jacobsson, 2021).

PTB is associated with about 70% of neonatal mortality, 36% of infant mortality, and 25–50% of long-term neurologic damage in children (American College of Obstetricians & Gynecologists [ACOG], 2016/2022). Long-term consequences of prematurity can include learning disabilities, lung disease, blindness, hearing impairment, cerebral palsy, and developmental delay. The lower the birthweight, the more likely an infant is to die or suffer serious impairment.

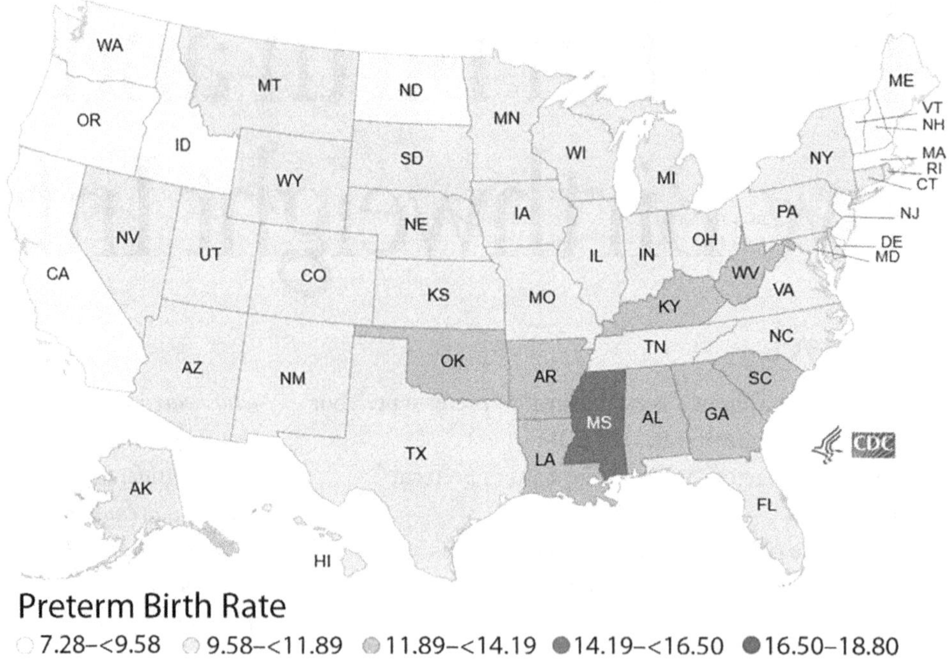

Figure 14-1. Preterm birth (PTB) rates by state, 2021. From "Percentage of Births Born Preterm by State," by Centers for Disease Control and Prevention, 2022 (https://www.cdc.gov/nchs/pressroom/sosmap/preterm_births/preterm.htm). In the public domain.

In the United States, about 550,000 preterm infants are born annually (Mandy, 2022b). The rate of preterm live births in the United States peaked in 2006 at 12.8% of live births, reached a low of 9.57% in 2014, then increased more or less steadily to 10.49% in 2021 (Osterman, Hamilton, Martin, Driscoll, & Valenzuela, 2023). About 84% of these preterm infants are born between 32 0/7 and 36 6/7 weeks of gestation, 10% are born between 28 0/7 and 31 6/7 weeks, and 5% are born before 28 0/7 weeks (Mandy, 2022b).

In the United States, the rate of PTB among black mothers is 52% higher than the rate among all other mothers (March of Dimes, 2022). Moreover, well-educated non-Hispanic black mothers have higher rates of PTB than less-educated Asian, Hispanic, or non-Hispanic white women (ACOG, 2021b). One possible explanation for this disparity is that many black mothers have endured lifelong exposure to institutional and interpersonal biases that create health disparities unrelated to wealth, achievement, or social standing (ACOG, 2021b).

Pathophysiology

PTL appears to be a long-term, multifactorial process rather than an acute condition. It is diagnosed when a pregnant client has regular uterine contractions accompanied by dilation and thinning of the cervix and descent of the fetus. Although PTB can be attributed to cervical insufficiency, genetic factors, or other issues, it is usually related to one or more of four primary processes. These processes are

- **Stress-induced premature activation of the maternal or fetal hypothalamic-pituitary-adrenal (HPA) axis.** The fetus plays a role in the initiation of labor and appears to respond to adverse intrauterine conditions by prematurely activating the HPA axis and initiating PTL. Conditions that cause fetal stress include uteroplacental ischemia, maternal psychosocial stress, placental or fetal vascular damage, preeclampsia, or abnormal maternal/fetal placental interface (Lockwood, 2022).
- **Inflammation, infection, or altered genital tract microbiome.** Systemic and genitourinary tract pathogens such as asymptomatic bacteriuria, bacterial vaginosis, aerobic vaginitis intraamniotic infection (IAI), and periodontal disease can increase the risk of PTB. PTB is less common when *Lactobacillus* is the predominant flora of the vaginal microbial community during pregnancy and more common when *Mobiluncus*, *Mageeibacillus*, *Gardnerella*, or *Ureaplasma* heavily colonize the vagina. Some bacteria species directly degrade the fetal membranes, increase the risk of preterm PROM (PPROM), and produce precursors to prostaglandin synthesis that stimulate uterine contractions (Lockwood, 2022). Researchers have found that 20–60% of PTL before 34 weeks of gestation is associated with bacteria in the amniotic fluid

The 4 Primary Mechanisms for PTB

- Premature activation of the maternal or fetal hypothalamic-pituitary-adrenal axis
- Infection or exaggerated inflammatory response
- Decidual hemorrhage/abruption
- Pathological uterine distension

(Lockwood, 2022; Simhan & Romero, 2021).

- **Placental abruption (decidual hemorrhage).** Maternal spiral artery hemorrhage and vascular damage may disrupt the maternal/fetal placental interface and increase the frequency, intensity, and strength of uterine contractions, leading to PTB (Lockwood, 2022).
- **Pathological uterine distension.** Multiple gestation, polyhydramnios, fetal macrosomia, and other conditions that overly distend the uterus are associated with PTL. Excessive stretching of the myometrium and fetal membranes can affect gap junctions and oxytocin receptors and lead to the production of inflammatory substances such as cytokines and prostaglandins (Lockwood, 2022).

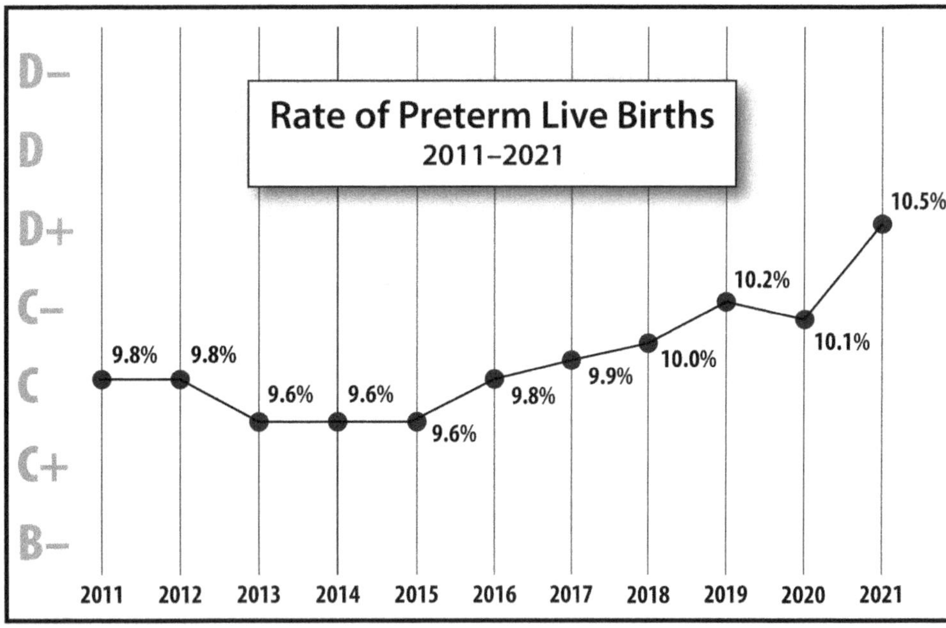

Figure 14-2. Almost failing. The percentage of preterm live births in the United States is high enough to earn a grade of D+ from the March of Dimes. Adapted from *2022 March of Dimes Report Card*, by March of Dimes, 2022 (https://www.marchofdimes.org/sites/default/files/2022-11/March-of-Dimes-2022-Full-Report-Card.pdf). Copyright 2022 by author.

Risk Factors

Any pregnant client can give birth preterm. Spontaneous PTB occurs in about 5% of nulliparas (ACOG, 2021b). The strongest predictors of PTB are prior PTB, prior prelabor rupture of membranes, multiple gestation, and short cervical length on routine second trimester screening (ACOG, 2021b). Pregnant clients who present with painless advanced cervical dilation and give birth preterm are at increased risk of doing the same in future pregnancies. Mothers who give birth to early preterm infants in their first pregnancies have a 35% risk of spontaneous PTB in their next pregnancies (ACOG, 2021b).

Other risk factors include (Robinson & Norwitz, 2023)

- Vaginal bleeding in early pregnancy.
- Strong family history of PTB, first-degree relative born preterm, and/or the client herself was born preterm.
- Uterine anomalies, cervical insufficiency (tendency of the cervix to painlessly open in the second or third trimester), and certain cervical surgeries such as loop electrosurgical excision procedure (LEEP) and cone biopsy.
- Infection—especially asymptomatic bacteriuria, genital tract infections, or periodontal disease.
- Low socioeconomic status, lack of adequate prenatal care, domestic violence.
- Tobacco, cocaine, or alcohol abuse.
- Short interval between pregnancies.
- Inadequate prenatal care. Conversely, low-risk clients who participate in CenteringPregnancy® group prenatal care programs appear to have a lower rate of PTB than low-risk nonparticipants (Picklesimer, Billings, Hale, Blackhurst, & Covington-Kolb, 2012).
- Fetal anomalies.
- Chronic health problems such as hypertension, diabetes, or clotting disorders.

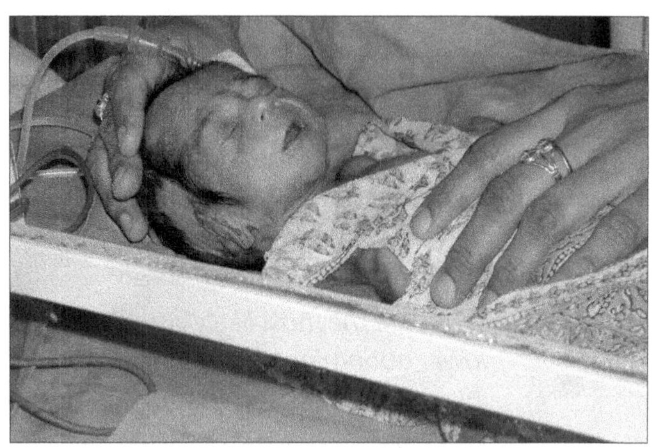

Figure 14-3. Infant aged 19 days in a neonatal intensive care unit (NICU) in Jaipur, India, in 2006. She was born at 28 weeks of gestation. She is held by the ungloved hands of her pediatrician. The risk of PTB is higher in low-resource areas, which tend to have less access to care for premature infants.

- Poor nutrition, poor weight gain, and being underweight or obese at the beginning of the pregnancy.
- Emotional stress, depression.
- Physically strenuous work, long working hours, prolonged standing.
- Age less than 17 or greater than 35.
- Shorter maternal stature. Taller stature is protective against PTB.
- Uterine overdistension.
- Frank vaginal bleeding at any point in pregnancy, especially if chronic.
- Placental abruption.
- Large or multiple fibroids, especially submucosal.
- Previous infant with sudden infant death syndrome (SIDS).
- Assisted reproduction techniques such as *in vitro* fertilization.
- Shortened cervical length measured by transvaginal ultrasound at 16–28 weeks of gestation.
- Cervix dilated to 1 cm or more before 24 weeks of gestation.

Assessment of Threatened PTL

Signs and Symptoms of PTL

Childbirth requires the cervix to change from firm, thick, high, and closed to open, anterior, thin, and soft. Often subclinical inflammation causes the cervix to shorten or dilate before the mother experiences symptoms of PTL. Cervical change that occurs over days or weeks is considered cervical ripening, whereas changes that take place over minutes or hours are considered labor (Lockwood, 2023).

PTL is diagnosed clinically when the client has regular uterine contractions and a change in cervical dilation, effacement, or both, *or* presents with regular contractions and cervical dilation of at least 2 cm (ACOG, 2016/2022). PTL is more likely to result in PTB if the client has at least 6 contractions per hr, cervical dilation more than 3 cm, and effacement is at least 80% (Iams, 2003; Rundell & Panchal, 2017; Simhan & Romero, 2021). The likelihood of PTB is further increased if membranes are ruptured or if there is vaginal bleeding.

First Thought, Worst Thought

What are the most likely causes of lower abdominal cramping between 24 and 36 weeks of gestation?

Musculoskeletal pain, urinary tract infection, or bacterial vaginosis.

What is the worst it could be?

PTL progressing to PTB.

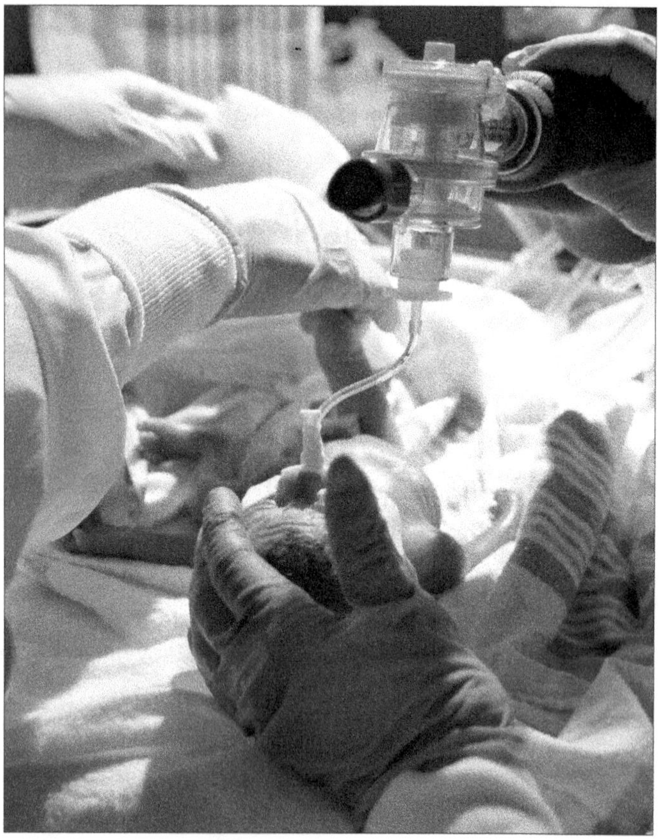

Figure 14-4. The premature infant of very low birthweight faces steep odds against survival with normal neurologic function. This baby girl, born at 26 weeks of gestation, struggled for more than 3 months against hypothermia, hypoglycemia, respiratory distress syndrome, apnea, fluid and electrolyte imbalances, jaundice, anemia, impaired nutrition, and infection. Ultimately, she beat the odds and survived without impairment.

Signs and symptoms of early PTL may be vague and nonspecific. Prodromal signs and symptoms may begin hours or days before they meet the diagnostic criteria for PTL (Lockwood, 2023). The client may experience menstrual-like cramping or pressure in the lower abdomen, pelvis, or lower back. The client may also notice a change in vaginal discharge or bloody spotting, diarrhea, or intestinal cramping. Signs and symptoms may become more pronounced during sexual activity (including breast stimulation and orgasm), long-distance travel, prolonged standing, or strenuous physical activity.

Signs and symptoms suggestive of PTL can be caused by or mistaken for other conditions. Urinary-tract infections, appendicitis, and gastroenteritis can both cause and mimic PTL. A trickle of fluid soaking the undergarments may indicate rupture of membranes, but more often is related to normal

Criteria for Diagnosis of PTL

20 0/7–36 6/7 weeks of gestation

and

Regular uterine contractions

and

Change in cervical dilation

and/or

Change in cervical effacement by digital examination or transvaginal assessment of cervical length

or

Initial presentation with regular contractions and cervical dilation ≥2 cm

Adapted from "Management of Preterm Labor" (Practice Bulletin 171), by American College of Obstetricians and Gynecologists, 2016/2022 (https://www.acog.org/clinical/clinical-guidance/practice-bulletin/articles/2016/10/management-of-preterm-labor). Copyright 2022 by ACOG.

vaginal discharge or bladder incontinence. Diarrhea, abdominal cramping, or a change in vaginal discharge can occur with many conditions unrelated to PTL. The presence of uterine contractions does not necessarily indicate PTL, even when they occur 6 or more times per hr. About 1 in 4 healthy mothers earlier than 32 weeks of gestation have 4 or more contractions per hr (Hedriana et al., 2013).

When clients present with signs and symptoms suggesting PTL, it can be exceedingly difficult to determine which will give birth early. Fewer than 10% of clients hospitalized with a clinical diagnosis of PTL give birth within 7 days of presentation, and 50% have term births (ACOG, 2016/2022). Consequently, providers may overtreat some clients with potentially harmful tocolytics, corticosteroids, or antibiotics, and undertreat others who subsequently have unexpected PTB.

Encourage your clients to report persistent contractions or cramping so they can be properly assessed by a provider. Clients who are evaluated for PTL and then sent home may hesitate to call again if contractions reoccur. They may express worry about overreacting to bodily sensations or bothering the provider unnecessarily. Validate clients' concerns and emphasize that discomforts suggestive of PTL must always be taken seriously.

Evaluation of the Client with Preterm Contractions

Any client with signs and symptoms consistent with PTL requires prompt evaluation, ideally at a hospital capable of

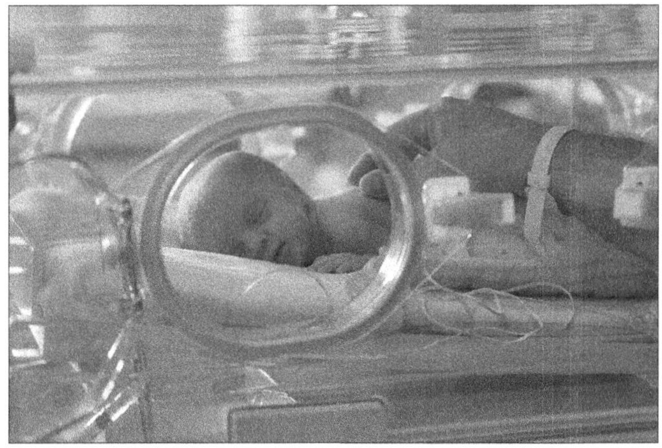

Figure 14-5. Iatrogenic PTB occurs when induction of labor or cesarean section is necessary because of maternal or fetal pathology. This late-preterm infant naps in her enclosure in the NICU while her father gently strokes her back. Labor was induced because her mother developed severe preeclampsia. The infant also had severe fetal growth restriction (FGR).

caring for an immature infant. Destination matters as much as time, particularly for infants less than 28 weeks of gestation. Extremely preterm infants have much better outcomes when they are born in a tertiary-care facility when compared to infants born in lower-level facilities that transfer after birth (Helenius, Longford, Lehtonen, Modi, & Gale, 2019). The following framework is intended to guide assessment in a hospital. It can be modified for emergency assessment in community settings.

The client with signs or symptoms of PTL requires timely and thorough physical assessment. Findings and management strategies are discussed in detail later in the chapter, but the initial steps of assessment are as follows:

1. **Consider medical and obstetric risk factors.**
2. **Consider the accuracy of the estimated due date.** Did the client have a first-trimester ultrasound? Is the recollection of the last menstrual period definite or just an approximation? Did the client have regular menstrual cycles? Was the pregnancy conceived while breastfeeding? Have fundal height measurements been consistent with weeks of gestation and with fundal heights in other pregnancies? Did the client experience quickening at the usual time?
3. **Take a GOLDCART history.** Assess for signs and symptoms of PTL.
4. **Assess vital signs:** Maternal temperature, blood pressure (BP), heart rate, and respiratory rate; fetal heart rate (FHR).
5. **Apply an external fetal monitor.** Evaluate the fetal heart pattern and uterine activity.
6. **Palpate the abdomen.** Assess the frequency, duration, and intensity of uterine contractions. Estimate fetal size, position,

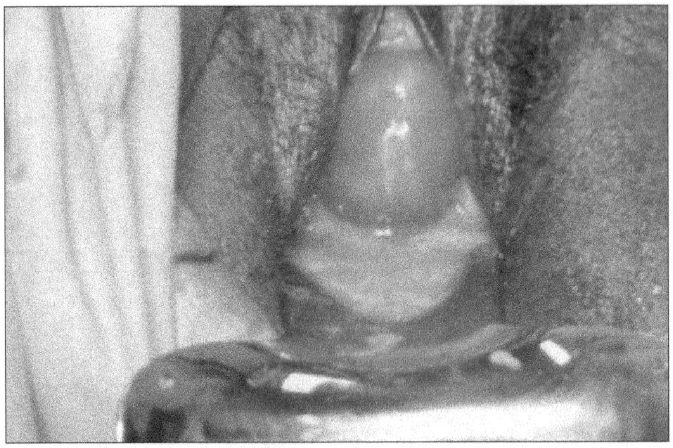

Figure 14-6. Amniotic sac prolapsed and bulging to the introitus on speculum examination. Membranes can protrude hourglass-fashion through a cervix that is less than 4 cm dilated, giving the impression of complete dilation. Image from "Outcome of Late Second Trimester Emergency Cerclage in Patients with Advanced Cervical Dilatation . . . ," by T. O. Egbe et al., 2013, *ISRN Obstetrics and Gynecology, 2013*, 834158. CC BY 2.0.

and station. Evaluate for indications of multiple gestation. Palpate all abdominal quadrants for tenderness and rigidity and consider alternative causes of abdominal pain.

7. **Examine the vagina.** Insert a nonlubricated speculum wet only with water (Lockwood, 2023). Assess for the presence of amniotic fluid pooling in the vaginal vault or trickling through the cervix. Note frank bleeding or bloody mucus. Visually estimate cervical dilation and effacement. It is easier to visually estimate dilation if you measure and memorize the width of the speculum ahead of time and use it as a guide. The blade of a Pederson medium speculum is usually 1 in. (2.5 cm) wide. If the cervix is 3 or more cm dilated and/or 75% cervical effacement with intact membranes, or if membranes have spontaneously ruptured, the client is likely to progress to giving birth preterm (Lyon, Bello, & Stevermer, 2017).
8. **If the cervix is open,** the amniotic sac may appear as a translucent water balloon bulging against the cervical opening. When membranes prolapse through a somewhat dilated and effaced cervix (hourglass membranes), the sight of the amniotic sac filling the vagina is easily mistaken for complete dilation. It may not be possible to distinguish between hourglass membranes and complete dilation on speculum examination, but ultrasound assessment of the cervix can clarify the diagnosis (Lockwood, 2023).
9. **Consider collecting a fetal fibronectin (fFN) swab during the speculum examination if the client is between 22 and 34 weeks of gestation.** The role of fFN testing in the client with suspected PTL is controversial (Lyons & McLaughlin, 2020). Fetal fibronectin is a protein glue produced by fetal cells found at the interface of the chorion and the decidua that binds the amnion to the uterine lining. A positive fFN test may indicate that the interface has been disturbed and the risk of PTB may be elevated.

A negative fFN test is reassuring: 99.2% of people with a negative result remain pregnant at least two more weeks (Hologic, 2017; Peaceman et al., 1997). The meaning of a positive test is less certain because of a high false-positive rate. One study suggests that fFN has a role in identifying people at risk for PTB when combined with cervical length assessment (van Baaren et al., 2014). More recent research indicates that fFN testing in singleton gestations with threatened PTL does not prevent PTB or improve perinatal outcome, but is associated with higher costs, more intervention, and longer hospital stays (Berghella & Saccone, 2016; Chiossi, Saade, Sibai, & Berghella, 2018). A positive fFN test result should not exclusively guide management of the client presenting with clinical symptoms of PTL (ACOG, 2016/2022).

Collect the fFN sample first, before inserting any other object in the vagina. Avoid collecting an fFN sample when the client has recent vaginal intercourse with a male partner; semen contains fFN and can produce a 22.2% false-positive rate at 12–24 hr, 11.8% at 24–48 hr. and 5.6% at 48–72 hr (Shimoya, Hashimoto, Shimizu, Saji, & Murata, 1998). A negative result, however, is valid even if the client has had recent coitus. Digital or transvaginal ultrasound examination, cervical culture swab, or pap smear before collection of the sample can cause a false-positive result, as can the presence of infection, cervical and/or vaginal lesions, blood or bacteria, cervical dilation more than 3 cm, and/or bulging or ruptured fetal membranes. False positive results may also occur in the presence of soaps, lubricants, antimicrobials, and disinfectants.

To perform an fFN test:

- *Insert swab into vagina.* Perform a sterile speculum examination. Insert the polyester-tipped swab and gently rotate across the posterior fornix or the ectocervical region of the external cervical os for 10 sec to absorb secretions.
- *Place swab in tube.* Remove the swab from the vagina and place it in the tube, saturating the tip with buffer solution. Immerse the tip in the solution. Snap the shaft where the scored area aligns with the top of the tube. Cover the tube so that the end of the shaft fits into the designated hole on the inner surface of the tube cap. Press firmly to close tightly. Label and send the sample to the appropriate laboratory.

Table 14-1
Sample GOLDCART History for a Client with Signs and Symptoms of Preterm Labor (PTL)

General situation and history—How many weeks pregnant are you? Do you have any health issues or pregnancy complications? How old are you? How many babies and pregnancies have you had? Do you have a history of PTL? Have you felt the baby move normally?
Onset—How did your signs and symptoms begin? What were you doing? What time did it start? Was gradual or abrupt? Have you had this before? How did you feel before it started?
Location—Where is your pain? Does it start in one place and radiate to somewhere else? Where?
Duration—How long have you had the symptoms? How have they changed over time? How far apart are the contractions? How long do they last?
Characteristics—Is the pain stabbing, shooting, crampy or dull? Does it come and go? Is your belly tight when you are having the pain? Do you feel pressure? On a scale of 1–10, 10 being the worst pain you ever had and 1 being hardly there at all, what number would you give this pain?
Associated symptoms—Are you having vaginal discharge? If so, what does it look like—color, consistency, amount? Any bleeding or leaking? Any other pain, weakness, headache, sweating, visual changes, numbness, shortness of breath, nausea, vomiting, fever, diarrhea, dizziness, or fainting?
Relieving/aggravating factors—What makes it better or worse? Did your symptoms improve when you changed position?
Treatment—Have you tried any treatment or remedy to manage your signs or symptoms? What have you tried? Did it help?

10. **Check for ruptured membranes.** Observe pooling, microscopic ferning, positive nitrazine (phenaphthazine) test, or immunoassay tests (ROM Plus®, AmniSure®).
11. **Collect swabs for laboratory evaluation.** Consider collecting a Group B *Streptococcus* (GBS) vaginal-rectal swab (if not done within the previous five weeks), gonorrhea/chlamydia cultures, and wet mount to screen for bacterial vaginosis, trichomonas, and candida infections.
12. **Conduct a digital examination.** Consider performing a digital cervical examination after excluding placenta previa and rupture of membranes. If it appears that birth is imminent or if the FHR is abnormal, consider performing a digital examination before or instead of a speculum examination (Lockwood, 2023).
13. **Consider a transvaginal ultrasound examination.** When performed correctly, measurement of cervical length in clients presenting with threatened PTL can give insight into whether PTB is likely to occur. Fewer than 5% of symptomatic clients give birth within 7 days if the cervical length is 30 mm or more when assessed by transvaginal ultrasound (Fuchs, Henrich, Osthues, & Dudenhausen, 2004; Lim, Butt, Nevo, & Crane, 2020; Lockwood, 2023; Parfitt, 2020; Simhan & Romero, 2021; Vafaei et al., 2017). A short cervical length is usually defined as less than 25 mm when the asymptomatic client is screened between 16 and 24 weeks of gestation (ACOG, 2021b). When the client is symptomatic, a transvaginal cervical length measurement of less than 15 mm (Lockwood, 2023; van Baaren et al., 2014) or less than 20 mm (Chiossi et al., 2018; Society for Maternal-Fetal Medicine [SMFM], n.d.) is associated with a higher risk for PTL. There is evidence, however, that individuals have unique cervical lengths (Gudicha et al., 2021). ACOG advises against using cervical-length measurements alone to build a management plan for the client with threatened PTL (ACOG, 2016/2022).
14. **Obtain a transabdominal obstetrical ultrasound evaluation.** Ultrasound examination is useful for confirming presentation; assessing amniotic fluid volume; estimating fetal weight and age; and evaluating fetal anatomy, placental location and morphology, and maternal anatomic abnormalities (Lockwood, 2023).
15. **Collect a clean-catch urine sample.** Screen the client for urinary tract infection. Urine drug screening may be performed for people with risk factors for substance abuse or if institutional guidelines specify drug screening for all cases of PTL. Gonorrhea/chlamydia screening may be performed from a urine sample.
16. **Consider collecting a complete blood count with differential** if you suspect intrauterine infection.

Management of PTL

The cornerstones of PTL management are timely detection, transfer to an appropriate facility for birth, and swift administration of corticosteroid and neuroprotection therapies to improve neonatal outcomes. Tocolysis is unlikely to stop progressive labor but may delay birth to allow for the administration of corticosteroids and magnesium sulfate. The client in PTL requires management in a hospital. In some cases, the midwife transfers care; in others, a midwife with hospital privileges manages the client collaboratively with a physician. The providers must develop a management plan appropriate for gestational age, presentation, availability of specialized neonatal care, any maternal or fetal morbidities, planned mode of birth, family preferences, and other important aspects of care.

Maternal Transfer

In many locations, high-acuity perinatal care is regionalized (ACOG, 2019/2021). A hospital with a level II neonatal intensive care unit (NICU) is staffed and equipped to manage most infants with birthweights over 1,500 g (Simhan & Romero, 2021). Level III centers can provide specialized care for the sickest and smallest newborns and intensive care for complex maternal conditions. Learn about the available resources in your community and make a transport plan for every contingency.

For the best chance to survive, a very small preterm infant requires a hospital with skilled providers, specialized equipment, and surgical and laboratory capabilities (Perry, 2021). If the infant requires intensive support, sometimes the recovering mother is left behind while the infant is transported to a distant facility or even to another state. Ideally, the mother may be transported to a higher level of care with the fetus still *in utero*. Early preterm infants born at a tertiary center have much lower rates of morbidity and mortality and shorter lengths of stay than infants born elsewhere and transported to definitive care (Perry, 2021). *In utero* transfer also reduces the likelihood of separation of mother and infant (Martin, 2022).

Pharmacological Treatment of PTL

Acute PTL may be difficult to arrest if the cervix is dilated beyond 3 cm. The therapies most clearly associated with improved neonatal outcomes include antenatal corticosteroids such as betamethasone for accelerated lung maturation and magnesium sulfate for fetal neuroprotection. Tocolytics can forestall birth long enough to administer antenatal steroids. Antibiotic therapy may be recommended in some clinical situations.

Antenatal Corticosteroids

Maternal treatment with antenatal corticosteroids benefits the preterm newborn more than any other intervention, primarily by accelerating fetal organ maturation (ACOG, 2016/2022, 2017/2020). Treatment with antenatal corticosteroids raises 5-min Apgar scores, improves lung function,

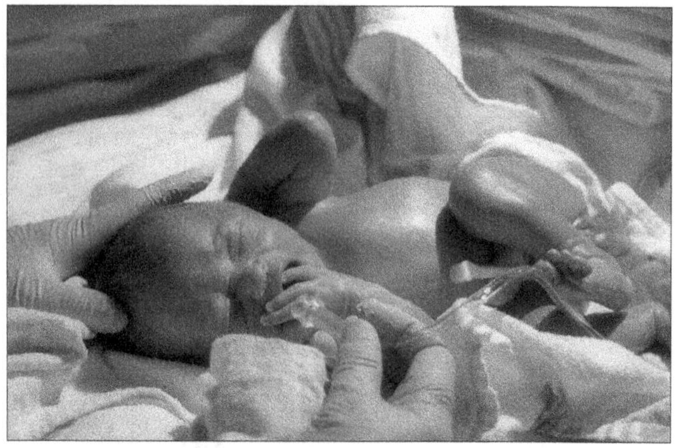

Figure 14-7. This neonate was born at 32 weeks of gestation, 6 days after her mother completed a course of antenatal corticosteroids. This treatment reduces the risk of perinatal and newborn death, respiratory distress syndrome, intraventricular hemorrhage, and necrotizing enterocolitis. Infants born after their mothers have received corticosteroid therapy have less need for respiratory support and prolonged NICU admission.

and reduces perinatal and neonatal mortality (McGoldrick, Stewart, Parker, & Dalziel, 2020). It probably reduces the risk of systemic infection in the first 48 hr of life, intraventricular hemorrhage, necrotizing enterocolitis, and developmental delay in later childhood (ACOG, 2017/2024; McGoldrick et al., 2020; Roberts, Brown, Medley, & Dalziel, 2017; Skoll et al., 2018). It also appears to decrease the need for mechanical ventilation or continuous positive airways pressure (CPAP), duration of oxygen supplementation, and surfactant use (ACOG, 2017/2024; McGoldrick et al., 2020; Mwansa-Kambafwile, Cousens, Hansen, & Lawn, 2010; Roberts et al., 2017; Skoll et al., 2018). The infant derives maximal benefit if antenatal steroids are administered between 2 and 7 days before birth (Gulersen et al., 2021). Because of the unpredictable nature of PTL, sometimes babies are born outside this window of ideal benefit.

While administration of antenatal steroids does not increase the risk of infection or endometritis in the mother (McGoldrick et al., 2020), they should not be given to clients with IAI (ACOG, 2017/2024). In cases of maternal diabetes, hyperglycemia commonly develops after antenatal corticosteroid administration, and maternal hyperglycemia shortly before birth increases the risk of neonatal hypoglycemia (Tuohy, Bloomfield, Crowther, & Harding, 2021). Even in the nondiabetic mother, antenatal steroids given in the late preterm period can increase the risk for neonatal hypoglycemia (Daskalakis et al., 2023; Fee, Stock, & Kemp, 2023; McElwee et al., 2022), especially when there are 12–71 hr between steroid administration and birth (McElwee et al., 2022). Delayed cord clamping in late PTB appears to give some protection against early neonatal hypoglycemia in infants who have received antenatal betamethasone (Hitchings, Rodriguez, Persaud, & Gomez, 2022).

24 0/7–33 6/7 Weeks of Gestation: Of Confirmed Benefit

Evidence strongly supports giving a single course of corticosteroids from 24 0/7 to 33 6/7 weeks of gestation to pregnant clients who are at high risk of PTB within the next week (ACOG, 2017/2024; Daskalakis et al., 2023; Lee & Guinn, 2023; NICE, 2015/2022; Skoll et al., 2018; Society of Obstetricians & Gynaecologists of Canada [SOGC], 2021).

22 0/7–23 6/7 Weeks of Gestation: Consider Clinical Situation

When a baby is born on the cusp of viability, the decision to pursue or withhold resuscitation is largely based on the preference of informed parents (Mercurio & Drago, 2022). If the family wishes full resuscitation, consider administering antenatal corticosteroids from 22 0/7 to 23 6/7 weeks of gestation if birth is likely to occur (ACOG et al., 2021/2022; Daskalakis et al., 2023; NICE, 2015/2022; Skoll et al., 2018). Neonates born at 22 0/7–22 6/7 weeks of gestation are twice as likely to survive if exposed to antenatal steroids (38.5% versus 17.7%) than those without steroids, and they are more than four times as likely (4.4% versus 1%) to survive without major morbidity (Ehret et al., 2018). Similarly, infants born at 23 0/7–23 6/7 weeks of gestation show a reduction in mortality and neurodevelopmental impairment when antenatal steroids are given (Carlo et al., 2011). Most surviving infants born before 26 0/7 weeks of gestation develop one or more significant morbidities including bronchopulmonary dysplasia, intraventricular hemorrhage, necrotizing enterocolitis, periventricular leukomalacia, retinopathy of prematurity, neurosensory deficits such as blindness, neurodevelopmental and cognitive impairment, cerebral palsy, or behavioral problems (Anderson et al., 2016; Lee & Guinn, 2023; Mercurio & Drago, 2022). The family should be counseled that even with the best of care, mortality is high for children born near the limit of viability. Because there is no evidence of benefit, ACOG does not recommend antenatal steroids before 22 0/7 weeks of gestation (ACOG et al., 2021/2022).

34 0/7–36 6/7 Weeks of Gestation: Controversial

The administration of late preterm antenatal steroids is controversial. Giving corticosteroids from 34 0/7 to 36 6/7 weeks of gestation appears to improve lung function and decreases other morbidities in late-preterm neonates (ACOG, 2017/2024). Corticosteroids reduce the incidence of transient tachypnea of the newborn but do not affect the incidence of respiratory distress syndrome and can increase the likelihood of neonatal hypoglycemia (Daskalakis et al., 2023). ACOG and others recommend giving a single course of betamethasone to mothers in the late preterm period who are at risk of birth within 7 days if they have not previously received a course of antenatal corticosteroids (ACOG, 2017/2024; SMFM Pub. Cmte., 2016). The United Kingdom's National Institute for Health and Care Excellence (NICE) recommends consideration of corticosteroids for mothers between 34 0/7 and 35 6/7 weeks of gestation who are in suspected or established PTL, are having a planned PTB or have preterm prelabor rupture of membranes (NICE, 2015/2022).

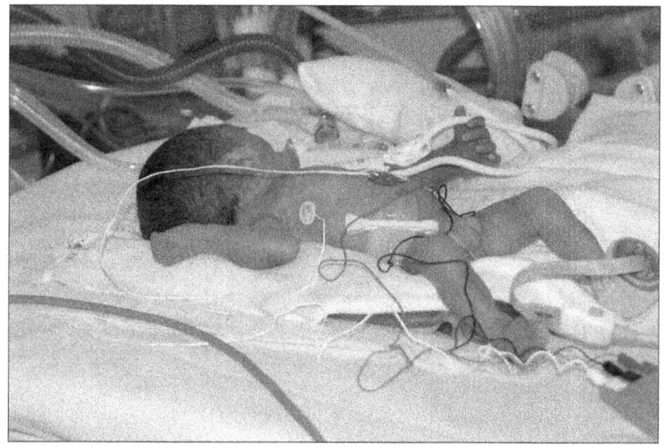

Figure 14-8. The purpose of tocolysis in PTL is not to prolong pregnancy indefinitely, but to pause PTL until corticosteroids reach their maximum effect. This 28-week infant has a better chance for survival because he was born 5 days after finishing a course of betamethasone.

The newest European guidelines, however, recommend offering antenatal steroids between 34 0/7 and 34 6/7 weeks only to selected cases and restricting use between 35 0/7 and 36 6/7 to prospective randomized trials because of the absence of long-term safety data and the perception that risks outweigh benefits in the short term (Daskalakis et al., 2023). Likewise, SOGC recommends against administering antenatal corticosteroids after 35 0/7 weeks of gestation (Skoll et al., 2018). International Federation of Gynecology and Obstetrics (FIGO) recommends against the *routine* administration of antenatal corticosteroids in the late preterm period, suggesting instead that the provider consider the balance of risks and benefits of this therapy for each client (Norman, Shennan, Jacobsson, & Stock, 2021).

Administration of Antenatal Corticosteroids

Betamethasone and dexamethasone are the most extensively studied corticosteroids, so they are preferred for antenatal treatment. The usual regimen is intramuscular (IM) betamethasone suspension 12 mg every 24 hr for a total of two doses or four doses of 6 mg dexamethasone IM every 12 hr (ACOG, 2017/2024; Lee & Guinn, 2023). Some benefit is achieved when the baby is born within a few hours of corticosteroid administration, but maximum efficacy occurs

2–7 days after administration of the first dose (Lee & Guinn, 2023). Efficacy begins to wane about a week after the first injection. Antenatal steroids still benefit the infant if birth occurs less than 24 hr after administration, so the medication should be given even if it is uncertain whether the baby will be born before the course can be completed (ACOG, 2017/2024).

Repeat (Rescue) Corticosteroids

ACOG advises a single repeat course of antenatal corticosteroids in clients less than 34 0/7 weeks of gestation who are likely to give birth in the next 7 days if the prior course ended more than 14 days previously (ACOG, 2017/2024). The World Health Organization (WHO) and FIGO suggest that a single repeat course of corticosteroids be considered 7 days after the initial course for the client who is less than 34 0/7 weeks of gestation if there is a high risk of PTB in the following week (Norman et al., 2021; WHO, 2015).

Tocolytic Medications

Uterine contractions are the most obvious sign of any labor. Historically, providers have believed that if they could just stop preterm contractions, they could arrest labor, and the client would carry to term (ACOG, 2015/2022). As discussed previously, however, PTL is usually a process involving stress-related premature activation of the fetal hypothalamic-pituitary-adrenal axis, infection/inflammation, placental abruption, cervical insufficiency, and/or pathologic uterine distension (Lockwood, 2022). Arresting contractions will not halt the underlying causes of PTL (Simhan & Romero, 2021).

Magnesium sulfate, calcium channel blockers, oxytocin antagonists, nonsteroidal antiinflammatory drugs (NSAIDs), and beta-adrenergic receptor agonists have been variously used to stop the contractions of PTL (ACOG, 2015/2022). Prolonging pregnancy through the use of tocolytic therapy does not appear to directly improve neonatal outcomes (ACOG, 2015/2022). Evidence supports the use of beta-adrenergic receptor agonists, calcium channel blockers, or NSAIDs to prolong pregnancy for up to 48 hr to allow for administration of antenatal steroids, magnesium sulfate for neuroprotection and transport, if necessary, to a tertiary facility (ACOG, 2015/2022).

Tocolysis is contraindicated if the risks of prolonging pregnancy or the risks associated with these drugs are greater than the risks associated with PTB (Simhan & Caritis, 2023). Contraindications to tocolysis include maternal or fetal conditions that necessitate expedited delivery, such as preeclampsia with severe features, hemorrhage with maternal cardiovascular instability, IAI, or evidence of fetal compromise (Simhan & Caritis, 2023). Tocolytics are withheld if spontaneous PTL occurs before 22 0/7 weeks of gestation because potential harm to the mother from the medications appears to outweigh any benefit to the fetus (ACOG, 2016/2022; Raju, Mercer, Burchfield, & Joseph, 2014). Clients with preterm contractions *without* cervical change, especially those with cervical dilation less than 2 cm, generally are not candidates for tocolytic therapy (ACOG, 2016/2022).

Calcium Channel Blockers

Calcium channel blockers (commonly used for treatment of hypertension, angina, and arrhythmias) effectively inhibit contractions and have a reasonable side-effect profile. Nifedipine is the agent most used because it selectively inhibits uterine contractions compared with other calcium blockers such as verapamil (Simhan & Romero, 2021), but some protocols favor nicardipine (Flenady et al., 2014). Calcium channel blockers suppress contractions more effectively than other oxytocic agents and with less serious neonatal morbidity and fewer maternal adverse effects (Flenady et al., 2014; Simhan & Romero, 2021).

Calcium channel blockers relax the smooth muscle of arterial walls, which decreases total vascular resistance. In response, the mother experiences a compensatory increase in heart rate and stroke volume to maintain BP. Consequently, side effects can include tachycardia, hypotension, palpitations, flushing, headaches, dizziness, and nausea (Simhan & Caritis, 2023).

Maternal contraindications include liver disease, heart failure, and use of other antihypertensive agents. Do not use together with magnesium or beta-mimetics. Avoid in cases of intrauterine infection, maternal hypertension, or cardiac disease.

Common dosing regimens for nifedipine:

Initial therapy

- Loading dose 20 mg orally, follow with 20 mg orally in 90 min,

  OR
- 10 mg orally every 20 min for up to four doses,

For persistent contractions:

- 20 mg orally every 3–8 hr for up to 72 hr to a maximum dose of 180 mg/day (Simhan & Romero, 2021),

  OR
- Initial loading dose of 20–30 mg orally, then 10–20 mg orally every 3–8 hr for up to 48 hr or a maximum dose of 180 mg/day (Simhan & Caritis, 2023).

COX-2 Enzyme Inhibitor (Indomethacin)

Indomethacin is an NSAID and a cyclooxygenase (COX-2) inhibitor that reduces uterine contractions and impedes cervical ripening by decreasing prostaglandin synthesis (Griggs, Hrelic, Williams, McEwen-Campbell, & Cypher, 2020). It is easily administered and usually has few maternal side effects. Indomethacin may be considered as a tocolytic in pregnancies less than 32 weeks of gestation for up to 48 hr.

Side effects: Exposure to COX-2 inhibitors may cause adverse effects in the fetus and newborn, including constriction of the fetal ductus arteriosus, renal insufficiency, oligohydramnios, neonatal pulmonary hypertension (Simhan & Romero, 2021). These complications are rare when the drug is used judiciously. Ductal constriction is unlikely to occur to a significant degree (and is usually reversible) if indomethacin is administered earlier than 31–32 gestational weeks and is limited to no more than 48 hr in duration (Simhan & Caritis, 2023). Because indomethacin can reduce fetal urine output, it is sometimes preferred to other tocolytic options when PTL is associated with polyhydramnios (Simhan & Romero, 2021). Indomethacin is also an option when degenerating uterine fibroids in pregnancy cause uterine contractions and pain in a pregnancy before 32 weeks of gestation (Simhan & Romero, 2021). Serious maternal side effects are uncommon (gastrointestinal bleeding, prolonged bleeding time, thrombocytopenia, and asthma in aspirin-sensitive clients), but about 4% of mothers treated develop minor side effects such as nausea and vomiting, esophageal reflux, and gastritis (Simhan & Caritis, 2023).

Maternal contraindications: Renal or hepatic disease, IAI, active peptic ulcer disease, poorly controlled hypertension, asthma, platelet disorders.

Fetal contraindications: Renal anomalies, oligohydramnios, ductal-dependent cardiac defects, twin-to-twin transfusion syndrome.

Usual dosing: 50–100 mg by mouth or rectally followed by 25 mg orally every 4–6 hr for 48 hr. Dosing protocol must be followed carefully to avoid injury to the fetus (Simhan & Caritis, 2023).

Beta-Mimetics

Beta-mimetic (beta-agonist) medications, including terbutaline and ritodrine, relax the smooth muscle of the uterus and suppress contractions. Beta-mimetics are structurally related to epinephrine and norepinephrine and so stimulate adrenergic receptors, causing an increase in maternal heart rate and stroke volume, peripheral vasodilation, release of insulin and bronchial relaxation (Simhan & Caritis, 2023). Terbutaline, a drug marketed for asthma, is the beta-mimetic most commonly used as a tocolytic in the United States (Simhan & Romero, 2021).

Safety Concerns

Beta-mimetics are associated with a high incidence of side effects ranging from unpleasant (common) to life-threatening (rare). Although most side effects are mild and brief, a black box warning for terbutaline cautions providers of the potential for serious maternal heart problems and death, particularly if it is used for more than 48–72 hr or as an oral outpatient therapy (U.S. Food & Drug Administration [FDA], 2011).

The administration of terbutaline to a pregnant client may cause palpitations, tremors, nausea, vomiting, headaches, tachycardia, chest pain, anxiety, shortness of breath, hyperglycemia, hypokalemia, or pulmonary edema. Terbutaline crosses the placenta and can cause fetal tachycardia, neonatal hypoglycemia, and elevated neonatal insulin levels (Neilson, West, & Dowswell, 2014). Terbutaline can also mask signs of shock in people with antepartum hemorrhage.

Maternal contraindications include known or suspected cardiac disease, diabetes requiring insulin; maternal tachycardia over 120 beats per min (bpm), preeclampsia with severe features or eclampsia, diabetes requiring insulin, or hyperthyroidism (Simhan & Romero, 2021). Do not use terbutaline for more than 72 hr. Do not use oral terbutaline (FDA, 2011). The use of beta-mimetics for tocolysis is waning in many higher-income countries, but they are still used widely where other tocolytic medications are not available (Coler et al., 2021).

Common dosing regimens for terbutaline:

- Subcutaneous (SC) injection of 0.25 mg (250 mcg), which may be repeated every 4 hr as indicated (Simhan & Romero, 2021)

  OR
- 0.25 mg SC every 20–30 min for up to four doses or until tocolysis is achieved (Marowitz & Vines, 2024; Simhan & Caritis, 2023)

  OR
- Continuous intravenous (IV) infusion. Consult local protocols for guidance. (Simhan & Caritis, 2023).

Oxytocin Receptor Antagonists

Oxytocin receptor antagonists (typically atosiban) inhibit the hormones oxytocin and vasopressin and suppress production of PGs. Atosiban is not available in the United States, but it commonly used in Europe and elsewhere (Simhan & Caritis, 2023). A 2014 Cochrane meta-analysis found that atosiban offered no benefit over placebo, beta-mimetics, or calcium channel blockers when used as a tocolytic agent (Flenady et al., 2014). The FDA chose not to approve atosiban for tocolysis because of possible safety concerns when used in fetuses at less than 28 weeks of gestation (Coler et al., 2021).

Side effects: The most common side effects of atosiban are hypersensitivity and injection-site reactions (Simhan & Caritis, 2023).

Usual dose: Atosiban is given via IV bolus of 6.75 mg followed by a 300 mcg/min infusion for 3 hr, and then 100 mcg/min for up to 48 hr (Simhan & Caritis, 2023).

Magnesium Sulfate ($MgSO_4$)

Magnesium sulfate has been used as a tocolytic for PTL since the 1970s (Cunningham et al., 2022, ch. 45). Its presumed efficacy, however, is *not* supported by data. In a 2014 Cochrane meta-analysis of randomized trials found that $MgSO_4$ was *ineffective* at delaying or preventing PTB and offered no improvement in mother or infant when used as a tocolytic agent (Crowther, Brown, McKinlay, & Middleton, 2014; Simhan & Romero, 2021).

Other Therapies

Magnesium for Neuroprotection

Fetal exposure to magnesium sulfate before early PTB decreases the incidence and severity of cerebral palsy, intraventricular hemorrhage, and neonatal mortality (ACOG, 2010/2023; Bachnas, Akbar, Dachlan, & Dekker, 2019; Crowther, Hiller, Doyle, & Haslam, 2003; Gentle et al., 2020; Marret et al., 2007; Rouse et al., 2008; Wolf et al., 2020). This neuroprotective effect is most beneficial to infants less than 32 weeks of gestation, and the earliest babies derive the greatest benefit (Simhan & Himes, 2023). $MgSO_4$ crosses the placenta quickly and is most effective when infused within 4 hr before birth (Shennan, Suff, & Jacobsson, 2021). Do not delay birth to administer $MgSO_4$.

Magnesium sulfate and antenatal steroids appear to have a synergistic benefit when used with early gestations. Infants born between 22 0/7 and 26 6/7 weeks of gestation have lower rates of severe neurodevelopmental impairment or death when exposed to both than infants exposed to steroids alone (Gentle et al., 2020). FIGO recommends use of $MgSO_4$ for neuroprotection of the fetus for clients at risk of imminent early PTB from viability to 30 0/7 weeks of gestation and recommends that the provider consider use of $MgSO_4$ for those less than 32–34 weeks of gestation (Shennan et al., 2021).

Dosage

Low dose: 4 g loading dose IV in normal saline solution over 20–30 min through an infusion pump, followed by a maintenance dose of 1 g/hr for maximum of 24 hr (Simhan & Himes, 2023).

High dose: 6 g loading dose IV, followed by a 2 g/hr maintenance dose for a maximum of 12 hr (Simhan & Himes, 2023).

Continue the infusion until birth or stop after 24 hr if undelivered. Limit IV fluid to 125 ml/hr. Measure intake and output every 2–4 hr. An indwelling urinary catheter is recommended to better assess fluid output. Hourly assessments include deep tendon reflexes and vital signs. Magnesium levels should be monitored only in people who have abnormal kidney function or those with signs of magnesium toxicity. Keep calcium gluconate by the bedside and administer if respiratory depression occurs.

Antibiotics

If a pregnant client has not been tested for GBS colonization in the previous 5 weeks, collect a vaginal/rectal swab during your initial assessment. Administer IV penicillin or ampicillin for GBS prophylaxis until culture results are available. If a GBS test was found to be negative within the past 5 weeks, repeat testing is unnecessary. Continue antibiotics for known GBS carriers, or if the culture is positive for GBS (ACOG, 2020b/2022). If a client reports a penicillin allergy with low risk of anaphylaxis or of uncertain severity, first-generation cephalosporins (e.g., cefazolin) may be used (ACOG, 2020b/2022). The penicillin-allergic client with a high risk of anaphylaxis should be treated with clindamycin if the culture shows the GBS strain is susceptible to it. IV vancomycin (at a dose determined by weight and baseline renal function) is used when the client is allergic to penicillin and the GBS organism is resistant to clindamycin.

Restrict the use of antibiotics to cases where there is clear benefit. A client in PTL with intact membranes who is not a GBS carrier does not require antibiotic therapy and does not benefit from it (ACOG, 2018/2021) except in the case of an overt infection such as pyelonephritis or IAI. Fetal exposure to perinatal antibiotics has been associated with bronchopulmonary dysplasia, obesity, asthma, eczema, inflammatory bowel disease, antibiotic resistance, long-term functional impairment, abnormal immune development (Zimmermann & Curtis, 2020), and cerebral palsy (Kenyon et al., 2008).

Moreover, antibiotic use in PTL causes dysbiosis of the infant's intestinal microbiota (Zimmermann & Curtis, 2020). Microbial colonization of fetal gut begins *in utero* and continues until about age 2 (Singh & Mittal, 2019). Shortly after birth, colonizing commensal microbes interact with the mucosal surface of the gut and begin to program the immune system (Dierikx et al., 2020). Antibiotic medications appear to change the flora in ways that can contribute to colic and alter digestion and metabolism (Ouald Chaib, Levy, Ouald Chaib, & Vandenplas, 2020).

Cervical Shortening and Insufficiency

Cervical length assessment in the second trimester can identify people at high risk for PTB and allow the provider to start treatment that can delay PTL, or in the case of cerclage, prevent it entirely (ACOG, 2021b). Progesterone supplementation benefits pregnant clients with a history of previous spontaneous preterm singleton birth and those with a short cervix noted on ultrasound examination (Berghella, 2023b; Norwitz, 2023a). There is no benefit to bed rest, limited work, or avoidance of vaginal intercourse (ACOG, 2021b). In fact, activity restriction appears to *increase* the risk of spontaneous PTB while increasing stress and inconvenience in the client's family life (ACOG, 2021b).

Cervical Length Screening

Cervical shortening can precede labor by several weeks (Berghella, 2023b). Cervical effacement begins at the internal cervical os and progresses outward; therefore, a shortened cervix may be detected by ultrasound before it becomes evident upon digital examination (Berghella, 2023b). Before 24 weeks of gestation, a short cervix is diagnosed when transvaginal ultrasound cervical length is 25 mm or less (Berghella, 2023b).

Endovaginal sonography of the cervix is the standard for cervical length assessment. A shortened cervix is strongly associated with a higher risk of PTB in people with a singleton pregnancy who have had a previous PTB (ACOG, 2021b). In these clients, ACOG recommends serial endovaginal ultrasound measurements of cervical length beginning at 16 weeks of gestation and repeated until 24 weeks of gestation (Norwitz, 2023a). Clients who had a prior medically indicated PTB do not require serial cervical length surveillance. Instead, the focus should be on avoiding the conditions that necessitated birth, such as the use of low-dose aspirin to reduce risk for people who gave birth early because of severe preeclampsia (Norwitz, 2023a).

Although transabdominal imaging of cervical length is less accurate and can be affected by maternal obesity or fetal position, it has been used for initial screening (ACOG, 2021b). ACOG advises that clients at low risk for PTB should be assessed with transabdominal or endovaginal sonography as part of the routine anatomy scan at 18–22 weeks of gestation (ACOG, 2021b). If a short cervix is detected or suspected using transabdominal sonography, the client should undergo endovaginal evaluation for a more accurate assessment (ACOG, 2021b).

Progesterone Supplementation

Progesterone helps to maintain the pregnancy by maintaining uterine quiescence and cervical integrity through anti-inflammatory effects and by preventing degradation of the fetal membranes (Norwitz, 2023a). Early in pregnancy, the corpus luteum produces progesterone until the placenta assumes this function at 7–9 weeks of gestation (Norwitz, 2023a). Supplemental progesterone can prolong pregnancy in some clients at risk for PTB (ACOG, 2021b; Stewart et al., 2021).

Vaginal Progesterone

Vaginal progesterone treatment has been shown to reduce the risk of PTB in people who are found to have a shortened cervix upon routine screening (ACOG, 2021b, 2023). Vaginal progesterone and cerclage (see "Cerclage," below) have been found to be equally effective for preventing PTB and improving perinatal outcomes in people with a singleton gestation, previous spontaneous PTB, and a short cervix on ultrasound in the second trimester (Conde-Agudelo et al., 2018).

A meta-analysis of 40 trials on PTB (Jarde, Lutsiv, Beyenne, & McDonald, 2019) found that vaginal progesterone was the only intervention that consistently prevented PTB in high-risk singleton pregnancies overall and in subjects with a previous PTB. Vaginal progesterone has not been proven effective in the absence of shortened cervical length (Zahn, 2023). ACOG recommends vaginal progesterone for asymptomatic mothers with singleton gestations, no prior PTB, and cervical length under 20–25 mm at less than 24 gestational weeks (ACOG, 2021b). Progesterone can be prescribed as a vaginal suppository (100 or 200 mg), vaginal gel (90 mg) or as a 100 mg micronized vaginal tablet (ACOG, 2021b; Norwitz, 2023a; SMFM Pub. Cmte. & Berghella, 2012).

17-Alpha Hydroxyprogesterone Caproate (17-OHPC, Makena®)

IM injections of 17-OHPC were once considered the standard of care for the prevention of recurrent PTB among high-risk clients and reduction of complications in their infants (Meis et al., 2003). More recently, however, the PROLONG study, a large international trial, showed 17-OHPC to be ineffective in reducing PTB before 35 weeks of gestation (Blackwell et al., 2020). In 2023, the FDA withdrew approval of Makena® and its generic, 17-OHPC (FDA, 2023). ACOG no longer recommends IM 17-OHPC for the primary prevention of PTB in clients with a history of spontaneous PTB (ACOG, 2023).

Side effects Progesterone injections can cause irritation or inflammation at the injection site. In a large retrospective study, adults exposed to 17-OHPC as fetuses between 1959 and 1966 were found to be at higher risk of any cancer (30 versus 14 per 100,000) by middle age (Murphy, Cirillo, Krigbaum, & Cohn, 2022). These exposures were in the first trimester; it is unclear whether the association is relevant to second- or third-trimester exposures. Vaginal progesterone supplementation appears to slightly increase the risk of intrahepatic cholestasis of pregnancy but does not affect its severity (Farago et al., 2020).

Cervical Insufficiency

Cervical insufficiency is the inability of the uterine cervix to retain a pregnancy in the second trimester and involves painless cervical dilation without contractions or labor in the absence of other identifiable pathology (ACOG, 2014/2024). People with cervical insufficiency often give birth unexpectedly before 24 weeks of gestation after a short interval of mild symptoms or no symptoms at all. Cervical insufficiency remains poorly understood, but it may be related to congenital changes in the internal structure of the cervix, mechanical injuries, or inflammatory processes (Wierzchowska-Opoka, Kimber-Trojnar, & Leszczyńska-Gorzelak, 2021). Risk factors for structural cervical weakness include surgical trauma to the cervix from cone biopsy, loop electrosurgical excision procedures (LEEP), mechanical dilation of the cervix during pregnancy termination, obstetric lacerations, congenital Müllerian duct anomalies, deficiencies in cervical collagen and elastin, and *in utero* exposure to diethylstilbestrol (ACOG, 2014/2024).

People with cervical insufficiency may be asymptomatic or may present with ambiguous symptoms such as pelvic pressure, mild contractions, premenstrual-like cramping, backache, or a change in vaginal discharge (Berghella, 2023a). Sometimes a shortened cervix is an incidental finding on a routine ultrasound. Clinical diagnosis of acute cervical insufficiency in the second trimester is made when cervical dilation is detected on speculum or digital examination or when membranes are visible at or beyond the external os in the absence of signs of labor or intrauterine infection (Simhan & Romero, 2021). In some cases, suprapubic or fundal pressure or the Valsalva maneuver may cause the fetal membranes to bulge into the endocervical canal or vagina (Berghella, 2023a). External uterine monitoring may show irregular, sporadic contractions or none.

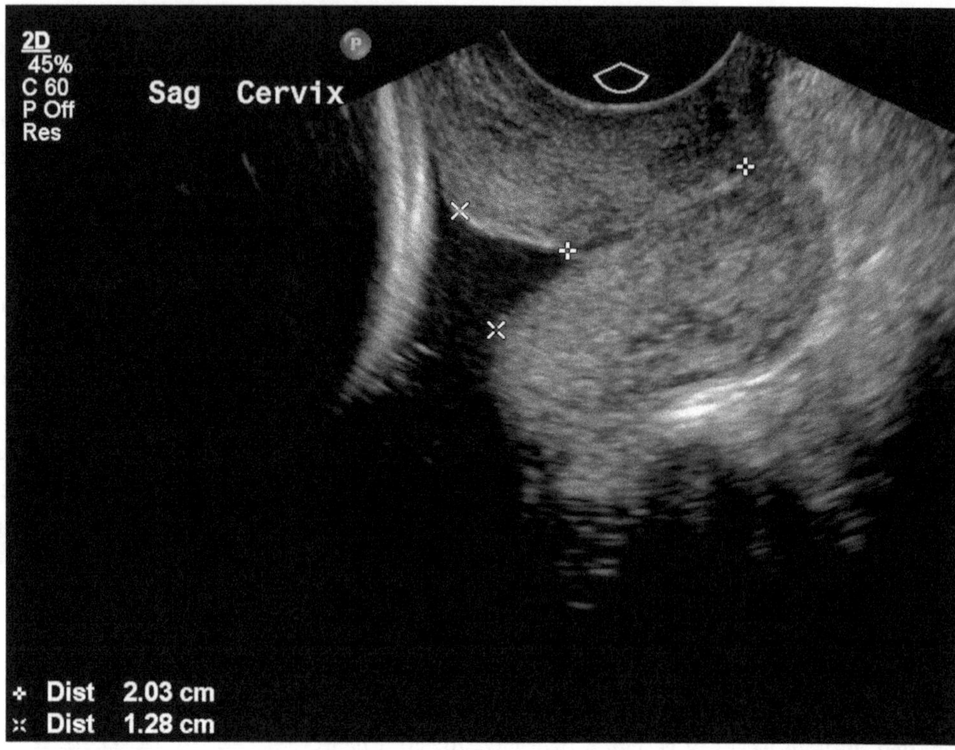

Figure 14-9. Transvaginal sonography of a cervix with a dilated internal os and funneling. The fetal skull is to the left of the image. Effacement progresses from the inner cervical os to the outer. The cervical length is shortened to 2.03 cm. Funneling is associated with a higher risk of PTB, especially if the funnel is U-shaped. (This funnel is V-shaped.)

First Thought, Worst Thought

What is the most likely cause of watery vaginal discharge in the preterm period?

Urinary incontinence or vaginal infection.

What is the worst it could be?

Preterm PROM (PPROM).

Cerclage

Cervical cerclage is a surgical procedure in which a synthetic suture or tape is used to reinforce the cervix (Norwitz, 2023b). The procedure is typically performed by an obstetrician or maternal-fetal medicine specialist. Structural support from a cerclage can successfully treat structural weakness of the cervix and allow a term delivery (Berghella, 2023a). Most cerclages are placed transvaginally. A McDonald cerclage is a purse-string stitch placed at the proximal cervix to cinch it closed. Shirodkar cerclage is also a drawstring loop, but the sutures are buried in the tissue, not exposed. The obstetrician may use the Shirodkar procedure to place a permanent stitch around the cervix, which necessitates a cesarean section. An abdominal cerclage allows a more proximal stable placement of the suture that can remain in place for future pregnancies. Abdominal cerclage is considered if the client has a deeply traumatized or amputated cervix (for example, from a severe laceration, cancer-related surgery, or failed transvaginal cerclages) or to address cervical incompetence before conception. Indications for cervical cerclage for clients with singleton pregnancies include (ACOG, 2014/2024)

- Painless cervical dilation in the second trimester of the current pregnancy.

- Prior PTB and a cervical length less than 25 mm before 24 weeks of gestation.
- History of one or more second-trimester pregnancy losses involving painless cervical dilation in the absence of labor or placental abruption.
- Prior cerclage due to painless cervical dilation in the second trimester.

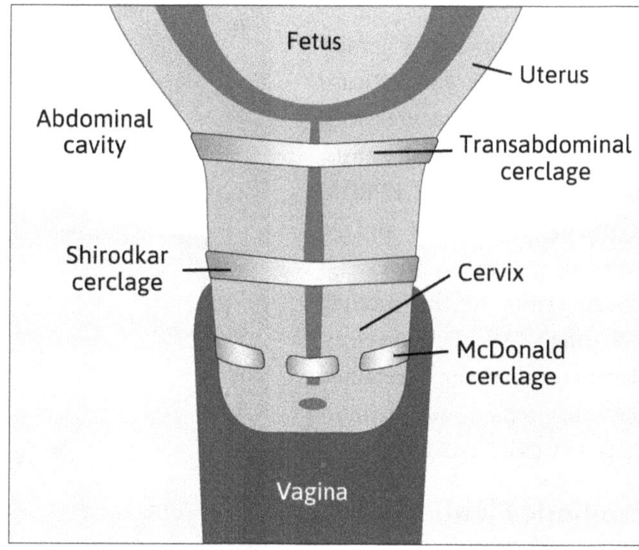

Figure 14-10. McDonald, Shirodkar, and transabdominal are the three most common cerclage procedures (©Анастасия Красавина/Adobe Stock).

Preterm Prelabor Rupture of Membranes (PPROM)

PPROM occurs in approximately 10% of all PTB in the United States and more than 20% in certain high-risk populations such as people with PTB or PPROM in prior pregnancies (Simhan & Romero, 2021). The strength and integrity of fetal membranes derive from extracellular membrane proteins, including collagens, fibronectin, and laminin (Duff, 2022). At term, PROM may result from normal physiologic weakening of the membranes together with shearing forces produced by uterine contractions (ACOG, 2018/2021). In contrast, PPROM is usually related to a pathological process such as infection, inflammation, mechanical stress, or abruption (Duff, 2022).

Individuals who suffered PPROM in a previous pregnancy are 3 times more likely to have PPROM in the current pregnancy (Duff, 2022). About 15–25% of people with PPROM have signs of IAI upon presentation, especially when membranes rupture at an early date (ACOG, 2020a/2023). Whereas first-trimester vaginal bleeding slightly increases the risk of PPROM, antepartum bleeding in more than one trimester increases the risk of PPROM 200–600% (Duff, 2022). Other risk factors include short cervical length, genital tract infection (especially bacterial vaginosis), polyhydramnios, acute trauma, genetic conditions, low body mass index, low socioeconomic status, smoking, and illicit drug use (ACOG, 2020a/2023; Duff, 2022).

PPROM increases the risk of PTB, neonatal sepsis, placental abruption (occurring in 4–12% of PPROM cases), fetal distress from cord compression, and long-term neurodevelopmental impairment (ACOG, 2020a/2023; Simhan & Romero, 2021). At earlier gestational ages, malpresentation is common, and the incidence of cord prolapse can be up to 11% (Lewis et al., 2007). When latency (time between PPROM and birth) is prolonged, especially early in gestation, the fetus is at risk for growth restriction, pulmonary hypoplasia, malformations of face and limbs from compression, scoliosis, hip dislocation, limb reduction, and body-wall defects. The mother is also at

Table 14-2

Sample GOLDCART History for Preterm Prelabor Rupture of Membranes

General situation and history—How many weeks pregnant are you? Do you have any health issues or pregnancy complications? How many pregnancies and babies have you had? Is the baby moving? Have you had any cesarean sections or other uterine surgeries? **Onset**—When do you think your water broke? Did it start as a gush or trickle? How much? What were you doing when you felt the leaking? Were you having cramps or contractions before you began to leak?
Location—Are you sure the fluid is coming from your vagina and not your bladder?
Duration—How long have you been leaking? Are you leaking more or less than when you started?
Characteristics—Is the fluid clear? Is there an odor to the fluid? Is there any blood? Is the fluid thin like water or urine or thick like mucus?
Associated symptoms—Are you having contractions? Do you have a backache? Do you have loose stools? Fever or signs of illness? Are you feeling increased pressure in your pelvis?
Relieving/aggravating factors—Do you notice a gush of fluid when you bear down or when you have a contraction? Do you leak more fluid when the baby is moving?
Treatment—Did you need an extra-large sanitary pad, adult diaper or towel to control the flow of fluid, or is the flow light enough to use a panty liner or no protection at all?

higher risk for hypovolemia/anemia from placental abruption, retained placenta with hemorrhage, maternal sepsis, and death. Periviable PPROM occurring between 14 and 24 weeks of gestation carries significant risks to the mother, including IAI, endometritis, placental abruption, retained placenta, sepsis, and hemorrhage (ACOG, 2020a/2023).

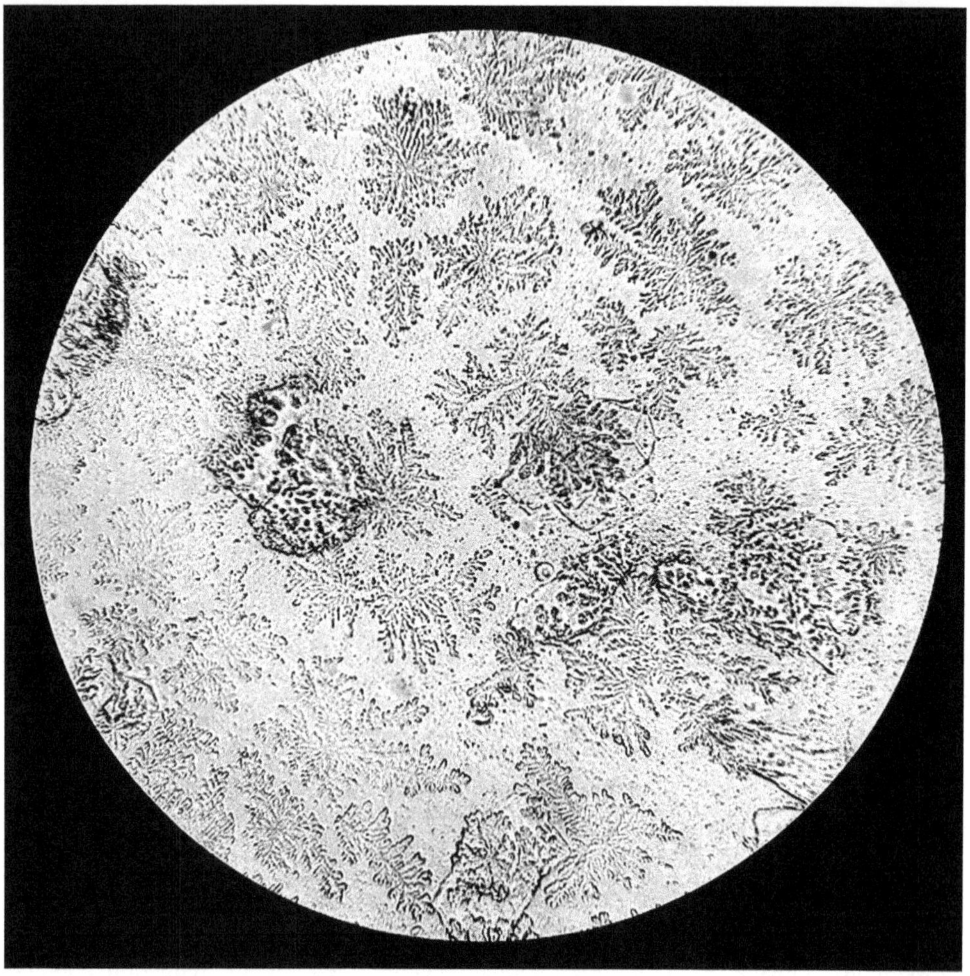

Figure 14-11. Under a microscope, dried amniotic fluid shows a distinctive fernlike pattern.

Amniotic Fluid

Amniotic fluid is vital to healthy gestation. It has antibacterial properties, equalizes pressure, cushions the fetus against trauma and the umbilical cord against compression, allows for movement and musculoskeletal development, and promotes the growth of healthy respiratory, gastrointestinal and urinary tracts. The risk of a poor outcome increases if the fetus is surrounded by insufficient or excessive quantities of fluid. Between 10 and 20 weeks of gestation, the average volume of amniotic fluid increases from about 25 ml to 400 ml (Tripathi, Khatod, & Agrawal, 2015). Volume continues to increase, peaking at roughly 1 L at 34–38 weeks. After 38 weeks, it decreases about 125 ml/week to an average of 800 ml at 40 weeks (Fischer, 2008).

Late in pregnancy, on average 1,000 ml of amniotic fluid moves into and out of the amniotic cavity daily, circulating and renewing itself while maintaining a relatively constant volume (Ross & Beall, 2023). It is resorbed by fetal swallowing and by crossing the amnion into the placental vasculature and is regenerated largely by the fetus (Ross & Beall, 2023). Fetal swallowing filters the fluid by moving particulate matter such as fetal hair and skin cells into the digestive tract to form meconium. The fetus then replaces the volume through urination. Near term, the daily amniotic flow in and around the fetus is estimated as follows (Ross & Beall, 2023):

- Fetal urine production: 800–1,200 ml/day
- Fetal lung liquid secretion: 170 ml/day
- Fetal swallowing: 500–1,000 ml/day
- Intramembranous flow: 200–400 ml/day
- Oral-nasal secretions: 25 ml/day
- Transmembranous flow: 10 ml/day

Abnormalities in fluid quantity can complicate a pregnancy. Oligohydramnios (low amniotic fluid) in the second half of pregnancy can be caused by rupture of membranes, diminished fetal urine flow (resulting from fetal urinary-tract obstruction or fetal-growth restriction, for example), or maternal dehydration (Ross & Beall, 2023). Oligohydramnios is associated with fetal malformation, stillbirth, abnormal heart rate pattern, and meconium aspiration (Ross & Beall, 2023). If fluid volume is inadequate for a long period, the fetus may suffer compression deformities and underdeveloped lungs. Polyhydramnios (excessive amniotic fluid) may result from increased fetal urine flow or less fetal swallowing. Other causes of polyhydramnios are alloimmunization; congenital infection, maternal diabetes; or fetal renal, neurologic, or gastrointestinal abnormalities. More than half of cases are of unknown etiology (Kazemi et al., 2019). Risks of polyhydramnios include fetal growth abnormalities (both macrosomia and

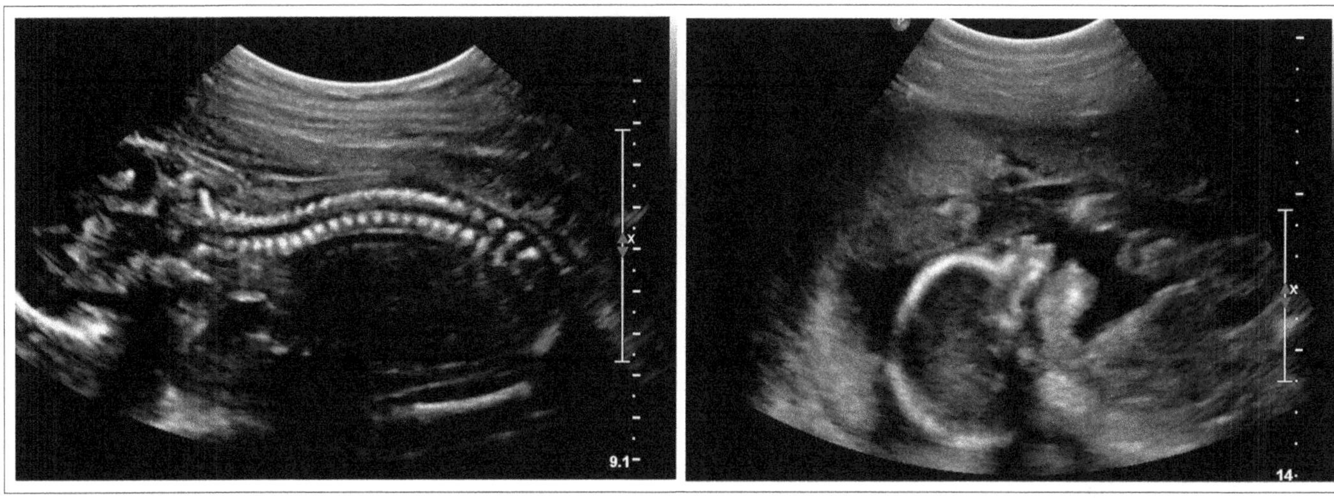

Figure 14-12. Twenty-two weeks of gestation with severe oligohydramnios following PPROM at 20 0/7 weeks. The small amount of remaining fluid was pooled around the head, and in the second image the fetus is seen drinking it. The baby survived.

growth restriction), low Apgar scores, abnormal FHR, PTB, unstable lie, malpresentation, cord prolapse, and placental abruption (Ross & Beall, 2023).

Evaluation of PPROM

Suspect PPROM when the client reports a gush or trickle of clear or straw-colored fluid that soaks through clothes. Sometimes there is a history of questionable leakage for hours, days, or weeks. You can diagnose most cases of PPROM by asking questions and performing a physical examination.

1. **Take a GOLDCART history** to establish time and circumstances of presumed membrane rupture.
2. **Obtain maternal vital signs** and conduct a physical examination, including abdominal assessment and Leopold's maneuvers.
3. **Monitor FHR and uterine activity.** Attach the client to an electronic fetal monitor. Evaluate the FHR pattern and any uterine activity.
4. **Assess evidence of leaking fluid.** Evaluate the fluid on the sanitary pad and note the color, consistency, odor, and amount.
5. **Perform a sterile speculum examination.** (Avoid performing a digital examination, which can increase risk of infection, unless the client is clearly in active labor.) Assess for pooling of amniotic fluid in the posterior vaginal vault. Pooling or visualization of fluid flowing through the cervical os establishes the diagnosis of PPROM. Take note of any dilation. Occasionally the umbilical cord or a fetal limb may be visualized coming through the cervix. Ask the client to press on the fundus, to cough, and to bear down to determine whether increased intraabdominal pressure causes fluid to trickle through the cervix. Collect a vaginal-rectal swab to screen for GBS carrier status. Consider testing for gonorrhea and chlamydia if the client has not been tested recently.
6. **Perform a nitrazine, fern, or commercial test.**

   Nitrazine test: Collect a swab from the posterior vaginal fornix and check the pH of the vaginal fluid with nitrazine paper. Nitrazine is a pH indicator dye incorporated into paper strips for testing vaginal fluid. Amniotic fluid has a pH of 7.1–7.3 and turns the test strip blue. Normal vaginal secretions have a pH of 4.5–6.0 and turn the test strip yellow. A positive result is not specific for PPROM; any liquid with an alkaline pH will turn the paper blue. False-positive results may occur in the presence of blood, semen, alkaline antiseptics, or bacterial vaginosis. False-negative results may occur with a very slow leak or prolonged rupture (ACOG, 2018/2021). NICE guidelines specify that the provider should *not* use nitrazine alone to diagnose PPROM (NICE, 2015/2022).

   Fern test: Swab the posterior vaginal fornix and paint a glass microscope slide with vaginal discharge. Let it dry for at least 10 min. Amniotic fluid dries to form a fern-like pattern visible under a microscope. Ferning is 98% sensitive and 88.2% specific for rupture of membranes during labor and 51.3% sensitive and 70.5% specific in the nonlaboring client (Gaddey, Bailey, & Smith, 2011). This test is unaffected by meconium or vaginal discharge, but more than 10% blood content can produce a false negative (Gaddey et al., 2011). False negative results can also occur if the sample is insufficient. Antiseptic solutions, semen, fingerprints, and cervical mucus can cause a false positive, although their crystallization patterns differ from that formed by undiluted amniotic fluid.

   Commercial immunoassay tests such as ROM Plus® and AmniSure® screen for substances abundant in amni-

Management of PPROM can hinge on accurate gestational-age dating.

otic fluid. They are reasonably accurate and can be performed at the bedside. Because they can give false positives and negatives, the results should not solely determine the course of care. A vaginal swab for one of these substances, fFN, will test positive if the membranes are ruptured, but it is nonspecific and nondiagnostic for PPROM (ACOG, 2020a/2023; Duff, 2022). A negative fFN test, however, is an indication that the client probably does not have ruptured membranes. An insufficient sample can cause a false negative. In the United Kingdom, an absorbent pad (AmnioSense™) changes color at pH greater than 5.2. *Candida albicans* (yeast) infection can cause false-positive results (Duff, 2022).

7. **Sonographic assessment.** When the clinical assessment fails to determine whether the amniotic membranes are ruptured, an ultrasound examination may be indicated. Many people with PPROM show oligohydramnios, which is defined as a maximum vertical pocket of amniotic fluid less than 2 cm in depth or an amniotic fluid index (AFI) of 5 cm or less. An AFI greater than 7 cm largely excludes the diagnosis of PPROM (Duff, 2022). If the AFI was in the upper ranges of normal before membranes ruptured, however, the fluid level may appear adequate even in PPROM. Sonographic assessment can also provide useful information about gestational age, size, wellbeing, presentation, and the presence or absence of anomalies.

Diagnosis of PPROM

The diagnosis may be obvious if the client arrives sitting on a soaked towel or ambiguous if the report involves a vague sensation of abnormal wetness. When findings are ambiguous, the midwife makes the diagnosis of PPROM in collaboration with the obstetrician. Findings suggestive or indicative of PPROM include

- Pooling of amniotic fluid in the vaginal vault or visualization of fluid flowing through the cervix (definitive). This fluid might contain particles of vernix or meconium.
- A positive nitrazine test (suggestive).
- The ferning of vaginal fluid on a microscope slide (suggestive).
- A positive ROM Plus® or AmniSure® test (suggestive).
- Oligohydramnios (strongly suggestive, especially if a recent amniotic fluid measurement was normal).
- The obstetrician can confirm PPROM by instilling indigo carmine dye into the amniotic sac through the abdominal wall then observe for the passage of blue-dyed fluid into the vagina (definitive).

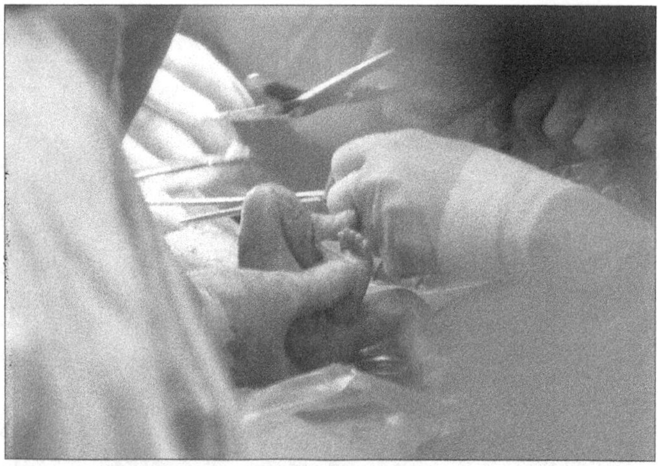

Figure 14-13. Extremely preterm infants are born by cesarean section for the same indications as in a term pregnancy, including breech or transverse presentation, cord prolapse, placental abruption, abnormal fetal heart rate (FHR), and preeclampsia with severe features.

Management of PPROM

Most clients with preterm prelabor rupture of membranes give birth within 1 week (ACOG, 2020a/2023). The latency period tends to be longer if membranes rupture long before term and shorter if they rupture near term. About 40–50% of clients with PPROM in the mid-second trimester give birth within 7 days and about 70–80% give birth within 2–5 weeks after membrane rupture (ACOG, 2020a/2023). In some cases, latency lasts for months. Rarely, ruptured fetal membranes appear to reseal spontaneously to allow the pregnancy to continue, usually with good outcomes (Mercer, 2021).

The community midwifery client with PPROM should be transferred to a hospital for physician management or physician-midwife collaborative care. Initial management proceeds down one of two major paths, toward (1) vaginal or cesarean birth or (2) expectant management. The provider determines the course of action with consideration of gestational age, the presence or absence of maternal/fetal infection, the presence or absence of labor, fetal presentation, fetal wellbeing, amount of cervical dilation, the client's preferences, and the availability of a facility capable of providing appropriate neonatal care (Duff, 2022). Prompt delivery is indicated if there is advanced labor, significant bleeding, any signs of intrauterine infection, or nonreassuring fetal testing. In some cases, malpresentation or unstable lie with a high risk of cord prolapse (for example, transverse lie with the fetal back toward the fundus) may be an indication for planned birth (Duff, 2022).

Expectant Management of PPROM

If no maternal or fetal contraindications exist (such as IAI or abnormal FHR), manage clients with PPROM before 34 weeks of gestation expectantly (ACOG, 2020a/2023). Prolonged latency after PPROM between 23 and 34 weeks of gestation does not worsen newborn outcomes, and the immature fetus benefits from every additional day or week in the uterus (Duff, 2022). The client with PPROM is typically managed with inpatient admission because of the potential for rapid birth, the risk of infection, and concerns for fetal compromise (Lauder, Sciscione, Biggio, & Osmundson, 2020). ACOG does not recommend outpatient management of PPROM with a viable fetus, but the client with periviable PROM may be considered for home care after evaluation in a hospital (ACOG, 2020a/2023).

Assess fetal wellbeing with some combination of kick counts, fetal monitoring, and/or biophysical profile. There is no data demonstrating that activity restriction improves perinatal outcome in pregnancies complicated by PPROM, and there is evidence that restricting activity can be harmful; therefore, SMFM recommends that clients with PPROM avoid bed rest and continue normal activities (SMFM, 2020b).

Table 14-3

ACOG Management Guidelines for Prelabor Rupture of Membranes with Normal Antenatal Testing

Term (37 0/7 weeks of gestation or more)
Group B *Streptococcus* (GBS) prophylaxis as indicated. Treat IAI if present. Proceed toward planned birth (induction or cesarean as appropriate/indicated).
Late preterm (34 0/7–36 6/7 weeks of gestation)
Expectant management or proceed toward planned birth as appropriate or indicated. Single course of corticosteroids, if steroids not previously given, if proceeding with planned birth in no less than 24 hr and no more than 7 days, and no evidence of IAI. Do not delay birth to administer steroids. GBS screening and prophylaxis as indicated. If amniotic infection is present, treat and proceed toward planned birth.
Preterm (24 0/7–33 6/7 weeks of gestation)
Expectant management. Neonatology and maternal–fetal medicine consultation for earlier gestational ages. Antibiotics are recommended to prolong latency if there are no contraindications. Single course of corticosteroids; insufficient evidence for or against rescue course. If an amniotic infection is present, treat and proceed toward planned birth. A vaginal–rectal swab for GBS culture should be obtained at the time of initial presentation and GBS prophylaxis administered as indicated. Magnesium sulfate for neuroprotection before anticipated birth for pregnancies less than 32 0/7 weeks of gestation if there are no contraindications.
Periviable (less than 23–24 weeks of gestation)
Client counseling; consider neonatology and maternal–fetal medicine consultation. Expectant management or induction of labor. Antibiotics may be considered as early as 20 weeks of gestation. GBS prophylaxis is not recommended before viability. Corticosteroids are not recommended before viability. Tocolysis is not recommended before viability. Magnesium sulfate for neuroprotection is not recommended before viability.
From "Prelabor Rupture of Membranes" (Practice Bulletin 217), by American College of Obstetricians and Gynecologists, 2020/2023, *Obstetrics & Gynecology, 135*(3), e80–e97. Copyright by ACOG.

Late Preterm PROM

Emerging evidence suggests that expectant management benefits the fetus with late preterm PROM. The 2016 PPROMT trial, a study of prelabor rupture of membranes close to term, found that expectant management between 34 0/7 and 36 6/7 weeks of gestation reduces neonatal morbidity (Morris et al, 2016). Similarly, the authors of a 2017 meta-analysis of randomized trials of management of PPROM (which included the PPROMT trial) determined that if mother and infant are not compromised, expectant management yields better neonatal outcomes (Bond et al., 2017). ACOG advises that expectant management and immediate birth are both reasonable options when PPROM occurs between 34 0/7 weeks of gestation and 36 6/7 weeks of gestation (ACOG, 2020a/2023). The benefit of additional time to mature *in utero* must be balanced against the risks of intrauterine infection, placental abruption, and cord prolapse/compression. Provider and parents should use shared decision-making to devise a plan. Expectant management should not extend beyond 37 weeks of gestation.

Components of Expectant Management

Consider the components of expectant management as follows:

- **Antenatal corticosteroids.** In cases of PPROM, corticosteroid treatment reduces the rate of neonatal

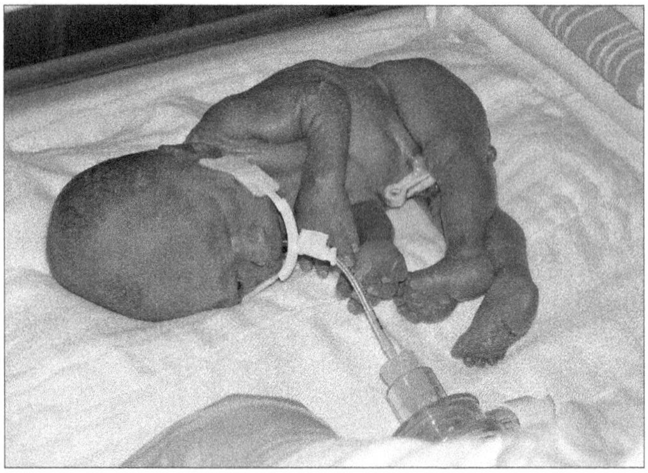

Figure 14-14. Compression deformities. This genetically normal infant remained in utero for about 9 weeks after spontaneous rupture of the membranes at 19 weeks of gestation. He was finally born via cesarean at 28 weeks of gestation when the mother began to hemorrhage from placental abruption. He survived, though he contended with many orthopedic and respiratory issues.

death, respiratory distress syndrome, intraventricular hemorrhage and necrotizing enterocolitis, and it shortens the duration of neonatal respiratory support by 30–60% without an increase in maternal or neonatal infection (Park, Isayama, & McDonald, 2016; Roberts et al., 2017). ACOG and others recommend a course of corticosteroids for clients with PPROM between 23 0/7 and 33 6/7 weeks of gestation and for clients with PPROM at 34 0/7–36 6/7 weeks who are expected to give birth in more than 24 hr and less than 7 days and have not received a previous course of steroids (ACOG, 2020a/2023; Duff, 2022; Sreedhar, Rathore, Benjamin, Gowri, & Mathews, 2020). Antenatal steroids may be given as early as 22 0/7 weeks of gestation if birth is anticipated within 7 days and the parents desire aggressive neonatal resuscitation (ACOG, 2020a/2023).

- **Magnesium sulfate for neuroprotection.** Clients with PPROM before 32 0/7 weeks of gestation at risk for imminent birth are candidates (ACOG, 2020a/2023).
- **Screening for infection.** Consider testing for HIV, syphilis, chlamydia, gonorrhea, hepatitis B, and hepatitis C if clinically appropriate. Collect a vaginal-rectal swab to screen for GBS. Consider performing a wet mount to screen for bacterial vaginosis (BV) and Trichomonas vaginalis (Duff, 2022).
- **Prophylactic antibiotics.** ACOG recommends a 7-day course of antibiotics to prolong latency in PPROM less than 34 0/7 weeks of gestation using a combination of IV ampicillin and erythromycin followed by oral amoxicillin and erythromycin (ACOG, 2020a/2023). Other authors recommend azithromycin rather than erythromycin (Duff, 2022). Other antibiotic regimens may be utilized per institutional protocol. ACOG does not recommend prophylactic antibiotics for pregnancies with PPROM 34 0/7 weeks or more of gestation unless a GBS culture result is positive or unknown (ACOG, 2020a/2023).

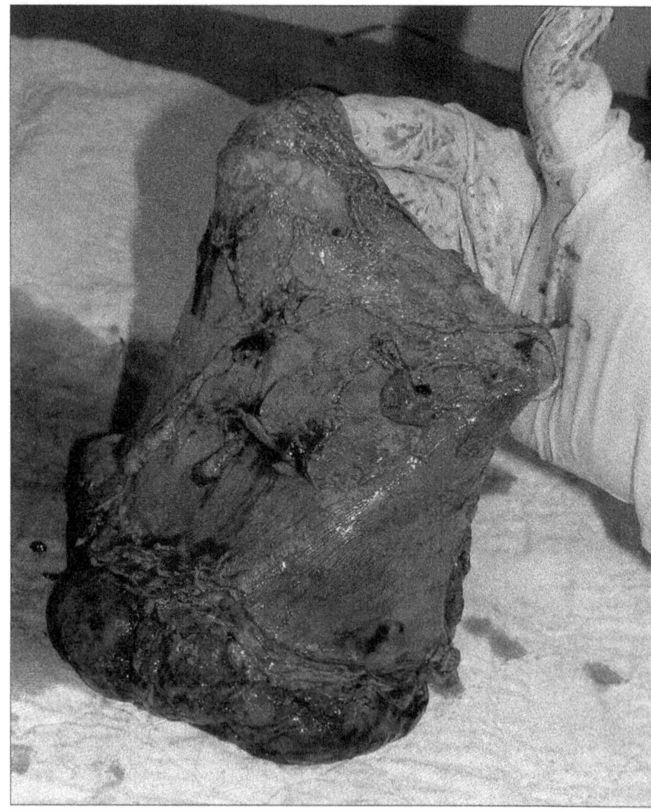

Figure 14-15. The placenta tells the story. Examination of the placenta from the baby in Figure 14-14 shows evidence of IAI and acute abruption.

- **Tocolytics.** In late preterm PROM, tocolysis is sometimes used to delay birth for up to 48 hr to allow administration of corticosteroids or to facilitate maternal transport, but the practice is controversial (ACOG, 2020a/2023). Delaying birth can increase the risk of intrauterine infection without proven maternal or neonatal benefit (ACOG, 2020a/2023). ACOG recommends against tocolytic therapy in late preterm PROM between 34 0/7 and 36 6/7 weeks of gestation (ACOG, 2020a/2023). Do not administer tocolytics if the client has signs or symptoms of IAI or placental abruption.
- **Anticoagulants.** If the client is at high risk of thromboembolism, sequential compression devices can be used to discourage venous stasis, and prophylactic enoxaparin (Lovenox®) or heparin can be administered.

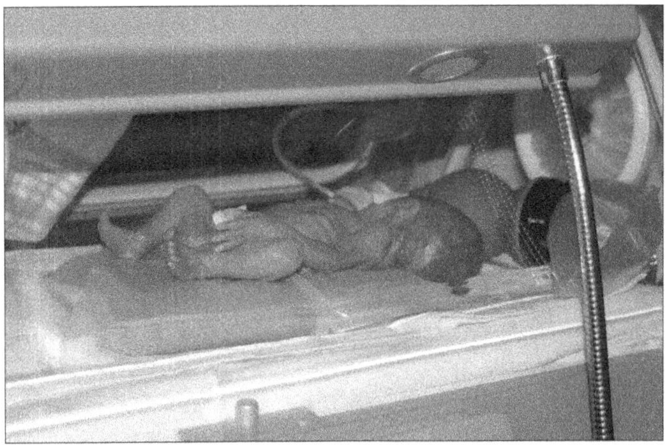

Figure 14-16. Even within a hospital, premature infants are usually moved in a specialized neonatal transport device. This 26-week infant is being transferred from the birth room to the NICU.

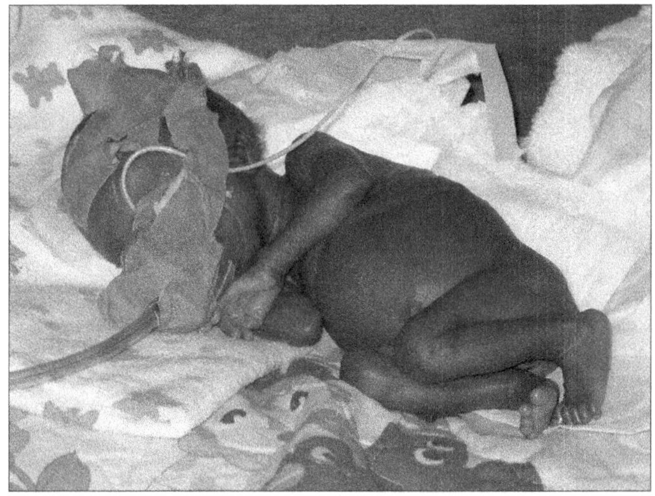

Figure 14-17. In low-resource locations, it can be a challenge to keep a preterm infant alive. A neonatal care provider at ECWA Evangel Hospital in Jos, Nigeria, improvised an oxygen mask from a medication cup and tape. "Premature Baby with Improvised Oxygen Mask," by M. Blyth, 2006 (https://commons.wikimedia.org/wiki/File:Premature_baby_with_improvised_oxygen_mask.jpg). CC BY 3.0.

Managing Unplanned PTB

Preterm infants can be born with unexpected swiftness. People in PTL may have vague or nonspecific symptoms until labor is advanced. The baby may arrive shortly after the water breaks and is more likely to assume a nonvertex position for birth. Premature infants are extremely delicate, and the birth attendant can easily damage fragile skin and organs. Allow the baby to emerge with as little assistance as possible. Preterm infants tend to emerge very rapidly and are extremely slippery.

Transport Considerations

Being born outside a hospital is a significant disadvantage to the preterm infant (Pirneskoski, Peräjoki, Nuutila, & Kuisma, 2016). In a study of live-born infants of 24–35 weeks of gestation in and around Paris, France, Jones et al. (2011) found that those born in-hospital had a lower mortality rate (8%) than those born at home and transported by skilled transport teams (18%). Most newborns that died were between 28 and 31 weeks of gestation and arrived at the hospital hypothermic. The surviving babies who had required transport were more likely than hospital-born infants to have persistent cardiorespiratory difficulties and require intubation (Jones et al., 2011). Late preterm infants born in community settings also seem to have higher rates of adverse neonatal outcomes, including Apgars lower than 7 at 5 min and infant death, the latter of which was statistically significant but still very low (Meuchel, Zwelling, Shields, Cheng, & Caughey, 2017). Transfer to a regional neonatal care facility before birth decreases risk to the infant and allows the mother to recover in the same hospital (Agostino, Aufieri, & Gente, 2016).

If a preterm infant is born unexpectedly outside a hospital, arrange rapid transport to an appropriate facility. Infants at low gestational age, those with congenital anomalies, or those otherwise at risk for decompensation may have better outcomes when a neonatal transport specialty team is used for transfer rather than a standard ambulance. These neonatal transportation experts, usually based at a receiving hospital, typically arrive with full-featured equipment such as a portable heated incubator fitted with ventilator; oxygen blender; suction; monitors for cardiac and respiratory function; pulse oximetry and capnography; a defibrillator; and even point-of-care laboratory testing for blood samples (Perry, 2017). Helicopter or airplane transport subjects the critically ill neonate infant to less shock, vibration, and noise than ambulance transport and may be considered if a tertiary-care facility is distant (Bouchut, Van Lancker, Chritin, & Gueugniaud, 2011).

Portable Thermal Mattresses

The TransWarmer® infant transport mattress reaches the optimal temperature of 100.4–107.6°F (38°–42°C) within 90 sec and stays warm for 2 hr. **Caution!** The gel temperature of the TransWarmer® must be 66.6°–82.9°F (9.2°–28.3°C) when activated to achieve the target temperature. Beyond this range, the infant risks burns, insufficient warming, or even induced hypothermia.

Characteristics of Preterm Infants

A preterm infant is at risk for complications related to anatomic or functional immaturity, including hypothermia, respiratory distress, patent ductus arteriosus, intracranial hemorrhage, hypoglycemia, necrotizing enterocolitis, infection, and retinopathy of prematurity (Mandy, 2023). The risk of these disorders increases with decreasing gestational age. Because infection and abnormal placentation can lead to PTL, the premature infant is often born compromised from intrauterine infection and/or growth restriction. Even late preterm infants, however, can have a complicated course.

Habitus: Below 32 weeks of gestation, the infant is thin-skinned and gaunt because of minimal subcutaneous fat. Preterm infants of low gestational age are weak and inactive with flaccid muscle tone. Reflexes may be only partially developed, and sucking may be uncoordinated and ineffective. Early preterm infants are easily overstimulated and may respond to noise or rough handling with apnea or bradycardia.

Vital sign instability: Apnea and bradycardia may be the first signs of abnormal body temperature, blood gases, electrolytes, blood sugar, or blood acid levels (Weiner & Zaichkin, 2021).

Glucose regulation: Very premature infants have little stored glucose. If resuscitation is needed or if the infant becomes cold, hypoglycemia may result.

Thermoregulation: Small infants become chilled easily through conduction, convection, radiation, and evaporation. Premature infants have thin skin, minimal subcutaneous fat, and a relatively large body surface area. They lose heat quickly and cannot produce enough to balance what is lost. Hypothermia can start a spiral of complications ending in cardiovascular collapse.

Intraventricular hemorrhage: The delicate web of capillaries in the brain of the neonate are especially vulnerable to damage in babies born before 32 weeks of gestation. A decrease in venous drainage from the head or sudden changes in blood CO_2 levels, BP, or blood volume may cause them to break. The result is intraventricular hemorrhage (bleeding into the ventricles of the brain). To decrease the risk of intraventricular hemorrhage, handle the newborn with extreme gentleness. *Do not raise the infant's legs higher than the head. It may increase cerebral venous pressure and risk of bleeding* (Weiner & Zaichkin, 2021). Avoid ventilating with excessive pressure and use a pulse oximeter to guide oxygen delivery. Providers must administer fluids very slowly, over 5–10 min, to avoid sudden changes in blood volume.

Lungs: Spontaneous breathing efforts are inefficient because of weak chest muscles and a supple rib cage. Surfactant is a substance made by the lungs that keeps the alveoli open between breaths. A lack of surfactant may cause the lungs to collapse after each breath. The lungs of the very immature infant may be stiff and require more pressure when using a bag and mask—but too much pressure can damage delicate lung tissues. Excessive ventilatory pressure may also interfere with venous return from the head and increase the risk of intraventricular hemorrhage (Weiner & Zaichkin, 2021). Supplementary oxygen may damage immature lung tissue but is often necessary to maintain adequate oxygen saturation when resuscitating a preterm infant.

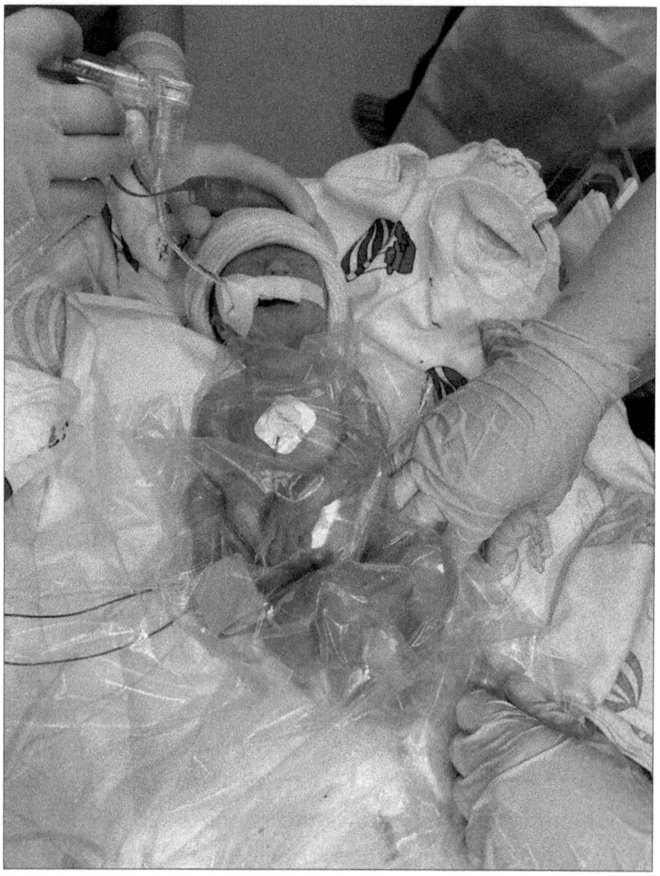

Figure 14-18. The mother of this baby girl unexpectedly experienced rupture of membranes at 27 3/7 weeks of gestation and presented to a community hospital with a NICU that did not manage babies below 28 weeks. While the mother awaited transfer to a higher-level facility, the fetus began having variable FHR decelerations to 60 beats per min (bpm) and developed minimal heart-rate variability. The mother underwent an emergency cesarean section under general anesthesia. The baby weighed 2 lb 8 oz (1,130 g), and per NRP guidelines was covered in plastic wrap to reduce heat loss. She was transferred to the tertiary hospital shortly after birth and thrived in the higher-level NICU. After 89 days, she was discharged home. At this writing, she is a healthy child with no apparent deficits. Photograph by Angela Cassel.

Delayed Cord Clamping

Delayed cord clamping provides life-changing benefits to preterm infants, including cardiovascular stability, improved BP, less need for blood transfusions, and possibly improved survival (Weiner & Zaichkin, 2021). The Neonatal Resuscitation Program (NRP) recommends delaying cord clamping until

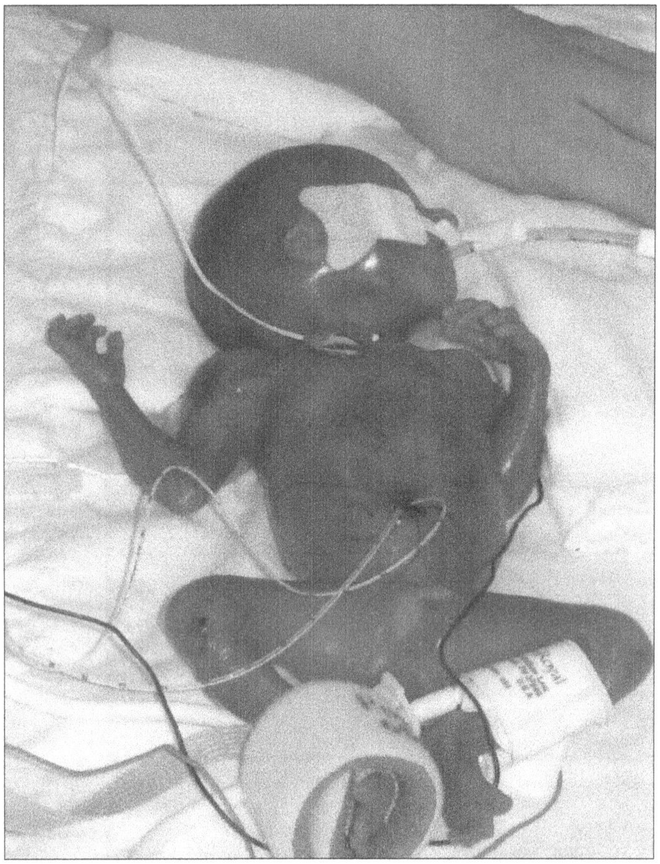

Figure 14-19. Cusp of viability. This infant was born at about 22 weeks of gestation. His parents wanted "everything" done for him. He was born kicking and even tried to cry, but he was too immature to survive. Despite the best technology had to offer, he died in the NICU after 18 hr.

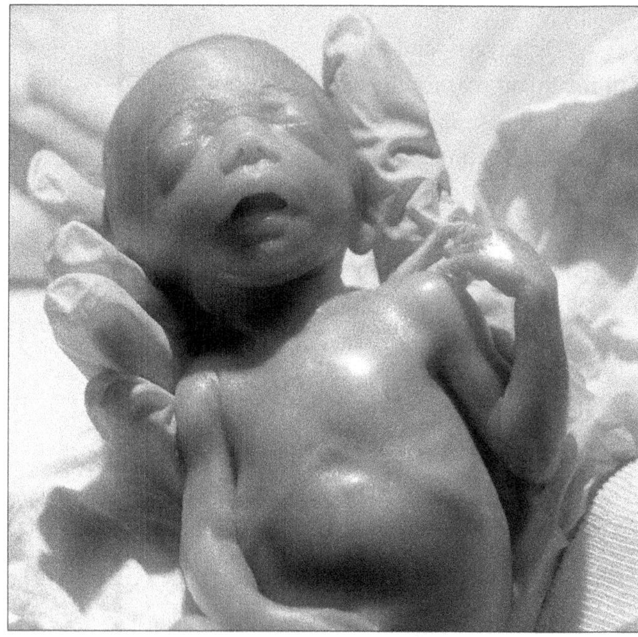

Figure 14-20. This infant was also born about 22 weeks of gestation. After the neonatologist explained options to the parents, they decided to keep her comfortable until she died. She survived about 5 min.

30–60 sec after birth for the vigorous preterm infant and opines that with a nonvigorous infant it may be reasonable to delay cord clamping briefly while the provider stimulates the infant to breathe and suctions the mouth and nose with a bulb syringe (Weiner & Zaichkin, 2021). Delayed cord clamping is only recommended if placental circulation is intact and is contraindicated in cases of placental abruption (Weiner & Zaichkin, 2021).

Resuscitation Considerations for the Preterm Infant

Preterm infants are at higher risk of complications because of rapid heat loss, immature organ systems, low blood volume, and vulnerability to hypoglycemia. Although resuscitation of a preterm infant proceeds much like that of a term infant, some guidelines differ. See Chapter 13 for a comprehensive discussion of the resuscitation of term and preterm newborns.

For term newborns, drying with warm cloths, skin-to-skin contact with mother, and early breastfeeding foster optimal thermoregulation. Preterm infants need aggressive intervention to remain warm. Increasing room temperature to 77–82.4°F (25–28°C) can help (Sultan, Habib, & Carvalho, 2017). NRP guidelines recommend using a thermal mattress for infants less than 32 weeks of gestation (Weiner & Zaichkin, 2021). Activate a portable thermal mattress by squeezing it 5 min before the baby is born (Weiner & Zaichkin, 2021). Cover the thermal mattress with a thin blanket so the surface is not in contact with the infant's fragile skin. The TransWarmer® infant transport mattress (a gel-filled, self-heating device) reaches the optimal temperature of 100.4–107.6°F (38°–42°C) within 90 sec and stays warm for 2 hr. **Caution!** Protect the TransWarmer® from extremes of heat and cold. To provide optimal warmth, the gel must be at room temperature, 66.6°–82.9°F (19.2°–28.3°C), when activated. Outside this range, the infant risks thermal burns, insufficient warming, or even induced hypothermia (Carmichael, McCullough, & Kempley, 2007).

Do not dry a newborn less than 32 weeks of gestation. Place the wet neonate into a polyethylene bag, wrap it in plastic wrap, or place it between two sheets of plastic food wrap. You may use a reclosable 1-gallon (3.8-L) plastic bag by slicing the bottom open, sliding the infant's head through the incision as if it were a shirt, and closing the bag under the feet (Weiner & Zaichkin, 2021). Ventilation with a bag mask and unheated gases can drop the newborn's temperature quickly. In low-resource settings where a NICU is unavailable and preterm infants must remain with their mothers, skin-to-skin kangaroo care is the most effective way to provide warmth (Mandy, 2023).

Avoid ventilating with excessive pressure and use a pulse oximeter to guide oxygen delivery. For infants less than 35 weeks of gestation, if an oxygen blender is available, set the percentage to 21–30% oxygen and titrate until the infant reaches the oxygen saturation range recommended by NRP guidelines (see Chapter 13, "Neonatal Resuscitation in Community Settings"). An infant with labored respirations or low oxygen saturation and a heart rate of 100 or greater may benefit from CPAP, if available (Weiner & Zaichkin, 2021). If a volume expander is required, administer fluids very slowly, over 5–10 min, to avoid sudden changes in blood volume.

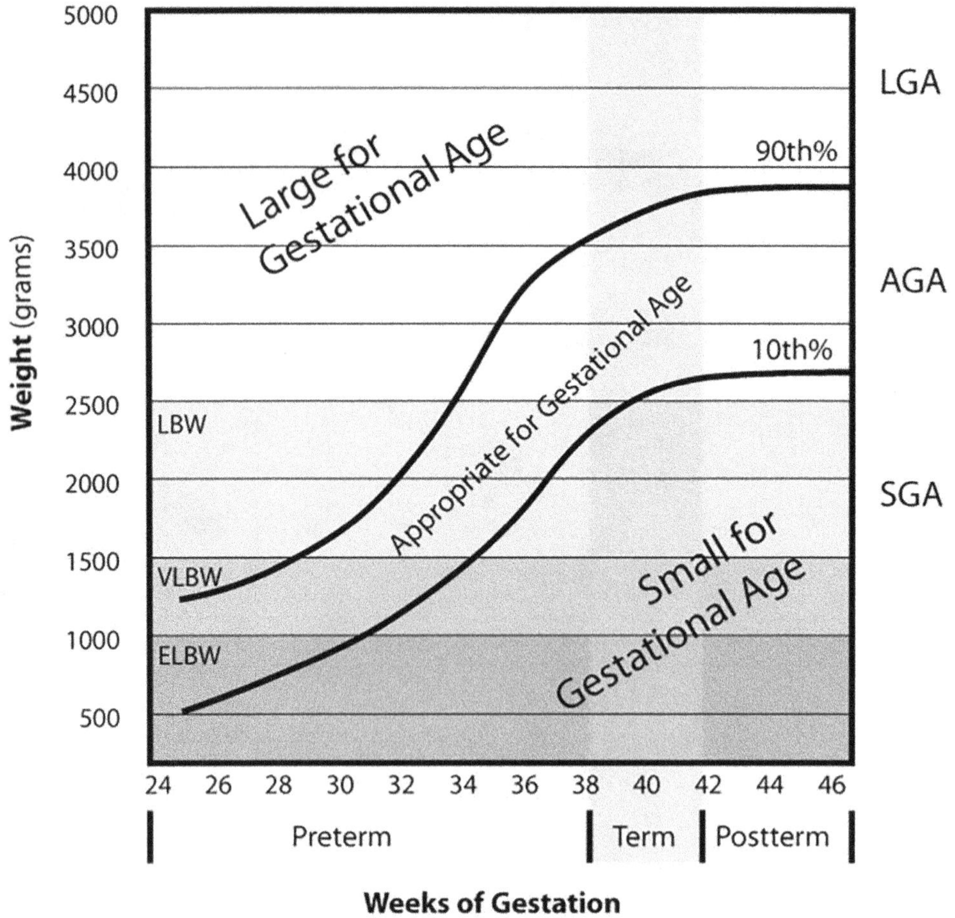

Figure 14-21. Gestational age and weight graph. The infant who is small for gestational age (SGA) is below the 10th percentile for weeks of gestation. "Weight vs Gestational Age," by Yehudamalul, 2010 (https://commons.wikimedia.org/wiki/File:Weight_vs_gestational_Age.jpg). CC BY-SA 3.0.

Late Preterm Infants

Birth between 34 0/7 and 36 6/7 weeks of gestation is considered late preterm. Although the late preterm newborn is often similar in appearance and weight to a term newborn, physiologic immaturity can complicate transition to extrauterine life (Rohan, 2021). In the first days after birth, late preterm newborns are at 600% greater risk of complications than term newborns (Barfield, & Lee, 2023). These complications include hypothermia, hypoglycemia, abnormal breathing, apnea, jaundice, feeding difficulties, low Apgar scores, seizure, and perinatal asphyxia (Karlsen, 2019). These risks are greatly increased by maternal risk factors such as hypertensive disorders of pregnancy, diabetes, antepartum hemorrhage, lung disease, infection, cardiac disease, renal disease, or genital herpes (Barfield, & Lee, 2023). Late preterm infants have a 200% higher mortality than term infants, and survivors are more likely to have neurodevelopmental abnormalities (Karlsen, 2019).

Birth at the Limit of Viability

The limit of viability is the point of development where the fetus has a reasonable chance of survival. Any infant has a right to lifesaving treatment, but also a right to mercy if painful heroic procedures are extremely unlikely to succeed (Mercurio & Drago, 2022). The likelihood of surviving without long-term major neurodevelopmental impairment increases with increasing gestational age. When born in a hospital with expert pediatricians in attendance and a capable NICU, most infants born at 26 weeks of gestation and beyond are likely to survive. Below 22 weeks of gestation, virtually none survive.

Each infant has its own set of variables that influence prognosis, including accuracy of gestational dating; birthweight; sex; plurality (number of fetuses in a multiple pregnancy); availability of tertiary care; and the presence or absence of infection, fetal abnormalities, or maternal disease (Mercurio & Drago, 2022). One large study estimated the probability of surviving to age 25 years without significant disability (intellectual impairment, autism spectrum disorder, cerebral palsy) as follows (Bourke et al., 2019):

- Infants born at 22 weeks of gestation—4%
- Infants born at 23 weeks—20%
- Infants born at 24 weeks—42%
- Infants born at 25 weeks—53%
- Infants born at 28 weeks—78%
- Full-term infants (39 0/7–40 6/7 weeks)—97%

For infants born at the cusp of viability, survival requires many months of specialized care. Even with the best possible treatment, they are at very high risk of long-term sensory, respiratory, motor, or neurological damage. Parents of extremely preterm infants must be carefully counseled to help them decide whether to provide supportive care only or attempt resuscitation and aggressive life support in the NICU.

Small and Growth-Restricted Infants

ACOG uses the term *fetal growth restriction* (FGR, also known as intrauterine growth restriction or IUGR) to describe *fetuses* with an estimated weight or abdominal circumference below the 10th percentile for gestational age and the term *small for gestational age* (SGA) to describe *newborns* with birthweight below the 10th percentile for gestational age (ACOG, 2021a). Any infant that is smaller than average is at higher risk for neonatal complications.

Small for gestational age. Neonates born after FGR often appear thin and wasted with loose, peeling skin, low skeletal muscle mass, and little subcutaneous fat tissue. The anterior fontanel may seem unusually large because of decreased membranous bone formation, and the cranial sutures may be widened (Mandy, 2022b). Neonatal gestational age assessment may be less accurate with an FGR infant because of more peeling and wrinkling of the skin, especially on the soles of the feet.

Although some SGA infants are pathologically growth-restricted, others may be constitutionally small, usually because of genetic factors (Moreira & Méio, 2022). Compromised growth and reduced energy reserves put the SGA neonate at risk for developing hypoglycemia, jaundice, hypothermia, intraventricular hemorrhage, necrotizing enterocolitis, seizures, sepsis, respiratory distress syndrome, and death (ACOG, 2021a). If an SGA infant is born in a community setting, consult with a pediatrician or transfer to a facility able to manage high-risk newborns, as appropriate.

Fetal (intrauterine) growth restriction describes a fetus who does not reach full potential for growth due to genetic or environmental factors. Growth failure can occur early in pregnancy, resulting in underdeveloped organs, or later in pregnancy, resulting in normal organs that are smaller than usual. FGR may be related to multiple gestation, maternal smoking or substance abuse, chronic maternal disease (especially hypertension, diabetes, or other chronic vascular disease), high altitude, excessive exercise, abnormal placentation, certain antepartal infections, exposure to teratogens, and/or fetal chromosomal abnormalities. FGR detected in early gestation or associated with polyhydramnios is associated with a higher risk for chromosomal anomalies (ACOG, 2021a).

The fetus with FGR, lacking nutrients to support normal growth, increases its chance for survival by growing slowly, preserving brain growth, accelerating lung maturation, and increasing red blood cell production (Tudehope, Vento, Bhutta, & Pachi, 2013). FGR can be symmetric or asymmetric. Symmetric FGR (20–30% of cases) affects all organ systems with the head and length in proportion with the rest of the body (Mandy, 2022a). Symmetric FGR can be associated with congenital infections or chromosomal abnormalities (Mandy, 2022a). Asymmetric FGR (70–80% of cases) involves disproportionate constraint of growth causing the baby to have a normal-sized head, somewhat shorter body length, and reduced abdominal circumference due in part to decreased liver size (Mandy, 2022a; Stephens, Bentley, Taylor, & Arbuckle, 2015). The fetus with asymmetric FGR sends blood flow away from less-vital organs such as the liver to improve perfusion to the brain, heart, adrenal glands, and placenta (Stephens et al., 2015). Asymmetric FGR usually results from acute compromise in placental circulation caused by conditions such as placental infarctions and pregnancy-induced hypertension (Mandy, 2022a).

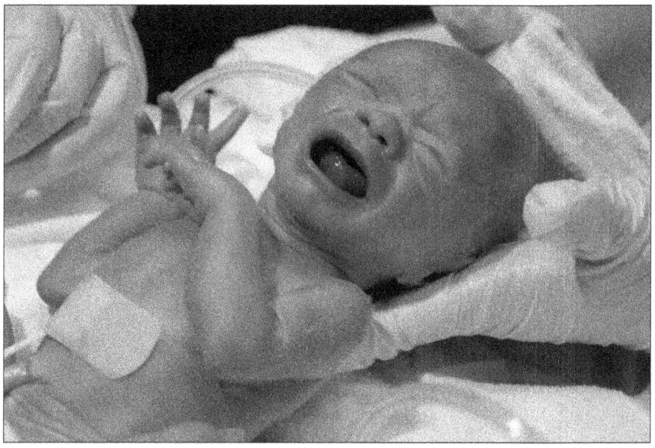

Figure 14-22. Asymmetric FGR. This baby weighed 4 lb 10 oz (2,100 g) at 39 weeks of gestation. His head had grown at a near-normal rate, but he had little subcutaneous fat and a disproportionately small abdomen.

FGR is often suspected when the provider notices a lag in fundal height measurement during a routine prenatal visit and is confirmed by sonographic evaluation or fetal growth. If the estimated weight or the abdominal circumference is below the 10th percentile for gestational age, ACOG recommends amniotic fluid assessment and Doppler blood flow studies of the umbilical artery (ACOG, 2021a). If not already assessed, fetal anatomy should be evaluated because growth-restricted fetuses commonly have structural and genetic abnormalities.

FGR involves high incidence of neonatal complications and increases the risk of stillbirth, so the growth-restricted fetus is not a candidate for birth outside a hospital. Management requires balancing the benefits of allowing the fetus to mature *in utero* and planning birth before it is severely compromised. Doppler velocimetry should be used together with serial growth imaging, nonstress tests, and biophysical profiles to monitor fetal wellbeing (ACOG, 2021a). SMFM guidelines state that for fetuses with estimated weight between the 3rd and 10th percentile and normal umbilical artery Doppler studies, birth may be planned for between 38 and 39 weeks of gestation (SMFM, 2020a). If the estimated fetal weight is below the 3rd percentile, birth is recommended at 37 weeks of gestation if Doppler flow is normal or upon diagnosis in cases of absent or reverse umbilical artery flow (SMFM, 2020a).

Topics for Discussion

1. List three things to consider while resuscitating a preterm infant.
2. Stella experienced PPROM at 32 0/7 weeks of gestation and is not in labor. Discuss the benefits that betamethasone could provide for her unborn baby.
3. During Amelia's 34-week prenatal appointment, you find that she is 5 cm dilated with a bulging bag of water. She strongly desires to give birth to this baby at home. What would you tell her?
4. List five risk factors for PTB.
5. Name and describe three health conditions that commonly develop in premature infants.
6. Michelle is 34 weeks pregnant with a fetus measuring in the 2nd percentile for gestational age. She consulted with a maternal fetal medicine specialist, who recommended induction of labor at 37 weeks of gestation. Michelle had been planning a home birth. Explain to Michelle why a 37 week induction of labor in a hospital with a NICU is the safest plan for her baby's birth.

References

Agostino, R., Aufieri, R., & Gente, M. (2016). Neonatal transport services. In G. Buonocore, R. Bracci, & M. Weindling (Eds.), *Neonatology: A practical approach to neonatal diseases* (2nd ed., pp. 1–13). Cham, Switzerland: Springer International.

American College of Obstetricians and Gynecologists. (2010, reaffirmed 2023). *Magnesium sulfate before anticipated preterm birth for neuroprotection* (Committee Opinion 455). Retrieved from https://www.acog.org/clinical/clinical-guidance/committee-opinion/articles/2010/03/magnesium-sulfate-before-anticipated-preterm-birth-for-neuroprotection

American College of Obstetricians and Gynecologists. (2014, reaffirmed 2024). Cerclage for the management of cervical insufficiency (Practice Bulletin 142). *Obstetrics & Gynecology, 123*(2, Pt. 1), 372–379. https://doi.org/10.1097/01.AOG.0000443276.68274.cc

American College of Obstetricians and Gynecologists. (2016, reaffirmed 2022). *Management of preterm labor* (Practice Bulletin 171). Retrieved from https://www.acog.org/clinical/clinical-guidance/practice-bulletin/articles/2016/10/management-of-preterm-labor

American College of Obstetricians and Gynecologists. (2017, corrected and reaffirmed 2024). *Antenatal corticosteroid therapy for fetal maturation* (Committee Opinion 713). Retrieved from https://www.acog.org/clinical/clinical-guidance/committee-opinion/articles/2017/08/antenatal-corticosteroid-therapy-for-fetal-maturation

American College of Obstetricians and Gynecologists. (2018, reaffirmed 2021). *Use of prophylactic antibiotics in labor and delivery* (Practice Bulletin 199). Retrieved from https://www.acog.org/clinical/clinical-guidance/practice-bulletin/articles/2018/09/use-of-prophylactic-antibiotics-in-labor-and-delivery

American College of Obstetricians and Gynecologists. (2019, reaffirmed 2021). *Levels of maternal care* (Obstetric Care Consensus 9). Retrieved from https://www.acog.org/clinical/clinical-guidance/obstetric-care-consensus/articles/2019/08/levels-of-maternal-care

American College of Obstetricians and Gynecologists. (2020a, reaffirmed 2023). *Prelabor rupture of membranes* (Practice Bulletin 217). Retrieved from https://www.acog.org/clinical/clinical-guidance/practice-bulletin/articles/2020/03/prelabor-rupture-of-membranes

American College of Obstetricians and Gynecologists. (2020b, reaffirmed 2022). *Prevention of Group B streptococcal early-onset disease in newborns* (Committee Opinion 797, interim update). Retrieved from https://www.acog.org/clinical/clinical-guidance/committee-opinion/articles/2020/02/prevention-of-group-b-streptococcal-early-onset-disease-in-newborns

American College of Obstetricians and Gynecologists. (2021a). *Fetal growth restriction* (Practice Bulletin 227). Retrieved from https://www.acog.org/clinical/clinical-guidance/practice-bulletin/articles/2021/02/fetal-growth-restriction

American College of Obstetricians and Gynecologists. (2021b). *Prediction and prevention of spontaneous preterm birth* (Practice Bulletin 234). Retrieved from https://www.acog.org/Clinical/Clinical-Guidance/Practice-Bulletin/Articles/2021/08/Prediction-and-Prevention-of-Spontaneous-Preterm-Birth

American College of Obstetricians and Gynecologists. (2023). *Updated clinical guidance for the use of progesterone supplementation for the prevention of recurrent preterm birth* (Practice Advisory). Retrieved from https://www.acog.org/clinical/clinical-guidance/practice-advisory/articles/2023/04/updated-guidance-use-of-progesterone-supplementation-for-prevention-of-recurrent-preterm-birth

American College of Obstetricians and Gynecologists, Society for Maternal-Fetal Medicine, Cahill, A. G., Kaimal, A. J., Kuller, J. A., & Turrentine, M. A. (2021, reaffirmed 2022). *Use of antenatal corticosteroids at 22 weeks of gestation* (Practice Advisory). Retrieved from https://www.acog.org/clinical/clinical-guidance/practice-advisory/articles/2021/09/use-of-antenatal-corticosteroids-at-22-weeks-of-gestation

Anderson, J. G., Baer, R. J., Partridge, J. C., Kuppermann, M., Franck, L. S., Rand, L., . . . Rogers, E. E. (2016). Survival and major morbidity of extremely preterm infants: A population-based study. *Pediatrics, 138*(1), e20154434. https://doi.org/10.1542/peds.2015-4434

Bachnas, M. A., Akbar, M. I. L., Dachlan, E. G., & Dekker, G. (2019). The role of magnesium sulfate ($MgSO_4$) in fetal neuroprotection. *Journal of Maternal-Fetal & Neonatal Medicine, 34*(6), 964–978. https://doi.org/10.1080/14767058.2019.1619688

Barfield, W. D., & Lee, K. G. (2023). Late preterm infants. In C. Armsby (Ed.), *UpToDate*. Retrieved October 30, 2023, from https://www.uptodate.com/contents/late-preterm-infants

Berghella, V. (2023a). Cervical insufficiency. In V. A. Barss (Ed.), *UpToDate*. Retrieved October 30, 2023, from https://www.uptodate.com/contents/cervical-insufficiency

Berghella, V. (2023b). Short cervix before 24 weeks: Screening and management in singleton pregnancies. In V. A. Barss (Ed.), *UpToDate*. Retrieved October 30, 2023, from https://www.uptodate.com/contents/short-cervix-before-24-weeks-screening-and-management-in-singleton-pregnancies

Berghella, V. & Saccone, G. (2016). Fetal fibronectin testing for prevention of preterm birth in singleton pregnancies with threatened preterm labor:

A systematic review and metaanalysis of randomized controlled trials. *American Journal of Obstetrics & Gynecology, 215* (4), 431–438. https://doi.org/10.1016/j.ajog.2016.04.038

Blackwell, S. C., Gyamfi-Bannerman, C., Biggio, J. R., Jr., Chauhan, S. P., Hughes, B. L., Louis, J. M, . . . Krop, J. (2020). 17-OHPC to prevent recurrent preterm birth in singleton gestations (PROLONG Study): A multicenter, international, randomized double-blind trial. *American Journal of Perinatology, 37*(2), 127–136. https://doi.org/10.1055/s-0039-3400227

Blyth, M. (2006). *Premature baby with improvised oxygen mask.* Retrieved from https://commons.wikimedia.org/wiki/File:Premature_baby_with_improvised_oxygen_mask.jpg

Bond, D. M., Middleton P., Levett, K. M., van der Ham, D. P., Crowther, C. A., Buchanan, S. L., & Morris, J. (2017). Planned early birth versus expectant management for women with preterm prelabour rupture of membranes prior to 37 weeks' gestation for improving pregnancy outcome. *Cochrane Database of Systematic Reviews*. https://doi.org/10.1002/14651858.CD004735.pub4

Bouchut, J. C., Van Lancker, E., Chritin, V., & Gueugniaud, P.-Y. (2011). Physical stressors during neonatal transport: Helicopter compared with ground ambulance. *Air Medical Journal, 30*(3), 134–139. https://doi.org/10.1016/j.amj.2010.11.001

Bourke, J., Wong, K., Srinivasjois, R., Pereira, G., Shepherd, C. C. J., White, S. W., . . . Leonard, H. (2019). Predicting long-term survival without major disability for infants born preterm. *Journal of Pediatrics, 215*, 90–97. https://doi.org/10.1016/j.jpeds.2019.07.056

Carlo, W. A., McDonald, S. A., Fanaroff, A. A., Vohr, B. R., Stoll, B. J., Ehrenkranz, R. A., . . . Higgins, R. D. (2011). Association of antenatal corticosteroids with mortality and neurodevelopmental outcomes among infants born at 22 to 25 weeks' gestation. *JAMA, 306* (21), 2348–2358. https://doi.org/10.1001/jama.2011.1752

Carmichael, A., McCullough, S., & Kempley, S. T. (2007). Critical dependence of acetate thermal mattress on gel activation temperature. *Archives of Disease in Childhood—Fetal and Neonatal Edition, 92*(1), F44–F45. https://doi.org/10.1136/adc.2006.096297

Centers for Disease Control and Prevention. (2022). *Percentage of births born preterm by state.* Retrieved from https://www.cdc.gov/nchs/pressroom/sosmap/preterm_births/preterm.htm

Chiossi, G., Saade, G. R., Sibai, B., & Berghella, V. (2018). Using cervical length measurement for lower spontaneous preterm birth rates among women with threatened preterm labor. *Obstetrics & Gynecology, 132*(1), 102–106. https://doi.org/10.1097/AOG.0000000000002695

Coler, B. S., Shynlova, O., Boros-Rausch, A., Lye, S., McCartney, S., Leimert, K. B., . . . Adams Waldorf, K. M. (2021). Landscape of preterm birth therapeutics and a path forward. *Journal of Clinical Medicine, 10*(13), 2912. https://doi.org/10.3390/jcm10132912

Conde-Agudelo, A., Romero, R., Da Fonseca, E., O'Brien, J. M., Cetingoz, E., Creasy, G. W., . . . Nicolaides, K. H. (2018). Vaginal progesterone is as effective as cervical cerclage to prevent preterm birth in women with a singleton gestation, previous spontaneous preterm birth, and a short cervix: Updated indirect comparison meta-analysis. *American Journal of Obstetrics & Gynecology, 219*(1), 10–25. https://doi.org/10.1016/j.ajog.2018.03.028

Crowther, C. A., Brown, J., McKinlay, C. J. D., & Middleton, P. (2014). Magnesium sulphate for preventing preterm birth in threatened preterm labour. *Cochrane Database of Systematic Reviews*. https://doi.org/10.1002/14651858.CD001060.pub2

Crowther, C. A., Hiller, J. E., Doyle, L. W., & Haslam, R. R. (2003). Effect of magnesium sulfate given for neuroprotection before preterm birth: A randomized controlled trial. *JAMA, 290*(20), 2669–2676. https://doi.org/10.1001/jama.290.20.2669

Cunningham, F. G., Leveno, K. J., Dashe, J. S., Hoffman, B. L, Spong, C. Y., & Casey, B. M. (Eds.). (2022). *Williams obstetrics* (26th ed., Kindle version). New York, NY: McGraw-Hill.

Daskalakis, G., Pergialiotis, V., Domellöf, M., Ehrhardt, H., Di Renzo, G. C., Koç, E., . . . Jacobsson, B. (2023). European guidelines on perinatal care: Corticosteroids for women at risk of preterm birth. *Journal of Maternal-Fetal & Neonatal Medicine, 36*(1), 2160628. https://doi.org/10.1080/14767058.2022.2160628

Dierikx, T. H., Visser, D. H., Benninga, M. A., van Kaam, A. H. L. C., de Boer, N. K. H., de Vries, R., . . . de Meij, T. G. J. (2020). The influence of prenatal and intrapartum antibiotics on intestinal microbiota in infants: A systematic review. *Journal of Infection, 81*(2), 190–204. https://doi.org/10.1016/j.jinf.2020.05.002

Duff, P. (2022). Preterm prelabor rupture of membranes: Clinical manifestations and diagnosis. In V. A. Barss (Ed.), *UpToDate*. Retrieved October 30, 2023, from https://www.uptodate.com/contents/preterm-prelabor-rupture-of-membranes-clinical-manifestations-and-diagnosis

Egbe, T. O., Njamen, T. N., Ekane, G. H., Tsingaing, J. K., Tchente, C. N., Beyiha, G., . . . Nyemb, E. (2013). Outcome of late second trimester emergency cerclage in patients with advanced cervical dilatation with bulging amniotic membranes: A report of six cases managed at the Douala general hospital, Cameroon. *ISRN Obstetrics and Gynecology, 2013*. https://doi.org/10.1155/2013/843158

Ehret, D. E., Edwards, E. M., Greenberg, L. T., Bernstein, I. M., Buzas, J. S., Soll, R. F., & Horbar, J. D. (2018). Association of antenatal steroid exposure with survival among infants receiving postnatal life support at 22 to 25 weeks' gestation. *JAMA Network Open, 1*(6), e183235. https://doi.org/10.1001/jamanetworkopen.2018.3235

Farago, N., Bachar, G., Lauterbach, R., Weissman, A., Weiner, Z., Beloosesky, R., & Zipori, Y. (2020). Vaginal progesterone increases the risk of intrahepatic cholestasis of pregnancy. A case-control study. *American Journal of Obstetrics & Gynecology, 222*(1, Suppl.), S701–S702. https://doi.org/10.1016/j.ajog.2019.11.1151

Fee, E. L., Stock, S. J., & Kemp, M. W. (2023). Antenatal steroids: Benefits, risks, and new insights. *Journal of Endocrinology, 258*(2), e220306. https://doi.org/10.1530/joe-22-0306.

Fischer, R. (2008). Amniotic fluid: Physiology and assessment. *Global Library of Women's Medicine*. https://doi.org/10.3843/GLOWM.10208

Flenady, V., Wojcieszek, A. M., Papatsonis, D. N. M., Stock, O. M., Murray, L., Jardine, L. A., & Carbonne, B. (2014). Calcium channel blockers for inhibiting preterm labour and birth. *Cochrane Database of Systematic Reviews*. https://doi.org/10.1002/14651858.CD002255.pub2

Fuchs, I. B., Henrich, W., Osthues, K., & Dudenhausen, J. W. (2004). Sonographic cervical length in singleton pregnancies with intact membranes presenting with threatened preterm labor. *Ultrasound in Obstetrics & Gynecology, 24*(5), 554–557. https://doi.org/10.1002/uog.1714

Gaddey, H., Bailey, J., & Smith, R. (2011). Ferning in amniotic fluid: Is it a useful indicator of ruptured membranes? *Journal of Family Practice, 60*(12), 769–771. Retrieved from https://www.mdedge.com/jfponline/article/64563/womens-health/ferning-amniotic-fluid-it-useful-indicator-ruptured-membranes

Gentle, S. J., Carlo, W. A., Tan, S., Gargano, M., Ambalavanan, N., Chawla, S., . . . Higgins, R. (2020). Association of antenatal corticosteroids and magnesium sulfate therapy with neurodevelopmental outcome in extremely preterm children. *Obstetrics & Gynecology, 135*(6), 1377–1386. https://doi.org/10.1097/AOG.0000000000003882

Griggs, K. M., Hrelic, D. A., Williams, N., McEwen-Campbell, M., & Cypher, R. (2020). Preterm labor and birth. *MCN, The American Journal of Maternal/Child Nursing: 45*(6), 328–337. https://doi.org/10.1097/NMC.0000000000000656

Gudicha, D. W., Romero, R., Kabiri, D., Hernandez-Andrade, E., Pacora, P., Erez, O., . . . Tarca, A. L. (2021). Personalized assessment of cervical length improves prediction of spontaneous preterm birth: A standard and a percentile calculator. *American Journal of Obstetrics & Gynecology, 224*(3), 288.e1–288.e17. https://doi.org/10.1016/j.ajog.2020.09.002

Gulersen, M., Gyamfi-Bannerman, C., Greenman, M., Lenchner, E., Rochelson, B., & Bornstein, E. (2021). Practice patterns in the administration of late preterm antenatal corticosteroids. *AJOG Global Reports, 1*(3), 100014. https://doi.org/10.1016/j.xagr.2021.100014

Hedriana, H., Byrne, J., Campbell Bliss, M., Kowalewski, L., Georges, M., Lombardo, V. L., . . . Clark, S. L. (2013). *March of Dimes preterm labor assessment toolkit*. White Plains, NY: March of Dimes. Retrieved from https://www.ihconline.org/media/cms/MOD_Pre-Term_Labor_Toolkit.pdf

Helenius, K., Longford, N., Lehtonen, L., Modi, N., & Gale, C. (2019). Association of early postnatal transfer and birth outside a tertiary hospital with mortality and severe brain injury in extremely preterm infants: Observational cohort study with propensity score matching. *BMJ, 367*, l5678. https://doi.org/10.1136/bmj.l5678

Hitchings, L., Rodriguez, M., Persaud, R., & Gomez, L. (2022). The effect of delayed cord clamping on blood sugar levels on 34–36 week neonates exposed to late preterm antenatal steroids. *Journal of Maternal-Fetal & Neonatal Medicine, 35*(18), 3587–3594. https://doi.org/10.1080/14767058.2020.1832074

Hologic, Inc. (2017). *Fetal fibronectin enzyme immunoassay and rapid fFN® for the TLiIQ® system*. Retrieved from https://www.hologic.com/sites/default/files/2018-05/AW-04196-002_004_02.pdf

Iams, J. D. (2003). Prediction and early detection of preterm labor. *Obstetrics & Gynecology, 101*(2), 402–412. https://doi.org/10.1016/s0029-7844(02)02505-x

Jarde, A., Lutsiv, O., Beyenne, J., & McDonald, S. J. (2019). Vaginal progesterone, oral progesterone, 17-OHPC, cerclage, and pessary for preventing preterm birth in at-risk singleton pregnancies: An updated systematic review and network meta-analysis. *BJOG, 126*(5), 556–567. https://doi.org/10.1111/1471-0528.15566

Jones, P., Alberti, C., Julé, L., Chabernaud, J. L., Lodé, N., Sieurin, A., & Dauger, S. (2011). Mortality in out-of-hospital premature births. *Acta Paediatrica, 100*(2), 181–187. https://doi.org/10.1111/j.1651-2227.2010.02003.x

Karlsen, K. (2019). *The S.T.A.B.L.E. Program: Post-resuscitation/pre-transport stabilization care of sick infants: Guidelines for neonatal healthcare providers* (6th ed., Kindle version). Park City, UT: S.T.A.B.L.E. Program.

Kazemi, S., Soleimani, F., Kazemi, S., Kazemnezhad, A., Kiani, Z., Pazandeh, F., & Azimi, N. (2019). Perinatal outcomes of idiopathic polyhydramnios with normal ultrasound: A systematic review and meta-analysis. *International Journal of Pediatrics, 7*(5), 9349–9362. https://doi.org/10.22038/ijp.2018.36148.3155

Kenyon, S., Pike, K., Jones, D. R., Brocklehurst, P., Marlow, N., Salt, A., & Taylor, D. J. (2008). Childhood outcomes after prescription of antibiotics to pregnant women with spontaneous preterm labour: 7-year follow-up of the ORACLE II trial. *Lancet, 372*(9646), 1319–1327. https://doi.org/10.1016/S0140-6736(08)61203-9

Lauder, J., Sciscione, A., Biggio, J., & Osmundson, S. (2020). The role of activity restriction in obstetric management (Society for Maternal-Fetal Medicine Consult Series 50). *American Journal of Obstetrics & Gynecology, 223*(2), B2–B10. https://doi.org/10.1016/j.ajog.2020.04.031

Lee, M.-J., & Guinn, D. (2023). Antenatal corticosteroid therapy for reduction of neonatal respiratory morbidity and mortality from preterm delivery. In V. A. Barss (Ed.), *UpToDate*. Retrieved October 30, 2023, from https://www.uptodate.com/contents/antenatal-corticosteroid-therapy-for-reduction-of-neonatal-respiratory-morbidity-and-mortality-from-preterm-delivery

Lewis, D. F., Robichaux, A. G., Jaekle, R. K., Salas, A., Canzoneri, B. J., Horton, K., . . . Stedman, C. (2007). Expectant management of preterm premature rupture of membranes and nonvertex presentation: What are the risks? *American Journal of Obstetrics & Gynecology, 196*(6), 566.e1–566.e5. https://doi.org/10.1016/j.ajog.2007.02.023

Lim, K. I., Butt, K., Nevo, O., & Crane, J. M. (2020). Guideline no. 401: Sonographic cervical length in singleton pregnancies: Techniques and clinical applications. Guideline 401. *Journal of Obstetrics and Gynaecology Canada, 42*(11), 1394–1413.e1. https://doi.org/10.1016/j.jogc.2019.06.002

Lockwood, C. J., (2022). Spontaneous preterm birth: Pathogenesis. In V. A. Barss (Ed.), *UpToDate*. Retrieved October 30, 2023, from https://www.uptodate.com/contents/spontaneous-preterm-birth-pathogenesis

Lockwood, C. J., (2023). Preterm labor: Clinical findings, diagnostic evaluation, and initial treatment. In V. A. Barss (Ed.), *UpToDate*. Retrieved October 30, 2023, from https://www.uptodate.com/contents/preterm-labor-clinical-findings-diagnostic-evaluation-and-initial-treatment

Lyon, C., Bello, J. K., & Stevermer, J. J. (2017). Steroids during late preterm labor: Better later than never. *Journal of family practice, 66*(2), 104–106. Retrieved from https://www.mdedge.com/jfponline/article/129931/pediatrics/steroids-during-late-preterm-labor-better-later-never

Lyons, P., & McLaughlin, N. (2020). Preterm labor. In P. Lyons & N. McLaughlin (Eds.), *Obstetrics in family medicine: A practical guide* (3rd ed., pp. 63–71). Cham, Switzerland: Humana Press. https://doi.org/10.1007/978-3-030-39888-0_8

Mandy, G. T. (2022a). Infants with fetal (intrauterine) growth restriction. In C. Armsby (Ed.), *UpToDate*. Retrieved October 30, 2023, from https://www.uptodate.com/contents/infants-with-fetal-intrauterine-growth-restriction

Mandy, G. T. (2022b). Preterm birth: Definitions of prematurity, epidemiology, and risk factors for infant mortality. In C. Armsby (Ed.), *UpToDate*. Retrieved October 30, 2023, from https://www.uptodate.com/contents/preterm-birth-definitions-of-prematurity-epidemiology-and-risk-factors-for-infant-mortality

Mandy, G. T. (2023). Overview of short-term complications in preterm infants. In C. Armsby (Ed.), *UpToDate*. Retrieved October 30, 2023, from https://www.uptodate.com/contents/overview-of-short-term-complications-in-preterm-infants

March of Dimes. (2022). *2022 March of Dimes report card*. Retrieved from https://www.marchofdimes.org/peristats/reports/united-states/report-card

Marowitz, A., & Vines, S. (2024). Complications during labor and birth. In J. Phillippi & I. Kantrowitz-Gordon (Eds.), *Varney's midwifery* (7th ed., Kindle version, ch. 30). Burlington, MA: Jones & Bartlett Learning.

Marret, S., Marpeau, L., Zupan-Simunek, V., Eurin, D., Lévêque, C., Hellot, M.-F., . . . PREMAG Trial Group. (2007). Magnesium sulphate given before very-preterm birth to protect infant brain: The randomised controlled PREMAG trial. *BJOG, 114*(3), 310–318. https://doi.org/10.1111/j.1471-0528.2006.01162.x

Martin, S. R. (2022). Inter-facility maternal transport. In V. A, Barss (Ed.), *UpToDate*. Retrieved October 30, 2023, from https://www.uptodate.com/contents/inter-facility-maternal-transport

McElwee, E. R., Wilkinson, K., Crowe, R., Hardy, K. T., Newman, J. C., Chapman, A., . . . Finneran, M. M. (2022). Latency of late preterm steroid administration to delivery and risk of neonatal hypoglycemia. *American Journal of Obstetrics & Gynecology MFM, 4*(5), 100687. https://doi.org/10.1016/j.ajogmf.2022.100687

McGoldrick, E., Stewart, F., Parker, R., & Dalziel, S. R. (2020). Antenatal corticosteroids for accelerating fetal lung maturation for women at risk of preterm birth. *Cochrane Database of Systematic Reviews*. https://doi.org/10.1002/14651858.CD004454.pub4

Meis, P. J., Klebanoff, M., Thom, E., Dombrowski, M. P., Sibai, B., Moawad, A. H., . . . Peaceman, A. M. (2003). Prevention of recurrent preterm delivery by 17 alpha-hydroxyprogesterone caproate. *New England Journal of Medicine, 348*(24), 2379–2385. https://doi.org/10.1056/NEJMoa035140

Mercer, B. M. (2021). Protocol 45: Premature rupture of the membranes. In J. T. Queenan, C. Y. Spong, & C. J. Lockwood (Eds.). *Protocols for high-risk pregnancies: An evidence-based approach* (7th ed., pp. 461–474). Hoboken, NJ: John Wiley & Sons.

Mercurio, M. R., & Drago, M. (2022). Periviable birth (limit of viability). In C. Armsby (Ed.), *UpToDate*. Retrieved October 30, 2023, from https://www.uptodate.com/contents/periviable-birth-limit-of-viability

Meuchel, L., Zwelling, B., Shields, M., Cheng, Y. W., & Caughey, A. B. (2017). Late preterm delivery: Comparison of outcomes in hospital vs. out-of-hospital birth. *American Journal of Obstetrics & Gynecology, 216*(1, Suppl.), S273. https://doi.org/10.1016/j.ajog.2016.11.721

Moreira, M. E. L., & Méio, M. D. B. B. (2022). Small for gestational age. In R. A. Moreira de Sá & E. B. Fonseca (Eds), *Perinatology: Evidence-based practices in perinatal medicine* (pp. 1151–1157). Cham, Switzerland: Springer. https://doi.org/10.1007/978-3-030-83434-0_59

Morris, J. M., Roberts, C. L., Bowen, J. R., Patterson, J. A., Bond, D. M., Algert, C. S., . . . Crowther, C. A. (2016). Immediate delivery compared with expectant management after preterm pre-labour rupture of the membranes close to term (PPROMT trial): A randomised controlled trial. *Lancet, 387*(10017), 444–452. https://doi.org/10.1016/S0140-6736(15)00724-2

Murphy, C. C., Cirillo, P. M., Krigbaum, N. Y., & Cohn, B. A. (2022). In utero exposure to 17α-hydroxyprogesterone caproate and risk of cancer in offspring. *American Journal of Obstetrics & Gynecology, 226*(1), 132.e1–132.e14. https://doi.org/10.1016/j.ajog.2021.10.035

Mwansa-Kambafwile, J., Cousens, S., Hansen, T., & Lawn, J. E. (2010). Antenatal steroids in preterm labour for the prevention of neonatal deaths due to complications of preterm birth. *International Journal of Epidemiology, 39*(Suppl. 1), i122–i133. https://doi.org/10.1093/ije/dyq029

Neilson, J. P., West, H. M., & Dowswell, T. (2014). Betamimetics for inhibiting preterm labour. *Cochrane Database of Systematic Reviews*. https://doi.org/10.1002/14651858.CD004352.pub3

[NICE] National Institute for Health and Care Excellence. (2015, revised 2022). *Preterm labour and birth: Maternal corticosteroids* (NICE Guideline NG25, pp. 15–17). Retrieved from https://www.nice.org.uk/guidance/ng25/resources/preterm-labour-and-birth-pdf-1837333576645

Norman, J., Shennan, A., Jacobsson, B., & Stock, S. J. (2021). FIGO good practice recommendations on the use of prenatal corticosteroids to improve outcomes and minimize harm in babies born preterm. *International Journal of Gynecology & Obstetrics,155*(1), 26–30. https://doi.org/10.1002/ijgo.13836

Norwitz, E. R. (2023a). Progesterone supplementation to reduce the risk of spontaneous preterm labor and birth. In V. A. Barss (Ed.), *UpToDate*. Retrieved October 30, 2023, from https://www.uptodate.com/contents/16560

Norwitz, E. R. (2023b). Transvaginal cervical cerclage. In V. A, Barss, (Ed.), *UpToDate*. Retrieved October 30, 2023, from https://www.uptodate.com/contents/transvaginal-cervical-cerclage

Osterman, M. J. K., Hamilton, B. E., Martin, J. A., Driscoll, A. K., & Valenzuela, C. P. (2023). Births: Final data for 2021. *National Vital Statistics Reports, 72*(1). Retrieved from https://stacks.cdc.gov/view/cdc/122047

Ouald Chaib, A., Levy, E. I., Ouald Chaib, M., & Vandenplas, Y. (2020). The influence of the gastrointestinal microbiome on infant colic. *Expert Review of Gastroenterology & Hepatology, 14*(10), 919–932. https://doi.org/10.1080/17474124.2020.1791702

Parfitt, S. E. (2020). Preterm labor and birth. In K. R. Simpson, P. A. Creehan, N. O'Brien-Abel, C. K. Roth, & A. J. Rohan (Eds.), *AWHONN's perinatal nursing* (5th ed., pp. 142–174). Philadelphia, PA: Wolters Kluwer.

Park, C. K., Isayama, T., & McDonald, S. D. (2016). Antenatal corticosteroid therapy before 24 weeks of gestation: A systematic review and meta-analysis. *Obstetrics & Gynecology, 127*(4), 715–725. https://doi.org/10.1097/AOG.0000000000001355

Peaceman, A. M., Andrews, W. W., Thorp, J. M., Cliver, S. P., Lukes, A., . . . Pietrantoni, M. (1997). Fetal fibronectin as a predictor of preterm birth in patients with symptoms: A multicenter trial. *American Journal of Obstetrics & Gynecology, 177*(1), 13–18. https://doi.org/10.1016/S0002-9378(97)70431-9

Perry, S. E. (2017). A historical perspective on the transport of premature infants. *Journal of Obstetric, Gynecologic & Neonatal Nursing, 46*(4), 647–656. https://doi.org/10.1016/j.jogn.2016.09.007

Perry, S. E. (2021). Fifty years of progress in neonatal and maternal transport for specialty care. *Journal of Obstetric, Gynecologic & Neonatal Nursing, 50*(6), 774–788. https://doi.org/10.1016/j.jogn.2021.04.013

Picklesimer, A. H., Billings, D., Hale, N., Blackhurst, D., & Covington-Kolb, S. (2012). The effect of CenteringPregnancy group prenatal care on preterm birth in a low-income population. *American Journal of Obstetrics & Gynecology, 206*(5), 415.e1–415.e7. https://doi.org/10.1016/j.ajog.2012.01.040

Pirneskoski, J., Peräjoki, K., Nuutila, M., & Kuisma, M. (2016). Urgent EMS managed out-of-hospital delivery dispatches in Helsinki. *Scandinavian Journal of Trauma, Resuscitation and Emergency Medicine, 24*(1), 94. https://doi.org/10.1186/s13049-016-0285-5

Raju, T. N. K., Mercer, B. M., Burchfield, D. J., & Joseph, G. F., Jr. (2014). Periviable birth: Executive summary of a joint workshop by the Eunice Kennedy Shriver National Institute of Child Health and Human Development, Society for Maternal-Fetal Medicine, American Academy of Pediatrics, and American College of Obstetricians and Gynecologists. *Obstetrics & Gynecology, 123*(5), 1083–1096. https://doi.org/10.1097/AOG.0000000000000243

Roberts, D., Brown, J., Medley, N., & Dalziel, S. R. (2017). Antenatal corticosteroids for accelerating fetal lung maturation for women at risk of preterm birth. *Cochrane Database of Systematic Reviews*. https://doi.org/10.1002/14651858.CD004454.pub3

Robinson, J. N., & Norwitz, E. R. (2023). Spontaneous preterm birth: Overview of risk factors and prognosis. In V. A. Barss (Ed.), *UpToDate*. Retrieved October 30, 2023, from https://www.uptodate.com/contents/spontaneous-preterm-birth-overview-of-risk-factors-and-prognosis

Rohan, A. J. (2021). Common neonatal complications. In K. R. Simpson, P. A. Creehan, N. O'Brien-Abel, C. K. Roth, & A. J. Rohan (Eds.), *AWHONN's perinatal nursing* (5th ed., pp. 651–688). Philadelphia, PA: Wolters Kluwer.

Ross, M. G., & Beall, M. H. (2023). Physiology of amniotic fluid volume regulation. In V. A. Barss (Ed.), *UpToDate*. Retrieved October 30, 2023, from https://www.uptodate.com/contents/physiology-of-amniotic-fluid-volume-regulation

Rouse, D. J., Hirtz, D. G., Thom, E., Varner, M. W., Spong, C. Y., Mercer, B. M., . . . Roberts, J. M. (2008). A randomized, controlled trial of magnesium sulfate for the prevention of cerebral palsy. *New England Journal of Medicine, 359*, 895–905. https://doi.org/10.1056/NEJMoa0801187

Rundell, K., & Panchal, B. (2017). Preterm labor: Prevention and management. *American Family Physician, 95*(6), 366–372. Retrieved from https://www.aafp.org/afp/2017/0315/p366.html

Shennan, A., Suff, N., & Jacobsson, B. (2021). FIGO good practice recommendations on magnesium sulfate administration for preterm fetal neuroprotection. *International Journal of Gynecology & Obstetrics, 155*(1), 31–33. https://doi.org/10.1002/ijgo.13856

Shimoya, K., Hashimoto, K., Shimizu, T., Saji, F., & Murata, Y. (1998). Effect of sexual intercourse on fetal fibronectin concentration in cervicovaginal secretions. *American Journal of Obstetrics & Gynecology, 179*(1), 255–256. https://doi.org/10.1016/S0002-9378(98)70280-7

Simhan, H. N., & Caritis, S. (2023). Inhibition of acute preterm labor. In V. A. Barss (Ed.), *UpToDate*. Retrieved October 30, 2023, from https://www.uptodate.com/contents/inhibition-of-acute-preterm-labor

Simhan, H. N., & Himes, K. P. (2023). Neuroprotective effects of in utero exposure to magnesium sulfate. In V. A. Barss (Ed.), *UpToDate*. Retrieved October 30, 2023, from https://www.uptodate.com/contents/neuroprotective-effects-of-in-utero-exposure-to-magnesium-sulfate

Simhan, H. N., & Romero, R. (2021). Preterm labor and birth. In M. B. Landon, H. L. Galan, E. R. M. Jauniaux, D. A. Driscoll, V. Berghella, W. A. Grobman, . . . A. G. Cahill (Eds.), *Gabbe's obstetrics: Normal and problem pregnancies* (8th ed., Kindle version, ch. 36). Philadelphia, PA: Elsevier

Singh, A., & Mittal, M. (2020). Neonatal microbiome—a brief review. *Journal of Maternal-Fetal & Neonatal Medicine, 33*(22), 3841–3848. https://doi.org/10.1080/14767058.2019.1583738

Skoll, A., Boutin, A., Bujold, E., Burrows, J., Crane, J., Geary, M., . . . Joseph, K. S. (2018). Antenatal corticosteroid therapy for improving neonatal outcomes. *Journal of Obstetrics and Gynaecology Canada, 40*(9), 1219–1239. https://doi.org/10.1016/j.jogc.2018.04.018

Society for Maternal-Fetal Medicine. (n.d.). *SMFM preterm birth toolkit*. Retrieved from https://web.archive.org/web/20221127061858/https://www.smfm.org/publications/231-smfm-preterm-birth-toolkit

Society for Maternal-Fetal Medicine. (2020a). *Diagnosis and management of fetal growth restriction* (SMFM Consult Series 52). Retrieved from https://www.smfm.org/news/smfm-consult-series-52-diagnosis-and-management-of-fetal-growth-restriction

Society for Maternal-Fetal Medicine. (2020b). *The role of activity restriction in obstetric management* (SMFM Consult Series 50). Retrieved from https://www.smfm.org/news/smfm-consult-series-50-the-role-of-activity-restriction-in-obstetric-management

Society for Maternal-Fetal Medicine Publications Committee. (2016). Implementation of the use of antenatal corticosteroids in the late preterm birth period in women at risk for preterm delivery. *American Journal of Obstetrics & Gynecology, 215*(2), B13–B15. https://doi.org/10.1016/j.ajog.2016.03.013

Society for Maternal-Fetal Medicine Publications Committee & Berghella, V. (2012). Progesterone and preterm birth prevention: translating clinical trials data into clinical practice. *American Journal of Obstetrics & Gynecology, 206*(5), 376–386. https://doi.org/10.1016/j.ajog.2012.03.010

Society of Obstetricians and Gynaecologists of Canada. (2021). *Twelve tests and treatments to question*. Retrieved from https://choosingwiselycanada.org/recommendation/obstetrics-and-gynaecology/

Sreedhar, S., Rathore, S., Benjamin, S., Gowri, M., & Mathews, J. E. (2020). Expectant versus immediate delivery in women with PPROM between 34 and 35+6 weeks: A Retrospective cohort. *Journal of Family Medicine and Primary Care, 9*(7), 3225–3229. https://doi.org/10.4103/jfmpc.jfmpc_146_20

Stephens, A. S., Bentley, J. P., Taylor, L. K., & Arbuckle, S. M. (2015). Diagnosis of fetal growth restriction in perinatal deaths using brain to liver weight ratios. *Pathology, 47*(1), 51–57. https://doi.org/10.1097/PAT.0000000000000188

Stewart, L. A., Simmonds, M., Duley, L., Llewellyn, A., Sharif, S., Walker, R. A., . . . Walley, T. (2021). Evaluating Progestogens for Preventing Preterm birth International Collaborative (EPPPIC): Meta-analysis of individual participant data from randomied controlled trials. *Lancet, 397*(10280), 1183–1194. https://doi.org/10.1016/S0140-6736(21)00217-8

Sultan, P., Habib, A. S., & Carvalho, B. (2017). Ambient operating room temperature: Mother, baby or surgeon? *British Journal of Anaesthesia, 119*(4), 839. https://doi.org/10.1093/bja/aex307

Tripathi, U., Khatod, N., & Agrawal, V. (2015). Evaluation of amniotic fluid volume and its relation to perinatal outcome. *Journal of Evolution of Medical and Dental Sciences, 4*(37), 6451–6455. Retrieved from https://www.jemds.com/abstract.php?at_id=7700

Tudehope, D., Vento, M., Bhutta, Z., & Pachi, P. (2013). Nutritional requirements and feeding recommendations for small for gestational age infants. *Journal of Pediatrics, 162*(3, Suppl.), S81–S89, https://doi.org/10.1016/j.jpeds.2012.11.057

Tuohy, J. F., Bloomfield, F. H., Crowther, C. A., & Harding, J. E. (2021). Maternal and neonatal glycaemic control after antenatal corticosteroid administration in women with diabetes in pregnancy: A retrospective cohort study. *PloS One, 16*(2), e0246175. https://doi.org/10.1371/journal.pone.0246175

U.S. Food and Drug Administration. (2011, February 17). *FDA Drug Safety Communication: New warnings against use of terbutaline to treat preterm labor.* Retrieved from https://www.fda.gov/drugs/drugsafety/ucm243539.htm

U.S. Food and Drug Administration. (2023, April 6). *FDA commissioner and chief scientist announce decision to withdraw approval of Makena.* Retrieved from https://www.fda.gov/news-events/press-announcements/fda-commissioner-and-chief-scientist-announce-decision-withdraw-approval-makena

Vafaei, H., Rahimirad, N., Hosseini, S. M., Kasraeian, M., Asadi, N., Raeisi Shahraki, H., & Bazrafshan, K. (2017). Triage by cervical length sonographic measurements for targeted therapy in threatened preterm labor: A double blind randomized clinical trial. *International Journal of Reproductive Biomedicine, 15*(11), 697–702. Retrieved from https://pubmed.ncbi.nlm.nih.gov/29404531/

Valencia, C. M., Mol, B. W., & Jacobsson, B. (2021). FIGO good practice recommendations on modifiable causes of iatrogenic preterm birth. *International Journal of Gynecology & Obstetrics, 155*(1), 8–12. https://doi.org/10.1002/ijgo.13857

van Baaren, G. J., Vis, J. Y., Wilms, F. F., Oudijk, M. A., Kwee, A., Porath, M. M., . . . Mol, B. W. J. (2014). Predictive value of cervical length measurement and fibronectin testing in threatened preterm labor. *Obstetrics & Gynecology, 123*(6), 1185–1192. https://doi.org/10.1097/AOG.0000000000000229

Weiner, G. M., & Zaichkin, J. (Eds.). (2021). *Textbook of neonatal resuscitation* (8th ed.). Itasca, IL: American Academy of Pediatrics.

Wierzchowska-Opoka, M., Kimber-Trojnar, Ż., & Leszczyńska-Gorzelak, B. (2021). Emergency cervical cerclage. *Journal of Clinical Medicine, 10*(6), 1270. https://doi.org/10.3390/jcm10061270

Wolf, H. T., Huusom, L. D., Henriksen, T. B., Hegaard, H. K., Brok, J., & Pinborg, A. (2020). Magnesium sulphate for fetal neuroprotection at imminent risk for preterm delivery: a systematic review with meta-analysis and trial sequential analysis. *BJOG, 127*(10), 1180–1188. https://doi.org/10.1111/1471-0528.16238

World Health Organization. (2015). *WHO recommendations on interventions to improve preterm birth outcomes*. Geneva, Switzerland: WHO. Retrieved from https://www.who.int/reproductivehealth/publications/maternal_perinatal_health/preterm-birth-guideline/en/

Yehudamalul [Screen name]. (2010, January 15). *Weight vs gestational age*. Retrieved from https://commons.wikimedia.org/wiki/File:Weight_vs_gestational_Age.jpg

Zahn, C. M. (2023, April 7). *ACOG statement on the FDA withdrawal of 17-OHPC*. Retrieved from https://www.acog.org/news/news-releases/2023/04/acog-statement-on-the-fda-withdrawal-of-17-ohpc

Zimmermann, P., & Curtis, N. (2020). Effect of intrapartum antibiotics on the intestinal microbiota of infants: A systematic review. *Archives of Disease in Childhood—Fetal and Neonatal Edition, 105*, 201–208. https://doi.org/10.1136/archdischild-2018-316659

Multiple Gestation 15

Objectives

- Give a step-by-step description of how to manage the birth of undiagnosed twins.
- Discuss differences among monochorionic, mono-amniotic, and diamniotic twins.
- Discuss the pathophysiology and management of twin-to-twin transfusion syndrome (TTTS).
- List five complications that are more likely to occur during a twin birth.

Composite Case Study

Ruby R. was at the end of a mostly hands-off labor at the free-standing birth center, and her blonde-haired baby was crowning in the gentle ripples of the tub. It was not a planned pregnancy, but Ruby and Jon had soon grown excited over the prospect welcoming their child following a low-intervention gestation and a natural birth. The labor was all she had hoped for, and she was about to meet her precious child. Sally, the nurse, set a tray of instruments on a table beside the tub.

Brynna White, CM, did a double take as the petite newborn slipped out into the water and into her gloved hands. This baby was tiny! Ruby's fundal height measurements had been 2–3 cm higher than expected on antenatal visits, and Brynna had estimated the fetal weight at 9 lb. This baby girl was only about 6 lb (2.7 kg). With a nagging sense of having missed something important, Brynna unwrapped the encircling cord loops and placed the little wriggler into her mother's reaching hands. Something was not right. Brynna swiftly, skillfully palpated Ruby's abdomen and reached for a Doppler. The regular cadence of a fetal heartbeat filled the room. TWINS!

"Ruby, I need you to get out of the tub. You are having two babies today!"

"Another one? How is that possible?" asked Ruby.

"I told you we should have had that ultrasound!" lamented Jon.

Because she did not know whether the babies shared a blood supply, Brynna clamped the umbilical cord upon diagnosis to reduce the chance of acute peripartum twin-to-twin transfusion syndrome. Knowing that there was a higher potential for complications with the second birth and that the birth center regulations prohibited twin births, Sally called emergency medical services. Brynna and Sally draped warm towels over Ruby's shoulders and helped her to walk to the bed, babe in arms. Brynna performed a careful abdominal and cervical exam and determined that Twin B was vertex and at -2 station. With every contraction, the fetus was having prolonged heart rate decelerations to 60 beats per min from a metronomic baseline of 165. EMS arrived in time to witness the birth of a second small baby girl, who required 5 min of assisted respirations to establish spontaneous breathing. The infant remained tachypneic and tachycardic after resuscitation. After the delivery of a very large shared placenta, Ruby experienced profound uterine atony and had a quantified blood loss of 1,854 ml. Mother and infants were transferred to the hospital via EMS, and all three ultimately did well.

Multifetal Pregnancy

Fertility treatments and a rising average maternal age at childbirth have increased the incidence of multiple gestation

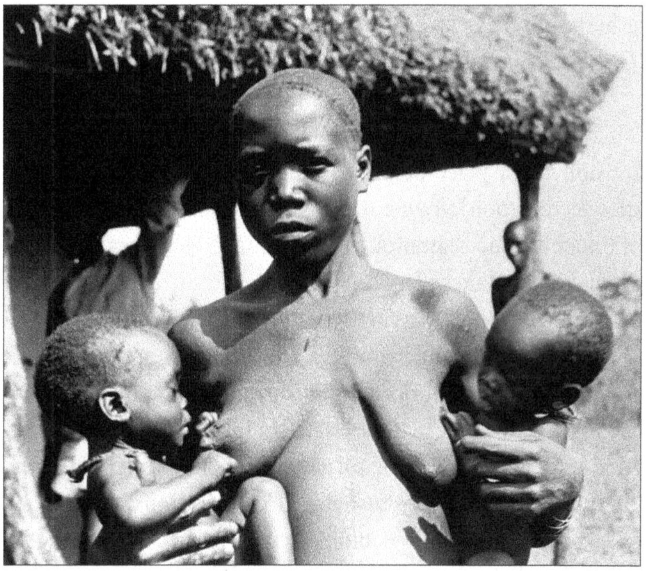

Figure 15-1. Unexpected twin births at home occur more frequently where home births are more common and ultrasound equipment is less accessible. "A Woman Suckling Twins, Lango People," n.d., (https://wellcomecollection.org/works/s3th7t7z). CC BY 4.0.

in the economically developed world (American College of Obstetricians & Gynecologists [ACOG], 2021/2024). The twinning rate rose from 18.9 per 1,000 live births in 1980 to 33.3 per 1,000 live births in 2009, then declined to 32.6 twins per 1,000 live births in 2018 (ACOG, 2021/2024). The number of triplet and higher-order multifetal births increased more than 400% from 1980 to 1998 with more-frequent use of assisted reproductive technology, then sharply decreased with changes in infertility management. Before the routine use of ultrasound, only about half of twin pregnancies were recognized before labor (Simpson, 2015).

Mechanism of Multiple Gestation

Multiple conceptions occur through one of two mechanisms. "Identical," or monozygotic, twins (31%) arise when a single fertilized ovum divides into two separate clusters of cells that give rise to two separate individuals with identical genes (Cunningham et al., 2022, ch. 48). Although they have the same genes, there may be differences in gene expression. Conditions in the uterus can alter physical characteristics such as size and head shape. They are always of the same sex, except in the rare case of a divided trisomy, for example, a male embryo with 47 XXY chromosomes divides and becomes a male embryo with 46 XY chromosomes and a female embryo with 45 XO chromosomes (Edwards, Dent, & Kahn, 1966).

Fraternal, or dizygotic, twins (69%) originate from separate ova fertilized at about the same time (Cunningham et al., 2022, ch. 48). Genetically, they are as closely related as any siblings. They can be of different sexes, they can have different fathers, and they can be conceived as much as two weeks apart (Ciebiera & Jakiel, 2017).

Identical twins with separate chorions and amnions (dichorionic-diamniotic placentation or "di-di") arise when division takes place before the morula stage (within 3 days after fertilization). Twins with one chorion and two amnions (monochorionic-diamniotic or "mono-di") typically occur when division takes place 4–8 days after fertilization. Virtually all monochorionic twins are monozygotic.

Twins within the same sac, sharing both a chorion and an amnion (monochorionic-monoamniotic or "mono-mono") occur with division between days 8 and 12. All are monozygotic and may be mirror-image twins, with different dominant hands and opposite hair-whorl directions. If division takes place after day 12, conjoined twins occur. Approximately 80–90% of dichorionic pregnancies involve dizygotic twins; the remainder are monozygotic (Chasen, 2023a).

An ultrasound examination in early pregnancy is the most accurate way to determine whether fetuses share a placenta, a chorion, and/or an amnion. When first-trimester ultrasound

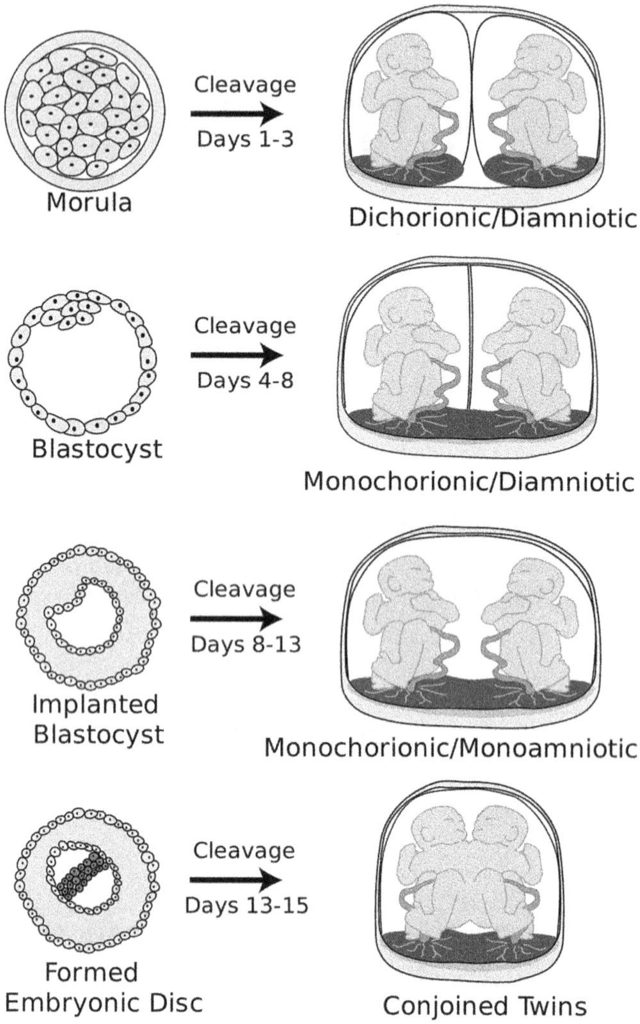

Figure 15-2. Whether identical twins share membranes, placenta, or body parts is determined by the timing of their separation. "Placentation," by K. Dufendach, 2008, December 1 (https://commons.wikimedia.org/wiki/File:Placentation.svg). CC BY 3.0.

identifies two discrete placentas, the provider can feel confident that the twins are dichorionic (Chasen, 2023a). An ultrasound performed between 7 and 14 weeks of gestation identifies the shared and separate sacs with greater than 98% accuracy (Chasen, 2023a). Second-trimester ultrasound examination is at least 90% accurate (Chasen, 2023a). By the third trimester, fetal membranes are more difficult to assess, and conclusions are less reliable. Later in pregnancy, dichorionic placentas can be so close to each other, they appear fused.

Although 1 birth in 80 is multifetal, it is estimated that 1 in 8 pregnancies begins as a multifetal conception resulting in the spontaneous loss or reduction of one or more embryos or fetuses (Cunningham et al., 2022, ch. 48). A triplet, quadruplet, or higher-order pregnancy can include monochorionic, dichorionic, or monoamniotic fetuses. Even in the first trimester, it is difficult for the sonographer or provider to accurately evaluate

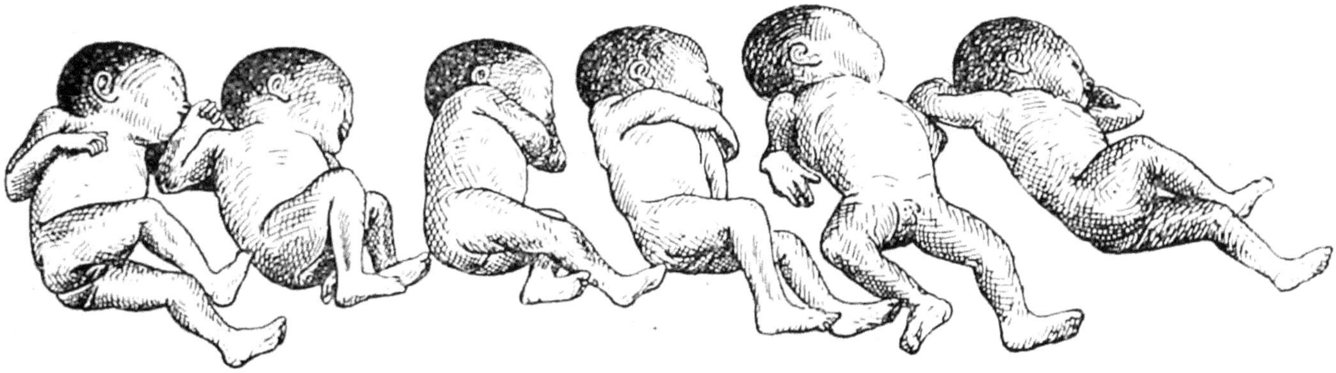

Figure 15-3. In 1903, an astonishing woman in present-day Ghana, who already had quadruplets and two sets of triplets, gave birth to sextuplets—16 children in four labors. The solitary girl and one of the boys had separate placentas; the other four boys were attached pairwise to two other placentas. The preterm infants were born alive; but in the absence of neonatal intensive care, unfortunately, all died within 4 days. From *A Manual of Midwifery for Students and Practitioners* (p. 809), by H. Jellett, 1905, London, United Kingdom: Baillière, Tindall & Cox. In the public domain.

the number of fetuses, chorionicity, and fetal presentations with higher-order multifetal gestations.

Maternal Adaptations to Multiple Pregnancy

Twin gestation makes greater demands on a mother's body than does a singleton gestation. To meet the metabolic needs of each fetus and placenta, the mother must take in more nutrients and fluids, and is likely to feel fatigued. It is common to feel increasingly short of breath because of an oversized uterus pressing on the diaphragm. Maternal cardiac output is 20% higher and plasma volume is 10–20% greater with twins than with singletons (Chasen, 2023a). Physiologic anemia often develops despite red-cell mass greater than that of a singleton pregnancy. Early in pregnancy, elevated serum levels of human chorionic gonadotropin (β-hCG; see Chapter 5) can trigger nausea and vomiting beyond that experienced by a mother carrying a singleton, impairing nutrition and hydration.

Risks of Multiple Gestation

Multifetal pregnancies place mother and fetuses at greater risk for almost every potential complication of pregnancy except postterm pregnancy and macrosomia (Unal & Newman, 2022). Gestational hypertension and preeclampsia occur in twin pregnancies at about twice the rate of that in singleton pregnancies (13% in twins versus 5–6% in single gestations for each condition; Chasen, 2023a). Preeclampsia with severe features and HELLP syndrome (Hemolysis, Elevated Liver enzymes, and Low Platelets) tend to occur earlier and more frequently in twin pregnancies than in singletons, regardless of zygosity or chorionicity (Unal & Newman, 2022). Acute fatty liver of pregnancy, albeit rare, occurs more frequently in twins than in singletons. Other disorders more common in multiple gestation include pruritic urticarial papules and plaques of pregnancy (PUPPP), gestational diabetes mellitus (GDM), intrahepatic cholestasis of pregnancy, abruption, and thromboembolism (Chasen, 2023a). Antenatal and postnatal hemorrhage are more likely in multiple gestations, and the risk of emergency cesarean—sometimes after the vaginal birth of the first twin—is high. The risk of placental abruption is twice as high in twin gestations as in singletons (Hubinont et al., 2015).

The greatest risk to multiple fetuses is premature birth. Multiples are 13 times more likely than singletons to be born before 32 weeks of gestation (ACOG, 2021/2024). Preterm twins have a higher risk of intracranial hemorrhage than singletons of the same gestational age and are more vulnerable to cerebral palsy (ACOG, 2021/2024). Multiples are more likely to have congenital malformations than children born singularly, especially if monochorionic. Multiple gestation increases the risk of stillbirth fivefold and neonatal death sevenfold (ACOG,

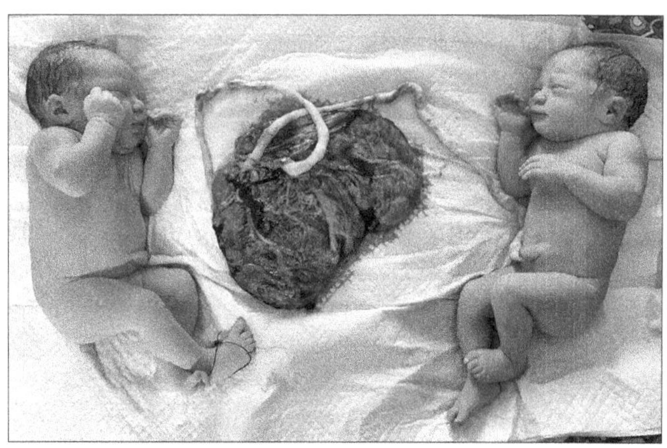

Figure 15-4. Newborn twins with intact cords. These monochorionic-diamniotic twins born in a community setting are still connected to their shared placenta with unclamped umbilical cords. A string around one baby's foot allows for accurate identification of both infants. Photograph by Amy DeSorgher.

2021/2024). Potential intrapartum complications include malpresentations (especially breech), cord prolapse, abruption, locked twins, dysfunctional or obstructed labor, and postpartum hemorrhage.

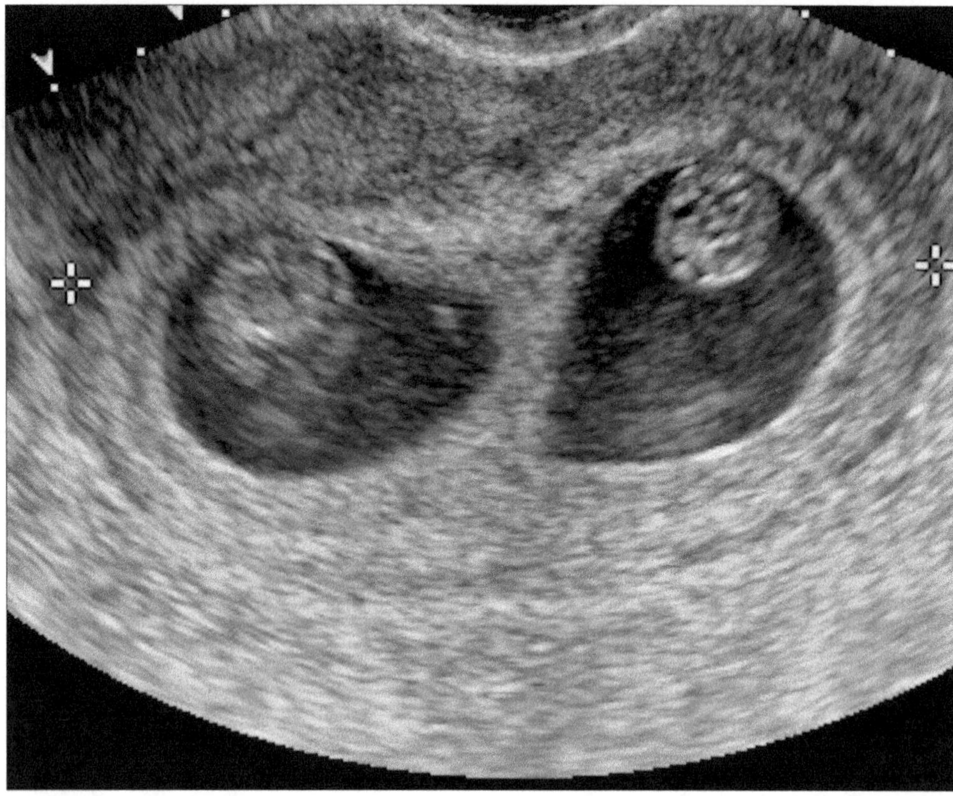

Figure 15-5. Dichorionic-diamniotic twins. These 11-week twins are in separate sacs and are not at risk for twin-to-twin transfusion syndrome (TTTS).

Multiple gestation can be emotionally taxing. The mother usually requires more fetal surveillance and other assessments than would be recommended for a singleton pregnancy, and this testing can be burdensome, expensive, and anxiety-provoking. The client with multiple gestation is more likely to require continuous monitoring and intrapartum intervention including induction, oxytocin augmentation, epidural anesthesia, and instrumental or surgical birth. These interventions can limit both privacy and choices while generating maternal fear and tension. Postpartum exhaustion, anxiety, and depression are more common in families caring for multiple newborns, more so when the support network is insufficient or if one or more infants are in a neonatal intensive care unit (NICU).

Fetal Growth Restriction (FGR) and Discordance

In dichorionic twins, there are several reasons for discordant growth. Like any siblings, dizygotic fetuses may be genetically programmed to reach different sizes, as when they are opposite sexes (Cunningham et al., 2022, ch. 48). Intrauterine crowding can limit the normal placental expansion necessary to support third-trimester fetal growth. In monochorionic twins, discordant growth is usually caused by unequal placenta sharing (Cunningham et al., 2022, ch. 48).

FGR of one or both twins is a significant cause of morbidity and mortality. Twins usually grow at a normal rate through the first and second trimesters. In the third trimester, especially after 30–32 weeks of gestation, the demands of the rapidly growing fetuses accelerate placental maturation and reduce placental sufficiency.

Because fundal-height measurements do not accurately identify FGR or growth discordance in multiple gestations, serial ultrasound imaging should be used to monitor fetal growth in the second and third trimesters (Chasen, 2023b). The ability of ultrasound assessment to identify twins at risk of adverse perinatal outcome is limited, however. If abnormal growth is suspected in either twin, refer the client to a maternal-fetal medicine (MFM) specialist for close fetal surveillance.

Congenital Anomalies

Congenital anomalies occur more frequently in multiple gestations than in singleton pregnancies and most frequently in monozygotic gestations. Typically, only one twin is affected. Malformations associated with monozygotic gestations include anencephaly (parts of brain and skull are missing), holoprosencephaly (abnormal division of brain hemispheres, often with severe facial abnormalities), exstrophy of the cloaca malformation sequence (a complex abdominal-wall defect involving an externalized bladder, imperforate anus, and often omphalocele, spinal defects, and renal malformations), VACTERL (or VATER) association (Vertebral, Anal, Cardiac, Tracheoesophageal, Renal, and Limb defects), sacrococcygeal teratoma (tumor at base of the coccyx), and sirenomelia (fusion of legs), and others (Mandy, 2023).

Placental Vascular Anastomoses

The placentas of almost all monochorionic twins have anastomoses (abnormal connections between blood vessels)

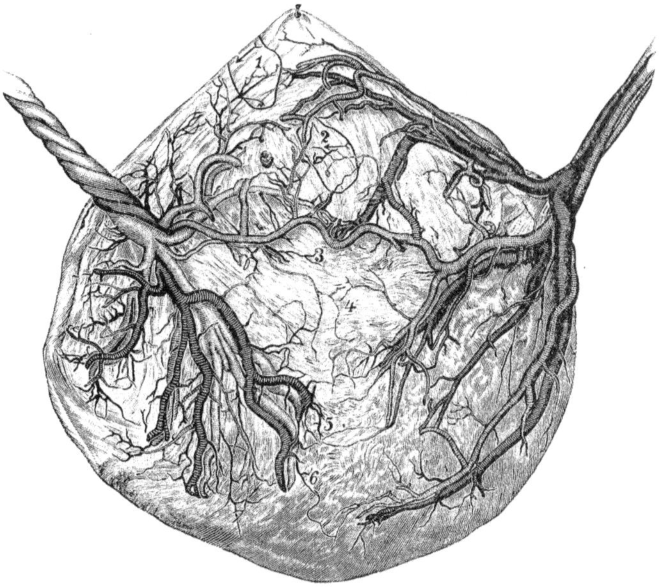

Figure 15-6. Six vascular anastomoses on the surface of the shared placenta of monozygotic twins. Each numeral on the drawing marks a vessel shared by both fetuses, setting the stage for TTTS or twin anemia polycythemia sequence (TAPS). From *The Science and Art of Midwifery* (4th ed., p. 229), by W. T. Lusk, 1892, New York, NY: Appleton. In the public domain.

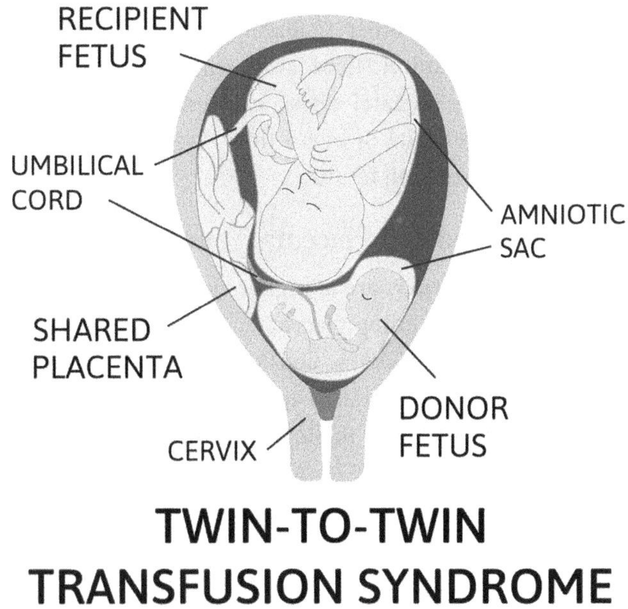

Figure 15-7. TTTS can cause one twin to engorge with blood and develop excess amniotic fluid while the other becomes circulation-deprived with insufficient amniotic fluid. The plethoric twin is at risk for lethal hydrops and heart failure. The anemic twin risks growth restriction. Both risk fetal and neonatal death (©Анастасия Красавина/Adobe Stock).

that result in blood being shared between the two fetuses (Papanna & Bergh, 2022). There are four kinds of vascular connection: artery-to-vein (arteriovenous), vein-to-artery (venoarterial), artery-to-artery (arterioarterial), and vein-to-vein (venovenous). If the number and size of anastomoses sending blood between twins in one direction is equal to the number and size of those sending blood in the other direction, the shared circulation is balanced (Papanna & Bergh, 2022). If the direction of flow through the placental anastomoses is unbalanced, the fetuses are at risk for TTTS or twin anemia polycythemia sequence (TAPS).

Twin-to-Twin Transfusion Syndrome (TTTS)

In TTTS, an imbalance in placental anastomoses gives one twin, the recipient twin, excessive blood and amniotic fluid volumes and leaves the donor twin deficient in both. In progressive TTTS, the recipient twin becomes hypervolemic (has excessive blood volume) and develops polyhydramnios (excessive amniotic fluid volume) while the donor twin becomes hypovolemic (has inadequate blood volume) and develops oligohydramnios (inadequate amniotic fluid volume). The donor twin becomes anemic and growth restricted. Decreased amniotic fluid volume can cause the donor twin to have abnormal lung development and contractures due to restriction of movement. The hypervolemic recipient twin can develop more-viscous blood, polycythemia (excess red blood cells), hydrops, thrombosis, and/or fetal congestive heart failure. Abnormalities of the skull and brain such as cerebral palsy and microcephaly can also develop in twin fetuses with shared placental circulation, probably because of blood pressure fluctuations that lead to ischemia. Likewise, if one twin dies, the survivor risks brain damage from acute hypotension (Cunningham et al., 2022, ch. 48).

Even with expert management, morbidity and mortality remain high. If the twins are close to term when significant TTTS is identified, the provider, usually an MFM specialist, will likely administer corticosteroids and expedite birth. TTTS that develops remote from term may be managed at a regional obstetrical medical center by removing fluid from the sac of the recipient twin by amniocentesis. Reducing the pressure within the sac, thus releasing pressure on placental vessels, can normalize blood flow to both twins. Laser ablation of placental anastomoses can seal the vascular connections between the twins. In some (rare) cases, an MFM provider may cause the death of one fetus to save the other or create a window between the two amniotic sacs (amniotic septostomy) to equalize fluid volume (Cunningham et al., 2022, ch. 48).

Twin Anemia Polycythemia Sequence (TAPS)

TAPS is a chronic form of TTTS in monochorionic twins caused by unbalanced flow through very small placental anastomoses, resulting in anemia of one twin and polycythemia of the other (Papanna & Bergh, 2022). In TAPS, however, amniotic fluid levels remain normal. TAPS is diagnosed via prenatal ultrasound examination using Doppler measurements of blood flow through the middle cerebral arteries of both fetuses.

Umbilical Cord and Placenta Abnormalities

Multiple gestations are at higher risk for placenta and cord anomalies, including placenta previa, abnormal cord insertion, bilobed placenta, and single umbilical artery. Velamentous cord insertion is eight times more common in twin pregnancies than in singletons (Ismail, Hannigan, O'Donoghue, & Cotter, 2017). Without a protective coating of Wharton's jelly, velamentous vessels are at risk for compression and rupture. Fetuses with velamentous cord insertion are more likely to develop tachycardia, bradycardia, and abnormal variability (Baumfeld, Gutvirtz, Shoham, & Sheiner, 2016).

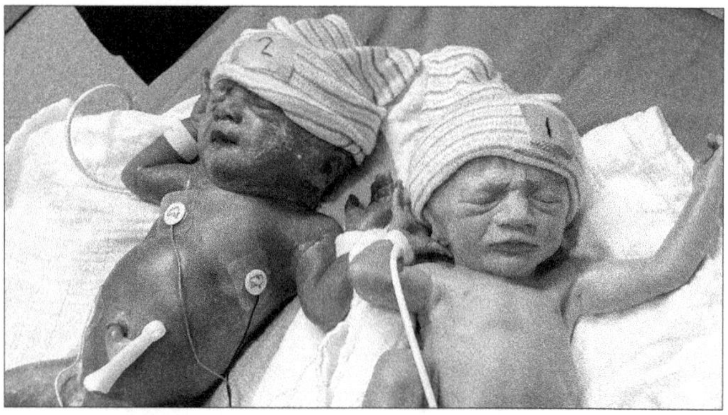

Figure 15-8. Twin anemia polycythemia sequence (TAPS) is a condition caused by an imbalance of shared placental blood vessels. One twin becomes polycythemic, the other becomes anemic. The amniotic fluid volume is not affected, as it is in TTTS. "Photo of Twins [*sic*] Legs with TAPS Color Difference," by FetalTherapyLUMC, 2013, October 11 (https://commons.wikimedia.org/wiki/File:TAPS_legs_twins.jpg). CC BY-SA 3.0.

Death of One Fetus

When one fetus in a multiple gestation dies in early in pregnancy, an empty sac can appear on ultrasound if the embryo is partially or completely reabsorbed (Senapati, Behera, Nayak, & Chinara, 2015). "Vanishing twins" are common, especially with use of assisted reproduction technology. Dickey and colleagues found that spontaneous loss of one or more sacs occurred in 36% of twins, 53% of triplets, and 65% of quadruplets, usually before 9 weeks of gestation (Unal & Newman, 2022). Although the surviving twin sometimes weighs slightly less or arrives slightly sooner than a singleton, the outcome is usually a healthy term or near-term infant.

When early fetal death occurs after a twin has developed a skeleton, the fetus is either expelled or retained *in utero* as a *fetus papyraceous*, a pale, mummified, parchmentlike devascularized corpse. After the first trimester, intrauterine demise of one fetus in a multiple gestation complicates 2.4%–6.8% of twin pregnancies and 4.3%–17% of triplets (Unal & Newman, 2022). The survivor(s) are at risk for preterm birth (PTB), neurologic impairment, and death. Very rarely, a dead twin retained *in utero* causes maternal coagulopathy.

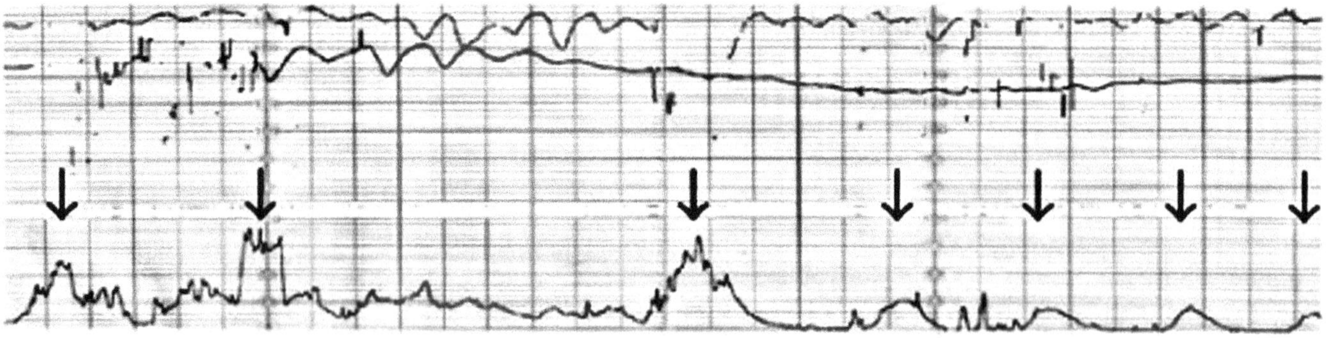

Figure 15-9. Acute TTTS. A primiparous mother carrying monochorionic-diamniotic twins at 31 4/7 weeks of gestation called to report decreased fetal moment for one twin and the onset of contractions. Electronic fetal monitoring (EFM) showed that the donor twin was critically tachycardic and the nonmoving recipient twin had absent variability. The male infants were delivered emergently by cesarean section. The plethoric twin weighed 4 lb 9 oz (2,060 g) and had hemoglobin of 20.7 g/dl and Apgar sores of 1 (1min) and 5 (5 min). The anemic twin weighed 3 lb 8 oz (1,580 g) and had hemoglobin of 10.8 g/dl and Apgars of 1 (1 min) and 6 (5 min). Maternal-fetal medicine (MFM) specialists in a tertiary facility had followed the pregnancy closely but TTTS had not been evident earlier. Both twins survived. The recipient infant had heart failure, which was still present at the age of one month. From "Maternal Perception of Decreased Fetal Movement in One Twin: A Clue Leading to the Early Detection of Absent Variability Due to Acute Twin-to-Twin Transfusion Syndrome," by H. Suzuki et al., 2013, *Case Reports in Obstetrics and Gynecology*, 345808, CC BY 3.0.

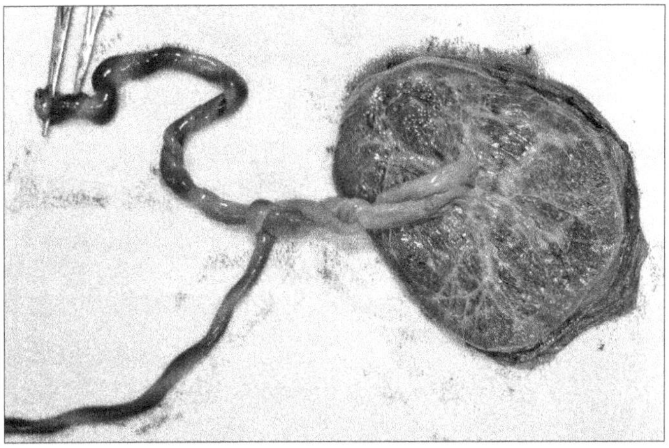

Figure 15-10. Monochorionic-monoamniotic twins are extremely vulnerable to cord entanglement, which this placenta clearly shows. These twins died *in utero* at 30 weeks of gestation.

Monoamniotic Twin Pregnancy

Monoamniotic twins share a placenta, amnion, chorion, and placental circulation. The twins are connected to the placenta by two separate cords, which usually insert within 6 cm of each other. Historically, monoamniotic twins have had perinatal mortality rates as high as 50% (mostly due to umbilical cord entanglement), premature birth, TTTS, and growth restriction. Major congenital anomalies, especially cardiac malformations, occur in 7–28% of monochorionic-monoamniotic twins, compared with 6% of monochorionic-diamniotic twins (Lockwood & Odibo, 2021). These anomalies are usually found in one twin or the other; both twins have the same malformation in fewer than 25% of cases (Lockwood & Odibo, 2021). More recently, improvements in prenatal diagnosis, increased fetal surveillance, use of antenatal corticosteroids, and elective PTB have decreased mortality to about 16.3% at 11 weeks of gestation and 5.1% from 32 to 34 weeks (Lockwood & Odibo, 2021).

Umbilical cord entanglement occurs in most monoamniotic twin pregnancies (Lockwood & Odibo, 2021). It can be identified with Doppler ultrasound studies as early as the first trimester, or three-dimensional ultrasound may show a knotted mass of cord. Intermittent reduction of blood flow through the cord can cause fetal neurologic damage, and prolonged occlusion can cause death (Lockwood & Odibo, 2021).

Outpatient management of third trimester monoamniotic twins, even with a rigorous schedule of nonstress testing and biophysical profiles, appears to result in fetal death rates almost twice as high as with inpatient monitoring (Lockwood & Odibo, 2021). Often, the mother is admitted to a hospital with a NICU and the capacity for emergency cesarean section after reaching viability, usually at 24–28 weeks of gestation (Unal & Newman, 2022). Antenatal corticosteroids are usually given at the time of admission to reduce newborn respiratory morbidity and mortality in case of PTB (Lockwood & Odibo, 2021). ACOG (2021) advises that monoamniotic twin gestations undergo birth by cesarean section.

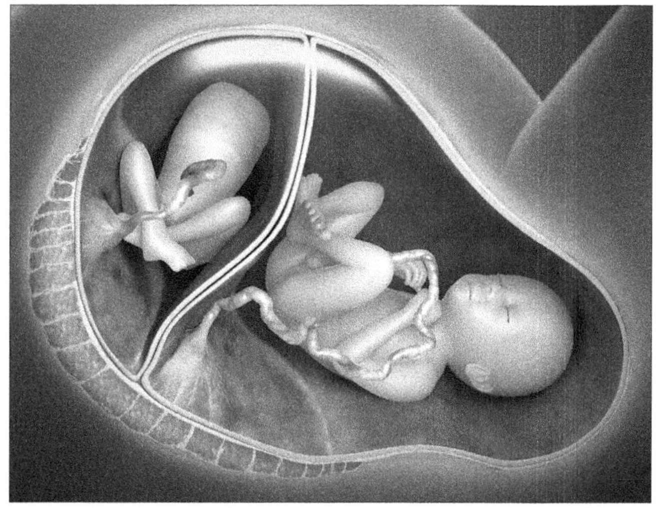

Figure 15-11. Acardiac twin. Acardiac twinning, or twin reversed arterial perfusion (TRAP) sequence, involves a normally formed donor twin with a recipient twin that lacks a heart and other upper-body structures. Often, the donor twin develops an enlarged heart and cardiac failure. "[Acardiac Twin]," by Scientific Animations, Inc., 2020 (https://commons.wikimedia.org/w/index.php?title=File:Acardiac_twin.jpg&oldid=458260093). CC-BY-4.0.

Rare Complications

Acardiac Twin Pregnancy—Twin-Reversed Arterial Perfusion (TRAP) sequence

Acardiac twin pregnancy is a rare condition (occurring in 1% of monochorionic twins) in which a normally formed fetus shares circulation with an abnormally formed recipient twin that lacks a heart and other structures (ACOG, 2021/2024). This condition can be caused by a large shunt in placental circulation that sends the outflow of oxygen-poor arterial blood from the donor twin directly into the recipient twin. This blood flows preferentially into the iliac vessels of the recipient twin and perfuses only the lower half of the body, disrupting the development of the upper body, including the heart. Often the head, torso, and limbs fail to develop as well. Because the recipient twin lacks a heart, the heart of the pump twin must maintain circulation through its own body, the body of the acardiac twin, and their shared placenta. The donor twin often develops cardiomegaly (enlarged heart) and heart failure.

Conjoined and Heteropagus Twins

Conjoined twin embryos are rare, and most do not survive until birth. Only 1 in 50,000 to 1 in 100,000 live births involve conjoined twins (ACOG, 2021/2024). Conjoined twins are classified into three major groups (Takrouney et al., 2020):

- Twins attached at the front (head, thorax, abdomen, or pelvis)
- Twins attached at the back (sacrum, spine, head)
- Twins attached at the side of the body

A heteropagus (parasitic) twin pregnancy involves conjoined twins. One relatively normal fetus (autosite) provides circulation to an attached nonviable twin (parasite) with severe anomalies (Fierling et al., 2021). Parasitic twins are generally attached in the same manner as other conjoined twins; but presentations differ widely and can include legs sprouting from the autosite twin's chest, a head and rudimentary torso emerging from the ribcage, or a stump with limb buds and rudimentary genitals projecting from the spine. The incidence of heteropagus twins is 1 in 1 million births (Djibrine et al., 2022). Fetus *in fetu* is an extremely rare variation of heteropagus twin in which the parasitic twin is entirely enclosed within its co-twin, usually within the retroperitoneal area of the host but sometimes within the cranium, scrotum, mouth, or adrenal gland (Traisrisilp et al., 2018).

Higher-Order Multiple Pregnancies

Each additional fetus increases the risks of perinatal morbidity and mortality, largely by increasing the likelihood of PTB (ACOG Cmte. on Ethics, 2017/2020). Higher-order multiple gestations (pregnancies with three or more fetuses) accounted for 79.6 per 100,000 births in the United States in 2020 but only 32.3 per 100,000 births in 1977, before *in vitro* fertilization (Hayes, 2023). Before 1999, only 128 quadruplet pregnancies were reported worldwide (Hafizi, Asgarieh, Taheri, & Ghomian, 2018). Higher-order multiple gestations are at greater risk for numerous complications.

Intrauterine demise/vanishing embryo. In one study of triplet pregnancies diagnosed in the first trimester, the loss of one or more sacs and/or embryos occurred in more than half, and loss of all three gestations occurred in 6% (Dickey et al., 2002). Most deaths occurred before the 9th gestational week. Multifetal pregnancies increase the risk of stillbirth about fivefold and the risk of neonatal death sevenfold when compared to singleton pregnancies: the more fetuses in the pregnancy, the greater the risk. The rate of fetal loss increases with each gestational sac counted in the first trimester and is as high as 53% in triplet pregnancies and 65% in quadruplet pregnancies diagnosed before 12 weeks of gestation (Hayes, 2023).

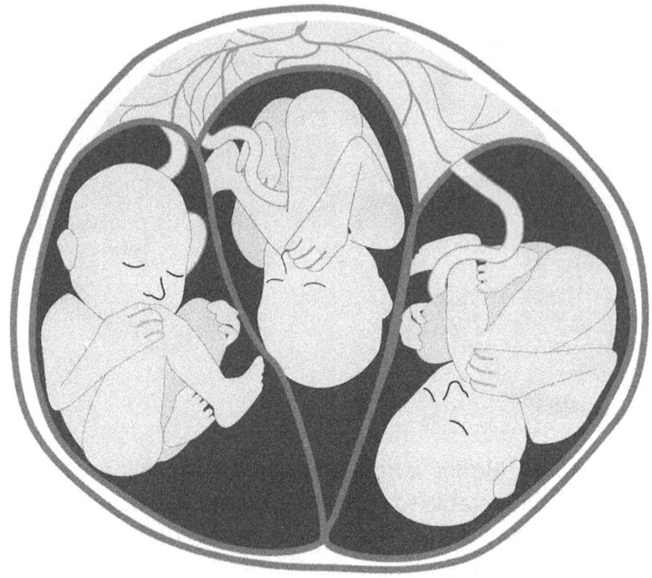

Figure 15-12. Monochorionic-triamniotic triplet pregnancy. When three fetuses share a placenta, the risks of preterm birth (PTB), growth abnormalities, and abnormal connections between placental blood vessels are much greater (©Анастасия Красавина/Adobe Stock).

Preterm Birth. The risk of PTB is greater with multiple than with singleton gestation. In the United States in 2018, the percentage of infants born preterm was 8.2% for singletons, 60.3% for twins and over 98% for triplet and quadruplet births (Martin, Hamilton, Osterman & Driscoll, 2019). About 82% of triplets are born before 34 weeks of gestation (Martin et al., 2019). PTB (iatrogenic or spontaneous) is the most common cause of death and morbidity in higher-order multiple gestations. PTB increases risk for cerebral palsy, learning disabilities, slow language development, behavioral difficulties, chronic lung disease, developmental delay, and death (ACOG Cmte. on Ethics, 2017/2020).

Pregnancy loss. The risk of spontaneous loss of the entire pregnancy is 8% for twins, 15% for triplets, and 25% for quadruplets (ACOG Cmte. on Ethics, 2017/2020).

Late fetal demise. Kawaguchi et al. (2013), found that after 22 weeks of gestation, fetal demise occurred in 0.8% of trichorionic triplet pregnancies (three separate placentas and sacs) versus 2.7% of monochorionic-triamniotic triplet pregnancies (one placenta, three separate sacs).

Growth abnormalities and discordance. In multiple gestation, growth abnormalities can have any of these manifestations (Chasen, 2023b):

- One or more (but not all) fetuses are small for gestational age (SGA).
- All fetuses are SGA.
- One or more fetuses significantly smaller than the rest, though none is SGA.

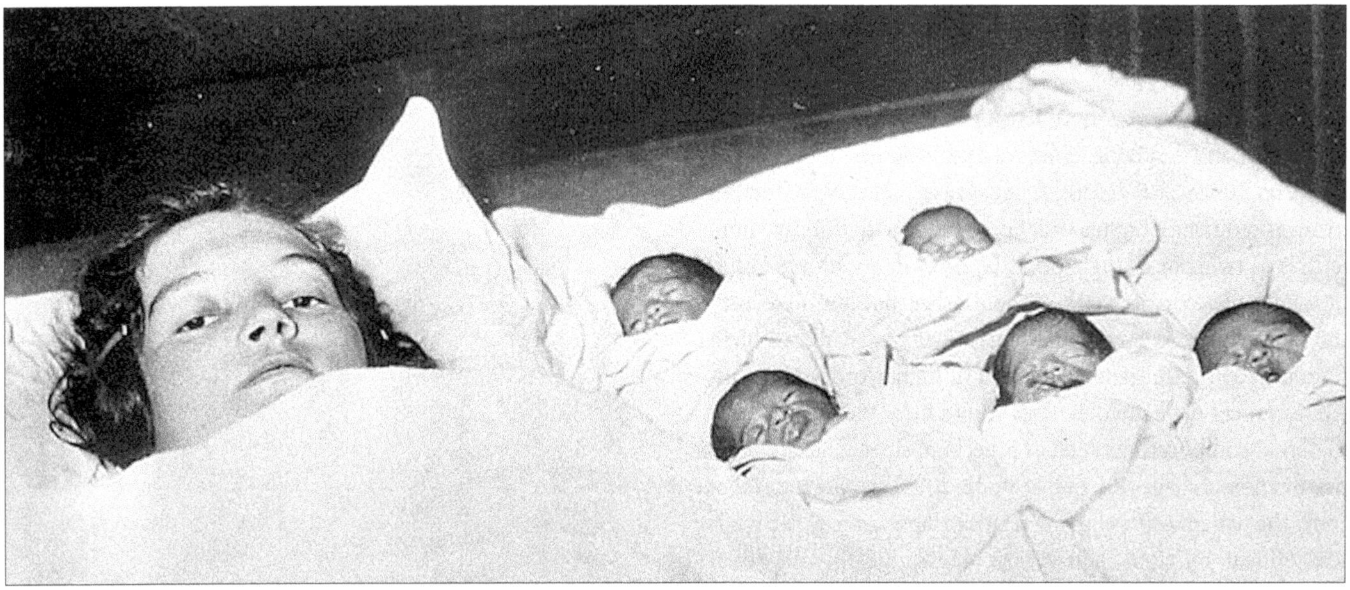

Figure 15-13. The Dionne Quintuplets were born unexpectedly in an Ontario farmhouse in 1934. It is astonishing that they and their mother survived. Before their birth, there had been only 32 recorded cases of quintuplet births, and none of these infants survived as long as 2 months. Elzire Dionne, age 25, had given birth to her 6 prior children at home with no prenatal care, including an impacted frank breech presentation. In May 1934 she was approximately 29 weeks of gestation when she experienced what would be diagnosed today as preeclampsia with severe features (systolic blood pressure over 200 mm Hg, proteinuria, severe pitting edema, vomiting, blurred vision, oliguria). Dr. Allen Roy Dafoe evaluated her and recommended strict bed rest. He did not suspect multiple gestation.

Sixteen days later, Dr. Dafoe (who had been up all night with another obstetric case), was summoned to the farmhouse. He arrived to find that two infants had been born, a third was emerging, and two neighbors were serving as impromptu attendants. Dr Dafoe attended the births of infants four and five, both of whom were born *en caul*. The placenta was single with no separation into sections and sprouted five cords of various lengths (the girls were later determined to be monozygotic). Elzire had a massive postpartum hemorrhage and went into shock with "the appearance of a dying woman" (Dafoe, 1934, p. 675). Because the father "had disappeared" (Dafoe, 1934, p. 674), Dafoe went to fetch a priest for last rites, "reluctantly leaving the midwife holding the fundus" (Dafoe, 1934, p. 675); but when he returned, Elzire's condition was improving.

The infants were wrapped in old napkins and bed sheeting, placed in a basket on the corner of the bed, and covered with a warm blanket. They were not expected to live. Neonatal intensive care units were not yet an option, and the first antibiotics were not available until the 1940s. There were no scales that could weigh the infants individually, but together they weighed 13 lb 6 oz. (6,100 g). Before the third day, there was no incubator available, so hot water bottles were used to maintain warmth. The infants were fed nothing for the first 25 hr but drops of warm water from an eyedropper. Then they were started on a mixture of cow's milk, boiled water, corn syrup, and rum. By day 5 they were drinking donated breast milk.

When the girls were a year old, the Ontario provincial government removed them from their home (ostensibly to protect them from germs, kidnappers, and exploitation) and placed them on public exhibition in a sideshow-like exhibit, Quintland. They earned the province $500 million (about $10.4 billion today) in less than 10 years (Gaffney, 2009, n.d.). Their names and images were used to sell products that included Quaker Oats™, Lysol® disinfectant, Libby's® Homogenized Baby Food, Palmolive® Soap, Colgate® Dental Cream, Karo® corn syrup, Five Flavor Life Savers®, and Baby Ruth® chocolate bars (Wood, 2019). This exploitation generated large incomes for many people—but not for the quintuplets themselves. "Dionne_quintuplets1934.jpg, May 28, 1934 (https://commons.wikimedia.org/wiki/File:Dionne_quintuplets1934.jpg). In the public domain.

Serial ultrasound examinations with MFM specialists should be used to closely monitor fetal growth. Discordant fetal growth is defined as a 20% difference in estimated fetal weight among fetuses. Although there is no clear evidence of higher neonatal morbidity or mortality with growth discordance alone, discordance can be associated with adverse perinatal outcomes if the pregnancy is also complicated by FGR, fetal anomalies, or oligohydramnios (ACOG, 2021/2024).

Maternal risks. In multifetal pregnancies, the maternal risk of hypertension, preeclampsia, GDM, and postpartum hemorrhage is elevated; each fetus increases the risk (ACOG Cmte. on Ethics, 2017/2020).

Multifetal Pregnancy Reduction

Multifetal pregnancy reduction is a procedure to selectively terminate one or more fetuses to improve outcomes for the mother and surviving fetuses of a multiple gestation (ACOG Cmte. on Ethics, 2017/2020). In most cases, selective reduction involves reducing a higher-order pregnancy with three or more fetuses to twins or a singleton. Each fetus in a multiple gestation not only increases risk to the mother, but also decreases the likelihood that any of the fetuses will survive until birth (Serour, 2006). Multifetal reduction of higher-order pregnancies improves neonatal outcomes and reduces the likelihood of maternal complications such as preeclampsia and severe postpartum hemorrhage (Rochon & Stone, 2022). ACOG states that "only the patient can weigh the relative importance of the medical, ethical, religious, and socioeconomic factors and determine the best course of action for her unique situation" (ACOG Cmte. on Ethics, 2017/2020).

Intrapartum Considerations of Multiple Pregnancy

Considerations for Birth

Timing of Birth

For multifetal pregnancies, optimal timing of planned birth depends on the number of fetuses, whether the fetuses share a chorion or amnion, and whether there are maternal or fetal conditions complicating pregnancy. Often, the care team must balance the risk of neonatal mortality and morbidity inherent with planned PTB against the risk of stillbirth with continued expectant management. In general, unless complications necessitate earlier birth,

- Mothers can expect to give birth to uncomplicated dichorionic-diamniotic twins at 38 0/7–38 6/7 weeks of gestation (ACOG 2021).
- Mothers can plan to give birth to uncomplicated monochorionic-diamniotic twins between 34 0/7 weeks and 37 6/7 weeks (ACOG 2021).
- Mothers can plan to give birth to uncomplicated monochorionic-monoamniotic twins at 32 0/7–34 0/7 weeks (ACOG 2021).
- Mothers can plan to give birth to uncomplicated triplets with three amniotic sacs, whether mono-, di-, or trichorionic, between 35 0/7 and 35 6/7 weeks (Hayes, 2023).
- Mothers can plan to give birth to triplets with fewer than three amniotic sacs by cesarean section between 32 0/7 and 32 6/7 weeks (Hayes, 2023).
- Cesarean birth is usually planned for just over 29 weeks for quadruplets and about 29 weeks for quintuplets (Fiorentzis et al., 2018). There is not enough data to guide expectant management (Fiorentzis et al., 2018).

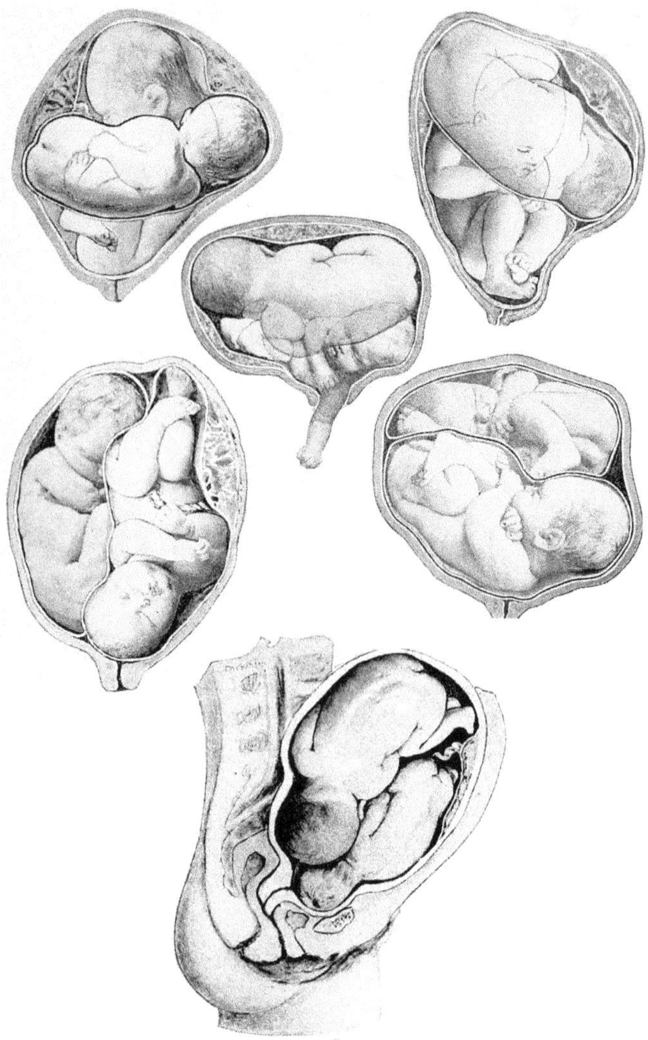

Figure 15-14. The fetuses of a multiple gestation can present in various combinations of breech, vertex, and transverse. From *An American Text-Book of Obstetrics for Practitioners and Students* (plate 40), by J. C. Cameron et al., 1897, Philadelphia, PA: W. B. Saunders. In the public domain.

Multiple Birth in the Hospital

Twins have a perinatal mortality rate seven times higher that of singletons (Cruikshank, 2007) and are at greater risk for poor outcomes regardless of the mode of birth (Barrett et al., 2013). In a hospital, the planned birth of multiples usually involves a multidisciplinary team that can include obstetricians, pediatricians, anesthesiologists, neonatal nurse-practitioners, nurse midwives, nurse anesthetists, and obstetrical and neonatal nurses. The likelihood of NICU admission is higher for twin newborns with prelabor rupture of membranes, intraamniotic infection, preeclampsia, chronic hypertension, diabetes mellitus, or meconium-stained amniotic fluid and for

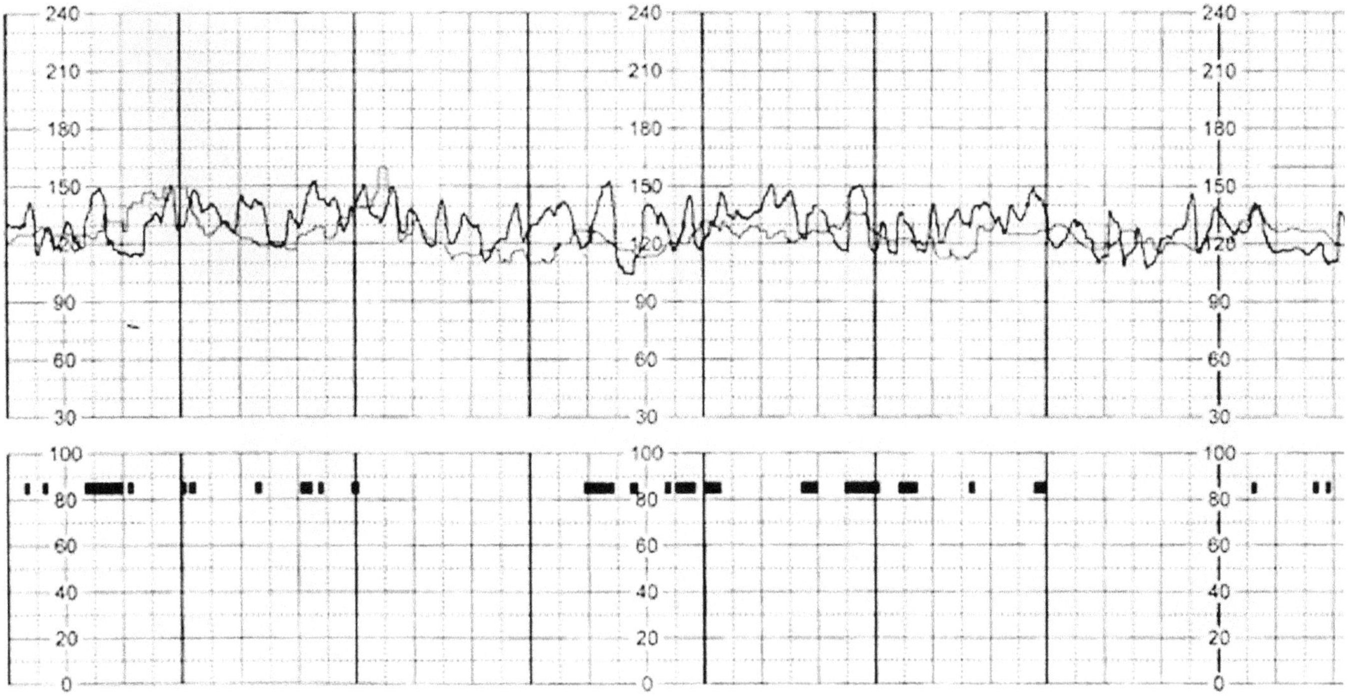

"Figure 15-15. Healthy twins on external fetal-monitor tracing. It can be hard to distinguish between twins if the rates are not assessed simultaneously. Rates can be similar, and the movements of one fetus stimulate the other. A tachycardic maternal heart rate can further confuse the picture. Tocometry was not in use at the time this tracing was recorded.

male newborns born by cesarean section (Chelliah, Vilchez, Dai, Bahado-Singh, & Sokol, 2014). Midwives have privileges to attend the birth of twins in some hospitals, often with the proviso that a physician be present or readily available during the birth.

Mode of Twin Birth

Using shared decision-making, the provider and client should work together to determine the timing and mode of twin birth. The rate of cesarean births among mothers with twin gestations increased from 53% in 1995 (ACOG Cmte. on Clinical Practice Guidelines—Obstetrics, Cahill, Raghuraman, & Kaimal, 2024) to about 75% in 2011 (Easter, Robinson, Carusi, & Little, 2018). Vaginal birth, however, does not worsen perinatal outcomes for twin gestations in which the first twin is in cephalic presentation (ACOG Cmte. on Clinical Practice Guidelines et al., 2024), even when remote from term (Sentilhes et al., 2015) or when the second twin is noncephalic (Sibony, Touitou, Luton, Oury, & Blot, 2003). Nonetheless, physicians who lack training or experience with vaginal breech delivery may recommend cesarean if the second twin is breech or perform one in preference to vaginal breech delivery if malpresentation develops intrapartum. Induction of twin pregnancies is generally considered safe, and intrapartum cesarean section rates are similar in spontaneous and induced labors (Mikaelsen, Johansen, Tappert, & Eggebø, 2022). In a study in Ireland of 441 mothers with twin pregnancies attempting a trial of labor (TOL), 77% achieved successful vaginal birth (Breathnach et al., 2011). Having found that even mothers at the highest risk for cesarean birth have a 50% success rate for vaginal birth, Fox et al. (2015) recommended TOL for twin gestations if the mother desires vaginal birth and it is not otherwise contraindicated.

At the onset of labor in a hospital, the portable ultrasound machine should be brought to the bedside and used to confirm the position of each fetus, locate each fetal heart to ensure accurate placement of the external monitor, and distinguish each heart rate. Continuous fetal monitoring is typically used throughout labor. A pulse oximeter should be placed on the mother to isolate her heart rate from that of the fetuses. Many electronic fetal monitors distinguish the heart rates of two or three fetuses with tracings of different widths and densities. A fetal scalp electrode can improve accuracy of monitoring the presenting twin. National Institute for Health and Care Excellence [NICE] guidelines recommend proceeding to cesarean if one of the twins cannot be accurately monitored because of the risk of undetected intrapartum hypoxia to the unmonitored twin (NICE, 2019).

About 4–10% of planned vaginal twin labors result in combined vaginal-cesarean birth, usually because of malpresentation, cord prolapse, failure to progress, abnormal fetal heart rate (FHR) pattern, or maternal complications (Aviram et al., 2015; Breathnach et al., 2011). Breech extraction or internal or external version are sometimes necessary to complete a vaginal birth. If these maneuvers fail, emergent cesarean may be required to rescue the second twin (Chasen, 2022). In a hospital, epidural analgesia can benefit the client undergoing TOL by improving the success rate of external version in case the second twin requires manipulation (Cruikshank, 2007; Hao et al., 2022). It can also serve as anesthesia if the mother requires intrauterine manipulation or emergency cesarean (Cruikshank, 2007).

Mode of Triplet Birth

In the United States, more than 90% of mothers with triplet gestations give birth via cesarean (Peress, Dude, Peaceman, & Yee, 2019). ACOG considers data insufficient for making recommendations on the route of birth for triplet pregnancies, but it suggests that a TOL be considered if the obstetrician has experience in vaginal birth of multiple gestations (ACOG, 2021/2024). The success rate of mothers carrying triplets who choose a TOL range from about 16% (Lappen, Hackney, & Bailit, 2016) to about 57% (Peress et al., 2019).

Risks of Multifetal Vaginal Birth

When compared to clients with singleton pregnancies, those with twin gestations tend to be older, have a higher pre-pregnancy body mass index, give birth at an earlier gestational age, and have smaller newborns (Leftwich, Zaki, Wilkins, & Hibbard, 2013). Studies disagree about whether labor length is longer, shorter, or progresses similarly to labor with a singleton gestation (Chasen, 2022). Postpartum hemorrhage related to atony from uterine overdistension commonly follows the birth of multiples.

Malpresentation in Labor

In about 42% of twin gestations, Twin A (closer to the cervix) and Twin B are both in cephalic presentation at the beginning of labor. About 38% of twins are cephalic (A)/noncephalic (B), 7% are noncephalic/cephalic, and 13% are noncephalic/noncephalic (Chasen, 2022; Chasen, Spiro, Kalish, & Chervenak, 2005). Noncephalic presentations can be any combination of breech, oblique, and transverse. About 11% of cephalic-presenting second twins change to noncephalic during the birth process (Easter et al., 2018).

Abnormal FHR

As with singletons, risk factors for an abnormal fetal heart tracing in multiple gestations include primiparous pregnancy, FGR, antepartum hemorrhage, and preterm labor (Kohli, Singh, Dey, Bal, & Seth, 2017). Continuous electronic fetal monitoring (EFM) is recommended for multiple gestation in active labor because omitting it can increase adverse perinatal outcomes (Chasen, 2022; Cruikshank, 2007; NICE, 2019). In the United Kingdom, NICE guidelines recommend dual-channel continuous EFM to ensure simultaneous assessment of the heart rates of both twins, together with pulse oximetry to distinguish the maternal pulse (NICE, 2019). Complicated multiple gestations, such as those with monoamniotic fetuses or those involving TTTS/TAPS, may require continuous monitoring before and throughout labor.

Surprisingly, there is minimal data comparing EFM to intermittent monitoring in labor with twin pregnancy (NICE, 2019). Intermittent auscultation can be time-consuming and difficult to accomplish with multiple gestations, and it carries the risk of inadvertently monitoring the same fetus twice. Twins often have heart rates in the same ranges and

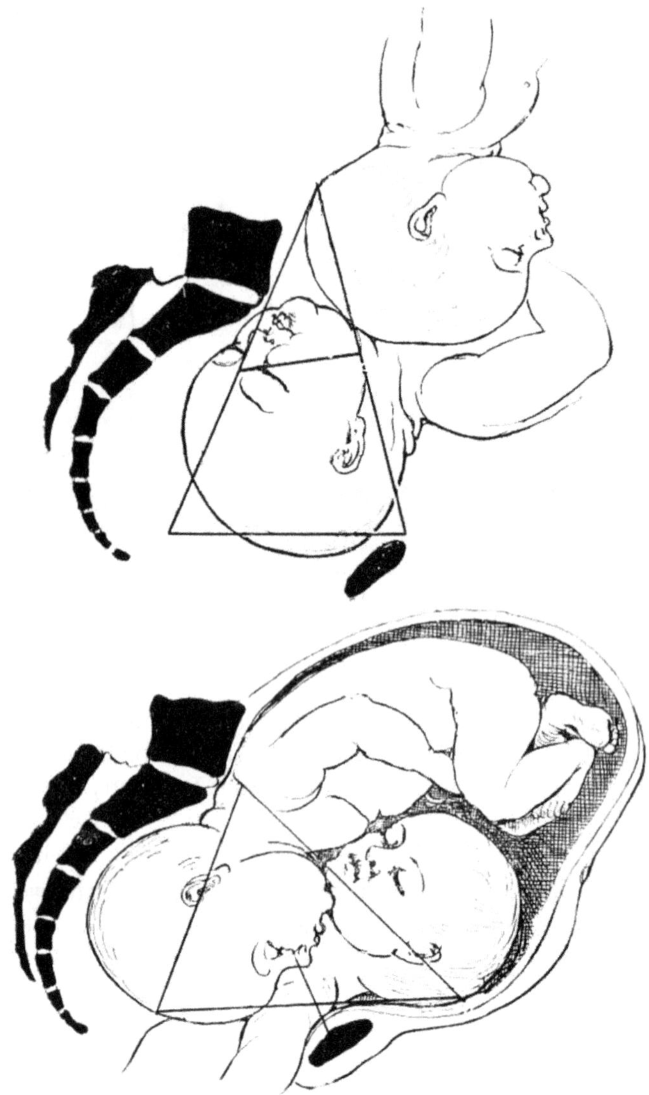

Figure 15-16. Impacted twins (above) and locked twins (below) can prevent vaginal birth, raising the risk of injury and death for both fetuses. Adapted from *A Text-Book of Obstetrics* (8th ed., p. 529, figs. 429–430), by B. C. Hirst, 1918, Philadelphia, PA: W. B. Saunders. In the public domain.

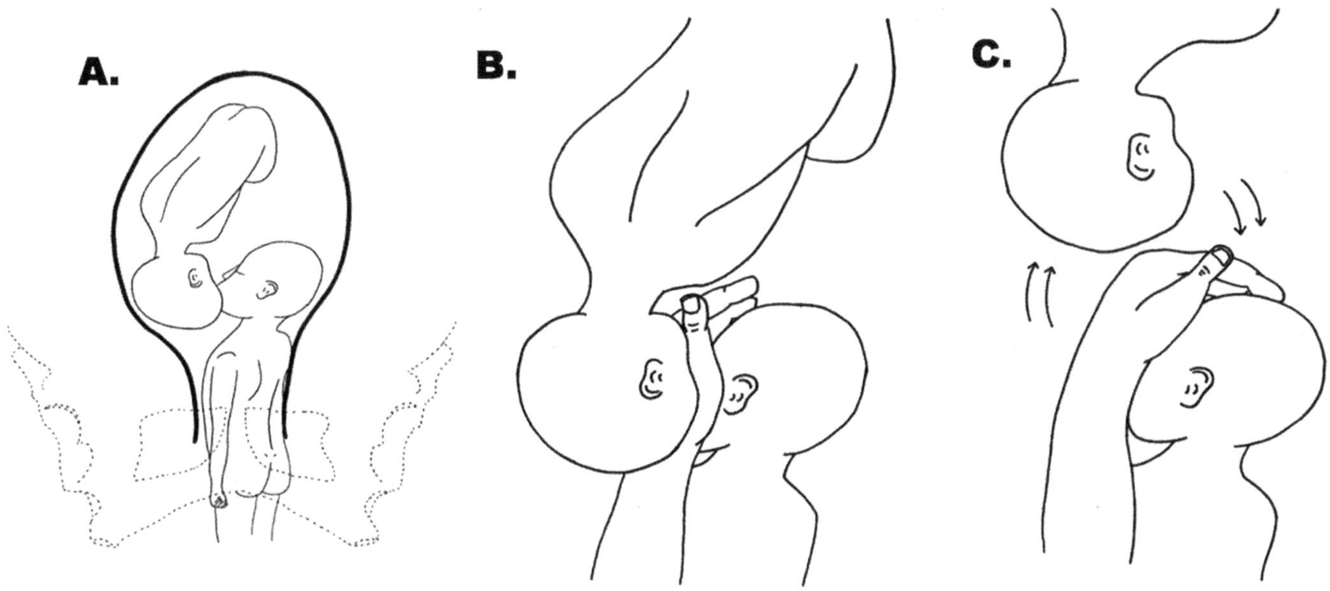

Figure 15-17. Fischbein's maneuver for locked twins. In this case study, pushing was initiated on hands and knees, but the mother shifted to a semireclining position because of fatigue. Descent and rotation stopped for breech-presenting Twin A (born to the waist), and breech maneuvers failed. The head of cephalic Twin B was evident in the maternal right lower quadrant, and a diagnosis of locked twins was made. The provider's left hand was inserted along Twin A's body, cupped the head of Twin A with the palm, and used the back of the hand as a fulcrum to elevate Twin B's head (B and C). This maneuver immediately freed Twin A, who was delivered easily with the Mauriceau–Smellie–Veit maneuver. Twin A weighed 5 lb 10 oz (2,550 g), and Apgar scores were 7 and 9. Three minutes after the birth of Twin A, Twin B descended to -1 station in the direct occiput posterior (OP) position and FHR fell to 80–90 beats per min (bpm). Uterine contractions had diminished, and maternal pushing was ineffective. Twin B, delivered with low Tucker-McLane forceps, weighed 6 lb 1 oz (2,750 g) and had Apgar scores of 7 and 9. From "A Maneuver for Head Entanglement in Term Breech/Vertex Twin Labor," by S. J. Fischbein, 2018, *Journal of Case Reports and Images in Obstetrics and Gynecology, 4, 100042Z08SF2018CR*. CC BY 4.0.

simultaneous accelerations and decelerations, and the ideal locations for monitoring each fetus can be inches apart. When intermittent monitoring is undertaken for intrapartum assessment of twins, one study showed that the use of a fetoscope such as a Pinard or Laennec device was associated with a lower rate of cesarean section due to fetal distress than in intermittent EFM and use of a hand-held Doppler, though there was no difference in neonatal outcomes (Martis, Emilia, Nurdiati, & Brown, 2017).

Locked Twins

Locked twins preventing vaginal birth is a rare complication occurring in 1 in 140 to 1 in 1,000 vaginal multiple births (Sinha, 2018). This condition can be prevented by identifying fetuses at risk for locking through ultrasound assessment and choosing cesarean birth. In the absence of ultrasound, locked twins often remain unidentified until labor becomes obstructed, increasing the likelihood of fetal demise and maternal infection, hemorrhage, and death. Twins become locked in any of four ways:

- **Vertex/vertex.** The skull of the second fetus impacts into the thorax of the first, preventing descent.
- **Breech/vertex.** As the first fetus descends in breech presentation, its chin interlocks with the chin of the vertex second fetus.
- **Breech/breech.** Two breech fetuses present simultaneously with as many as four legs and two loops of cord descending together.
- **Vertex/breech.** A part of the second twin snags a part of the first twin, preventing birth (Sinha, 2018).

Because locked breech/vertex twins are usually identified when the first twin is partially born, asphyxia and death of the leading twin is likely, especially in a community setting. Often the second twin also dies. If locked twins are diagnosed before labor is advanced, both fetuses can often be safely delivered by cesarean (Gueye et al., 2021).

Fischbein (2018) offers a maneuver to disengage locked breech/vertex twins, illustrated in Figure 15-17, which involves using the back of the hand as a fulcrum to dislodge the second twin. Sometimes one or both twins can be saved by Zavanelli's maneuver, pushing the presenting twin back into the uterus and delivering both by cesarean (Kerbage, Coulon, Subtil, & Garabedian, 2016; Swartjes, Bleker, & Schutte, 1992). This technique carries a significant risk of uterine rupture. If the presenting breech twin has died and there is no other way to resolve the issue, in some cases the first twin must be decapitated to complete the birth (Sharma, Anand, & Khajuria, 2014).

Postpartum Hemorrhage (PPH)

Overdistension of the uterus in multiple gestation increases the risk of postpartum hemorrhage. One study found that the incidence of postpartum hemorrhage of at least 1,000 ml was 18 times higher with the birth of twins than that during a singleton birth (S. Suzuki et al., 2007). In this study, 24% of the mothers having a vaginal twin birth had significant postpartum hemorrhage, and 4% required blood transfusion. Secondary postpartum hemorrhage is also more common in multiple gestation. Mothers of twins are more likely to require manual removal of the placenta and/or evacuation of retained products (Chasen, 2022).

Unexpected Twins in Community Settings

Birth Setting for Twins

The appropriateness of planned birth of twins in community settings is controversial. Some state laws permit midwives to attend clients with multiple gestation at home, others prohibit it, and the remainder do not address the issue (Midwifery Scope of Practice by State, n.d.). One Australian study found that perinatal mortality in home births was 1 in 14 for breech presentations and 1 in 7 for twins, largely because of underestimation of the significance of abnormal FHR readings (Bastian, Keirse, & Lancaster, 1998). When twin births are planned at home, it appears that outcomes are better if a physician attends the birth instead of or in addition to a midwife (Mehl-Madrona & Madrona, 1997).

The Commission for the Accreditation of Birth Centers considers known multiple gestation an absolute contraindication for birth at an accredited birth center (CABC, 2023). ACOG and the American Academy of Pediatrics (AAP) consider multiple gestation a contraindication for home births due to the lack of continuous fetal monitoring; an experienced obstetrical, neonatal, anesthesiology, and nursing team; a readily available operating room; and sonography (AAP Cmte. on Fetus & Newborn, 2013; ACOG Cmte. on Obstetric Practice, 2017/2023). The Society of Obstetricians and Gynaecologists of Canada specifically recommends hospital birth with continuous FHR monitoring for both fetuses and access to ultrasound and anesthesia. Conversely, the American College of Nurse-Midwives considers known multiple gestation a risk factor suggesting hospital birth, but not an absolute indication for transfer to a hospital (ACNM, 2016).

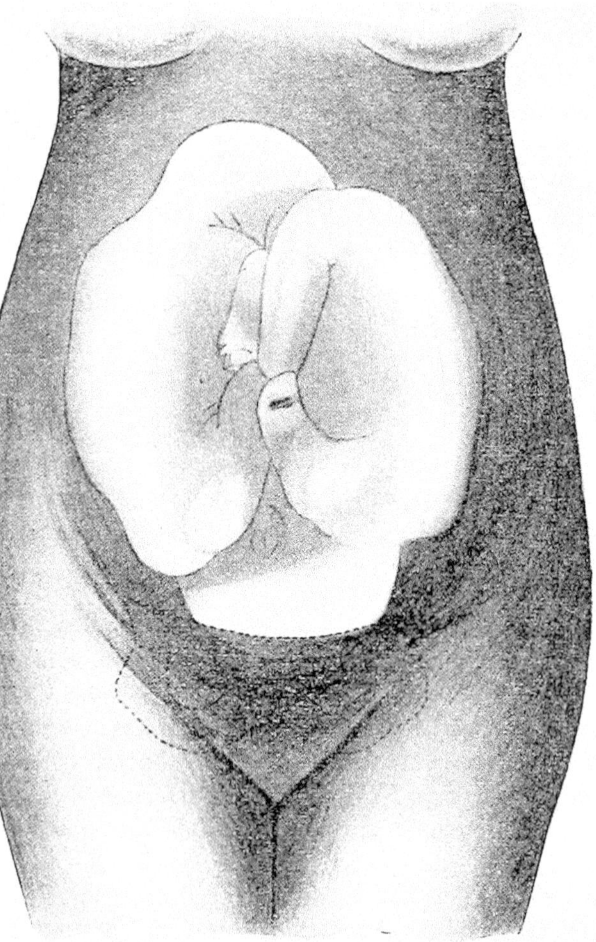

Figure 15-18. The lightest-colored parts of the image indicate hard prominences felt when palpating the abdomen of a mother at term where Twin A is vertex and Twin B is breech. From *A Manual of Midwifery for Students and Practitioners* (p. 816), by H. Jellett, 1905, London, United Kingdom: Baillière, Tindall & Cox. In the public domain.

Clinical Diagnosis of Twins

In high-resource areas, most twins are discovered on ultrasound examination in the first half of the pregnancy. When routine second-trimester ultrasound examination is unavailable or declined, 38% of twin pregnancies are diagnosed after 26 weeks of gestation and 13% are diagnosed at birth (Chasen, 2023a; Ewigman et al., 1993). The client often reports feeling large for dates, more fetal movement, persistent nausea and vomiting, or significant fatigue. The midwife may suspect twins if the client's fundal height is more than 5 cm greater than expected at 20–30 weeks of gestation or if the abdominal contour is irregular and fetal parts are palpable in all quadrants. Two large fetal poles may be in the fundus, or two backs may be palpable. Abdominal palpation is often inconclusive if

Table 15-1

Management of Undiagnosed Twin Birth

- Call emergency medical services (EMS).
- Initiate your transfer protocol.
- Explain the situation to the client and family.
- Prepare the room with additional instruments, towels or blankets, clamps, postpartum hemorrhage kit, etc.
- If Twin A has a nuchal cord, avoid clamping and cutting it. It may belong to Twin B.
- Attend the birth of the first twin as usual.
- If a shared placenta is a possibility, clamp and cut the cord immediately.
- Do not give uterotonics (oxytocin, misoprostol, et al.) after the birth of the first twin.
- Monitor the heart rate of Twin B continuously.
- Palpate the maternal abdomen carefully to determine the position of Twin B.
- With your hands on the abdomen, gently assist Twin B into a longitudinal lie, if necessary.
- Perform a vaginal examination for presentation and cervical dilation and to check for cord prolapse.
- Expect 2–20 min delay before birth of Twin B.
- Obtain maternal intravenous (IV) access.
- Avoid rupturing membranes if the presenting part is not in the pelvis.
- Prepare for postpartum hemorrhage and neonatal resuscitation.
- If possible, expedite birth for Twin B if
  The heart rate pattern is nonreassuring
  The mother is hemorrhaging
- Clamp the cord of Twin B with two clamps.
- Use uterotonics for active third stage management.
- Assist the mother's efforts to deliver the placenta.

one twin overlies the other, if the client is obese, or if there is polyhydramnios (Cunningham et al., 2022, ch. 48). The finding of two definite heartbeats with rates differing by 10 or more beats per min is diagnostic of twins. It can be difficult to isolate two separate heart rhythms using a Doppler device because either twin can be heard over much of the abdominal wall and because twin heart rates often coincide. Two distinct fetal heart sounds can be heard with an amplified fetal stethoscope around 18–20 weeks of gestation (Cunningham et al., 2022, ch. 48).

Although most multiple gestations are obvious by term, some thwart easy diagnosis in community settings where ultrasound is not readily available. Occasionally, multiple gestation is discovered during intrapartum assessment or when the uterus remains large and lumpy after the birth of an infant. In some cases, a provider might perform a digital examination to investigate a retained placenta and encounter another fetus. Obesity, polyhydramnios, and/or the presence of fibroid tumors can mimic twins. Conversely, some clients, usually tall ones with small fetuses, carry twins to term with few indications and normal fundal heights.

Suspect surprise twins at birth if the newborn is much smaller than the uterine size and shape would suggest. The client sometimes has an unrelieved urge to push, and the uterus may remain large and high, above the umbilicus. Fetal heart tones (FHT) and movement can be present, and a presenting part or intact amniotic sac may be felt upon vaginal examination.

Considerations for Unexpected Twin Birth

The midwife who attends the birth of unexpected twins must adapt quickly to the situation at hand. Typically, the midwife has no way of knowing whether one or both twins have abnormal growth or congenital anomalies or whether the fetuses share a placenta, amnion, or chorion. Often the presentation of the first twin is more obvious than that of the second.

Project calm. If you are composed and confident, others in the room will often follow your lead. Gently inform the parents that there are two fetuses. As in any momentous event, their first response may be shock or disbelief. A laboring client absorbed in bodily sensation may not fully comprehend your words unless you use short, simple phrases repeated as often as necessary. Quickly state the risks of certain complications and propose a plan of care. As always, ask the client's permission before any intervention.

Care in labor involves considering the same issues that are important in a singleton labor. Continually ask yourself "How is the mother? How are the babies? How is the labor?" If birth is imminent, summon emergency medical services (EMS) and proceed with birth in place. If it would be safer to initiate transport, move the mother quickly to the hospital.

Get Help

Call EMS. If the infants are born and all is well when the ambulance arrives, the mother can decline transport, but it is important to summon EMS in case of complications. If you are at a birth center, call for assistance from every available employee. Even secretarial staff can be put to work giving information to EMS, copying records, and faxing the chart to the receiving facility. Assign family members tasks as necessary. Birth may proceed smoothly, but prepare for the possibility that one or both infants will need resuscitation and that the mother will experience postpartum hemorrhage or retained placenta. Obstructed birth for one or both fetuses is also possible.

As many as three ambulances may be necessary if both infants and the mother require resuscitation. Give a report to the receiving hospital. If you are unsure whether the nearest hospital can safely manage a high-risk mother and/or newborns, ask the on-call physician where you should transport.

Prepare for Birth

For *each* infant, you will need a resuscitation kit including cord clamps, airway adjuncts, suction catheters, oxygen delivery equipment, neonatal resuscitation bags, blankets, and towels. Ensure that the room is warm. Establish intravenous (IV) access in the mother's arm or hand. Open your postpartum-hemorrhage medications and prepare them for use. Consolidate your equipment so you can bring it with you in the ambulance. Clear unnecessary people and clutter from the room.

If waterbirth had been planned, the client should exit the tub and move to the bed in case manipulations or resuscitation is needed. Assess the position of both fetuses. Often, at least one is breech. When compared with vaginal breech birth in a dorsal position, vaginal breech birth in an upright position (on knees, on all fours, or standing) can reduce the length of second-stage labor and the likelihood of neonatal injuries (Bogner, Strobl, et al., 2015; Bogner, Wallner, et al., 2018; Louwen, Daviss, Johnson, & Reitter, 2017; Reitter, Halliday, & Walker, 2020).

Assist the Birth of the First Twin

Attend the birth of the first twin as you would any infant, breech or vertex. If second-stage labor is delayed, consider locked twins, especially if the first fetus is breech and the second is vertex. If the first twin has a nuchal cord, do not clamp or cut it. If the twins are monoamniotic, Twin B's cord may be wrapped around the neck of Twin A.

Because it is not known whether unexpected twins are monochorionic, clamp and cut the cord without delay after birth; failing to do so can cause blood volume imbalances if the fetuses shared placental circulation (Winter, Crofts, Draycott, & Muchatuta, 2017, ch. 13). If circulation is shared, large quantities of blood can suddenly transfuse between twins during labor and birth (acute peripartum TTTS), and the direction of transfusion is unpredictable (Chasen, 2022a). Signs of acute transfusion include bradycardia and a sinusoidal FHR pattern (Emery et al., 2015). If the cord is not promptly clamped after birth, as many as 2.5% of first-born monochorionic twins delivered vaginally develop acute anemia (Lopriore et al., 2014). Second-born twins are at risk for not only anemia but also hypovolemic shock from exsanguinating into the placenta and/or into the

CARESS Mnemonic for Surprise Second Twin

Call for help

Assess the fetus

Ready your equipment

Ensure maternal-fetal-neonatal well-being

Support second birth

Support placental delivery

unclamped cord of the first twin (Chasen, 2022a). Delayed cord clamping is recommended for known dichorionic twins, but if the twins are unexpected, chorionicity would be unknown.

Do not give uterotonics for active third-stage management after the first infant is born. Place a single cord clamp on the placental end of the first twin's umbilical cord for identification. Ensure that the newborn is breathing normally, warm and dry, and in a safe location. If the infant is premature, proceed as recommended in Chapter 14, "Managing Unplanned PTB." If the infant does not require resuscitation, place him or her skin-to-skin with the mother. Monitor maternal status and vital signs as indicated.

Evaluate the Second Fetus

Once the first twin has vacated the uterus, the second is at significant risk for cord prolapse, placental abruption, or undeliverable malpresentation such as transverse lie. Auscultate the FHR continuously after the birth of the first twin (Winter et al., 2017). If it is abnormal, change maternal position and infuse a bolus of IV fluids. Perform Leopold's maneuvers to assess fetal presentation, then a digital vaginal examination to verify presenting part and fetal position. Sometimes the cervix partially closes between twins. Note whether the second fetus has intact membranes and, if they have ruptured, the color of the amniotic fluid. If the presentation of the second twin is unstable, it can change from cephalic to transverse, oblique, breech, or limb. You may place both hands on the mother's abdomen and hold the cephalic fetus in a longitudinal lie to reduce the chance of malpresentation (Winter et al., 2017).

Usually, the second twin emerges in 2–20 min, after the uterus accommodates itself to its diminished contents and resumes expulsion. In some cases, contractions stop or become irregular, and the cervix starts to close. If the second twin is larger than the first, the cervix may need to dilate further to accomplish birth. If the FHR is normal, allow the normal process of birth to continue with the fetus in either vertex or breech presentation (Winter et al., 2017). If amniotomy is required, wait until the presenting part is well engaged.

In the hospital, it appears that a longer interval between twin births is acceptable if the FHR is reassuring with continuous monitoring (Chasen, 2022). The community-based provider must balance the risks of rapid intervention against the risks of expectant management, taking into consideration the experience of the provider, distance and availability of definitive care, fetal heart pattern, characteristics of labor, other risk factors and conditions, number of providers present to assist, any resuscitation requirements of the firstborn infant, and the preferences and expectations of the client (Tal et al., 2018). A delay in the birth of a second twin or an abnormal FHT can signify an urgent need for an intervention unavailable in a community setting, such as cesarean section, breech extraction, vacuum extraction, forceps assistance, or breech version.

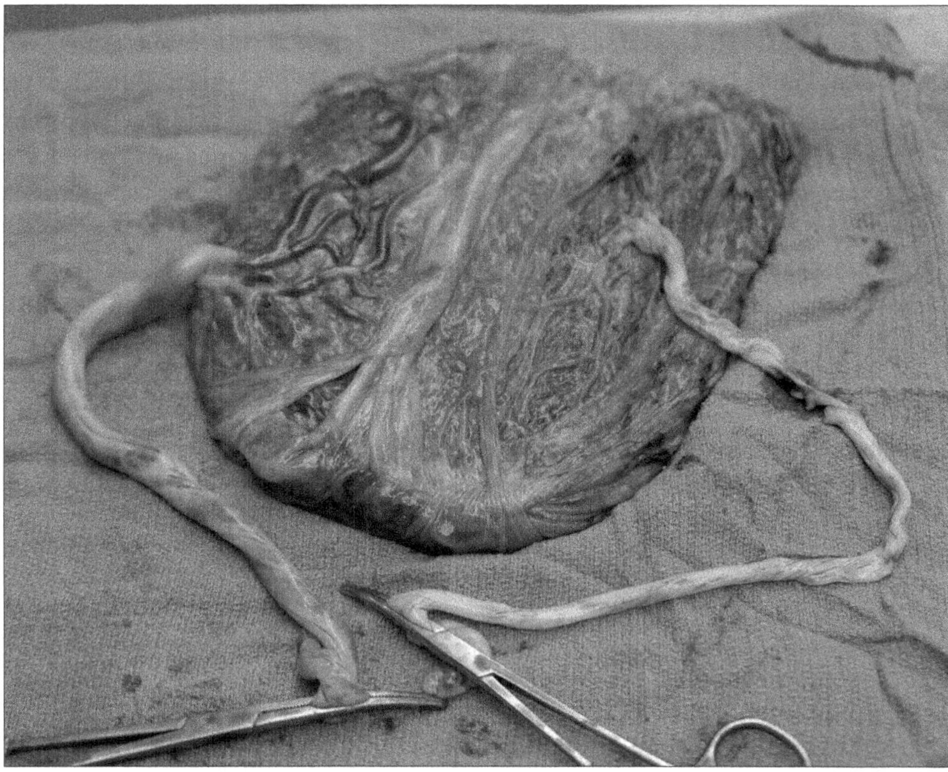

Figure 15-19. Placenta of preterm monochorionic-diamniotic twins with TTTS. Note that on the left, the cord and placenta are thick and the veins are engorged. On the right, the cord and placenta are thin and the veins are small and collapsed. The twin on the left had polyhydramnios, the twin on the right had oligohydramnios.

Assist Second Birth

Allow maternal effort to expel the baby with the same techniques that would support the birth of a vertex or breech singleton. Expedite birth for Twin B if the FHR is abnormal, if the mother is hemorrhaging, or if the mother is involuntarily pushing. Apply three clamps to the cord before cutting. Place two clamps on the placental end of the cord to identify it as belonging to the second twin to facilitate accurate assessment of placental structure. It is important to maintain accurate identification of each twin. In the absence of identification bracelets, in a community setting you may tie a ribbon or string securely around a newborn's ankle, paint one twin's toenail with nail polish, or place two plastic cord clamps on the navel stump of one baby.

Document infants as Twin A (or Twin 1) and Twin B (or Twin 2) according to birth order. Be aware that the fetus that was labeled Twin A on ultrasound might not be the twin that emerges first (Chasen, 2022). Attend to each of your three clients in turn: mother, newborn, and fetus. Delegate care of one member of the triad to another provider if present. Otherwise, maintain situational awareness and focus on each as issues arise.

Third Stage Labor

During the third stage of labor following the birth of twins, the uterus may feel unusually large. The fundus may be palpable above the umbilicus. The risk of postpartum hemorrhage is higher with multiple gestation because of uterine overdistension and the larger surface area occupied by multiple placentas. Administer oxytocin prophylactically. Ensure that the bladder is empty. If infants are stable, keep them skin-to-skin with the mother and cover mother and infants with a warm blanket. Assist the mother's efforts to expel the placenta as indicated. Confirm all products of conception have delivered.

Carefully examine the placenta for missing pieces and count the number of chorionic and amniotic sacs. Note whether the placentas are separate or fused. Document the site of insertion and number of vessels in each umbilical cord. In dichorionic-diamniotic twins, there are either two separate placentas or a fused mass of two placentas and two amniotic sacs separated by thick membranes (Hubinont et al., 2015). In monochorionic-diamniotic twins, there is a single placental mass, and the intertwin membrane is thin and translucent. In monochorionic-monoamniotic twins, there is no membrane between the twins, and the cords may be tangled or knotted.

Topics for Discussion

1. List four intrapartum complications that can follow birth of the first twin in a monochorionic-diamniotic twin pregnancy.
2. Why are monochorionic-monoamniotic twins at very high risk for fetal demise and stillbirth?
3. Chava R. just delivered her first twin. She is having a significant stream of vaginal bleeding. What do you suspect? How would you proceed?
4. You just attended the birth of Madelyn K.'s surprise twins, and everything went well. She is declining transport to the hospital. You do not carry infant identification bands in your birth bag. List three methods you can use to distinguish one baby from the other for identification purposes.

References

American Academy of Pediatrics Committee on Fetus and Newborn. (2013). Planned home birth. *Pediatrics, 131*(5), 1016–1020. https://doi.org/10.1542/peds.2013-0575

American College of Nurse-Midwives. (2016). Midwifery provision of home birth services (Clinical Bulletin 14). *Journal of Midwifery & Women's Health, 61*(1), 127–133. https://doi.org/10.1111/jmwh.12431

American College of Obstetricians and Gynecologists. (2021, reaffirmed 2024). *Multifetal gestations: Twin, triplet, and higher-order multifetal pregnancies* (Practice Bulletin 231). *Obstetrics & Gynecology, 137*(6), e145–e162. https://doi.org/10.1097/AOG.0000000000004397

American College of Obstetricians and Gynecologists Committee on Clinical Practice Guidelines—Obstetrics, Cahill, A. G., Raghuraman, N., Gandhi, M., & Kaimal, A. J. (2024). *First and second stage labor management* (Clinical Practice Guideline 8). *Obstetrics & Gynecology, 143*(1), 144–162.

American College of Obstetricians and Gynecologists Committee on Ethics. (2017, reaffirmed 2020). *Multifetal pregnancy reduction* (Committee Opinion 719). Retrieved from https://www.acog.org/clinical/clinical-guidance/committee-opinion/articles/2017/09/multifetal-pregnancy-reduction

American College of Obstetricians and Gynecologists Committee on Obstetric Practice. (2017, reaffirmed 2023). *Planned home birth* (Committee Opinion 697, interim update). Retrieved from https://www.acog.org/clinical/clinical-guidance/committee-opinion/articles/2017/04/planned-home-birth

Aviram, A., Weiser, I., Ashwal, E., Bar, J., Wiznitzer, A., & Yogev, Y. (2015). Combined vaginal-cesarean delivery of twins: Risk factors and neonatal outcome—A single center experience. *Journal of Maternal-Fetal & Neonatal Medicine, 28*(5), 509–514. https://doi.org/10.3109/14767058.2014.927430

Barrett, J. F., Hannah, M. E., Hutton, E. K., Willan, A. R., Allen, A. C., Armson, B. A., . . . Asztalos, E. V. (2013). A randomized trial of planned cesarean or vaginal delivery for twin pregnancy. *New England Journal of Medicine, 369*(14), 1295–1305. https://doi.org/10.1056/NEJMoa1214939

Bastian, H., Keirse, M. J. N. C., & Lancaster, P. A. L. (1998). Perinatal death associated with planned home birth in Australia: Population based study. *BMJ, 317*(7155), 384–388. https://doi.org/10.1136/bmj.317.7155.384

Baumfeld, Y., Gutvirtz, G., Shoham, I., & Sheiner, E. (2016). Fetal heart rate patterns of pregnancies with vasa previa and velamentous cord insertion. *Archives of Gynecology and Obstetrics, 293*(2), 361–367. https://doi.org/10.1007/s00404-015-3819-6

Bogner, G., Strobl, M., Schausberger, C., Fischer, T., Reisenberger, K., & Jacobs, V. R. (2015). Breech delivery in the all fours position: A prospective observational comparative study with classic assistance. *Journal of Perinatal Medicine, 43*(6), 707–713. https://doi.org/10.1515/jpm-2014-0048

Bogner, G., Wallner, V., Fazelnia, C., Strobl, M., Volgger, B., Fischer, T., & Jacobs, V. R. (2018). Delivery of the second twin: Influence of presentation on neonatal outcome, a case controlled study. *BMC Pregnancy and Childbirth, 18*, 176. https://doi.org/10.1186/s12884-018-1815-0

Breathnach, F. M., McAuliffe, F. M., Geary, M., Daly, S., Higgins, J. R., Dornan, J., . . . Perinatal Ireland Research Consortium. (2011). Prediction of safe and successful vaginal twin birth. *American Journal of Obstetrics & Gynecology, 205*(3), 237e1–e7. https://doi.org/10.1016/j.ajog.2011.05.033

Cameron, J. C., Davis, E. P., Dickinson, R. L., Earle, C. W., Etheridge, J. H., Garrigues, H. J., . . . Schwarz, J. (1897). *An American text-book of obstetrics for practitioners and students*. Philadelphia, PA: W. B. Saunders. Retrieved from https://archive.org/details/americantextbook00norr/

Chasen, S. T. (2022). Twin pregnancy: Labor and delivery. In V. A. Barss (Ed.), *UpToDate*. Retrieved October 30, 2023, from https://www.uptodate.com/contents/twin-pregnancy-labor-and-delivery

Chasen, S. T. (2023a). Twin pregnancy: Overview. In V. A. Barss (Ed.), *UpToDate*. Retrieved October 30, 2023, from https://www.uptodate.com/contents/twin-pregnancy-overview

Chasen, S. T. (2023b). Twin pregnancy: Routine prenatal care. In V. A. Barss (Ed.), *UpToDate*. Retrieved October 30, 2023, from https://www.uptodate.com/contents/twin-pregnancy-routine-prenatal-care

Chasen, S. T., Spiro, S. J., Kalish, R. B., & Chervenak, F. A. (2005). Changes in fetal presentation in twin pregnancies. *Journal of Maternal-Fetal & Neonatal Medicine, 17*(1), 45–48. https://doi.org/10.1080/14767050400028592

Chelliah, A. M., Vilchez, G., Dai, J., Bahado-Singh, R. O., & Sokol, R. J. (2014). Risk factors for neonatal intensive care unit admission after term twin deliveries. *Obstetrics & Gynecology, 123*, 141S. https://doi.org/10.1097/01.AOG.0000447119.93694.1d

Ciebiera, M. & Jakiel, G. (2017). "Two weeks younger sister": A case of monopaternal superfecundation after clomifene citrate ovulation induction. *Ultrasound in Obstetrics & Gynecology, 50*(51), 356–356. https://doi.org/10.1002/uog.18660

Commission for the Accreditation of Birth Centers. (2023). *CABC indicators of compliance with standards for birth centers* (reference ed. 2.3). Hamburg, PA: Author. Retrieved from https://www.birthcenteraccreditation.org/wp-content/uploads/2023/09/CABC_IndicatorsRefEd-2.3_2023-0915.pdf

Cruikshank, D. P. (2007). Intrapartum management of twin gestations. *Obstetrics & Gynecology, 109*(5), 1167–1176. https://doi.org/10.1097/01.AOG.0000260387.69720.5d

Cunningham, F. G., Leveno, K. J., Dashe, J. S., Hoffman, B. L., Spong, C. Y., & Casey, B. M. (Eds.). (2022). *Williams obstetrics* (26th ed., Kindle version). New York, NY: McGraw-Hill.

Dafoe, A. R. (1934). The Dionne quintuplets. *JAMA, 103*(9), 673–677. https://doi.org/10.1001/jama.1934.72750350003011

Dickey, R. P., Taylor, S. N., Lu, P. Y., Sartor, B. M., Storment, J. M., Rye, P. H., . . . Matulich, E. M. (2002). Spontaneous reduction of multiple pregnancy:

Incidence and effect on outcome. *American Journal of Obstetrics & Gynecology, 186*(1), 77–83. https://doi.org/10.1067/mob.2002.118915

Djibrine, M. N. A., Ngaringuem, O., Hagré, Y. D., Adam, A., Attimer, K., & Choua, O. (2022). Heteropagus conjoined twins: Five cases. *Journal of Pediatric Surgery Case Reports, 76*. https://doi.org/10.1016/j.epsc.2021.102086

Dufendach, K. (2008, December 1). *Placentation* [Illustration]. Retrieved from https://commons.wikimedia.org/wiki/File:Placentation.svg

Easter, S. R., Robinson, J. N., Carusi, D., & Little, S. E. (2018). The U.S. twin delivery volume and association with cesarean delivery rates: A hospital-level analysis. *American Journal of Perinatology, 35*(4), 345–353. https://doi.org/10.1055/s-0037-1607316

Edwards, J. H., Dent, T., & Kahn, J. (1966). Monozygotic twins of different sex. *Journal of Medical Genetics, 3*(2), 117. https://doi.org/10.1136%2Fjmg.3.2.117

Emery, S. P., Bahtiyar, M. O., Dashe, J. S., Wilkins-Haug, L. E., Johnson, A., Paek, B. W., . . . Simpson, L. L. (2015). The North American Fetal Therapy Network consensus statement: Prenatal management of uncomplicated monochorionic gestations. *Obstetrics & Gynecology, 125*(5), 1236–1243. https://doi.org/10.1097/aog.0000000000000723

Ewigman, B. G., Crane, J. P., Frigoletto, F. D., LeFevre, M. L., Bain, R. P., McNellis, D., & RADIUS Study Group. (1993). Effect of prenatal ultrasound screening on perinatal outcome. *New England Journal of Medicine, 329*(12), 821–827. https://doi.org/10.1056/NEJM199309163291201

FetalTherapyLUMC [screen name]. (2013, October 11). *Photo of twins [sic] legs with TAPS color difference.* Retrieved from https://commons.wikimedia.org/wiki/File:TAPS_legs_twins.jpg

Fierling, R. M., Lüthy, M. H., Gobet, R., Aufdenblatten, C. A., Dreher, T., Zweifel, N., . . . Moehrlen, U. (2021). Anatomical features and challenges in separation and reconstruction of heteropagus twins. *Journal of Pediatric Surgery Case Reports, 67*. https://doi.org/10.1016/j.epsc.2021.101814

Fiorentzis, S., Salta, S., Pargianas, M., Pontikaki, A., Koutsoulis, D. P., Akrivis, C., . . . Kosmas, I. (2018). Quadruplets and quintuplets. In J. Elito, Jr. (Ed.), *Multiple pregnancy—New challenges*. London, United Kingdom: IntechOpen. https://doi.org/10.5772/intechopen.80338

Fischbein, S. J. (2018). A maneuver for head entanglement in term breech/vertex twin labor. *Journal of Case Reports and Images in Obstetrics and Gynecology, 4*. https://doi.org/10.5348/100042Z08SF2018CR

Fox, N. S., Gupta, S., Melka, S., Silverstein, M., Bender, S., Saltzman, D. H., . . . Rebarber, A. (2015). Risk factors for cesarean delivery in twin pregnancies attempting vaginal delivery. *American Journal of Obstetrics & Gynecology, 212*(1), 106.e1–106.e5. https://doi.org/10.1016/j.ajog.2014.07.056

Gaffney, D. (n.d.). In B. Cosgrove (Ed.), The Dionne quintuplets: Little girls lost in the harsh glare of fame. *Life*. (Original work published 2009.) Retrieved from https://www.life.com/history/the-dionne-quintuplets-little-girls-lost-in-the-harsh-glare-of-fame/

Gueye, M., Wade, M., Mbodji, A., Ndiaye, M. D., Mbaye, N., Ndiaye, M. T., . . . Mbaye, M. (2021). Report of a new case of interlocking heads in a breech-vertex twin delivery: A conversation with my residents. *Open Journal of Obstetrics and Gynecology, 11*(1), 40–47. https://doi.org/10.4236/ojog.2021.111005

Hafizi, L., Asgarieh, E. R., Taheri, N., & Ghomian, N. (2018). Successful management of spontaneous quadruplet pregnancy: A case report. *Journal of Family & Reproductive Health, 12*(3), 173–176. Retrieved from https://www.ncbi.nlm.nih.gov/pmc/articles/PMC6571448/

Hao, Q., Hu, Y., Zhang, L., Ross, J., Robishaw, S., Noble, C., . . . Zhang, X. (2020). A systematic review and meta-analysis of clinical trials of neuraxial, intravenous, and inhalational anesthesia for external cephalic version. *Anesthesia & Analgesia, 131*(6), 1800–1811. https://doi.org/10.1213/ANE.0000000000004795

Hayes, E. J. (2023). Triplet pregnancy. In V. A. Barss (Ed.), *UpToDate*. Retrieved October 30, 2023, from https://www.uptodate.com/contents/triplet-pregnancy

Hirst, B. C. (1918). *A text-book of obstetrics* (8th ed.). Philadelphia, PA: W. B. Saunders. Retrieved from https://archive.org/details/b29818242

Hubinont, C., Lewi, L., Bernard, P., Marbaix, E., Debiève, F., & Jauniaux, E. (2015). Anomalies of the placenta and umbilical cord in twin gestations. *American Journal of Obstetrics & Gynecology, 213*(4, Suppl.), S91–S102. https://doi.org/10.1016/j.ajog.2015.06.054

Ismail, K. I., Hannigan, A., O'Donoghue, K., & Cotter, A. (2017). Abnormal placental cord insertion and adverse pregnancy outcomes: A systematic review and meta-analysis. *Systematic Reviews, 6*(1), 242. https://doi.org/10.1186/s13643-017-0641-1

Jellett, H. (1905). *A manual of midwifery for students and practitioners*. London, United Kingdom: Baillière, Tindall & Cox. Retrieved from https://archive.org/details/b21932670

Kawaguchi, H., Ishii, K., Yamamoto, R., Hayashi, S., Mitsuda, N., & Perinatal Research Network Group in Japan. (2013). Perinatal death of triplet pregnancies by chorionicity. *American Journal of Obstetrics & Gynecology, 209*(1), 36.e1–e7. https://doi.org/10.1016/j.ajog.2013.03.003

Kerbage, Y., Coulon, C., Subtil, D., & Garabedian, C. (2016). Locked twins: Successful vaginal delivery of both twins after Zavanelli manoeuvre of Twin B. *European Journal of Obstetrics & Gynecology and Reproductive Biology, 207*, 236–237. https://doi.org/10.1016/j.ejogrb.2016.10.035

Kohli, U. A., Singh, S., Dey, M., Bal, H. K., & Seth, A. (2017). Antenatal risk factors in emergency caesarean sections done for fetal distress. *International Journal of Reproduction, Contraception, Obstetrics and Gynecology, 6*(6), 2421–2426. https://doi.org/10.18203/2320-1770.ijrcog20172324

Lappen, J. R., Hackney, D. N., & Bailit, J. L. (2016). Maternal and neonatal outcomes of attempted vaginal compared with planned cesarean delivery in triplet gestations. *American Journal of Obstetrics & Gynecology, 215*(4), 493.e1–493.e6. https://doi.org/10.1016/j.ajog.2016.04.054

Leftwich, H. K., Zaki, M. N., Wilkins, I., & Hibbard, J. U. (2013). Labor patterns in twin gestations. *American Journal of Obstetrics & Gynecology, 209*(3), 254.e1–254.e5. https://doi.org/10.1016/j.ajog.2013.06.019

Lockwood, C. J., & Odibo, A. (2021). Monoamniotic twin pregnancy (including conjoined twins). In V. A. Barss (Ed.), *UpToDate*. Retrieved October 30, 2023, from https://www.uptodate.com/contents/monoamniotic-twin-pregnancy-including-conjoined-twins

Lopriore, E., Holtkamp, N., Sueters, M., Middeldorp, J. M., Walther, F. J., & Oepkes, D. (2014). Acute peripartum twin-twin transfusion syndrome: Incidence, risk factors, placental characteristics and neonatal outcome. *Journal of Obstetrics and Gynaecology Research, 40*(1),18–24. https://doi.org/10.1111/jog.12114

Louwen, F., Daviss, B.-A., Johnson, K. C., & Reitter, A. (2017). Does breech delivery in an upright position instead of on the back improve outcomes and avoid cesareans? *International Journal of Gynecology & Obstetrics, 136*(2), 151–161. https://doi.org/10.1002/ijgo.12033

Lusk, W. T. (1892). *The science and art of midwifery* (4th ed.). New York, NY: Appleton. Retrieved from https://babel.hathitrust.org/cgi/pt?id=mdp.39015053093715

Mandy, G. T. (2023). Neonatal complications of multiple births. In C. Armsby (Ed.), *UpToDate*. Retrieved October 30, 2023, from https://www.uptodate.com/contents/neonatal-complications-of-multiple-births

Martin, J. A., Hamilton, B. E., Osterman M. J. K., & Driscoll, A. K. (2019). Births: Final data for 2018. *National Vital Statistics Reports, 68*(13), 1–47. Retrieved from https://www.cdc.gov/nchs/data/nvsr/nvsr68/nvsr68_13-508.pdf

Martis, R., Emilia, O., Nurdiati, D. S., & Brown, J. (2017). Intermittent auscultation (IA) of fetal heart rate in labour for fetal well-being. *Cochrane Database of Systematic Reviews*. https://doi.org/10.1002/14651858.CD008680.pub2

Mehl-Madrona, L., & Madrona, M. M. (1997). Physician- and midwife-attended home births. Effects of breech, twin, and post-dates outcome data on mortality rates. *Journal of Nurse-Midwifery, 42*(2), 91–98. https://doi.org/10.1016/s0091-2182(96)00153-x

Midwifery scope of practice by state: VBAC, multiple births, breech births in non-hospital settings. (n.d.). Retrieved from https://azdhs.gov/documents/licensing/special/midwives/committees/mspac/additional-resources/state-laws-chart-vbac-br-mg.pdf

Mikaelsen, I., Johansen, A. N., Tappert, C., & Eggebø, T. M. (2022). Induction of labor in twin pregnancies—A retrospective cohort study. *Sexual & Reproductive Healthcare, 32*. https://doi.org/10.1016/j.srhc.2022.100724

[NICE] National Institute for Health and Care Excellence. (2019). *Twin and triplet pregnancy* (NICE Guideline NG137). Retrieved from https://www.nice.org.uk/guidance/ng137/resources/twin-and-triplet-pregnancy-pdf-66141724389829

[NICE] National Institute for Health and Care Excellence. (2023). *Intrapartum care* (NICE Guideline NG235). Retrieved from https://www.nice.org.uk/guidance/ng235

Papanna, R., & Bergh, E. (2022). Twin-twin transfusion syndrome: Screening, prevalence, pathophysiology, and diagnosis. In V. A. Barss (Ed.), *UpToDate*. Retrieved October 30, 2023, from https://www.uptodate.com/contents/twin-twin-transfusion-syndrome-screening-prevalence-pathophysiology-and-diagnosis

Peress, D., Dude, A., Peaceman, A., & Yee, L. M. (2019). Maternal and neonatal outcomes in triplet gestations by trial of labor versus planned cesarean delivery. *Journal of Maternal-Fetal & Neonatal Medicine, 32*(11), 1874–1879. https://doi.org/https://doi.org/10.1080/14767058.2017.1421931

Reitter, A., Halliday, A., & Walker, S. (2020). Practical insight into upright breech birth from birth videos: A structured analysis. *Birth, 47*(2), 211–219. https://doi.org/10.1111/birt.12480*67*

Rochon, M., & Stone, J. (2022). Multifetal pregnancy reduction and selective termination. In K. Eckler (Ed.), *UpToDate*. Retrieved October 30, 2023, from https://www.uptodate.com/contents/multifetal-pregnancy-reduction-and-selective-termination

Scientific Animations, Inc. (2020, September 13). [Acardiac twin] [Illustration]. Retrieved from https://commons.wikimedia.org/w/index.php?title=File:-Acardiac_twin.jpg&oldid=458260093

Senapati, S., Behera, S. S., Nayak, L., & Chinara, P. K. (2015). Fetus papyraceous in twin pregnancy: Incidental finding during caesarean section. International Journal of Scientific Study, 3(4), 168–169. https://doi.org/10.17354/ijss/2015/32

Sentilhes, L., Oppenheimer, A., Bouhours, A.-C., Normand, E., Haddad, B., Descamps, P., . . . Kayem, G. (2015). Neonatal outcome of very preterm twins: Policy of planned vaginal or cesarean delivery. American Journal of Obstetrics & Gynecology, 213(1), 73.e1–73.e7. https://doi.org/10.1016/j.ajog.2015.02.020

Serour, G. (2006). Ethical recommendations on multiple pregnancy and multifetal reduction. International Journal of Gynecology & Obstetrics, 92(3), 331–332. https://doi.org/10.1016/j.ijgo.2005.12.019

Sharma, S., Anand, A., & Khajuria, R. (2014). Interlocked twins: A case report. *JK Science, 16*(4), 188–189. Retrieved from https://www.jkscience.org/archives/Dr Sudhaa.pdf

Sibony, O., Touitou, S., Luton, D., Oury, J. F., & Blot, P. H. (2003). A comparison of the neonatal morbidity of second twins to that of a low-risk population. *European Journal of Obstetrics & Gynecology and Reproductive Biology, 108*(2), 157–163. https://doi.org/10.1016/s0301-2115(02)00435-9

Simpson, L. L. (2015). What you need to know when managing twins: 10 key facts. *Obstetrics and Gynecology Clinics of North America, 42*(2), 225–239. https://doi.org/10.1016/j.ogc.2015.01.002

Sinha, T. (2018). True interlocking twins: The lessons learnt. *Indian Obstetrics & Gynaecology, 7*(4), 24–26. Retrieved from https://www.iog.org.in/index.php/iog/article/view/338/616

Suzuki, H., Kuwata, T., Ohkuchi, A., Yada, Y., Matsubara, S., & Suzuki, M. (2013). Maternal perception of decreased fetal movement in one twin: A clue leading to the early detection of absent variability due to acute twin-to-twin transfusion syndrome. *Case Reports in Obstetrics and Gynecology, 2013*. https://doi.org/10.1155/2013/345808

Suzuki, S., Kikuchi, F., Ouchi, N., Nagayama, C., Nakagawa, M., Inde, Y., . . . Miyake, H. (2007). Risk factors for postpartum hemorrhage after vaginal delivery of twins. *Journal of Nippon Medical School, 74*(6), 414–417. https://doi.org/10.1272/jnms.74.414

Swartjes, J. M., Bleker, O. P., & Schutte, M. F. (1992). The Zavanelli maneuver applied to locked twins. *American Journal of Obstetrics & Gynecology, 166*(2), 532. https://doi.org/10.1016/0002-9378(92)91664-V

Takrouney, M. H., Ibrahim, I. A., Abdel-Ghaffar, H. S., Abdel-Wahhab, A. I., Mostafa, M. M., Ali, W. N., & Abd-Elaal, M. S. (2020). Conjoined twins: A report of four cases. *International Journal of Surgery Case Reports, 73*, 289–293. https://doi.org/10.1016/j.ijscr.2020.06.072

Tal, A., Peretz, H., Garmi, G., Zafran, N., Romano, S., & Salim, R. (2018). Effect of inter-twin delivery interval on umbilical artery pH and Apgar score in the second twin. *Birth, 45*(1), 37–42. https://doi.org/10.1111/birt.12317

Traisrisilp, K., Srisupundit, K., Suwansirikul, S., Norasetthada, T., Kosarat, S., & Tongsong, T. (2018). Intracranial fetus-in-fetu with numerous fully developed organs. *Journal of Clinical Ultrasound, 46*(7), 487–493. https://doi.org/10.1002/jcu.22566

Unal, E. R., & Newman, R. B. (2022). Multiple gestations. In M. B. Landon, H. L. Galan, E. R. M. Jauniaux, D. A. Driscoll, V. Berghella, W. A. Grobman, . . . A. G. Cahill (Eds.), *Gabbe's obstetrics: Normal and problem pregnancies* (8th ed., Kindle version, ch. 39). Philadelphia, PA: Elsevier.

Winter, C., Crofts, J., Draycott, T., & Muchatuta, N. (Eds.). (2017). *PROMPT course manual* (3rd ed.). Cambridge, United Kingdom: Cambridge University Press.

A woman suckling twins, Lango people [photograph]. (n.d.). Retrieved from https://wellcomecollection.org/works/s3th7t7z

Wood, S. (2019, March 20). The story of the Dionne Quintuplets is a cautionary tale for the age of 'kidfluencers.' Time. Retrieved from https://time.com/5555131/dionne-quintuplets-kidfluencers/

Safer Practice, Healthier Midwife 16

Objectives

- Describe how provider sleep deprivation can affect client safety.
- Describe how a midwife might be affected by a traumatic event.
- Describe how client safety can be compromised by racial inequities in care.
- Discuss the role of root-cause analysis in determining factors related to a bad client outcome.
- List three self-care activities that can improve a midwife's physical and mental health.
- Define resilience and discuss how a midwife can cultivate it.

Composite Case Study

Marisol G. was having a long, arduous labor with baby number six. Her previous labors had been easy and fast, and she hadn't considered the possibility that she could labor from dawn to dusk or beyond. Embree, a certified nurse-midwife relatively new to birth-center practice, rubbed Marisol's back as she began to grunt, then push with contractions. When time had passed and no head appeared, Embree performed a cervical exam. Marisol's cervix was 50% effaced and 7 cm dilated, hanging in front of the fetal head like an empty sock. The fetal head was at -3 station. The baby was asynclitic and occiput posterior, so Embree continued to coach Marisol on positioning and movement and showed her how to redirect the pushing urge.

Four hours later, Marisol was 8 cm, 80% effaced, and -2 station with the fetus still occiput posterior, asynclitic, and not well applied to the cervix. Contractions were 5–9 min apart and mild to moderate to palpation. The fetal heart rate was 140 with accelerations and no decelerations. The amniotic sac was intact, but Embree was not inclined to perform an amniotomy with the baby in such an unfavorable position. Embree estimated fetal weight at about 9 lb (4 kg), about the size of Marisol's previous newborns. The mother was well hydrated and not exhausted, though she was discouraged. Marisol resumed her regimen of abdominal support, side lying releases, stair climbing, and position changes to shift fetal position and stimulate labor.

Embree explained to Marisol and her family in everyday terms that labor was not progressing normally, probably because the position of the baby was causing a relative cephalopelvic disproportion. The contraction pattern and slow progress suggested obstructed labor. Embree went on to say that if the baby changed position, labor might progress normally. Continuing without medical intervention, however, increased Marisol's risk for complications including postpartum hemorrhage and exhaustion. In this situation, oxytocin augmentation with or without epidural anesthesia sometimes offers the best chance of avoiding a cesarean. On the other hand, Marisol had made a small amount of progress over 4 hr, so transport was not yet mandatory according to the birth center's practice guidelines.

Marisol flatly declined transport unless there was no other way. Embree recommended establishing a saline well for intravenous access to facilitate treatment of postpartum hemorrhage should it occur, but Marisol declined this as well. Embree honored her wishes and suggested repositioning the fetus with a rebozo and stimulating contractions with a breast pump. Marisol agreed to try her midwife's suggestions and also chose to encourage contractions with a black cohosh blend that her herbalist had recommended. She then downed a strong cup of chamomile tea for relaxation and stress relief. She lay on her side in an exaggerated Sims' position and fell deeply asleep. In accordance with the birth center practice guidelines, Embree called her collaborating physician and apprised him of the situation, putting Marisol on his radar in case transport was necessary later.

Two hours later, Marisol's amniotic membranes broke with a gush, startling her awake. She began involuntarily pushing, and Embree scrambled to don sterile gloves. The baby's head emerged occiput anterior, its pink skin coated in greenish meconium. It did not restitute. Embree and her nurse moved the mother to hands and knees, and the baby was born easily, followed by a gush of particulate green fluid. The baby boy had poor tone and no obvious breathing efforts after drying and stimulation, but his heart rate was 120. The nurse called emergency medical services. Keeping the umbilical cord intact, Embree resuscitated the infant with a bag valve mask for the first 4 min of life while the parents touched and talked to him. The baby's 1- and 5-min Apgar scores were 4 and 6, respectively. At 6 min after birth, the newborn began to cry vigorously and regained normal tone and movement. The nurse called EMS to cancel the ambulance. The newborn's 10-min Apgar was 9, with one point deducted for color.

The midwives offered Marisol 10 units of IM oxytocin after the birth, considering that the slow, dysfunctional labor was a risk factor for hemorrhage, but Marisol declined the medication. The placenta delivered easily, but then Marisol began to bleed briskly secondary to uterine atony. While the nurse massaged the uterus, Embree examined the placenta and found that about half of the chorion was missing. She performed a digital vaginal exam and felt membranes protruding through the cervix. She twisted them with her fingers and teased them out; they emerged in one piece. She dislodged some clots from the lower segment, and the uterus contracted firmly. Marisol, unsettled by the 1,000 ml of blood that had pooled beneath her, agreed to an injection of oxytocin. Her uterus responded with a sustained contraction and Marisol's bleeding slowed. The infant's physical examination was normal, and he remained vigorous with excellent tone, a loud cry, and a voracious appetite. He weighed 8 lb, smaller than Marisol's previous babies. Marisol and her son were discharged home with normal vital signs at 4 hr postpartum.

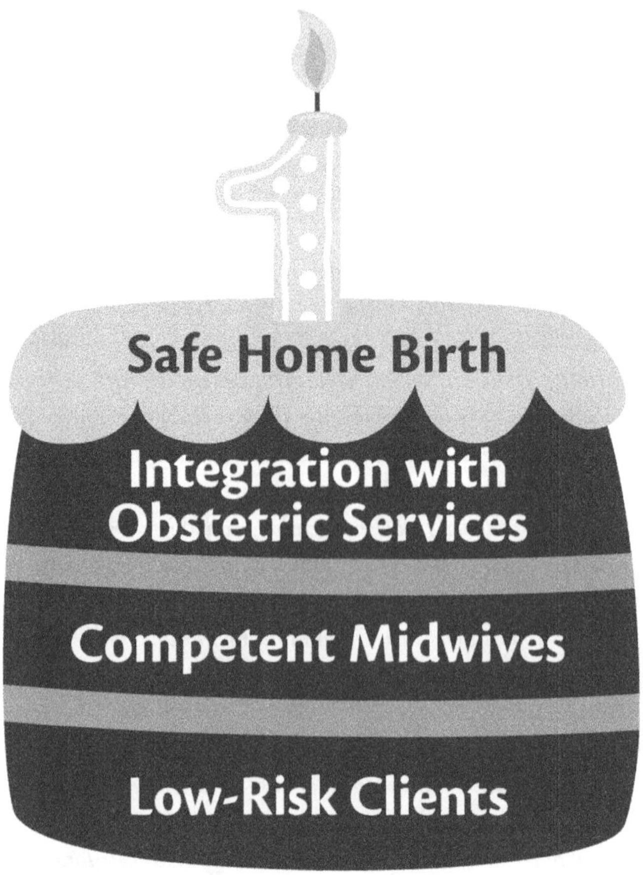

Figure 16-1. Home birth is the safest when only low-risk clients are accepted into the practice, midwives are well educated and uphold the standard of care for community birth, and when obstetric backup is readily available in case of complications.

Because of the baby's low 1- and 5-min Apgar scores, the clinical director of the birth center flagged the case for a group debriefing session at a monthly staff meeting. The group discussed the events and considered what management practices had been effective and what had not. Participants concluded that Embree and the nurse were correct to call EMS when the baby emerged depressed but should not have canceled the ambulance. The baby had been ventilated for 4 min before he sustained effective respirations, was covered in particulate meconium fluid, and did not achieve an Apgar score of 9 until 10 min of life. These characteristics put the baby at risk for abnormal neonatal transition, and the baby could not yet be considered stable at the time when the ambulance was canceled. The group discussed the practice guidelines that specified any baby needing resuscitation requires blood-glucose testing. Neither Embree nor her nurse had remembered this requirement, and they did not test the baby's glucose. Practice guidelines also specified if a baby has a 5-min Apgar score less than 7, the midwife must call the pediatrician before discharge and arrange for short-term follow-up. Although this was not done, the nurse had paid a home visit to the family 24 hr later and confirmed that the baby was doing well. All staff members agreed on these points. This feedback was intended to improve performance and not meant as reproach. Two months later, the birth center used a similar scenario for its emergency drill, so all staff members could practice managing these complications.

Building a Safer Practice

Professional Responsibility

Midwives have a responsibility to continuously align their practice's goals and guidelines with the profession's expectations (American College of Nurse-Midwives [ACNM], 2015; International Confederation of Midwives [ICM], 2011; Midwives Alliance of North America [MANA], 2005). Any successful midwifery practice is dynamic, growing and evolving as it improves policies and performance. The community midwife can foster continuous improvement by participating in peer-review and debriefing sessions, using error-reduction techniques such as checklists and improving communication, and integrating evidence-based professional standards into the provision of care (Nethery et al., 2021). Birth in a community setting is safest when midwives meet or surpass the ICM educational standards, accept only low-risk clients, and have ready access to consultation and seamless transfer (American College of Obstetricians & Gynecologists [ACOG] Cmte. on Obstetric Practice, 2017/2023; Nethery et al., 2021). It is safest when the midwife engages in drills and simulations to keep skills sharp and feels confident to manage unexpected complications. Safe practice also hinges on the midwife's ability to do the job, which is influenced by sleep duration and quality, health issues, stress, or burnout and is enhanced by self-care.

Midwifery is built on trust in physiologic birth, client autonomy, collaboration, and shared decision-making. The community midwife promotes health and safety to the greatest degree by adhering to the midwifery model of care:

- Screening to identify low-risk clients likely to have normal pregnancy, birth, and postpartum course.
- Providing comprehensive care and support through the antepartum, intrapartum, and postpartum periods.
- Providing individualized education and counseling, providing choices, and facilitating shared decision-making.
- Supporting the physical, psychological, and social wellbeing of the mother.
- Avoiding routine interventions that can produce needless complications.
- Recognizing deviations from normal and referring mothers who experience complications to definitive care.

The community midwife is responsible (and accountable) for determining whether out-of-hospital birth is risk-appropriate (ACOG Cmte. on Obstetric Practice, 2017/2023). Screening to identify low-risk clients must be based on current scientific knowledge, accepted medical practice, applicable laws and regulations, professional standards, and available resources (ACNM, 2016). At intake into the practice and at every subsequent encounter, the midwife should evaluate risk factors and discuss them candidly with the client (ACNM, 2016). Shared decision-making involves discussing the benefits and drawbacks of various management options; exploring reasonable alternatives; soliciting the client's opinions, requirements, and preferences; modifying plans as needed within the bounds of safety; and intervening, consulting, collaborating and/or referring when necessary. (ACNM, 2016).

Midwives have a moral obligation to honor the human rights and dignity of all people (ACNM, 2015). By virtue of their humanity, midwives also have worth and must safeguard their own dignity and professional integrity just as they strive to protect the dignity of others (ACNM, 2015). Midwives must respect their own values, knowledge, and beliefs in interaction with others and avoid compromising important professional principles, values, and goals (ACNM, 2015). Exercising personal and professional integrity is the best way to show respect for clients who place their trust in midwives (ACNM, 2015).

All health care professionals have an ethical mandate to take care of themselves by observing, emphasizing, and attending to their own needs (Egan et al., 2019; Linton & Koonmen, 2020; Wright, 2020). Clinicians *must* adopt self-care practices that nurture or restore their physical, mental, and spiritual wellbeing so that they can provide high-quality care for others (Linton & Koonmen, 2020). Providers who are exhausted, stressed, unfocused, or unmotivated are more likely to be poor teammates, commit medical errors, have poor client outcomes, and to be named in medical malpractice suits (Wright, 2020).

Strategies for Safe Practice

Each practice has a unique culture and modes of care delivery that can differ depending on provider, client, and setting. Despite these differences, most midwifery practices can benefit from incorporating proven principles to improve client safety. These include

- Building an intentional, deliberate approach to safety (Liberati et al., 2019). Safe practice requires constant vigilance and purposeful organization.
- Mitigating risk to clients by anticipating problems; seeking to identify them in their early stages, before they become critical; maintaining situational awareness; and being vigilant for subtle signs of complications. (Liberati et al., 2019).
- Building habits of continuous improvement, excellence in clinical practice, and avoidance of error.
- Building a culture of transparency in which staff can raise safety concerns without fear of embarrassment or retaliation.
- Adhering to core ethical standards, including those that safeguard dignity and support a satisfying, empowering childbirth experience.
- Holding everyone to the highest standard of proficiency in performing clinical tasks and responding to crises.
- Improving knowledge through training programs and continuing education and improving readiness through simulations and drills.
- Striving for effective communication, interdependency, and mutual respect across roles and disciplines.

Simulations and Drills

Acute complications can occur with suddenness that shocks the attending midwife into immobility. Simulation workshops and emergency drills allow providers to practice critical response skills, overcome fears, build muscle memory for procedures, and increase accuracy and speed of response (Burns, Duff, Leggett, & Schmied, 2021; Dillon, 2021; Dillon et al., 2021). Birth centers accredited by the Commission for Accreditation of Birth Centers must hold simulation drills to assess staff proficiency and appropriateness of policies and to identify areas for improvement (American Association of Birth Centers, 2017).

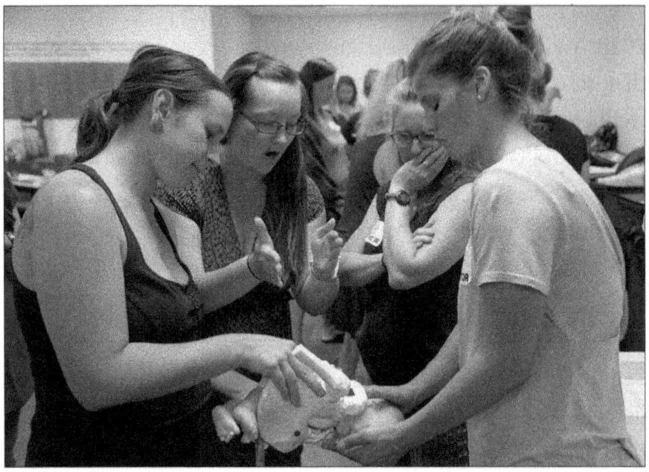

Figure 16-2. Research validates the effectiveness of simulation-based skills practice, like those offered at Birth Emergency Skills Training live workshops.

Collaborative drills with emergency medical services (EMS) and hospital-based providers offer opportunities to sharpen skills and build trust between disciplines (Wallace et al., 2021).

Clinical Practice Guidelines

Variations and differences inevitably occur among practices (practice A does this, practice B does that) or within practices (midwife C does one thing, midwife D does another). Variation also occurs in individual behavior (midwife E does something when she is alert and something else when she is exhausted). Mothers and infants have better outcomes and quality of care when processes are standardized and care is as near uniform as possible (Lavelle, Schast, & Keren, 2015). In recent years, quality-improvement programs have demanded evidence-based universal guidelines to improve care and to standardize practice (Lincoln, 2015).

Practice guidelines foster best practices by interpreting the evidence base and applying it clinically (Shekelle, 2018). When evidence is lacking, the carefully considered opinions of experts, boards, and panels (for example, ACNM, ACOG, or the National Institute for Health and Care Excellence) should inform clinical practice. Not only does standardization improve quality of care, it also decreases costs and improves consistency in practice (ACOG, 2019; Lincoln, 2015). Guidelines and checklists are useful in managing the requirements of most clients, but not all. The provider who has clinically valid reasons for deviating from established guidelines should document them carefully in the client's chart (ACOG, 2019).

Standardizing Care with Checklists and Bundles

Clear guidelines based on sound science can improve health care outcomes. The use of checklists improves client safety by ensuring that providers follow all steps in a procedure or workflow and by improving consistency and task completion (Govindappagari et al., 2020; Hales & Pronovost, 2006). Numbered checklists are easier to follow than the bulleted kind and easier to return to without skipping after someone interrupts.

A safety bundle is not a physical kit, but a set of evidence-based practices that can improve client outcomes when all team members use them reliably (Lavallée, Gray, Dumville, Russell, & Cullum, 2017). For example, to reduce risk for the client with postpartum hemorrhage, the care team can use a bundle that includes:

- Assessment of PPH risk for every client and reassessment of risk throughout the course of labor. The midwife can obtain intravenous (IV) access and plan for active management of the third stage of labor for clients at higher risk. Clients at high risk for PPH benefit from intrapartum care in a hospital where surgical management and blood products are readily available.
- Easy access to key emergency telephone numbers, including those for emergency medical service responders, the collaborating physician, and the labor and delivery (L&D) and emergency departments of all potential receiving facilities.
- A postpartum hemorrhage (PPH) kit within easy access at every birth. This kit would contain uterotonic medications (oxytocin and misoprostol at room temperature, methylergonovine and carboprost retrieved from the refrigerator); gauze packing and/or an intrauterine tamponade balloon; equipment to obtain IV access and bags of crystalloid fluids; a suture kit with local anesthetic, needle driver, scissors, tissue forceps, Allis clamps, and an assortment of suture material; and other essential equipment. Any equipment that cannot be packaged into the kit should be stored in a readily accessible location.
- A readily available instruction card or checklist that outlines the steps of management for postpartum hemorrhage. Individual components of the PPH equipment kit can also contain checklists. For example, the uterine tamponade kit can include an instruction chart to remind the midwife how to correctly use the equipment and to ensure that every step is performed correctly and in sequence. Each medication used to control PPH can be packaged with a card that clearly lists the proper dose, route of administration, contraindications, and how often the dose can be repeated.
- A policy for quantifying blood loss at every birth by weighing pads and frequently announcing the cumulative total.

Eliminating Biases

Every health care provider has an ethical and moral responsibility to uncover personal and systemic biases and combat them (Vela et al., 2022). The first step is to examine personal beliefs and make changes to improve care for marginalized individuals. Examine yourself for bias in the way you approach your clients. Midwives and other health care providers devote their lives to improving the health of others and can be strongly resistant to acknowledging their roles in supporting structural racism (Bingham, Jones, & Howell, 2019). Bias training may raise your awareness of assumptions that can affect how you provide care to clients from minority backgrounds (Bingham et al., 2019).

The Implicit Association Test (IAT) is a tool that measures the strength of associations between concepts and evaluations or stereotypes. Several free IAT tests available online assess attitudes toward race, skin tone, age, gender, religion, weight, disability, and other areas of potential bias. You can take them anonymously to learn about your own hidden or subconscious preconceptions while helping researchers gather data on this subject. The IAT, first published in 1998 by Project Implicit, a nonprofit organization, is now administered through Harvard University. You can test yourself at https://implicit.harvard.edu/implicit/takeatest.html The results of this test can be surprising, disturbing, and life-changing. Understanding your personal biases can influence the care you provide and your social interactions going forward.

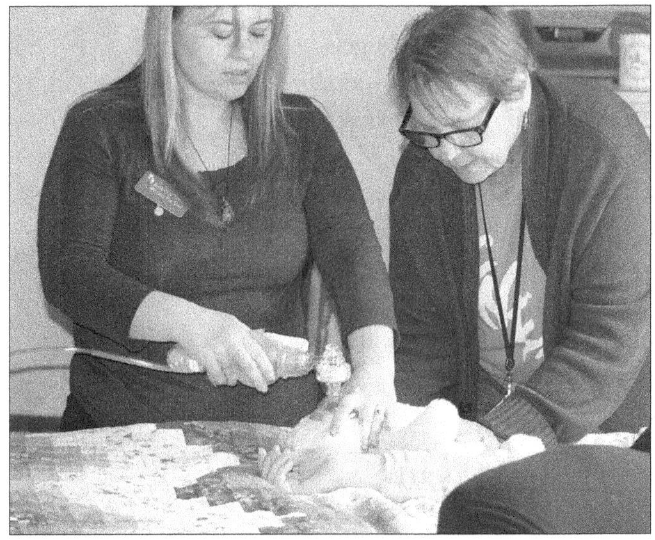

Figure 16-3. Monthly emergency drills prepare birth attendants to respond efficiently in real emergencies. In this case, a nurse and a midwife at a freestanding birth center resuscitate a teddy bear while another midwife pretends to hemorrhage. Sometimes EMS personnel participate in these drills.

Peer Review

ACNM Standards for the Practice of Midwifery (2011) and the MANA *Core Competencies for Basic Midwifery Practice* (2011) require all certified nurse-midwives (CNMs) and certified professional midwives (CPMs) to participate in peer review. Peer and chart reviews expose the strengths and weaknesses of a midwifery service and facilitate continual improvement in safety and quality of care in an atmosphere of mutual trust and respect (Dahlen, 2012). When deficiencies are discussed with sensitivity and diplomacy, a root-cause analysis can help determine how best to avoid future concerns. Certain hospital quality improvement and quality assurance activities may be immune to discovery in many legal actions (Benson, Benson, & Stein, 2016). For providers who are not part of an organized health system, however, errors and misjudgments disclosed at peer review or in other situations can have legal repercussions (North American Registry of Midwives, 2022).

Root-Cause Analysis

Because no one performs perfectly all the time, errors occur. Root-cause analysis is a comprehensive review process used to identify the fundamental elements that underpin mistakes and omissions (Klein, 2019). When the root cause is understood, the provider can take steps to change the process so that the errors do not reoccur. It takes courage to report or admit to errors, but transparency allows you to build a safer practice by correcting inefficient or risky processes (Boulanger, Keohane, & Yeats, 2019).

One way to explore the root causes of sentinel events, near-miss events, and errors is to ask "why?" (Klein, 2019). For example, if a client loses 1,800 ml of blood, ask yourself and your team "why?" The answer may be atony. *Why else?* Because the client was a grand multipara with a very long labor. *Why else?* Because oxytocin was not in the midwife's birth kit, and the nurse had to hunt for it while the client was bleeding. *Why else?* Because the nurse and midwife were involved with resuscitating the baby and did not notice the mother was bleeding until 1,000 ml of blood was lost. From this conversation, the nurse and midwife can determine that risk factors for PPH should be reassessed throughout labor, all equipment should be checked before responding to home births, a fully stocked postpartum hemorrhage kit should be readily available at the bedside, and the mother should be observed carefully postpartum, even when providers are busy with the infant.

Debriefing

Team debriefing after an emergency can improve performance and assist cognitive and emotional processing. It can be "hot," immediately after the event; "warm," minutes to hours afterwards; or "cold," days to weeks later (Kessler, Cheng, & Mullan,

2014). It should be a friendly, nonjudgmental dialogue in which every member of the team has a voice. Team members should get a chance to tell their stories and to gain insights from the perspective of others. Debriefing can identify performance improvements for client safety without accusation or blame.

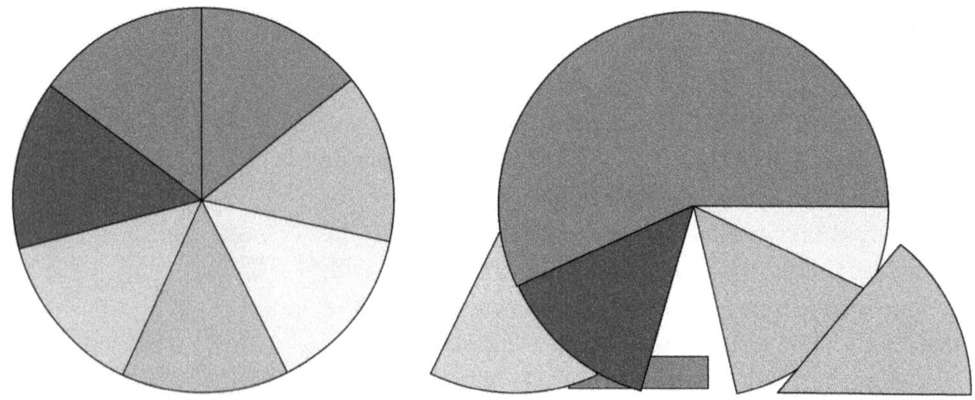

Figure 16-4. Maintaining a balanced life. Health care providers are healthiest when each dimension of a balanced life receives adequate time and attention: work; family; social interactions; spirituality; creativity and play; wellness and fitness; and sleep, rest, and downtime. When work dominates, it puts pressure on the remainder of providers' lives and impairs their health and effectiveness.

Self-Care for a Safer Practice

Like rivers that change course in an ever-changing landscape, exemplary midwives continuously refine and reshape the way they practice with the goal of becoming better clinicians and care providers. It can be a humbling and unsettling experience to critically examine how we think and how it relates to our practice. Every midwife wants to be a "good" provider. Exposing our weaknesses and limitations can make us feel vulnerable and inadequate.

All health care professionals give better care to clients when they first ensure that their own needs are met (Linton & Koonmen, 2020). The World Health Organization (WHO) describes self-care as promoting and maintaining one's own health, preventing disease, and coping with illness and disability (WHO, 2021). Yet many providers who are excellent at caring for clients neglect their own wellbeing, perceiving self-care as unimportant or self-indulgent (Linton & Koonmen, 2020). They may be unwilling to complain about or expose their overburdened condition to avoid imposing more work on equally overburdened colleagues or to avoid appearing incapable or weak (Egan et al., 2019).

Work-Life Balance

People called to midwifery often make sacrifices and compromises in other areas of their lives to attend to their clients. Ironically, putting the mission first can create imbalances that complicate the mission. It also makes midwives vulnerable to exploitation, undercompensation, and disrespect. Fulfillment can be compromised by destabilizers such as overwork, family or social drama, spiritual crisis, or simple lack of sleep.

For a community midwife, sometimes it seems that the deck is stacked against maintaining physical and mental health. A bad night at work for a midwife can involve life-and-death issues, sleep deprivation, uncooperative clients, meddlesome bystanders, and hostile staff at a receiving hospital. The unpredictability and suddenness of obstetric emergencies can cause the midwife to feel off-balance and out of control in all areas of life. An understaffed practice must cover call shifts by extending provider hours, leading to overwork and life imbalance. A midwife working in a dysfunctional group practice may find aspects of personal life undervalued by coworkers. Midwives with solo home-birth practices are sometimes on call all day, all night, all year, with no time off. Being on perpetual call with no personal time can lead to physical and emotional exhaustion.

Many professional organizations emphasize the need to engage in self-care and uphold self-respect. For example, the International Council of Nurses states that the nurse should "seek a work-life balance, ongoing personal growth, and . . . a healthy lifestyle" (ICN, 2021, p. 13). The American Medical Association declares that "to preserve the quality of their performance, physicians have a responsibility to maintain their health and wellness, broadly construed as preventing or treating acute or chronic diseases, including mental illness, disabilities, and occupational stress" (AMA, 2022). So do all health care professionals. The International Confederation of Midwives goes farther, encouraging midwives to "support and sustain each other in their professional roles, and actively nurture their own and others' sense of self-worth" (ICM, 2014, p. 2), and it asserts that midwives have an ethical duty to uphold self-respect and integrity (ICM, 2014), which are essential to health and wellbeing. The ACNM Code of Ethics states that midwives have equal status with other human beings and should respect their own values, competencies, and dignity (ACNM, 2015). It should go without saying that health care providers should not look away when they observe colleagues floundering, suffering, or deteriorating.

A balanced life has many overlapping parts that mesh to create a resilient and contented unity, such as

- *Health*: Physical fitness, proper nutrition, and adequate sleep promote health. So does stress reduction, which can include yoga, breath control, mindfulness meditation, biofeedback, hypnosis, guided imagery, acupuncture, massage, or therapy for the development of self-reflection and evaluation (Wright, 2020).

- *Intellectual growth*: Examining old assumptions, developing new interests, and cultivating curiosity can stimulate the mind.
- *Spirituality*: Seeking higher power, truth or meaning can cultivate a feeling of peace, purpose, and forgiveness.
- *Connections:* Developing and maintaining relationships with family, friends, acquaintances, pets, community, and organizations can open the heart.
- *Creativity and play*: Participation in sports or games, painting, journaling, playing music, making crafts, and engaging in hobbies can reduce stress and improve mood and focus.
- *Downtime*: Like sleep, relaxation is essential to wellbeing. Meditate, connect with nature, read for pleasure, and take vacations.
- *Work*: Work and life are not opposites; they are inextricable complements. Most midwives love what they do throughout their careers. Work provides meaningful interactions with other people, the opportunity to do good, and intellectual challenge. Meaningful work also builds identity and self-worth.

Self-compassion is viewing yourself with the same consideration, forgiveness, and mindfulness with which you would view a client in your care (Egan et al., 2019). It is treating oneself kindly, viewing shortcomings with understanding, and recognizing that every person has difficult experiences and limitations. Missing the mark does not mean that one is a failure. When midwives cultivate a healthy work-life balance and practice self-nurturing and self-compassion, they can avoid the burnout that can prematurely end a career. Providers who take a holistic approach to themselves will find the beneficial effects synergistic and cumulative.

Burnout

Professional burnout is a condition in which a person responds to chronic work stressors with pathologic levels of emotional exhaustion, cynicism, depersonalization, or a sense of inadequacy (Thumm, Smith, Squires, Breedlove, & Meek, 2021). In the United States, burnout may affect 40% of midwives in clinical practice (Thumm et al., 2021). By comparison, 25% of maternity nurses and 46% of obstetricians experience burnout (Thumm et al., 2021). In general, community midwives have a lower rate of burnout than hospital-based midwives (Thumm et al., 2021).

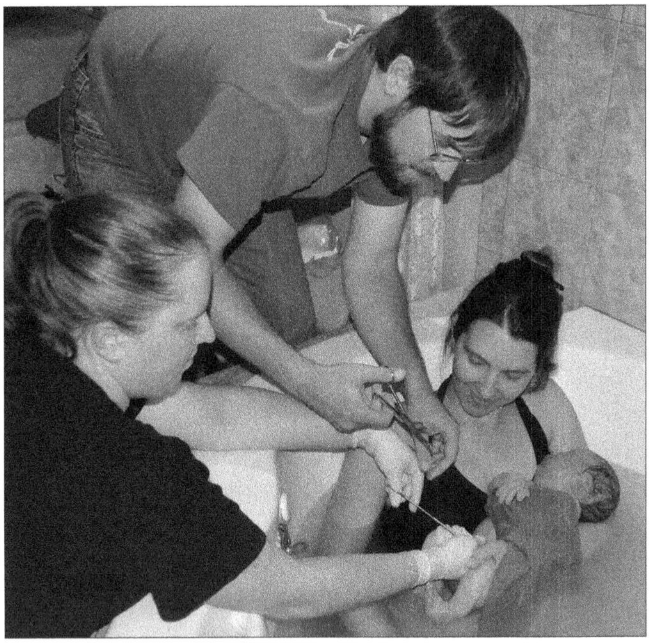

Figure 16-5. Clients count on midwives to bring their best selves to work and to be capable, caring, and competent at any time, day or night.

Stress and burnout can develop when midwives work excessive hours with insufficient recovery time or contend with unsafe staffing ratios, heavy caseloads, lack of autonomy, litigation fears, insufficient pay, inadequate training, lack of support, and conflict in relationships with colleagues (Wright, 2020). Providers experiencing burnout are more likely to fail to provide necessary client care, to make medical errors, and to have adverse client outcomes (Thumm et al., 2021). They are also unhappy at work and more likely to leave their current jobs or profession (Sidhu, Su, Shapiro, & Stoll, 2020).

Burnout involves three major components, each a mechanism to protect the psyche against severe stress:

Emotional exhaustion occurs when providers become overwhelmed and drained from overinvesting in the lives of others. Eventually, they may disengage from clients and colleagues and become so emotionally depleted that they do not recover with time off.

Depersonalization involves distancing oneself from work by becoming negative, callous, or cynical. A midwife who depersonalizes clients begins to see them as burdens and may become increasingly resentful of the demands they make on time or energy. Depersonalization behaviors can include complaining and making unprofessional comments to coworkers. Some midwives lose the ability to empathize or grieve when a client experiences a bad outcome.

Reduced personal accomplishment involves decreased motivation and drive. Over time, the midwife frequently develops feelings of incompetence, ineffectiveness, or incapability, which further degrade performance.

Provider Impairment

Midwives must protect themselves and others from harmful, unethical, and incompetent behavior, including those resulting from a lack of knowledge and skill, impairment of judgment or function, or deliberate violation of standards (ACNM, 2015). Provider impairment is the physical or mental inability to carry out client-care responsibilities with reasonable skill and safety. Impaired midwives must either take action to regain their ability to practice safely or stop working (ACNM, 2015). All providers have an ethical duty to seek help when they are unable to provide safe care and to address or report possible impairment in others (Candilis, Kim, & Sulmasy, 2019). Ignoring an impairment problem not only puts clients in danger, but also jeopardizes the midwife's license, livelihood, and reputation.

Illness, injury, medication, substance abuse, and emotional distress can impair the midwife's ability to provide optimal care. The provider who goes to work compromised by acute illness such as influenza is more likely to make bad decisions and basic errors while exposing others to the disease. A provider with rotator cuff tendinitis may be unable to perform the maneuvers necessary to resolve a shoulder dystocia. Muscle relaxants, antihistamines, painkillers, steroids, and other preparations can cloud judgment and reduce mental acuity. Complications related to diabetes, arrhythmias, or head trauma can cause mental status changes and foggy thinking. An aging provider may experience gradual or intermittent loss of mental clarity or motor skill.

Sleep Deprivation

In midwifery, there is often no rest for the weary. Providers in group practices can be on call for days at a time and often find little opportunity for sleep. Midwives in solo practices commonly take call around the clock and around the calendar. When labors cluster, the fatigued birth attendant can develop cognitive impairment very similar to that caused by alcohol intoxication (Sugden, Athanasiou, & Darzi, 2012).

Sleep is a universal physiological and psychological need. Although we do not fully understand all the purposes of sleep, it clearly restores higher brain function. People *must* sleep. The body fulfills this biological mandate as faithfully as it sustains breathing and heartbeat, and it inevitably responds to prolonged wakefulness with involuntary episodes of sleep.

Inadequate sleep increases the risk of traffic accidents, work-related injuries, and medical errors. Chronic sleep deprivation increases the risk for cardiovascular disease, stroke, obesity, type 2 diabetes, cancer, and neurodegenerative disease (Garbarino, Lanteri, Bragazzi, Magnavita, & Scoditti, 2021). It can also cause immunosuppression, which makes exhausted providers more vulnerable to colds, influenza, COVID-19 (SARS-CoV-2), or other illnesses (Ishikura et al., 2021). Vaccines administered to sleep-deprived people may be less effective due to inadequate immune response (Cirelli, 2023).

Sleep deprivation has also been associated with psychosis, anxiety, suicidal behavior, and the risk for depression (Garbarino et al., 2021). It can cause emotional instability and lead to poor decision-making. Preventable disasters such as the partial nuclear-reactor meltdowns at Three Mile Island and Chernobyl and the loss of the space shuttle *Challenger* have been attributed to early-morning human errors related to sleep deficit (Horne, 2012).

The body clock promotes wakefulness at usual times of activity and sleep at usual times of rest (Sugden et al., 2012). The main circadian biologic low point occurs from 2 a.m. to 6 a.m. A less-pronounced trough occurs from 2 p.m. to 6 p.m. (Howard, 2005). As sleep debt builds up, the brain struggles harder to sustain wakefulness through a typical 16 hr day. Around usual bedtime, these alerting signals cease and allow sleep to occur (Luyster, Strollo, Zee, & Walsh, 2012). The circadian system also aligns the daily rhythms of many metabolic activities, such as maintenance of core body temperature and production of the hormones melatonin and cortisol.

Restorative sleep requires adequate duration (quantity) and depth (quality) to support alertness, performance, and health (Cirelli, 2023). Sleep cycles last approximately 90 min and typically reoccur four to six times during a normal sleep period. Consolidated sleep is much more restorative than sleep obtained in fragmented intervals (Worley, 2018). Those with circadian sleep rhythm disruption develop patterns of persistent and recurrent sleep disturbance that can impair brain functioning in insidious ways (Sugden et al., 2012).

When working at night during the circadian trough, it can be difficult to remain alert. A midwife who must sleep during the day, when the body clock is promoting alertness, tends to have disrupted and shortened sleep (Cheng & Drake, 2023). A fatigued midwife may cope well with routine situations but have difficulty responding to unforeseen, uncertain, or quickly changing circumstances (Horne, 2012). Irrelevant information or emotional drama can draw attention away from key issues, and the midwife sometimes finds it difficult to weigh the risks and consequences of management options. If a crisis develops, the midwife may show poor judgment and continue familiar but inappropriate or ineffective routines (Cheng & Drake, 2023). The effect of 18 hr of wakefulness on hand-eye coordination is comparable to that produced by 0.05% blood alcohol concentration; 24 hr is equivalent to 0.1% BAC (Dawson & Reid, 1997; Gluck, 2007)—well above the legal threshold of intoxication in every U.S. state. Most of us would never dream

Table 16-1

Queensland Health Fatigue Assessment

1. Sleep in previous 24 hr						**Score**
Hours	≤2	3	4	≥5		
Points	12	8	4	0		
2. Sleep in previous 48 hr						
Hours	≤8	9	10	11	≥12	
Points	8	6	4	2	0	
3. Projected time awake						
Hours you will have been awake at the end of your shift (minus any expected sleep during the shift). For each hour of wakefulness in excess of your hours of sleep in part 2, add 1 point						
Total score		**1–4**	**5–8**	**9+**		
Fatigue risk		**Moderate**	**High**	**Very high**		

It is difficult to assess one's own level of impairment after prolonged wakefulness. The Queensland Health Fatigue Assessment is a tool that allows providers to estimate fatigue risk and take steps to improve safety if the score is very high. Adapted from *Fatigue Risk Management System Resource Pack* (p. 45), by Queensland Health, 2009, Brisbane, Australia: Queensland Government. Copyright by the State of Queensland.

of working intoxicated, but many midwives struggle with comparable sleep deprivation on a regular basis.

Moreover, fatigue affects the ability to judge our own impairment. A tired midwife might feel alert and competent while losing threads of conversations or misinterpreting clinical information. In a profession where providers largely monitor their own performances, the discrepancy between subjective assessment and objective functioning can pose a significant safety risk.

Sleep inertia is the transitional state between sleep and wakefulness, characterized by grogginess, disorientation, drowsiness, cognitive impairment, and a strong desire to return to sleep (Trotti, 2017). The prefrontal cortex, which is involved in planning, outcome prediction, judgment, and other complex activities, needs about 20–30 min of wakefulness to counteract sleep inertia and fully engage. A midwife on call may feel groggy and disoriented when awakened to speak with clients or confront a challenging task. Sleep inertia can impair reasoning and short-term memory; speed of processing information; and retrieval of numbers, words, or facts (Howard, 2005). It can also reduce the likelihood of remembering details in the morning.

A sleep-deprived midwife can struggle to remain alert, but inevitably the brain overrides attempts to remain awake. The exhausted midwife who resists sleep while driving or attending a client will eventually experience "microsleeps" lasting 3–30 sec, which can go unnoticed (Luyster et al., 2012). Chronic sleep deprivation appears to cause long-term neural changes that require many nights of good sleep to reverse (Cirelli, 2023).

Clinicians working long shifts appear more likely to harm clients. A study of intern physicians found that those on call every third night, working 24 hr or more per shift, made 36% more serious surgical errors than those limited to 17-hr shifts and 65-hr work weeks (Howard, 2005). In another study, residents working recurrent 24-hr shifts made five times as many serious diagnostic errors, suffered 61% more needle sticks, and showed measurable deterioration in overall performance when compared to colleagues working 16-hr shifts (Joint Commission, 2011/2018). Their clients are 36% more likely to suffer an adverse event and 300 times more likely to die because of the provider's error or omission (Joint Commission, 2011/2018). Other research noted that nurses who worked 12.5 hr or longer per shift were less vigilant and three times more likely to make an error in client care (Joint Commission, 2011/2018).

Sleep deprivation and fatigue create inequalities in the care provided to clients (Sugden et al., 2012). The client who gives birth at 4 a.m. with a midwife who has been awake for 28 hr is more likely to receive substandard care than if the same midwife had been well-rested. Most clients would be concerned about their safety if they knew that their provider was sleep deprived; 80% would request a different provider (Nurok, Czeisler, & Lehmann, 2010).

Midwives often find themselves caught between the need to take care of clients and their own physiological limits. When they manage labors in a functionally impaired state, they risk violating the ethical mandate to do no harm to clients. An accident or misjudgment involving a sleep-deprived obstetrical provider can result not only in adverse outcomes, but also in lawsuits or even criminal charges. When possible, providers should avoid assuming client care or holding office hours after being awake all night. Midwifery practice guidelines should include a plan for relieving providers of duty should they become unable to provide safe care.

Optimizing Alertness

Fatigue-related impairment is a seemingly unsolvable problem for midwives. The nature of the work requires midwives to attend clients through long labors that often outlast normal wakefulness. Yet the only way to counteract the severe consequences of sleep disruption is to sleep when necessary for as long as necessary (Joint Commission, 2011/2018).

Naps taken before or during the night shift improve functioning, though providers who nap on duty should sleep for less than 45 min to decrease disorientation from sleep inertia upon awakening (ACOG Cmte. on Patient Safety, 2018). On day shift, a short nap during the midafternoon circadian slump restores alertness, improves performance, and decreases errors (Faraut, Boudjeltia, Vanhamme, & Kerkhofs, 2011).

Midwives who must provide around-the-clock coverage do well to get as much high-quality sleep as possible whenever it is available. Midwives who work inconsistent hours should try not to compromise sleep to meet family and social responsibilities. Night-shift workers can make the best use of fragmented sleep time by sleeping in two periods—an inviolable 4-hr "anchor" sleep that takes priority and a second period of sleep that can vary with circumstances (Cheng & Drake, 2023).

Mental relaxation techniques can dispel anxiety before each sleep period. A white-noise machine, fan, ionizer, or other device can lengthen sleep by masking ambient noise. Darkness is conducive to sleep. When ambient light is unavoidable, room-darkening shades and sleep masks can reduce disruption.

Dark nights and bright days optimize the diurnal clock. In one study, nurses working rotating shifts had less insomnia, anxiety, and depression when exposed to short periods of high intensity light during the first half of the evening/night shift and darkness during daytime sleep (Huang, Tsai, Chen, & Hsu, 2013). In other studies, light exposure increased alertness and reaction times (Cheng & Drake, 2023). On the other hand, exposure to artificial light after sundown decreases the body's production of melatonin, a hormone produced nocturnally by the pineal gland, that not only regulates the sleep wake cycle but also slows the growth of certain cancers (Figueiro, Levent, Wood, & Plitnick, 2015).

The fatigued midwife can shift gears by taking a short walk, climbing stairs, or doing yoga. Social interaction and activity breaks promote alertness. Share your thoughts with colleagues to ensure that you are considering all possibilities. Have low-calorie, high-energy snacks on hand to stabilize blood sugar and settle the nausea that often accompanies sleep deprivation.

Small doses of caffeine (approximately 75–100 mg) taken throughout the shift can help sustain alertness (Cheng & Drake, 2023) and improve work performance. Caffeine is also effective when taken strategically before the circadian low point, followed by a nap of up to 20 min (that is, until the caffeine takes effect) and exposure to bright light upon waking (Faraut et al., 2011).

Exhausted midwives should nap before attempting to drive home if they cannot arrange transportation. Fatigue is a factor in up to 20% of traffic accidents and can be fatal (Luyster et al., 2012). During a 3-sec microsleep, a vehicle traveling 55 mph (89 kph) covers more than 240 ft (773m), out of control by definition, and may cross into oncoming traffic or leave the roadway. Evidence of fatigue or sleeping at the wheel can expose drivers (and perhaps others) to civil or criminal action.

Regular exercise enhances sleep quality, but vigorous exercise should be done at least 3 hr before bedtime so that it will not interfere with falling asleep. Alcohol can decrease the time required to fall asleep, but it is also associated with sleep disturbances, upper-airway instability, and sleep apnea. Mental relaxation techniques, acupuncture, yoga, and meditation can promote sleep after prolonged wakefulness. Cognitive therapy can address anxiety and worries that prevent restful sleep.

When taken as a supplement, melatonin can promote sleep and resynchronize a disrupted circadian rhythm (Alizadeh Feremi, Alipoor, & Esmaeili, 2021; Biggio et al., 2021; Zisapel, 2018). Melatonin has a low potential for dependence and there is little evidence of substantial adverse events from long-term use (Fatemeh et al., 2022). Some people find herbs such as valerian, chamomile, hops, and kava useful for encouraging sleep.

Substance-Use Disorders

The prevalence of substance-use disorders in health care professionals is like that of the general population: about 10–15% of all health care professionals misuse drugs or alcohol at some point during their careers (Baldisseri, 2007). Substance-use disorders can affect the clinician's ability to function at work and at home (Fitzgerald, 2021). Signs of a substance-use disorder include (Ross, 2003)

Issues at work:

- Lateness to appointments; frequent tardiness or absence; unknown whereabouts
- Numerous client complaints
- Secrecy
- Poor decisions, declining quality of care
- Inaccurate charting
- Inappropriate prescribing of controlled substances
- Decreased productivity
- Increased irritability, conflicts with colleagues, aggression
- Smell of alcohol, obvious intoxication, needle marks

- Erratic job history

Issues at home:

- Withdrawal from family, friends, and community, erratic behavior, disordered relationships
- Increase in accidents, arrests
- Increase in medical issues and use of medical care
- Increased aggression, agitation, and conflict
- Financial difficulties
- Decline in personal hygiene
- Depression, anxiety, and mood instability

Table 16-2

Trauma and Stress-related Conditions That Affect Midwives

Compassion fatigue is the physical, emotional, or spiritual exhaustion that can develop after caring for many clients in significant emotional pain or physical distress. Over time the caregiver shuts down emotionally and exhibits decreased capacity for empathy and personal connection. *Example:* A midwife withdraws emotionally and frequently leaves the room while laboring with an anxious primigravida with a history of childhood rape and a strong need for support.
Posttraumatic stress disorder (PTSD) is an anxiety disorder that can develop after direct exposure to a traumatic event. *Example:* A midwife tripped over an electrical cord and fell to her knees, dropping the newborn on the floor. When she picked the baby up, she saw that he had sustained a depressed skull fracture. The midwife has intrusive thoughts and dreams about the event, is quick to tears and anger, and develops palpitations and panic whenever she hears a baby cry.
Secondary traumatic stress (secondary trauma, indirect trauma, vicarious trauma) produces similar symptoms to PTSD and can follow involvement with those who have been traumatized. Vicarious traumatization can arise from merely hearing or reading about the traumas of others. *Example:* A home-birth client who values gentle birth transfers to the hospital and encounters a brusque, disrespectful physician. She has a vacuum-assisted birth and sustained a third-degree laceration which resulted in a postpartum hemorrhage. Upon hearing of the client's ordeal, the midwife experiences anger, guilt, heartbreak, and frustration that interferes with work and personal life.
Burnout, a state of emotional, mental, and often physical exhaustion, can result from prolonged or repeated stress, usually in relation to a demanding workplace. A midwife with burnout feels emotionally depleted, detached, and negative and develops a sense of futility about work that does not improve with time off. *Example*: A midwife who once took every opportunity to meet her clients' needs becomes resistant to returning client telephone calls. She reschedules afternoon appointments if it appears she will not get home on time and argues with the support staff. She finds herself increasingly critical of her clients' choices and beliefs.

Midwifery and Traumatic Stress

Although births are usually healthy and joyous events, most midwives also encounter complications, emergencies, and tragedies. Helping professionals such as midwives, therapists, nurses, physicians, psychologists, psychiatrists, clergy, and first responders are at risk for developing stress responses after traumatic events. Trauma can drastically alter one's worldview, religious faith, relationships, health, or mode of living. It can be more difficult to cope when the trauma is severe, when other life stresses are present, or when social support is lacking.

Other helping professions such as medicine and psychology encourage providers to set emotional boundaries and to avoid friendships with clients. Midwifery, however, was founded on the intimate support women provide one another—the word *midwife* means "with woman" (Rice & Warland 2013). Empathy (experiencing the circumstances of others from their perspectives and sharing their feelings) is a key value in midwifery. Midwives bond strongly to clients, and both the mother and the midwife are likely to experience intense emotion during the birth process (Aydın & Aktaş, 2021). Midwives grasp that emotional live wire and willingly feel the bite of its current, over and over. This heightened empathy, however, leaves midwives especially vulnerable to stress reactions after traumatic birth.

Mothers and their infants arouse powerful protective and nurturing instincts in midwives, and what befalls their clients can weigh as heavily as personal bereavement (Leinweber & Rowe, 2010; Rice & Warland 2013). Like the clients they serve, midwives can feel unsupported, unprepared, or overwhelmed by their own emotional reactions to traumatic events. These reactions are normal responses to abnormal occurrences, but they can erode self-confidence and hurt professional performance (Substance Abuse and Mental Health Services Admin. [SAMHSA], 2014).

The American Psychiatric Association (APA) defines posttraumatic stress disorder (PTSD) as an anxiety problem that can develop after extremely traumatic events such as combat, crime, actual or threatened death, serious injury, or sexual violation (APA, 2022). The trauma can involve direct experience of the event, witnessing the event, being emotionally close to someone who was involved, or being exposed to disturbing details of the event (Bisson et al., 2021). PTSD is diagnosed when symptoms not attributable to a medical condition, a medication, a nonmedicinal substance, or alcohol cause distress or impairment or interfere with work for at least one month (APA, 2022). Symptoms of PTSD include (APA, 2022)

- *Reexperiencing the event*: Recurrent intrusive memories of the event, nightmares, flashbacks, or intense anxiety triggered by situations that resemble the event. For example, a midwife who experienced the death of a baby caused by shoulder dystocia becomes anxious whenever there is a delay after the birth of a baby's head, when attending a birth in the room where the death occurred, or when a client resembles the one who suffered the loss.
- *Alterations in arousal*: Irritability; aggressive, reckless, or self-destructive behavior; sleep disturbances; hypervigilance (continuously assessing the environment for potential threats); or an exaggerated startle response. For example, the midwife provokes an argument at shift change and drives home at excessive speeds.
- *Avoidance*: Distancing from people, places, conversations, or activities that summon distressing memories or feelings about the event. For example, the midwife who experienced a maternal death due to eclampsia avoids attending drills on the topic because of the flood of memories and emotions they may unleash.
- *Negative alterations in cognition and mood*: Developing a distorted or exaggerated self-concept; perceptions of blame, guilt, shame, or fear; diminished interest in activities; or inability to experience happiness, satisfaction, or love. For example, a midwife concludes that a client experienced preterm prelabor rupture of membranes in the second trimester because she is a bad midwife who cannot be trusted to take care of clients.

Secondary traumatic stress (STS) is the emotional distress that results from helping or wanting to help a traumatized or suffering person (Beck, LoGiudice, & Gable, 2015). It can develop from witnessing maltreatment, such as when another provider coerces a client into an unnecessary cesarean, or from involvement in a catastrophic event, such as a uterine rupture. After a difficult transfer to the hospital, a community midwife may feel traumatized by conflicts with hospital personnel or the use of interventions that the mother wished to avoid. Often midwives feel personally responsible, as if they had failed the client, leading them to question their clinical skills and knowledge (Charmer, Jefford, & Jomeen, 2021; Christoffersen, Teigen, & Rønningstad, 2020).

Symptoms of STS are like those of PTSD and are comparable in severity to symptoms experienced by those who directly experience traumatizing events (Beck et al., 2015). The impact of the event is greatest when the provider feels a personal connection with the client or family (McDaniel & Morris, 2020). Symptoms consistent with STS are very common in nurses, affecting 26% of hospice nurses, 25% of forensic nurses, 7% of emergency-department nurses, and 35% of L&D nurses (Beck et al., 2015).

Trauma, like grief, comes in waves, periods of distress followed by return to balance. Immediately after a traumatic event, the victim's emotions might include shock, numbness, confusion, sadness, anxiety, agitation, self-recrimination, and guilt (SAMHSA, 2014). A midwife with an abnormally severe response to trauma can experience continuous distress without intervals of relative calm or rest, an inability to attend to daily activities and roles, or disabling flashbacks. Feeling misunderstood and ashamed of their emotional volatility, some victims withdraw from social contact. Survivors of childhood trauma can find it especially difficult to regulate emotions such as anger, anxiety, sadness, and shame.

Although most midwives recover relatively quickly, others feel the effects of an emotional blow for weeks, months, or a lifetime. Some become suicidal. Situations with similarities to the traumatic event—a client with the same name or a labor with similar characteristics—can trigger a barrage of guilt, anxiety, self-doubt, or shame as upsetting as the original event. Survivors sometimes have flashbacks that increase anxiety for hours afterward, reexperiencing the trauma as if it were happening in that moment like a few seconds of movie footage spliced into ordinary life (SAMHSA, 2014).

When traumatic emotions are not processed, they can emerge as concentration difficulties, an exaggerated startle response, anxiety, or insecurity. They can also cause physical complaints such as sleep disturbances, nausea or bowel issues, palpitations, hypertension, headaches, weakness, vision problems, and pain (SAMHSA, 2014). Untreated, persistent traumatic stress leads to burnout, and burnout leads to higher rates of medical errors, which in turn create more stress, more burnout, and more errors in a destructive spiral (SAMHSA, 2014).

A midwife coping poorly with trauma may attempt to regain emotional control through substance abuse, compulsive behavior such as gambling or overwork, or denial of emotions. Defense or coping mechanisms are conscious or unconscious psychological strategies used to regulate emotion and cope with stress (Di Giuseppe et al., 2021). Use of maladaptive defense mechanisms (e.g., passive aggression, acting without regard for consequences, distortions of self-image, repression of difficult thoughts or emotions, or indulging obsessive thoughts about the incident) can increase stress levels, lower resilience, and lead to burnout (Di Giuseppe et al., 2021).

Healthy coping mechanisms include turning to others for help or support; rededicating oneself to fulfilling the needs of others; planning future responses; embracing the amusing or ironic aspects of the situation; directly expressing feelings or wishes; observing one's own thoughts, feelings, motivations, and behavior; and channeling potentially maladaptive impulses into beneficial activities. Individuals who use these adaptive defense mechanisms to enhance coping are better able to withstand and recover from stress, and they can maintain a greater sense of personal accomplishment and ability than those who do not (Di Giuseppe et al., 2021). Midwives who were emotionally stable before the trauma tend to be highly resilient and usually find ways to heal and cope (SAMHSA, 2014).

Effective interventions during the first days and weeks after trauma can reduce the likelihood that long-term posttraumatic stress will develop (SAMHSA, 2014). To heal from trauma, one must learn to manage triggers, memories, and feelings without becoming agitated or, at the other extreme, emotionless and withdrawn (SAMHSA, 2014). A trauma therapist can help a traumatized individual to manage difficult emotions through therapies such as cognitive behavioral therapy, cognitive restructuring therapy, and stress-inoculation training. Eye movement desensitization and reprocessing therapy (EMDR) uses eye movements or bilateral tapping to help people process emotional experiences that they cannot yet discuss (Wilson et al., 2018). Sometimes medications are prescribed to benefit the healing process.

Midwives should support one another after a bad outcome, even (perhaps especially) in the case of clear negligent error (Sheehy & Baird, 2022). Social supports and personal relationships can mitigate the damage of emotional trauma and can be essential to healing. Simply spending time with a sympathetic listener helps to restore equilibrium. Respite from duty can improve recovery, decrease the burden of stress, and prevent the affected midwife from harming a client while emotionally distracted.

Fortunately, most midwives who develop symptoms of traumatic stress are highly resilient. Like physical wounds, most emotional traumas heal in time, especially if the midwife seeks help from a qualified mental health professional. Traumatic experiences are not always detrimental to the midwife but can contribute to resilience and growth. After working through the emotional aftermath of a difficult situation, many midwives ultimately become stronger and more confident, experiencing growth in personal, spiritual, and professional dimensions (Aydın & Aktaş, 2021). Posttraumatic growth can decrease fear and increase trust (Aydın & Aktaş, 2021). Some midwives report that healing from a traumatic event improves their ability to solve problems and their capability to manage painful emotions (Aydın & Aktaş, 2021).

Table 16-3

Cognitive Changes That Commonly Follow Traumatic Stress

Cognitive errors Misinterpreting a current situation as dangerous because it resembles the trauma. *Example:* The midwife anxiously checks vital signs of a normal newborn more frequently than necessary, sometimes disturbing breastfeeding to do so. A few weeks before, the midwife was unable to resuscitate a newborn who had stopped breathing an hour after birth.
Excessive or inappropriate guilt Attempting to gain control over a traumatic experience by assuming responsibility. *Example:* A preterm infant is born unexpectedly at home to a low-risk mother and does not survive. Although the mother's prenatal course had been normal until the day she went into labor, the midwife feels she is to blame and concludes that she could have prevented the tragedy through better assessment, better teaching, or doing a pelvic examination at the last prenatal visit.
Intrusive thoughts and memories Experiencing, without warning or desire, thoughts and memories associated with the trauma. *Example:* A midwife helps a baby to the breast after a satisfying birth. Looking at the loving, joyful family, she is suddenly overwhelmed by the memory of a mother who gave birth to a stillborn and is consumed with a feeling of heartbreak and loss that overrides all other emotions.

Coping with Fear

Virtually all midwives, even those who fundamentally trust and respect themselves and the birth process, have fears (Dahlen & Caplice, 2014). Situations that midwives fear most include the death of a mother or infant, being watched and criticized, being the cause of a negative birth outcome or experience, being unprepared for the unknown, and losing passion for and confidence in normal birth (Dahlen & Caplice, 2014). Most midwives also fear obstetric emergencies such as shoulder dystocia, postpartum hemorrhage, fetal distress, neonatal resuscitation, umbilical cord prolapse, antepartum hemorrhage, uterine rupture, and eclampsia (Dahlen & Caplice, 2014). Over time, fear can elevate stress and lead to burnout.

Stress, anxiety, uncertainty, and fear can influence how midwives manage labors and the kinds of labors they choose to support (Page & Mander, 2014). An experience that generates fear can essentially rewire the brain. Even after the situation has resolved, neurons fire in the newly established pattern if the situation arises again (Dahlen & Caplice, 2014).

Midwives can acquire fear from hearing frightening birth stories, witnessing traumatic events, or even from working in environments where there are high levels of fear (Dahlen & Caplice, 2014). Fearful midwives may care less effectively for their clients and exude anxiety that negatively affects the birth

Common Fears Associated with Hospital Transfers

- Fear of poor client outcome
- Fear of making the wrong decision
- Fear of peer disapproval for a poor decision
- Fear of client disapproval for a poor decision
- Fear of being unjustifiably criticized, disrespected, or dismissed by hospital staff
- Fear of hospital staff undermining the midwife's credibility with the client
- Fear of unnecessary (or necessary) interventions
- Fear of clients' emotional trauma from complicated birth
- Fear of unfamiliar environments, rules, priorities, and procedures

Adapted from "The Hierarchy of Defense Mechanisms: Assessing Defensive Functioning with the Defense Mechanisms Rating Scales Q-Sort," by M. Di Giuseppe and J. C. Perry, 2021, *Frontiers in Psychology, 12*, 718440. CC BY 4.0.

process (Dahlen & Caplice, 2014). Fear can spread quickly to other members of the birth team.

Midwives can decrease their own fears by facing them head-on and seeking to disempower them, one by one. Discuss your fears with someone you can trust. Consider counseling if fears are intrusive, overwhelming, or limiting. Prepare yourself for emergencies, especially those that frighten you the most. Read the latest research and participate in simulations and drills.

When you face a situation that frightens you, focus on what you would like to happen, not on what you fear. Quiet your mind, focus on your breath, relax your shoulders, feel your feet on the ground. On the way to a birth, conduct emergency drills in your mind and give them all good outcomes. See yourself resolving a tricky shoulder dystocia or resuscitating an infant.

Clients often have their own fears about childbirth or mirror those held by providers (Dahlen & Caplice, 2014). Mothers who fear childbirth may be more accepting of medical interventions that paradoxically increase their risk of a bad outcome. The partner of the laboring client can also experience fear and emotional trauma from observing invasive procedures, perceiving danger, or standing helpless as mother or infant suffers serious complications (Rice & Warland, 2013). Midwives earn trust through integrity and reliability, by not making empty promises or giving false reassurances, and by helping clients feel safe and powerful.

Cultivating Resilience

Good health is multidimensional and involves a lack of physical and mental illness together with a sense of happiness and wellbeing (Karime, Zaheri, Shahoie, Roshani, & Olyaie, 2018). Mental health is a crucial part of the foundation of well-being and effective performance (WHO, 2004). Mental, physical, and social functioning are interdependent, and none is superior to the others (WHO, 2004).

Resilience is the ability to bounce back from hardship, setbacks, and frustrations. It is intimately related to one's sense of competence, stress tolerance, and ability to accept and incorporate change (Andersen, Mintz-Binder, Sweatt, & Song, 2021). It is not a static attribute but a skill that can be developed by perseverance and by actively facing challenges (Reyes, Andrusyszyn, Iwasiw, Forchuk, & Babenko-Mould, 2015). Resilience allows the midwife to overcome daily problems, professional challenges, and major life changes (Sabzevari & Rad, 2019). Professionally, resilient providers appear to be less susceptible to burnout and compassion fatigue (Olson, Kemper, & Mahan, 2015).

Resilience-building habits include

- Cultivating optimism and cognitive flexibility
- Self-care: sleep, exercise, and good nutrition
- Honing active coping skills
- Learning to face fears
- Engaging in spiritual practices
- Maintaining a sense of humor
- Writing about stressful and traumatic events as a way of confronting them
- Following passions
- Nurturing personal and professional relationships
- Befriending feelings and accepting emotions
- Practicing loving-kindness meditation and forgiveness
- Spending time in nature
- Connecting with loved ones
- Deliberately filling life with what is valued the most

The practices of mindfulness and self-compassion appear to increase resilience more than any other intervention (Barratt, 2017; Biber, 2021). Mindfulness involves developing a nonjudgmental awareness of the present moment in an attitude of openness, acceptance, and patience (Barratt, 2017). Mindfulness practice can reduce stress levels and improve a provider's ability to engage effectively with clients no matter whether it is an informal addition to daily activities or a formal part of meditation (Sulosaari, Unal, & Cinar, 2022).

Mindfulness is an important part of self-compassion. Many health care providers easily and instinctively extend tremendous compassion to others but have little consideration for their own vulnerabilities. Negative views of oneself generate anxiety and depression, which increase the likelihood of making errors on the job and impede the delivery of sustained compassionate care (Tawfik et al., 2018; Barratt, 2017). By becoming more aware of one's own self-talk and emotions, one can learn to recognize harsh internal judgment and potentially destructive self-criticism within the daily flow of thought (Barratt, 2017).

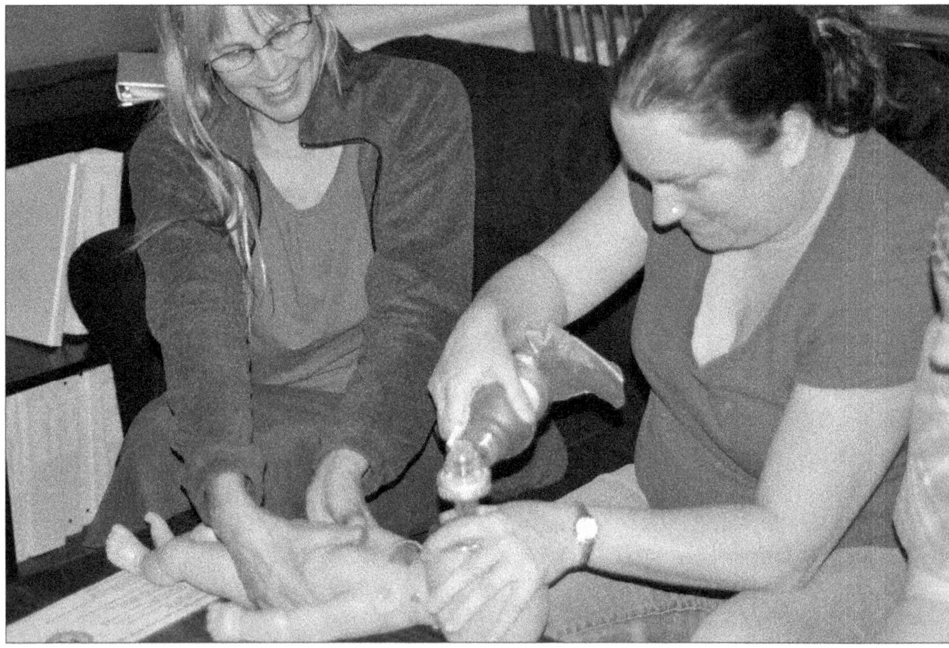

Figure 16-6. The author and another midwife practice neonatal resuscitation at a Birth Emergency Skills Training workshop. Learning skills in an atmosphere of camaraderie and good humor improves retention of knowledge, minimizes fear and dread, and enables midwives to respond fluidly in an actual emergency. Photograph by Andrea Dixon.

Compassion is the ability to care for and show concern for others. Self-compassion involves treating oneself with non-judgmental kindness, respect, understanding, and forgiveness during periods of hardship and stress. It involves gently bearing witness to one's own discomfort and learning to tolerate uncomfortable feelings such as distress, anger, or fear. Self-compassion recognizes that everyone has a unique experience of life, faces trials and triumphs, makes mistakes, falls short, and fails to reach goals. This awareness can alleviate feelings of shame and isolation and keep healthy self-compassion from becoming self-pity or self-indulgence. Cultivating self-compassion builds resilience and mental health (Andersson, Stenfors, Lilliengren, Einhorn, & Osika, 2021; Kotera, Cockerill, Chircop, Kaluzeviciute, & Dyson, 2021).

Loving-kindness meditation is a technique that can increase one's feelings of social connection, empathy, and compassion (Kearney, Malte, Storms, & Simpson, 2021; Seppala, Hutcherson, Nguyen, Doty, & Gross, 2014; Wang et al., 2021; Zhao, 2022). Among veterans with PTSD, loving-kindness meditations were about as effective as group cognitive processing therapy in reducing PTSD symptoms (Kearney et al., 2021). There are many types of loving-kindness meditation. One technique begins with centering yourself by noticing your breathing and consciously relaxing your muscles. Imagine two loved ones standing on either side of you, bathing you in their love. Hold this love within you, then send it back to them in a warm, loving glow that surrounds the three of you. Expand that warm glow to include other loved ones, colleagues, and acquaintances. Increase the glow to bring warmth and healing to any disturbing, difficult people in your life. Extend the flow of warmth and love to the people in your community, and finally the entire world. As you radiate love, wish each person or group health, happiness, and wellbeing (Seppala et al., 2014). Practicing this technique regularly can feed the flame of your passion for midwifery and help you to bring your best self into every life you touch.

Topics for Discussion

1. A safety bundle is a small set of evidence-based practices that can improve client outcomes when all team members use them reliably. What aspect of your practice would benefit from a safety bundle? What changes can you make to improve safety in this area?
2. Discuss how you might uncover your own hidden biases toward race, gender, social status, or other characteristics. If you uncover a bias, how might you take steps to improve your objectivity?
3. Diana used to be a passionate, engaged midwife, but lately she often makes cynical comments, arrives late for work, and complains about sleepless nights and needy clients. Discuss possible reasons for the changes in Diana's behavior and how she might get herself back on track.
4. Julio, who has been a midwife for 5 years, brags about being able to work 40 hr without sleep. Mindy, a colleague, is concerned that Julio is working at the edge of his biological limits and may be providing unsafe care. Julio may also be endangering other motorists on the drive home from work. How might Mindy address these concerns?

References

Alizadeh Feremi, K., Alipoor, L., & Esmaeili, R. (2021). Effect of melatonin on the sleep quality: A systematic review. *Reviews in Clinical Medicine, 8*(2), 60–68. https://doi.org/10.22038/rcm.2021.55887.1356

American Association of Birth Centers. (2017). *Standards for birth centers* (12th ed.). Perkiomenville, PA: Author. Retrieved from https://www.birthcenters.org/resource/resmgr/AABC-STANDARDS-RV2017.pdf

American College of Nurse-Midwives. (2011). *Standards for the practice of midwifery*. Retrieved from http://www.midwife.org/ACNM/files/ACNMLibraryData/UPLOADFILENAME/000000000051/Standards_for_Practice_of_Midwifery_Sept_2011.pdf

American College of Nurse-Midwives. (2015). *Code of ethics with explanatory statements*. Retrieved from https://www.midwife.org/acnm/files/ACNMLibraryData/UPLOADFILENAME/000000000293/Code-of-Ethics-w-Explanatory-Statements-June-2015.pdf

American College of Nurse-Midwives. (2016). Midwifery provision of home birth services (Clinical bulletin 14). *Journal of Midwifery & Women's Health, 61*(1), 127–133. https://doi.org/10.1111/jmwh.12431

American College of Obstetricians and Gynecologists. (2019). *Clinical guidelines and standardization of practice to improve outcomes* (Committee Opinion 792). Retrieved from https://www.acog.org/clinical/clinical-guidance/committee-opinion/articles/2019/10/clinical-guidelines-and-standardization-of-practice-to-improve-outcomes

American College of Obstetricians and Gynecologists Committee on Obstetric Practice. (2017, reaffirmed 2023). *Planned home birth* (Committee Opinion 697, interim update). Retrieved from https://www.acog.org/clinical/clinical-guidance/committee-opinion/articles/2017/04/planned-home-birth

American College of Obstetricians and Gynecologists Committee on Patient Safety and Quality Improvement. (2018). *Fatigue and patient safety* (Committee Opinion 730). Retrieved from https://www.acog.org/-/media/project/acog/acogorg/clinical/files/committee-opinion/articles/2018/02/fatigue-and-patient-safety.pdf

American Medical Association (2022). *Code of medical ethics opinion 9.3.1*. Retrieved from https://www.ama-assn.org/delivering-care/ethics/physician-health-wellness

American Psychiatric Association. (2022). *Diagnostic and statistical manual of mental disorders* (5th ed., text revision). Arlington, VA: Author.

Andersen, S., Mintz-Binder, R., Sweatt, L., & Song, H. (2021). Building nurse resilience in the workplace. *Applied Nursing Research, 59*. https://doi.org/10.1016/j.apnr.2021.151433

Andersson, C., Stenfors, C. U. D., Lilliengren, P., Einhorn, S., & Osika, W. (2021). Benevolence—Associations with stress, mental health, and self-compassion at the workplace. *Frontiers in Psychology, 12*. https://doi.org/10.3389/fpsyg.2021.568625

Aydın, R., & Aktaş, S. (2021). Midwives' experiences of traumatic births: A systematic review and meta-synthesis. *European Journal of Midwifery, 5*, 1–10. https://doi.org/10.18332/ejm/138197

Baldisseri, M. R. (2007). Impaired healthcare professional. *Critical Care Medicine, 35*(2, Suppl.), S106–S116. Retrieved from https://pubmed.ncbi.nlm.nih.gov/17242598/

Barratt, C. (2017). Exploring how mindfulness and self-compassion can enhance compassionate care. *Nursing Standard, 31*(21), 55–63. https://doi.org/10.7748/ns.2017.e10671

Beck, C. T., LoGiudice, J., & Gable, R. K. (2015). A mixed-methods study of secondary traumatic stress in certified nurse-midwives: Shaken belief in the birth process. *Journal of Midwifery & Women's Health, 60*(1), 16–23. https://doi.org/10.1111/jmwh.12221

Benson, M., Benson, J., & Stein, M. (2016). Hospital quality improvement: Are peer review immunity, privilege, and confidentiality in the public interest? *Northwestern Journal of Law and Social Policy, 11*(1). Retrieved from http://scholarlycommons.law.northwestern.edu/njlsp/vol11/iss1/1

Biber, D. (2021). Mindful self-compassion for nurses: A systematic review. *Nursing Management, 29*(3), 18–24. https://doi.org/10.7748/nm.2021.e2028

Biggio, G., Biggio, F., Talani, G., Mostallino, M. C., Aguglia, A., Aguglia, E., & Palagini, L. (2021). Melatonin: From neurobiology to treatment. *Brain Sciences, 11*(9), 1121. https://doi.org/10.3390/brainsci11091121

Bingham, D., Jones, D. K., & Howell, E. A. (2019). Quality improvement approach to eliminate disparities in perinatal morbidity and mortality. *Obstetrics and Gynecology Clinics of North America, 46*(2), 227–238. https://doi.org/10.1016/j.ogc.2019.01.006

Bisson, J. I., Wright, L. A., Jones, K. A., Lewis, C., Phelps, A. J., Sijbrandij, M., . . . Roberts, N. P. (2021). Preventing the onset of post traumatic stress disorder. *Clinical Psychology Review, 86*. https://doi.org/10.1016/j.cpr.2021.102004

Boulanger, J., Keohane, C., & Yeats, A. (2019). Role of patient safety organizations in improving patient safety. *Obstetrics and Gynecology Clinics of North America, 46*(2), 257–267. https://doi.org/10.1016/j.ogc.2019.02.001

Burns, E. S., Duff, M., Leggett, J., & Schmied, V. (2021). Emergency scenarios in maternity: An exploratory study of a midwifery and medical student simulation-based learning collaboration. *Women and Birth, 34*(6), 563–569. https://doi.org/10.1016/j.wombi.2020.10.005

Candilis, P. J., Kim, D. T., & Sulmasy, L. S. (2019). Physician impairment and rehabilitation: Reintegration into medical practice while ensuring patient safety: A position paper from the American College of Physicians. *Annals of Internal Medicine, 170*(12), 871–879. https://doi.org/10.7326/M18-3605

Charmer, L., Jefford, E., & Jomeen, J. (2021). A scoping review of maternity care providers experience of primary trauma within their childbirthing journey. *Midwifery, 102*. https://doi.org/10.1016/j.midw.2021.103127

Cheng, P., & Drake, C. L. (2023). Sleep-wake disturbances in shift workers. In A. F. Eichler (Ed.), *UpToDate*. Retrieved October 30, 2023, from http://www.uptodate.com/contents/sleep-wake-disturbances-in-shift-workers

Christoffersen, L., Teigen, J., & Rønningstad, C. (2020). Following-up midwives after adverse incidents: How front-line management practices help second victims. *Midwifery, 85*. https://doi.org/10.1016/j.midw.2020.102669

Cirelli, C. (2023). Insufficient sleep: Definition, epidemiology, and adverse outcomes. In A. F. Eichler, (Ed.), *UpToDate*. Retrieved October 30, 2023, from https://www.uptodate.com/contents/insufficient-sleep-definition-epidemiology-and-adverse-outcomes

Dahlen, H. (2012). Homebirth: Ten tips for safety and survival. *British Journal of Midwifery, 20*(12), 872–876. https://doi.org/10.12968/bjom.2012.20.12.872

Dahlen, H. G., & Caplice, S. (2014). What do midwives fear? *Women and Birth, 27*(4), 266–270. https://doi.org/10.1016/j.wombi.2014.06.008

Dawson, R., & Reid, K. (1997). Fatigue, alcohol and performance impairment. *Nature, 388*, 235. https://doi.org/10.1038/40775

Di Giuseppe, M., Nepa, G., Prout, T. A., Albertini, F., Marcelli, S., Orrù, G., & Conversano, C. (2021). Stress, burnout, and resilience among healthcare workers during the COVID-19 emergency: The role of defense mechanisms. *International Journal of Environmental Research and Public Health, 18*(10), 5258. https://doi.org/10.3390/ijerph18105258

Di Giuseppe, M., & Perry, J. C. (2021). The hierarchy of defense mechanisms: Assessing defensive functioning with the defense mechanisms rating scales Q-sort. *Frontiers in Psychology, 12*. https://doi.org/10.3389/fpsyg.2021.718440

Dillon, S. (2021). Simulation in obstetrics and gynecology: A review of the past, present, and future. *Obstetrics and Gynecology Clinics of North America, 48*(4), 689–703. https://doi.org/10.1016/j.ogc.2021.07.003

Dillon, S. J., Kleinmann, W., Fomina, Y., Werner, B., Schultz, S., Klucsarits, S., . . . Nelson, D. B. (2021). Does simulation improve clinical performance in management of postpartum hemorrhage? *American Journal of Obstetrics & Gynecology, 225*(4), 435.e1–435.e8. https://doi.org/10.1016/j.ajog.2021.05.025

Egan, H., Keyte, R., McGowan, K., Peters, L., Lemon, N., Parsons, S., . . . Mantzios, M. (2019). 'You before me': A qualitative study of health care professionals' and students' understanding and experiences of compassion in the workplace, self-compassion, self-care and health behaviours. *Health Professions Education, 5*(3), 225–236. https://doi.org/10.1016/j.hpe.2018.07.002

Faraut, B., Boudjeltia, K. Z., Vanhamme, L., & Kerkhofs, M. (2011). Immune, inflammatory and cardiovascular consequences of sleep restriction and recovery. *Sleep Medicine Reviews, 16*(2), 139–147. https://doi.org/10.1016/j.smrv.2011.05.001

Fatemeh, G., Sajjad, M., Niloufar, R., Neda, S., Leila, S., & Khadijeh, M. (2022). Effect of melatonin supplementation on sleep quality: A systematic review and meta-analysis of randomized controlled trials. *Journal of Neurology, 269*, 205–216. https://doi.org/10.1007/s00415-020-10381-w

Figueiro, M. G., Levent, S., Wood, B., & Plitnick, B. (2015). Light at night and measures of alertness: Implications for shift workers. *Biological Research for Nursing*, 2015, in press. https://doi.org/10.1177/1099800415572873

Fitzgerald, R. M. (2021). Caring for the physician affected by substance use disorder. *American Family Physician, 103*(5), 302–304. Retrieved from https://www.aafp.org/pubs/afp/issues/2021/0301/p302.html

Garbarino, S., Lanteri, P., Bragazzi, N. L., Magnavita, N., & Scoditti, El. (2021). Role of sleep deprivation in immune-related disease risk and outcomes. *Communications Biology, 4*, 1304. https://doi.org/10.1038/s42003-021-02825-4

Gluck, P. A. (2007). Patient safety in women's health care: A framework for progress. *Best Practice & Research Clinical Obstetrics & Gynaecology, 21*(4), 525–536. https://doi.org/10.1016/j.bpobgyn.2007.01.012

Govindappagari, S., Guardado, A., Goffman, D., Bernstein, J., Lee, C., Schonfeld, S., . . . Bernstein, P. (2020). Is communication improved with the implementation of an obstetrical version of the World Health Organization Safe Surgery Checklist? *Journal of Patient Safety, 16* (4), 279–283. https://doi.org/10.1097/PTS.0000000000000327

Hales, B. M., & Pronovost, P. J. (2006). The checklist—A tool for error management and performance improvement. *Journal of Critical Care, 21*(3), 231–235. https://doi.org/10.1016/j.jcrc.2006.06.002

Horne, J. (2012). Working throughout the night: Beyond 'sleepiness'—impairments to critical decision making. *Neuroscience & Biobehavioral Reviews, 36*(10), 2226–2231. https://doi.org/10.1016/j.neubiorev.2012.08.005

Howard, S. K. (2005). Sleep deprivation and physician performance: Why should I care? *Baylor University Medical Center Proceedings, 18*(2), 108–112. https://doi.org/10.1080/08998280.2005.11928045

Huang, L. B., Tsai, M. C., Chen, C. Y., & Hsu, S. C. (2013). The effectiveness of light/dark exposure to treat insomnia in female nurses undertaking shift work during the evening/night shift. *Journal of Clinical Sleep Medicine, 9*(7), 641–646. https://doi.org/10.5664/jcsm.2824

International Confederation of Midwives. (2011). *Global standards for midwifery regulation.* (2011). Retrieved from https://www.internationalmidwives.org/assets/files/general-files/2018/04/global-standards-for-midwifery-regulation-eng.pdf

International Confederation of Midwives. (2014). *International code of ethics for midwives*. Retrieved from https://www.internationalmidwives.org/assets/files/definitions-files/2018/06/eng-international-code-of-ethics-for-midwives.pdf

International Council of Nurses. (2021). *The ICN code of ethics for nurses*. Geneva, Switzerland: Author. Retrieved from https://www.icn.ch/system/files/2021-10/ICN_Code-of-Ethics_EN_Web_0.pdf

Ishikura, I. A., Rosa, D. S., Hachul, H., Pires, G. N., Tufik, S., & Andersen, M. L. (2021). Sleep deficit in COVID-19 health-care workers may increase the infection risk. *Scandinavian Journal of Public Health, 49*(7), 697–699. https://doi.org/10.1177/14034948211007679

Joint Commission. (2011, revised 2018). *Health care worker fatigue and patient safety* (Sentinel Event Alert 48). Retrieved from https://www.jointcommission.org/-/media/tjc/documents/resources/patient-safety-topics/sentinel-event/sea_48_hcw_fatigue_final_w_2018_addendum.pdf

Karime, R., Zaheri, F., Shahoie, R., Roshani, D., & Olyaie, N. (2018). The relationship between mental health and resilience in midwives working in Kurdistan province, 2017–2018. *Journal of Advanced Pharmacy Education & Research, 8*(4), 83–88. Retrieved from https://japer.in/en/article/the-relationship-between-mental-health-and-resilience-in-midwives-working-in-kurdistan-province-2017-2018

Kearney, D. J., Malte, C. A., Storms, M., & Simpson, T. L. (2021). Loving-kindness meditation vs cognitive processing therapy for posttraumatic stress disorder among veterans: A randomized clinical trial. *JAMA Network Open, 4*(4), e216604. https://doi.org/10.1001/jamanetworkopen.2021.6604

Kessler, D. O., Cheng, A., & Mullan, P. C. (2014). Debriefing in the emergency department after clinical events: A practical guide. *Annals of Emergency Medicine, 65*(6), 690–698. https://doi.org/10.1016/j.annemergmed.2014.10.019

Klein, V. R. (2019). Risk management in obstetrics and gynecology. *Clinical Obstetrics and Gynecology, 62*(3), 550–559. https://doi.org/10.1097/GRF.0000000000000473

Kotera, Y., Cockerill, V., Chircop, J., Kaluzeviciute, G., & Dyson, S. (2021). Predicting self-compassion in UK nursing students: Relationships with resilience, engagement, motivation, and mental wellbeing. *Nurse Education in Practice, 51*. https://doi.org/10.1016/j.nepr.2021.102989

Lavallée, J. F., Gray, T. A., Dumville, J., Russell, W., & Cullum, N. (2017). The effects of care bundles on patient outcomes: A systematic review and meta-analysis. *Implementation Science, 12*, 142. https://doi.org/10.1186/s13012-017-0670-0

Lavelle, J., Schast, A. & Keren, R. (2015). Standardizing care processes and improving quality using pathways and continuous quality improvement. *Current Treatment Options in Pediatrics 1*, 347–358. https://doi.org/10.1007/s40746-015-0026-4

Leinweber, J. Rowe, H. (2010). The costs of "being with the woman": Secondary traumatic stress in midwifery. *Midwifery 26*(1), 76–87. https://doi.org/10.1016/j.midw.2008.04.003

Liberati, E. G., Tarrant, C., Willars, J., Draycott, T., Winter, C., Chew, S., & Dixon-Woods, M. (2019). How to be a very safe maternity unit: An ethnographic study. *Social Science & Medicine, 223*, 64–72. https://doi.org/10.1016/j.socscimed.2019.01.035

Lincoln, T. (2015). *Solutions in sight: Safety initiatives have dramatically reduced harms during childbirth but are unevenly implemented.* Washington, DC: Public Citizen. Retrieved from http://www.citizen.org/documents/obstetrics-healthcare-safety-report.pdf

Linton, M., & Koonmen, J. (2020). Self-care as an ethical obligation for nurses. *Nursing Ethics, 27*(8), 1694–1702. https://doi.org/10.1177/0969733020940371

Luyster, F. S., Strollo, P. J., Zee, P. C., & Walsh, J. K. (2012). Sleep: A health imperative. *Sleep, 35*(6), 727–734. https://doi.org/10.5665/sleep.1846

McDaniel, L. R., & Morris, C. (2020). The second victim phenomenon: How are midwives affected? *Journal of Midwifery & Women's Health, 65*(4), 503–511. https://doi.org/10.1111/jmwh.13092

Midwives Alliance of North America. (2005). *Standards and qualifications for the art and practice of midwifery*. Retrieved from https://mana.org/pdfs/MANAStandardsQualificationsColor.pdf

Midwives Alliance of North America. (2011). *Core competencies for basic midwifery practice*. Retrieved from https://mana.org/pdfs/MANACoreCompetenciesColor.pdf

Nethery, E., Schummers, L., Levine, A., Caughey, A. B., Souter, V., & Gordon, W. (2021). Birth outcomes for planned home and licensed freestanding birth center births in Washington State. *Obstetrics & Gynecology, 138*(5), 693–702.

North American Registry of Midwives. (2022). *Community peer review*. Retrieved from http://narm.org/accountability/community-peer-review/

Nurok, M., Czeisler, C. A., & Lehmann, L. S. (2010). Sleep deprivation, elective surgical procedures, and informed consent. *New England Journal of Medicine, 363*(27), 2577–2579. https://doi.org/10.1056/NEJMp1007901

Olson, K., Kemper, K. J., & Mahan, J. D. (2015). What factors promote resilience and protect against burnout in first-year pediatric and medicine-pediatric residents? *Journal of Evidence-Based Integrative Medicine, 20*(3), 192–198. https://doi.org/10.1177/2156587214568894

Page, M., & Mander, R. (2014). Intrapartum uncertainty: A feature of normal birth, as experienced by midwives in Scotland. *Midwifery, 30*(1), 28–35. https://doi.org/10.1016/j.midw.2013.01.012

Queensland Health. (2009). *Fatigue risk management system resource pack*. Brisbane, Australia: State of Queensland. Retrieved from http://www.apex.org.nz/wp-content/uploads/Risk-Assessment-Tool.pdf

Reyes, A. T., Andrusyszyn, M.-A., Iwasiw, C., Forchuk, C., & Babenko-Mould, Y. (2015). Resilience in nursing education: An integrative review. *Journal of Nursing Education, 54*(8), 438–444. https://doi.org/10.3928/01484834-20150717-03

Rice, H., & Warland, J. (2013). Bearing witness: Midwives experiences of witnessing traumatic birth. *Midwifery 29* (9), 1056–1063. https://doi.org/10.1016/j.midw.2012.12.003

Ross, S. (2003). Identifying an impaired physician. *Virtual Mentor, 5*(12), 420–422. Retrieved from https://journalofethics.ama-assn.org/sites/journalofethics.ama-assn.org/files/2018-07/cprl1-0312.pdf

Sabzevari, M. T., & Rad, M. (2019). Resilience strategies against working pressures in midwives: A qualitative study. *Journal of Education and Health Promotion, 8*(1), 33. Retrieved from https://www.ncbi.nlm.nih.gov/pmc/articles/PMC6432840/

Seppala, E. M., Hutcherson, C. A., Nguyen, D. T., Doty, J. R., & Gross, J. J. (2014). Loving-kindness meditation: A tool to improve healthcare provider compassion, resilience, and patient care. *Journal of Compassionate Health Care, 1*(1), 1–9. https://doi.org/10.1186/s40639-014-0005-9

Sheehy, A., & Baird, K. (2022). A qualitative study of early career Australian midwives' encounters with perinatal grief, loss and trauma. *Women and Birth*. In press. https://doi.org/10.1016/j.wombi.2022.01.009

Shekelle, P. (2022). Overview of clinical practice guidelines. In J. Givens (Ed.), *UpToDate*. Retrieved July 30, 2023, from https://www.uptodate.com/contents/overview-of-clinical-practice-guidelines

Sidhu, R., Su, B., Shapiro, K. R., & Stoll, K. (2020). Prevalence of and factors associated with burnout in midwifery: A scoping review. *European Journal of Midwifery, 4*. https://doi.org/10.18332/ejm/115983

Substance Abuse and Mental Health Services Administration. (2014). *Trauma-informed care in behavioral health services* (Treatment Improvement Protocol (TIP) Series 57). HHS Publication No. (SMA) 13-4801. Rockville, MD: Author. Retrieved from http://www.ncbi.nlm.nih.gov/books/NBK207201/pdf/Bookshelf_NBK207201.pdf

Sugden, C., Athanasiou, T., & Darzi, A. (2012). What are the effects of sleep deprivation and fatigue in surgical practice? *Seminars in Thoracic and Cardiovascular Surgery, 24*(3), 166–175. https://doi.org/10.1053/j.semtcvs.2012.06.005

Sulosaari, V., Unal, E., & Cinar, F. I. (2022). The effectiveness of mindfulness-based interventions on the psychological well-being of nurses: A systematic review. *Applied Nursing Research, 64*. https://doi.org/10.1016/j.apnr.2022.151565

Tawfik, D. S., Profit, J., Morgenthaler, T. I., Satele, D. V., Sinsky, C. A., Dyrbye, L. N., . . . Shanafelt, T. D. (2018). Physician burnout, well-being, and work unit safety grades in relationship to reported medical errors. *Mayo Clinic Proceedings, 93*(11), 1571–1580. https://doi.org/10.1016/j.mayocp.2018.05.014

Thumm, E. B., Smith, D. C., Squires, A. P., Breedlove, G., & Meek, P. M. (2021). Burnout of the US midwifery workforce and the role of practice environment. *Health Services Research, 57*(2), 351–363. https://doi.org/https://doi.org/10.1111/1475-6773.13922

Trotti L. M. (2017). Waking up is the hardest thing I do all day: Sleep inertia and sleep drunkenness. *Sleep Medicine Reviews, 35*, 76–84. https://doi.org/10.1016/j.smrv.2016.08.005

Wallace, J., Hoehn-Velasco, L., Jolles, D., Stapleton, S., Flynn, C., Bauer, K., & Wright, J. (2021). Assessment of interprofessional collaboration at free-standing birth centers: Does collaboration influence outcomes? *Journal of Interprofessional Education & Practice, 25*. https://doi.org/10.1016/j.xjep.2021.100479

Wang, Y., Fu, C., Liu, Y., Li, D., Wang, C., Sun, R., & Song, Y. (2021). A study on the effects of mindfulness-based cognitive therapy and loving-kindness mediation on depression, rumination, mindfulness level and quality of life in depressed patients. *American Journal of Translational Research, 13*(5), 4666–4675. Retrieved from https://pubmed.ncbi.nlm.nih.gov/34150046/

Wilson, G., Farrell, D., Barron, I., Hutchins, J., Whybrow, D., & Kiernan, M. D. (2018). The use of eye-movement desensitization reprocessing (EMDR) therapy in treating post-traumatic stress disorder—A systematic narrative review. *Frontiers in Psychology, 9*. https://doi.org/10.3389/fpsyg.2018.00923

World Health Organization. (2004). *Promoting mental health: Concepts, emerging evidence, practice: Summary report*. Geneva, Switzerland: Author. Retrieved from https://apps.who.int/iris/bitstream/handle/10665/42940/9241591595.pdf

World Health Organization. (2021). *WHO guideline on self-care interventions for health and well-being*. Geneva, Switzerland: Author. Retrieved from https://apps.who.int/iris/rest/bitstreams/1356501/retrieve

Worley, S. L. (2018). The extraordinary importance of sleep: The detrimental effects of inadequate sleep on health and public safety drive an explosion of sleep research. *P&T, 43*(12), 758–763. Retrieved from https://www.ncbi.nlm.nih.gov/pmc/articles/PMC6281147/

Wright, E. M. (2020). The ethical imperative of self-care: A call to action. *Journal of Midwifery & Women's Health, 65*(6), 733–736. https://doi.org/10.1111/jmwh.13150

Zhao, Z. (2022). The influence of loving-kindness meditation on mental health—A systematic review. In C. Allen, S. Hertz, W. H. Greene, G. J. D. Hewings, & K. Lovell (Eds.), *Proceedings of the 2021 International Conference on Social Development and Media Communication (SDMC 2021)* (pp. 957–961). Dordrecht, Netherlands: Atlantis Press. https://doi.org/10.2991/assehr.k.220105.176

Zisapel, N. (2018). New perspectives on the role of melatonin in human sleep, circadian rhythms and their regulation. *British Journal of Pharmacology, 175*(16), 3190–3199. https://doi.org/10.1111/bph.14116

Index

A

D

E

I

J

K

L

M

R

S

T

U

V

W–Z

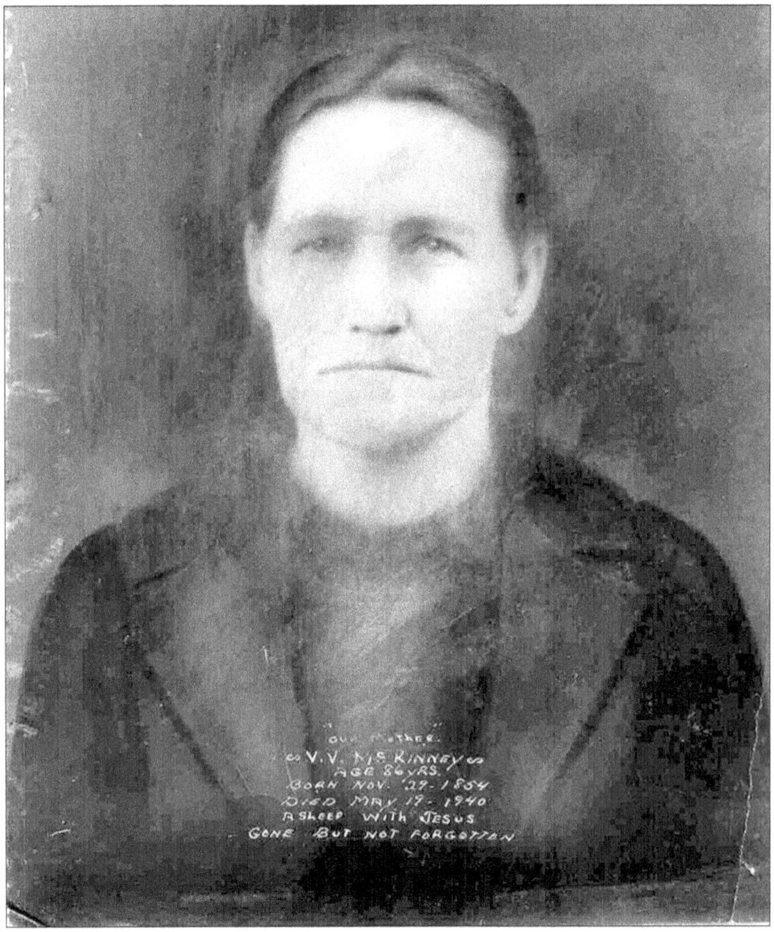
"OUR MOTHER"
V.V. McKINNEY
AGE 86 YRS.
BORN NOV. 29-1854
DIED MAY 17-1940
ASLEEP WITH JESUS
GONE BUT NOT FORGOTTAN

The author's great-great grandmother, Victoria Virginia Blankenship Mckinney Cunningham (1854–1940), was a "granny-woman" midwife and skilled herbalist in West Virginia. Known as Granny Vic, she was greatly respected by her community of impoverished mountain people. Her granddaughter Minnie Ethel Mitchem Whitt (1893–1982) was also a granny-woman, who traveled on horseback to attend births in remote cabins.

www.ingramcontent.com/pod-product-compliance
Lightning Source LLC
Chambersburg PA
CBHW061150240926
51846CB00006B/973
* 9 7 8 1 9 4 1 7 0 0 4 2 6 *